D1163546

SKELETAL TRAUMA

Fractures • Dislocations • Ligamentous Injuries

Medical Illustrators

Philip Ashley and Denis Lee in association with
Leona Allison
Marie Chartrand
Megan Costello
Charles Curro
Glenn Edelmayer
Theodore Huff
Christine Jones
John Klausmeyer
Valerie Loomis
Larry Ward

SKELETAL TRAUMA

Fractures • Dislocations • Ligamentous Injuries

V O L U M E   T W O

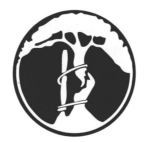

Bruce D. Browner, M.D.

Professor and Director, Division of Orthopaedic Surgery
The University of Texas Medical at Houston
Chief of Orthopaedics, Hermann Hospital
Houston, Texas

Jesse B. Jupiter, M.D.

Associate Professor of Orthopaedic Surgery
Harvard Medical School, Massachusetts General Hospital
Boston Massachusettes

Alan M. Levine, M.D.

Associate Professor of Orthopaedics, Surgery, and Oncology
Division of Orthopaedic Surgery and Oncology
University of Maryland School of Medicine
Baltimore, Maryland

Peter G. Trafton, M.D.

Surgeon-in-Charge, Division of Trauma, Department of Orthopaedics,
Rhode Island Hospital
Associate Professor of Orthopaedics, Brown University
Providence, Rhode Island

W.B. SAUNDERS COMPANY

Hartcourt Brace Jovanovich, Inc.

Philadelphia • London • Toronto • Montreal • Sydney • Tokyo

W. B. Saunders Company
Harcourt Brace Jovanovich, Inc.

The Curtis Center
Independence Square West
Philadelphia, PA 19106

Library of Congress Cataloging-in-Publication Data

Skeletal trauma / [edited by] Bruce Browner . . . [et al.]. — 1st ed.
    p. cm.
   ISBN 0-7216-2726-9
    1. Musculoskeletal system — Wounds and injuries. 2. Fractures.
I. Browner, Bruce D.
   [DNLM: 1. Bone and Bones — injuries. 2. Dislocations.
3. Fractures. 4. Ligaments — injuries.   WE 175 S627]
   RD731.S564   1992
   617.4′71044 — dc20
   DNLM/DLC
                                90-8922

Editor: W. B. Saunders Staff

Developmental Editor: Kathleen McCullough

Designer: Karen O'Keefe

Production Manager: Carolyn Naylor

Manuscript Editors: Lorraine Zawodny and Kendall Sterling

Mechanical Illustrator: Megan Costello

Illustration Coordinator: Brett MacNaughton

Indexer: Dennis Dolan

Cover Designer: W. B. Saunders Staff

Skeletal Trauma: Fractures, Dislocations,
and Ligamentous Injuries

ISBN 0-7216-2727-7 Volume 1
0-7216-2728-5 Volume 2
0-7216-2726-9 1 Set

Copyright © 1992 by W. B. Saunders Company

All rights reserved.   No part of this publication may be reproduced or transmitted in any form or by any means, electronic or mechanical, including photocopy, recording, or any information storage and retrieval system, without permission in writing from the publisher.

Printed in the United States of America

Last digit is the print number: 9   8   7   6   5   4   3   2   1

We dedicate this book to our wives and children for their patience, support, and sacrifices while we have been occupied with skeletal trauma and *Skeletal Trauma*.

Barbara Thea Browner

Jeremy Todd Browner

Nicole Shannan Browner

Beryl Stephanie Abrams Jupiter

Stacy Deborah Jupiter

Benjamin Scott Jupiter

Barbara Gwen Levine

Dana Ari Levine

Alissa Leigh Levine

Andrea Naomi Levine

Frances Conkey Trafton

Katherine Shane Trafton

Theodore Grier Trafton

Elizabeth Fairbank Trafton

Contributors

Jean-Jacques Abitbol, M.D.
Assistant Professor, Surgery, University of California, San Diego, School of Medicine; Attending Staff, UCSD Medical Center; VA Medical Center, San Diego, CA
Thoracic and Upper Lumbar Spine Injuries

Jesse R. Ada, M.D.
Former Fellow in Orthopaedic Trauma, University of Alabama Medical Center, Birmingham, AL; Orthopaedic Surgeon, Guam Memorial Hospital, Tamuning, Guam
Fractures of the Scapula, Clavicle, and Glenoid

Richard Barth, M.D.
Resident, Department of Orthopaedic Surgery, University of Pennsylvania School of Medicine, Philadelphia, PA
Pathologic Fractures: Neoplasia and Metabolic Fracture

Fred Behrens, M.D.
Professor, Orthopaedic Surgery, Case Western Reserve University; Director, Department of Orthopaedic Surgery, MetroHealth Medical Center; Cleveland, OH
Fractures with Soft Tissue Injuries

Mark R. Belsky, M.D.
Associate Clinical Professor, Orthopaedic Surgery, Tufts University School of Medicine, Boston, MA; Chief, Orthopaedic Surgery, Newton-Wellesley Hospital, Newton, MA
Fractures and Dislocations of the Hand

Daniel R. Benson, M.D.
Professor, University of California, Davis, School of Medicine, Davis, CA; Chief, Spine Service, University of California, Davis, Medical Center, Sacramento, CA
Initial Evaluation of the Spine-Injured Patient

Lawrence B. Bone, M.D., F.A.C.S.
Assistant Professor, Orthopaedic and General Surgery, State University of New York at Buffalo School of Medicine and Biomedical Sciences; Director, Trauma Service, Erie County Medical Center; Buffalo, NY
Emergency Treatment of the Injured Patient

Timothy J. Bray, M.D.
Assistant Clinical Professor, Orthopaedic Surgery, University of California, Davis, Medical Center, Sacramento, CA; Associate, Reno Orthopaedic Clinic, Reno, NV
Fractures and Soft Tissue Injuries of the Ankle

Christopher W. Bryan-Brown, M.D.
Professor, Albert Einstein College of Medicine of Yeshiva University; Vice Chairman, Clinical Affairs, Anesthesiology/Critical Care, Montefiore Medical Center; Bronx, NY
Anesthetic Management of the Trauma Patient

Thomas M.E. Brushart, M.D.
Assistant Professor, Orthopaedic Surgery and Neurology, Johns Hopkins University; Attending Surgeon, Raymond M. Curtis Hand Center, Union Memorial Hospital; Baltimore, MD
Brachial Plexus and Shoulder Girdle Injuries

Robert W. Bucholz, M.D.
Professor and Chairman, Department of Orthopaedic Surgery, University of Texas Southwestern Medical Center at Dallas Southwestern Medical School, Dallas, TX
Lower Cervical Spine Injuries

Andrew R. Burgess, M.D., F.A.C.S.
Assistant Professor, Orthopaedic Surgery, University of Maryland School of Medicine; Assistant Professor, Orthopaedic Surgery, Johns Hopkins University School of Medicine; Director, Orthopaedic Traumatology, Maryland In-

stitute for Emergency Medical Services Systems (Shock Trauma Center); Baltimore, MD
Principles of External Fixation

Aaron Calodney, M.D.
Assistant Professor, Department of Anesthesiology, The University of Texas Health Science Center at Houston Medical School; Staff Anesthesiologist, University Center for Pain Medicine at The Hermann Hospital; Houston, TX
Useful Nerve Blocks for Pain Relief and Surgery
Perioperative Pain Management of the Injured
Reflex Sympathetic Dystrophy

Jeffrey Cannella, M.D.
Assistant Professor, Department of Anesthesiology, University of Texas Medical School at Houston; Staff Anesthesiologist, University Center for Pain Medicine at The Hermann Hospital; Houston, TX
Useful Nerve Blocks for Pain Relief and Surgery
Perioperative Pain Management of the Injured
Reflex Sympathetic Dystrophy

James D. Capozzi, M.D.
Associate Clinical Professor of Orthopaedics, Mount Sinai School of Medicine of the City University of New York; Attending Orthopaedic Surgeon, The Mount Sinai Hospital; Attending Orthopaedic Surgeon, Doctors Hospital; New York, NY
Intertrochanteric Hip Fractures

Edward J. Cheal, Ph.D.
Assistant Professor, Orthopaedic Surgery, Harvard Medical School; Senior Research Associate, Beth Israel Hospital; Senior Research Associate, Brigham and Women's Hospital; Co-director, Biomechanics Laboratory, Rehabilitation Research and Development, West Roxbury VA Medical Center; Boston, MA
Biomechanics of Fractures

Christopher L. Colton, F.R.C.S., F.R.C.S.E.
Clinical Teacher and Consultant, Nottingham University Hospital Medical School; Consultant Orthopaedic Surgeon and Senior Orthopaedic Traumatologist, Nottingham University Hospital; Nottingham, England
The History of Fracture Treatment

John F. Connolly, M.D., F.A.C.S.
Director, Orthopedic Training, Orlando Regional Medical Center; Attending staff, Orlando Regional Medical Center, and Arnold Palmer Hospital; Orlando, FL
Principles of Closed Management of Common Fractures

Charles N. Cornell, M.D.
Assistant Professor, Surgery, Cornell University Medical College; Assistant attending staff, Orthopaedic Surgery, Hospital for Special Surgery; Assistant attending staff, Orthopaedic Surgery, The New York Hospital; New York, NY; Chief, Orthopaedic Surgery Section, VA Hospital; Bronx, NY
Metabolic Bone Disease

Jeffrey Ecker, M.B.
Microsurgical Fellow, University of Southern California School of Medicine; Fellow, Los Angeles County Hospital, Los Angeles, CA; Consultant, Royal Perth Hospital, Perth, Australia
Soft Tissue Coverage

Frank J. Eismont, M.D.
Professor, Departments of Orthopaedics and Rehabilitation, University of Miami School of Medicine; Co-director, Acute Spinal Cord Injury Unit, University of Miami–Jackson Memorial Hospital Medical Center; Director, Residency Education Program; Miami, FL
Thoracic and Upper Lumbar Spine Injuries

David V. Feliciano, M.D.
Professor and Vice-Chairman, Department of Surgery, University of Rochester School of Medicine and Dentistry Medical Center; Attending Surgeon and SICU Director, The Strong Memorial Hospital; Rochester, NY
Evaluation and Treatment of Vascular Injuries

Kenneth R. First, M.D.
Orthopaedic Surgeon, Lankenau Hospital, Philadelphia, PA
Principles of External Fixation

F. Barry Florence, M.D.
Instructor, Department of Anesthesiology, University of Texas Medical School at Houston, Houston, TX
Anesthetic Management of the Trauma Patient

Bruce E. Frederickson, M.D
Associate Professor, Orthopedic and Neurological Surgery, State University of New York Health Science Center at Syracuse College of Medicine; Attending staff, SUNY Health Science Center and Crouse-Irving Memorial Hospital; Active Staff at VA Hospital; Head, Back Rehabilitation Program, St. Camillus Health and Rehabilitation Center; Syracuse, NY
Nonoperative Treatment of the Spine: External Immobilization

Steven R. Garfin, M.D.
Professor, Division of Orthopaedics and Rehabilitation, University of California, San Diego, School of Medicine; Attending staff, UCSD Medical Center; San Diego, CA
Thoracic and Upper Spine Lumbar Injuries

Harris Gellman, M.D.
Associate Clinical Professor, Department of Orthopedic Surgery, University of Southern California, School of Medicine; Attending staff, Cedars-Sinai Medical Center, Los Angeles, CA; Chief, Spinal Cord Injury Hand Clinic, Rancho Los Amigos Medical Center; Downey, CA
Gunshot Wounds to the Musculoskeletal System

Gregory E. Gleis, M.D.
Associate Professor, Department of Orthopedics, University of Louisville School of Medicine; Chief, Orthopedics, Louisville VA Medical Center; Staff, Norton's Hospital, Children's Hospital, Methodist Hospital, Jewish Hospital, and Humana Hospital–University of Louisville; Louisville, KY
Diagnosis and Treatment of Complications

Stuart A. Green, M.D.
Clinical Professor, Orthopaedic Surgery, University of California, Irvine, College of Medicine, Irvine, CA; Director, Problem Fracture Service, Rancho Los Amigos Medical Center, Downey, CA
The Ilizarov Method

Edward N. Hanley, Jr., M.D.
Chairman, Department of Orthopaedic Surgery, Carolinas Medical Center, Charlotte, NC
Operative Treatment of Spinal Injuries: Surgical Management

Sigvard T. Hansen, Jr., M.D.
Professor, Department of Orthopaedics, University of Washington School of Medicine; Orthopaedist-in-Chief, Harborview Medical Center; Seattle, WA
Foot Injuries

John H. Harris, Jr., M.D., D.Sc.
Professor and John S. Dunn Chairman, Department of Radiology, University of Texas Medical School at Houston; Radiologist-in-Chief, The Hermann Hospital; Houston, TX
Spinal Imaging

Wilson C. Hayes, Ph.D.
Maurice Edmond Mueller Professor of Biomechanics, Harvard Medical School; Director, Orthopaedic Biomechanics Laboratory, Beth Israel Hospital; Boston, MA
Biomechanics of Fractures

David L. Helfet, M.D., M.B., Ch.B.
Associate Professor of Orthopaedics Clinical Department, University of South Florida College of Medicine; Director, Orthopaedic Trauma Service, Tampa General Hospital; Tampa, FL
Fractures of the Distal Femur

John A. Hipp, Ph.D.
Instructor, Orthopaedic Surgery, Harvard Medical School; Senior Research Associate, Orthopaedic Biomechanics Laboratory, Beth Isreal Hospital; Boston, MA
Biomechanics of Fractures

James L. Hughes, M.D.
Professor, University of Mississippi School of Medicine; Chairman, Department of Orthopaedic Surgery, University Hospital; Jackson, MS
Fractures of the Diaphyseal Humerus

Tom Janisse, M.D.
Clinical Instructor, Department of Anesthesiology, University of Texas Medical School at Houston; Attending staff, University Center for Pain Medicine at the Hermann Hospital; Houston, TX
Perioperative Pain Management of the Injured
Reflex Sympathetic Dystrophy

P. Jeffrey Jarrett, M.D.
Clinical Assistant Professor, Orthopaedic Surgery, Emory University School of Medicine, Atlanta, GA
Injuries of the Cervicocranium

Kenneth D. Johnson, M.D
Associate Professor, Department of Orthopaedic Surgery, Vanderbilt University School of Medicine; Director, Division of Orthopaedic Trauma, Vanderbilt University Medical Center; Nashville, TN
Femoral Shaft Fractures

Timothy L. Keenen, M.D.
Assistant Professor, Division of Orthopaedics, Oregon Health Sciences University School of Medicine, Portland, OR
Initial Evaluation of the Spine-Injured Patient

James F. Kellam, M.D., F.R.C.S.(C.), F.A.C.S.
Associate Professor, Department of Surgery, University of Toronto; Consultant, Sunnybrook Hospital; Toronto, Ontario, Canada; Vice Chairman and Director of Orthopedic Trauma, Department of Orthopedics, Carolinas Medical Center, Charlotte, NC
Fractures of the Pelvic Ring; Diaphyseal Fractures of the Forearm

Joseph M. Lane, M.D.
Professor, Orthopaedic Surgery, Cornell University Medical College; Chief, Orthopaedic Surgery, Memorial Sloan-Kettering Cancer Center; Chief, Metabolic Bone Disease and Director of Research, Hospital for Special Surgery; New York, NY
Metabolic Bone Disease

David Leffers, M.D.
Florida Orthopaedic Institute, Tampa, FL
Dislocations and Soft Tissue Injuries of the Knee

Paul E. Levin, M.D.
Assistant Professor and Chief, Division of Orthopaedic Trauma, State University of New York at Stony Brook Health Sciences Center School of Medicine, University Hospital, Stony Brook, NY
Hip Dislocations

Roger N. Levy, M.D.
Clinical Professor of Orthopaedics, Mount Sinai School of Medicine of the City University of New York; Attending Orthopaedic Surgeon, Mount Sinai Hospital; Chief, Arthritis Service, Mount Sinai Hospital; New York, NY
Intertrochanteric Hip Fractures

Robert Y. McMurtry, M.D.
Professor and Head of Surgery, University of Calgary Faculty of Medicine; Chief of Surgery, Foothills Hospital; Calgary, Alberta, Canada
Fractures of the Distal Radius

Jeffrey Mast, M.D.
Associate Clinical Professor, Department of Orthopedic Surgery, Wayne State University College of Medicine; Attending staff, Orthopedic Department, Hutzel Hospital; Detroit, MI
Principles of Internal Fixation

Joel M. Matta, M.D.
Associate Professor of Clinical Orthopaedics, University of Southern California School of Medicine; Active staff: Hospital of the Good Samaritan, LAC/USC Medical Center, Orthopaedic Hospital, California Medical Center, and St. Vincent's Medical Center; Los Angeles, CA
Surgical Treatment of Acetabulum Fractures

David K. Mehne, M.D.
Assistant Professor, Orthopedic Surgery, University of Puerto Rico, San Juan, Puerto Rico; Chief, Department of Orthopedic Surgery, Hospital General Menonita, Aibonito, Puerto Rico
Trauma to the Adult Elbow and Fractures of the Distal Humerus

Michael Mendes, M.D.
Attending Staff Physician, Department of Orthopedics, Geisinger Medical Center, Danville, PA
Principles of Closed Management of Common Fractures
Principles of Internal Fixation

Michael E. Miller, M.D.
Associate Professor, Orthopaedic Surgery, Emory University School of Medicine; Chief, Orthopaedic Surgery, Grady Memorial Hospital; Atlanta, GA
Fractures of the Scapula, Clavicle, and Glenoid

Michael A. Mont, M.D.
Assistant Professor, Orthopaedic Surgery, Johns Hopkins University School of Medicine, Baltimore, MD
Intertrochanteric Hip Fractures

Michael L. Nerlich, M.D.
Assistant Professor, Trauma Surgery, Department of Trauma Surgery, Hannover Medical School, Hannover, Germany
Biology of Soft Tissue Injuries

Tom R. Norris, M.D.
Attending staff, Departments of Hand and Orthopaedic Surgery, Pacific Presbyterian Medical Center, San Francisco, CA
Fractures of the Proximal Humerus and Dislocations of the Shoulder

Attila Poka, M.D.
Assistant Professor, Orthopaedic Surgery, University of Maryland School of Medicine; Attending Orthopaedic Traumatologist, Maryland Institute for Emergency Medical Services Systems/Shock Trauma Center, University of Maryland Medical System; Baltimore, MD
Principles of External Fixation

P. Prithvi Raj, M.D.
Professor, Department of Anesthesiology, The University of Texas Medical School at Houston; Director, The University Center for Pain Medicine at Hermann Hospital
Useful Nerve Blocks for Pain Relief and Surgery
Perioperative Pain Management of the Injured
Reflex Sympathetic Dystrophy

Cecil H. Rorabeck, M.D., F.R.C.S.(C.)
Professor of Surgery, Division of Orthopaedic Surgery, University of Western Ontario; Chief, Division of Orthopaedic Surgery, University Hospital; London, Ontario, Canada
Compartment Syndromes

Howard Rosen, M.D.
Clinical Professor, Orthopaedics Mount Sinai School of Medicine; Chief, Fracture Trauma Service, Hospital for Joint Diseases Orthopaedic Institute; New York, NY
Nonunion and Malunion

Leonard Ruby, M.D.
Professor, Orthopedic Surgery, Tufts University School of Medicine; Chief, Division of Hand Surgery, Department of Orthopaedic Surgery, New England Medical Center Hospitals; Boston, MA
Fractures and Dislocations of the Carpus

Thomas A. Russell, M.D.
Assistant Professor, Department of Orthopaedics, University of Tennessee Center for the Health Sciences, College of Medicine
Subtrochanteric Fractures of the Femur

Roy Sanders, M.D.
Clinical Assistant Professor, Department of Orthopedics, University of South Florida; Associate Director, Orthopedic Trauma Service, Tampa General Hospital; Tampa, FL
Patella Fractures and Extensor Mechanism Injuries

Richard A. Saunders, M.D.
Chief Resident, Department of Orthopedic Surgery, George Washington University Medical Center, Washington, D.C.
Physical Impairment Ratings for Fractures

Felix H. Savoie, M.D.
Assistant Professor, Department of Orthopaedic Surgery, University of Mississippi Medical Center; Attending staff, University Hospital, Veterans Administration Hospital, Mississippi Methodist Rehabilitation Center; Jackson, MS
Fractures of the Diaphyseal Humerus

Joseph Schatzker, M.D., F.R.C.S.(C.)
Professor, Orthopaedic Surgery, University of Toronto; Orthopaedist-in-Chief, Sunnybrook Health Science Centre; Toronto, Ontario, Canada
Tibial Plateau Fractures

Robert K. Schenk, M.D.
Professor Emeritus, Anatomy, Histology, and Embryology, University of Berne; Head, Bone Histology Laboratory, Institute of Pathophysiology, University of Berne; Berne, Switzerland
Biology of Fracture Repair

David Seligson, M.D.
Professor, Division of Orthopaedic Surgery; Chief, Fracture Service, University of Louisville School of Medicine; Attending staff: VA Medical Center, Methodist Hospital, Baptist East Hospital, and Humana Hospital-University of Louisville, Louisville, KY
Diagnosis and Treatment of Complications

Randolph Sherman, M.D., F.A.C.S.
Assistant Professor, Plastic and Orthopedic Surgery, University of Southern California School of Medicine; Chief: Section of Plastic Surgery Service, Los Angeles County Hospital/USC; Microsurgical Service, Hospital of the Good Samaritan; Plastic Surgery Service, K.H. Norris/USC Cancer Center; Los Angeles, CA
Soft Tissue Coverage

Albert Simpkins, Jr., M.D.
Active Staff, Parkview Community Hospital, Riverside, CA
Operative Treatment of Spinal Injuries: Surgical Management

Lex A. Simpson, M.D.
Partner, Reno Orthopedic Clinic, Reno, NV
Fractures and Soft Tissue Injuries of the Ankle

Marc F. Swiontkowski, M.D.
Associate Professor, University of Washington School of Medicine; Attending Orthopaedic Surgeon: Harborview Medical Center, University of Washington Medical Center, Children's Hospital and Medical Center; Seattle, WA
Intracapsular Hip Fractures

J. Charles Taylor, M.D.
Assistant Professor of Orthopaedics, University of Tennessee, Memphis, College of Medicine; Staff, Campbell Clinic; Memphis, TN; Chief, Orthopaedics, Regional Medical Center at Memphis, Elvis Presley Memorial Trauma Center; Attending staff: Baptist Memorial Hospital (Central, East, and DeSoto), LeBonheur Children's Medical Center, William F. Bowld Hospital; Memphis, TN
Subtrochanteric Fractures of the Femur

Harald Tscherne, M.D.
Professor and Chairman, Department of Trauma Surgery, Hannover Medical School, Hannover, Germany
Biology of Soft Tissue Injuries

E. Frazier Ward, M.D.
Associate Professor, Orthopaedic Surgery, University of Mississippi School of Medicine; Department of Orthopaedic Surgery, University of Mississippi Medical Center; VA Medical Center; Jackson, MS
Fractures of the Diaphyseal Humerus

Joanne Werntz, M.D.
Attending staff, Florida Hand and Microsurgery Center, in association with Matthews Orthopaedic Clinic, P.A., Orlando, FL
Metabolic Bone Disease

Thomas E. Whitesides, Jr., M.D.
Professor, Department of Orthopaedic Surgery, Emory University School of Medicine; Active Staff: Emory University Hospital, Grady Memorial Hospital, Henrietta Eggleston Hospital for Children; Atlanta, GA
Injuries of the Cervicocranium

Sam W. Wiesel, M.D.
Professor and Chairman, Department of Orthopedic Surgery, Georgetown University School of Medicine; Attending staff, Georgetown University Hospital; Washington, DC
Physical Impairment Ratings for Fractures

E.F. Shaw Wilgis, M.D.
Associate Professor, Plastic Surgery and Orthopedic Surgery, Johns Hopkins University; Chief, Division of Hand Surgery, Union Memorial Hospital; Baltimore, MD
Brachial Plexus and Shoulder Girdle Injuries

Donald A. Wiss, M.D.
Associate Professor, Orthopedic Surgery, University of Southern California School of Medicine; Director, Orthopedic Trauma Service, Los Angeles County-USC Medical Center; Los Angeles, CA
Gunshot Wounds to the Musculoskeletal System

Hansen A. Yuan, M.D.
Professor, State University of New York Health Science Center at Syracuse College of Medicine; Attending staff: SUNY Health Science Center at Syracuse, Crouse-Irving Memorial Hospital; Active Staff, VA Hospital; Consultant, St. Joseph's Hospital, Syracuse, NY
Nonoperative Treatment of the Spine: External Immobilization

Foreword

Bruce D. Browner, Jesse B. Jupiter, Alan M. Levine, and Peter G. Trafton have assembled a comprehensive text on fracture management. This up-to-date work covers the most recent trends in fracture treatment and summarizes methods of fracture care.

There is no doubt that the technology explosion of the last two decades has resulted in improved care of musculoskeletal injuries. However, the negative aspect of this burgeoning technology has been the increased cost in this country of health care delivery, which has reached critical levels. We orthopedic surgeons have a responsibility to participate in the solution of those problems. The government is addressing this issue very forcefully. One can anticipate that major changes in the way medical care is delivered and reimbursed will take place in the near future.

Some have indiscriminately used expensive technology and have misguidedly emphasized the need to restore to perfect anatomy all injured bones and joints. Many deviations from normal anatomy are easily compensated by the human body without adverse sequelae. Surgical intervention to correct deviations should be reserved for those instances in which experience and documented knowledge dictate their use.

The fragmentation of orthopedics into multiple subspecialties and the growing compartmentalization into areas of special interest may be threatening the future viability of orthopedic surgery. In addition, parallel to the fragmentation process, orthopedists limit their interest or concentrate their practice on narrow areas of specialization, and some have limited their involvement in the treatment of injury. Although fracture management has always been a basic concern of orthopedists, the withdrawal of many of us from trauma care has weakened this cohesive factor in our profession. The role of the orthopedist in trauma care has changed. That role as a coordinator in the management of the acutely injured patient has been assumed by others in varying degrees. Attempts are also being made by other disciplines, including some composed of individuals with limited licenses, to seek involvement in the care of fractures. These developments require that we reinforce our commitment to excellence in our profession and that we emphasize our comprehensive knowledge of the musculoskeletal system and our orthopedic training, which uniquely qualify us to be the best providers of fracture care.

Books such as this one should remind us of the importance of maintaining the highest standards of education for orthopedic surgeons during residency and practice. With a careful presentation of indications, techniques, and pitfalls, this text establishes the appropriate use of technology by emphasizing the basis for management of skeletal trauma. As orthopedists, we must rededicate ourselves to preserving this foundation, which has made Western Medicine great.

AUGUST SARMIENTO, M.D.
Professor and Chairman
Department of Orthopaedics
University of Southern California
School of Medicine

Preface

The preface to the first edition of each major fracture text published in the last 70 years indicates that the new book was created because there had been significant evolution in the understanding and treatment of musculoskeletal injuries and the new knowledge was not reflected in existing texts. In each case, a new book was written by a new generation of fracture surgeons who had actively participated in helping to establish the new methods of fracture treatment and teach others about them. The editors and authors of *Skeletal Trauma: Fractures, Dislocations, and Ligamentous Injuries* represent a continuation of this tradition. Many have concentrated their clinical practice and research in the new subspecialty of orthopedic traumatology that has developed in North America over the last ten years. Under the influence of the AO (Arbeitsgemeinshaft für Osteosynthesefragen, The Association for the Study of Internal Fixation), these surgeons have adopted a more operatively oriented approach to fracture management. These surgeons have staffed the fracture services at large trauma centers in the United States and Canada. They have been presented with a large number of patients with high-energy injuries resulting from blunt and penetrating trauma. This extensive contemporary experience has allowed them to contribute actively to the development of the latest methods of treating skeletal injuries. These individuals have helped to form the *Orthopaedic Trauma Association,* which has provided an important forum for the further development of the science of orthopedic traumatology.

The decision to go forward with the writing of this new book was made in the summer of 1987. The editors agreed with the publisher that existing fracture texts did not reflect the contemporary approach to skeletal trauma management that had become the standard of practice. This new text has been constructed to serve the needs of both the practicing orthopedist and the orthopedic resident. It was our aim to provide a problem-solving resource to tell the orthopedist both "what" to do with each injury as well as "how" to perform specific operations. Radiographs and two-color illustrations have been used extensively to present the patho-anatomy, classifications, and operative techniques. In addition to large sections on the upper and lower extremity, a vastly expanded section on spine and pelvic trauma is presented. The spine section represents one of the most detailed references available concerning management of spinal injuries.

Although orthopedic surgeons are increasingly concentrating their practices in subspecialty areas, trauma still represents a major portion of orthopedic activity. During their training, all orthopedists must receive a thorough education in the treatment of skeletal injuries. The general section of this textbook was designed as a comprehensive educational resource for orthopedic residents. It opens with a beautifully written and colorful history of fracture surgery. This is followed by three authoritative chapters on basic science. Chapters on emergency treatment of the injured patient and anesthetic management of the trauma patient present general information concerning trauma care. Chapters on regional anesthesia and perioperative pain management provide detailed information from anesthesiologists on techniques that can be used by orthopedists. This section also includes chapters on the principles of closed management, internal fixation, external fixation, and an overall coverage of fractures with soft tissue injury, including closed and open fractures. Chapters are provided on the evaluation and treatment of associated injuries and complicatons. This section also includes discussions of gunshot injuries and pathologic fractures. There is an overview of the treatment of malunions and nonunions and a separate discussion on the applications of the Ilizarov method. The section closes with the consideration of disability analysis. Much of this information was not available in previous fracture texts and could only be gleaned from multiple outside references.

In the four years it has taken to produce this book, the editors have worked assiduously to ensure that the new information and concepts are incorporated in the text. We are indebted to our colleagues who have contributed chapters. All are busy, overcommitted academicians who invested significant time in this project. We have been impressed by their devotion and clarity of thought and presentation. As fracture surgeons, we believe that it is our turn to chronicle methods of the day. We hope that what we have written will aid orthopedic surgeons for many years in the vital work of caring for patients with skeletal injuries.

BRUCE D. BROWNER, M.D.

Acknowledgments

We would like to acknowledge the role played by the senior editorial staff at W.B. Saunders. Edward Wickland, Senior Editor throughout most of the project, was the driving force who functioned as executive producer. Kitty McCullough, our Developmental Editor, pulled together the many manuscripts and individual illustrations that had to be combined for this two volume text. Her equanimity and cheerful but persistent communications were helpful in collecting the material and soothing tempers. John Cooke, Executive Vice President, and Carolyn Naylor, Assistant Director, Book Production, and their staff did a marvelous job transforming our raw material into a beautiful printed textbook.

No staff was hired by the editors for the production of this text. This was only possible because we were able to rely on the extraordinary talents, devotion, and hard work of our own personal staffs.

Bruce Browner gratefully acknowledges the work of Debbie Moore, his executive secretary, who labored tirelessly in helping him to communicate with the editors, authors, artists, and W.B Saunders staff. In addition, she spent countless hours transcribing, proofreading, and editing the manuscripts, galley proofs, and page proofs. Doug Heidemann, Administrative Specialist, collected manuscripts and illustrations received from authors in many sections, keeping this material catalogued and filed, and then ensuring that it was promptly and efficiently transmitted to the publisher. Dr. Browner would like to thank the orthopaedic residents for their understanding of the demands placed on their Chief by this project, and for their assistance in the proofreading and the refinement of the general section.

Jesse Jupiter would like to thank his executive secretary, Sue Ann Humin, for helping him communicate with the authors and illustrators, and keeping him focused on the task at hand. He expresses his gratitude as well to Michel Tresfort, transcriptionist, for proofreading all of the manuscripts in addition to his regular duties.

Alan Levine extends his appreciation to Cindy Dubois, his secretary, for assisting him in communicating with the authors and illustrators, and transcribing the manuscripts. He would also like to thank Martha Keltz, his research assistant, for preparing copies of articles pertinent to each chapter and for extensive efforts in proofreading.

Peter Trafton recognizes his administrative secretary, Robin Morin, for her assistance throughout the project with correspondence, copying, mailing, and telephone calls.

The unique appearance of this fracture text and a major component of its message is transmitted by the beautiful illustrations that have been created for these two volumes. These talented artists worked closely with the authors and editors to assure anatomic and technical accuracy and clarity of presentation. We are indebted to them for helping us to transmit essential information regarding the diagnosis and treatment of skeletal injuries.

Finally, we must pay tribute to those who have gone before us, who have taught us the principles and techniques of trauma management, and who have stimulated us to follow in their footsteps. We hope that what we have done and what we have written will give them pride. They have passed the torch to us, and we have attempted to pass the light on to others through our writing.

Introduction

*E*xtremely timely, important, and well-conceived, *Skeletal Trauma* reflects the revolutionary advances that have taken place in orthopedic surgery over the last 25 years. These advances have come about in response to changes in society that have greatly increased the incidence of skeletal trauma injuries from high-speed or high-energy violence and to progress in technology that has dramatically improved the treatment of these injuries.

Prior to 1965, skeletal trauma consisted mainly of low- or moderate-energy, closed fractures. Common injuries such as wrist, ankle, hip, and osteoporotic spinal compression fractures were treated by general practitioners and general surgeons as often as by orthopedic surgeons. However, beginning approximately in 1965, several seemingly unrelated events reshaped the traditional approach to fracture care.

First, young people who were born at the peak of the "baby boom" generation began to drive. Large numbers of young drivers, who were often fueled by alcohol or later by recreational drugs, took to our deteriorating highways in high-powered, fast-moving vehicles.

Second, fields of specialization and even subspecialization pervaded the practice of medicine. Physicians confined their practices to specific body systems: for example, orthopedics, urology, or neurosurgery, and these specialties became distinct practices apart from general surgery. Specialists eventually acquired most of the patient care within their areas of expertise. Consequently, orthopedists started to take over the care of virtually all musculoskeletal injuries, including even minor fractures.

Having established a narrower focus and mirroring societal progress in general, surgical specialists turned to high technology to achieve better treatment results and to justify specialization. Each specialty developed implants and artificial parts to repair or replace damaged or worn-out body parts.

In orthopedics, implants included total joints, which were originally and most successfully used in the hip and the knee. The most revolutionary advances pertinent to skeletal trauma were promoted by the Arbeitsgemeinshaft für Osteosynthesefragen (AO). Founded in Switzerland in 1958, the AO Group developed a system of fracture-repair instruments and implants that had started to gain international recognition by 1965, although they were not widely used in North America until approximately 1975.

Finally, accusations of malpractice were becoming a notorious consequence of unsatisfactory results following surgery, and patients and their attorneys were demanding better anatomic and functional restoration, even after severe injury.

The combination of rapidly increasing numbers and severity of musculoskeletal injuries, a burgeoning technology, and a demand for better treatment has helped to reshape orthopedics since 1965. However, at the same time these positive changes were occurring, there emerged a large class of underprivileged and unemployed people whose lifestyle revolved around violence. As a result, automobile and motorcycle accidents were no longer the only causes of high-energy trauma. Gunshot wounds accounted for large numbers of skeletal trauma injuries and for trauma associated with other life-threatening injuries. Most victims of this type of violence lived primarily in the decaying centers of our largest cities, usually near our largest and most prestigious teaching hospitals, and were brought to these hospitals for treatment.

Orthopedic surgery, neurosurgery, anesthesiology, and the specialties within general surgery, including thoracic and vascular surgery, responded to the growing numbers of severely injured patients by branching into subgroups with major interest in trauma, and thus developed the new subspecialty of traumatology, the study and treatment of high-energy injury. Today, we have general surgery traumatologists, orthopedic traumatologists, neurosurgical traumatologists, and anesthesiology and general surgery intensivists, who run surgical intensive care units. In addition, traumatology encompasses specialists in urology, pulmonary care, radiology, and many others who have developed special interest and expertise in trauma.

Skeletal Trauma will appeal to both the general orthopedist, whose practice consists of fracture care, and the orthopedic traumatologist, who treats fewer patients but those who are severely injured. The material presented here is exceptionally well organized. General Principles provides the latest information in basic science, bone healing, soft-tissue response to injuries, biomechanic characteristics of bone, implants, and the pathophysiology of the injured patient. The principles that are used in treating various types of injuries and the basic treatment modalities are discussed in detail. The clinical sections are divided into three classic areas: Spine and Pelvis, edited by Alan Levine; the Upper Extremity, edited by Jesse Jupiter; and the Lower Extremity, edited by Peter Trafton.

The main strength of this book lies in the selection of the authors, all of whom have devoted a great part if not all of their careers to a special interest in musculoskeletal traumatology. Many have subspecialized even further in their areas of interest in the musculoskeletal system and have become superspecialists in upper extremity and hand trauma, pelvic and acetabular trauma, long-bone trauma, and foot and ankle trauma. Of special note is that each author has a currently active practice in the area of interest he was asked to discuss. In many cases, these authors are responsible for the recent advances that have been made in their particular areas.

Some chapters are necessarily long in order to include all the contributions that have been made to a topic. Because injuries resulting from high-energy violence can occur in numerous variations and combinations, their diagnoses and treatments are presented in detail.

Treating patients with modern techniques and treatment protocols is enormously important for socioeconomic reasons. Trauma in all its aspects costs the United States nearly $150 billion every year. If the latest technology and surgical expertise were available in well-organized regional trauma centers, that cost could be cut in half, saving society $75 billion per year. Some of these resources could be used to improve the quality of education, deteriorating highways, substandard vehicles and driver training, unsafe conditions in the workplace, and poor living conditions in our central cities. However, sparing society the expenses due to disability and a diminished work force is less important than improving the quality of life of individuals who are victims of unfortunate injuries. Modern traumatology techniques have significantly lessoned the disability, disfigurement, and loss of life that was routinely expected after high-energy injuries just a generation ago.

SIGVARD T. HANSEN, JR., M.D.

Contents

II

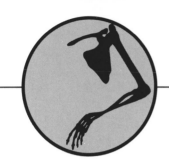

Section Editor

JESSE B. JUPITER, M.D.

III

Upper Extremity

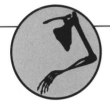

Jesse B. Jupiter, M.D.
Mark R. Belsky, M.D.

33

Fractures and Dislocations of the Hand

*T*he hand is man's most exquisite organ of direct interaction with the surrounding universe. Each digit of the hand can be viewed in a manner analogous to an entire limb, given its complement of structures; yet nowhere else in the body does function follow form as closely as in the hand. The precision and stability of its small articulations, the fine balance between its extrinsic and intrinsic motors, and the complex tendon mechanisms gliding on their diaphanous beds demand a stable, aligned supporting skeleton. These gliding structures intimately enveloping the tubular skeleton of the phalanges prove in many cases to be the ultimate determinants of the functional outcome following skeletal trauma. Charnley recognized this when he stated that "the reputation of a surgeon may stand as much in jeopardy from this injury (phalangeal fracture) as from any fracture of the femur."[38]

Fractures involving the tubular bones of the hand represent the most frequent of all skeletal injuries.[60,143,204,224] Although failure to gain union with phalangeal and metacarpal fractures is unusual,[102] the prevention of angular or rotational deformity, tendon adhesion, or articular dysfunction continues to challenge even the most experienced surgeon. The economic costs of injuries to the hand are staggering (Table 33–1). Each year in the United States more than one third of all injuries involve the upper extremity, affecting more than 16 million Americans and requiring more than 500,000 hospitalizations and more than 6 million emergency room visits.[111] In America the hand suffers more than 1.5 million fractures and almost 6 million open wounds each year.[128] These injuries result in 16 million lost days of work, 2 billion dollars in lost earnings, and almost 4 billion dollars in individual costs to industry.[90] The economic burden

has been equally documented in Europe. Boehler noted that compensation paid out for hand injuries in Austria proved to be almost twice that for fractures of the long bones.[20] Tubiana reported that in 1975 in France hand injuries were responsible for 27% of the total amount paid in disability benefits for all work-related accidents, and the number of lost work days approached 8 million.[209]

Functional Anatomy

Extending out from the carpal arch of the wrist, the four digital metacarpals form the breadth of the hand (Fig. 33–1). The longitudinal and distal transverse arches of the hand pass through the metacarpals, having a common "keystone" in the metacarpophalangeal joints (Fig. 33–2). The rigid central pillar of the hand projects through the second and third metacarpals, whereas the thumb, fourth, and fifth metacarpals and their carpometacarpal articulations provide the mobile borders of the palm. The deep transverse metacarpal ligaments interconnect the four metacarpals, adding to their internal support.

The metacarpals are tubular bones structurally divided into a base, shaft, neck, and head (Fig. 33–3). The base is designed like a footing at the base of a foundation, being nearly twice as wide as the shaft when viewed in the coronal plane. Strong supporting ligaments and the congruent articulations of the trapezoid and capitate make the second and third carpometacarpal joints nearly immobile. This is in contrast to the modified saddle joint that articulates the hamate with the base of the fourth and fifth metacarpals, and

925

Table 33–1.

Epidemiology of Injuries of the Tubular Bones in the Hand (1975–1976)

Injury	Number	Days Lost From Work	Restricted Activity (Days)
Metacarpal	150,000	1,157,000	3,421,000
Phalanges	856,000	711,000	6,244,000
Multiple hand fractures	22,000	—	67,000
Dislocation of the finger	67,000	—	156,000

Source: Compiled from Kelsey, J. L.; Pastides, H.; Kreiger, N.; et al. Upper extremity disorders. A survey of their frequency and cost in the United States. St. Louis, C. V. Mosby, 1980.

affords considerable mobility in the anteroposterior plane.

The metacarpal shaft extends distally with a gentle dorsal convexity. The concave palmar cortex is denser than the dorsal cortex,[124] supporting the hypothesis that with functional loading the palmar side of the metacarpal will experience compressive forces in contrast to the tensile stresses dorsally.[100]

When viewed in the sagittal plane the metacarpal head represents a curve of increasing diameter, beginning dorsally and extending along the articular surface to the palmar side. When viewed in the coronal plane, the metacarpal head is pear-shaped, with the palmar surface extending out of each side (Fig. 33–4). The collateral ligaments of the metacarpophalangeal joint originate dorsal to the axis of flexion to insert broadly along the palmar aspects of the proximal phalanges. It is partly because of this eccentric origin of the collateral ligaments on the oddly shaped metacarpal head that the metacarpophalangeal joint is more lax in extension and more stable in flexion. The distal metacarpals are subject to flexion and adduction forces from both the extrinsic flexor muscles and the interosseous muscles in the hand.[104]

The thumb metacarpal is shorter and stouter than others and is positioned on the trapezium in palmar abduction and pronation to allow for its prehensile functioning. The thumb carpometacarpal joint is unique in functioning as nature's universal joint. Some have described it as a reciprocally biconcave saddle joint,[81,116,149] whereas others have described it as a saddle for a "scoliotic horse."[105] The natural relationship of these reciprocal convex and concave arcs oriented close to 90° apart provides a path for the thumb to abduct, pronate, and flex during its movements in opposition to the digits. Likewise, this complex articulation with its surrounding capsular ligaments provides stability to the powerful thenar and extrinsic muscles that insert onto the thumb (Fig. 33–5).

The thumb metacarpophalangeal articulation is more concentric than the adjacent digital metacarpophalangeal joints, affording nearly equal stability throughout its arc of flexion and extension. The metacarpal head is bicondylar, with the radial condyle slightly larger. This provides the thumb proximal pha-

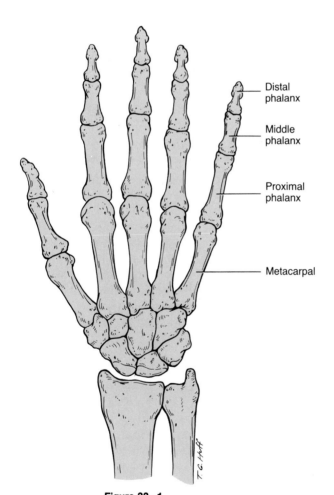

Distal
phalanx

Middle
phalanx

Proximal
phalanx

Metacarpal

Figure 33–1

Tubular skeleton of the hand.

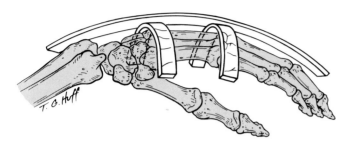
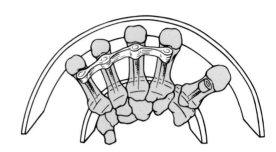

Figure 33–2

The longitudinal and transverse arches of the hand pass through the metacarpals. The metacarpals are interconnected at their bases by a complex network of ligaments and distally by the deep transverse metacarpal ligament.

lanx with a modest degree of pronation at the final point of pinch.

In distinct contrast to the interconnected metacarpals, the phalanges represent isolated skeletal units. The skeletal length of the three phalangeal segments follows closely the ratio of 1 : 1.618 (the golden mean) of the Fibonacci series discovered by Leonardo de Pisa (1202 A.D.).[130] Thus from distal to proximal, the length of each phalanx is the sum of the length of the more distal two segments. The proximal phalangeal length thus closely equals the sum of the middle and distal phalanges, with the proximal interphalangeal joint axis located exactly at the mathematical center of the digit, making it truly the nucleus of digital anatomy and function.[131] This normal skeletal relationship and alignment will keep the intrinsic and extrinsic muscle-

tendon units in equilibrium, thereby requiring only a minimal amount of force to move the digit as well as maintain a specific locus in space. Alteration in length, rotation, or angular alignment can upset this fine balance, accentuating the dysfunction.

The proximal and middle phalanges can be structurally divided into the base, shaft, neck, and head (condyles), whereas the distal phalanx differs in having a base, shaft, and tuft (Fig. 33–6). The dorsal surface of the proximal and middle phalanges is straight, and the palmar surface is concave. In contrast to the metacarpal, the phalangeal cortex is thicker dorsally.[187] In normal functional use, the powerful flexor forces suggest that the dorsal side is mechanically subjected to tensile stresses. In certain phalangeal fractures, however, this concept may not be applicable, as the deformities sec-

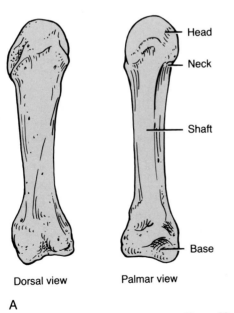
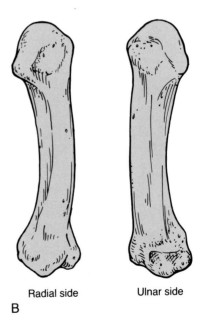

Dorsal view   Palmar view

A

Head

Neck

Shaft

Base

Radial side   Ulnar side

B

Figure 33–3

Surgical anatomy of the metacarpal.

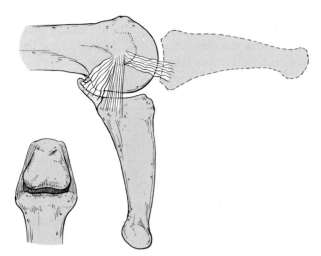

Figure 33-4

Metacarpophalangeal joint. The metacarpal head is wider on its volar projection and has a curve of increasing diameter from dorsal to palmar. Both explain why the collateral ligament is lax in extension and taut in flexion.

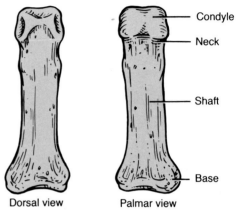

Condyle

Neck

Shaft

Base

Dorsal view   Palmar view

Figure 33-6

Surgical anatomy of the proximal phalanx.

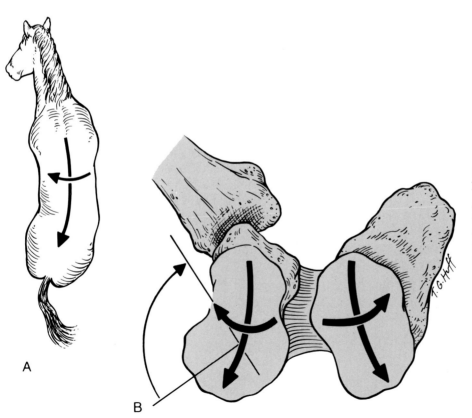

A

B

Figure 33-5

The thumb metacarpal and its complex "universal joint" articulation with the trapezium. Some have considered this to be a saddle, whereas others have described it as a saddle for a "scoliotic horse."

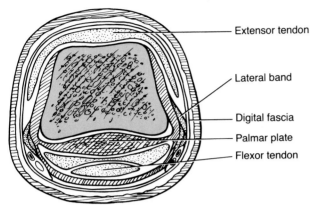

Figure 33–7

The inherent relationship of the gliding structures to the phalangeal skeleton is seen in this cross-sectional representation of a digit at the proximal phalangeal joint.

ondary to muscle imbalance may subject the dorsum to compressive forces.[87,179]

Also in contrast to the metacarpals, the digital skeleton is enveloped by the gliding surfaces of the overlying intrinsic and extrinsic tendons. There is no overlying muscle, and the subcutaneous fat is minimal, adding to the propensity for tendon dysfunction following skeletal trauma, as well as the complexity of securely stabilizing the phalangeal skeleton with internal fixation (Fig. 33–7).

The small interphalangeal articulations are complex both in their form and in their function. These will be discussed in detail in the section on proximal interphalangeal joint fracture-dislocations.

General Principles

Regardless of how innocent a hand fracture may appear, the physician should take care to evaluate pertinent historical factors and perform a complete physical and radiologic examination. The mechanism of injury, when and where it occurred, symptoms of sensory and motor disturbance, important associated medical illness, allergy history, and tetanus vaccination status all are fundamental questions to be asked.

In patients with an open fracture or complex hand trauma, the entire limb must be inspected for more proximal injury. Clothing should be removed to permit both visual and manual inspection of the proximal articulations and skeleton of the upper limb.

Both closed and open skeletal trauma in the hand may have associated trauma to nerves, blood vessels, or tendons. Sensibility is documented by response not only to light touch but also to two-point discrimination. Circulation can be determined by visual inspec-

tion and documented by timed capillary refill, comparing the capillary refill of the injured digit tested along its paronychial ridge to an adjacent digit or corresponding digit on the other hand. The integrity of the extensor and flexor tendons to the digit is individually determined, and the physician should palpate along ligament insertions to ensure their integrity.

The tubular skeleton of the hand requires three x-ray views—anteroposterior (AP), lateral, and oblique—to accurately assess the position and integrity of these small skeletal units and their articulations (Fig. 33–8). The phalanges must be seen in a true lateral projection and the injured digit isolated to avoid superimposition of the skeletal units of the adjacent digits. A number of specialized radiographic projections have been developed to aid in visualizing specific areas of the skeleton. These will be discussed in specific fracture sections.

When evaluating fractures of the metacarpals and phalanges, the examiner must determine the alignment of the digits, both on initial presentation and, if required, after fracture reduction. Alignment is determined clinically by viewing the relationship of the fingernails with the digits in full extension. The nails should be almost parallel, although in many individuals the distal phalanges of the index and little fingers will angle toward the long finger. Importantly, skeletal alignment must also be assessed with the digits flexed fully. In this position the fingertips should all point toward the scaphoid tuberosity (Fig. 33–9). The contralateral hand will serve as an excellent control for angulation and rotation.

In many cases anesthesia is required to permit painless assessment of alignment and also to permit a closed reduction, if indicated. Wrist block anesthesia offers several advantages for this purpose, as it can effectively provide complete sensory anesthesia without blocking the extrinsic flexor and extensor muscles. These are necessary to provide voluntary extension and flexion to allow the examiner to determine deformity and assess fracture stability.[12]

The nerves to be blocked include the median, ulnar, dorsal sensory ulnar, and superficial radial, either selectively or completely dependent on the bone fractured. Five to eight milliliters of either mepivacaine (Carbocaine) or 1% xylocaine are mixed with 0.5% bupivacaine (Marcaine), both without epinephrine. A $\frac{5}{8}$-in 25-gauge needle is used. The median nerve is blocked 1.5 cm proximal to the carpal canal, with the injection just radial and beneath the antebrachial fascia and palmaris longus tendon. This block, used in conjunction with a superficial radial nerve block, is effective for fractures involving the thumb and the index and long fingers and for some fractures involving the ring finger. The superficial branch of the radial nerve is blocked

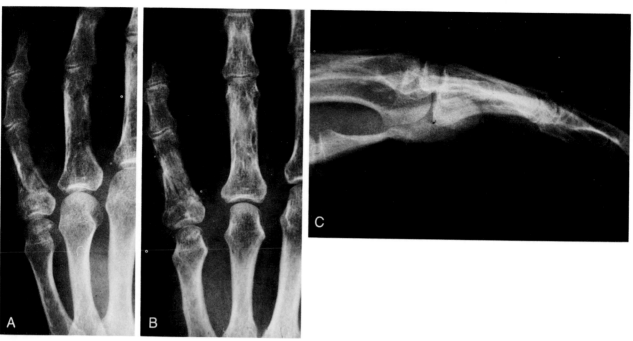

Figure 33-8

The tubular skeleton in the hand requires three x-ray projections to determine the alignment and joint relationships. This phalangeal fracture was best seen in the oblique projection *(A)*.

three fingerbreadths above the radial styloid; a transverse wheal will be raised subcutaneously over the radial side of the distal forearm.

The ulnar nerve can be anesthetized with a transverse injection under the flexor carpi ulnaris tendon proximal to the wrist crease. Aspiration is necessary prior to injection, as the ulnar artery runs adjacent to the nerve. To block the dorsal sensory branch of the ulnar nerve, the needle is passed subcutaneously and directed dorsally toward the base of the fifth metacarpal. Ulnar nerve blocks are used for fractures of the little finger ray and in conjunction with median and radial sensory blocks for ring finger ray fractures (Fig. 33-10).

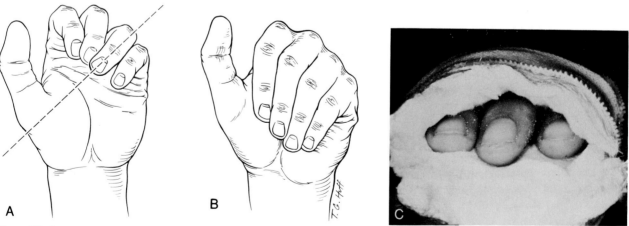

Figure 33-9

To determine rotational and angular alignment of the hand skeleton, the nails should be parallel with the digits in extension. In flexion *(B)*, the digits should all point to the scaphoid tuberosity. *C*, This 22-year-old male sustained a short oblique fracture of the proximal phalanx of his long finger. Visible malrotation is seen with the digits in extension.

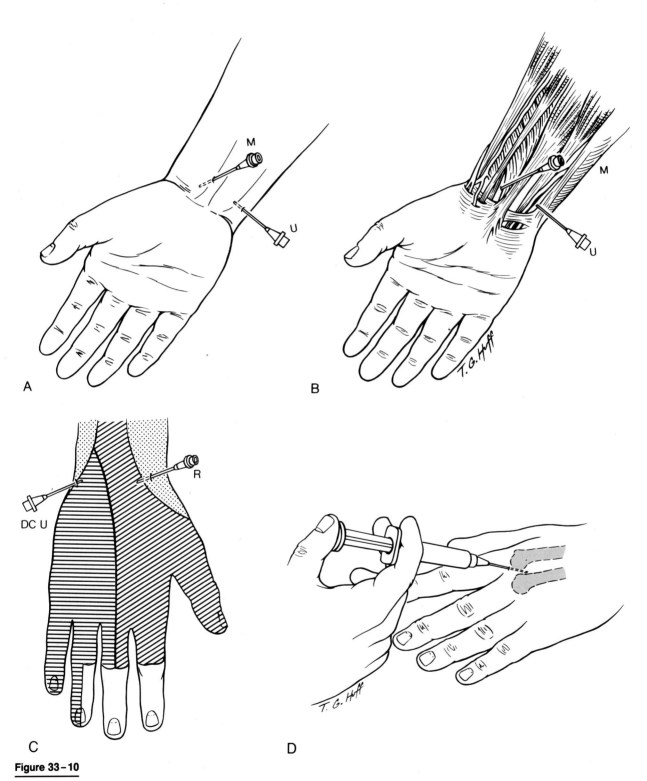

Figure 33–10

Four types of nerve block at the wrist. A and B, Sites of injection to block the median (M) and ulnar (U) nerves at the wrist. C, Sites of injection to block the dorsal cutaneous ulnar nerve (DCU) and radial sensory nerve (R) at the wrist. D, The common digital nerves can be blocked with an injection through the dorsal web space.

Table 33-2.

Goals in Treatment: Fractures in the Hand

Restoration of articular congruity
Reduction of malrotation and angulation
Maintenance of reduction with minimal surgical intervention
Surgically acceptable wound
Rapid mobilization

Table 33-4.

Stable Metacarpal and Phalangeal Fractures

Impacted fractures
Fractures with little or no displacement
Many isolated metacarpal shaft fractures
Distal phalanx fractures
Fractures without displacement through arc of digital motion

Metacarpal and Phalangeal Fracture Treatment: Concepts and Goals

Hand fractures can be complicated by deformity from no treatment, stiffness from overtreatment, and both deformity and stiffness from poor treatment.

ALFRED SWANSON[204]

The goal of treatment of fractures of the metacarpals and phalanges includes the restoration or preservation of function (Table 33-2). Inherent in this goal is the repositioning of a fractured or dislocated bone to a position that will be consistent with function. Whenever possible, articular congruity should be restored. To accomplish this goal, the physician must select a method that will offer the least soft tissue damage and accelerate the mobilization of the injured part as soon as fracture stability permits. This should be determined on the basis of information gained from the clinical and radiologic assessment of the fracture.[52,210]

The vast majority of fractures involving the tubular skeleton in the hand can be effectively treated by an organized, careful, nonoperative approach. The determination of the individual fracture's stability or "personality" is of paramount importance in closed hand fractures, as it has become increasingly evident that many stable aligned phalangeal and metacarpal fractures require only limited immobilization and fare bet-

ter with early return to mobility.[7,8,98] Studies by Borgeskov[22] (485 fractures), Wright[221] (809 fractures), and Pun et al.[161] (284 fractures) have documented the improved results with limited (one to two weeks) immobilization of stable metacarpal and phalangeal fractures of the hand.

A number of factors that can be determined from the initial examination and radiographs will help identify the fracture personality. A functional classification should take into account the fracture location, pattern, soft tissue injury, deformity, and intrinsic stability (Table 33-3). Other pertinent factors include the patient's age, medical condition, socioeconomic status, and motivation.

Hand splintage should always be in the position of immobilization rather than rest.[99,114] This involves splinting the wrist in 20° of extension, the metacarpophalangeal joints in 60° to 70° of flexion, and the interphalangeal joints in extension. The thumb metacarpal must be kept in palmar abduction to maintain the functional web space (Fig. 33-11).

In general, stable fractures include closed impacted shaft fractures, fractures with little or no displacement, most distal phalangeal fractures, many isolated metacarpal shaft fractures, and those well-aligned fractures that remain in position through a full arc of motion (Table 33-4). Pun et al.'s radiographic criteria of acceptable alignment of phalangeal and metacarpal fractures include the following[161]:

Table 33-3.

Functional Fracture Parameters: Phalangeal and Metacarpal Fracture Characteristics

Location	Pattern	Skeleton	Deformity	Soft Tissue	Associated Injury	Reaction to Motion
Base	Transverse	Simple	Angulation	Closed	Skin	Stable
Shaft	Oblique	Impacted	Dorsal	Open	Tendon	Unstable
Neck	Spiral	Comminuted	Palmar	—	Ligament	—
Head (condyle)	Avulsion	Bone loss	Rotation	—	Nerve	—
Epiphysis			Shortening	—	Blood vessel	—

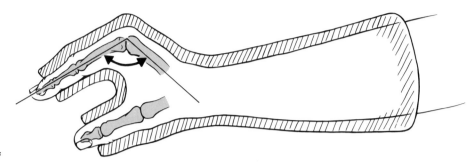

Figure 33-11

The position of immobilization of the hand involves splinting the wrist in 20° of extension, the metacarpophalangeal joints in 60° to 70° of flexion, and the interphalangeal joints in extension.

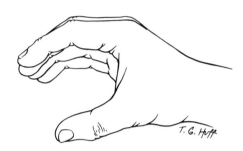

10° angulation in both sagittal and coronal planes except in the metaphysis, where 20° angulation in the sagittal plane is accepted

Up to 45° angulation in the sagittal plane in the neck of the fifth metacarpal

50% overlap at the fracture site

No rotational deformity

Similarly, certain fracture patterns tend to be unstable even when anatomically restored by closed manipulation (Table 33-5). These fractures will generally require some form of stabilization, but their outcome will often be determined as much by the violence of the original injury, associated soft tissue damage, and contamination as by the method of skeletal reconstruction.[9,94,98,161,198]

Thus to achieve the goal of functional restoration, the surgeon must take into account a number of factors related to the fracture and associated injuries and develop a logical treatment approach. The surgeon can choose from a number of treatment methods, including the following[52]:

1. Early motion with limited support
2. Closed reduction followed by external support
3. Closed reduction and percutaneous pins
4. Closed reduction and traction or external fixation
5. Open reduction and internal or external fixation

The treatment must be tailored to the demands of the specific fracture personality, the surgeon's experience, and patient motivation.

Table 33-5.
Unstable Metacarpal and Phalangeal Fractures

Rotated spiral fractures
Comminuted fractures
Severely displaced fractures
Some short oblique fractures
Multiple fractures
Subcondylar proximal phalanx fractures
Palmar base middle phalanx fractures
Fractures with associated extensive soft tissue injury
Displaced articular fractures: Bennett's and reverse Bennett's

Fracture Immobilization Techniques

The fingers are certainly very precious for everybody, but for certain individuals (musicians, artists, etc.) the loss of a finger is perhaps more consequential than the loss of a thigh. In my present opinion, the osteosynthesis of phalangeal fractures must be performed by one of the following techniques: cerclage in the long oblique fractures and transarticular nailing for transverse fractures.

ALBIN LAMBOTTE[120]

During the past quarter century, increasingly sophisticated advances have been made in operative techniques of the skeleton of the hand. However, there remains no general agreement as to the appropriate method of skeletal stabilization for even the simplest of fractures. The development of stable fixation with screws and plates has expanded the application of internal fixation but has by no means replaced plaster splints, casts, or Kirschner wires. The surgeon dealing with hand trauma should be well versed in many of these methods to more effectively tailor the treatment to the specific needs of the fracture.

FUNCTIONAL CASTING

Functional casting, popularized by Burkhalter and Reyes, takes advantage of the stabilizing forces of the flexor and intrinsic muscles on the phalanges with the metacarpophalangeal joint held in 90° of flexion.[32,164] It is particularly applicable with closed, dorsally angulated transverse or short oblique phalangeal shaft fractures or impacted base phalangeal fractures that prove stable on reduction. Anatomic reduction and mobilization of the digits neutralize the imbalance of the flexors and extensors, and the intact dorsal extensor mechanism functions as a "tension band" to the palmar cortex.[28,44] Digital rotation and angulation are largely controlled by having the four digits move together.

Technique

Following metacarpal or wrist block, the fracture is reduced with longitudinal traction. Angulation and rotation are checked in extension and flexion, and a short-arm plaster cast is applied, holding the wrist in 30° of extension and the metacarpophalangeal joints in 90° of flexion, leaving the proximal interphalangeal joints free. Active digital motion is encouraged from the onset (Fig. 33–12).

The patient should be followed preferably weekly for three weeks, at which time the cast can be discontinued and buddy straps applied for an additional two to three weeks (Fig. 33–13). Lateral tomography may be required to ensure maintenance of reduction during functional casting, as lateral radiographs are often difficult to interpret (Table 33–6).

This technique requires careful attention to detail to maintain the metacarpophalangeal joints in flexion, allow and encourage full proximal interphalangeal motion, and arrange adequate follow-up examinations.

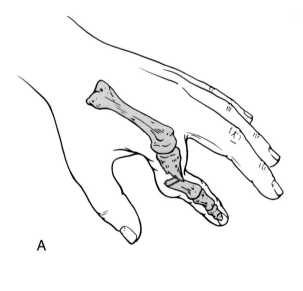

A

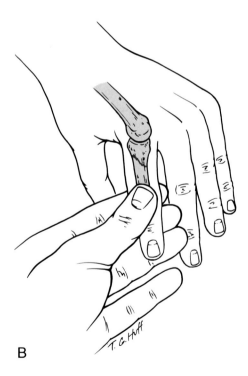

B

Figure 33–12

Technique of fracture reduction and stabilization with extension block casting. *A,* A displaced proximal phalangeal fracture. *B,* Following metacarpal block, the fracture is reduced by longitudinal traction with the metacarpophalangeal joint in maximal flexion.

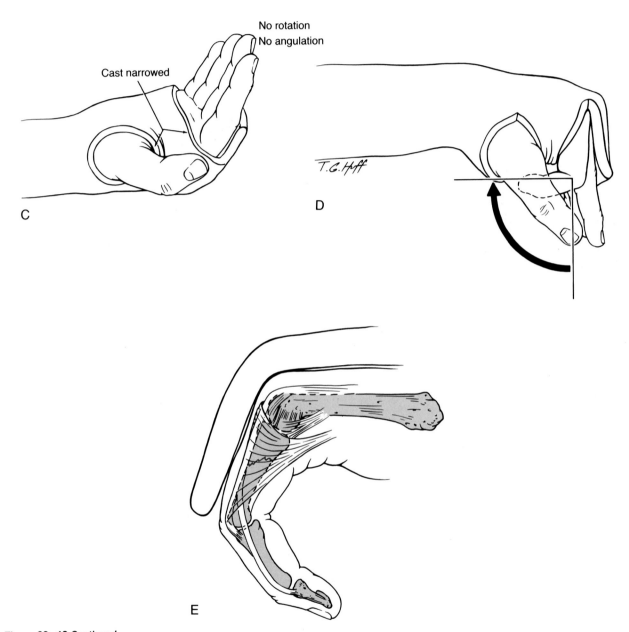

Figure 33–12 *Continued*

C and *D*, A short-arm plaster cast is applied with the metacarpophalangeal (MCP) joints in maximal flexion. The plaster is extended to the proximal interphalangeal joint. The cast must cut just proximal to the MCP joints to permit full flexion. *E*, Extension block splinting utilizes the intact dorsal structures to help maintain the reduction.

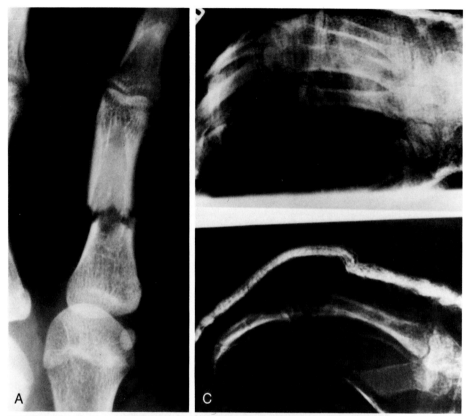

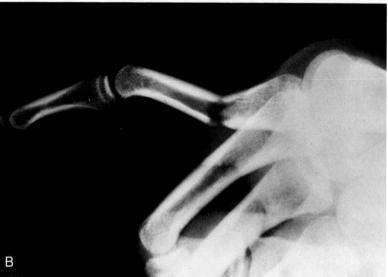

Figure 33–13

A 19-year-old female sustained a closed displaced proximal phalangeal fracture of the midshaft of her dominant index finger (*A* and *B*). Closed reduction and extension block casting were performed. Fracture union was clinically apparent in four weeks and full mobility in six weeks (*C*).

Table 33–6.	
Extension Block Casting	
Indications:	Closed dorsally angulated transverse and short oblique shaft fractures and impacted base proximal phalangeal fractures
Advantages:	Nonoperative
	Technically simple
	No instrumentation
	Encourages functional motion
Disadvantages:	Application limited to certain fracture types
	Control radiographs difficult to assess

KIRSCHNER WIRES

Pin fixation of a hand fracture was first reported in the American literature by Tennant in 1924.[205] He used a steel phonograph needle for the fixation of a metacarpal fracture. Remarkably, more than a half century later, wire fixation is still considered by many to be the "gold standard" against which other methods of skeletal fixation must be compared.[10,74,101,200] However, a number of real and potential problems exist with the use of Kirschner wires in the hand. These implants are subject to loosening and migration and may require additional plaster immobilization.[18,135,138,212] When the

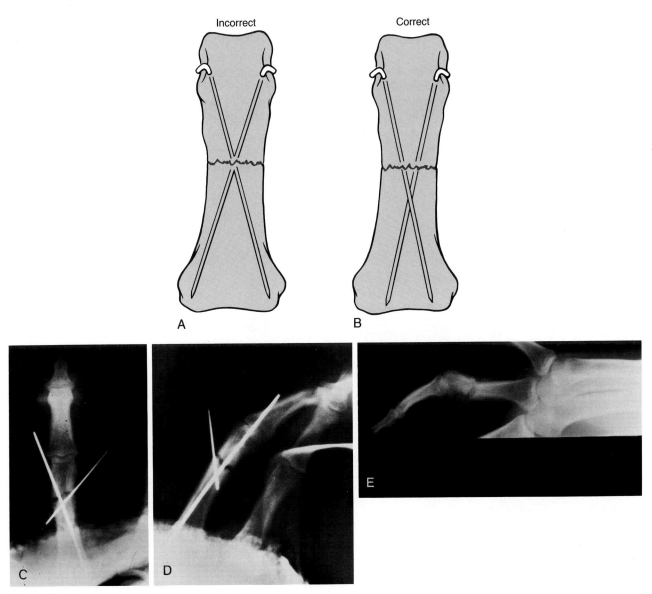

Figure 33–14

A and *B*, Crossed Kirschner wires are best applied by crossing proximal or distal to the fracture level. *C* to *E*, This 28-year-old male had an open proximal phalangeal fracture treated with crossed Kirschner wires, which held the fracture distracted. A nonunion resulted.

wires are applied in a crossing manner, they can serve to distract the fracture site and delay union. In a study of 23 nonunions of the tubular bones of the hand, the most common etiology was improper or ineffective Kirschner wire fixation.[102] Crossed Kirschner wires, commonly performed openly using retrograde pinning,[57] can distract the fracture. When this technique is used, the Kirschner wires should cross either proximal or distal to the fracture and gain firm anchorage in the proximal and distal metaphysis (Fig. 33–14).[176]

Namba and co-workers have identified mechanical factors that influence the holding power of these wires.[148] They found increased penetration ability and holding power with trocar tips, when compared with a diamond tip or a wire cut by hand in the operating room (Fig. 33–15). They also noted improved holding power when the wires were inserted while drilling at lower speeds.

Despite its mechanical and technical shortcomings, the Kirschner wire offers the distinct advantage of percutaneous application, thus avoiding surgical exposure and its attendant soft tissue trauma.[10,74,101] In the phalanges, this technique has its widest application in closed unstable diaphyseal, base, and neck fractures. In metacarpal fractures, it can be used effectively for isolated shaft, neck, or base fractures. Wires are inserted either longitudinally or transversely depending on the location of the fracture.

Technique

In the proximal phalanges, the technique of closed reduction and percutaneous Kirschner wire fixation involves reduction under wrist block anesthesia using longitudinal traction on the middle phalanx while flexing the metacarpophalangeal joint to 80° and the proximal interphalangeal joint to 45°. For transverse fractures, a 0.035-in or 0.045-in Kirschner wire is passed down the metacarpal head just eccentric to the extensor tendon to avoid tendon adhesion and is directed across the flexed metacarpophalangeal joint down the shaft of the proximal phalanx to the subchondral bone in the head of the phalanx. Some neck fractures are more unstable and can be treated with two or three 0.028-in Kirschner wires (Fig. 33–16).

After manipulation, the reduction of spiral and oblique fractures is maintained by a towel clamp or pointed reduction clamp holding the fracture percutaneously. Two or three 0.028-in Kirschner wires spaced evenly along the fracture's length are directed perpendicular to the long axis of the phalanx, engaging both cortices of the phalanx. The wires should be placed as far as possible from each other along the length of the fracture line.

In both pin applications, the pins are left out of the skin, well padded, and a plaster cast is applied with the metacarpophalangeal joint held in flexion. The cast is removed at three weeks, and the patient is encouraged to begin digital motion. The longitudinal pins are removed at the time of cast removal, and motion is started. Transverse-oriented pins may remain for one additional week, with motion begun with the pins in place (Table 33–7).

INTRAOSSEOUS WIRES

The technique of intraosseous wiring, popularized by Lister,[129] has proven effective in certain transverse phalangeal fractures as well as in avulsion and intraarticular fractures.[72] Its primary application has been in transverse fractures associated with soft tissue injuries,

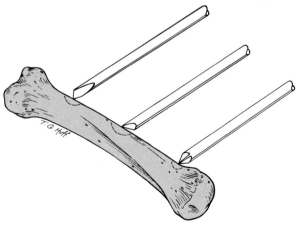

Figure 33–15

The trocar-tipped Kirschner wire penetrates the phalangeal cortex more readily than the diamond-tipped wire or self-cut wire.

Table 33–7.	
Kirschner Wire Fixation	
Indications:	Primary: percutaneous fixation of unstable, closed fractures
	Secondary: internal fixation of operatively treated fractures
Advantages:	Ease of application
	Inexpensive; available in different sizes
	Requires minimal equipment
	Can be applied percutaneously
Disadvantages:	Weak implant—requires additional support
	Subject to loosening and migration
	Can distract a fracture

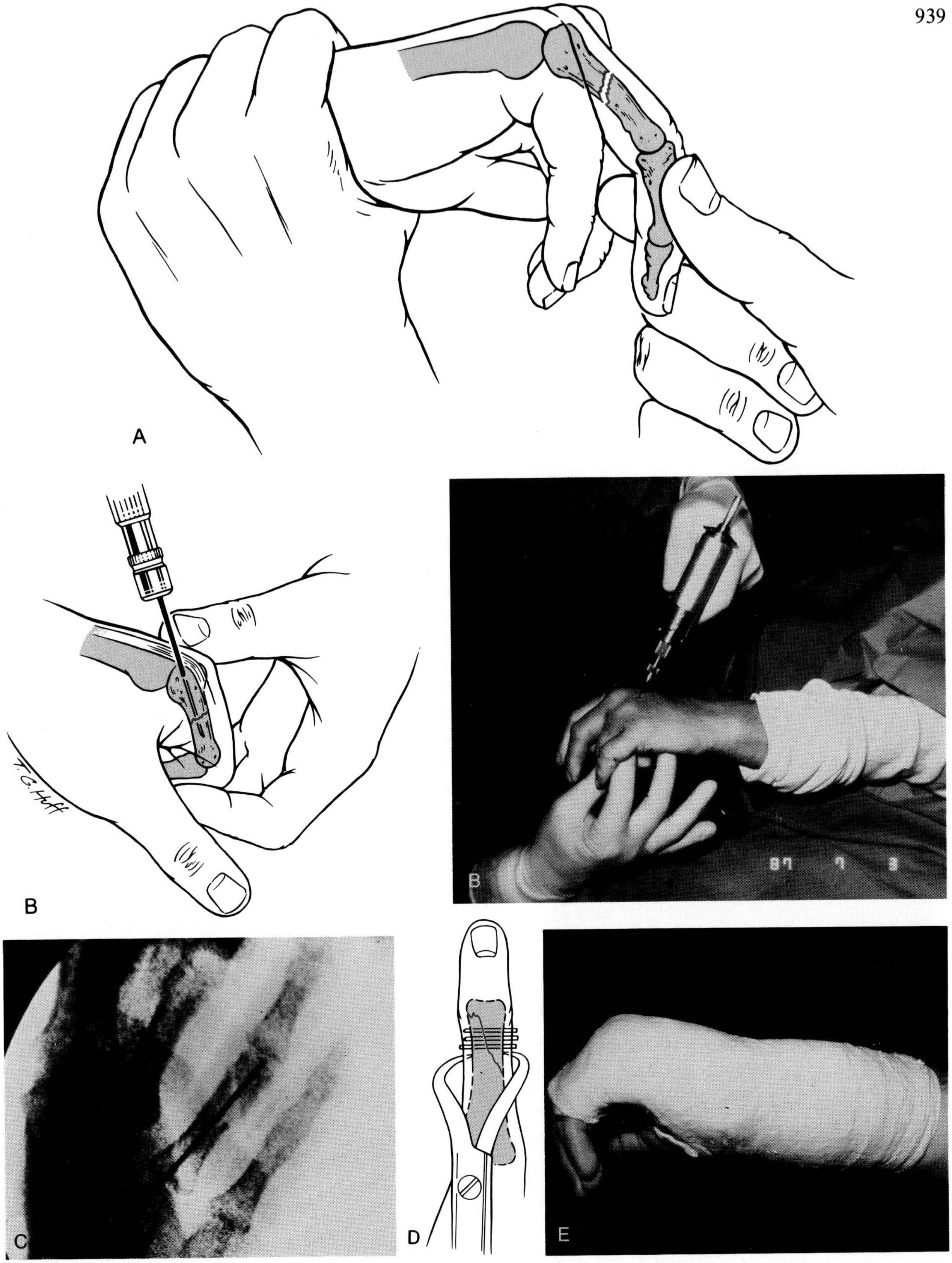

Figure 33-16

Techniques of closed percutaneous fixation of phalangeal fractures. *A,* The fracture is reduced by longitudinal traction on the middle phalanx with the metacarpophalangeal joint flexed 80° and the proximal interphalangeal joint flexed 45°. *B* and *C,* With transverse fractures, a 0.035-in or 0.045-in Kirschner wire is introduced using image intensification into the metacarpal head eccentric to the extensor tendon and is driven down to the subchondral bone in the neck. The picture on the image intensifier shows the fracture reduced and held with the longitudinal Kirschner wire. *D,* With oblique fractures, the fracture is reduced with a pointed reduction forceps, and two or three 0.028-in Kirschner wires are passed across the fracture site. *E,* The wires are cut outside the skin and well padded, and a short-arm cast is applied with the metacarpophalangeal joint flexed 80°.

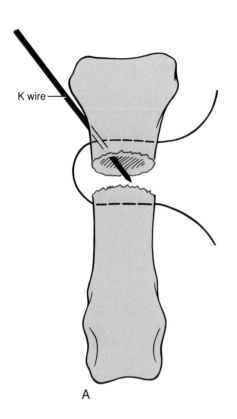

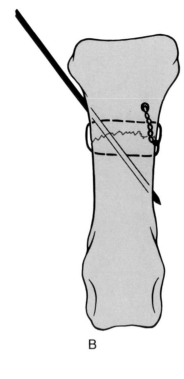

Figure 33–17

Lister type A intraosseous wiring technique. *A*, A 26-gauge stainless steel wire is passed transversely proximal and distal to the fracture line and just dorsal to the midaxis of the phalanx. A 0.035-in Kirschner wire is passed obliquely into the distal fragment until the tip is in the fracture line. *B*, The fracture is reduced, the Kirschner wire is passed into the proximal fragment, and the stainless steel wire is tightened. The twisted end can be placed into a drill hole in the cortex.

replantations, or arthrodeses. The technique involves a small stainless steel loop of wire (26-gauge) passed transversely across the fracture line just dorsal to the midaxis along with an oblique Kirschner wire to neutralize rotational forces (Fig. 33–17). Although the fixation is stable enough to permit controlled mobilization, the oblique Kirschner wire can cause tendon or skin irritation and limit motion (Table 33–8). Zimmerman and Weiland[223] modified this technique by placing two 26-gauge wires perpendicular to each other (Fig. 33–18). This modification, although requiring the same surgical exposure, is significantly more stable in mechanical testing. In fact, in Vanik et al.'s study of comparative strengths of internal fixation techniques,

the 90-90 wire technique compared favorably in rigidity to plate fixation (Table 33–9).[212]

Technique

The intraosseous wiring technique, described by Lister as type A wiring, involves making two drill holes with a 0.035-in Kirschner wire parallel to and 5 mm from the fracture ends and slightly dorsal to the midaxis of the bone. A 26-gauge (no. 0) stainless steel wire is passed through the holes in such a way that the twisted end of the wire will lie on the noncontact side of the digit. Prior to fracture reduction, a 0.035-in Kirschner wire is driven obliquely out through the distal cortex until the

Table 33–8.	
Intraosseous Wiring: Lister Type A Technique	
Indications:	Open transverse phalangeal fractures
	Replantation
Advantages:	Technically straightforward
	Minimal equipment
	Stable fixation for early mobilization
Disadvantages:	Limited clinical application
	Requires surgical exposure
	Kirschner wire can limit tendon gliding

Table 33–9.	
Intraosseous Wiring: 90-90 Technique	
Indications:	Open transverse fractures
	Replantations
	Arthrodesis
Advantages:	Biomechanically strong
	Low-profile implant
	Equipment minimal
Disadvantages:	Technically demanding
	Limited applications
	Poor in osteopenic bone

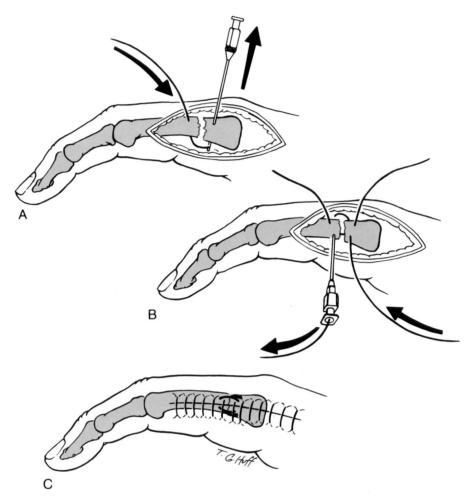

Figure 33–18

The 90-90 intraosseous wire technique. *A*, One wire is passed from dorsal to palmar using a 20-gauge hypodermic needle. *B*, A second 26-gauge wire is introduced in a similar manner but at a 90° angle to the first. *C*, The fracture is reduced and held, ensuring rotational alignment; both wires are tightened and the twisted ends cut short.

tip protrudes slightly at the fracture site. The fracture is reduced, and preferably a second surgeon drives the wire into the proximal fragment. The ends of the stainless steel wire are twisted around each other, grasped with a heavy needle holder, and tightened in two steps: the first is to pull on the wire to make it lie snug on the far cortex; the second step is to twist the wire to tighten it (see Fig. 33–17).

In patients with intraarticular fractures or smaller avulsion fragments attached to the collateral ligaments,

the monofilament wire is passed through soft tissue around the fragment (or through parallel drill holes into larger fragments) and brought to the opposite cortex across the fracture line. The fracture is then reduced and held while the wire is tightened. This approach (type B) avoids devascularization of these small fragments, but its disadvantage is that the tightening of the wire occurs against the opposite cortex, thus indirectly at the fracture line (Fig. 33–19 and Table 33–10).

The technique of 90-90 wiring is somewhat more

Figure 33–19

Type B intraosseous wire technique of Lister. *A*, A 26- or 28-gauge stainless steel wire is passed through or around the small fragments and brought across the fracture line through the opposite cortex. *B*, The wire is tightened by pulling on the wire to make it lie snug against the fragment and then twisting it.

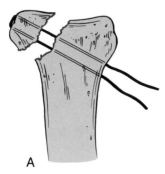

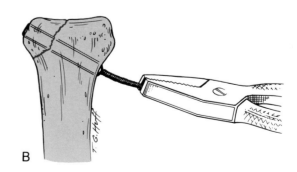

Table 33–10.	
Intraosseous Wiring: Lister Type B Technique	
Indications:	Intraarticular fractures
	Avulsion fractures
Advantages:	Limited exposure of the fracture fragment
	Maintains vascularity to the fragment
	Low-profile implant
	Technically straightforward
Disadvantages:	Indirect wire tightening can limit security of fixation
	Poor rotational control
	Wire can devascularize ligament

demanding, as two sets of holes parallel to the fracture line and 90° apart are made. This requires precise rotational alignment prior to tightening of each wire. A 20-gauge hypodermic needle is recommended as a "carrier" for the passage of the 26-gauge stainless steel wire. When passing the wire from dorsal to palmar, hyperflexion at the fracture site will improve surgical access. This technique, although more demanding and requiring somewhat greater surgical exposure surrounding the fracture, does offer enhanced stability to permit functional loading of the digit during the rehabilitation (see Fig. 33–18).

TENSION BAND WIRING

Intraosseous wiring techniques have been expanded by Belsole and colleagues to take advantage of the inherent mechanical forces that occur in functional loading of the digital skeleton.[13,14,77] In a stable state, the phalanges and metacarpals are mainly stressed by bending forces, with less stress occurring as a result of extension, torsion, or axial loading. This results in compressive forces on the palmar side and distraction or tensile forces dorsally. With a dorsally placed implant, not only are bending and distraction forces neutralized, but also the functional loading forces convert these forces into compressive loads that are active within the plane of the fracture.[100,179] For any implant to be successful, it must resist torsional and shearing loads. The tension band wiring technique accomplishes these mechanical requirements by placing the small-gauge stainless steel wire above the cortex and strategically wrapped around Kirschner wires, which also serve to interlock the fracture fragments.

Technique

The tension band wiring technique is performed through surgical exposure and therefore is indicated only in those unstable fractures not amenable to percutaneous techniques (see Table 33–5). The fracture is reduced and held while 0.035-in Kirschner wires are inserted. For transverse or short oblique fractures, crossed Kirschner wires are used while 0.035-in Kirschner wires are inserted. For transverse or short oblique fractures, crossed Kirschner wires are used, whereas for long oblique or spiral fractures, the Kirschner wires are placed perpendicular to the fracture plane. The wires are cut so that only 1 to 2 mm protrude from the cortex on both sides. Whenever possible the wires should be placed so as to avoid interference with tendon gliding. The 26- or 28-gauge monofilament stainless steel wire is woven about the ends of the Kirschner wires in a modified figure of 8 and twisted tightly (Fig. 33–20). If the fracture is comminuted, several Kirschner wire–stainless steel wire constructs can be made. If cortical defects are present opposite the tension wire, cancellous bone grafting is recommended prior to tightening of the wire. Active motion should be encouraged within a few days postoperatively, as the functional loading will promote fracture healing and, importantly, limit postoperative adhesions (Table 33–11).

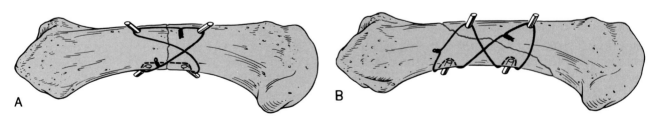

Figure 33–20

Tension band wiring technique. *A*, For a transverse or short oblique fracture, Kirschner wires are placed in a crossed pattern, and the stainless steel 26-gauge wire is passed around the tips in a modified figure of 8. *B*, For spiral or long oblique fractures, parallel Kirschner wires are placed perpendicular to the fracture plane.

Table 33–11.
Tension Band Wiring

Indications:	Unstable phalangeal and metacarpal fractures requiring open reduction and internal fixation
	Failed plates and screws
	Diaphyseal fractures with three or four fragments
Advantages:	Very stable
	Biomechanically sound
	Low profile
	Simple instruments
Disadvantages:	Operative exposure may be significant
	Technically difficult with certain fracture patterns

COMPRESSION SCREWS

In concept and form, small screws and miniscrews and plates represent a natural evolution from those used successfully in the larger skeleton (Fig. 33–21). However, unique anatomic considerations in the hand demand knowledge and experience when applying these implants to the tubular skeleton in the hand. The gliding structures enveloping the digital skeleton are easily compromised by the implant bulk, and their location often restricts the optimal mechanical placement of the internal fixation. The meager cortical thickness and often small and tenuously vascularized fracture fragments present other challenges to the achievement of stable internal fixation without devascularization or fragmentation of these fragile fragments.

In spite of their technical complexities, the precision, rigidity, and relatively low profile afforded by these miniscrews have added significantly to the surgeon's ability to manage complex fractures in the hand.[45,66,89,172] In the metacarpals and phalanges, displaced long oblique or spiral fractures or articular fractures involving greater than 25% of the articular surface are excellent indications for screw fixation (Fig. 33–22). In addition, unicondylar and large avulsion fractures are often able to be secured with screws alone. The stability provided by interfragmentary fixation allows for functional rehabilitation even in the most complex of hand injuries (Table 33–12).

The techniques of interfragmentary lag screw fixation are presented in chapter 11. In the hand, several points should be emphasized. The 2.7-mm screws are best used in the metacarpal base and, in large adults, in the metacarpal shaft. The 2.0-mm screws can be used in smaller metacarpals and in conjunction with 2.7-

mm screws, placing the smaller screws near the apices of the fracture. In the phalanges, 1.5-mm screws are preferable, with 2.0-mm screws used if the threads of the smaller screw "strips," thus denying adequate cortical purchase.

The following technical points of application are worth highlighting[29,87]:

1. Diaphyseal fractures to be fixed by screws alone should present a fracture line at least twice the diameter of the bone.

2. The fracture should be opened and the fracture line inspected to determine the optimal positions of the screws and to seek out hidden fracture lines or comminution that will offset screw purchase.

3. The fracture should be anatomically reduced to achieve interlocking of the fracture lines and to maximize the zone of compression.

4. Avoid repeated drilling, as the lag screw is dependent on the grasp of the screw in the threaded hole.

5. Avoid placing screws where technically convenient. Instead, place them in the location that is mechanically most desirable (Fig. 33–23).

6. Screw fixation of a single fragment should be considered only if the fragment is at least three times the thread diameter of the screw.

PLATE FIXATION

Although the bulk of a plate is less well tolerated in the hand than elsewhere in the axial skeleton, there remain a number of complex fractures in which fixation with a plate has provided sufficient stability with which to initiate functional rehabilitation. These include metacarpal fractures with soft tissue loss, comminuted intra- or periarticular fractures, comminuted fractures with shortening or malrotation, and fractures with segmental bone loss. In the phalanges with their enveloping gliding structures, plate application should be limited to fractures with substance loss, intraarticular T condylar fractures, and some fractures with periarticular comminution.

A number of plates have been designed specifically for use in the hand.[66,87] Metacarpal shaft fractures are stabilized with one-quarter tubular plates using 2.7-mm screws unless bone loss is present, thus necessitating the use of a stronger 2.7-mm dynamic compression plate.[47] Periarticular fractures are amenable to 2.0-mm condylar plates or 2.7-mm L or T plates.[30] Similar plate designs are available for 2.0-mm screws for the phalanges. However, the most versatile plate in the phalanges is the 1.5-mm condylar plate.

In contrast to interfragmentary screws, plates will often require removal, as their bulk commonly interferes with overlying tendons. If, however, their applica-

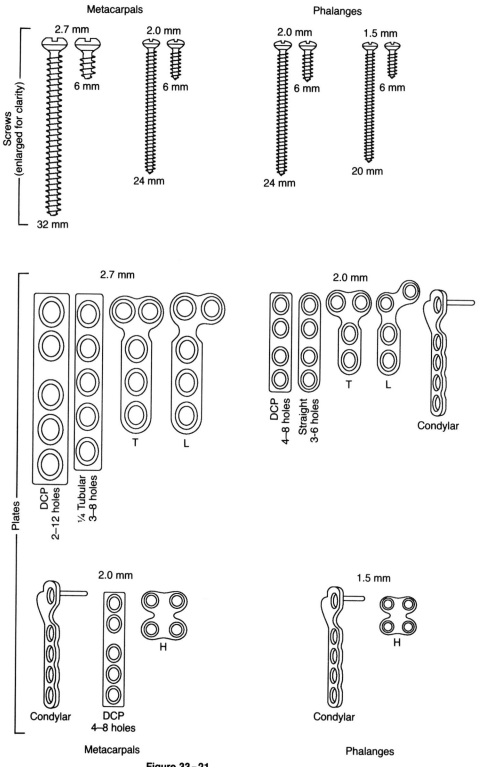

Figure 33–21

Minifragment implants for hand surgery.

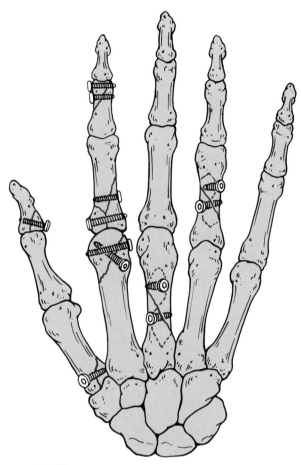

Figure 33-22

Optimal fracture patterns for interfragmentary screw fixation in the hand.

plication, particularly in the phalanges, for only the most complex fracture patterns.

The small condylar plate has expanded the application of plates in the hand as a result of its versatility, lower profile, and design features (Table 33-13).[30] In the distal metacarpal, the plate is applied on the dorsolateral aspect corresponding to the dorsal tubercle of the origin of the collateral ligaments; in the phalanges, sagittal placement of the implant is preferred. The technique of condylar plate application in a bicondylar fracture of the proximal phalanx is discussed in the following section.

Technique

The fracture site is exposed through a lateral approach, and the transverse retinacular ligament is reflected, allowing skeletal access slightly below the lateral band. An area is exposed on the proximal phalangeal condyle for the distal blade and screw insertion. The intercondylar fracture is reduced and provisionally secured with a 0.028-in transverse Kirschner wire placed dorsal or palmar to where the blade will be inserted and used as a guide for later placement of the blade. The joint axis is defined with a Kirschner wire, after which the blade hole is drilled with a 1.5-mm drill through a protective sleeve. The depth is measured and the standard 14-mm blade cut to the required length. The blade is inserted in the drill hole, the subcondylar part of the fracture is reduced, and the plate's location on the phalangeal shaft is observed. Frequently the plate will require contouring, which can only be done by removing the plate. The plate is reapplied and an interfragmentary 1.5-mm screw placed through the distal hole of the plate adja-

tion permits rapid mobilization and thereby minimizes adhesions, this removal should be put into the perspective of allowing for a functional restoration along with skeletal healing. The surgeon should reserve plate ap-

Table 33-12. Interfragmentary Screw Fixation	
Indications:	Displaced spiral or long oblique fractures
	Intraarticular fractures > 25% of articular surface
	Avulsion fractures
Advantages:	Stable fixation for functional rehabilitation
	Predictable union when properly applied
	Low-profile implant without need for removal
Disadvantages:	Technically demanding
	Requires operative exposure
	Implant and equipment are complex

Table 33-13. Plate Application	
Indications:	Complex metacarpal and phalangeal fractures with soft tissue injury or bone loss
	Unstable short oblique or comminuted diaphyseal fractures with shortening or malrotation
	Complex intra- or periarticular fractures
Advantages:	Stable skeletal fixation
	Maintains or restores length
	Condylar plate lateral position permits extraarticular placement
Disadvantages:	Extreme technical difficulty
	Little room for error
	Bulk of implant a problem with overlying tendons

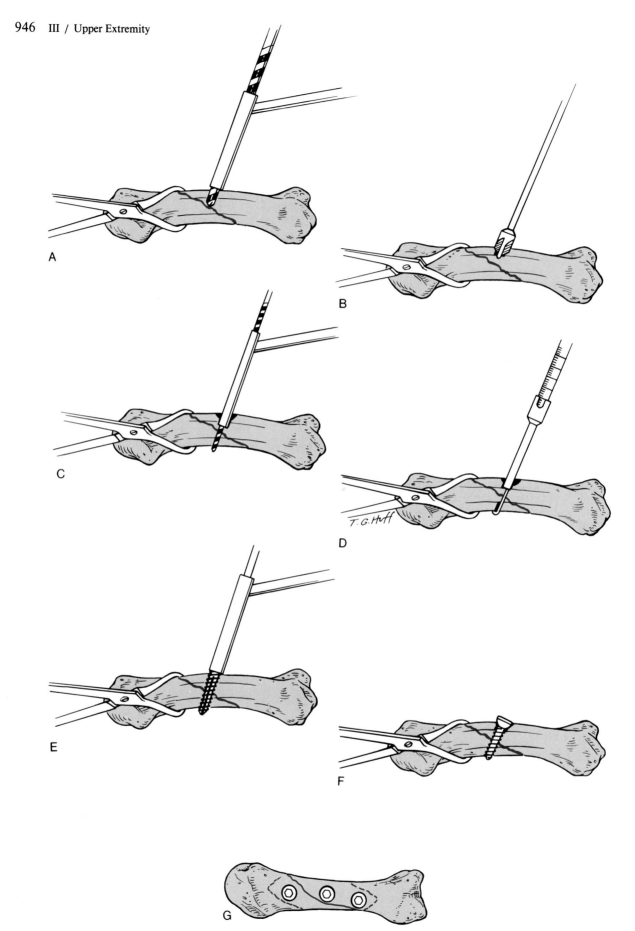

See legend on opposite page

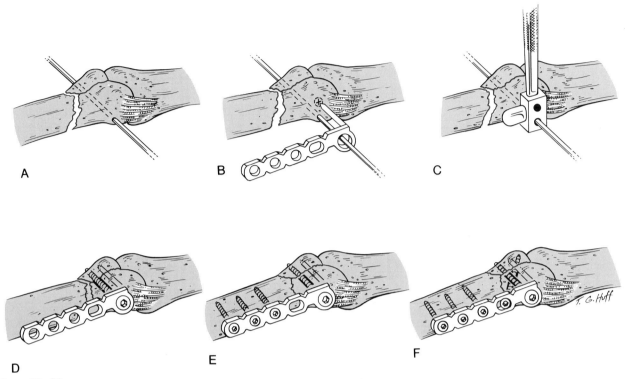

Figure 33-24

Technique of application of a 1.5-mm condylar plate for a T condylar phalangeal fracture. *A*, The condylar fragments are reduced and held with a 0.028-in Kirschner wire passed parallel to the line of the joint. *B*, The blade plate is seated over the Kirschner wire and a seating hole marked ideally to sit just proximal and dorsal to the collateral ligament origin. *C*, Using a guide, a 1.5-mm drill is used to make a seating hole for the blade. *D*, After contouring the plate to fit the shaft, the blade is introduced and a 1.5-mm screw placed into the condyle in a lag fashion. *E*, The condyles are reduced onto the shaft and the most proximal screws placed through the plate. *F*, A final interfragmentary lag screw is introduced obliquely through the most distal plate hole for added compression of the articular fragments.

cent to the blade. The condyles are now again reduced onto the shaft and the plate secured to the shaft with 1.5-mm screws. An additional interfragmentary lag screw can be introduced through the oblique hole in the plate just proximal to the blade (Fig. 33–24).

EXTERNAL SKELETAL FIXATION

External skeletal fixation of the hand is by no means a new concept.[46,159] However, small external fixation frames have been developed that offer not only stability but also versatility and the ability to make adjustments easily both intra- and postoperatively.[166,202] Blunt-tipped pins that are predrilled; swiveling, adjustable

pin-holding clamps; and compression and distraction units are now available. External fixation was traditionally viewed as applicable only to complex composite injuries in the hand,[64,181] but the improved design and pin applications have enabled its application in such complex injuries as proximal interphalangeal joint fracture-dislocations or highly comminuted diaphyseal fractures (Table 33–14).[3,85,86]

Simple fixators have been constructed with Kirschner wires and acrylic cement. Although adequate for emergency stabilization, their lack of stability has led to pin track problems and loss of position. The miniature external fixator designed by Henri Jacquet in 1976 has, to a large degree, solved these problems (Fig. 33–25).

Figure 33-23

Sequence of steps in interfragmentary screw fixation of a spiral metacarpal fracture with 2.0-mm screws. *A*, Overdrill gliding hole with 2.0-mm drill; do not drill beyond first cortex. *B*, Countersink. *C*, Drill across fracture with 1.5-mm drill bit and appropriate drill guide used as insert sleeve. *D*, Measure depth. *E*, Tap with 2.0-mm tap and tap sleeve. *F*, Insert 2.0-mm lag screw. *G*, Insert second or third screws like the first, adjusting their positions with the rotational changes in fracture configuration.

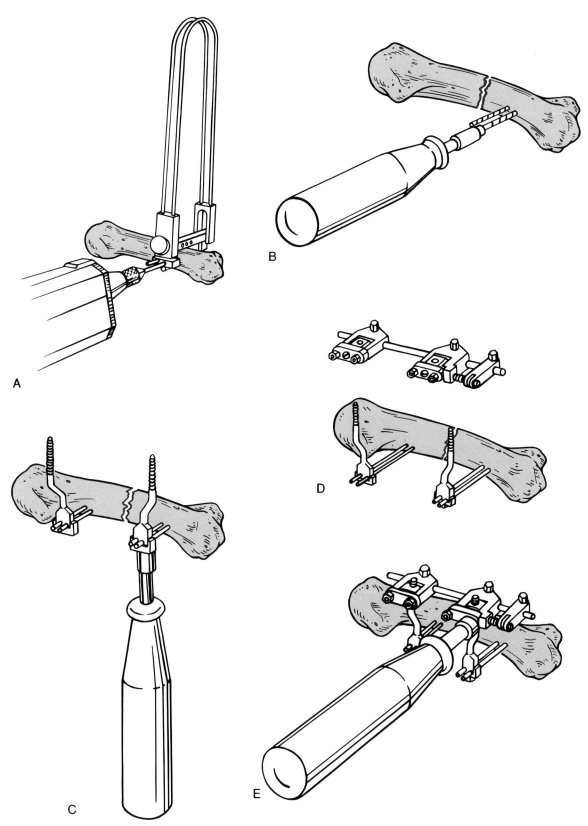

Figure 33–25

Technique of application of miniature external fixator of Jacquet. *A*, A drill guide is used to accurately direct the minipins. *B*, A hand chuck is utilized to place the pins. *C*, The primary connection between the pins and frame is with offset or straight pinholders. *D*, Simple or sliding swivel clamps link the pinholders to the connecting rod of the frame. *E*, The bolts that connect the clamps to the pinholders and connecting rods are tightened with a socket wrench.

Table 33–14.

External Skeletal Fixation

Indications:	Highly comminuted fractures
	Fractures with bone loss
	Fractures with extreme soft tissue trauma
	Infected fractures
	Thumb web space maintenance
	Complex articular fracture-dislocations of the proximal interphalangeal joint
Advantages:	Avoids operative manipulation of fracture fragments
	Maintains length and alignment with traction without crossing joints
	Access to soft tissue care advantageous
	Can be applied percutaneously
Disadvantages:	Complex application
	Pins can inhibit gliding structures
	Pin track infection
	Traction can delay skeletal healing

Table 33–15.

Incidence of Metacarpal Fractures and Dislocations (N = 421)

Type	Number
Neck	110
Shaft	
Spiral/oblique	55
Transverse	94
Longitudinal	1
Comminuted	7
Base	55
Articular	
Head	32
Condyles (proximal)	4
Dorsal base	4
Palmar base	6
Lateral base	50*
Comminuted	3

*Thirty-seven of these were Bennett's fractures.
Source: Compiled from Dobyns, J. H.,; Linscheid, R. L.; Cooney, W. P. J Hand Surg 8:687–692, 1983.

Technique

The pinholes are predrilled with 1.5-mm drill bits through a guide. A hand chuck inserts the blunt-tipped, self-tapping 2.0-mm pins. These are attached to pin holders, which can be offset to create more space for the connecting frame in the small skeleton of the phalanges. The pin holders are linked by a connecting rod held onto the pin holders with swiveling clamps that are adjustable in all planes. This is particularly effective in the digits, allowing the pins to be placed prior to reduction of the fracture. The swiveling clamps can have a sliding clamp to permit distraction or compression through the frame. A socket wrench is needed to secure the clamps and pin holders.

Metacarpal Fractures

Injury to the second through fifth metacarpals, which are interconnected at their bases and necks, can result in significant swelling, pain, and early or late hand dysfunction. The treatment of metacarpal fractures has progressed considerably during the past 50 years, when nearly all metacarpal fractures were treated by bandaging over a roller bandage with little attempt at fracture reduction.[215] The current approach should be based on fracture location, inherent stability, associated soft tissue trauma, and the functional demands of the patient.

Treatment goals specific to the metacarpals include preservation of the longitudinal and transverse arches and prevention of rotational deformity, which will manifest as overlapping of the digit. Shortening, when 3 mm or less, may only be appreciated by the loss of contour of the metacarpal head during flexion of the metacarpophalangeal joint. When shortening exceeds this, however, an imbalance between the intrinsic and extrinsic tendons will arise.

Metacarpal fractures are conveniently grouped according to the anatomic division of the bone: base, shaft, neck, and head. Dobyns et al., in their series of 1621 fracture-dislocations of the hand and wrist, documented 421 metacarpal fractures (Table 33–15).[52]

EXTRAARTICULAR FRACTURES

Extraarticular Base Injuries

As a general rule, the interosseous muscles and intrinsically strong carpometacarpal capsular and interosseous ligaments provide intrinsic stability to extraarticular fractures at the metacarpal bases.[80] When resulting from direct trauma, extraarticular fractures are frequently impacted and clinically stable. In these cases, supportive splints are indicated. In the setting of more violent trauma, these fractures may be associated with complex soft tissue injuries, and internal fixation with Kirschner wires may be advisable. More stable fixation can be gained with the 2.0-mm or 2.7-mm condylar plates (Fig. 33–26).

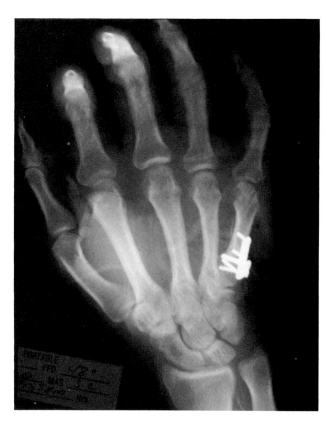

Figure 33-26

A 28-year-old male sustained a rollover injury to his hand with extensive soft tissue trauma. A 2.0-mm condylar plate was used to stabilize a fracture at the base of the metacarpals. (Courtesy of Alan Freeland, M.D.)

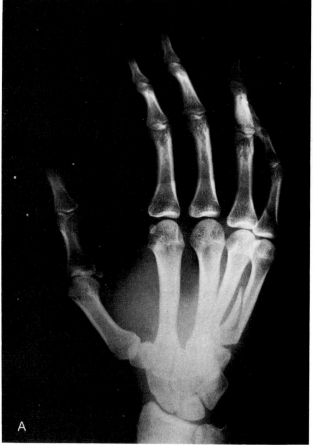

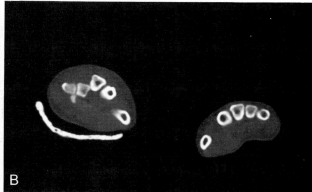

Figure 33-27

A, An oblique radiograph of a fracture-dislocation of the fourth and fifth carpometacarpal joints. The injury is difficult to interpret on routine lateral radiograph. *B*, CT scan clearly demonstrates the injury when compared with the contralateral side.

Carpometacarpal Fracture-Dislocations

The carpometacarpal (CMC) fracture-dislocation can be more difficult to treat than the extraarticular base fracture. These injuries are commonly the sequelae of high-energy trauma and are accompanied by soft tissue swelling. A number of combinations of CMC fracture-dislocations have been reported,[19,84,88,113,162] although fracture-dislocations of the fifth CMC joint have been reported most extensively in the literature.[21,49,73,147]

Severe swelling, pain, and crepitation on examination should alert the physician to the possibility of injury to the CMC joints. Three x-ray views are mandatory, as the dislocation may not be visible on the anteroposterior view, and the lateral radiograph may be difficult to interpret because of overlap of the adjacent CMC joints. For this reason, 30° oblique radiographs with the forearm both supinated and pronated will accentuate the second and fifth CMC joints, respectively.[110] Lateral tomography or computed axial tomography will be especially helpful in confirming the presence of a fracture-dislocation and, more importantly, the extent of the articular disruption (Fig. 33–27).

Fracture-dislocations of the fifth CMC joint, and less so of the fourth, are of particular importance, given the mobility of these joints. The fifth and fourth metacarpals articulate with the distal articular surface of the

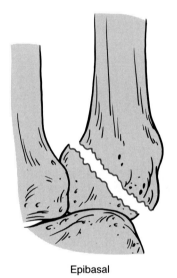

Epibasal

A

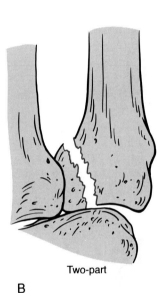

Two-part

B

Figure 33–28

Four types of fractures of the base of the fifth metacarpal.

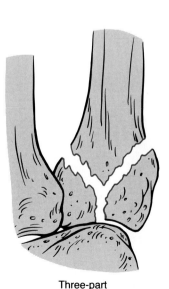

Three-part

C

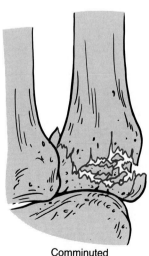

Comminuted
with impaction

D

hamate, which is divided by a ridge into two distinct facets. The fifth metacarpal articulation is that of a concave-convex "saddle" type joint resembling the thumb trapezial metacarpal joint. This provides the fifth CMC articulation with not only a flexion-extension arc of between 20° and 30° but also a slight rotatory motion that functions to aid the little finger in contact with the thumb.[80,162] The more radial facet of the hamate is flatter, providing only 10° to 15° of mobility with the fourth metacarpal.

Injuries to these two joints can be the result of a combination of forces, with axially directed forces producing the more comminuted fracture patterns. The extensor carpi ulnaris, which inserts on the base of the fifth metacarpal, acts as a deforming force and accounts to some degree for the instability of these "reverse Bennett's" fractures. The deep motor branch of the ulnar nerve passes adjacent to the hook of the hamate and can be traumatized with these fractures.[48,156]

As with fractures at the base of the thumb metacarpal, these fractures can be divided into four fracture patterns (Fig. 33–28): epibasal, two-part (reverse Bennett's), three-part, and comminuted with impaction. Displaced epibasal and two-part fracture-dislocations are readily reduced using longitudinal traction on the fifth metacarpal followed by manual pressure on the base of the metacarpal. Adequate anesthesia is essential, and finger trap traction may be required to gain skeletal length and maintain the reduction while radiographs are obtained. Because these are unstable fractures, once they are reduced they should be stabilized with two 0.045-in Kirschner wires placed percutaneously. One pin should be directed across the metacarpohamate joint and the other into the base of the fourth metacarpal. Using a large-bore hypodermic needle as a pin guide will greatly facilitate the placement of the pins into the tubular fifth metacarpal. The pins are left out of the skin, and plaster immobilization with an ulnar gutter cast is applied for a duration of six weeks (Fig. 33–29).

The three-part or comminuted fracture may not reduce as easily with longitudinal traction. It is not uncommon for these fracture-dislocations to be comminuted, particularly when associated with high-energy trauma.[48,88,179] Tomography is essential to define the fracture anatomy, as impacted articular fragments are not always readily reduced by longitudinal traction. If these are left untreated, symptomatic posttraumatic arthritis can prove problematic, especially in patients who rely on their hands for their livelihood.[39]

Displaced articular fragments are small and exceptionally difficult to reduce and stabilize. For that reason, it is advisable to attempt to reduce the fracture fragments by "ligamentotaxis" using an external fixation device applied to the hamate and metacarpal shaft (Fig. 33–30). If radiographs demonstrate continued displacement of the articular surface, the fragments can be manipulated into place through a limited dorsoulnar incision and secured with 0.028-in or 0.035-in Kirschner wires. As with the reduction of impacted

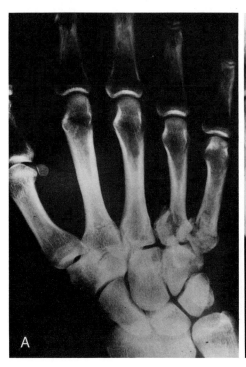
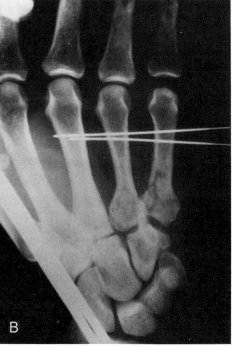

Figure 33–29

A three-part fracture-dislocation of the fifth carpometacarpal joint was effectively reduced by longitudinal traction and manipulation and stabilized with 0.045-in Kirschner wires. An epibasal fracture of the fourth metacarpal was also present.

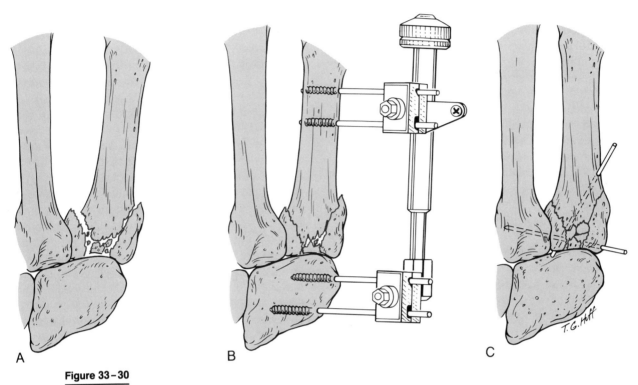

Figure 33–30

Three steps in reduction and fixation of impacted fifth carpometacarpal fracture-dislocation using a minidistractor.

Figure 33–31

Using a minilengthener, a severely comminuted fracture-dislocation of the fifth metacarpal was successfully reduced and held with the minidistractor which was incorporated into a cast.

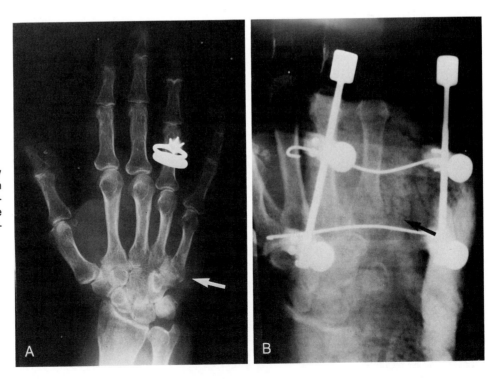

articular fractures elsewhere, a metaphyseal defect will exist that should be packed with a small amount of cancellous bone graft obtained from the distal radius (Fig. 33–31). The fixator is left in place for six weeks and protected with an ulnar gutter cast or splint.

Multiple Carpometacarpal Fracture-Dislocations

When recognized early, multiple CMC fracture-dislocations are usually reducible either by direct manipulation alone or with added longitudinal traction. They are, for the most part, unstable and require percutaneous Kirschner wire fixation using 0.045-in Kirschner wires placed obliquely across the CMC joints into the proximal carpal row. Soft tissue swelling is normal. Therefore a circular plaster cast should be used with caution in the initial postoperative period and is preferably applied once the swelling begins to subside. However, when seen more than five to seven days after injury, these complex fracture-dislocations may no longer be amenable to successful closed reduction. Open reduction is best accomplished through longitudinal incisions, which interfere less with venous and lymphatic drainage (Fig. 33–32). The reduction of multiple CMC fracture-dislocations begins with the "keystone" third CMC joint. Again, the reductions are stabilized with Kirschner wires. The patient should be cautioned that these joints may spontaneously fuse or require surgical arthrodesis if painful posttraumatic arthritis ensues.

METACARPAL SHAFT FRACTURES

Displacement of isolated closed metacarpal shaft fractures is often limited,[100,162] as the four metacarpal shafts of the intrinsic muscles are linked together proximally and distally by interosseous ligaments. Transverse fractures will angulate with the apex dorsal fragment and the distal fragment pulled palmarward because of the pull of the interosseous muscles (Fig. 33–33). Increased palmar displacement of the metacarpal heads can disturb grip, and angulation can result in muscle imbalance, with hyperextension at the metacarpophalangeal joint and reduced extension at the proximal interphalangeal joint. The mobile carpometacarpal joints of the fourth and fifth metacarpals can accommodate some dorsal-palmar angulation, whereas those of the fixed second and third metacarpals cannot. For metacarpal shaft fractures, up to 20° of dorsal angulation can be accepted for the fourth and fifth metacarpals, but not more than 10° for the second and third.[151,190] The amount of acceptable angulation for the fourth and fifth metacarpals will be greater when the fracture occurs more distally in the neck.

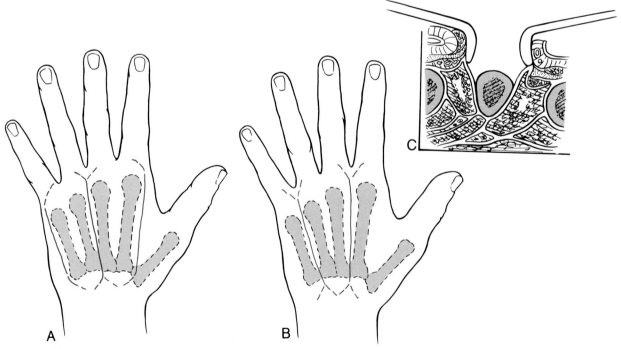

Figure 33–32

Surgical approaches to the metacarpals. A, Incisions for individual metacarpal exposure. B, Incisions for exposure of all four metacarpals. C, Exposure of the metacarpal is subperiosteal on the dorsal surface, with care taken to minimize elevation of the interosseous muscles.

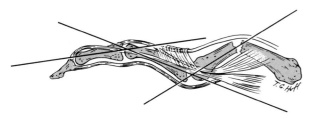

Figure 33-33

Transverse metacarpal shaft fractures will angulate, with the apex pointing dorsally, because of the pull of the interosseous muscles.

Oblique fractures tend to shorten, whereas spiral fractures will rotate (Fig. 33-34). Shortening of up to 3 mm is well tolerated and may be apparent only by the loss of the normal contour of the metacarpal head with metacarpophalangeal joint flexion. Less tolerance is acceptable with rotational deformity. As little as 5° of metacarpal rotation can lead to more than 1.5 cm of digital overlap.[66] In general, border metacarpal fractures are less stable than those of the central two metacarpals as a result of the increased interosseous support of the latter.

Isolated Metacarpal Shaft Fractures

Transverse closed metacarpal shaft fractures with little or no displacement are intrinsically stable and readily treated with a plaster splint or cast for three to four weeks.[151] The cast is applied with the metacarpophalangeal joint flexed 60° to 70° and carefully molded to provide three points of contact: one over the dorsal apex of the fracture and the other two on the palmar side proximal and distal to the fracture.

If the initial displacement is substantial or the fracture displaces in the cast, percutaneous Kirschner wire fixation should be considered. Several techniques of wire placement are available, and a 0.045-in smooth Kirschner wire is the wire of choice. A technique particularly suited to the border metacarpals is that of placing one wire proximal and one wire distal to the fracture in a transverse direction into the adjacent metacarpal (Fig. 33-35).[119] This particular configuration was demonstrated by Massengill and co-workers[138] to have significant strength when subjected to a biomechanical evaluation. An alternative method is a longitudinal wire placement with the Kirschner wire introduced

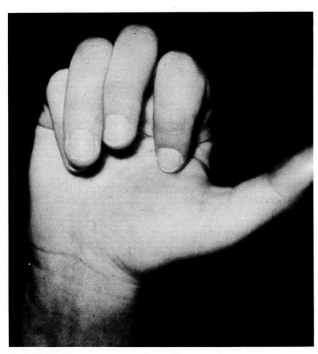

Figure 33-34

A malrotated spiral metacarpal shaft fracture can result in disabling digital overlap.

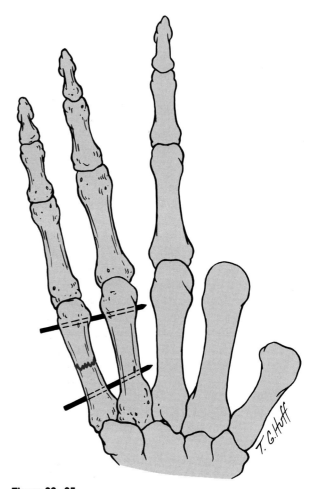

Figure 33-35

A displaced transverse metacarpal shaft fracture specifically involving the border metacarpals can be stabilized with 0.045-in Kirschner wires placed transversely into the adjacent intact metacarpal.

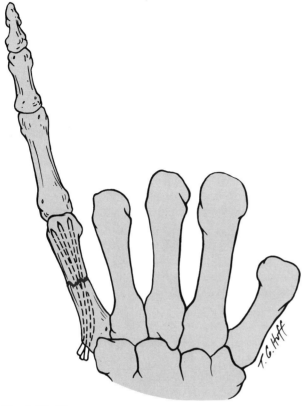

Figure 33–36

The flexible intramedullary rod technique of Hall is based on filling the medullary canal with curved, smooth-tipped rods passed into the metacarpal through drill holes distant from the fracture site.

through a tuberosity of the metacarpal head with the metacarpophalangeal joint held in flexion. This approach carries the potential problem of the wire interfering with metacarpophalangeal joint motion. A third wire technique is that described by Hall,[82] which he termed "flexible intramedullary rodding" (FIR). This technique employs a specially designed rod 0.8 mm in diameter and 10 cm long with a rounded tip. Through a 1-cm incision over the base of the metacarpal, several unicortical drill holes are made with a 0.045-in Kirschner wire. The fracture is reduced using image control, and the flexible rods are introduced through the previously drilled holes and passed across the fracture site into the distal subchondral bone. The position within the shaft is confirmed with the image intensifier. Additional rods are then introduced in a similar manner until the canal is packed with the wires. The rods are cut close to the bone, leaving only 1 to 2 mm protruding from the bone. Hall cautions that the portal of entry for the flexible rods should be as far from the fracture as possible to minimize the possibility of the fracture displacing along the path of the rods. This technique is also applicable to displaced metacarpal neck fractures

(Fig. 33–36). With all three percutaneous wire techniques, the patient is protected in a plaster cast for three to four weeks, followed by wire removal and active assisted motion.

Isolated closed oblique or spiral shaft fractures, if malaligned, will prove unstable following an attempt at closed reduction. Although percutaneous Kirschner wire fixation offers the advantage of closed fracture technique, it is often exceedingly difficult to obtain adequate fixation to control the rotatory malalignment. In these cases, operative treatment should be considered if there is angular or rotatory malalignment (Fig. 33–37).

Multiple Metacarpal Shaft Fractures

Multiple displaced metacarpal shaft fractures, especially when associated with soft tissue trauma, are an indication for open reduction and internal fixation.

Surgical Approach to the Metacarpals

Longitudinal extensile incisions are preferable to serpentine or transverse incisions on the dorsum of the hand. The border metacarpals can be approached individually through longitudinal incisions between the second and third or the fourth and fifth metacarpals. The third and fourth metacarpals are approached with a longitudinal incision between the metacarpals with Y-shaped extensions if needed to gain more proximal or distal extensions. When all four metacarpals require exposure, two incisions are made: one between the second and third metacarpals and another between the fourth and fifth (see Fig. 33–32).

The juncturae tendinum interconnecting the common extensor tendons over the distal metacarpals can be split to enhance exposure and then repaired at wound closure. The metacarpals are approached by incising the periosteum longitudinally and exposing the fracture subperiosteally. This will minimize disruption of the origins of the interosseous muscles. The exposure should be limited to the extent needed to accommodate the required implant. Small retractors and sharp-pointed fixation clamps are essential to minimize trauma to the soft tissues (see Fig. 33–32C). The periosteum can at times be closed over the implant.

The skeletal fixation of multiple metacarpal fractures is based on the preference and experience of the surgeon (see Fracture Immobilization Techniques). Our philosophy has been to provide internal fixation that is stable enough to permit functional loading postoperatively and to avoid cast immobilization.

Interfragmentary lag screw fixation is the choice of implant for spiral metacarpal fractures. Attention to detail is vital when using these small screws (see Frac-

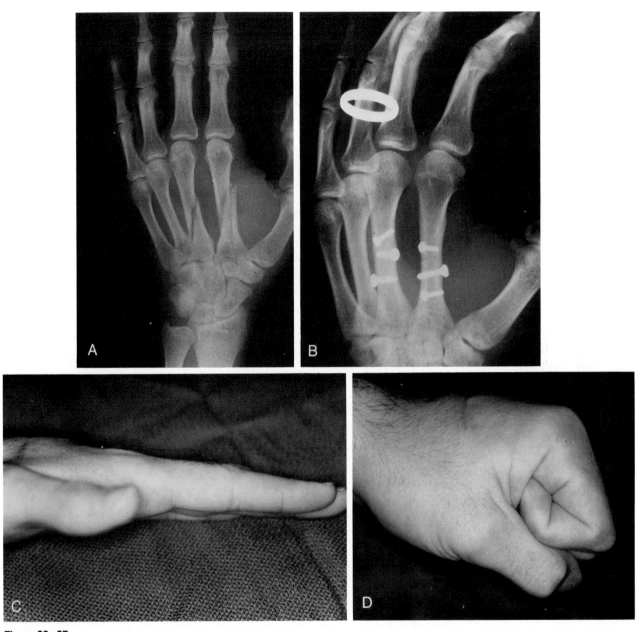

Figure 33-37

A 23-year-old male sustained two displaced spiral metacarpal fractures in a rugby match. He presented with a swollen hand and shortening and malrotation of the involved rays. Secure fixation was achieved with interfragmentary lag screw fixation. *A*, Preoperative radiograph demonstrates the long spiral fracture lines. *B*, Anatomic reduction and stable fixation were achieved with carefully placed 2.7-mm and 2.0-mm lag screws. *C* and *D*, Full motion was gained.

ture Immobilization Techniques). In large adults, 2.7-mm screws are used, and in smaller individuals, 2.0-mm screws are used. Screw fixation alone will be successful only if the fracture length is at least twice the diameter of the metacarpal and at least two screws are used. Screw placement is determined by the anatomy of the fracture plane. With two screws, effective resistance to shear and torsional stresses is best achieved with one screw placed perpendicular to the fracture line and

another placed perpendicular to the metacarpal shaft. With stable fixation, patients can begin active movement as soon as they are comfortable (see Fig. 33-37).

If problems are noted intraoperatively with the stability of the screw fixation, the tension band wire technique advocated by Belsole and Greene should be considered, as this can provide fixation that is stable enough to permit functional rehabilitation without the requirements of a plaster cast.[13,14]

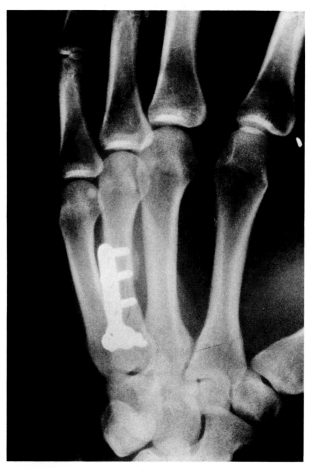

Figure 33–38

A displaced, malrotated, short oblique fracture of the proximal third of the fourth metacarpal was secured with a T plate. An interfragmentary screw was placed through the plate across the oblique fracture line. (From Jupiter, J.; Silver, M.A. In: Chapman, M., ed. Operative Orthopaedics. Philadelphia, J.B. Lippincott, 1988.)

Short oblique fractures provide an excellent fracture line for interfragmentary screw fixation, but the single screw must be "neutralized" against rotational and shear stresses by a plate. The choice of plate must be individualized for the specific location on the shaft. However, as a general rule the plate should permit two screws (four cortices) proximal and distal to the fracture. In the midshaft, a one-quarter tubular plate applied dorsally with 2.7-mm screws is appropriate for most adult metacarpals. If the fracture is at the proximal third of the metacarpal, a T or L plate may be the best implant. It is important first to place the screws through the T or L portion and then to fix the screws through the straight portion. If done in a reverse manner, rotational deformity will likely occur as the screws are tightened in the T or L portion (Fig. 33–38). Depending on the fracture line, the lag screw may be placed either through or independent of the plate.

Multiple transverse shaft fractures are frequently associated with soft tissue trauma and are well suited to plate fixation (Fig. 33–39). In the absence of comminution and with an intact palmar cortex, a one-quarter tubular plate with 2.7-mm screws is adequate. In this instance, the plate can function as a tension band plate. It should be contoured to sit slightly above the dorsal cortex, because when the screws are applied and tightened, the anterior cortex will be compressed. As such, the plate will be under "tensile" stress and will be protected from bending stress.[87]

When faced with comminution, a stronger implant such as the 2.7-mm dynamic compression (DC) plate should be chosen, and consideration should be given to placing some cancellous bone graft from the distal radius on the anterior aspect of the metacarpal. If the fractures consist of one or two butterfly fragments, an alternative to plate fixation is the tension band wire technique. This will permit each fragment to be individually assembled back onto the diaphysis in a secure fashion. Some caution should be exercised, as this technique, although effective, demands particular attention to detail (Fig. 33–40). Kirschner wire fixation alone with these fractures is difficult, often does not provide rotational stability, and requires plaster immobilization. The last, in particular, can be unfortunate, given the all too common soft tissue component of these injuries.

Metacarpal Fractures with Bone Loss

Metacarpal shaft fractures associated with bone loss are generally only one part of a complex composite skeletal and soft tissue injury. A traditional approach has consisted of maintaining skeletal length with external fixation or intermetacarpal wires, gaining soft tissue closure, and restoring skeletal continuity at a later stage when the soft tissue stability is ensured and some mobility is regained in the digital joints.[152]

Along with improvements in the techniques of stable skeletal fixation and soft tissue reconstruction has come a recognition that early reconstruction of the skeleton presents a decided advantage in accelerating rehabilitation efforts and minimizing the overall duration of the associated disability. Freeland et al. have demonstrated excellent results with metacarpal skeletal restoration performed within ten days of the initial injury.[65] Their protocol is based on extensive wound debridement of all nonviable tissue while maintaining skeletal length and alignment with a number of techniques, including spacer wires, transfixation Kirschner wires, and external fixation devices. A second debridement is performed three to seven days after the first. If the wound appears clean, definitive skeletal recon-

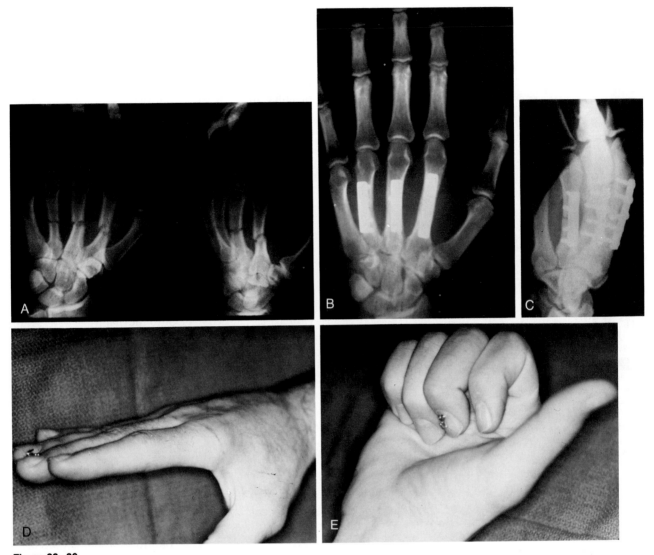

Figure 33-39

A laborer sustained blunt trauma to his dominant right hand. Massive swelling was associated with three transverse metacarpal fractures. *A*, AP *(left)* and oblique *(right)* radiographs reveal three transverse metacarpal shaft fractures. Minimal comminution was present. *B* and *C*, Through two longitudinal incisions, the swelling was decompressed and the fractures stabilized with four-hole one-quarter tubular plates. *D* and *E*, Active-assisted motion was begun on the first postoperative day along with Coban wraps to diminish swelling. At two weeks, the patient had regained nearly full motion. The fracture healed, and the patient returned to his job within eight weeks postoperatively. (From Jupiter, J.; Silver, M.A. In: Chapman, M., ed. Operative Orthopaedics. Philadelphia, J.B. Lippincott, 1988.)

struction with autogenous iliac crest graft and stable internal fixation is performed in conjunction with full-thickness soft tissue reconstruction (see chapter 15). Freeland et al. reported a high rate of skeletal union without clinical infection. This approach offers distinct advantages in the management of these severe complex injuries. Skeletal length and alignment are more easily ensured without the problems of operating in a contracted, less compliant soft tissue envelope.[37,171] Union is accomplished by the bone grafts being placed in a well-vascularized environment and being securely fixed with more stable internal fixation.[178] Finally,

rapid restoration of the skeleton with secure fixation offers the opportunity to start functional rehabilitation, thus minimizing the potential for joint contracture and tendon adhesion.

METACARPAL NECK FRACTURES

Fractures at the level of the metacarpal neck are among the most common of all fractures in the hand. Not infrequently, they are the result of a direct impact on the metacarpal head with the hand in a clenched fist position. Fracture of the fifth metacarpal is by far the

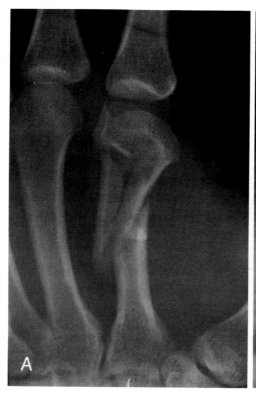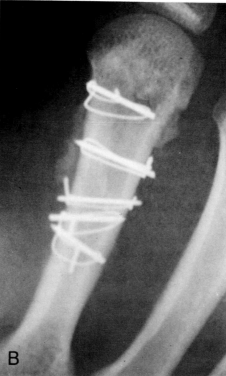

Figure 33–40

A comminuted metacarpal shaft fracture is reassembled and secured fixed with an arrangement of tension band wires. (Courtesy of Robert Belsole, M.D.)

most frequent and has become known as the "boxer's fracture." This description is somewhat misleading, as professional fighters are more likely to sustain a second or third metacarpal neck fracture.

Metacarpal neck fractures are impacted and, when displaced, angulate with dorsal angulation at the fracture line and the distal metacarpal head displaced palmarward. This palmar displacement can lead to an imbalance of the extrinsic tendons presenting as a claw deformity (Fig. 33–41). Physical examination should also assure that no rotational deformity is present. If the angulation is substantial, the metacarpal head palmar prominence may present a problem with grip.

A true lateral radiograph is necessary with these fractures in order to measure the angle of displacement of

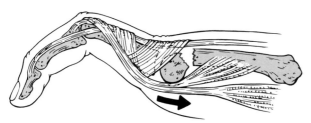

Figure 33–41

Excess palmar displacement of a metacarpal neck fracture will lead to imbalance of the extrinsic tendons and a claw deformity. The metacarpal head may be felt in the palm and may interfere with grip.

the distal fragment. Given the mobility of the fifth and, to a lesser extent, the fourth CMC joints, some angulation at the fracture is acceptable in these two metacarpals. Some authors believe that more than 30° of palmar displacement necessitates an attempt at reduction,[190] whereas others will accept up to 50° of angulation before a reduction is considered.[8,58,91,95]

Less disagreement can be found regarding the second and third metacarpals, as little if any compensatory motion is present at their CMC joints. Thus angulation beyond 10° will likely prove symptomatic. Lateral tomography is of great help when evaluating fractures of these two metacarpals. Metacarpal neck fractures that require no manipulation can be protected in a gutter splint for two weeks with the metacarpophalangeal joints flexed beyond 60°.

In the event that the patient presents with an unacceptable palmar displacement of the metacarpal head, a closed reduction under wrist block anesthesia is advisable with the metacarpophalangeal joint flexed to 90°. The proximal phalanx is grasped and used to correct any rotational deformity as well as palmar angulation; the latter is readily corrected by pushing up on the metacarpal head with the proximal phalanx (Fig. 33–42).[61,97] A short-arm cast or gutter splint is applied with care to mold the cast to maintain the metacarpophalangeal joint in 90° of flexion but leave the proximal interphalangeal joint in extension. The splint should be

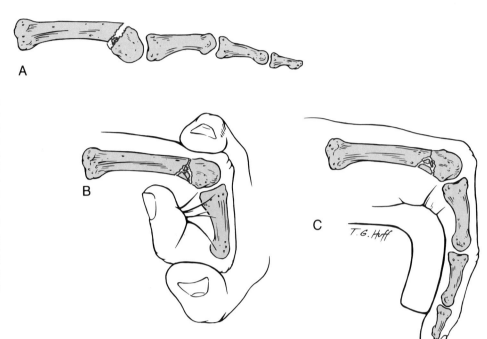

Figure 33–42

A displaced metacarpal neck can be reduced by flexing the metacarpophalangeal joint to 90° and using the proximal phalanx to control rotation and as a lever to push up the metacarpal head. *A,* A displaced neck fracture is generally associated with comminution on the volar surface. *B,* Fracture reduction used the proximal phalanx to push up the metacarpal head. *C,* Immobilization in plaster should place the metacarpophalangeal joint in 70° to 90° of flexion and the proximal interphalangeal joints close to full extension.

left in place for three weeks with a check radiograph obtained at seven to ten days postreduction. It has become well accepted that the proximal interphalangeal joint should not be held in flexion as recommended initially by Jahss,[97] as it can result in disastrous flexion contracture and even skin loss from pressure necrosis over the joint (Fig. 33–43).

If a patient is seen with a severely angulated neck fracture of > 50° or is seen initially five to seven days or more after the injury, it is not likely that the closed reduction will be effectively held in plaster support. Under these circumstances percutaneous wire fixation is recommended. A number of techniques for wire placement exist, as illustrated in Figure 33–44. Our preference is to avoid, if possible, pins being placed in or near the gliding structures that envelope the metacarpal head. The stacked wire technique advocated by Hall[82] allows the pins to be placed through a site distant from the fracture and is recommended for this situation (Fig. 33–45). The metacarpal should be immobi-

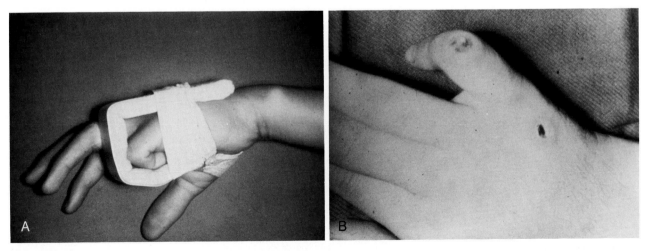

Figure 33–43

A 40-year-old female had a displaced boxer's fracture of the fifth metacarpal neck. *A,* The fracture was reduced and held in a splint with the proximal interphalangeal and metacarpophalangeal joints in extreme flexion. *B,* A severe flexion contracture of the proximal interphalangeal joint resulted, along with an area of pressure necrosis over the joint. An unsatisfactory functional outcome was the result.

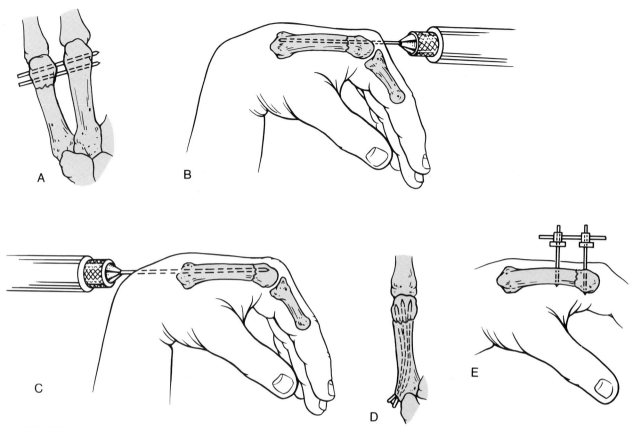

Figure 33–44

There is a variety of closed methods of percutaneous pin fixation of metacarpal neck fractures. *A*, Transverse pinning into the intact adjacent metacarpal. *B*, A longitudinal proximally directed pin placed eccentrically into the metacarpal head. *C*, A longitudinal distally directed pin. *D*, Multiple stacked pins directed from a proximal window in the base of the phalanx. *E*, Two external fixation pins used to aid in and maintain reduction.

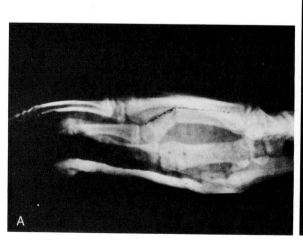

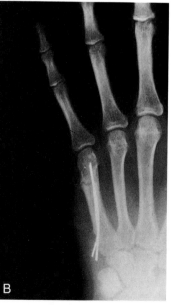

Figure 33–45

A 15-year-old with a fifth metacarpal neck fracture of 60° angulation *(A)* was treated by closed reduction and pin fixation introduced from a site proximal to the fracture in the base of the metacarpal *(B)*. (From Jupiter, J.; Silver, M.A. In: Chapman, M., ed. Operative Orthopaedics. Philadelphia, J.B. Lippincott, 1988.)

Figure 33–46

A 40-year-old female was thrown from her horse and sustained a closed displaced fifth metacarpal neck fracture that was discovered three weeks after injury. An open reduction was performed and the fracture stabilized with a tension band wire passed around two Kirschner wires. Early motion was encouraged, as the fixation was mechanically sound.

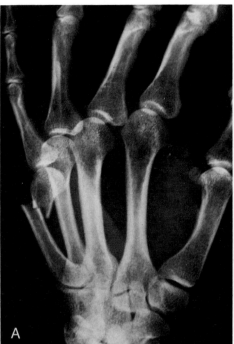
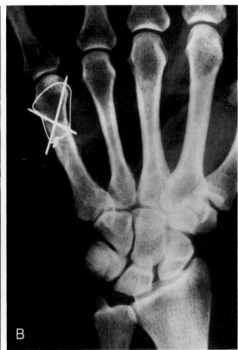

lized for two to three weeks, followed by a removable splint for one week.

Rarely is open reduction necessary. On occasion a patient presents at three to four weeks after injury, and closed manipulation is unsuccessful. In these cases, the fracture is approached through a longitudinal skin incision. The fracture site is also exposed through a longitudinal incision in the extensor mechanism. Our preference for internal fixation is a tension band wire placed around two Kirschner wires (Fig. 33–46).

Plates in this anatomic region are best reserved for those complex injuries combining soft tissue and skeletal loss. The 2.7-mm T or L plate combined with a compact cancellous bone graft has been the implant most often utilized (Fig. 33–47). The bulk of the implant and screws lying under the extensor tendon mechanism has presented some difficulty for the rehabilitation of these gliding structures. This problem has been solved to a large degree with the 2.0-mm and 2.7-mm condylar plates, which can be applied along the lateral surface of the metacarpal neck and shaft along with a bone graft.

An additional approach in these cases involves external fixation. The technique described by Pritsch and colleagues[160] of placing one pin in the metacarpal head and one in the shaft has been effectively used by these authors even for some closed fractures. Pin loosening and interference with tendon excursion are the pitfalls with this technique.

METACARPAL HEAD FRACTURES

Intraarticular fractures involving the head of the metacarpal are uncommon injuries. In a review of 250 open and closed articular fractures, Hastings and Carroll found only 16 that involved the metacarpal head, and only five were closed injuries.[85] A comprehensive review of 103 such fractures by McElfresh and Dobyns[140] revealed an array of fracture patterns ranging from collateral ligament avulsion fractures to extensive comminuted fractures associated with loss of bony substance. McElfresh and Dobyns divided two-part head fractures into oblique (sagittal) fractures of the metacarpal shaft entering the joint, vertical (coronal) fractures, and horizontal (transverse) fractures (Fig. 33–48). The most common fracture pattern was a comminuted head fracture found in 31 of 103 fractures. The most common metacarpal involved was the second, and these authors postulated this to be the result of its border position and lack of mobility at the CMC joint. The increased mobility of the fifth CMC joint puts its metacarpal head in a more flexed position at the moment of a direct axial blow, resulting in the neck fracture being much more common in this metacarpal.

These injuries may be exceptionally difficult to appreciate on routine radiographs. The lateral radiograph, in particular, is often unrewarding because of overlapping of adjacent metacarpophalangeal joints. Therefore the Brewerton view has been advocated for

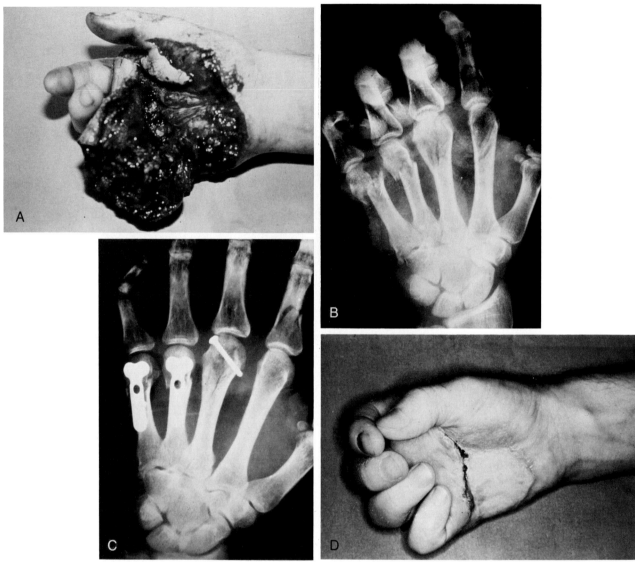

Figure 33–47

A 27-year-old male sustained a complex injury in an industrial machine. *A*, An extensive zone of soft tissue injury was present on the palmar surface. *B*, The radiograph revealed three complex metacarpal neck fractures. *C*, Stable internal fixation was provided with 2.7-mm T plates and a lag screw in the third metacarpal. *D*, Functional rehabilitation was initiated at five days following stabilization of the soft tissue injury.

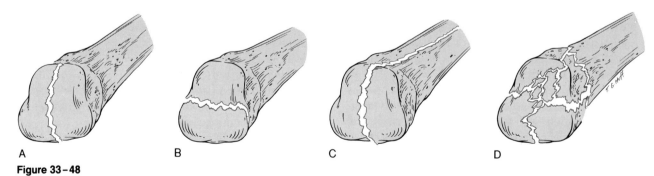

Figure 33–48

Fractures of the metacarpal head present several distinct patterns. *A*, Vertical (coronal). *B*, Horizontal (transverse). *C*, Oblique (sagittal). *D*, Comminuted.

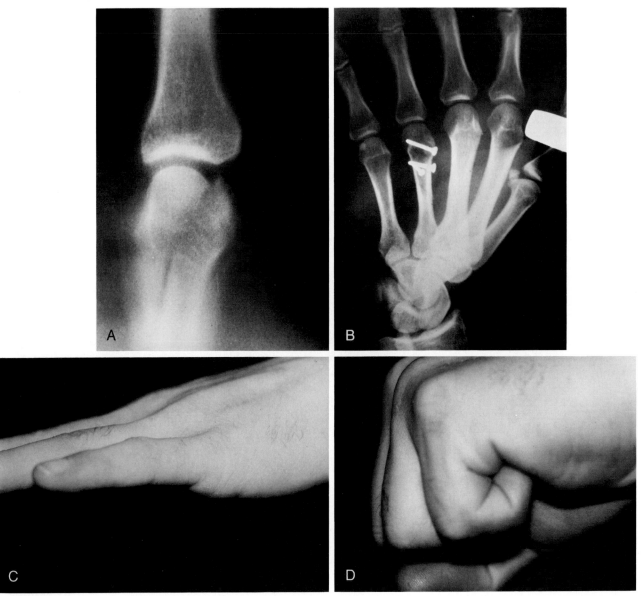

Figure 33–49

A 38-year-old male sustained a sagittal metacarpal head fracture of his fourth metacarpal as an extension of a more proximal shaft fracture. *A,* The AP tomogram demonstrates clearly the articular congruity. *B,* Stable fixation was achieved with carefully placed interfragmentary lag screws. *C* and *D,* Functional mobility returned within five weeks following injury.

these injuries.[123] This is performed with the metacarpophalangeal joints flexed between 60° and 70° and the dorsal surfaces of the digits lying flat on the x-ray cassette. The x-ray tube is angled 15° from ulnar to radial. Anteroposterior and lateral tomography has an important role not only in confirming the presence of these fractures but also in identifying the specific fracture pattern (Fig. 33–49).

The goal of treatment of these fractures, as with most intraarticular fractures, involves anatomic restoration and fixation that is stable enough to permit active mo-

bilization. The operative approach to these complex fractures should be considered only if preoperative planning suggests that these goals can be accomplished. Thus with extensively comminuted fractures, distraction fixation with an external fixation device or early mobilization may be preferable to surgical intervention, which generally will offer little hope of success.

The operative approach is through a dorsal incision with an interval developed between the extensor tendon and sagittal band. The fracture fragments are gently manipulated, leaving soft tissue attachments in

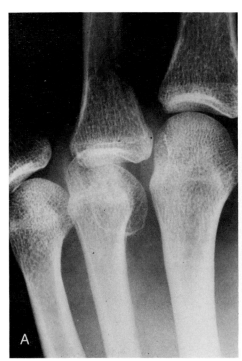
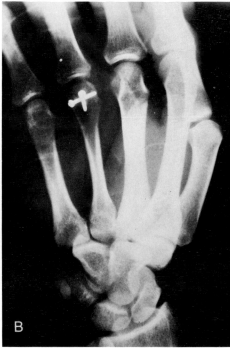

Figure 33-50

An impacted metacarpal head fracture was operatively reduced and securely fixed with two interfragmentary screws that were carefully countersunk into the dorsal cortex.

place to minimize the risk of devascularizing these tenuous fragments. Kirschner wires, although effective in holding the fragments in place, fail to provide sufficient stability to allow early mobilization. In addition, the pins themselves can irritate the surrounding soft tissues, also limiting mobilization. For those reasons, the miniscrews and self-compressing Herbert screw, which can be sunk beneath the chondral surface, have added significantly to the effective operative management of certain of these fractures (Fig. 33-50).[112] Placing the screw heads dorsally and cautiously countersinking them will minimize their impeding tendon mobility. The interfragmentary compression that is achieved results in more predictable union in the restored anatomic position.

A metacarpal head fracture resulting from penetrating trauma from a fistfight should be viewed as a highly contaminated wound. Extensive irrigation and debridement are essential, and some may consider leaving the wound open for 24 hours, followed by a second debridement with definitive internal fixation and wound closure.

The most serious complication intrinsic to this unusual fracture is loss of joint motion, despite careful operative techniques.[136] Avascular necrosis may occur as a result of the initial trauma or from operative intervention.

THUMB METACARPAL FRACTURES

Fractures of the thumb metacarpal are second in frequency only to those involving the fifth metacarpal, comprising nearly 25% of all metacarpal fractures.[67] Furthermore, of all thumb metacarpal fractures, more than 80% involve the base.[67,143] These fractures can be divided into four groups, similar to fractures at the base of the fifth metacarpal (Fig. 33-51 and Table 33-16): epibasal extraarticular, Bennett's, Rolando's, and comminuted. The mechanism of injury in all four types is

Table 33-16.	
Incidence of Thumb Metacarpal Fractures	

Type	%
Bennett's	34
Basal	44
Y/T	9
Oblique extraarticular	6
Transverse extraarticular	29
Diaphysis	10
Neck/head	12

Source: Gedda, K. O. Acta Chir Scand (Suppl 193):5, 1954.

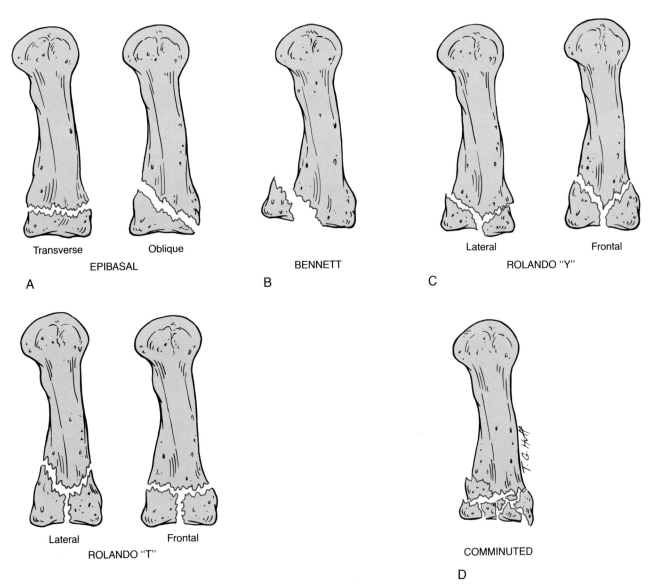

Figure 33-51

Fractures of the base of the thumb metacarpal can be grouped into four types: epibasal (A), Bennett's (B), Rolando's (C), and comminuted (D).

very similar, being that of an axially directed force through a partially flexed metacarpal shaft.

Epibasal Fractures

Epibasal extraarticular fractures are more commonly transverse rather than oblique. The mobility of the trapeziometacarpal will allow as much as 30° of angulation at this level without significant loss of mobility or strength.[76] The vast majority of transverse fractures are stable and require protective cast immobilization in a thumb spica cast for four to six weeks. If the angulation

is greater than 30°, closed reduction and percutaneous Kirschner wire fixation are recommended.

The epibasal oblique fracture can be confused with the intraarticular Bennett's fracture, and tomography may be required to define any articular involvement. If displaced, closed reduction and Kirschner wire fixation (as with transverse fractures) should be considered.

Bennett's (Two-Part) Fracture

Intraarticular fractures involving the thumb carpometacarpal joints comprise the most frequent of all thumb fractures[38,67,143] yet have been the source of continued discussion since Bennett first described the fracture in 1882.[15] The mere fact that the literature offers an exhaustive list of treatment options during the past century reflects the fact that no one method is ideal for all cases.[26,35,69,76,158,173,191,208]

The CMC joint of the thumb represents two reciprocally interlocked saddles that permit both flexion and extension as well as abduction and adduction.[81,149,155,157] Cooney and co-workers characterized the articular surface as a universal joint with its longitudinal axial rotation limited by its capsule, ligaments, and extrinsic muscle-tendon units.[41,42] The intracapsular volar oblique ligament is essential as a stabilizing unit of the metacarpal, as it inserts onto the ulnar articular margin of the volar beak on the ulnar aspect of the metacarpal base. Maximum tension occurs in this ligament with the metacarpal in flexion, abduction, and supination. With Bennett's fracture, the medial volar beak of the first metacarpal is split off. Attached to this fracture fragment is this critical restraining ligament. The result is displacement of the metacarpal base dorsally and rotation into supination by the pull of the abductor pollicis longus. The metacarpal head is also displaced into the palm by the pull of the adductor pollicis.[155]

Bennett's fracture, along with other fractures at the base of the metacarpal, is the result of an axially directed force on the thumb metacarpal while it is partially flexed. Males predominate in almost a 10:1 ratio to females, and two-thirds of these fractures occur in the dominant hand.[155] In Gedda's exhaustive study, nearly 50% of all Bennett's fractures occurred in patients younger than 30 years.[67]

Because of the thumb metacarpal's oblique orientation in reference to the plane of the palm, routine radiographs of the hand may be difficult to interpret and will often fail to reveal the true extent of the fracture anatomy as well as subluxation of the metacarpal. A true anteroposterior view of this joint can be obtained by the x-ray view described by Roberts.[168] This is accomplished by taking an anteroposterior view of the thumb with the forearm in maximal pronation and the dorsum of the thumb resting on the x-ray cassette. Perhaps of even greater value is the true lateral view advocated by Billing and Gedda.[16] This is obtained with the forearm flat on the table, the hand pronated approximately 20° with the thumb flat on the cassette, and the x-ray tube angled 10° from the vertical in a distal-to-proximal direction (Fig. 33–52). This view will enable (1) a more exact judgment of the metacarpal displacement, (2) an estimate of the size and position of the volar fragment, and (3) an estimate of the existing gap between the fragment and the metacarpal base. Tomography is often considered, particularly if there is a suggestion of impaction at the articular surface.

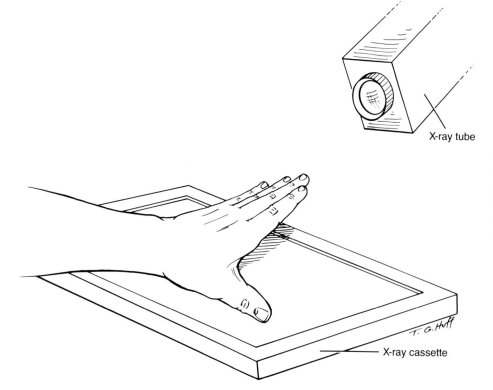

X-ray tube

X-ray cassette

Figure 33–52

A true lateral radiograph of the first metacarpal trapezial joint is taken with the thumb flat on the cassette, the hand pronated 20° to 30°, and the x-ray tube positioned 10° in a distal-to-proximal direction.

There appears to be no general consensus regarding the optimal method of treatment of Bennett's fracture, despite a vast number of surgeons who used different methods, with all reporting good results.[15,26,35,67,76,158,173,191,208] This may well be a result of a lack of agreement as to the relationship of articular anatomy and late results. Although Gedda's data strongly suggested a correlation with persistent fracture displacement and the development of radiographically evident arthritis,[67,68] this has not been the case in a number of other series.[35,38,78,155,158,173,213] Pellegrini and Burton have noted a low incidence (2.8%) of patients who had a past history of a fracture at the base of the thumb and required subsequent surgery for symptomatic osteoarthritis.[154] These authors explained that the weak correlation between anatomic fracture reduction and good functional results was largely the result of the relatively unconstrained nature of this joint. Yet they, too, recommended closed reduction and percutaneous pin fixation if there was < 3 mm of fracture displacement and open reduction and internal fixation if there was > 3 mm of fracture displacement.

The solution to this problem may well be found in the description of the fracture patterns by Gedda in 1954[67] and more recently by Buechler (Fig. 33–53).[29] Gedda noted that there were wide variations in the size of the volar ulnar metacarpal beak fragment and the extent of displacement of the metacarpal on the trape-

zium, even to the point of complete dislocation. In some instances he described intraarticular impaction fractures. Buechler[29] has identified three features that distinguish one fracture from another. These include the following:

1. The location and displacement of the fracture.

2. The extent of crush or impaction at the metacarpal base.

3. The presence or absence of shearing or impaction injury to the radial side of the articular surface of the trapezium.

Buechler has also divided the base of the metacarpal into three zones, with the middle zone being the area that will normally be loaded (see Fig. 33–53). If the fracture occurs in the other two zones, there will rarely be later problems. Furthermore, if it lies in the central zone but there is no impaction of the articular surface, it will also fare well, provided the metacarpal subluxation is reduced. Only the subgroup of Bennett's fracture that is associated with a zone of impacted articular surface will be subject to greater shearing forces at the trapezial articulation and later develop posttraumatic changes.[121]

The approach to the displaced Bennett's fracture should therefore be based on the specific nature of the fracture pattern. For the vast majority of fractures in Buechler's zones I and III, as well as those in zone II without evidence of impaction, closed reduction and percutaneous pin fixation are our preference (Fig. 33–54). The reduction is accomplished with longitudinal traction on the end of the thumb, coupled with abduction and extension of the thumb metacarpal. The metacarpal is pronated to bring it into opposition with the nondisplaced palmar fragment, and the base of the metacarpal is manually reduced (Fig. 33–55). The Kirschner wires can be placed through the metacarpal into the carpus or index metacarpal. It is not necessary to try to secure the small fracture fragment (Fig. 33–56). Although there have been studies suggesting that cast immobilization alone is effective,[158] some distinct problems exist with this treatment. These include the following:

1. The complexity of providing accurate three-point fixation over the thumb metacarpal and of maintaining this contact pressure when soft tissue swelling has diminished.

2. The difficulties of following the adequacy of the reduction with radiographs through the cast.

3. The poor results reported with cast treatment for those fractures initially seen four or more days following injury.[38,78]

Open reduction and internal fixation of displaced Bennett's fractures are indicated (1) when there is residual displacement of the joint surface of 2 mm or more

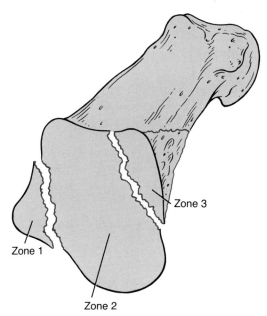

Figure 33–53

Three zones of articular involvement in Bennett's fractures as proposed by Buechler. If the fracture involves a displaced impacted articular surface in zone 2, there will be potential for later posttraumatic arthritis. This is unlikely in such fractures in zones 1 and 3.

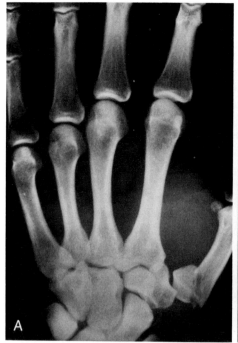
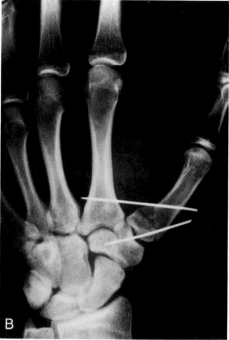

Figure 33–54

A 36-year-old male sustained a displaced oblique epibasal fracture of his dominant thumb metacarpal *(A)*. The fracture was reduced with traction and manual pressure on the base of the metacarpal and stabilized with 0.045-in Kirschner wires placed percutaneously *(B)*.

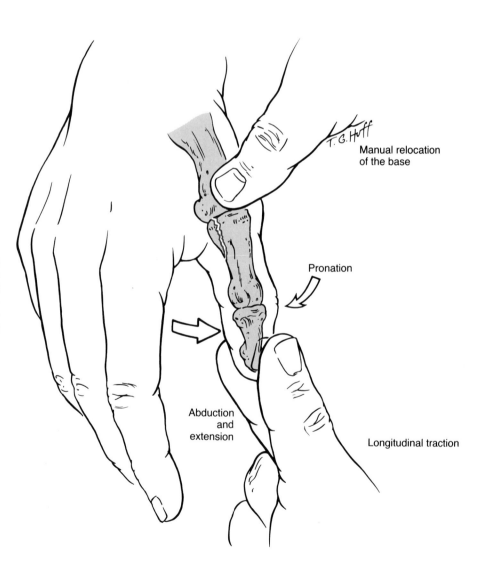

Manual relocation of the base

Pronation

Abduction and extension

Longitudinal traction

Figure 33–55

Reduction of a displaced Bennett's fracture-dislocation includes longitudinal traction on the end of the thumb coupled with abduction, extension, and pronation of the metacarpal. Manual pressure on the base will aid in its relocation.

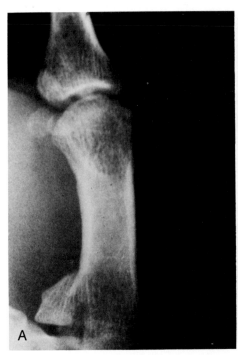
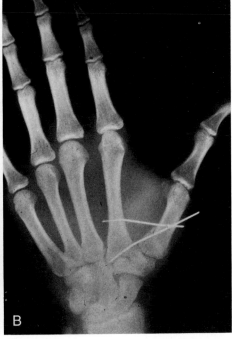

Figure 33-56

A displaced Bennett's fracture-dislocation in a 24-year-old male was treated with closed reduction and percutaneous pin fixation. *A,* The radiograph reveals the Bennett's fracture-dislocation. *B,* Two 0.045-in Kirschner wires stabilize the reduced metacarpal on the trapezium.

after closed manipulative reduction; (2) when there is radiographic evidence of impaction of the fracture, particularly in Buechler's zone II (best identified on tomography); or (3) for individual socioeconomic reasons. A volar incision is used. Care is taken to observe and protect branches of the radial sensory nerve, which can pass toward the palmar side at the base of the thumb. The origins of the abductor pollicis brevis and opponens pollicis are elevated off the proximal aspect of the first metacarpal in a subperiosteal manner. The CMC joint capsule is identified and opened, and the fracture hematoma is evacuated. The joint is visually inspected to look for free fragments, areas of impaction, or injury to the trapezial cartilage. A dental pick is ideal to gently loosen the hematoma from the fracture site, and reduction can be accomplished with longitudinal traction and manipulation of the metacarpal. A 0.035-in Kirschner wire will provide for provisional fixation of the reduction. If the volar oblique fragment is very small, a second Kirschner wire is used to secure the metacarpal into the second metacarpal, and a cast is used for six weeks.

With larger fragments, such as those in zone II, screw fixation is indicated.[62] Any impaction of the trapezial articular surface is elevated. If a visible defect is observed in the subchondral bone, a small amount of cancellous bone obtained from the distal radius will be necessary to support the elevated articular surface. In judging the size of the screw to be used, the surgeon should bear in mind that the screw thread diameter should be 30% or less of the width of the cortical surface

of the fracture to minimize the risk of fracture of the fragment (see Fracture Immobilization Techniques).[62] The 2.7-mm screw is useful in most cases, and an additional 2.0-mm screw placed in a different direction is advised for large fragments (Fig. 33-57). Radiographs, including a true AP and lateral view, are obtained to confirm both the accuracy of the reduction as well as the screw position and length.

The thenar muscles are reattached and the wound closed after release of the tourniquet. A postoperative removable splint is made and active motion permitted as soon as comfort allows. Pinching is avoided for one month postoperatively, and a return to full functional use can be anticipated by six to eight weeks postoperatively.

Rolando's (Three-Part) Fracture

Although Rolando's original description was that of a three-part fracture, it seems that this eponymic description has been utilized by other authors for more comminuted variants (Fig. 33-58).[67] We reserve this description for the uncommon, true three-part intraarticular fracture of the thumb metacarpal. AP and lateral tomography may be required to confirm the anatomy of this fracture, particularly if nonoperative treatment is contemplated. If tomography is not available, radiographs of the thumb taken while longitudinal traction is applied to the metacarpal are advisable.

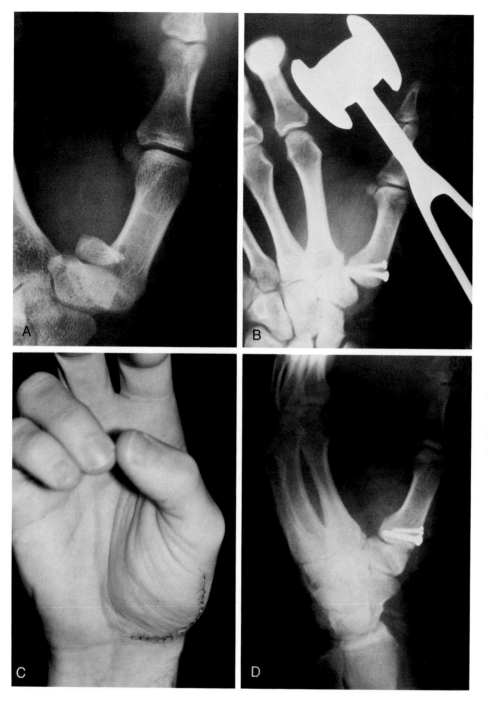

Figure 33–57

A 37-year-old male, a surgeon, sustained a displaced Bennett's fracture-dislocation of his dominant thumb. *A,* The radiograph reveals the fracture displacement. *B,* Intraoperatively, a large impacted central articular fragment was elevated and the fracture reduced and stabilized with a 2.7-mm and a 2.0-mm screw. *C,* Mobilization was initiated early postoperatively. *D,* An anatomic and full functional result was gained. The surgeon returned to work two weeks after injury.

We believe that this fracture is best treated by open reduction and internal fixation. The surgical approach is similar to that for Bennett's fracture. The fracture is reduced with longitudinal traction manipulating the two articular fragments into place. These are provisionally secured with a 0.035-in or 0.028-in Kirschner wire and secured with an interfragmentary 2.0-mm screw. The reconstructed articular fragments can then be secured to the metacarpal shaft with a 2.7-mm T or L

plate (Fig. 33–59).[62] On occasion, one fragment will be found impacted and will require elevation and support with cancellous bone graft from the distal radius. Postoperative management is similar to that for Bennett's fracture (Fig. 33–60).

An alternative method that can be considered is traction, either static (using an external fixation device) or dynamic (with traction wire passed through the base of the metacarpal out through the first web space and

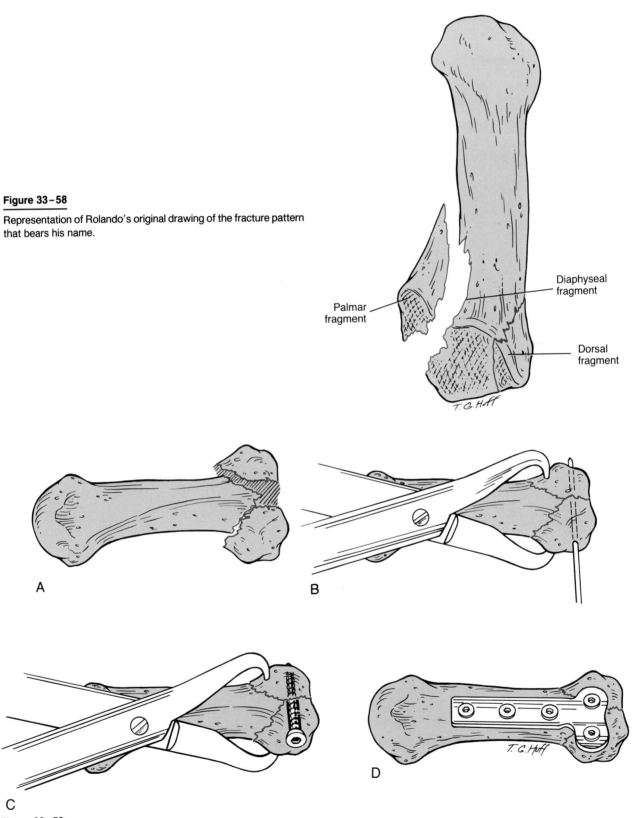

Figure 33–58

Representation of Rolando's original drawing of the fracture pattern that bears his name.

Palmar fragment

Diaphyseal fragment

Dorsal fragment

A

B

C

D

Figure 33–59

Operative technique of reduction and internal fixation of three-part Rolando fracture. *A,* The three-part T type fracture. *B,* Reduction is achieved by longitudinal traction and reduction of the articular fragments. *C,* The articular fragments are secured with an interfragmentary lag screw. *D,* The articular fragments are secured to the metacarpal shaft with a T or L plate.

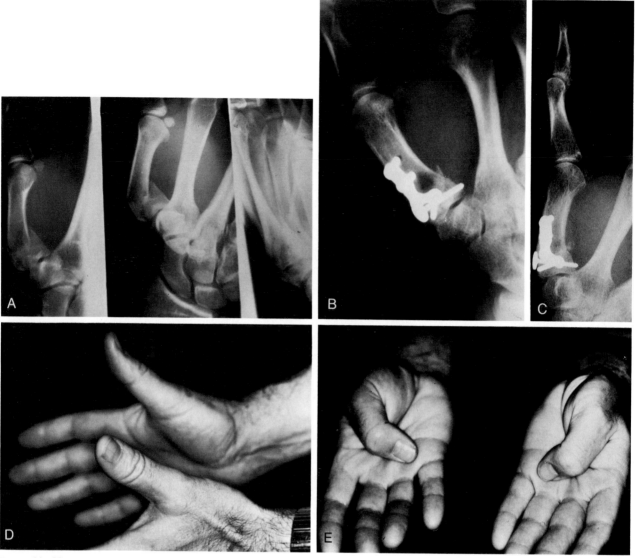

Figure 33–60

A 42-year-old male with a displaced three-part Rolando fracture at the base of his dominant right thumb. *A*, The radiographs demonstrate the fracture. *B* and *C*, Open reduction and internal fixation were accomplished. A 2.0-mm lag screw was placed over a washer to stabilize the articular fragments, and this was secured to the shaft with an L plate using 2.7-mm screws. Cancellous bone graft obtained from the distal radius was used to support the reduced articular surface. *D* and *E*, Full function resulted.

attached to outrigger traction).[69,208] Both of these methods can also be considered as a last resort if difficulty should ensue in applying internal fixation of these small fragments (Fig. 33–61).

Comminuted Fractures

Comminuted fractures are exceptionally difficult to treat. Gedda noted posttraumatic arthritis in more than 50% of 14 cases having an adequate follow-up.[67] As with the Rolando fracture, distraction has become an important factor in the approach to these fractures. Unless the comminution is excessive, involving multi-

ple small fragments, we prefer an open reduction using a distractor intraoperatively to provide a "ligamentotaxis" reduction of these small fragments.

The surgical approach is similar to that already described. Pins are placed directly into the body of the trapezium and distal metacarpal shaft and attached to a minidistractor. With longitudinal traction applied, the joint fragments can be manipulated into place, secured with 0.028-in Kirschner wires, and supported with cancellous bone graft. The distractor is left in place for four weeks and then removed, and a thumb spica splint or cast is applied for an additional two weeks (Fig. 33–62). An alternative to this is the traction method

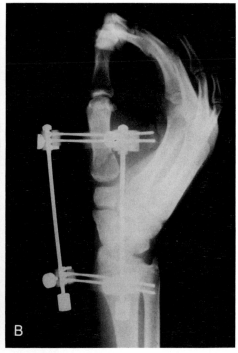

Figure 33–61

A three-part Rolando fracture was treated with closed reduction and distraction fixation with an external fixation device applied in the radius and thumb metacarpal.

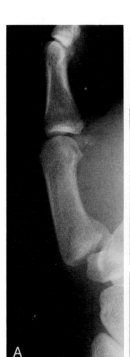

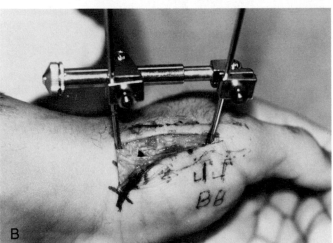

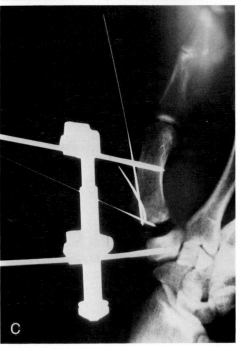

Figure 33–62

A 19-year-old male sustained a comminuted intraarticular fracture at the base of his dominant thumb. *A*, The radiograph reveals at least four major fragments. *B*, A minidistractor was applied with pins placed in the trapezium and first metacarpal. *C*, The fragments were manipulated into place, secured with small Kirschner wires, and supported with cancellous bone graft obtained from the distal radius.

975

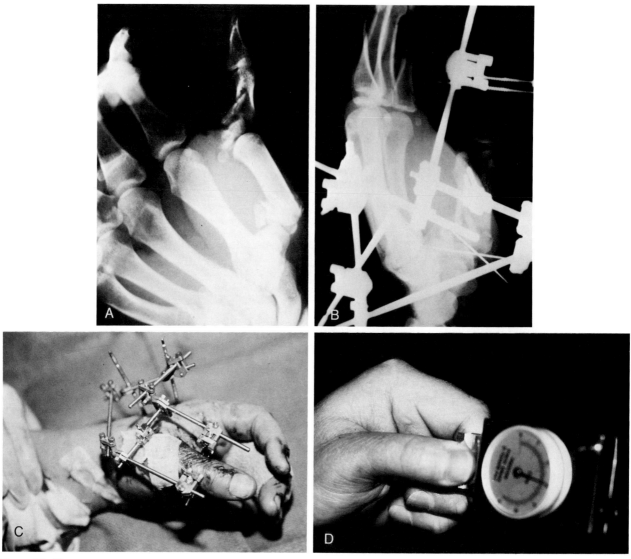

Figure 33–63

A 30-year-old male suffered a severe multilevel devascularizing injury to his dominant thumb in a press. *A*, The radiograph demonstrates the extensively comminuted intraarticular fractures at the base of both the metacarpal and proximal phalanx. *B*, Distraction fixation was applied to both comminuted fractures, and Kirschner wires were used to secure the fragments of the metacarpal fracture. Bone graft was obtained from the distal radius. *C*, The thumb was revascularized, and the external fixation was connected to pins placed in the second metacarpal. *D*, Excellent function resulted. (From Jupiter, J.; Silver, M. In: Chapman, M., ed. Operative Orthopaedics. Philadelphia, J.B. Lippincott, 1988.)

with a longitudinal Kirschner wire through the first web space as described by Thoren.[26,69,208]

At times these fractures are the result of high-energy trauma with associated soft tissue and other skeletal injuries. The miniature external fixator can be utilized not only as a distractor for the comminuted intraarticular fracture but also as an effective means of maintaining the span of the first web space by connecting the unit to similar pins placed in the second metacarpal (Fig. 33–63).[64,66]

Phalangeal Fractures

INCIDENCE

Phalangeal fractures are common. Gedda and Moberg, in a series of 2501 fractures in the hand, noted that more than 50% involved the proximal (P1) or middle (P2) phalanges.[68] In a series of 485 metacarpal and phalangeal fractures, Borgeskov found that 17.3% involved P1, 5.7% involved P2, and 45% involved the

Table 33-17. Relative Frequency of Phalangeal Fractures		
	Proximal (N = 106)	**Middle (N = 71)**
Head	18	12
Neck	11	16
Diaphysis	72	35
Base	5	8

Thumb	6%
Index	90%
Long	22%
Ring	15%
Little	17%

Source: Thomine, J. M. Les fractures ouvertes du squeulette digital dans les plaies de la main et des doigts. Actualites Chirugicales. Paris, Masson et Cie. 776–780, 1975.

distal phalanx (P3).[22] Thomine, in a series of 177 proximal and middle phalangeal fractures, noted that 60% involved P1 and 40% involved P2; the frequency of fracture by locations and digits is listed in Table 33–17.[206]

Although phalangeal fractures are common and in many instances require little care,[22,28,161,221] the potential for soft tissue adhesion, joint dysfunction, and malunion makes it necessary to define the "personality" of the individual fractures and tailor the treatment accordingly.[40,93,121,188,194,199,204]

PROXIMAL PHALANX FRACTURES

Extraarticular Base Fractures

Fractures at the base of P1 in adults can at times prove troublesome. When impacted, these will commonly angulate in a volar direction at the fracture. If allowed to unite with 25° or more of angulation, digital motion will be impaired, as the extensor mechanism becomes shortened, leading to loss of full extension at the proximal interphalangeal joint (Fig. 33–64).[44] The extent of angulation of these fractures may be difficult to accurately judge on radiographs; it may be difficult to see on the lateral projection because of overlap of adjacent digits, and the AP projection may not reveal much because of superimposition of the skeleton at the fracture line.

Coonrad and Pohlman found the most common problem with closed reduction and cast treatment was an inadequate degree of metacarpophalangeal joint flexion while in the cast, leading to loss of reduction.[44] If the fracture appears stable on reduction, cast immobilization should be considered, provided the metacar-

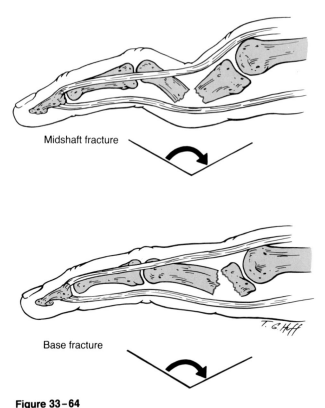

Midshaft fracture

Base fracture

Figure 33–64

Angulation of fractures of the proximal phalanx may be clinically less apparent at the base than at the middiaphyseal level.

pophalangeal joint is maintained in at least 60° to 70° of flexion (see Fracture Immobilization Techniques). If, however, the reduction is unstable or the patient is seen more than five to seven days after injury, closed manipulation and longitudinal percutaneous pinning are recommended (see Fracture Immobilization Techniques). In both cases the cast is maintained for three weeks and is followed by active motion, protecting the digit with a buddy strap to the adjacent digit for two weeks.

Those fractures associated with complex trauma, particularly flexor tendon lacerations, should be treated with stable internal fixation. The 1.5-mm condylar plate applied on the lateral aspect of the phalanx provides fracture stability with less interference to the extensor mechanism than a plate applied to the dorsal surface.[30]

Intraarticular Base Fractures

Intraarticular fractures of the base of the proximal phalanx can be subdivided into three types (Fig. 33–65): collateral ligament avulsion fractures, compression fractures, and vertical shaft fractures that extend into the joint. Avulsion fractures are most commonly seen

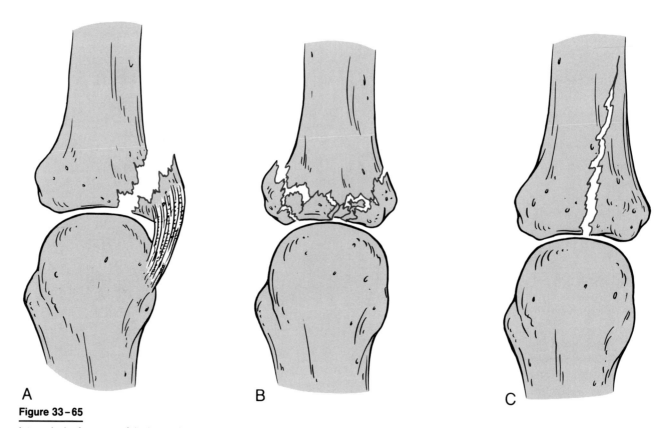

Figure 33–65

Intraarticular fractures of the base of the proximal phalanx can be classified into three main types: collateral ligament avulsion *(A);* compression *(B);* and vertical shaft *(C).*

associated with ulnar collateral ligament trauma to the thumb. Compression fractures are the result of an axial load and often have centrally impacted and rotated fragments. Vertical fractures can also have an impacted or split articular fragment.[85]

Those avulsion fractures with little or no displacement are readily treated with a buddy strap to the adjacent digit on the side of the injury. When they are displaced, anatomic reduction is important to prevent chronic instability or posttraumatic arthritis. Tension band wiring of these avulsion fractures has proven to have predictable results, offers the advantage of limited soft tissue dissection, and avoids the risk of fragmentation of the fragment.[103] The technique involves a dorsal approach that creates an interval between the extensor tendon and sagittal bands. The joint capsule is opened, and the fracture hematoma is removed. With gentle manipulation, the fracture fragment can be reduced and the articular surface anatomically aligned. Approximately 1 cm distal to the fracture, a drill hole is made in the proximal phalanx from dorsal to palmar using a 0.035-in Kirschner wire. A 26- or 28-gauge monofilament stainless steel wire is passed through the drill hole and retrieved with a curved hemostat from the palmar surface. A 20-gauge hypodermic needle is bent in a gentle curve and passed through the insertion of the collateral ligament onto the fragment. The wire is passed around the fragment in a figure-of-8 fashion and brought out through the ligament by passing it into the beveled end of the needle. With the fragment reduced, the wire is tightened and the twisted end cut short and bent along the phalanx (Fig. 33–66).

A similar approach is possible with comminuted fragments (Fig. 33–67). However, with a vertical shear fracture, an additional Kirschner wire is necessary or, preferably, an interfragmentary screw and Kirschner wire.

Postoperatively the patient can begin active motion, protecting the digit with a buddy strap to the adjacent digit (Fig. 33–68).

Compression fractures do not predictably reduce by longitudinal traction, as the impacted fragments may be devoid of soft tissue attachments. These require open reduction and gentle depression of the impacted articular fragments. The metacarpal head will effectively serve as a template on which the congruity of the articular surface of P1 can be built. Cancellous bone graft will be necessary to support the articular frag-

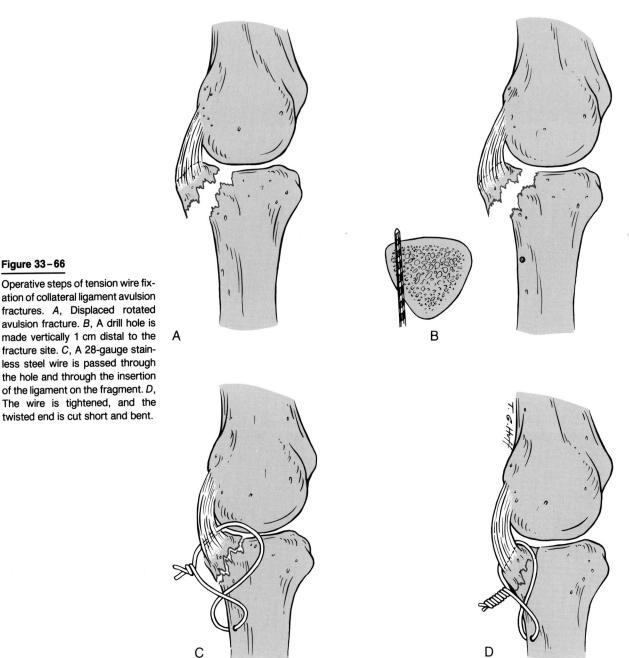

Figure 33–66

Operative steps of tension wire fixation of collateral ligament avulsion fractures. *A*, Displaced rotated avulsion fracture. *B*, A drill hole is made vertically 1 cm distal to the fracture site. *C*, A 28-gauge stainless steel wire is passed through the hole and through the insertion of the ligament on the fragment. *D*, The wire is tightened, and the twisted end is cut short and bent.

ments. In some instances, interfragmentary screw fixation can be applied, but the defect must be filled with compacted cancellous graft to prevent overcompression of the fragments and loss of the congruity of the articular reconstruction.[85] With some complex compression fractures, the minicondylar plate will be applicable, as it can serve both to buttress the articular reconstruction and to achieve interfragmentary compression through the plate holes (Fig. 33–69).

Vertical fractures can, on occasion, be successfully reduced with longitudinal traction on the phalanx with the metacarpophalangeal joint flexed. If both the articular and more distal shaft components reduce anatomically, then percutaneous wire fixation using image intensification should be considered. If reduction cannot be achieved, then open reduction and internal fixation with interfragmentary lag screws are advisable (Fig. 33–70).

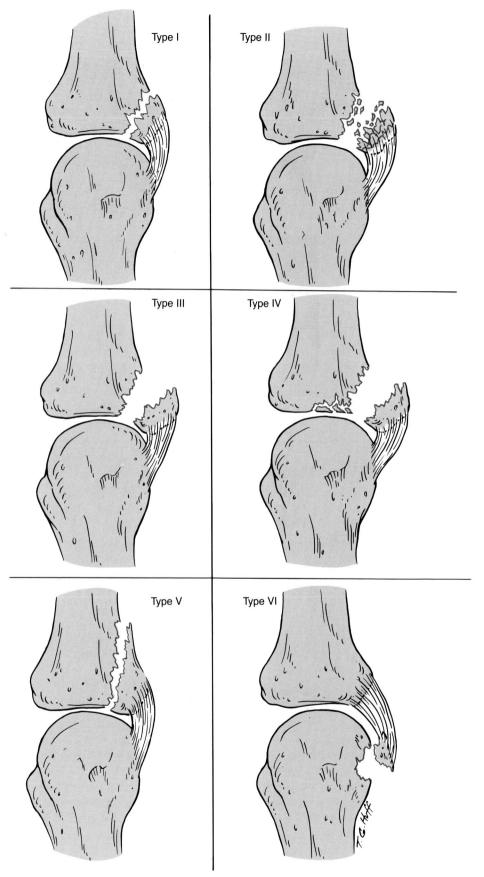

Figure 33–67

Avulsion fractures of the base of the proximal phalanx can be classified into six types.

Figure 33-68

A 15-year-old male sustained two rotated avulsion fractures at the base of the proximal phalanges of his long and ring fingers. *A*, The radiograph demonstrates the displacement of the avulsion fracture. *B*, The fractures were stably fixed with tension band wires. Full motion was recovered within two weeks, and rapid union was noted.

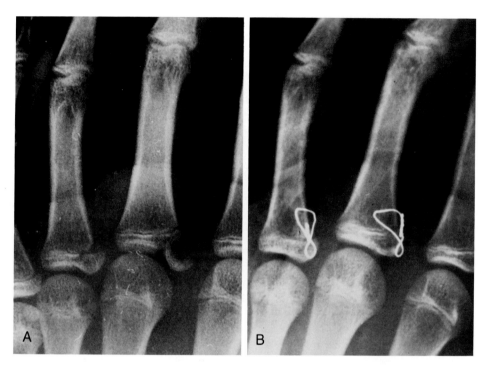

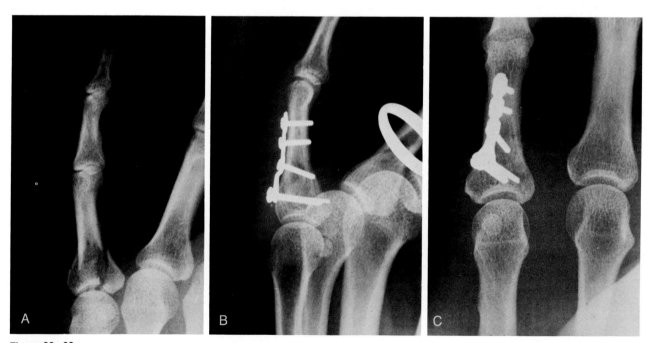

Figure 33-69

A 35-year-old male fell while skiing and sustained a complex compression fracture of the base of the proximal phalanx of his little finger. *A*, The radiograph demonstrates the disruption of the articular surface. A large impacted central fragment was found. *B* and *C*, Anatomic reduction, cancellous bone grafting, and a minicondylar plate applied on the lateral surface provided a stable skeletal and articular construct. Motion was begun on the first postoperative day.

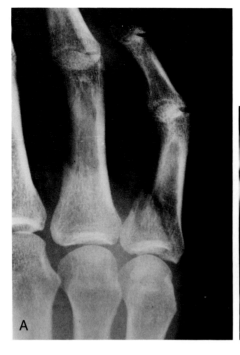
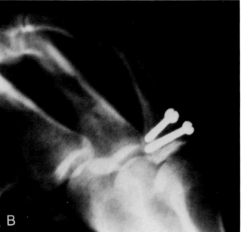

A

B

Figure 33-70

A vertically directed intraarticular fracture of the proximal phalanx of the finger was reduced operatively and fixed with several interfragmentary lag screws.

PROXIMAL AND MIDDLE PHALANX FRACTURES

Diaphyseal Fractures

Diaphyseal fractures of P1 and P2 are both subject to the deforming influences of intrinsic and extrinsic muscle forces. This as well as the mechanism of injury are the two major factors determining their fracture patterns.[143]

Transverse fractures will have a tendency to angulate with the apex pointed palmarward (Fig. 33-71). With P1 fractures, this is because of the insertion of the interosseous muscles on the proximal part of the phalanx; the distal part of P1 goes into extension as a result of the pull of the central slip and lateral bands of the extensor mechanism. With transverse P2 fractures, the apex of angulation may vary depending on the level of the fracture. Thus a transverse fracture at the proximal third of P2 may angulate with the apex dorsalward, whereas a fracture beyond the insertion of the flexor digitorum sublimis tendons will tend to angulate with its apex palmarward.

Spiral and long oblique fractures will tend to rotate along a longitudinal axis, whereas short oblique fractures may angulate. Rotational deformities will be evident by evaluation of the fingernails in digital extension and by deviation of the distal phalanges with digital flexion (see Fig. 33-9).

Comminuted diaphyseal fractures, often associated with a greater degree of soft tissue injury, will likely shorten, although this may be difficult to judge when the digit is swollen.

In assessing these fractures (see the section on general principles) for stability, deformity, and associated soft tissue injury, the physician must always bear in mind that stiffness, angular or rotatory deformity, or tendon adhesion will affect the function not only of the involved digit but also of adjacent digits as well as overall hand performance.

Fractures That Are Closed, Aligned, and Stable

Treatment options for stable well-aligned fractures are primarily directed at providing comfort and avoiding lengthy immobilization. Buddy straps to adjacent digits or gutter splints are generally adequate to achieve these intended goals.[8,161,198,221] If early motion is permitted, control radiographs should be obtained within

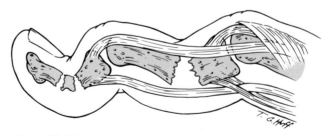

Figure 33-71

Transverse diaphyseal fractures of P1 and P2 tend to angulate as a result of the intrinsic and extrinsic muscle forces.

Table 33–18.

P1 and P2 Diaphyseal Fracture Treatment

Fracture Personality	Treatment Choice	Advantage
Closed; aligned; stable	Buddy strap	Mobility
Closed; malaligned; stable post-reduction		
Transverse/short oblique	Extension block casting	Maintains mobility and length of soft tissues
Spiral	Cast	Minimizes risk of displacement with motion
Closed; malaligned; unstable post-reduction		
Transverse, short oblique, spiral	Percutaneous Kirschner wires	Maintains length and soft tissue integrity
		High rate of success and low rate of complications
Highly comminuted	External fixation	Maintains length and soft tissue integrity
		Allows mobility of proximal and distal articulations
Closed; malaligned; reduction cannot be obtained	Open reduction and internal fixation	Direct control over fracture Anatomic alignment possible
Transverse/short oblique	Tension band wire	Stable fixation allows early motion
Long oblique/spiral	Lag screws	
Comminuted	Plate	

five to seven days to make certain displacement has not occurred. Healing will occur within three weeks clinically, although radiographically it may take as long as five weeks to see significant signs of bony union (Table 33–18).

Fractures That Are Closed, Malaligned, and Stable Post Reduction

For transverse or short oblique fracture patterns, the extension block casting method is effective and should be considered (see Fracture Immobilization Techniques). As it is mechanically sound, active digital flexion compressive forces are transmitted to the stable palmar cortex while the extensor mechanism and periosteum help to hold the fracture in place. This not only helps maintain fracture reduction but also maintains the length of the soft tissue envelope and prevents proximal interphalangeal joint stiffness.[32,164] Four weeks in this splint, followed by two weeks of protective buddy strapping, will be adequate for nearly all closed phalangeal fractures.

For spiral fractures that are stable to motion following reduction, dorsal and volar splints or cast are preferential. The distal phalanges and fingernails should be

visible, and radiographs are suggested at one and two weeks after casting to make certain malrotation has not occurred.

Fractures That Are Closed, Malaligned, and Unstable Post Reduction

For the vast majority of fractures that remain unstable following reduction, percutaneous pinning is indicated (see Fracture Immobilization Techniques). The advantages include preservation of the soft tissue envelope surrounding the fracture, maintenance of the resting length of the ligaments and tendons, and limited morbidity. Attention to detail in pin placement, plaster application over the pins, and postoperative management are consistent with efforts to achieve a successful outcome. In most series results were invariably good, with 90% good to excellent results (Table 33–18 and Figs. 33–72 and 33–73).[10,74,101]

Fractures That Are Closed, Malaligned, Comminuted, and Unstable Post Reduction

Very comminuted closed fractures are uncommon but can be most difficult to manage. They have a strong tendency to shorten, angulate, and rotate, and casting

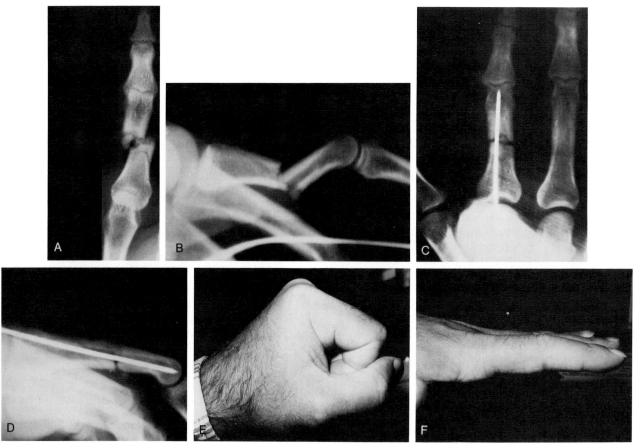

Figure 33–72

An unstable closed transverse fracture of P1 was treated with closed reduction and a longitudinal 0.045-in Kirschner wire. AP *(A)* and lateral *(B)* radiographs demonstrate the deformity. AP *(C)* and lateral *(D)* radiographs taken with the fracture reduced and held with a longitudinal Kirschner wire. *E* and *F*, Full functional recovery three weeks after Kirschner wire removal.

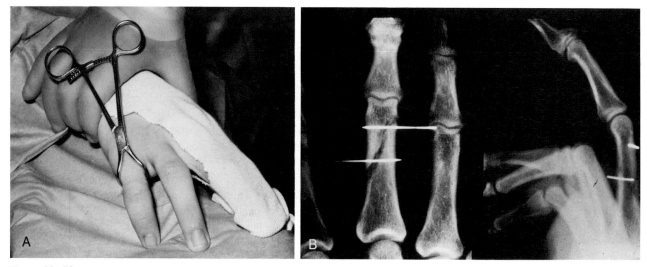

Figure 33–73

An unstable closed long oblique fracture of P1 was treated by closed reduction and transverse percutaneous wire fixation with 0.028-in Kirschner wires. *A*, Under image intensification, the fracture is reduced and held with a pointed reduction clamp. *B*, Stable fixation is achieved with transverse 0.028-in Kirschner wires.

alone or longitudinal percutaneous Kirschner wire fixation and casting may not sufficiently control the deforming tendencies. External traction through skin, pulp, or wire is unpredictable and fraught with potential problems, including pulp necrosis, pin track infection, and joint stiffness.

Similarly, operative treatment of these complex skeletal fractures risks destabilization and devascularization of the small fracture fragments, increased soft tissue trauma, and delayed union or nonunion. Soft tissue

adhesions and articular stiffness are common following most operative endeavors with these fractures. Stable fixation with plates will afford an opportunity to minimize these problems with early mobilization, but fixation with screws may be compromised by the extent of the diaphyseal comminution.

For all of the preceding reasons, distraction fixation with miniature external fixation devices is preferred in these unusual cases. They offer the advantages of maintaining the intact and well-perfused soft tissue en

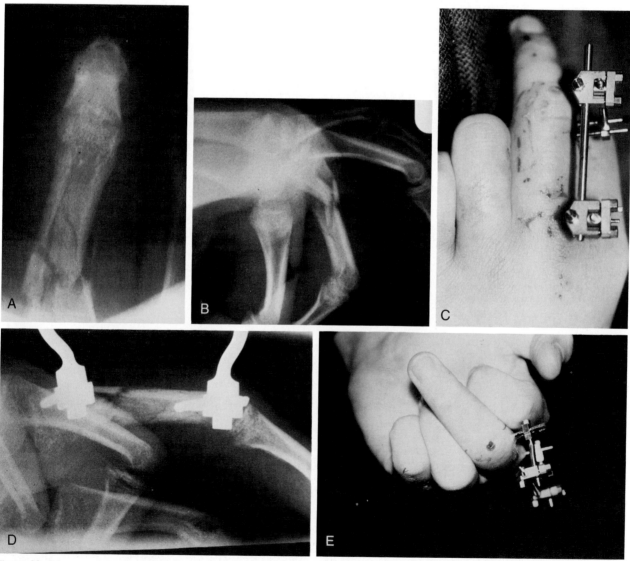

Figure 33-74

A 16-year-old male presented two weeks following injury with a displaced closed comminuted fracture of P1 of his dominant long finger. Limited motion existed. AP (A) and lateral (B) radiographs revealed an angulated comminuted fracture with early periosteal callus. C and D, Under image intensification, a miniature external fixator was applied, placing two pins in the base and two in the neck. The fracture was reduced, and the pins connected. E, The fixation was stable enough to permit mobilization of the metacarpophalangeal and interphalangeal joints. The fixator was removed four weeks after application.

Illustration continued on following page

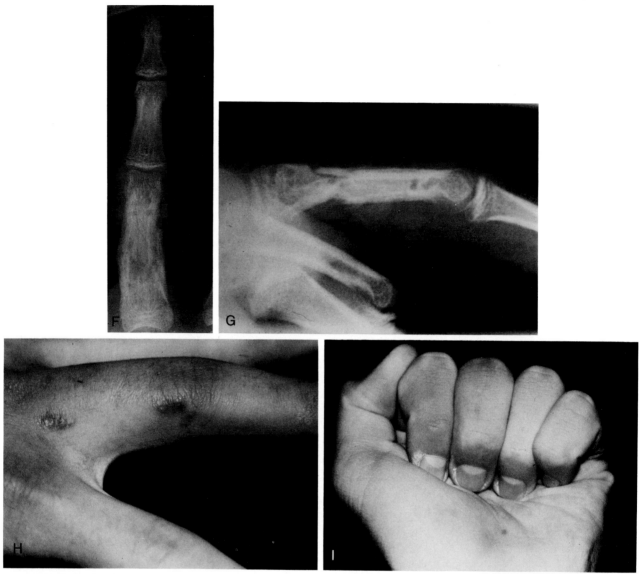

Figure 33–74 *Continued*

F and *G,* Radiographs taken at six weeks revealed a healed, well-aligned phalanx. *H* and *I,* Full functional motion was achieved six weeks following fixator application.

velope, of allowing for proximal and distal joint mobility, and of being much less technically demanding than internal fixation techniques (see Fracture Immobilization Techniques).[17,160,166] The fixator should remain in place at least four and possibly five weeks depending on radiographic evidence of callus formation. A protective splint is advisable for an additional two weeks, with only gentle active motion allowed out of the splint during this time (Fig. 33–74 and Table 33–18).

Closed and Malaligned Fractures in Which Reduction Cannot Be Obtained

It is uncommon not to be able to obtain an adequate reduction with most acute fractures. However, there

can be soft tissue interposition blocking some fractures. More commonly, this clinical dilemma will arise with a fracture seen two or more weeks post injury when callus is beginning to form but solid union has not developed. In these conditions, fracture reduction and stable internal fixation may be preferable to waiting and performing an osteotomy, often with additional needs for tenolysis or capsulotomy.

Surgical Exposure

The proximal and middle phalanges can be approached through either a dorsolateral or midaxial skin incision. The shaft can be approached either by split-

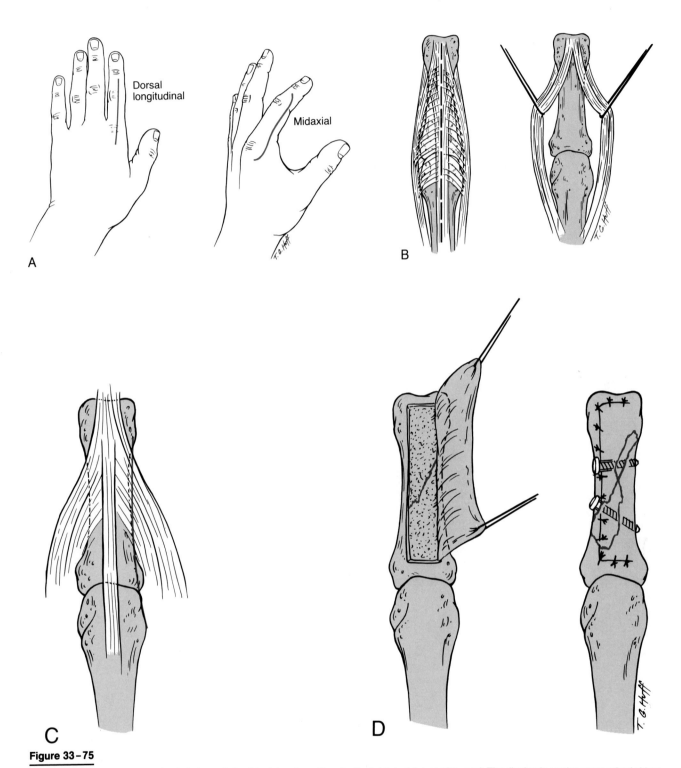

Figure 33-75

Surgical approach to the proximal phalanx. *A,* A midaxial or dorsal longitudinal skin incision can be used. The diaphysis can be approached either through *(B)* an extensor splinting or *(C)* an incision creating an interval between the common extensor and lateral band. *D,* The periosteum is elevated in a long wide flap that is sutured back into place to cover the implants.

ting the central extensor tendon longitudinally or by creating an interval between the lateral band and extensor tendon. In either case, the periosteum is elevated as a long, wide flap and preserved for later resuturing to

help serve as a gliding layer between the implants and the extensor mechanism (Fig. 33-75).

Closed transverse and short oblique fracture patterns involving P1 and P2 that require open reduction and

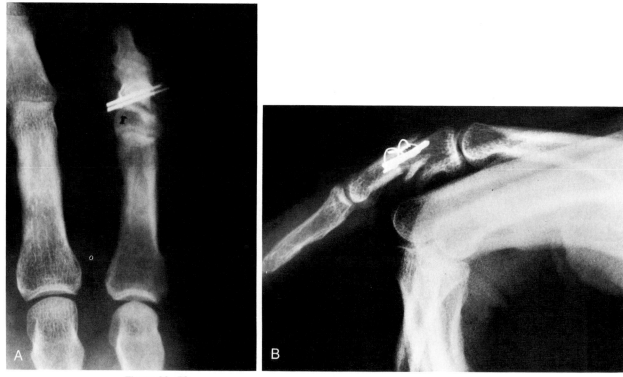

Figure 33-76

A complex closed shaft fracture of P2 stabilized with a tension band wire technique.

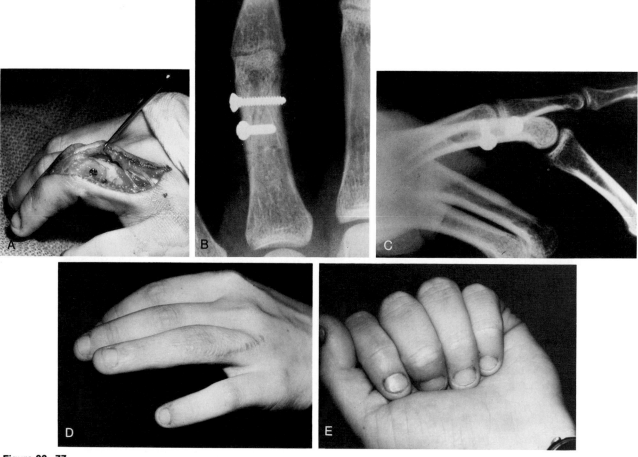

Figure 33-77

A 28-year-old female veterinarian presented two weeks after cast immobilization for a spiral fracture. Malrotation was evident along with soft tissue swelling and limited metacarpophalangeal and interphalangeal joint mobility. *A,* The fracture was exposed and fixed with two 2.0-mm screws. AP *(B)* and lateral *(C)* radiographs revealed the anatomic reduction and carefully placed screws. *D* and *E,* Early mobilization was begun, and full motion was regained by six weeks postoperatively.

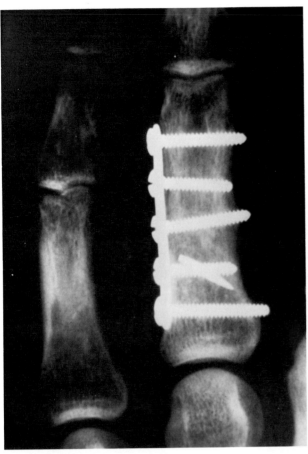

Figure 33–78

A malaligned proximal phalangeal fracture was stabilized with a mini-plate applied along the lateral surface of the phalanx to minimize implant interference with the extensor tendon mechanism. Note the broken drill bit within the bone.

internal fixation are amenable to tension band wiring. This technique offers sufficient stability to allow for early postoperative mobilization, yet presents a low profile (see Fracture Immobilization Techniques). This is particularly important, as the surrounding tendons and soft tissues of the phalanges have little ability to tolerate bulky implants (Fig. 33–76).

Long oblique and spiral fractures are preferably treated with 1.5-mm interfragmentary lag screws (see Fracture Immobilization Techniques).[89] These also offer stable fixation without undue bulk (Fig. 33–77). If comminution exists, a plate is indicated and can be applied along the lateral surface of the phalanx to again minimize interference with the dorsal gliding structures (Fig. 33–78 and Table 33–18).[30,47,87,104,178]

PHALANGEAL NECK FRACTURES

Closed fractures involving the phalangeal neck are extremely uncommon in adults, although they can

present a most difficult management problem in the pediatric age group. In the latter these fractures will often rotate dorsally, and it is not uncommon to have soft tissue interposition.[6,50,177]

In the adult, displaced fractures are readily reduced by closed means but are difficult to control with external splint or cast immobilization. For this reason, percutaneous Kirschner wire fixation is placed either across the metacarpophalangeal joint with the joint in 80° of flexion or through the lateral base of the proximal phalanx (see Fracture Immobilization Techniques).[10] Plaster support is necessary for a minimum of three weeks, and the pins should be left in for an additional week (Fig. 33–79).

PHALANGEAL CONDYLAR FRACTURES

Functional Anatomy

The condylar configuration of the head of the phalangeal skeleton forms an integral part of a unique hinge articulation. The stability of these joints is dependent on dynamic and passive factors. Dynamic stability results from joint compressive forces that increase with pinch and grip actions, increasing lateral stability. This in turn is dependent on the integrity of the articular configurations. If distorted by displaced articular fractures, the joint compressive forces no longer are directed perpendicular to the normal axis of motion, thereby contributing to instability.[25] Passive stability results from collateral ligament tension, which increases with flexion. The true collateral ligament is most important in flexion but is lax in extension, whereas the accessory collateral ligament and volar plate are major stabilizers with the joint in extension.[115,117]

When viewed "end on" the condyles resemble a grooved trochlea (pulley). However, they are asymmetric in shape and contour. The palmar aspect is nearly twice as wide as the dorsal margin. The base of the middle and distal phalanges has an intercondylar ridge and recesses that support articulating condyles, but this arrangement is not completely congruous. This feature allows some rotation and translation, which affords the digit the ability to better adapt to irregular shapes in grip (Fig. 33–80).[25]

Treatment Goals

Fractures of the condylar architecture of the head of the phalanges can result in pain, deformity, and loss of motion.[5,85,127,139] Flexion contracture following these injuries is common. Because the function of the interphalangeal joints is coordinated in part by a common extensor mechanism, dysfunction of one will nearly

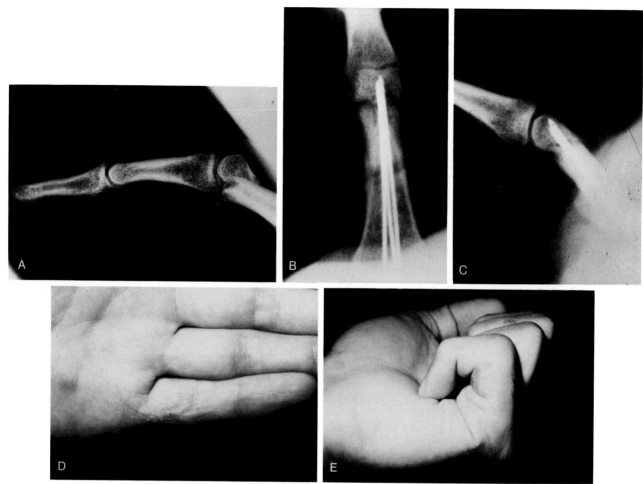

Figure 33–79

A displaced neck fracture of the proximal phalanx of the little finger was treated with a closed reduction and longitudinal percutaneous Kirschner wire fixation. *A,* The lateral radiograph demonstrates a displaced phalangeal neck fracture. AP *(B)* and lateral *(C)* radiographs of the fracture following closed reduction and percutaneous wire fixation. The Kirschner wires were left in place for four weeks. *D* and *E,* Nearly full digital motion was regained by two weeks following Kirschner wire removal.

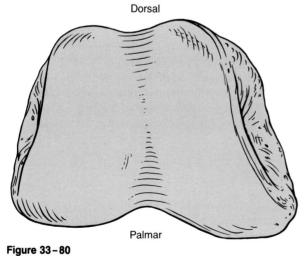

Dorsal

Palmar

Figure 33–80

Condylar arrangement of the head of the proximal phalanx. Note that, when viewed end on, the condyles are not symmetric.

always affect the other. Therefore anatomic repositioning is the goal. With displaced fractures, this can occasionally be accomplished nonoperatively. More often than not, however, an operative approach is required.[19,28,89,112,176,178,179,194] The ability to achieve stable internal fixation will add immeasurably to the final outcome.

Unicondylar Fractures

Unicondylar fractures are the result of a shearing force and tend to be unstable. Although the fracture may only be displaced in a lateral direction, the attached collateral ligament will frequently cause the condyle to rotate. The latter will lead not only to intraarticular incongruity but also to angular displacement of the more distal phalanx.

Figure 33–81

A 26-year-old female fell while skiing. *A,* The anteroposterior x-ray film reveals displacement of the articular surface. *B,* On the lateral film, displacement of the condyles and the interphalangeal joint is evident.

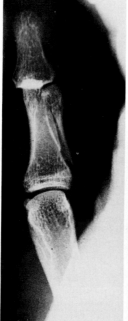
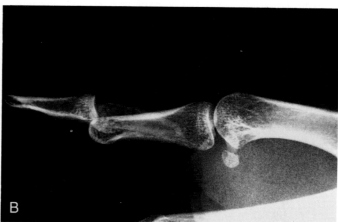

Nondisplaced fractures can be treated nonoperatively with a digital splint for seven to ten days, followed by protective mobilization (i.e., by buddy strapping the digit to the adjacent digits). Because of the obliquity of the fracture line, these patients should have repeat radiographs to confirm the anatomic position.

A closed reduction can be considered when the unicondylar fracture represents an isolated injury without associated skeletal or soft tissue trauma. This is accomplished by axial traction and by angulating the digit away from the injured condyle. The condyle is compressed with a pointed reduction clamp, and a transverse 0.028-in percutaneous Kirschner wire is placed into the opposite condyle. The reduction must be carefully confirmed with standard radiographs (three views) in the operating room, as the small size of these fragments can mislead the surgeon unless good quality radiographs are obtained. What may appear as a minimal asymmetry in the AP projection may, in fact, represent a malrotation that is more evident in a true lateral radiograph. When the reduction is anatomic, a true lateral radiograph will have both condyles projected on each other. With malrotation, each condyle will be evident (Fig. 33–81).

Displaced unicondylar fractures are, for the most part, approached operatively, as there can be little tolerance for a nonanatomic reduction. The surgical approach is dorsal, and the condyle is exposed by creating an interval between the extensor tendon and ipsilateral lateral band. Once the intraarticular hematoma is evacuated, the fracture anatomy can be appreciated. Prior to reduction, two features should be evaluated. The first is the dimensions of the condylar fragment, particularly in relationship to the thread diameter of the screw that is to be used (usually 1.5 mm). Second, the insertion of the collateral ligament is carefully identified so that it can be protected during the reduction and internal fixation. The vascularity to the condylar fragment is dependent in part on the collateral ligament. Thus undue surgical trauma can lead to avascular necrosis of the fragment.

Reduction is accomplished under direct vision, and provisional fixation is achieved with a transversely directed 0.028-in Kirschner wire. If the fragment is of sufficient size (see Fracture Immobilization Techniques), a 1.5-mm screw is placed. The entry point ideally should be just above and proximal to the origin of the collateral ligament to avoid injury to the ligament and potential avascular necrosis of the condylar fragment (Fig. 33–82). For larger fragments with a longer oblique fracture line, a Kirschner wire should also be used to neutralize shear forces on the screw. Alternatively, for smaller fragments, two 0.028-in Kirschner wires will be adequate to maintain the anatomic reduction.

With the stability afforded by interfragmentary lag screw fixation, mobilization can be started within a few days after surgery. The digit is protected with buddy

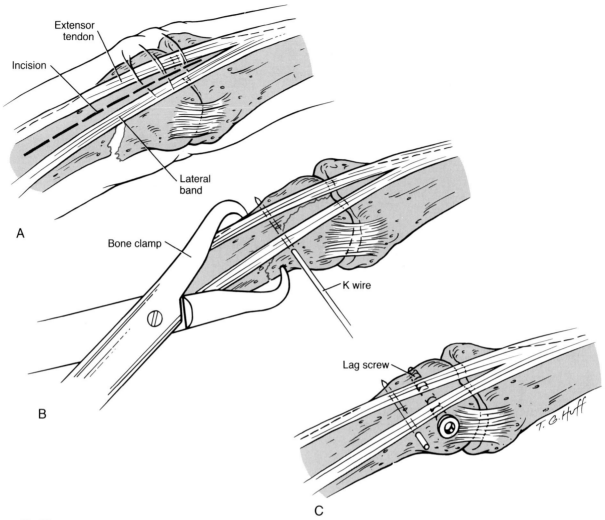

Figure 33–82

Operative approach to internal fixation of a unicondylar fracture of the head of the proximal phalanx. *A,* The approach is between the extensor tendon and lateral band. Prior to reduction, the fragment's dimensions are determined. The fragment must be at least three times the diameter of the intended screw to allow interfragmentary screw fixation to be safely used. *B,* The fragment is reduced and provisionally secured with a 0.028-in Kirschner wire. *C,* The placement of the screw should be slightly dorsal and proximal to the origin of the collateral ligament. With a large fragment, the Kirschner wire can be left in to add rotational control.

strapping to an adjacent digit for two to three weeks (Fig. 33–83).

Bicondylar Fractures

Bicondylar fractures result from compressive loads directly on the head of the phalanx, splitting the two condyles. The collateral ligament attachment to each fragment tends to separate and rotate each from the other, making closed reduction exceptionally difficult. However, a surgical approach must not be considered lightly, as the exposure may be limited, the fragments

small and unstable, and the fixation technically demanding. The 1.5-mm condylar plate has provided a stable implant that resides along the lateral surface of the phalanx, thus avoiding interference with the extensor tendon over the proximal interphalangeal joint (see Fracture Immobilization Techniques).

In some instances, the fracture lines extend more proximally (Fig. 33–84) to allow for stable fixation with interfragmentary screws alone.[132] An alternative technique is a modification of the tension band wire fixation. This technique is a particularly effective last resort if problems arise with plate fixation. Two sets of

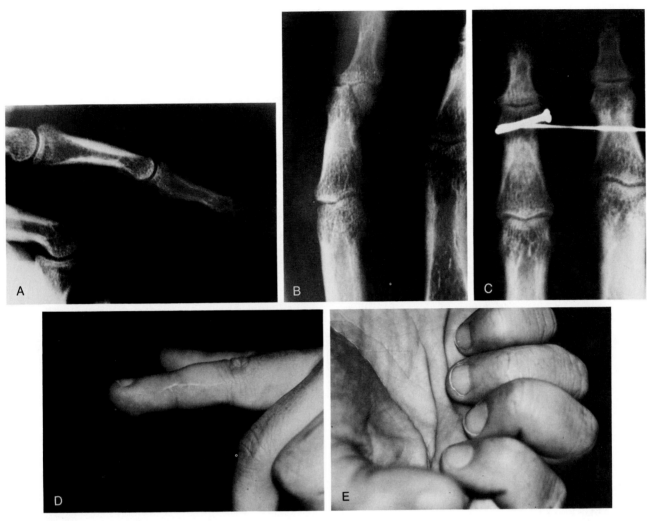

Figure 33–83

A neurosurgical resident sustained a displaced rotated condylar fracture of the middle phalanx of his dominant ring finger. Lateral *(A)* and oblique *(B)* radiographs reveal rotation of the condyle. *C*, Open reduction and internal fixation were achieved with a 1.5-mm interfragmentary screw and 0.028-in Kirschner wire. *D* and *E*, Full function resulted, and he returned to surgical duties two weeks postoperatively.

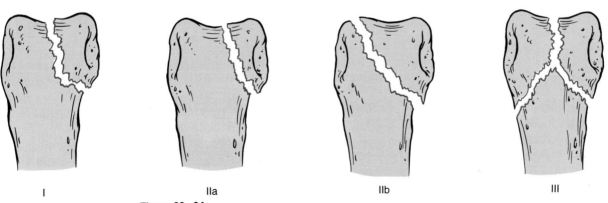

I   IIa   IIb   III

Figure 33–84

London's classification of condylar fractures of the interphalangeal joints.

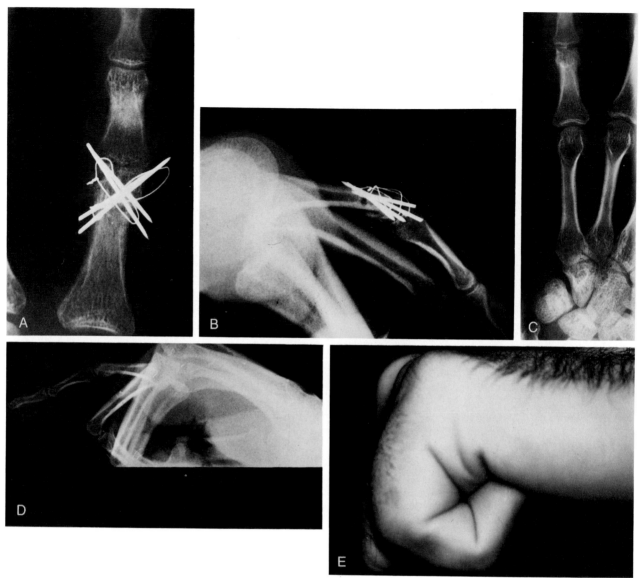

Figure 33–85

A 23-year-old male sustained a displaced bicondylar fracture of the proximal phalanx of his left little finger. *A* and *B,* An attempt to secure the fracture with a 1.5-mm condylar plate was unsuccessful, and a tension band wire technique was used instead. *C* and *D,* The fracture healed without evidence of avascular changes. *E,* Full flexion and a 5° extension lag were the functional outcomes.

0.028-in Kirschner wires are placed obliquely and distally from each condyle into the opposite, more proximal cortex. The wire placement should enter the condyles just above the true collateral ligaments but peripheral to the articular cartilage surfaces. A 30-gauge monofilament stainless steel wire is passed over the points of the Kirschner wire, brought around the condyles and over the dorsum of the phalanx in a figure of 8, and then brought around the proximal protrusion of the Kirschner wires. Each figure of 8 is tightened, holding the condyles to avoid rotational deformation. The stainless steel wire passes under the extensor mech-

anism sitting flat on the phalanx. The fixation gained by this approach is sufficient to permit mobility in the early postoperative period (Fig. 33–85).

Because of the complexity of these articulations, the meager size and vascularity of the fracture fragments, and the joints' close relationship to the extensor mechanism, these fractures are among the most difficult to manage in the hand. Unstable or improperly placed fixation, excessive soft tissue stripping, and unsupervised postoperative care can all result in an unsatisfactory outcome (Fig. 33–86).

The complexity of this articular injury increases

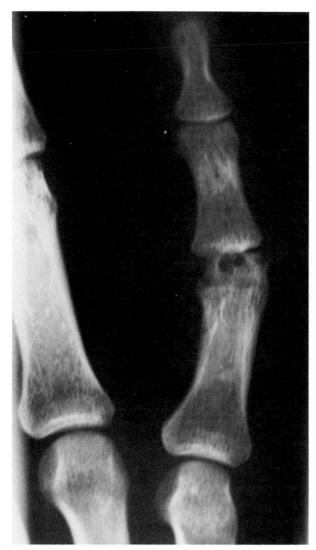

Figure 33–86

Excessive soft tissue stripping or a screw that is too large can lead to ischemic changes in condylar fractures. This radiograph reveals changes consistent with subchondral collapse resulting from avascular necrosis following open reduction and internal fixation of a unicondylar fracture.

when combined with soft tissue disruption. The ability to achieve articular restoration and stable fixation has a decided advantage in this setting (Fig. 33–87).

Fractures of the Proximal Interphalangeal Joint

FRACTURES OF THE BASE OF THE MIDDLE PHALANX

Fractures involving the articular base of the middle phalanx are the result of an axial load. The specific fracture pattern as well as the direction and degree of displacement will be determined by the nature of the deforming force.[53,133]

Fractures of the volar base at the site of attachment of the palmar plate are the most common of these injuries. These are often confined to only a small portion of the volar lip of the middle phalanx and result from a direct axial load (e.g., a "jammed" finger in a sporting event) (Fig. 33–88). Treatment is often only for comfort and protection. Coban wraps will keep swelling to a minimum, and a dorsal extension block splint will serve to prevent repeat injury. The splint is required for only two weeks, followed by buddy straps, which should be worn an additional two to four weeks.

Volar fractures associated with dorsal dislocation of the middle phalanx can be classified into those that are stable following closed reduction and those that are unable to be maintained by closed treatment. The stable volar fractures will be those comprising less than 30% to 40% of the articular surface. The stability is a reflection of the attachment of the dorsal part of the true collateral ligament onto the middle phalanx (Fig. 33–89).

The technique advocated by McElfresh et al.[141] involves a closed reduction followed by extension block splinting and is best suited for dorsal fracture-dislocations that are stable following reduction with the proximal interphalangeal joint held in a flexed position. It is easily performed under metacarpal block anesthesia. Longitudinal traction and flexion of the proximal interphalangeal joint will reduce the dislocation. A true lateral radiograph must confirm that the dorsal displacement has been eliminated. The digit is allowed to extend slowly until the dorsal subluxation recurs; this point is carefully noted. The joint is again reduced, holding it in flexion 5° to 10° beyond the point at which it redislocated. A short-arm cast is made, incorporating a contoured dorsal alumafoam splint extending dorsally onto the injured digit. The wrist is held in 30° of extension, the metacarpophalangeal joint in 60° to 80° of flexion, and the proximal interphalangeal joint in flexion just beyond its point of instability. Tape is applied to the splint over the proximal phalanx, allowing further active flexion of the injured joint. Again, a true lateral radiograph must confirm the reduction.

The patient is seen at weekly intervals and the splint slowly extended by 10° over the joint each week until full extension is achieved. As a rule this will be realigned by four to six weeks, at which time the splint is removed and buddy straps applied for an additional two to three weeks.

Strong suggested an ingenious method for splinting these fracture-dislocations that consists of two dorsal alumafoam splints bent toward each other over the

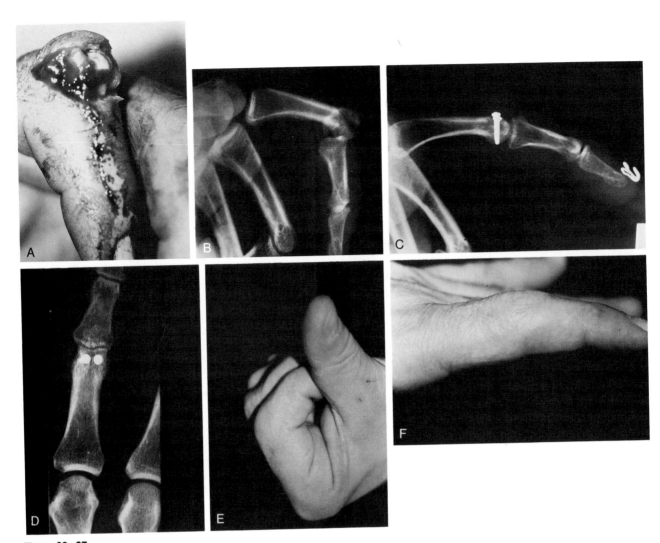

Figure 33–87

A, A 33-year-old male sustained a table saw injury to the dorsum of his left index finger. The extensor mechanism was disrupted, and there was a vertical and horizontal splitting of the articular condyles. *B*, The lateral radiograph demonstrates the articular disruption. *C* and *D*, Following thorough debridement, the condyles were reduced and internally fixed with two 1.5-mm interfragmentary screws. The extensor mechanism was reconstructed acutely. Radiographs taken at six weeks reveal the anatomic restoration without evidence of avascular necrosis. *E* and *F*, The patient regained nearly full extension and 80° of flexion. His postoperative mobilization was begun three weeks following injury to allow for healing of the extensor mechanism.

injured joint to keep the joint resting in the position of flexion, which maintains the reduction.[201] Both splints are taped to the digit, and active flexion exercise is begun. In a manner similar to that described by McElfresh et al., the joint is extended by 10° on a weekly basis. This technique, however, can only be considered in a compliant patient, as all digital splints can slip or loosen.

When the fracture involves between 30% and 50% of the base of the middle phalanx, the technique of dorsal block splinting may not be as predictable.[85] In McElfresh et al.'s series, only 4 of 17 patients had fracture fragments larger than 30%. For articular fragments that

are not comminuted, open reduction and internal fixation have had predictable results. A midaxial approach affords excellent exposure and with manual traction on the middle phalanx, the joint can be readily reduced. The internal fixation method optimally should allow early mobilization. Either single screw fixation or Lister's type B intraosseous wire technique should be considered (see Fracture Immobilization Techniques). Transarticular Kirschner wiring for three weeks followed by dorsal block splinting has been effective in some authors' experience.[85,139,219]

If the fragments are comminuted and unstable with dorsal block splinting, the available options include dynamic traction and volar plate arthroplasty. Several methods of dynamic traction have been devised and include (1) the dynamic force couple technique designed by Agee,[2] (2) dynamic traction and early passive movement in a circular traction splint (advocated by Schenk[175]), and (3) dynamic external fixation designed by Hastings and Ernst.[86] The first two options have been demonstrated to be effective in each author's hands but are complex to apply or cumbersome or both. However, they should be considered if an adequate reduction can be achieved. The dynamic external fixation of Hastings is preferable, as it controls the dorsal subluxation effectively by having skeletal pins on either side of the joint.[86]

Volar plate arthroplasty has been promoted by Eaton and Malerich for the acute management of this group of injuries.[56] This technique is performed through a palmar approach. The comminuted fracture fragments are resected, and the middle phalanx is reduced. A pullout wire is woven through the palmar plate and passed out through the fracture site and secured over the dorsum of the middle phalanx. In the presence of instability, the joint is held reduced, and an oblique 0.035-in Kirschner wire is passed across the joint. The wire is left in for two weeks, followed by motion in an extension block splint.

By far the most complex injury pattern is that in which articular comminution extends beyond 50% of the articular surface of the middle phalanx base. The fundamental problem in this subgroup of fracture-dislocations is the loss of the collateral ligament support to the middle phalangeal shaft (see Fig. 33–89). The more

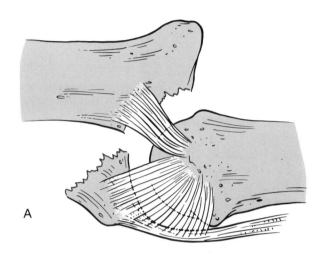
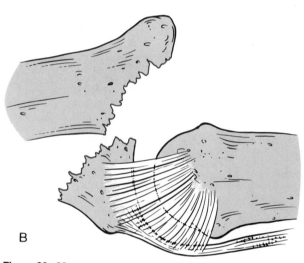

Figure 33–89

Stability of a displaced dorsal fracture-dislocation is dependent on the collateral ligament. With fragments involving more than 40% to 50% of the volar articular base of the middle phalanx, any attachment of the true collateral ligament is lost.

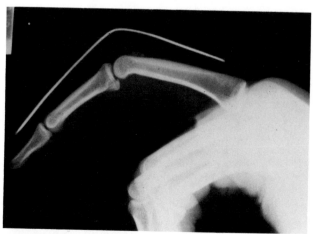

Figure 33–88

A 23-year-old female jammed her finger in a volleyball game. She presented with a painful swollen digit. Radiographs demonstrated a small nondisplaced avulsion fragment on the base of the middle phalanx. Coban wraps and early mobilization with a protective alumafoam extension block splint led to a rapid functional recovery.

distal attachments of the extrinsic flexor tendons add to the deforming pull on the middle phalanges.[85] Traction, external fixation with or without open reduction, internal fixation, and volar plate arthroplasty are all unpredictable, but the traction "arcuate" splint technique of Schenk has been shown to be effective for these fractures. Traction is applied to a horizontal transosseous wire through the middle or distal phalanx for six to eight weeks. For these complex fractures, Schenk reported an average arc of motion of 87° in ten patients.[175] The technique of osteotomy and grafting of the volar fragment to restore a more competent volar buttress as advocated by Zemel et al. may also have the most promise in these cases.[222]

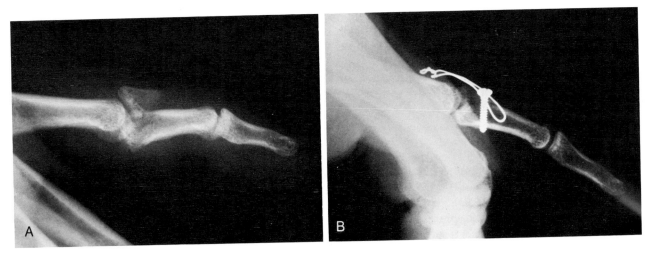

Figure 33–90

A 20-year-old male sustained a fracture of the dorsal base of the middle phalanx associated with a volar dislocation. Open reduction and internal fixation with an interfragmentary screw were accomplished. An additional tension band wire was directed through a dorsally placed drill hole in the middle phalanx and woven through the central slip to help neutralize the force on the screw.

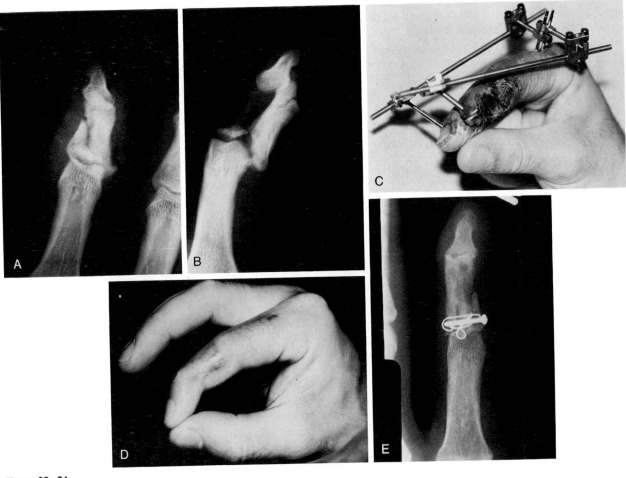

Figure 33–91

A 26-year-old male sustained a severe impaction injury of the middle phalanx of his dominant index finger. *A* and *B*, Radiographs demonstrate the unfortunate damage to the joint surface. *C*, A minidistractor was applied, and the joint was reduced and stabilized with internal fixation and a cancellous distal radius bone graft. *D*, The joint proved to be stiff, but was stable and pain free. *E*, Follow-up radiograph at six months.

Fractures of the base of the middle phalanx with or without dorsal dislocation are common injuries, but a favorable outcome is far from assured in even the most innocent of injuries. Proximal interphalangeal joint stiffness, flexion contracture, and redislocation have all been associated with these articular injuries.

Fractures of the Dorsum of the Middle Phalanx

Dorsal avulsion fractures represent a disruption of the attachment of the central slip of the extensor mechanism. These are considered as acute boutonniere fractures and treated with extension splinting for up to six weeks, leaving the distal interphalangeal joint free for active motion.

Much less commonly this injury is associated with a volar dislocation of the middle phalanx. An attempt at a closed reduction is advisable. If successful, transarticular Kirschner wire fixation is recommended for three weeks. The joint should also be splinted in extension, leaving the distal interphalangeal joint free. If the dorsal fragment is of sufficient size, an open reduction and internal fixation are preferential. Protected active motion can be initiated if the internal fixation is stable (Fig. 33–90).

Impaction Fractures

A number of specific impaction fracture patterns of the articular surface of the base of the middle phalanges have been outlined in a review by Hastings and Car-

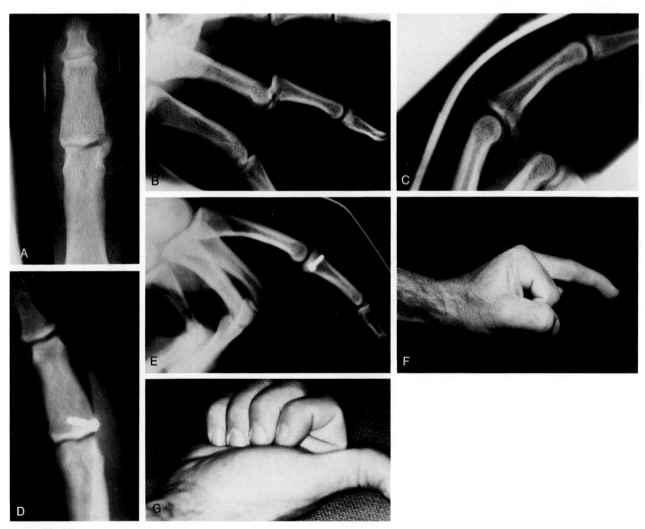

Figure 33–92

A 21-year-old male sustained a fracture-dislocation of his long finger in a sporting event. AP *(A)* and lateral *(B)* radiographs demonstrate the dislocation and presence of a large volar lateral plateau fracture. *C,* Closed reduction was unsuccessful in reducing the fragment as a result of displacement by its attached collateral ligaments. *D* and *E,* Open reduction and internal fixation of the fragment with a 1.5-mm screw achieved both an anatomic joint surface and a stable articulation. Early motion was achieved. *F* and *G,* Nearly full extension and flexion were regained.

roll.[85] A direct axial load will produce a central impaction fracture pattern. These are uncommon injuries but can be suitable, in some cases, to operative treatment. As with comminuted articular fractures at the base of the thumb, distraction with an external fixation device will help define the fracture fragments, and it may prove possible to elevate the larger impacted articular fragments and mold them to the corresponding articular surface of the head of the proximal phalanx. Cancellous bone graft must be placed under the elevated joint surface. Unfortunately, some of these are high-energy injuries that offer little hope of functional restoration. Even so, reassembly of the fracture fragments can provide an easier skeletal anatomy on which to perform arthrodesis or arthroplasty (Fig. 33–91).

Lateral Plateau Fractures

Fractures with eccentric loading will result in disruption of the volar side of one of the articular fossae of the base of the middle phalanx. The fragment can be rotated and displaced by the attached collateral ligament.

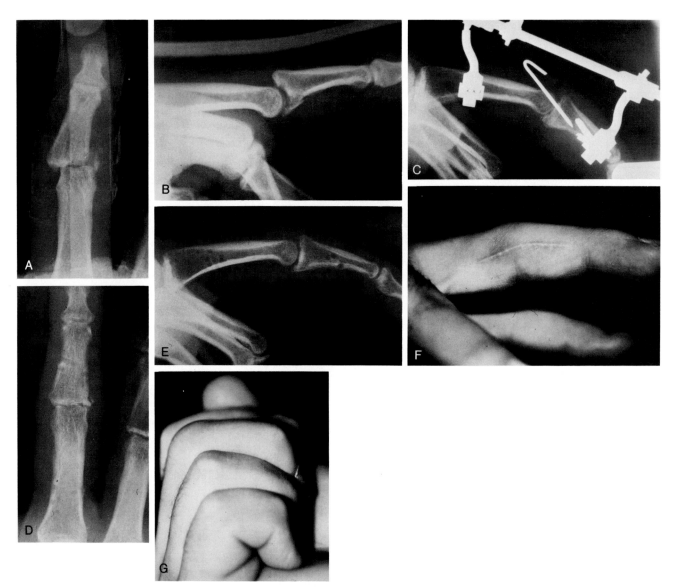

Figure 33–93

A 33-year-old male was referred for treatment of an unstable volar lateral plateau fracture with associated articular impaction. AP (A) and lateral (B) radiographs demonstrate the fracture-dislocation. C, A miniature external fixator was applied, and distraction was achieved across the joint. Through a midaxial incision, the compressed articular fragment was elevated and the volar lateral plateau fragment reduced. D and E, AP and lateral radiographs, respectively, taken at nine weeks postoperatively. F and G, The fixator was removed six weeks postoperatively, and the patient regained nearly full motion by nine weeks postoperatively.

It is not uncommon to find impaction of some part of the articular surface. Instability may be present dorsally or rotational instability of the digit may be present around the contralateral intact collateral ligament. A surgical approach can achieve restoration of both joint stability and articular anatomy. With larger volar fragments, stable internal fixation is possible with 1.5-mm screws (Fig. 33–92). Another fixation option involves Kirschner wire and monofilament stainless steel wire (no. 28 or 30-gauge) passed through the attached collateral ligament and around the fragment. If a part of the articular surface should require elevation, cancellous graft can be placed in support of the articular surface (Fig. 33–93).

Fractures of the Middle Phalanges

The outcome of fractures of the middle phalanges in general is more favorable than that for fractures of the proximal phalanges. This is mostly because disturbance of distal interphalangeal joint motion is not nearly as great a functional problem as are similar disturbances of the proximal interphalangeal or metacarpophalangeal joint motion.

These fractures are often readily reduced, as the stable proximal interphalangeal joint makes manipulative reduction straightforward. With unstable fractures, Kirschner wire fixation is the best choice if the fracture line is amenable. Only with widespread soft tissue trauma should open reduction and stable internal fixation be considered.

Unicondylar and bicondylar fractures are similar to those of the head of the proximal phalanx, and treatment considerations should mirror those already discussed (see Phalangeal Condylar Fractures).

Fractures of the Distal Phalanx

ANATOMY

The unique architecture of the human distal phalanx plays an important role not only in overall digital form and function but also in the complexity of its fracture patterns. In addition, the relationship of the distal phalanx with its highly specialized overlying soft tissue envelope often forms the basis for treatment considerations in fractures of this bone.

The broad spadelike distal tuberosity is perhaps the distal phalanx's most distinguishing feature when compared with the structure of the middle phalanx. This so-called ungual tuberosity represents an evolutionary development of the early hominids, perhaps as

a result of a greater incorporation of pulp use in gripping as well as an increased reliance on tools.[184] This feature is lacking today in most primates.[203]

The palmar surface of the ungual tuberosity provides the site of attachment of well-defined fascial bands that separate the distal digital pulp into wedgelike compartments similar to the structure of the heel pad.[96] This particular anatomic arrangement diffuses contact pressures through the conical fat columns, thereby distributing pulp pressures more equally.[184] The overlying nail plate also plays a role in stabilizing the deforming forces on the terminal pulp.

Spinous processes project on both sides of the ungual tuberosity. These serve as anchors for the taut lateral interosseous ligaments arising from the lateral tubercles on either side of the base of the distal phalanx (Fig. 33–94). These ligaments, thought by Shrewsbury and Johnson to be extensions of the osteocapsular portions of the more proximal oblique retinacular ligament, function to protect the neurovascular bundles as they pass dorsally from the pulp to the nail bed.[184] These ligaments also serve to prevent displacement of comminuted tuberosity fractures (Fig. 33–95).

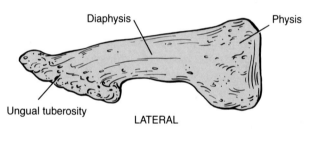

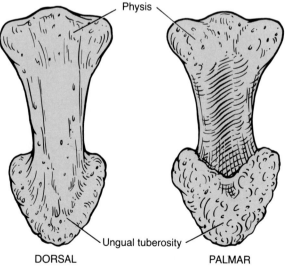

Figure 33–94

The structure of the distal phalanx is considerably different from that of the proximal and middle phalanges.

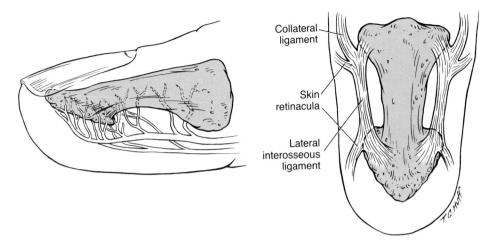

Collateral ligament

Skin retinacula

Lateral interosseous ligament

Figure 33–95

AP and lateral drawings of distal phalanx demonstrating lateral interosseous ligaments and neurovascular bundles. These ligaments function to protect the neurovascular bundles as they pass dorsally to the nail bed.

The diaphysis, or waist, of the distal phalanx is less well protected from contact stress than the ungual tuberosity, and the cortex is considerably thicker. Flat on the dorsal surface, the waist is concave palmarly to create the ungual fossa unique to hominids.

The base of the distal phalanx offers a prominent crest on the dorsal surface for the insertion of the terminal extensor tendon. The tendon firmly adheres to the dorsal joint capsule, extending from the dorsal aspect of one collateral ligament to that of the other. Its fibers blend into the capsule and periosteum and extend virtually to the root of the nail.[107] It is precisely because of these extensive attachments that there exist variations in the clinical presentations of the tendinous "mallet" finger. The lateral tubercles on either side of the base are situated near its palmar aspect, serving as the site of attachment for the collateral ligaments of the distal interphalangeal joint as well as for the lateral interosseous ligaments. The articular surface is divided into asymmetric concave radial and ulnar recesses separated by a convex intercondylar ridge.[71] This asymmetry corresponds to the asymmetric condyles of the head of the middle phalanx and accounts for the deviation seen particularly in the border digits.[71] On the palmar surface, the flexor digitorum profundus insertion extends distally out onto the midportion of the distal phalanx. The profundus therefore inserts into the entire width of the base of the distal phalanx, blending with the fibers of the palmar plate and periosteum.[107] The fibers of the tendon run in a spiral course, with the superficial fibers attaching to both the sides of the distal phalanx and the lateral tubercles, whereas the deep fibers pass more distally and centrally.[137,218]

The distal interphalangeal joint is especially noteworthy in its structural ability to allow passive hyperextension, something not found in any other Hominidae except in the gibbon's hand.[211] This is in part because of the fact that the palmar plate, unlike the proximal interphalangeal joint, has a flexible proximal attachment without any "check-reins" onto the middle phalanx.[71] This ability for passive hyperextension allows for pulp-to-pulp pinch, which is unique to man.

TYPES OF DISTAL PHALANX FRACTURES AND TREATMENT

The distal phalanx is by far the most commonly fractured bone in the hand, comprising as much as 50% of all hand fractures in some series.[34] This is not at all surprising when one considers how exposed the terminal parts of the digits are to local trauma. The vast majority of distal phalangeal fractures are the result of a crushing injury, frequently comminuting the bone and often associated with overlying soft tissue or nail bed trauma. The distal phalanx is well supported by fibrous septa and the overlying nail matrix and does not have any tendons spanning the bone as deforming forces.[34] Fractures of this bone will generally heal without undue complications, but the physician must avoid becoming too complacent when treating these injuries, as the potential complications can be disabling. These include pain, cold weather intolerance, altered sensibility, nail bed and nail deformity, malunion, and even nonunion.

Classification

Several useful classifications of distal phalangeal fractures exist. Kaplan has divided the fractures into three major categories (Fig. 33–96)[109]: (1) longitudinal split fractures; (2) comminuted fractures (most often associated with overlying soft tissue injury); and (3) transverse fractures, which may have angulatory deformity near the base.

Another and perhaps more useful classification, shown in Table 33–19, is that of Dobyns and coworkers, who subdivide the fractures anatomically as well as by soft tissue injury.[51]

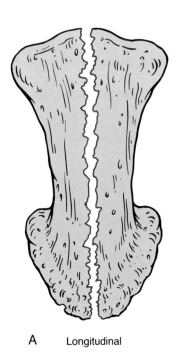

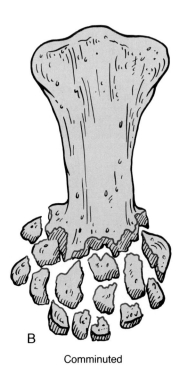

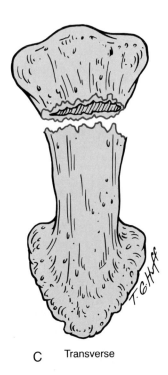

A   Longitudinal

B

Comminuted

C   Transverse

Figure 33–96

Kaplan's classification of distal phalanx fractures.

Treatment Considerations

Tuft Fractures

The closed tuft fracture can be exceptionally painful, as there is little room for the fracture hematoma within the compartmentalized pulp space. Release of the subungual hematoma with a heated paper clip or disposable cautery, followed by the application of ice and a protective splint, will provide comfort and support the fracture. A simple splint can be fashioned from the malleable aluminum rims on glass intravenous (IV) bottles, covered with adhesive tape, and bent around the distal phalanx to provide both support and protection. Generally most closed tuft fractures require no more than three weeks of splintage.[28]

Open tuft fractures are more likely to be unstable because of disruption of the supporting pulp and nail plate. Metacarpal block anesthesia is satisfactory to permit careful debridement, irrigation, and soft tissue repair. Most often repair of the soft tissue is sufficient to stabilize the tuft fracture, although occasionally a 0.028-in Kirschner wire will be needed to support a grossly displaced fracture. Oral antibiotics and tetanus prophylaxis are advisable. Despite the fact that the fracture has been exposed to the environment, these injuries are rarely complicated by sepsis when subject to an adequate irrigation and debridement, and hospital admission is not necessary.

It is important to bear in mind that splinting is solely for comfort. Care must be taken to avoid skin necrosis from splints that are too tightly applied. The fingertip will very likely be tender for a considerable number of months after the injury. Radiographic union may take

Table 33–19. Dobyns et al.'s Classification of Distal Phalanx Fractures		
	Closed	**Open**
Tuft	Inherently stable Union by six to eight weeks.	May be unstable with nail bed and pulp injury
Shaft	Nondisplaced fractures Union may take longer (8 to 12 weeks)	May be unstable Nail bed injury common Nonunion can occur
Base (physeal)	May be unstable; closed reduction often required Heals by six weeks	Eponychium injured May be angulated or malrotated; closed or open reduction often needed

Source: Compiled from Dobyns, J. H.; Beckenbaugh, R. D.; Bryan, R. S.; et al. In: Flynn, J. E., ed. Hand Surgery, Ed. 3. Baltimore, Williams & Wilkins, 1982, pp. 111–180.

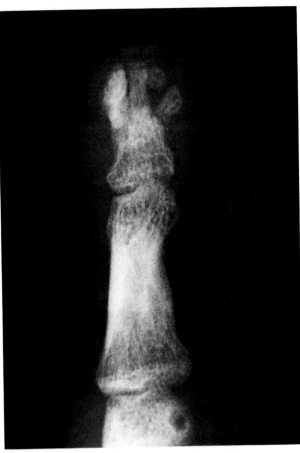

Figure 33–97

Following a crush injury, a comminuted tuft fracture will often demonstrate radiographically a delay in healing. Nonunion, however, is rare.

up to six months to a year,[51] and the surgeon should be wary of attributing discomfort to a delayed union or impending nonunion (Fig. 33–97). Extreme hypersensitivity is more likely the result of crushing of the multiple small terminal branches of the digital nerves. A trained hand therapist should be consulted to formulate a desensitization program for what can be a distressing problem.

Shaft Fractures

As with closed fractures of the tuft, the vast majority of closed distal phalangeal shaft fractures are minimally displaced, inherently stable, and require limited splintage. Although the longitudinal fractures generally heal within three to four weeks, transverse shaft fractures may take longer, and it is advisable to maintain support until clinical discomfort abates or radiographic union is evident.

Open shaft fractures can prove problematic and are often associated with disruption of the overlying nail bed. In concert with fracture irrigation and debridement, the nail itself should be uplifted and the nail bed inspected. On occasion, the sterile nail matrix may be displaced into the fracture line, providing a block to reduction as well as a potential cause for nonunion. The shaft fracture should be accurately aligned and, if unstable, supported by a longitudinal 0.035-in Kirschner wire (Fig. 33–98). The sterile matrix is repaired with 7-0 ophthalmic gut under loupe magnification. If the nail itself is in good condition, it can be cleansed with soap and povidone-iodine and replaced.

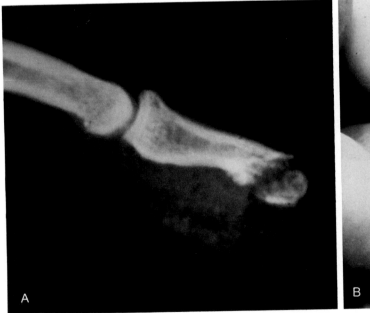

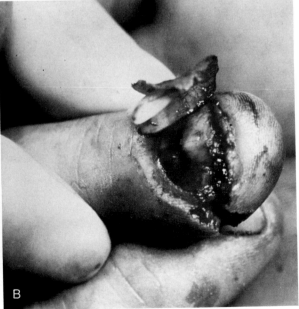

Figure 33–98

An open distal phalangeal shaft fracture (A) commonly will produce a laceration of the sterile nail matrix (B).

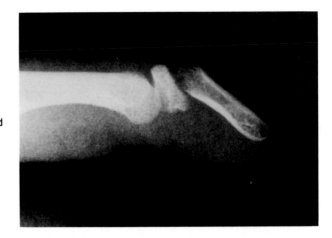

Figure 33-99

Fractures of the base of the distal phalanx tend to be unstable and will angulate with the apex pointing dorsally.

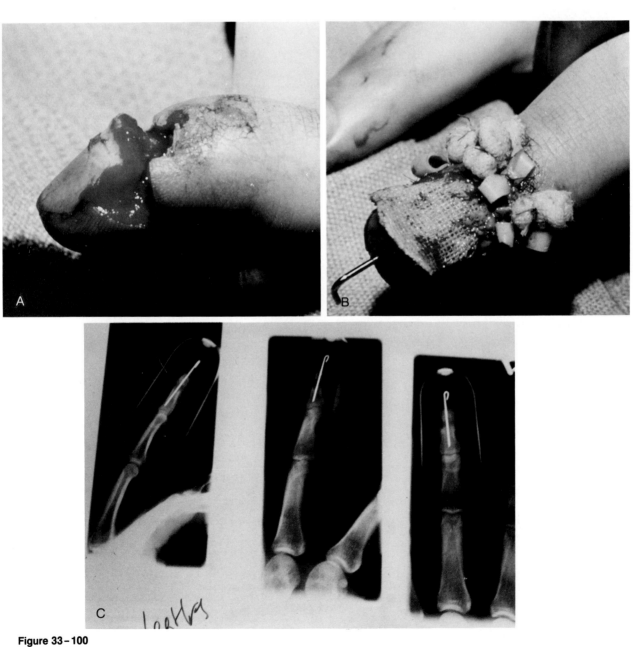

Figure 33-100

An incomplete amputation was treated with debridement, longitudinal Kirschner wire fixation of the distal phalanx, and nail bed repair.

This will serve to stabilize the fracture and soft tissue repairs as well as prevent scarring between the eponychium and nail matrix. A strip of petrolatum-impregnated gauze will also serve this purpose if the nail is not suitable. With either technique, the splint should be left in place for 10 to 14 days. Accurate axial alignment is of some importance to avoid late nail deformity.

Base (Physeal) Fractures

Regardless of the extent of overlying soft tissue involvement, fractures of the base of the distal phalanx tend to be unstable. Subject to the deforming pull of both the extensor and flexor tendons and not afforded the intrinsic support of the nail and nail plate, these fractures will tend to angulate with the apex pointing dorsally (Fig. 33–99).

In the adult, the closed fracture at the base of the distal phalanx is best treated by an alumafoam splint, keeping the distal fragment and distal interphalangeal joint in extension for a minimum of four weeks. Open fractures have the potential for rotational instability. These are commonly seen with severe soft tissue inju-

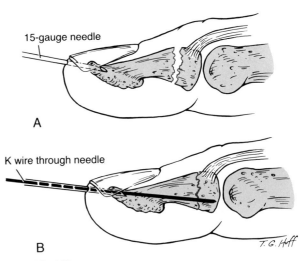

A

B

Figure 33–102

A 15-gauge hypodermic needle is an ideal drill guide for Kirschner wire placement into the tuft of the distal phalanx.

ries, such as incomplete amputations, and represent unstable fractures. A 0.035-in or a 0.045-in Kirschner wire placed in a retrograde manner will provide adequate internal splintage (Fig. 33–100). Crossing the distal interphalangeal joint should be avoided unless the proximal fragment is comminuted or fails to allow sufficient purchase of the wire.

When passing a Kirschner wire into the distal phalanx, several technical points are worth mentioning. Bear in mind that the tuft of the distal phalanx lies just beneath the sterile matrix. Introduce the wire just beneath the hyponychial fold when passing it in an antegrade fashion (Fig. 33–101). If the initial pass of the wire is unsatisfactory, do not withdraw the wire, as a second pass will quite possibly follow the same hole. Instead, with the initial wire in place, direct a second wire independently and then withdraw the initial wire. A 15-gauge hypodermic needle will serve as an effective guide for the Kirschner wire and will help prevent the tip of the wire from slipping off the rounded tip of the tuft (Fig. 33–102). Bending the exposed tip of the wire around and onto itself will create a blunt tip, thus avoiding catching the wire on an object and torquing the fracture site or soft tissue repair (Fig. 33–103).

In the pediatric age group, two distinct physeal injuries are found, depending on the age of the patient (Fig. 33–104). The preadolescent injury is most often an open fracture representing a Salter-Harris type I or II physeal separation.[174,182] These can be mistaken for distal interphalangeal joint dislocations or mallet injuries. The extensor tendon remains attached to the proximal epiphyseal fragment while the unopposed flexor digitorum profundus pulls the remainder of the

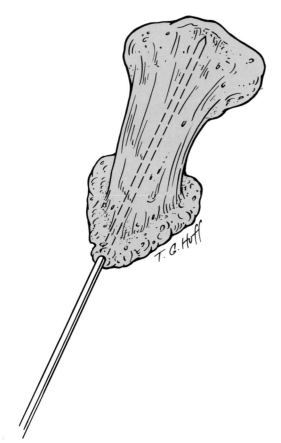

Figure 33–101

Kirschner wire fixation of the distal phalanx involves placement of the wire through the distal tuft just beneath the hyponychial fold.

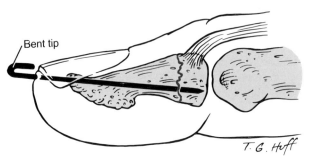

Figure 33–103

Bending of the protruding Kirschner wire in the distal phalanx will avoid catching the wire on objects and torquing the fracture.

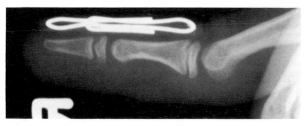

Figure 33–105

Following a closed reduction of an epiphyseal separation at the base of the distal phalanx, the digit was immobilized, incorporating a paper clip into the splint to augment the strength of the splint.

distal phalanx into the flexion. Not uncommonly, the base of the distal fragment protrudes through the wound, projecting over the eponychial fold while the nail and nail plate remain attached to the distal fragment. This injury should not be taken lightly, as the potential risks are substantial and include recurrent deformity, premature epiphyseal closure, sepsis, and residual nail deformity.[5,6,177,220]

Adequate anesthesia is mandatory, and general anesthesia is often required. The fracture site should be gently exposed and thoroughly irrigated. Reduction of the fracture can be accomplished with slight traction and manipulation of the distal fragment and nail into extension, placing the nail back under the eponychial fold. The nail itself will provide sufficient splintage for the fracture and is best preserved. Avoid, if possible, the use of Kirschner wires, as a higher incidence of infection has been reported with the use of Kirschner wires in these injuries.[165] Although as much as 30° of dorsal

or volar angulation can be accepted in the young child (as remodeling will occur), it is preferable to attempt to gain anatomic repositioning. The reduction can be effectively supported with an alumafoam splint incorporated into a plaster cast and maintained for four weeks.

In the older child, the physeal fracture more closely resembles a mallet injury. A closed reduction is done by gently extending the distal phalanx. Again, support with an alumafoam splint incorporated into a cast or with a cast alone may be needed for the active child and should be maintained for four weeks (Fig. 33–105; see Mallet Injuries).

Flexor Digitorum Profundus Avulsion Fractures

A relatively uncommon but potentially disabling injury is the avulsion fracture of the base of the distal phalanx caused by rupture of the insertion of the flexor digitorum profundus tendon. The mechanism gener-

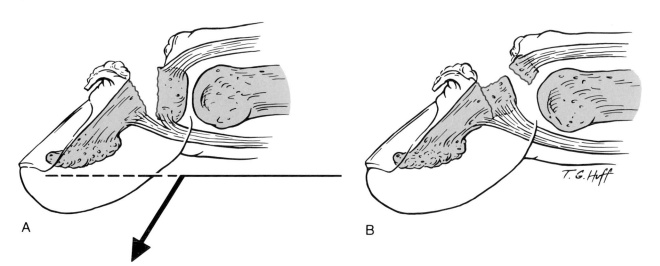

A   B

Figure 33–104

Two distinct physeal injuries of the pediatric distal phalanx include an open Salter-Harris type I or II physeal separation in the younger child *(A)* or a mallet type fracture in the older child *(B)*.

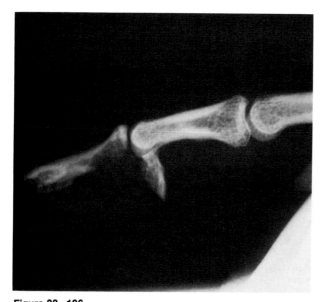

Figure 33–106

A flexor digitorum profundus avulsion fracture in a 19-year-old male.

ally will involve a hyperextension stress while the involved digit is actively flexed against an object. The ring finger is most often involved, with the classic example being that of a football player grabbing an opponent's jersey while attempting to make a tackle.[33,79,217]

The clinical presentation is that of a swollen, painful digit, particularly at the site of avulsion. Ecchymosis may be present. Because the patient can still actively flex at both metacarpophalangeal joints, the injury may be overlooked and considered only to be a "jammed" finger. Inability to initiate distal interphalangeal joint flexion should alert the examiner to the possibility of this lesion. Three radiographic views — anteroposterior, lateral, and oblique — must always be obtained, as the fracture fragment, when present, may be only a small flake of bone lying in the soft tissue plane just anterior to the proximal interphalangeal joint (Fig. 33–106).

Classification

Several authors have proposed classifications for flexor digitorum profundus avulsion injuries. Leddy and Packer[125,126] have established the following simple but clinically useful classification (Fig. 33–107):

Type I: The tendon has ruptured at its insertion without a bony fragment and has retracted into the palm. Both vincula supplying the tendon have ruptured, with considerable interruption to the vascular supply to the tendon.

Type II: The tendon has retracted to the level of the proximal interphalangeal joint and is held there by

the intact long vinculum. A flake of bone from the distal phalanx may be seen on radiograph.

Type III: A large bony fragment has been avulsed. Proximal retraction beyond the middle of the middle phalanx is ordinarily prevented by the fourth annular pulley.

Smith has suggested an additional type, type IV, in which a fragment of bone is fractured off the volar base of the distal phalanx with a simultaneous independent avulsion of the flexor profundus retracted to the base of the proximal phalanx.[189]

Robins and Dobyns have proposed the following classification based on the anatomic insertions of the profundus tendon[169]:

1. Profundus tendon avulsion without fracture.

2. Profundus tendon avulsion with a large fracture fragment. Either the superficial or the deep fibers of the tendon insertion, or both, may remain on the fragment or may be stripped off.

3. Profundus tendon avulsion with a small fracture fragment. The deep fibers strip off, but the superficial fibers usually remain attached and frequently displace the fragment more proximally.

4. Profundus avulsion with both large and small fragment fractures. The superficial fibers may remain with the small fragment, displacing it proximally. The large fragment, free of tendon attachments, remains distally held by the volar plate, collateral ligaments, or fourth annular pulley.

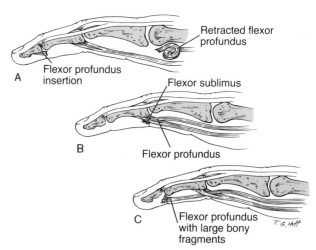

Figure 33–107

The classification system proposed by Leddy and Packer for flexor digitorum profundus (FDP) avulsion injuries. *A*, Type I: FDP rupture and retraction into the palm. *B*, Type II: The FDP ruptures and retracts to the level of the proximal interphalangeal joint. A flake of bone may be present. *C*, Type III: A large bony fragment is avulsed along with the FDP.

A different entity that could be confused with a profundus tendon avulsion fracture has been reported by Bowers and Fajgenbaum.[23] They described a case in which the volar plate of the distal interphalangeal joint was avulsed from its insertion onto the distal phalanx with a small fragment of bone. The mechanism of injury was a hyperextension force associated with dorsal subluxation of the distal phalanx. Open reduction of the joint and immobilization in 45° of flexion with a Kirschner wire for four weeks was recommended.

Treatment

The success of treatment often can be directly correlated with the accuracy of the diagnosis and the rapidity of surgical intervention. Additional factors that will influence the outcome include the level to which the tendon retracts, the remaining vascular supply to the avulsed tendon, and the presence and size of bony fragments on radiograph.[125,126]

With the Leddy and Packer type I injuries, the tendon must be retrieved and passed through an intact pulley system back to its point of insertion. This can only be considered if the diagnosis has been made within ten days after injury and before tendon swelling, collagen degeneration, and myostatic contracture occur. Reinsertion after this point could well lead to a significant flexion contracture of both the distal and proximal interphalangeal joints.

The tendon can be approached either through midaxial or volar zigzag incisions. A small flexible catheter or pediatric feeding tube is helpful in retrieving the tendon back under the intact pulley system and flexor sheath. A distally based osteoperiosteal flap is created in the base of the distal phalanx, and drill holes are made into the distal phalanx, exiting through the overlying nail. A no. 4 monofilament suture can be woven through the end of the tendon and through the drill holes with Keith needles and tied over a sponge and button.

Postoperative care is based, to some degree, on the individual surgeon's bias toward flexor tendon injuries. We have found the passive mobilization program advocated by Duran et al. to be effective in most cases.[54] The hand is maintained in a dorsal blocking splint, immobilizing the wrist in midflexion, the metacarpophalangeal joints in approximately 45° of flexion, and the proximal and distal interphalangeal joints in near extension. A program is designed to permit the patient to passively flex the proximal and distal interphalangeal joints at 2-hour intervals throughout the day, leaving the hand in the splint. This program must be closely monitored by a therapist as well as by the surgeon and probably is not applicable to an unreliable patient.

If the patient is seen more than ten days after injury,

the options include no treatment, a free graft or stage tendon reconstruction, or a terminal interphalangeal joint tenodesis or arthrodesis.

In contrast, when the tendon has retracted only to the level of the proximal interphalangeal joint (Leddy and Packer type II), it may be possible to reinsert these avulsions as late as six weeks following injury. The tendon is retrieved and passed under the fourth annular pulley and reinserted into the base of the distal phalanx in a manner similar to that described for type I injuries. The small flake fracture often associated with these injuries may be excised prior to inserting the tendon back into the distal phalanx. Postoperative treatment is similar to that for type I injuries.

In approaching Leddy and Packer type II avulsion fractures, one must bear in mind the variable fracture patterns as described by Robins and Dobyns.[169] Particular attention should be paid to the preoperative radiograph of the entire digit in order to recognize the occasional double fracture with the profundus tendon retracted proximally with a small flake of bone. Many of the injuries involving large bony fragments will have associated dorsal subluxation of the distal phalanx. It is not uncommon to find that the avulsed fragment involves a significant portion of the articular surface of the base of the distal phalanx. In general, the prognosis for functional recovery is poorer for those patients in whom the tendon insertion has separated from the bony fragment or in whom the base of the distal phalanx is comminuted.[54]

Considerable care is taken to maintain any soft tissue attachments to the fracture fragments, particularly if the profundus insertion is partially separated. The large fragments are prevented from migrating proximally by the fourth annular pulley, and attention should be paid to preserving the integrity of the pulley. Anatomic reduction of the articular surface is mandatory unless the joint surface has been fragmented. In these cases, more often seen in open injuries, consideration can be given to an immediate arthrodesis of the distal joint.

Internal fixation with two parallel 0.028-in Kirschner wires or a single 1.5-mm cortical screw is sufficient (Fig. 33–108). The wires can be removed in three to four weeks postoperatively. If the tendon has been avulsed, a 4-0 monofilament suture is woven through the tendon end and passed dorsally on either side of the distal phalanx through the overlying nail and sutured over a sponge and button. Sutures should also be placed between the tendon and any available periosteum or fibrous tissue from its original insertion site. Postoperative treatment is dependent on the extent of tendon disruption from the avulsed fragment. In those cases in which the tendon has completely separated from the bony fragment, the digit should be immobilized for

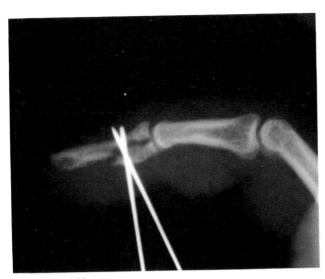

Figure 33-108

A type III profundus avulsion fracture has been reapproximated and secured with Kirschner wire fixation.

three weeks. Following this, motion can be started under the supervision of a therapist. Sutures can be removed two weeks later.

Mallet Injuries

The deformity that has come to be known as the "mallet finger" was first recognized in the literature in 1880 by Segond.[180] There remains, however, considerable disagreement regarding this injury, not the least of which concerns its descriptive terminology. Only rarely, in fact, does the digit resemble a mallet. The term "baseball finger" [106] is equally misleading, as this sport accounts for only a small percentage of mallet injuries.

The literature is replete with methods and devices for the treatment of the mallet injury. The role of surgical intervention is controversial in regard to the indications for surgery and the technique. Even what constitutes a "good" result and what should be the patient's expectations regarding any residual disability remain in question and are subject to continuous reevaluation. However, it is fundamental to establish the type of injury to the terminal extensor mechanism prior to considering treatment, as the underlying pathologic manifestations can be varied.

TENDINOUS MALLET

The tendinous mallet represents a loss of continuity of the extensor mechanism at the distal interphalangeal joint. This common injury results from forced flexion against an actively extended digit. This occurs not only in sports but also from such minor incidents as putting on socks, washing laundry, or bed making. Less common causes include lacerations on the dorsum of the middle and distal phalanx and a crushing injury over the distal joint that results in a zone of avascular necrosis in the tendon. The latter may manifest itself weeks following the initial trauma.[1]

Watson-Jones[214] further defined the extensor tendon injury as including the following three distinct patterns (Fig. 33-109):

1. Incomplete tendon injury caused by stretching of the tendinous fibers. The clinical presentation will be a less pronounced droop (15° to 30°) with some ability to actively extend. Extension against resistance, however, will be appreciably weaker than the adjacent digit and usually painful.

2. Complete disruption of the extensor mechanism at its insertion onto the distal phalanx, often with rupture of the dorsal joint capsule. The distal joint will have a more pronounced droop (30° to 60°) and is completely unable to extend actively against gravity. The fact that the distal joint is not pulled into more flexion with complete disruption of the extensor mechanism and dorsal capsule has been attributed by Stack to the presence of the oblique retinacular ligament.[122,193] This, however, has been questioned by Shrewsbury and Johnson, who were unable to consistently define the presence of an oblique retinacular ligament in anatomic dissections.[185,186] They felt that the collateral ligaments were more likely to be the supporting elements offsetting to some degree the pull of the flexor digitorum profundus.

3. Disruption of the extensor mechanism at its insertion onto the dorsum of the distal phalanx. A small "flake" of bone is avulsed along with the tendon and is visible on the lateral radiograph. This is not considered a mallet fracture and will be effectively treated as a tendinous injury.

Clinical Presentation

The closed tendinous mallet finger is more commonly seen in the middle-aged patient, frequently after innocent trauma. In a series of 92 cases, Abouna and Brown noted that 73% of these injuries occurred in the home, 20% at work, and 7% from a sports injury.[1] When seen soon after trauma, the patient's complaints are those of pain and inability to fully extend the terminal joint. Swelling is usually present and may in fact mask the flexed posturing of that joint. In some "loose-jointed" individuals, hyperextension will be noted at the proximal interphalangeal joint because of imbalance of the extensor mechanism, leading to increased pull of the extensor on the base of the middle phalanx.

MECHANISM

Forced flexion

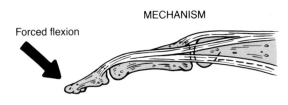

INJURY

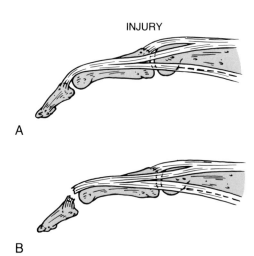

A

B

Figure 33–109

Tendinous mallet injuries have been defined by Watson-Jones[214] to include three distinct patterns: stretching of the common extensor at its insertion (A), complete disruption of the extensor mechanism (B), and complete disruption of the extensor mechanism with a small "flake" of bone avulsed from the distal phalanx (C).

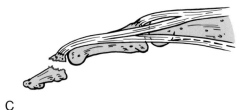

C

Treatment

It is now generally agreed by most authors that only the distal interphalangeal joint requires immobilization.[1,4,27,59,75,92,144,146,195] The treatment for the three types of tendinous mallet injuries differs only in a shorter duration of immobilization for type I incomplete ruptures.

A small malleable alumafoam splint contoured to provide three points of contact is recommended in the acute setting. Some authors choose to place the splint on the palmar surface, using tape over the terminal joint to maintain its position. A word of caution regarding positioning the distal joint in excessive hyperextension: the circulation of the skin over the joint can be precarious, and it is wise to make certain the skin is not blanched on application of the splint to minimize the risk of necrosis.[163] For type I injuries, continuous splinting for a minimum of four weeks and preferably six weeks is suggested. Six to eight weeks of continuous splinting, followed by nocturnal splinting for three to four weeks, is best for types II and III tendinous mallet fingers.

Successful treatment of tendinous mallet injuries can be obtained even when initially seen two to three months after injury.[1,4,83,146,167] In these situations, splintage is required for at least 8 to 12 weeks.

In unusual circumstances, the patient's occupation may be such that splinting is not practical. In these cases, one may consider passing a Kirschner wire across the distal interphalangeal joint with the wire cut off just below the skin.[36] The risks of pin track infection, joint sepsis, and osteomyelitis must be considered when making this decision.

BONY MALLET

Mallet deformity resulting from a bony injury occurs in association with a fracture of the dorsal articular surface of the distal phalanx (usually one third or greater). The terminal unit of the extensor tendon inserting onto this fracture fragment can no longer function to extend the distal phalanx (Fig. 33–110).

Although splint support of a tendinous mallet is generally agreed on, the treatment of a bony mallet remains subject to some debate. To better understand why this is so, it may be best to recognize that different anatomic considerations exist with bony mallet injuries. By individualizing each mallet fracture, the treatment approach can be simplified.

First, the mallet fracture may result from several different mechanisms of injury. Some occur in a manner similar to the tendinous mallet (i.e., forcible flexion of

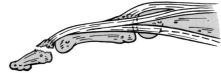

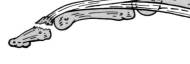

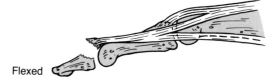

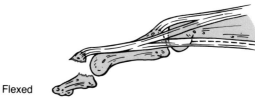

BONY MALLET

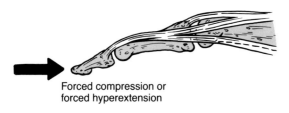

Forced compression or
forced hyperextension

Flexed

Flexed

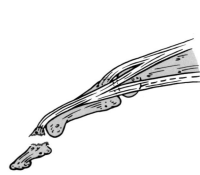

Figure 33–110

A bony mallet fracture may present in a variety of fracture patterns.

an extended digit avulsing a bony fragment of variable size along with its attached extensor mechanism). Others are quite different, resulting instead from direct trauma to the tip of the extended digit driving the base of the distal phalanx onto the head of the middle phalanx.[92,142] This injury may not present with much droop of the terminal phalanx.[5] Rather, this compression type of mallet fracture will have not only displacement of part of the base of the distal phalanx but also impaction of the subchondral bone. These fractures tend to be seen more often in younger individuals and are usually incurred while participating in sports.[92]

A third variant is that caused by a sudden hyperextension force that results in the dorsal aspect of the base of the distal phalanx being impacted against the head of the middle phalanx, resulting in a dorsal lip fracture and volar subluxation of the distal phalanx. These fractures will often involve more than 50% of the articular

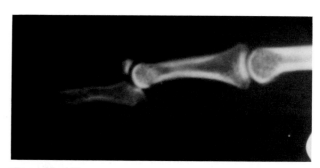

Figure 33–111

A bony mallet in the little finger of a 36-year-old female associated with subluxation of the distal phalanx. Operative treatment is indicated.

Table 33-20.

Wehbe and Schneider Classification of Mallet Fracture

Type 1:   Bony injury of varying extent without subluxation of the joint
Type 2:   Fractures associated with joint subluxation
Type 3:   Epiphyseal and physeal injuries
Each type is further subdivided into three types:
    A. Fracture fragment less than one third of articular surface of the distal phalanx
    B. Fracture from one third to two thirds of the articular surface
    C. Fracture more than two thirds of articular surface

Source: Wehbe, M. A.; Schneider, L. H. J Bone Joint Surg 66A:658–669, 1984.

surface. This injury pattern is particularly difficult to treat, as the routine immobilization position of hyperextension will accentuate the subluxation. Open reduction should be considered (Fig. 33–111).[87]

The classification proposed by Wehbe and Schneider identifies the variation in the bony mallet injuries, although it does not identify the impacted compression type of injury (Table 33–20).[216] These authors additionally were able to show excellent results with nonoperative treatment of all types of mallet fractures. Bone remodeling occurred in each case, and the articular surface remained preserved. A near-normal, painless range of motion was achieved in 21 of their 22 patients. They splinted all fractures for six to eight weeks continuously. The only drawback noted by the authors was a residual bump present on the dorsum of the joint.

Although many mallet fractures can be treated nonoperatively, certain fracture types are perhaps more

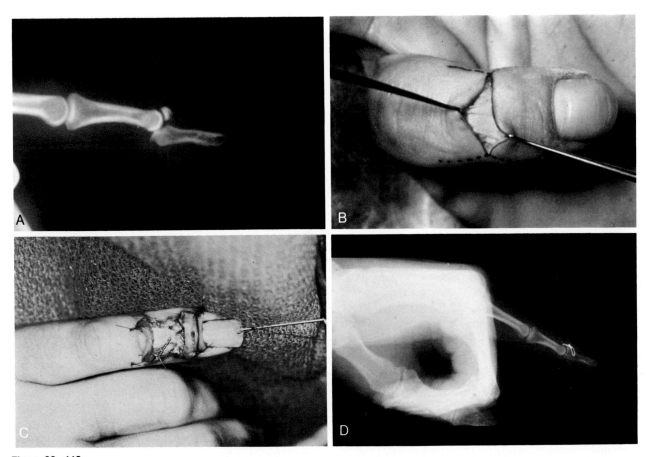

Figure 33–112

A 25-year-old graduate student sustained a closed displaced mallet fracture associated with displacement of the articular surface despite splint treatment. *A*, The lateral radiograph demonstrates the displaced articular fragment. *B*, Through a dorsal H incision, the extensor tendon and attached fragment are readily visible. *C*, Following debridement of the fracture hematoma, the articular fragment is reduced under direct vision. A drill hole is placed in the distal phalanx distal to the fracture and dorsal to the midaxis of the phalanx. A 30-gauge stainless steel wire is passed through the drill hole. The stainless steel wire is placed through the insertion of the extensor tendon into the bony fragment and tightened in a figure-of-8 fashion. *D*, Excellent fixation is achieved without the risk of fragmentation of the small bony fragment.

predictably treated operatively. These include widely displaced fractures involving 50% or more of the articular surface, those fractures associated with volar subluxation of the distal phalanx, and impaction injuries at the base of the distal phalanx. In addition, displaced mallet fractures of the thumb interphalangeal joint are likely better treated by operative means, given the potential for displacement by powerful extrinsic tendons.

A study by Stark et al. has shown excellent results using operative treatment.[196] These authors gained anatomic reduction and used small Kirschner wires. The technique of tension band wiring has been equally effective in the operative management of these precarious bony fragments.[103] Through a dorsal H incision the fragment is easily identified and reduced after debriding the fracture hematoma. A drill hole is made distal to the fracture line and dorsal to the midaxis of the phalanx, and a 30-gauge monofilament stainless steel wire is passed through the hole and through the insertion of the extensor tendon onto the fracture fragment. When the fragment has been reduced, the wire is tightened slowly, holding the fragment in place to control the possibility of dorsal rotation. Fractures associated with subluxation of the distal phalanx should have a longitudinal Kirschner wire placed across the distal joint for two to three weeks (Fig. 33–112).

The surgical approach to these fractures is difficult and fraught with complications. The soft tissue cover is tenuous, the fragment is small and easily fragmented, and joint stiffness is not uncommon. Before making the decision to approach this fracture operatively, one should carefully assess whether splint treatment is applicable.

Dislocations

Dislocations and ligamentous injuries in the hand are common.[11,53,55,150] Although the proximal interphalangeal joint is most often affected, all of the digital articulations as well as those of the thumb are vulnerable. The spectrum of injury to the ligaments extends from a minor stretch (sprain) to a complete disruption.

The deformity caused by a joint dislocation is classified by the position of the distal skeletal unit in relationship to its proximal counterpart. Thus a palmar proximal interphalangeal joint dislocation describes a dislocation in which the middle phalanx is displaced in a palmar direction relative to the proximal phalanx (Fig. 33–113).

Most digital dislocations are the result of an axial load combined with an angular vector of force. The magnitude and direction of the force combined with

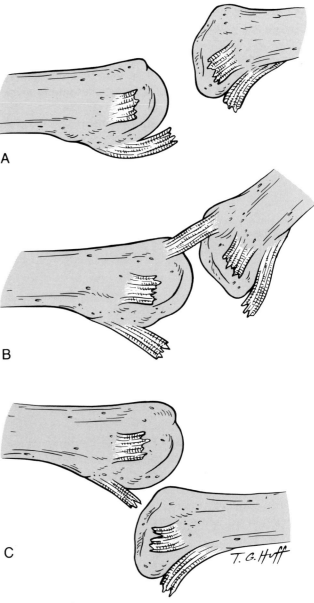

Figure 33–113

Dislocations in the hand are classified by the position of the distal skeletal unit in relationship to its proximal counterpart. *A,* A dorsal proximal interphalangeal (PIP) joint dislocation. *B,* A lateral PIP joint dislocation. *C,* A palmar PIP joint dislocation.

the position of the joint at the time of injury will determine the type and extent of the dislocation.

CLINICAL EVALUATION

A dislocation of a small articulation in the hand is ordinarily clinically apparent. Prior to physical examination, a true lateral radiograph must be viewed to determine if a fracture is present. The sensibility and circulation of the digit are confirmed, followed by a cautious examination of the involved joint. Any laceration must be inspected carefully, as a skin "tear" may reflect an open dislocation requiring treatment in the sterile environment of the operating room. If closed reduction or stress testing of the joint is required, metacarpal block or wrist block anesthesia should be given.

Following reduction, joint stability is determined. Eaton has suggested that stability be judged both actively and passively.[55] Redisplacement with active motion suggests significant ligamentous disruption. The examiner should gently stress each collateral ligament passively with a laterally directed force and should test the palmar plate with a dorsal-to-volar–directed force. Angulation or increased mobility, especially when compared with the same joint on the contralateral hand, reflects disruption of the involved structure(s).

PROXIMAL INTERPHALANGEAL JOINT

Often associated with a jamming injury, ligament injuries and dislocations of the proximal interphalangeal joints are common. Three types of pure dislocations are observed: dorsal, palmar, and lateral (see Fig. 33–113). Closed reduction is the treatment of choice. Following wrist block anesthesia, longitudinal traction and manipulation will reduce most proximal interphalangeal joint dislocations. A dislocation that presents with the distal component rotated suggests the possibility of an entrapped flexor tendon around the head of the proximal phalanx.

Once the dislocation is clinically reduced, radiographs are mandatory to confirm the position of the joint. Active and passive joint testing will help determine the presence and degree of any residual instability. If instability is observed, especially with active motion, interposition of the soft tissue should be suspected. Open reduction may be required in these instances.

Dorsal dislocation represents a complete tear of the palmar plate from its insertion on the base of the middle phalanx. Collateral ligament disruption is not uncommon. Following closed reduction, we prefer to immobilize the joint with a dorsally placed alumafoam splint in 10° to 15° of flexion. Once comfortable, the patient can start active flexion while in the splint (Fig. 33–114). In most cases, the splint can be discontinued after two weeks and replaced with Velcro buddy straps that hold the involved digit to adjacent digits for an additional two weeks. Buddy strapping is also advisable during athletic activities for at least six more weeks.

Lateral dislocations represent rupture of one collateral ligament as well as the palmar plate. The digit may present with both angular and rotational deformity, as the middle phalanx may pivot on the intact collateral ligament. Following closed reduction, active and passive testing will determine the intrinsic stability of the joint. We ordinarily splint these injuries for two to three weeks before allowing motion. Buddy straps are advisable for three to four weeks following removal of the splint.

If reduction cannot be achieved or the postreduction radiograph shows an asymmetric widening of the proximal interphalangeal joint space, a soft tissue interposition should be suspected. In these cases the condyle of the head of the proximal phalanx has "buttonholed" through a rent between the lateral band and central slip of the extensor tendon on the side of the disrupted

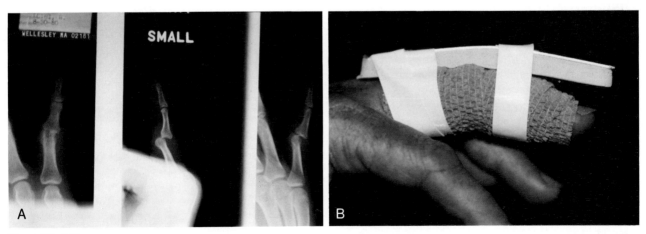

Figure 33–114

A dorsal dislocation of the proximal interphalangeal joint in an 18-year-old male. *A*, Lateral radiographs demonstrate the dorsal displacement of the middle phalanx on the proximal phalanx. *B*, Following metacarpal block and closed manipulative reduction, the digit is wrapped with an elastic crepe bandage, and a dorsal extension block alumafoam splint is applied.

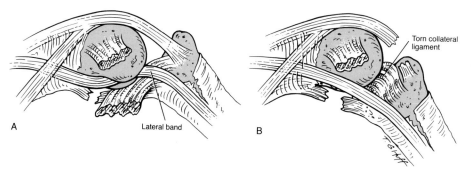

Figure 33–115

Palmar proximal interphalangeal joint dislocations injure the palmar plate, collateral ligaments, and central slip. *A*, Irreducible palmar dislocation caused by interposition of a lateral band in the joint. *B*, Irreducible palmar dislocation can be caused by interposition of the torn collateral ligament.

collateral ligament. Operative intervention is required.[53]

A volar proximal interphalangeal joint dislocation is rare and must be treated in a different manner.[153,192,207] In this case, the central slip of the extensor mechanism is injured along with the collateral ligaments and palmar plate. If reduction cannot be achieved or maintained, a boutonniere deformity will result, leading to significant joint dysfunction. Reduction should be performed with the metacarpophalangeal joint held in flexion along with traction and manipulation of the middle phalanx. If reduction is successful, the patient's ability to actively extend the joint is tested. If the patient is able to extend to within 30° of full extension, a dorsal splint is applied, keeping the proximal interphalangeal joint in full extension but allowing the distal interphalangeal joint to be mobile. If active extension is not possible, complete disruption of the central slip is probable, and surgical intervention is recommended (Fig. 33–115).[53,207]

DISTAL INTERPHALANGEAL JOINT

Dislocations of the distal interphalangeal joints are uncommon. When they do occur, they are more likely to be dorsal than palmar. Although these injuries often involve disruption of both collateral ligaments and the palmar plate, closed reduction can usually be achieved with metacarpal block anesthesia. Splint support for 7 to 14 days with the distal interphalangeal joint in slight flexion may be all that is needed, as these injuries tend to be stable after reduction.

Open injuries require thorough lavage, as the joint has been contaminated. Loose soft tissue closure and splinting for two weeks should allow for adequate soft tissue healing.

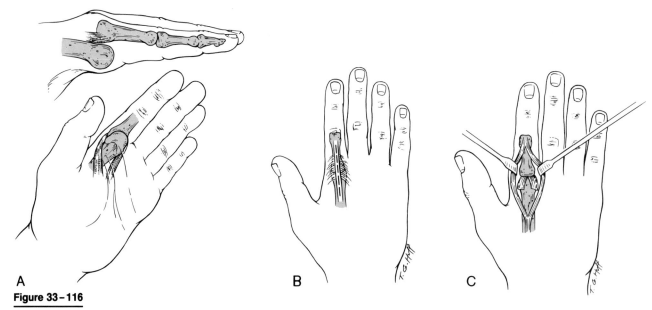

Figure 33–116

A dorsal dislocation of the metacarpophalangeal joint is considered "complex," as a closed reduction is rarely successful because of interposition of the palmar plate. *A*, The palmar plate displaces dorsal to the metacarpal head. In addition, the metacarpal head "buttonholes" between the flexor tendons and lumbrical muscle. *B*, Surgical reduction of the complex dislocation is readily accomplished through a dorsal approach splitting the common extensor. *C*, The palmar plate is splint longitudinally, followed by atraumatic reduction of the metacarpal.

Palmar distal interphalangeal joint dislocations are more difficult to manage, as the injury may involve disruption of the insertion of the terminal extensor tendon as well as of the collateral ligaments and the palmar plate. Postreduction splintage with the joint in extension will be required for a minimum of eight weeks to allow for healing of the extensor tendon.

METACARPOPHALANGEAL JOINT

Dorsal dislocations of the metacarpophalangeal joint are uncommon but can be difficult to manage if the reduction is blocked by soft tissue interposition (complex dislocation).[53,55,108,134,150] The clinical picture of a dislocated metacarpophalangeal joint with a dimple in the palmar skin over the metacarpal head should arouse suspicion of a complex dislocation. The index and little fingers are more commonly involved, as volar intermetacarpal ligament support is found on only one side of these digits.

Much has been written regarding the pathologic anatomy of the complex metacarpophalangeal dislocation. Kaplan and others have suggested that the metacarpal head has "buttonholed" between the flexor tendons and lumbrical muscle; they recommend a volar surgical approach.[108,134,150] However, it is the palmar plate, still attached to the dorsally displaced proximal phalanx, that becomes wedged between the joint surfaces and prevents closed manipulative reduction. It is for this reason that a dorsal surgical approach proves straightforward and safer, as there is little chance of injury to the digital nerves, which are displaced by the metacarpal head and lie just beneath the palmar skin. The palmar plate is split longitudinally, and the metacarpal head can be atraumatically reduced, as the two segments of the palmar plate fall to either side (Fig. 33–116). Postoperatively, the joint is immobilized in 60° to 75° of flexion for several days, followed by active mobilization in a splint applied dorsally to act as a block to prevent hyperextension. The splint is kept in place for three to four weeks.

THUMB

Carpometacarpal Joint

Complete dislocation of the carpometacarpal joint of the thumb without associated fracture is very uncommon.[183] It has been thought to be associated with complete disruption of the volar oblique ligament passing from the trapezium to the volar beak of the thumb metacarpal.[53,55] However, Burkhalter, following surgical exploration of several carpometacarpal dislocations, did not find complete rupture of this ligament; instead he found that the metacarpal rotated in supina-

tion out of the capsule of the joint.[31] He suggested that reduction should include maximal pronation of the thumb metacarpal. If this can be accomplished by closed means, the reduction is best maintained by percutaneous Kirschner wires passing from the metacarpal into the trapezium, along with a thumb spica cast for six weeks. The reduction must be confirmed radiographically by a true lateral and AP radiograph (see discussion of Bennett's fracture) (Fig. 33–117).

Metacarpophalangeal Joint

Acute ligament injuries to the metacarpophalangeal joint of the thumb are common and are notoriously associated with ski pole injuries.[70] Stability of this joint is related not only to the collateral ligaments, capsule, and palmar plate but also to the actions of the thenar muscles.[41,43] It is in part because of the thenar muscles' dynamic stabilizing influence that accurate examination of the injured thumb metacarpophalangeal joint may require anesthetic block of these muscles.

The ulnar collateral ligament is far more commonly injured than its radial counterpart. Avulsion fractures may be present in a number of different patterns (see Fig. 33–67). The cause of this injury is a sudden valgus stress, often in conjunction with hyperextension of the joint.

Joint stability is tested in full extension as well as in 30° of flexion.[24,41,53,55,63,118,150] The radial and median nerves should be anesthetized at the wrist to provide both analgesia and thenar muscle relaxation. A complete ligament disruption is suspected if the joint can be stressed in a radial direction 25° to 35° beyond a similar stress to the other thumb metacarpophalangeal joint. This should be demonstrated in both full extension and 30° of flexion. More often than not, the presence of ecchymosis will suggest a complete ligament tear as well as volar subluxation of the proximal phalanx seen on a true lateral radiograph. Arthrography and stress testing with radiographic control can be misleading, and we do not recommend these studies for acute injuries.[24]

In 1962 Stener observed at surgery that the completely torn ulnar collateral ligament is often found to be displaced proximally with adductor muscle aponeurosis interposed between the ligament and its point of insertion (Fig. 33–118).[197] These findings have been confirmed by others and indicate surgical exploration if a complete ligament disruption is suspected. Incomplete tears are treated with a thumb spica cast for four to six weeks, followed by a removable, hand-based orthoplast splint protecting against a valgus stress on the healing ligament.

The operative approach is accomplished through a dorsoulnar incision.[53,197] Care is taken to identify and

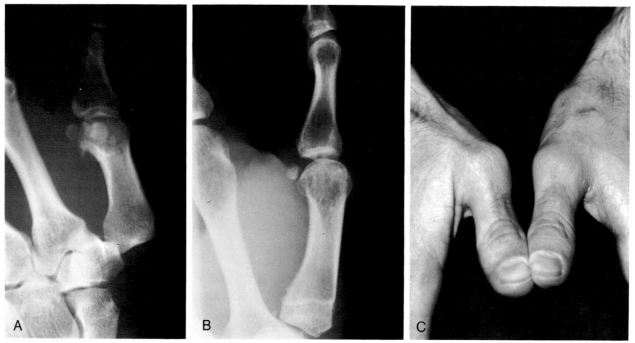

Figure 33–117

A 20-year-old gymnast presented with pain and limitation of motion in his right thumb four weeks following a fall from the parallel bars. *A*, The radiograph reveals complete dislocation of the carpometacarpal joint of the thumb. *B*, An open reduction and stabilization are performed using a strip of the flexor carpi radialis tendon. *C*, Excellent long-term stability was noted.

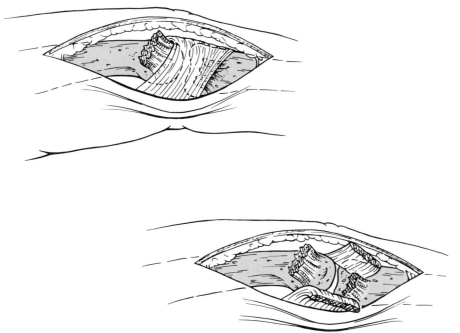

Figure 33–118

The Stener lesion represents a complex disruption of the thumb metacarpophalangeal joint ulnar collateral ligament. The ligament is displaced and rests proximal and superficial to the insertion of the adductor tendon.

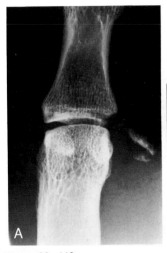
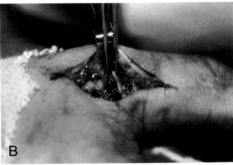
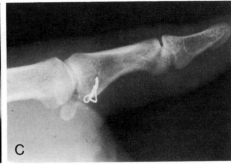

Figure 33–119

A 34-year-old male presented with a skiing injury to the metacarpophalangeal joint of his thumb. *A*, AP radiograph shows displacement of the bony attachment of the ulnar collateral ligament. *B*, At surgery, the comminuted fragments were found attached to the collateral ligament and displaced proximally to the adductor tendon. *C*, The ligament and its bony fragments were reapproximated and secured with tension wire applied in a figure-of-8 pattern.

protect dorsal radial sensory nerve branches. The adductor aponeurosis is opened and the joint capsule observed. Frequently a dorsal tear of the capsule will be observed. The ligament should be repaired not only to the base of the proximal phalanx at its normal insertion but also to the palmar plate.[53] Capsular closure will add to the stability of the repair and is followed by reapproximation of the adductor aponeurosis. The thumb should be immobilized in a thumb spica cast for four weeks, followed by protected mobilization allowing only flexion and extension exercises while maintained in a removable thumb splint.

Avulsion fractures can be determined on the initial radiographs and can be treated as described for intraarticular base fractures of the proximal phalanges (Fig. 33–119).[85,103]

REFERENCES

1. Abouna, J.M.; Brown, H. The treatment of mallet finger. The results in a series of 148 consecutive cases and a review of the literature. Br J Surg 55:653–667, 1968.
2. Agee, J.M. Unstable fracture-dislocations of the proximal interphalangeal joint of the fingers. Clin Orthop 214:101–112, 1987.
3. Asche, G. Possibility of the para-articular finger fractures with external minifixation. Handchir Mikrochir Plast Chir 16:195–195, 1984.
4. Auchincloss, J.M. Mallet finger injuries: A prospective controlled trial of internal and external splintage. Hand 14:168–173, 1982.
5. Barton, N.J. Intraarticular fractures and fracture-dislocations. In: Bowers, W, ed. The Interphalangeal Joints. New York, Churchill Livingstone, 1987, pp. 77–93.
6. Barton, N.J. Fractures of the phalanges of the hand in children. Hand 11:134–143, 1979.
7. Barton, N.J. Fractures and joint injuries of the hand. In: Wilson, J.W., ed. Watson-Jones Fractures and Joint Injuries, Ed. 6. Edinburgh, Churchill Livingstone, 1983, pp. 739–788.
8. Barton, N.J. Fractures of the hand. J Bone Joint Surg 66B:159–167, 1984.
9. Barton, N.J. Fractures of the shafts of the phalanges of the hand. Hand 11:110–133, 1979.
10. Belsky, M.R.; Eaton, R.G.; Lane, L.B. Closed reduction and internal fixation of proximal phalangeal fractures. J Hand Surg 9A:725–729, 1984.
11. Belsky, M.R.; Ruby, L.K.; Millender, L.H. Injuries of the finger and thumb joints. Contemp Orthop 7:39–48, 1983.
12. Belsky, M.R.; Eaton, R.G. Closed percutaneous wiring of metacarpal and phalangeal fractures. In: Tubiana, R., ed. The Hand, Vol. 2. Philadelphia, W.B. Saunders, 1985, p. 790.
13. Belsole, R.J.; Greene, T.L. Comparative strengths of internal fixation techniques. J Hand Surg 10A:315–316, 1985.
14. Belsole, R. Physiologic fixation of displaced and unstable fractures of the hand. Orthop Clin North Am 11:393–404, 1980.
15. Bennett, E.H. Fractures of the metacarpal bones. Dublin J Med Sci 73:72, 1882.
16. Billing, L.; Gedda, K.Q. Roentgen examination of Bennett's fracture. Acta Radiol 38:471–476, 1952.
17. Bilos, Z.J.; Eskestrand, T. External fixator use in comminuted gunshot fractures of the proximal phalanx. J Hand Surg 4:357–359, 1979.
18. Black, D.M.; Mann, R.J.; Constine, R.; et al. The stability of internal fixation in the proximal phalanx. J Hand Surg 11A:672–677, 1986.
19. Bloem, J.J. The treatment and prognosis of uncomplicated dislocated fractures of the metacarpals and phalanges. Arch Chir Neerl 23:55–65, 1971.
20. Boehler, L. Die Technik der Knockenbruchbehandlung. Wien, Aufl. Maudrich, 1951.
21. Bora, F.W. Jr.; Didizan, N.H. The treatment of injuries to the

carpometacarpal joint of the little finger. J Bone Joint Surg 56A:1459–1463, 1974.

22. Borgeskov, S. Conservative therapy for fractures of the phalanges and metacarpals. Acta Chir Scand 133:123–130, 1967.

23. Bowers, W.H.; Fajgenbaum, D.M. Closed rupture of the volar plate of the distal interphalangeal joint. J Bone Joint Surg 61A:146, 1979.

24. Bowers, W.H.; Hurst, L.C. Gamekeeper's thumb. Evaluation by arthroscopy and stress roentgenography. J Bone Joint Surg 59A:519–524, 1977.

25. Bowers, W.H. The anatomy of the interphalangeal joints. In: Bowers, W.H., ed. The Interphalangeal Joint. New York, Churchill Livingstone, 1987, pp. 2–13.

26. Breen, T.F.; Gelberman, R.H.; Jupiter, J.B. Intraarticular fractures of the basilar joint of the thumb. Hand Clin 4:491–501, 1988.

27. Brooks, D. Splint for mallet fingers. Br Med J 2:1238, 1964.

28. Brown, P. The management of phalangeal and metacarpal fractures. Surg Clin North Am 53:1393–1437, 1973.

29. Buechler, U. Personal communication, 1989.

30. Buechler, U.; Fischer, T. Use of a minicondylar plate for metacarpal and phalangeal periarticular injuries. Clin Orthop 214:53–58, 1987.

31. Burkhalter, W. Newsletter #18, American Society for Surgery of the Hand, 1981.

32. Burkhalter, W.; Reyes, P. Closed treatment of fractures in the hand. Bull Hosp Joint Dis 44:145–151, 1984.

33. Burton, R.I.; Eaton, R.G. Common hand injuries in the athlete. Orthop Clin North Am 4:809–838, 1973.

34. Butt, W.D. Fractures of the hand, II. Statistical review. Can Med Assoc J 86:775–779, 1962.

35. Cannon, S.; Dowd, G.; Williams, D.; et al. A long-term study following Bennett's fracture. J Hand Surg 11B:426–431, 1986.

36. Casscells, S.W.; Strange, T.B. Intramedullary wire fixation of mallet finger (follow-up note). J Bone Joint Surg 51A:1018–1019, 1969.

37. Chait, C.A.; Cort, A.; Brown, S. Metacarpal reconstruction in compound contaminated injuries of the hand. Hand 13:152–157, 1981.

38. Charnley, J. The Closed Treatment of Common Fractures, Ed. 3. Edinburgh, Churchill Livingtone, 1974, p. 150.

39. Clendenin, M.B.; Smith, R.J. Fifth metacarpal hamate arthrodesis for posttraumatic osteoarthritis. J Hand Surg 9A:374–378, 1984.

40. Clinkscales, G.S. Complications in the management of fractures in hand injuries. South Med J 63:704, 1970.

41. Cooney, W.; Chao, E. Biomechanical analysis of static forces in the thumb during hand function. J Bone Joint Surg 59A:27–36, 1977.

42. Cooney, W.; Lucca, M.; Chao, E.; et al. The kinesiology of the thumb trapezio-metacarpal joint. J Bone Joint Surg 63A:1371–1381, 1981.

43. Coonrad, R.N.; Goldner, J.L. A study of the pathological findings and treatment in soft tissue injury of the thumb metacarpophalangeal joint. J Bone Joint Surg 50A:439–451, 1968.

44. Coonrad, R.; Pohlman, M. Impacted fractures in the proximal portion of the proximal phalanx of the finger. J Bone Joint Surg 57A:1291–1296, 1969.

45. Crawford, G.P. Screw fixation for certain fractures of the phalanges and metacarpals. J Bone Joint Surg 58A:487–492, 1976.

46. Crockett, D.J. Rigid fixation of bone of the hand using K-wires bonded with acrylic resin. Hand 6:106–107, 1974.

47. Dabezies, E.J.; Schulte, J.P. Fixation of metacarpal and phalangeal fractures with miniature plates and screws. J Hand Surg 11A:283–288, 1986.

48. Dammisse, I.G.; Lloyd, G.J. Injuries to the fifth carpometacarpal region. Can J Surg 22:240–244, 1979.

49. Dennyson, W.G.; Stother, I.G. Carpometacarpal dislocations of the little finger. Hand 8:161–164, 1976.

50. Dixon, G.L. Jr.; Moon, N.F. Rotational supracondylar fractures of the proximal phalanx in children. Clin Orthop 83:151–156, 1972.

51. Dobyns, J.H.; Beckenbaugh, R.D.; Bryan, R.S.; et al. Fractures of the hand and wrist. In: Flynn, J.E., ed. Hand Surgery, Ed. 3. Baltimore, Williams and Wilkins, 1982, pp. 111–180.

52. Dobyns, J.H.; Linscheid, R.L.; Cooney, W.P. Fractures and dislocations of the wrist and hand, then and now. J Hand Surg 8:651–656, 1983.

53. Dray, G.; Eaton, R. Dislocation in the digits. In: Green, D.P., ed. Operative Hand Surgery, Ed. 2, Vol. 1. New York, Churchill Livingstone, 1988, p. 795.

54. Duran, R.J.; Houser, R.G.; Coleman, C.R.; Postelwaite, D.S. A preliminary report on the use of controlled passive motion following flexor tendon repairs in zones II and III. J Hand Surg 1:79, 1976.

55. Eaton, R.G. Joint Injuries of the Hand. Springfield, IL, Charles C Thomas, 1971, p. 23.

56. Eaton, R.G.; Malerich, M.M. Volar plate arthroplasty of the proximal interphalangeal joint: A review of 10 years' experience. J Hand Surg 5:260–268, 1980.

57. Edward, G.S.; O'Brien, E.T.; Hechman, M.M. Retrograde cross pinning of transverse metacarpal and phalangeal fractures. Hand 14:141–148, 1982.

58. Eigenholtz, S.N.; Rizzon, P.C. Fracture of the neck of the fifth metacarpal bone—is overtreatment justified? JAMA 178:425–426, 1961.

59. Elliott, R.A. Splints for mallet and boutonniere deformities. Plast Reconstr Surg 52:282–285, 1973.

60. Emmett, J.E.; Breck, L.W. A review and analysis of 11,000 fractures seen in a private practice of orthopaedic surgery. J Bone Joint Surg 40A:1169–1175, 1958.

61. Flatt, A.E. Closed and open fracture of the hand. Fundamentals of management. Postgrad Med 39:17–26, 1966.

62. Foster, R.J.; Hastings, H. II. Treatment of Bennett, Rolando, and vertical intraarticular trapezial fractures. Clin Orthop 214:121–129, 1987.

63. Frank, W.E.; Dobyns, J.H. Surgical pathology of collateral ligament injuries of the thumb. Clin Orthop 83:102–114, 1972.

64. Freeland, A.E. External fixation for skeletal stabilization of severe open fractures of the hand. Clin Orthop 214:93–100, 1987.

65. Freeland, A.E.; Jabaley, M.E.; Burkhalter, W.E.; Chaves, A.M.V. Delayed primary bone grafting in the hand and wrist after traumatic bone loss. J Hand Surg 9A:22–28, 1984.

66. Freeland, A.E.; Jabaley, M.E.; Hughes, J.L. Stable Fixation of the Hand and Wrist. New York, Springer Verlag, 1987.

67. Gedda, K.O. Studies on Bennett fractures: Anatomy, roentgenology, and therapy. Acta Chir Scand Suppl. 193:5, 1954.

68. Gedda, K.O.; Moberg, E. Open reduction and osteosynthesis of the so-called Bennett's fracture in the carpometacarpal joint of the thumb. Acta Orthop Scand 22:249–256, 1953.

69. Gelberman, R.H.; Vance, R.M.; Zakaib, G.S. Fractures at the base of the thumb: Treatment with oblique traction. J Bone Joint Surg 61A:260–262, 1979.

70. Gerber, C.; Senn, E.; Matter, P. Skier's thumb. Surgical treatment of recent injuries to the ulnar collateral ligament of the thumb metacarpophalangeal joint. Am J Sports Med 9:171–177, 1981.

71. Gigis, P.I.; Kuczynski, K. The distal interphalangeal joints of the human fingers. J Hand Surg 7:176–182, 1982.

72. Gingrass, R.P.; Fehring, B.H.T.; Matloub, H. Intraosseous wiring of complex hand fractures. Plast Reconstr Surg 66:383–394, 1980.

73. Gore, D.R. Carpometacarpal dislocation producing compression of the deep branch of the ulnar nerve. J Bone Joint Surg 53A:1387–1390, 1971.

74. Green, D.P.; Anderson, J.R. Closed reduction and percutaneous pin fixation of fractured phalanges. J Bone Joint Surg 55A:1651–1654, 1973.

75. Green, D.P.; Rowland, S.A. Fractures and dislocations in the hand. In: Rockwood, C.A.; Green, D.P., eds. Fractures and Dislocations. Philadelphia, J.B. Lippincott, 1984, pp. 317–323.

76. Green, D.; O'Brien, E. Fractures of the thumb metacarpal. South Med J 65:807–814, 1972.

77. Greene, T.L.; Noellert, R.C.; Belsole, R.J. Treatment of unstable metacarpal and phalangeal fractures with tension band wiring techniques. Clin Orthop 214:78–84, 1987.

78. Griffiths, J. Fractures at the base of the first metacarpal bone. J Bone Joint Surg 46B:712–719, 1964.

79. Gunter, G.S. Traumatic avulsion of the insertion of the flexor digitorum profundus insertion in athletes. J Hand Surg 4:461–464, 1979.

80. Gunther, S.F. The carpometacarpal joints. Orthop Clin North Am 15:259–277, 1989.

81. Haines, R.W. The mechanism of rotation at the first carpometacarpal joint. J Anat 78:44, 1944.

82. Hall, R.F. Treatment of metacarpal and phalangeal fractures in non-compliant patients. Clin Orthop 214:31–36, 1987.

83. Hallberg, D.; Lindholm, A. Subcutaneous rupture of the extensor tendon of the distal phalanx of the finger, mallet finger: Brief review of the literature and report on 127 cases treated conservatively. Acta Chir Scand 119:260–267, 1960.

84. Hartwig, R.H.; Louis, D.S. Multiple carpometacarpal dislocations. J Bone Joint Surg 61A:906–908, 1979.

85. Hastings, H. II; Carroll, C. IV. Treatment of closed articular fractures of the metacarpophalangeal and proximal interphalangeal joints. Hand Clin 4:503–528, 1988.

86. Hastings, H.; Ernst, J.M.J. Complex articular fractures of the base of the middle phalanx. Presented at American Society for Surgery of the Hand Meeting, San Antonio, TX, September 1987.

87. Hastings, H. II. Unstable metacarpal and phalangeal fracture treatment with screws and plates. Clin Orthop 214:37–52, 1987.

88. Hazlett, J.W. Carpometacarpal dislocations other than the thumb: A report of 11 cases. Can J Surg 11:315–322, 1968.

89. Heim, U.; Pfeiffer, K.M. Internal fixation of small fragments, Ed. 3. New York, Springer-Verlag, 1988.

90. Holbrook, T.L.; Grazier, K.; Kelsey, J.; Stauffer, R. The frequency of occurrence, impact, and cost of selected musculoskeletal conditions in the United States. Chicago, American Academy of Orthopaedic Surgeons, 1984, pp. 1–87.

91. Holst-Nielsen, F. Subcapital fractures of the four ulnar metacarpal bones. Hand 8:290–293, 1976.

92. Honner, R. Acute and chronic flexor and extensor mechanism injuries at the distal joint. In: Bower, W.H., ed. The Interphalangeal Joints. Edinburgh, Churchill Livingstone, 1987, pp. 111–118.

93. Howard, L.D. Jr. Fractures of the small bones of the hand. Plast Reconstr Surg 29:334–335, 1962.

94. Huffaker, W.H.; Wray, R.C.; Weeks, P.M. Factors influencing final range of motion in the fingers after fractures of the hand. Plast Reconstr Surg 63:83–87, 1979.

95. Hunter, J.M.; Cowen, N.J. Fifth metacarpal fracture in a compensation clinic population. J Bone Joint Surg 52A:1159–1165, 1970.

96. Itoh, Y.; Uchinishi, K.; Oka, Y. Treatment of pseudarthrosis of the distal phalanx with the palmar midline approach. J Hand Surg 8:80–84, 1983.

97. Jahss, S.A. Fractures of the proximal phalanges. A new method of reduction and immobilization. J Bone Joint Surg 20:178–186, 1938.

98. James, J.I.P. Fractures of the proximal and middle phalanges of the fingers. Acta Orthop Scand 32:401–412, 1962.

99. James, J.I.P. The assessment and management of the injured hand. Hand 2:97–105, 1970.

100. Jones, W.W. Biomechanics of small bone fixation. Clin Orthop 214:11–18, 1987.

101. Joshi, B.B. Percutaneous internal fixation of fractures of the proximal phalanges. Hand 8:86–92, 1976.

102. Jupiter, J.B.; Koniuch, M.; Smith, R.J. The management of delayed unions and nonunions of the tubular bones of the hand. J Hand Surg 4:457–466, 1985.

103. Jupiter, J.B.; Sheppard, J.E. Tension wire fixation of avulsion fractures in the hand. Clin Orthop 214:113–120, 1987.

104. Jupiter, J.B.; Silver, M.A. Fractures of the metacarpals and phalanges. In: Chapman, M.W., ed. Operative Orthopaedics. Philadelphia, J.B. Lippincott, 1980, pp. 1235–1250.

105. Kapanji, A.I. Selective radiology of the first carpometacarpal joint. In: Tubiana, R., ed. The Hand. Philadelphia, W.B. Saunders, 1985, pp. 635–644.

106. Kaplan, E.B. Mallet or baseball finger. Surgery 7:784–791, 1940.

107. Kaplan, E.B. Functional and Surgical Anatomy of the Hand, Ed. 2. Philadelphia, J.B. Lippincott, 1965.

108. Kaplan, E.B. Dorsal dislocation of the metacarpophalangeal joint of the index finger. J Bone Joint Surg 39:1081–1086, 1957.

109. Kaplan, L. The treatment of fractures and dislocations of the hand and fingers. Technic of unpadded casts for carpal, metacarpal, and phalangeal fractures. Surg Clin North Am 20:1695–1720, 1940.

110. Kaye, J.J.; Lister, G.D. Another use for the Brewerton view. J Hand Surg 3:603, 1978.

111. Kelsey, J.L.; Pastides, H.; Kreiger, N.; et al. Upper extremity disorders. A survey of their frequency and cost in the United States. St. Louis, C.V. Mosby, 1980.

112. Kilbourne, B.C.; Paul, E.G. The use of small bone screws in the treatment of metacarpal, metatarsal, and phalangeal fractures. J Bone Joint Surg 40A:375–383, 1958.

113. Kleinman, W.B.; Grantham, S.A. Multiple volar carpometacarpal joint dislocations. J Hand Surg 3:377–382, 1978.

114. Koch, S.L. Disabilities of the hand resulting from loss of joint function. JAMA 104:30–35, 1935.

115. Kuczynski, K. The proximal interphalangeal joint. J Bone Joint Surg 50B:656–663, 1968.

116. Kuczynski, K. Carpometacarpal joint of the human thumb. J Anat 118:119–126, 1974.

117. Kuczynski, K. Lesser-known aspects of the proximal interphalangeal joints of the human hand. Hand 7:31–34, 1975.

118. Lamb, D.W.; Angarita, G. Ulna instability of the metacarpophalangeal joint of the thumb. J Hand Surg 10B:113–114, 1985.

119. Lamb, D.W.; Abernathy, P.A.; Raine, P.A.M. Unstable fractures of the metacarpal (a method of treatment by transverse wire fixation to intact metacarpals). Hand 5:43–48, 1973.

120. Lambotte, A. Contribution to conservative surgery of the injured hand. Arch Franco-Belges Chir 31:759, 1928.

121. Lamphier, T.A. Improper reduction of fractures of the proximal phalanges of fingers. Am J Surg 94:926–930, 1957.

122. Landsmeer, J.M.F. The anatomy of the dorsal aponeurosis of the human finger and its functional significance. Anat Rec 104:31, 1949.

123. Lane, C.S. Detecting occult fractures of the metacarpal head: The Brewerton view. J Hand Surg 2:131–133, 1977.

124. Lazar, G.; Shulter-Ellis, F.P. Intramedullary structure of human metacarpals. J Hand Surg 5:477, 1980.

125. Leddy, J.P. Avulsions of the flexor digitorum profundus. Hand Clin 1:77–83, 1985.

126. Leddy, L.P.; Packer, J.W. Avulsion of the profundus insertion in athletes. J Hand Surg 4:461–464, 1979.

127. Lee, M.L.H. Intraarticular and peri-articular fractures of the phalanges. J Bone Joint Surg 45B:103–109, 1963.

128. Lipton, H.A.; Skoff, H.; Jupiter, J.B. The management of hand injuries. New Develop Med 3:5–42, 1988.

129. Lister, G. Intraosseous wiring of the digital skeleton. J Hand Surg 3:427–435, 1978.

130. Littler, J.W. On the adaptability of man's hand (with reference to the equiangular curve). Hand 5:187–191, 1973.

131. Littler, J.W.; Thompson, J.S. Surgical and functional anatomy. In: Bowers, W.H., ed. The Interphalangeal Joints. New York, Churchill Livingstone, 1987, pp. 14–20.

132. London, P.S. Sprains and fractures involving the interphalangeal joints. Hand 3:155–158, 1971.

133. Lubahn, J.D. Dorsal fracture-dislocations of the proximal interphalangeal joint. Hand Clin 4:15–24, 1988.

134. Malerich, M.M.; Eaton, R.G. Complete dislocation of a little finger metacarpophalangeal joint treated by closed technique. J Trauma 20:424–425, 1980.

135. Mann, R.J.; Black, D.; Constine, R.; et al. A quantitative comparison of metacarpal fracture stability with five different methods of internal fixation. J Hand Surg 10A:1024–1028, 1985.

136. Margles, S. Intraarticular fractures of the metacarpophalangeal and proximal interphalangeal joints. Hand Clin 4:67–74, 1988.

137. Martin, B.F. The tendons of the flexor digitorum profundus. J Anat 92:602–608, 1958.

138. Massengill, J.B.; Alexander, H.; Langrana, N.; et al. A phalangeal fracture model—quantitative analysis of rigidity and failure. J Hand Surg 7:264–270, 1982.

139. McCue, F.; Honner, R.; Marriott, C.; et al. Athletic injuries of the proximal interphalangeal joint requiring surgical treatment. J Bone Joint Surg 52A:937–956, 1970.

140. McElfresh, E.C.; Dobyns, J.H. Intraarticular metacarpal head fractures. J Hand Surg 8:383–393, 1983.

141. McElfresh, E.L.; Dobyns, J.H.; O'Brien, E.T. Management of fracture-dislocation of the proximal interphalangeal joint by extension-block splinting. J Bone Joint Surg 54(A):1705–1710, 1972.

142. McMinn, D.J. Mallet finger and fracture. Injury 12:477–479, 1981.

143. McNealy, R.W.; Lichtenstein, M.E. Fractures of the bones of the hand. Am J Surg 50:563–570, 1940.

144. Mikic, Z.; Helal, B. The treatment of the mallet finger by Oakley splint. Hand 6:76–81, 1974.

145. Moberg, E. Fractures and ligamentous injuries of the thumb and fingers. Surg Clin North Am 40:297, 1960.

146. Moss, J.G.; Steingold, R.F. The long-term results of mallet finger injury: A retrospective study of 100 cases. Hand 15:151–154, 1983.

147. Nalebuff, E.A. Isolated anterior carpometacarpal dislocation of the fifth finger: Classification and case report. J Trauma 8:1119–1123, 1968.

148. Namba, R.S.; Kabo, M.; Meals, R.A. Biomechanical effects of point configuration in Kirschner wire fixation. Clin Orthop 214:19–22, 1987.

149. Napier, J. The form and function of the carpometacarpal joint of the thumb. J Anat 89:362–369, 1955.

150. Neviaser, R.J. Dislocations and ligamentous injuries of the digits. In: Chapman, M.W., ed. Operative Orthopaedics. Philadelphia, J.B. Lippincott, 1989, pp. 1199–1212.

151. Opgrande, J.D.; Westphal, S.A. Fractures of the hand. Orthop Clin North Am 14:779–792, 1983.

152. Peimer, C.A.; Smith, R.J.; Leffert, R.D. Distraction fixation in the primary treatment of metacarpal bone loss. J Hand Surg 6:111–124, 1981.

153. Peimer, C.A.; Sullivan, D.J.; Wild, D.R. Palmar dislocation of the proximal interphalangeal joint. J Hand Surg 9A:39–48, 1984.

154. Pellegrini, V.D. Jr.; Burton, R.I. Surgical management of basal joint arthritis of the thumb: Part I. Long-term results of silicone arthroplasty. J Hand Surg 11A:309–324, 1986.

155. Pellegrini, V.D. Jr. Fractures at the base of the thumb. Hand Clin 4:87–102, 1988.

156. Peterson, P.; Sack, S. Fracture-dislocation of the base of the fifth metacarpal associated with injury to the deep motor branch of the ulnar nerve: A case report. J Hand Surg 11A:525–528, 1986.

157. Pieron, A.P. The mechanism of the first carpometacarpal (CMC) joint. An anatomical and mechanical analysis. Acta Orthop Scand 148:7–104, 1973.

158. Pollen, A. The conservative treatment of Bennett's fracture-subluxation of the thumb metacarpal. J Bone Joint Surg 50B:91–101, 1968.

159. Pritsch, M.; Engel, J.; Tsur, H.; Farin, I. The fractured metacarpal neck: New method of manipulation and external fixation. Orthop Rev 7:122–123, 1978.

160. Pritsch, M.; Engel, J.; Frian, I. Manipulation and external fixation of metacarpal fractures. J Bone Joint Surg 63A:1289–1291, 1981.

161. Pun, W.K.; Chow, S.P.; Luk, K.D.K.; et al. A prospective study on 284 digital fractures of the hand. J Hand Surg 14A:474–481, 1989.

162. Rawles, J.G. Jr. Dislocations and fracture-dislocations at the carpometacarpal joints of the fingers. Hand Clin 4:103–112, 1988.

163. Rayan, G.M.; Mullins, P.T. Skin necrosis complicating mallet finger splinting and vascularity of the distal interphalangeal joint overlying skin. J Hand Surg 12A:548–552, 1987.

164. Reyes, F.A.; Latta, L.L. Conservative management of difficult phalangeal fractures. Clin Orthop 214:23–30, 1987.

165. Rider, D.L. Fractures of the metacarpals, metatarsals, and phalanges. Am J Surg 38:549–559, 1947.

166. Riggs, S.A. Jr.; Cooney, W.P. 3d. External fixation of complex hand and wrist fractures. J Trauma 23:332–336, 1983.

167. Robb, W.A.T. The results of treatment of mallet finger. J Bone Joint Surg 41B:546–549, 1959.

168. Roberts, P. Bulletins et memoires de la Societe de Radiologie Medicale de France 24:687, 1936.

169. Robins, P.R.; Dobyns, J.H. Avulsion of the insertion of the flexor digitorum profundus tendon associated with fracture of the distal phalanx. In: AAOS Symposium on Flexor Tendon Surgery in the Hand. St. Louis, C.V. Mosby, 1975, p. 151.

170. Rolando, S. Fracture de la base du premier metacarpien et

principalement sur une variété non encore écrite. Presse Med 33:303–304, 1910.

171. Rose, E.H. Reconstruction of central metacarpal ray defects of the hand with a free vascularized double metatarsal and metatarsophalangeal joint transfer. J Hand Surg 9A:28–31, 1984.

172. Ruedi, T.P.; Burri, C.; Pfeiffer, K.M. Stable internal fixation of fractures of the hand. J Trauma 11:381–389, 1971.

173. Salgeback, S.; Eiken, O.; Carstam, N.; et al. A study of Bennett's fracture—special reference to fixation by percutaneous pinning. Scand J Plast Reconstr Surg 5:142–148, 1971.

174. Salter, R.B.; Harris, W.R. Injuries involving the epiphyseal plate. J Bone Joint Surg 45A:587–622, 1963.

175. Schenk, R.R. Dynamic traction and early passive movement for fractures of the proximal interphalangeal joint. J Hand Surg 11A:850–858, 1986.

176. Segmueller, G. Principles of stable internal fixation in the hand. In: Chapman, J.M., ed. Operative Orthopaedics. Philadelphia, J.B. Lippincott, 1988, pp. 1213–1218.

177. Segmueller, G.; Schonenberger, F. Fractures of the hand. In: Weber, B.G.; Gruner, C.; Fruehler, F., eds. Treatment of Fractures in Children and Adolescents. New York, Springer-Verlag, 1980, p. 340.

178. Segmueller, G. Indications for stable internal fixation in hand injuries. In: Chapman, M., ed. Operative Orthopaedics. Philadelphia, J.B. Lippincott, 1988, pp. 1219–1233.

179. Segmueller, G. Surgical Stabilization of the Skeleton of the Hand. Baltimore, Williams and Wilkins, 1977, pp. 18–22.

180. Segond, P. Note sur un cas d'arrachment du point d'insertion des deux languettes phalangettiennes de l'extenseur du petit doigt par flexion forcée del la phalangette sur la phalangine. Prog Med 8:534–535, 1880.

181. Seitz, W.H. Jr. Management of severe hand trauma with a mini-external fixateur. Orthopedics 10:601–610, 1987.

182. Seyman, N. Juxta-epiphyseal fractures of the terminal phalanx of the finger. J Bone Joint Surg 48B:347–349, 1966.

183. Shah, J.; Patel, M. Dislocation of the carpometacarpal joint of the thumb. A report of four cases. Clin Orthop 175:166–169, 1983.

184. Shrewsbury, M.M.; Johnson, R.K. Form, function, and evolution of the distal phalanx. J Hand Surg 8:475–479, 1983.

185. Shrewsbury, M.M.; Johnson, R.K. A systematic study of the oblique retinacular ligament of the human finger: Its structure and function. J Hand Surg 2:194–199, 1977.

186. Shrewsbury, M.M.; Johnson, R.K. Ligaments of the distal interphalangeal joint and the mallet position. J Hand Surg 5:214–216, 1980.

187. Shulter-Ellis, F.P.; Lazar, G. Internal morphology of human phalanges. J Hand Surg 9A:490–495, 1984.

188. Smith, F.L.; Rider, D.L. A study of the healing of one hundred consecutive phalangeal fractures. J Bone Joint Surg 17:91–105, 1935.

189. Smith, J.H. Jr. Avulsion of a profundus tendon with simultaneous intraarticular fracture of the distal phalanx—case report. J Hand Surg 6:600–601, 1981.

190. Smith, R.J.; Peimer, C.A. Injuries to the metacarpal bones and joints. Adv Surg 2:341–374, 1977.

191. Spangberg, O.; Thoren, L. Bennett's fracture: A method of treatment with oblique traction. J Bone Joint Surg 45B:732–739, 1963.

192. Spinner, M.; Choi, B.Y. Anterior dislocation of the proximal interphalangeal joint. J Bone Joint Surg 52A:1329–1336, 1970.

193. Stack, H.G. Mallet finger. Hand 1:83–89, 1969.

194. Stark, H.H. Troublesome fractures and dislocations of the hand. AAOS Instr Course Lect 19:130–149, 1970.

195. Stark, H.H.; Boyes, J.H.; Wilson, J.N. Mallet finger. J Bone Joint Surg 44A:1061–1068, 1962.

196. Stark, H.H.; Gainor, B.J.; Ashworth, C.R.; et al. Operative treatment of intraarticular fractures of the dorsal aspect of the distal phalanx of digits. J Bone Joint Surg 69A:892–896, 1987.

197. Stener, B. Displacement of the ruptured ulnar collateral ligament of the metacarpophalangeal joint of the thumb. J Bone Joint Surg 44B:869–879, 1962.

198. Strickland, J.W.; Steichen, J.B.; Kleinman, W.B.; et al. Phalangeal fractures, factors influencing digital performance. Orthop Rev 11:39–50, 1982.

199. Strickland, J.W.; Steichen, J.B.; Kleinman, W.B.; Flynn, N. Factors influencing digital performance after phalangeal fracture. In: Strickland, J.W.; Steichen, J.B., eds. Difficult Problems in Hand Surgery. St. Louis, C.V. Mosby, 1982, pp. 126–139.

200. Strickland, J.W.; Steichen, J.B.; Showalter, J.F. Phalangeal fractures in a hand surgery practice: A statistical review and in-depth study of the management of proximal phalangeal shaft fractures. J Hand Surg 4:285, 1979.

201. Strong, M.L. A new method of extension-block splinting of the proximal interphalangeal joint. Preliminary report. J Hand Surg 5:606–607, 1980.

202. Stuchin, S.A.; Kummer, F.J. Stiffness of small bone external fixation methods: An experimental study. J Hand Surg 9:718–724, 1984.

203. Susman, R.L. Comparative and functional morphology of hominid fingers. Am J Physiol Anthropol 50:215–236, 1979.

204. Swanson, A.B. Fractures involving the digits of the hand. Orthop Clin North Am 1:261–274, 1970.

205. Tennant, C.E. Use of a steel phonograph needle as a retaining pin in certain irreducible fractures of the small bones. JAMA 83:193, 1924.

206. Thomine, J.M. Les fractures ouvertes du squeulette digital dans les plaies de la main et des doigts. Actual Chir. Paris, Masson et Cie. 776–780, 1975.

207. Thompson, J.S.; Eaton, R.G. Volar dislocation of the proximal interphalangeal joint. J Hand Surg 2:232, 1977.

208. Thoren, L. A new method of extension treatment in Bennett's fracture. Acta Chir Scand 110:485–493, 1955.

209. Tubiana, R. Incidence and cost of injuries to the hand. In: Tubiana, R, ed. The Hand, Vol. II. Philadelphia, W.B. Saunders, 1985, pp. 159–164.

210. Tubiana, R. Evolution of bone and joint techniques in hand surgery. In: Tubiana, R, ed. The Hand, Vol. II. Philadelphia, W.B. Saunders, 1985. pp. 469–494.

211. Tuttle, R.H. Quantitative and functional studies on the hand of the anthropoidea. J Morphol 128:309–364, 1969.

212. Vanik, R.K.; Weber, R.C.; Matloub, H.S.; et al. The comparative strengths of internal fixation techniques. J Hand Surg 9A:216–221, 1984.

213. Wagner, C. Transarticular fixation of fracture-dislocation of the first metacarpal carpal joint. West J Surg Gynecol Obstet 59:362–365, 1951.

214. Watson-Jones, R. Fractures and Joint Injuries, Ed. 4. Edinburgh, E&S Livingstone, 1956, pp. 645–646.

215. Waugh, R.L.; Ferrazzano, G.P. Fractures of the metacarpals exclusive of the thumb. A new method of treatment. Am J Surg 59:186–194, 1943.

216. Wehbe, M.A.; Schneider, L.H. Mallet fractures. J Bone Joint Surg 66A:658–669, 1984.

217. Wenger, D.R. Avulsion of the profundus tendon insertion in football players. Arch Surg 106:145, 1973.
218. Wilkinson, J.L. The insertions of the flexor pollicis longus and digitorum profundus. J Anat 87:75–88, 1953.
219. Wilson, J.N.; Rowland, S.A. Fracture-dislocation of the proximal interphalangeal joint of the finger. Treatment by open reduction and internal fixation. J Bone Joint Surg 48A:493–502, 1966.
220. Wood, V.E. Fractures of the hand in children. Orthop Clin North Am 7:527–542, 1976.
221. Wright, T.A. Early mobilization in fractures of the metacarpals and phalanges. Can J Surg 11:491–498, 1968.
222. Zemel, N.P.; Stark, H.H.; Ashworth, C.R.; et al. Chronic fracture-dislocation of the proximal interphalangeal joint— treatment by osteotomy and bone graft. J Hand Surg 6:447–455, 1981.
223. Zimmerman, N.B.; Weiland, A.J. Ninety-ninety intraosseous wiring for internal fixation of the digital skeleton. Orthopaedics 12:99–104, 1989.
224. Zur Verth, M. Behandlung der Finger und Handverletzungen. Hefte Z Unfallh 6:1929–1930.

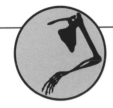

Leonard Ruby, M.D.

34

FRACTURES AND DISLOCATIONS OF THE CARPUS

Fractures of the Scaphoid

Scaphoid fractures comprise 60 to 70% of all carpal bone fractures[15] and are second only to fractures of the distal radius in frequency. Osterman and Mikulic[100] have estimated that there are 345,000 scaphoid fractures annually in the United States. If 90 to 95% unite (which can be expected with proper treatment), then there will be 17,250 to 34,500 nonunions per year. In spite of almost 100 years of experience and an extensive literature[15] there are still many areas of controversy in regard to treatment. The most frequently seen clinical picture is that of a young adult male who has sustained a dorsiflexion injury to his wrist and presents with radial side wrist pain classically in the anatomic snuffbox. Due to the importance of the scaphoid in wrist mechanics and because of the frequency of fracture in the young adult male, this injury has economic as well as physical significance.

MECHANISM OF INJURY

In order to better understand the pathomechanics, Weber and Chao[146] consistently produced scaphoid waist fractures in cadaver wrists by applying a dorsiflexion load to the radial half of the palm while the wrist was stabilized in 95 to 100° of extension. It is surmised that the proximal pole of the scaphoid is fixed in this position by the radius proximally, dorsally, and radially; by the capitate and lunate ulnarly; and by the radiolunate triquetrum ligament and the radioscaphocapitate ligament volarly. At the same time, the distal pole is free to translate dorsally with the distal row of carpals, which results in fracture, usually of the waist of

the scaphoid. The palmar aspect of the bone fails in tension and the dorsal aspect fails in compression. Smith and co-workers[119] showed that osteotomy of the waist of the scaphoid in cadaver specimens causes a 27° volar angulation of the scaphoid with consequent collapse deformity of the wrist with dorsiflexion of the proximal row of carpals. This study confirms the stabilizing link function of the scaphoid between the proximal and distal rows that has been assumed by most authors based on the anatomy of the scaphoid and clinical experience.[36,45,69,91,119]

DIAGNOSIS

As is often the case in clinical medicine, a strong index of suspicion is the key to early diagnosis. Therefore if a young adult male presents with a history of a fall on the palm of his hand and pain and tenderness in the anatomic snuffbox, the diagnosis of scaphoid fracture should be assumed until proven otherwise. Radiographic examination is still the best method for determining the presence of a fracture.[88] Indeed, before x-rays were discovered in 1895, fractures of the scaphoid were seldom recognized. At the turn of the century, Professor Stimpson of the Cornell University Medical School said that simple fractures of this bone were rare and disability the usual outcome.[88] Although many different views have been recommended, we find, in common with most authors, that a standard posteroanterior (PA), an ulnar deviation PA, true lateral (i.e., radius, lunate, capitate colinear), and 45° pronation PA view is a useful initial series. The lateral view is helpful in identifying carpal malalignment often seen in displaced scaphoid fractures. The ulnar deviation

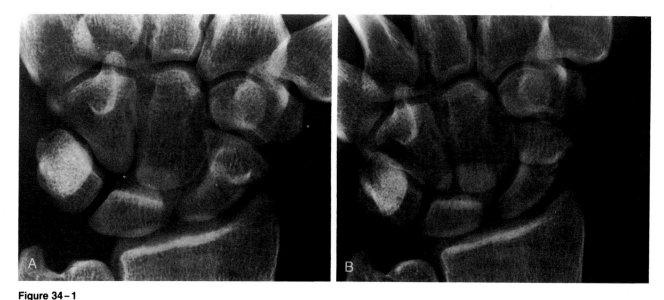

Figure 34-1

A, A posteroanterior radiograph showing a scaphoid fracture with no displacement. The fracture is difficult to visualize on this x-ray film. *B,* A posteroanterior radiograph of ulnar deviation in which the fracture line is apparent.

view positions the long axis of the scaphoid more parallel with the radiographic plate and thus the fracture line more parallel to the x-ray beam. Also, this maneuver tends to distract the fracture fragments (Fig. 34–1*A,B*). Both of these factors facilitate visualization of the fracture line.[74]

If these radiographs are equivocal or negative in the face of strong clinical suspicion, further oblique views can be taken. Stecher[127] recommends a PA view that is angled 20° from vertical from distal to proximal. This too has the effect of directing the x-ray beam more parallel to the fracture line. If uncertainty still exists after these maneuvers, the patient should be placed in a cast for 2 to 4 weeks and the examination repeated. There are instances in which even the second examination is equivocal in spite of the expected resorption at

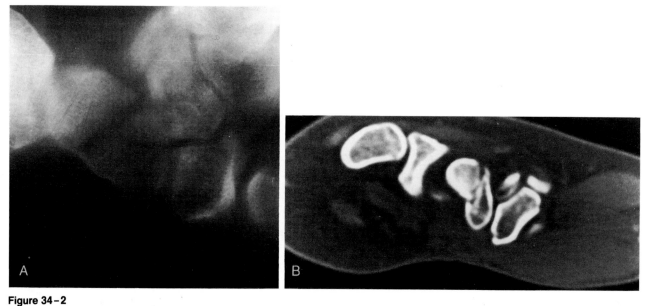

Figure 34-2

A, A lateral polytome showing an obvious fracture line across the waist of the scaphoid. *B,* Print of a computed tomographic scan showing scaphoid waist fracture, with angulation.

the fracture site,[63] and in these patients, radionuclide bone scan, polytomography, and/or computerized tomography can be helpful.[40,63,99] The scan is the most sensitive but least specific of these modalities. Thus if the scan is negative, a scaphoid fracture is ruled out. If the bone scan is positive, more specific studies such as polytomography or computerized tomography (CT) can be helpful. When ordering the tomographic study, it is essential to ask the radiologist for axial studies of the scaphoid, since cross-sectional views of the wrist are often routinely done and are very difficult to interpret. In other words, the same principles apply to tomographic views as to plain views. To be useful, the beam must be parallel to the suspected fracture line or perpendicular to the long axis of the scaphoid. Added information about intercarpal alignment can be seen on the lateral (sagittal) views as the radius-lunate-capitate relationship is well visualized (Fig. 34–2A,B).

TREATMENT

It is in this area that most of the controversy regarding scaphoid fracture still exists.[81,88] This is partly due to the fact that until recently it was not generally appreciated that these fractures may not be isolated injuries and often are only the most obvious sign of a more extensive injury to the wrist. Another confounding factor is the definition of a successful result. Some of the older studies especially have defined a successful result in clinical terms; i.e., adequate motion and no significant pain.[81] Although this is not an unreasonable point of view, the best available evidence suggests that the optimum result will more likely be obtained if the selected treatment results in a radiologically proven healed scaphoid with normal carpal alignment.

While there is no single universally agreed upon classification of scaphoid fracture, there are guidelines that help the surgeon design the best course of treatment in a given patient. The fracture can be classified according to the time since injury as (1) fresh fracture (less than 3 weeks old), (2) delayed union (4 to 6 months old), or (3) nonunion (greater than 4 to 6 months old).[129] These are, of course, arbitrary definitions and no one can say with certainty when a delayed union begins or ends. The fracture can also be defined anatomically into distal one-third, middle one-third, or proximal one-third, and this classification has prognostic implications. Proximal pole fractures are described as having a poorer rate of healing than more distal fractures, presumably due to interruption of the blood supply, which enters the bone at or distal to the middle third.[44,116,137] Gelberman and Menon[44] have shown that the major blood supply is from branches of the radial artery that enter the bone at or distal to the waist at the dorsal

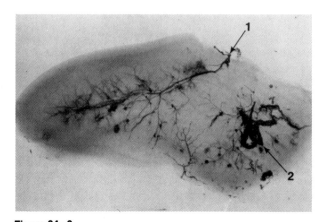

Figure 34–3

A sagittal section of the scaphoid with the proximal pole oriented to the left. The dorsal scaphoid branch of the radial artery (1); the volar scaphoid arterial branch (2). (From Gelberman, R.; et al. J Hand Surg 5:508–513, 1980.)

ridge. This blood supply comprises 70 to 80% of the total intraosseous vascularity and 100% of the proximal pole (Fig. 34–3).

Herbert and Fisher[57] have suggested that the plane of the fracture is important and have described oblique and transverse fractures. Cooney[24] and Weber[144] have distinguished between displaced and undisplaced fractures. Displacement was defined by Cooney as a 1 mm or more step-off on the anteroposterior or oblique scaphoid views or greater than 15° of lunate capitate angulation or greater than 45° of scapholunate angulation on the lateral views. Both authors have shown that the prognosis is adversely affected by displacement and angulation. We agree that displacement and angulation are more important indicators of prognosis than the plane of the fracture. In summary, negative prognostic factors are late diagnosis, proximal location, displacement or angulation, and possibly obliquity of the fracture line.

Nonoperative Treatment

There are two types of nonoperative treatment presently available: cast immobilization[88,140] and cast immobilization with electrical stimulation.[14,39] A great variety of casts have been described, and almost every position of the wrist has been advocated, including flexion,[65,146] extension,[39] radial deviation,[146] ulnar deviation,[65] neutral,[116] and various combinations. The proximal and distal extent of the cast also varies, with some authors recommending cast application to just above the elbow to prevent pronation and supination[140] while others include the index and middle fingers as well as the thumb.[29]

Part of this diversity in cast immobilization treatment may be due to the consistently successful results (94 to 98.5%) reported by several authors with cast treatment of fresh undisplaced fractures.[144] It appears that the exact type of cast is not a critical factor in successful treatment. The goal is to immobilize the fracture as well as possible, and in our experience this means a well-fitting cast starting just above the elbow with the wrist in neutral position and including the thumb tip. This allows some flexion and extension of the elbow. The cast is usually changed at two-week intervals in order to ensure that it fits snugly. Postero-anterior and lateral radiographs are performed at 6 weeks. If the fracture is not healed radiographically, regardless of the absence of pain, a below-elbow cast is applied for six more weeks. If after a total of 12 weeks of immobilization, radiographic examination fails to show unequivocal healing, then polytomography or CT scanning is performed.

Some authors have suggested that noninvasive electrical stimulation be applied at this point.[6,39] After a review of the experience with electrical stimulation, Osterman[100] concluded that noninvasive methods of electrical stimulation are most appropriately applied to those patients who have failed previous bone grafting, have well-aligned waist fractures, do not have significant collapse pattern, and do not have a small proximal fragment or significant arthritis. In the absence of controlled studies showing the efficacy of electrical stimulation, we prefer bone grafting as the next step after failure of cast treatment. Herbert and Fisher[57] have stated that nonoperative treatment has a 50% failure rate in their experience and for that reason and the fact that many patients, especially young manual laborers and professional athletes, will not tolerate prolonged cast immobilization, early internal fixation should be performed. This view is not presently shared by most authors but may be applicable in selected cases.

Operative Treatment

Surgical treatment may be thought of as an invasive means of obtaining union of the scaphoid in adequate position. Surgery is also a means of salvage of a patient with a painful wrist if there has been failure to obtain union or arthritis is severe. The accepted indications for surgery are failure of nonoperative treatment, displaced fresh fracture, and established nonunions. The question of advising surgery to the patient with an asymptomatic nonunion is a difficult one. The experience of Mack and colleagues[82] and Ruby and co-workers[115] has shown that scaphoid nonunion probably results in wrist malalignment and arthritis if left untreated for 5 to 10 years. If surgical treatment for the fracture is selected, the goals of obtaining good alignment of the wrist and scaphoid and adequate stabilization should be kept in mind. The techniques of operative treatment of the fracture presently include bone grafting with or without osteosynthesis. The salvage techniques are radial styloidectomy, the Bentzon procedure,[9] implant arthroplasty, proximal row carpectomy,[27,49,96] and either complete[18,48] or partial arthrodesis.[10,134,142]

Bone Grafting. This is the oldest technique[1] and has usually been used for established nonunion or delayed union. Several different methods of bone grafting have been described over the years.[5,34,84,94,116,121] Corticocancellous[116] or cancellous[84] interposition grafts and anterior wedge grafts[34] are the most commonly used at the present time. The original Matti technique as described in 1937[84] consisted of excavation of the proximal and distal fracture fragments through a dorsal approach and placement of a cancellous strut within these two cavities to act as an internal fixation device as well as a nidus for osteogenesis (Fig. 34–4). In 1960, Russe[116] described a volar approach also using cancellous graft, and more recently he performed a double corticocancellous graft (Fig. 34–5).[50] Because the blood supply of

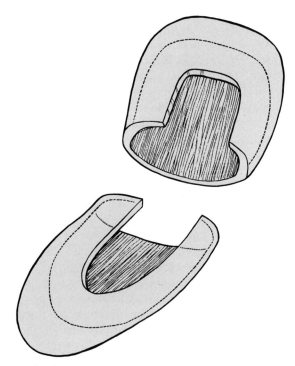

Figure 34–4

Reproduction of the original drawing of Matti (1937) showing the amount of excavation for a scaphoid nonunion bone graft. This cavity was filled with cancellous bone from the greater trochanter, and the bone graft was pressed carefully into the cavity as a dentist might pack gold into a tooth. (From Verdan, C.; Narakas, A. Surg Clin North Am 48:1083–1095, 1968.)

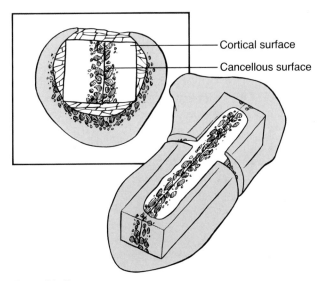

— Cortical surface

— Cancellous surface

Figure 34–5

Russe's latest technique using Matti's excavation concept but incorporating corticocancellous graft for improved fixation and a volar approach. (From Green, D.P. J Hand Surg 10A:597–605, 1985.)

the scaphoid is primarily dorsal-distal, the volar approach is the most popular today. The Matti-Russe type graft is indicated when the nonunion is not associated with significant dorsal intercalated segment instability (DISI) of the wrist. When DISI is present, an anterior wedge graft after the method of Fisk[36] and Fernandez[34] is the preferred option. Green[50] has pointed out that the Matti-Russe technique has a lower success rate when the proximal pole is avascular, as documented by no bleeding of the bone at surgery. In his experience, he had a failure rate of 100% in five patients in whom there was no bleeding of the proximal pole at the time of surgery. He and others have shown that radiographic vascularity is not a reliable indicator of actual vascularity.[50] Our favorable experience with the Matti-Russe method is consistent with that of most authors, and one can expect 80 to 90% healing rates.[50,116]

***Technique (Matti-Russe).**[84,116]* A 4 to 5 cm zigzag volar incision is made along the course of the flexor carpi radialis tendon ending at the tuberosity of the scaphoid. One should be careful in dividing the skin not to injure the palmar cutaneous branch of the median nerve, which often lies in the skin flap over the flexor carpi radialis tendon. The flexor carpi radialis is mobilized and retracted ulnarward, and the radial artery is retracted radialward. It is not necessary to isolate the radial artery, although at the distal end of the incision the superficial branch is often visualized and may have to be ligated if the scaphotrapezial joint is to be exposed. The posterior wall of the flexor carpi radialis sheath is divided longitudinally and the underlying

pericapsular fat is exposed. This too is divided and the multiple vessels in this layer are electrocauterized with a bipolar instrument. The exposed volar wrist capsule and volar capsular ligaments are divided sharply, beginning at the distal radius and continuing distally to the scaphoid tuberosity. At this point, the radioscaphoid joint and the entire volar surface of the scaphoid will be exposed. The fracture site is usually obvious, but if not, look for a wrinkle in the articular cartilage of the scaphoid and attempt forceful extension of the wrist. Once the fracture is exposed, create a hole in the volar nonarticular cortex of the scaphoid and excavate opposing cavities in the fragments. Russe advocated using only hand instruments for this step, but we have used the Midas Rex* with a 2x bit for the preliminary curettage and completed the excavation with straight and curved hand-held curettes. If the proximal pole is very small and avascular, then we carry the curettement to the subchondral bone level. In theory, this allows the cartilage to be nourished by synovial fluid, and the proximal pole is converted into an osteocartilaginous graft. Particular care must be taken not to penetrate the proximal pole if this maneuver is used. After adequate curettement (until bleeding cancellous bone is exposed) of both fragments, a properly shaped and sized cancellous graft harvested from the iliac crest is packed tightly into the defect by overdistracting the fragments. Any remaining defect is filled with cancellous bone chips. Stability is then checked by manipulation of the wrist in radioulnar deviation and flexion-extension. If unstable, then two parallel 0.045-in Kirschner wires can be inserted from the distal pole across the graft and into the proximal pole. Radiographs should then be taken to ensure proper placement of wires and alignment of the scaphoid and the rest of the wrist. The volar ligaments and capsule are closed with absorbable 2-0 suture in horizontal mattress fashion. The rest of the closure is routine. If Kirschner wires are used, they should be allowed to protrude from the skin and bent over to prevent migration or cut off under the skin. A U-shaped above-elbow splint is applied for 5 to 7 days. This is replaced by a solid short above-elbow cast for six weeks, which is changed every two to three weeks. If wires are used and left exposed, it is important that they be well padded and that the cast remain snug or they can become loose and infected. Six weeks postoperatively, radiographs are taken out of plaster and a short arm cast including the entire thumb is continued for six more weeks or until healing is complete by radiography.

If there is angulation at the fracture site with con-

---

* Midas Rex Pneumatic Tools, Inc., 2925 Race Street, Ft. Worth, TX 76111.

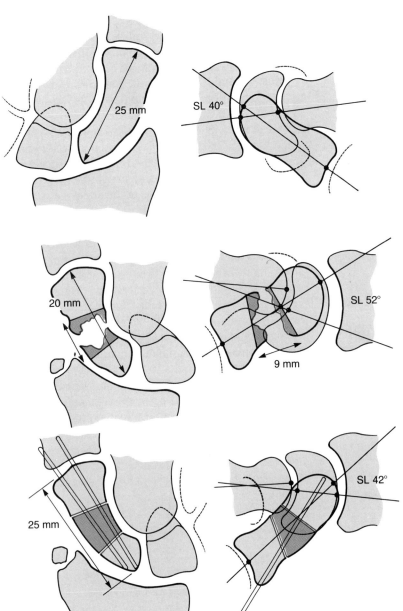

Figure 34–6

Line drawing illustrating the Fisk-Fernandez grafting technique. SL = scapholunate. (Redrawn from Fernandez, D.L. J Hand Surg 9A:733–737, 1984.)

comitant dorsal intercalated segment instability, then the Fisk-Fernandez[34,36] method is most appropriate.

Technique (Fisk-Fernandez). According to Fernandez,[34] it may be helpful to measure the normal scaphoid to determine the amount of bone to be resected and the size of the bone graft. A volar wrist approach similar to that in the Matti-Russe technique is used. Although volar angulation at the fracture site makes visualization difficult, wrist dorsiflexion and ulnar deviation will reveal the fracture. In order to reduce the dorsal intercalated segment deformity of the carpus, after dividing the capsule and volar ligaments, carry the dissection farther ulnarward to expose the capitate head and the lunate. This allows the capitate lunate joint to be reduced by releasing adhesions on the volar aspect of the midcarpal joint. Then place a laminar spreader in the scaphoid fracture site and open this as much as possible. This maneuver reliably reduces the fracture and the carpus. The fracture site is then curetted sufficiently to expose good bleeding cancellous bone on both surfaces. A corticocancellous wedge-shaped bone graft is harvested from the iliac crest. In some patients, the entire scaphoid is shortened and there is volar and ulnar angulation at the fracture site. This may be due to comminution dorsally at the time of fracture or erosion at the fracture site due to motion between the fragments.[36] In this situation, once reduction is obtained, there will be a dorsal gap as well as a larger volar defect. Therefore, a trapezoid-shaped graft is trimmed to fit snugly in the defect with the cortical surface anterior. The graft is then placed and two 0.045-in Kirschner wires are driven from the scaphoid tuberosity through the distal pole across the graft and into the proximal pole (Fig. 34–6). If the proximal fragment is very small or has to be extensively curetted because of avascularity, we attempt to place the wires into the lunate to improve fixation. Stability is checked by observing the fracture site while manipulating the wrist. Radiographs are then taken in the anteroposterior and lateral planes to check alignment and pin placement. An above-elbow U-shaped splint is applied incorporating the thumb for five to seven days. This is then changed to a short above-elbow thumb spica with the wrist in neutral position for six weeks, with the cast changed every two to three weeks. If necessary, a short arm cast including the entire thumb is continued for six to nine more weeks until solid union is established by radiographs. This cast is also changed every two to three weeks.

Internal Fixation. The indications for internal fixation have been mentioned and include displaced acute fractures, fractures associated with transscaphoid perilunate fracture, dislocation, delayed union, or nonunion when bone grafting is insufficient to provide adequate internal fixation. A relative indication is inability to tolerate long-term cast immobilization. The internal fixation techniques described include Kirschner wires,

screws,[21,42,57,58,71,85] and staples,[141] although the latter have not achieved much popularity and are not in general use. Small AO screws have been used for many years, but the reported results have been variable.[42,71,85]

Most recently, the Herbert screw system has attracted attention and is being used by several authors[17,122] with encouraging preliminary results. This device consists of a smooth shaft with threads at both ends with differing pitch. As the screw is advanced, compression is obtained across the fracture site by putting greater pitch in the leading end threads than the trailing end threads. There is no head on the screw so the end is countersunk under the cartilage. When the procedure is completed, both ends of the screw are buried and do not interfere with joint motion; thus the screw need not be removed. It has been shown that stable internal fixation is provided by this device. In comparison with Kirschner wires, however, the technique is demanding and unforgiving. Further, it is necessary to traumatize the scaphotrapezial joint to insert the jig. As noted, very small proximal or distal avascular fragments are not suitable for fixation with a screw. Herbert's reported results in his original 1984 paper[57] were excellent for acute fractures and delayed union, with sound union on radiography achieved in 30 of 33 patients (91%). He had an 80% success rate in nonunion cases (21 failures out of a total of 105). Thus in established nonunion cases, the Matti-Russe procedure with an 85% union rate reported by several authors[25,50,84,116] over the last 25 years is at least comparable. The proposed advantage of the Herbert screw is

Figure 34–7

The Herbert screw insertion technique. *A,* The pilot drill for the trailing end of the screw. *B,* The long drill for the leading end of the screw. *C,* The tap for the leading end of the screw. *D,* Inserting the screw. *E,* The screw in use, with a corticocancellous wedge graft to retain scaphoid alignment. (From Herbert, T.J.; Fisher, W.E. J Bone Joint Surg 66B:114–123, 1984.)

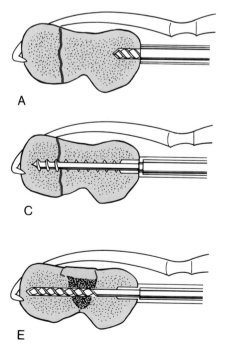
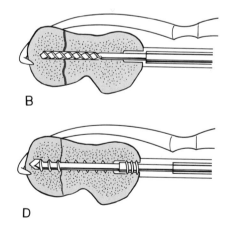

A

B

C

D

E

shorter immobilization time. Herbert recommends an average of four weeks in plaster. Although further experience with the Herbert screw will ultimately determine its place in the surgeon's armamentarium, at present it appears to be an excellent alternative in acute displaced fractures and fracture-dislocations when the prognosis is poor with closed treatment and Kirschner wires may not provide adequate fixation.

Technique (Modified Herbert).[57] A volar radial approach similar to that in the Russe technique is used and extended distally beyond the tuberosity of the scaphoid (Figs. 34–7; 34–8*A,B*). The superficial branch of the radial artery is ligated and divided and the scaphotrapezial joint is opened transversely. The fracture is then opened and the ends prepared by removing all sclerotic bone and fibrous tissue. If this leaves a large defect, a wedge-shaped corticocancellous graft is cut from the outer aspect of the iliac crest and inserted. The Herbert jig is then placed with the hook around the proximal pole of the scaphoid. The barrel is placed on the distal pole and the jig is clamped into place. Jig placement is both critical and difficult, with the most common error being placement too near the anterior surface of the scaphoid. To prevent this, it is important to place the proximal hook around to the dorsal surface of the proximal pole.[17] A second reported error is insufficient dissection of the scaphotrapezial joint, which

prevents proper placement of the jig barrel as far dorsal as possible.[17] Sometimes, removing bone from the anterior surface of the trapezium is necessary. If this configuration is unstable or difficult to align, we have found it helpful to place a Kirschner wire through both fragments and the graft (if any) before clamping the jig into place. Radiographs are taken to confirm proper alignment of the wrist, scaphoid, and jig. The large diameter drill is used, followed by the smaller one. The tap for the distal threads is used, followed by the proper length screw as read off the jig. The screw is then placed, and the jig is removed (Fig. 34–7). Stability is checked by moving the wrist and checking the fracture site. Closure is accomplished in layers and a U-shaped above-elbow splint applied. At 10 to 14 days the splint is taken off and sutures are removed. Herbert allows motion and a removable splint at this point until healing is complete by radiograph. If a bone graft is used, a short arm cast is applied for four to six weeks postoperatively. In the acute fracture or fracture-dislocation, we have found it technically easier and less traumatic to use a dorsal approach and reverse the screw direction using a Kirschner wire as a guide pin to ensure proper placement and length of the screw. The jig is not used for this approach (Fig. 34–8 *A,B*).

Salvage Procedures. If the decision is made not to attempt to achieve union of the scaphoid, there are

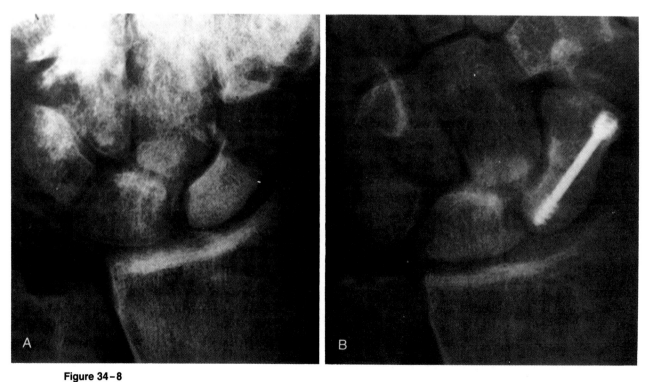

Figure 34–8

A, A preoperative x-ray film of a scaphoid waist fracture. *B,* Postoperatively, the fracture fixed with a Herbert screw.

several alternatives. It should be emphasized that these procedures are indicated after failure of primary treatment, which in most cases will have been an operative attempt to gain union. Given the high rate of success in obtaining union with bone grafting techniques, these methods are necessary in relatively few patients.

Bentzon's Procedure.[9] The rationale for the creation of a painless pseudarthrosis of the scaphoid is the assumption that the pain in nonunited scaphoid fractures is primarily due to the nonunion itself. A painless pseudarthrosis is obtained by introducing a soft tissue flap from the dorsoradial aspect of the wrist capsule into the fracture site. Boeckstyns[12] has reported the results on 26 patients with a mean follow-up of 27 years. Radiographs were available for 20 of these patients. Fifteen patients had no pain, eight had occasional pain, and three had moderate pain. Carpal collapse was present in 15 patients with dorsal intercalated segment instability pattern on radiography. Osteoarthritis was seen in seven patients. This procedure has not been popular outside of Scandinavia and is recommended by its namesake for its minor operative morbidity in patients with failed attempts at union. In our opinion, the Bentzon procedure is a good demonstration of the contention that the pain from scaphoid nonunion is due primarily to the nonunion. However, as the progression of arthritis shows, this technique does not restore normal wrist kinematics, and it may be important to do so to prevent radiocarpal arthritis. We have no experience with this procedure.

Radial Styloidectomy. This procedure may be indicated as an adjunct to bone grafting or internal fixation especially when there is osteoarthritis of the articulation between the distal pole and the radial styloid. The excised bone can be used as the graft, and its removal does provide increased exposure of the scaphoid if a radial approach is used. Of course, radial styloidectomy by itself does nothing for the scaphoid nonunion, and if the nonunion is the source of the patient's pain, other measures will have to be undertaken. If one is overzealous in performing radial styloidectomy, the wrist can be destabilized by detaching the origins of the radial scaphocapitate and radial lunate ligaments.[10] There have been no long-term follow-up reports demonstrating the efficacy of this procedure and we do not favor its routine use as an isolated procedure.

Proximal Row Carpectomy. For the patient who is not a suitable candidate for long periods of immobilization and has a low demand wrist or whose fracture has failed to heal after bone graft, excision of the proximal carpal row is an option. We prefer this in the older patient, although several authors have reported good results in young manual laborers.[51,60,62,90,96,123,125] Unfortunately, radiocarpal arthritis or capitate arthritis is

a contraindication to this procedure. The pattern of arthritis in longstanding scaphoid nonunion is first radius–distal scaphoid pole and then capitate head–proximal scaphoid pole.[115]

Green[51] has reported his personal series of proximal row carpectomies in 15 patients with an average age of 34. Follow-up was from 6 months to 6 years, averaging 30 months. Of these 15 patients, 2 had severe pain, 3 had moderate pain, 6 had mild discomfort, and 4 had no pain. Twelve patients returned to their previous or heavier work as compared to preoperatively. Range of motion in 13 patients was 39° dorsiflexion, 40° palmar flexion, 31° ulnar deviation, and 5° radial deviation. Strength averaged 83.5% of the opposite side in the dominant wrist in seven patients, and 41% of the opposite side in nondominant wrists in six patients. Therefore, Green concludes, quoting McLaughlin and Baab,[90] that "whenever motion, even at the price of some weakness and discomfort, is preferable to a strong, painless but stiff wrist," proximal row carpectomy should be considered as an alternative to wrist arthrodesis. We have limited experience with this procedure since very few of our patients have normal capitate articular surfaces after failed treatment for scaphoid nonunion.

TECHNIQUE. (Fig. 34–9*A,B*). To perform this operation use a longitudinal straight dorsal skin incision centered over Lister's tubercle. Unless indicated, do not expose the fourth compartment extensors but enter the wrist by exposing the extensor pollicis longus tendon, retract it radialward, osteotomizing Lister's tubercle and incising the periosteum of the distal radius and joint capsule in one layer. These layers are elevated radially and ulnarly as far as necessary to expose the entire carpus deep to all the other extensor tendons. The lunate and triquetrum are then removed. Using a curved ¼-in osteotome as a knife to divide the ligaments facilitates this dissection. We usually remove only the proximal two-thirds of the scaphoid unless there is impingement at the radial styloid on the distal remnant. The head of the capitate is then seated in the lunate facet. If there is instability, a 0.062-in Kirschner wire is driven transarticularly and kept in place for the first three to four weeks postoperatively. The wound is closed in layers over a drain, which is removed after 24 to 48 hours. A splint is applied for the first week until swelling subsides, followed by a short arm cast for four to six weeks. Finger motion is begun and encouraged immediately postoperatively.

There are a few points that deserve emphasis. First, if there are significant articular changes at the head of the capitate or the lunate facet of the radius, this procedure is contraindicated. Second, if there is impingement at the distal one third of the scaphoid on the radial styloid,

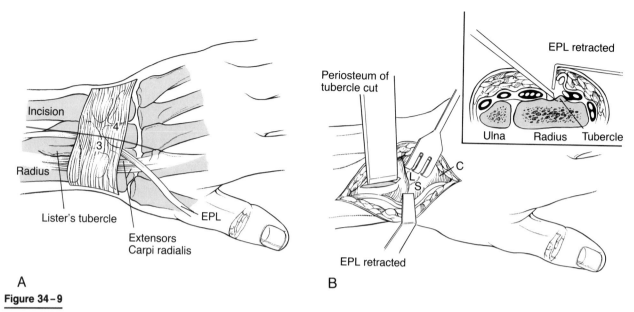

Figure 34-9

A and *B*, Schematic demonstration of a dorsal approach to the wrist for intercarpal arthrodesis. 3 = third dorsal compartment (EPL); 4 = fourth dorsal compartment (EDC); L = lunate; S = scaphoid; C = capitate. (Redrawn from Weil, C.; Ruby, L.K. J Hand Surg 11A:911–912, 1986.)

the distal portion of the scaphoid should be removed. If there is still impingement, a limited radial styloidectomy should be done. Third, it is important to preserve the radiocapitate ligament as this is the sole retaining structure to keep the carpus from displacing ulnaward.

Arthrodesis. Both partial and complete arthrodesis have been recommended for patients who have persistent nonunion, severe arthritis, or extensive avascular necrosis with collapse. Limited arthrodesis has been proposed for the radial scapholunate joint[18,134] when there is persistent nonunion and radioscaphoid arthritis. When arthritis is present only at the scaphocapitate joint or there is extensive sclerosis of the scaphoid fragments, Sutro[129] and Helfet[56] have suggested scaphocapitate fusion. We have no experience with these techniques and prefer total radiocarpal and midcarpal arthrodesis (though not including the carpometacarpal joints) for these patients.

TECHNIQUE. A straight longitudinal oblique incision is made centered over Lister's tubercle. The extensor pollicus longus tendon is mobilized, retracted radially and the tubercle is osteotomized. The capsule of the wrist and periosteum over the distal radius is incised and these layers are elevated subperiosteally to avoid exposing the fourth or fifth compartment extensor tendons. At this point, decorticate all joint surfaces to be fused using the power burr. We do not routinely include the carpometacarpal joints or the scaphotrapezial-trapezoid joints. Two or three parallel 3/32-in Steinmann pins are placed from the radius into the carpus. Cancellous bone graft is inserted from the

ileum and packed tightly into the joint spaces (Fig. 34–10A,B). Alternatively, if grafting is not desired, one can use a dorsal compression plate from the radius into the third metacarpal. The wound is closed in layers over a drain. A splint is applied for the first week followed by a short arm cast until radiographs show consolidation, which usually takes six weeks. A personal series of 28 patients attained 75% of normal grip strength and were pain-free at an average follow-up of four years postoperatively.

Special Situations

PROXIMAL POLE FRACTURES. Vascular studies by Gelberman and Menon[44] and Taleisnik and Kelly[137] have established that fractures through the proximal one-third of the scaphoid have a high likelihood of devascularizing the proximal fragment since most of the blood supply enters the bone distal to this level. The proximal pole is covered almost entirely with cartilage and has a poor blood supply apart from its connection to the rest of the scaphoid. Nonetheless, if seen early, these fractures can be treated nonoperatively with a cast until the outcome is obvious. The patient is cautioned that the fracture has a significant chance of nonunion. If nonunion or delayed union does occur, we recommend a cancellous bone graft through a volar approach (Matti-Russe technique). It is particularly important in such areas to perform a thorough and aggressive curettement of the proximal pole to bleeding cancellous bone if present or subchondral bone if not. This is followed by tight packing with cancellous graft (Matti technique). The same surgical treatment is rec-

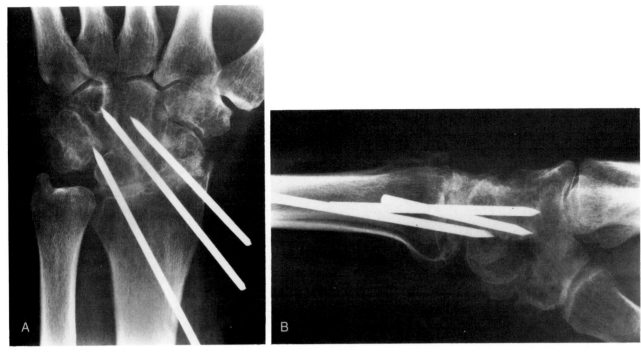

Figure 34-10

Anteroposterior (A) and lateral (B) x-ray films of wrist arthrodesis demonstrating the placement of parallel Steinmann pins.

ommended for avascular necrosis of the proximal pole if there is no collapse or significant arthritis, in spite of limited success in others' experience.[50]

In the setting of collapse of the proximal pole, significant arthritis, or a failed bone graft, several options are available. One can either repeat the bone graft or perform an excision of the proximal fragment with or without replacement with either a tendon[32] or a silicone spacer.[148] According to Zemel and colleagues,[148] 20 of 21 (95%) of these patients had a good clinical result at an average of five years postoperatively, although all patients showed some increase in the scapholunate angle and wrist collapse. No silicone synovitis was reported. We feel that this experience is evidence that the pain in the presence of a scaphoid nonunion is usually due to the nonunion. Therefore any procedure that deals with this aspect of the problem should be effective in achieving some degree of pain relief as evidenced in the Bentzon procedure. However, the altered wrist mechanics will inevitably cause arthiritis later, which may prove symptomatic. To this must be added the now well-known risk of silicone synovitis.[120] We have been reluctant to perform proximal pole excision based upon concern for scapholunate dissociation due to the necessary loss of the stabilizing effect of the scapholunate ligament. We therefore prefer a limited or complete wrist arthodesis as a salvage for failed bone graft of a proximal pole nonunion.

DISTAL POLE FRACTURES. These are often avulsion injuries of the tuberosity and can be expected to heal promptly with cast treatment. Distal third fractures of the body of the scaphoid, if fresh and undisplaced, should heal in four to eight weeks according to Russe.[116] A fracture that is difficult to diagnose is the distal pole vertical intraarticular fracture, which may show only on polytomography or CT scan. If undisplaced, these should be treated with a cast; if displaced, open reduction and internal fixation should be performed.

AUTHOR'S PREFERRED APPROACH. For the acute undisplaced fracture, an above-elbow cast including the thumb tip with the wrist in neutral position is applied for six weeks and changed at two to three week intervals. Radiographs are taken at six weeks, and if solid union is not evident, a short arm cast is applied and changed every two to three weeks until a total of three to four months have elapsed. Radiologic examination is done at three to four week intervals until solid union is evident and confirmed by polytomography or CT in questionable cases.

For the acute displaced fracture, open reduction and internal fixation are performed with either a Herbert bone screw or Kirschner wires through the dorsal approach.

For delayed union or nonunion of the undisplaced fracture, cancellous or corticocancellous bone grafting is done through an anterior approach. For displaced nonunion, open reduction is performed through an anterior approach with a wedge or trapezoidal shaped corticocancellous graft with or without internal fixation.

For a failed bone graft, total intercarpal arthrodesis, including scaphoid to capitate to lunate to triquetrum to hamate, is done.

For a symptomatic longstanding nonunion with significant osteoarthritis (usually not present until 10 years after the injury), the preferred salvage procedure is total wrist arthrodesis. If the arthritis is not particularly symptomatic, no surgery may be necessary.

Kienböck's Disease

Ever since Kienböck's original description of lunatomalacia (soft lunate) in 1910[64] the precise etiology and treatment have eluded the best efforts of many investigators.[43] By definition, Kienböck's disease is radiologic avascular necrosis of the lunate. It is well accepted that avascularity of the lunate is a part of the process, but whether the cause or the result of trauma or fracture is uncertain. Unfortunately, the clinician and patient are often faced with the necessity of treating what is often a painful and disabling condition.

Etiology

The loss of the blood supply to the lunate has been attributed to primary fracture,[7] repetitive trauma causing microfracture,[33,43] and traumatic injury to the ligaments that carry blood to the lunate.[64] In addition, Taleisnick has shown that not all fractures lead to avascular changes and that these fractures can heal with closed treatment.[135] It was noted by Hulten[59] in 1928 that there was a statistical association among patients whose ulna appeared shorter than the radius on a PA radiograph of the wrist (Fig. 34–11). This has been termed an ulnar negative variant. If the distal articular surface of the ulna is longer than the radius, this is an ulnar positive variant. An ulnar neutral variant exists if the articular surfaces of the radius and ulna are at the same level. Razemon[111] felt that because the radial part of the lunate is supported by the radius and the ulnar part rests on the compliant triangular fibrocartilage, shear stresses are created within the bone making it more susceptible to fracture. Thus, ulnar minus variance is thought to be etiologically related to Kienböck's disease by some authors.[59,105,111] It is likely that the cause of Kienböck's disease is multifactorial and that stress in combination with a precarious blood supply plays a role in some patients.[135]

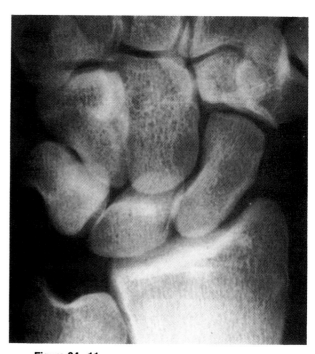

Figure 34–11

X-ray film showing a wrist with ulnar negative variance.

Diagnosis

By definition, the diagnosis is a radiologic one. Very early in the course the lunate may appear normal, but with time, one sees the typical pattern of sclerosis, loss of lunate height, fragmentation, and eventually wrist collapse and arthritis. Clinically, the physician can be suspicious if the patient is a young adult with central dorsal wrist pain and tenderness, swelling, loss of motion, and diminished grip strength. If there is clinical suspicion without radiographic findings, technetium bone scan or magnetic resonance imaging can be helpful. The presence of ulnar negative variance should raise the possibility of Kienböck's disease. Fractures, usually occurring in the coronal plane, are best seen on polytomography or CT scans.

Treatment

That there is no universally accepted treatment for Kienböck's disease is reflected by the large number of treatment options.[135] Nevertheless, some treatments are applied more commonly to this problem than others, and it is these that will be described.

Cast immobilization is no longer considered a useful method for treatment of Kienböck's disease.[124] In 1980, Beckenbaugh[7] discussed the natural history in 38 patients and came to the conclusion that operative treatment was better than cast immobilization. It appears at present that the modality selected should be based to some degree on the radiologic stage of the process. Both Stahl[124] and Lichtman[72] have proposed classifications. It is generally agreed that stage I represents slight sclerosis; stage II, sclerosis and fragmentation without collapse; stage III, fragmentation with collapse; and stage IV, fragmentation, collapse, and arthritis (Fig. 34–12). Most treatment modalities are based on stress reduction (unloading), revascularization, or replacement of the lunate. In addition, there

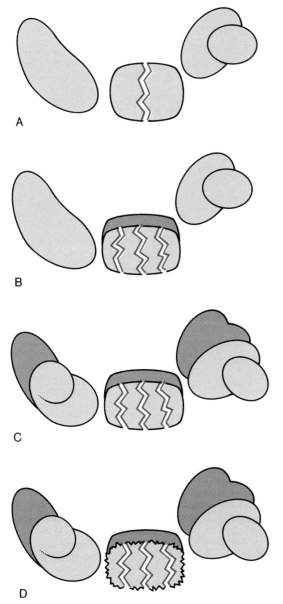

Figure 34–12

Illustration of the four stages of Kienböck's disease. *A*, Stage 1: sclerosis of the lunate; *B*, stage 2: sclerosis and fragmentation; *C*, stage 3: sclerosis and collapse; *D*, stage 4: sclerosis, collapse, and intercarpal arthritis. (From Taleisnik, J. The Wrist. Churchill Livingstone, 1985, p.190, by permission.)

are various combinations and, of course, salvage procedures. For stage I disease, treatment options include no treatment, cast application, unloading surgery, or open reduction if there is a recognized fracture. For stage II, unloading procedures, revascularization, and lunate excision with replacement or combinations have been advocated. For stage III, the same options apply, although most authors state that the prognosis is worse. For stage IV, salvage procedures such as wrist fusion or proximal row carpectomy are recommended for the sufficiently symptomatic patient.

A review of most current literature as well as the author's experience indicates that without treatment, progressive deterioration of the lunate and consequent wrist degeneration are the most likely outcome.[7] In addition, a lunate excision with silicone rubber replacement alone has been shown to involve significant complications, including dislocation of the prosthesis, progressive collapse of the carpus,[4] and silicone synovitis.[120] Therefore, for stages I, II, and III, we prefer unloading procedures, which include radial shortening,[105] ulnar lengthening,[4] and limited intercarpal arthrodesis.[23,143] Each of these has its advocates.

Almquist[3] has summarized the results of seven series, including his own, in which 69 of 79 patients achieved a successful clinical result with radial shortening.

Radial Shortening (Almquist)

A volar approach is performed at the junction of the middle and distal one third of the radius. A six-hole 3.5-mm dynamic compression plate is selected. Two screws are placed distally and the radius is marked for both rotational alignment and the proposed osteotomy. The plate is then removed and a predetermined section of radius is removed between the third and fourth screw holes to level the radial and ulnar articular surfaces. The plate is then replaced and the remainder of the screws placed. Almquist suggests that this procedure be used only for patients who have "no significant collapse" (i.e., stage I or II) and of course an ulnar negative variance.

Ulnar lengthening was originally described by Persson in 1950[105] because of problems with radius healing after shortening osteotomy. Armistead and Linscheid[4] have reported their experience with this technique and advocate its use in stage II and early stage III patients. They report good results in two series of patients, the second series consisting of 22 patients.[77] There was one failure, and three patients were lost to follow-up.

More time and experience will be necessary to define the role of "joint leveling" in the management of Kienböck's disease. In an editorial in the Journal of Hand

Surgery in 1985,[76] Linscheid sounded a cautionary note regarding joint leveling procedures based on his experience of increased wear and degeneration on the ulnar aspect of the lunate, the triangular fibrocartilage, and the triquetrum postoperatively.

Another unloading technique that has several advocates[23,142] is "limited" intercarpal arthrodesis. This procedure in theory limits the load on the lunate by transmitting it through the fused carpal bones. Watson[143] recommends scaphoid-trapezial-trapezoid arthrodesis, while Chuinard advocates capitate-hamate arthrodesis,[23] and Almquist has described a capitate shortening in conjunction with a capitohamate fusion.[3] All these procedures attempt to decrease the normal load on the lunate by transferring it to the other bones of the proximal carpal row. Trumble and co-workers[138] in an in vitro study have shown that the capitate-hamate fusion was not effective in decreasing lunate load. The joint leveling procedures, scaphoid-trapezium-trapezoid fusion, and scaphoid-capitate fusion were effective in reducing the lunate loading but resulted in significant decrease in range of motion. Again, Linscheid[76] cautions that limited wrist arthrodesis alters wrist kinematics extensively and may contribute to later arthritis.

For late stage III patients, a total intercarpal arthrodesis without excision of the lunate can be attempted. We prefer this to scaphoid-trapezium-trapezoid fusion since it is technically easier and the loss of wrist motion is not substantially greater.

Technique (Total Intercarpal Arthrodesis). Using a dorsal wrist approach, the intercarpal joints are denuded to cancellous bone using a power burr. The wrist is then distracted so as to correct the collapse deformity, and 0.054 or 0.062-in Kirschner wires are driven across the scaphocapitate, triquetrohamate, and capitate joints. Cancellous bone harvested from the iliac crest is packed tightly into the defects. The wrist is closed in layers and a U-shaped above-elbow splint applied. The splint is changed to a solid short above-elbow cast at one to two weeks and the sutures removed. The cast is removed at six to eight weeks and healing checked by radiography. If solid, the pins are removed and motion begun.

For stage IV disease, we prefer total radiocarpal and midcarpal arthrodesis. If the radius and capitate articular surfaces are intact, a proximal row carpectomy can be considered. Approximately 70% of patients will obtain adequate pain relief, motion, and strength with proximal row carpectomy.

Fractures of the Capitate

Fractures of the capitate are relatively rare, comprising 0.8% of 826 carpal injuries reported by Bohler,[13] yet they are often associated with unsatisfactory outcomes.[110] The association of a capitate fracture with a scaphoid fracture has been termed the scaphocapitate syndrome. The etiology of this lesion is hyperdorsiflexion of the wrist. The fracture occurs through the waist of the scaphoid and the neck of the capitate. The head of the capitate and the proximal fragment of scaphoid may rotate together, and unless reduced, the capitate

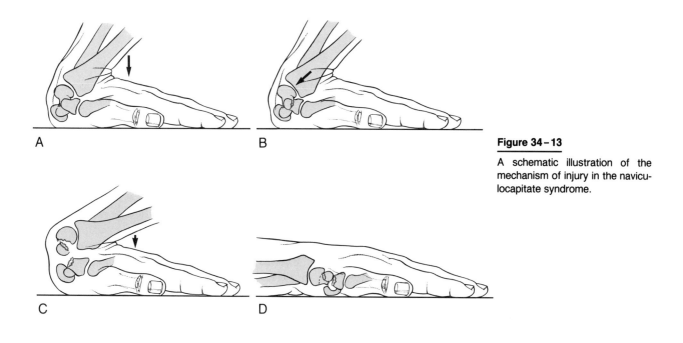

A   B

C   D

Figure 34-13

A schematic illustration of the mechanism of injury in the naviculocapitate syndrome.

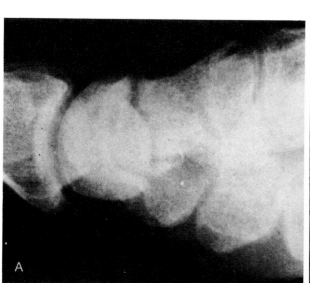
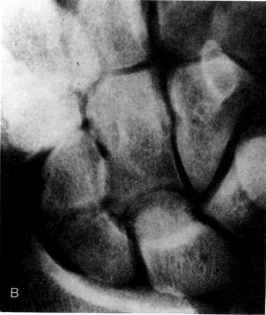

Figure 34–14

A, A lateral x-ray film of the carpus, demonstrating a naviculocapitate syndrome with the proximal pole of the capitate rotated 180° and the articular surface facing the fracture site. *B*, An anteroposterior view of the wrist demonstrating the naviculocapitate syndrome with the proximal pole of the capitate rotated. (From Monahan, P.R.W.; Galasto, C.S.B. J Bone Joint Surg 54B:122–124, 1972.)

will not unite. The head of the capitate can rotate 180° with the articular surface of the proximal pole facing the fracture surface of the distal pole. This is thought to occur when the dorsal ridge of the radius impinges on the dorsal aspect of the capitate, fracturing it at the neck junction. The wrist then continues to hyperdorsiflex and the distal pole of the capitate continues to dorsally displace on the proximal pole by presenting the fracture surface of the proximal pole to the articular surface of the proximal pole (Fig. 34–13). When the wrist is placed back in flexion, the proximal pole is rotated 180° so that its fracture surface comes to lie adjacent to the articular surface of the lunate. This is a difficult diagnosis to make and must be looked for carefully on radiographs (Fig. 34–14*A,B*). Once the diagnosis is made, open reduction and internal fixation must be performed.[16,35]

Isolated fractures of the capitate at the waist may also occur. If undisplaced, cast treatment should be adequate. Avascular necrosis of the proximal pole is a possible outcome just as it is in the proximal pole scaphoid fracture. The blood supply to the proximal pole of the capitate is derived exclusively from the intraosseous supply from the distal portion.[139] Some authors have recommended excision of the avascular proximal fragment and fusion to the scaphoid and lunate.[16]

Fractures of the Hamate

Fractures of the body of the hamate are uncommon and are often associated with fourth and fifth carpometacarpal fracture-dislocations. If undisplaced, closed treatment is used. If displaced or unstable, either closed reduction with percutaneous Kirschner wire pinning of the joint or open reduction and internal fixation should be performed. Only five cases of isolated hamate body fractures have been reported. Open reduction and internal fixation are recommended when there is displacement of the fragment.[98]

Hook of the hamate fractures are more common and have attracted attention in the literature as they are a significant and often missed source of disability.[22,126] They are especially common in golfers, and tennis, racquetball, and baseball players. The injury is thought to occur when the proximal end of the club or racquet strikes the hamate hook[126] in hitting an unyielding surface such as the ground or floor. The physician should suspect the diagnosis if the patient has deep, ill-defined pain in the volar ulnar half of the palm after such an injury. Other physical findings are tenderness over the hook of the hamate, ulnar nerve symptoms, and occasionally flexor tendon rupture.[28] Radiographs will

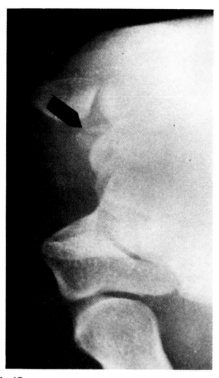

Figure 34 – 15

X-ray film of the carpal tunnel, demonstrating a split fracture of the hook of the hamate. Lateral tomography and oblique x-ray films would possibly not show this fracture. (From Carter, P.R., et al. J Bone Joint Surg 59A:583–588, 1977.)

show this fracture if they are taken in the correct plane, which may be difficult to do. Carpal tunnel views and 45° supination obliques may be helpful (Fig. 34–15). If these are not definitive, then polytomography or CT scans should be used. The generally agreed upon treatment is excision of the fractured hook.[22,126]

Technique

Make a short longitudinal palmar incision directly over the hook. Be careful to identify and protect the motor branch of the ulnar nerve, which lies just ulnar to the hook. Continue the dissection subperiosteally until the fracture site is encountered and remove the fractured fragment. Smooth the base of the fracture and close the periosteum over the raw surface. A splint is applied for one to two weeks until the patient is comfortable and gradual resumption of activities is allowed as tolerated. A padded glove may be helpful for the first four weeks after initiating grip activities.

Fractures of the Triquetrum

Isolated fractures of the triquetrum are the third most common carpal fracture after those of the scaphoid and lunate but do not usually cause symptoms in and of themselves. The most common type is probably a shear or chisel fracture caused by impingement of the ulnar

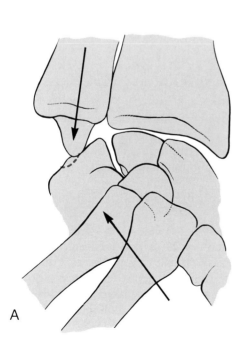

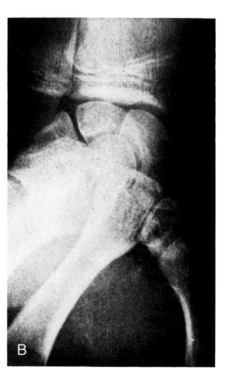

Figure 34 – 16

A, Diagram demonstrating the proposed mechanism of the "chisel" fracture of the triquetrum. The *arrow* along the ulna represents the weight of the torso; the *oblique arrow* represents the ground force during a fall with the wrist in dorsiflexion and ulnar deviation. *B,* An x-ray film demonstrating a chisel fracture of the triquetrum. (From Levy, M., et al. J Bone Joint Surg 61B:355–357, 1979.)

styloid on the dorsal proximal aspect of the triquetrum when the wrist is forcibly dorsiflexed and ulnarly deviated (Fig. 34–16A,16B). This is seen as a flake of bone on the lateral radiograph. Symptomatic closed treatment with a cast for 4 to 6 weeks is all that is usually required. The flake can be excised if symptomatic. If the much rarer body fracture occurs, this too can be treated by closed means if undisplaced, or if displaced, by open reduction and internal fixation. Avascular necrosis has never been reported.

Fractures of the Trapezium

Isolated trapezium fractures are uncommon injuries, occurring in about 5% of all carpal fractures.[26] There are two types. The first type is that of the body of the bone. These are either vertical in orientation or crush type with comminution. Since these are intraarticular, either open reduction and internal fixation or traction methods can be used for treatment.[15,26]

The second type is the trapezial ridge fracture. These rare injuries[101] result either from a direct blow as in a fall on the outstretched hand or from an avulsion of the flexor retinaculum when the palm contacts a hard surface and the transverse arch is forcibly spread. Diagnosis is suspected by joint tenderness and confirmed by carpal tunnel views or tomography. One must have a high index of suspicion since routine views will not show this fracture (Fig. 34–17). Treatment depends on the location of the fracture. If it is at the tip (type II), a cast for three to six weeks molding the first ray into abduction is sufficient. If it is at the base (type I), early excision of the fracture fragment is recommended since it frequently goes on to nonunion. If either type results in a painful nonunion, then excision should be performed as for ununited hook of the hamate fractures.[101] The results of excision are variable.

Fractures of the Pisiform

These too are relatively uncommon, comprising 1 to 3% of all carpal bone injuries. Approximately one-half are associated with fractures of the distal radius, hamate, or triquetrum. Diagnosis is suggested by local pain and tenderness and a history of a direct blow to the pisiform. A 30° supination oblique radiograph or CT or polytomographic views are confirmatory. Treatment is by short arm cast in 30° of wrist flexion and ulnar deviation for six weeks. If painful nonunion develops, the pisiform is approached through a longitudinal splitting of the flexor carpi ulnaris. Careful subperiosteal excision should be performed with repair of

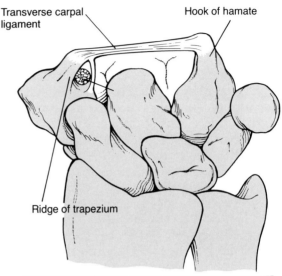

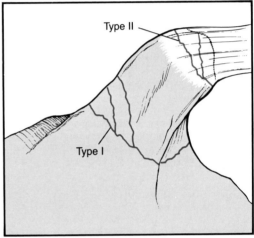

Figure 34–17

Diagram of type I (base) and type II (tip) fractures of the trapezial ridge. (From Palmer, A.K. J Hand Surg 6:561–564, 1981.)

the flexor carpi ulnaris tendon. One should not confuse the presence of an irregular ossification center in the immature patient for a fracture.[15,16]

Dislocation of the Carpus

GENERAL CONSIDERATIONS

Functional Anatomy

The wrist may be thought of as a mechanical system whose function is to provide motion to and transmit force between the hand distally and the forearm proximally. In order to accomplish the seemingly contradictory functions of mobility and stability with minimal bulk, the wrist has evolved into a complex of joints between seven bones (the pisiform is a sesamoid for the flexor carpi ulnaris) linked to each other by a complicated set of ligaments. It is the bony and ligamentous geometry that allows this unique joint complex to successfully provide for motion and force transmission. At present there are two major theories of wrist function.

Row Theory. This theory can be summarized as follows: the wrist consists of three proximal (scaphoid, lunate, triquetrum) and four distal (trapezium, trapezoid, capitate, hamate) row bones (Fig. 34–18). This arrangement creates two major joints, the radiocarpal and the midcarpal. The scaphoid, which bridges the two rows, provides a stabilizing link for the midcarpal joints.[30,35,37,79,114] The proximal row is an intercalated segment between the distal row and the radius–triangular fibrocartilage (TFC) proximally.[30,35,114] Although composed of rigid elements, the proximal row changes its external configuration by allowing motion between the scaphoid, lunate, and triquetrum, thus providing congruency in all wrist positions. Compressive forces are thought to be transmitted from the distal row to the intercalated segment proximal row and then to the radius-TFC. In Weber's opinion, most of the

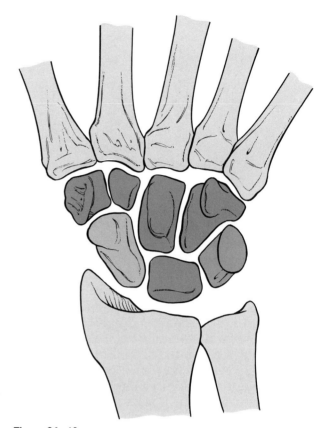

Figure 34–19

The columnar theory of the carpal anatomy. (Redrawn from Lichtman, D.M., et al.: J Hand Surg 6:522, 1981.)

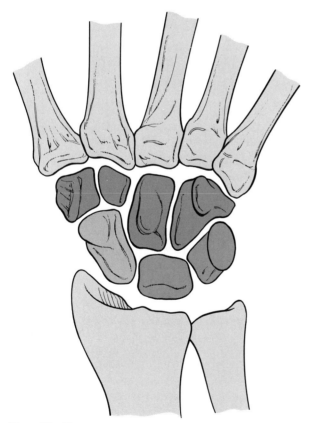

Figure 34–18

The row theory of carpal anatomy. (From Green, D.P. Operative Hand Surgery, Vol. 2. Churchill Livingstone, 1988, p. 876, by permission.)

force is transmitted from the second and third metacarpals to the trapezoid and capitate, then to the proximal two thirds of the scaphoid and lunate, and finally to the radius.[145] Palmer and Werner have shown that the amount of force transmitted to the radius is a function of ulnar variance.[104] Their studies have shown that in the ulnar negative variant wrist, 100% of force transmission is through the radius. In a wrist with positive ulnar variance, 70% of the force is transmitted through the radius, the remainder being borne by the TFC/ulnar head.

Columnar Theory. This theory depicts the carpus differently. According to Taleisnik,[132] who reintroduced and modified Navarro's theory,[95] the wrist consists of three columns (Fig. 34–19). The central column consists of the lunate proximally and the capitate and the rest of the distal row distally and is the primary flexion extension column. The mobile radial column is made up entirely of the scaphoid, and the ulnar or rotation column consists of the triquetrum. It is the author's opinion that the row theory best fits the available data.

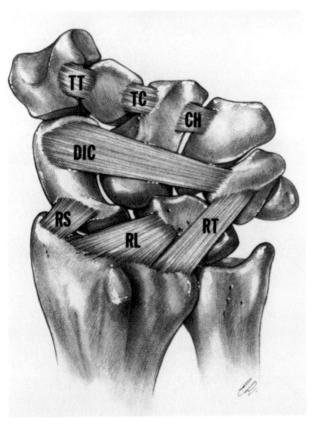

Figure 34-20

The extrinsic dorsal ligaments of the wrist. TT = trapeziotrapezoid; TC = trapeziocapitate; CH = capitohamate; DIC = dorsal intercarpal; RS = radioscaphoid; RL = radiolunate; RT = radiotriquetral. (Illustration by Elizabeth Roselius, © 1985. Reprinted with permission from Taleisnik, J. The Wrist. Churchill Livingstone, New York, 1985.)

Ligament Anatomy

The carpal bones are linked to each other and to the metacarpals and forearm by a complicated set of ligaments. Taleisnik[130] and Mayfield[86] and associates have studied this area extensively and their work forms the basis for our current understanding. In brief, there are three sets of ligaments: the dorsal capsular, volar capsular, and interosseous ligaments. The dorsal ligaments are relatively thin and are therefore not thought to be very important (Fig. 34-20). The volar ligaments are intracapsular and are best seen from inside the joint. They can be thought of as forming a V within a V with a weak area between them that overlies the capitolunate joint and is called the space of Poirier (Fig. 34-21A,B). The proximal V links the carpus to the forearm, and the distal V, or deltoid, ligament links the distal row to the proximal row and to the radius. The radioscaphocapitate ligament is the only ligament that spans both rows.

The most important of the volar ligaments are the radioscaphocapitate, the radiolunate, the radioscapholunate, the ulnolunate, and the ulnocarpal meniscus

homologue.[130] The distal V, or deltoid, ligament is composed of the scaphocapitate and triquetral-capitate ligaments. Collectively the volar ligaments are thought to be important in stabilizing the carpus with respect to the radius and ulna as well as stabilizing the midcarpal joint. It should be kept in mind that these ligaments are made up of thickenings of the volar wrist capsule and are difficult to identify as separate structures from the volar surface. The bones of the proximal row are further bound together by the scapholunate interosseous ligament and the lunate-triquetral interosseous ligament. The distal row bones are bound even more tightly by their interosseous ligaments. True collateral ligaments of the wrist probably do not exist as such and are represented by the tendon sheaths of the first dorsal extensor compartment and the sixth dorsal extensor compartment radially and ulnarly, respectively. There are also dorsal radiocarpal ligaments that can be summarized as the dorsal radiolunate triquetral and the dorsal intercarpal ligaments. The former may help stabilize the proximal row to the radius.

Wrist Kinematics

There is no general agreement on the exact amount of motion that occurs at the various carpal articulations.[114,117,145] This is because these motions are small in amplitude and occur primarily in rotation and are therefore very difficult to visualize by traditional means including radiography. While there is as yet no way to obtain precise measurements in vivo,[117] recent work on cadaver specimens has shed some light on this difficult area.[114] Total flexion and extension is made up approximately equally by motion at the midcarpal and radiocarpal joints. However, the midcarpal joint contributes more to flexion (62%) than the radiocarpal joint as the wrist moves from neutral to full flexion. Conversely, as the wrist moves from neutral to full extension the radiocarpal joint contributes more (62%) than the midcarpal joint. Further, wrist radial-ulnar deviation is contributed to by motion at the midcarpal and radiocarpal joints with the majority (55%) of this motion occurring at the midcarpal joint (Fig. 34-22). As the wrist moves from radial to ulnar deviation, the proximal row extends as well as deviates ulnarly. As the wrist moves from ulnar to radial deviation the proximal row flexes and deviates radially. The distal row also translates dorsally in ulnar deviation and volarly in radial deviation. This translation may be the cause of proximal row extension and flexion.[145] Simultaneously, there are small amplitude motions occurring between the bones of each row. All these motions are normally smooth and integrated, allowing total wrist motion to be synchronous and flowing.

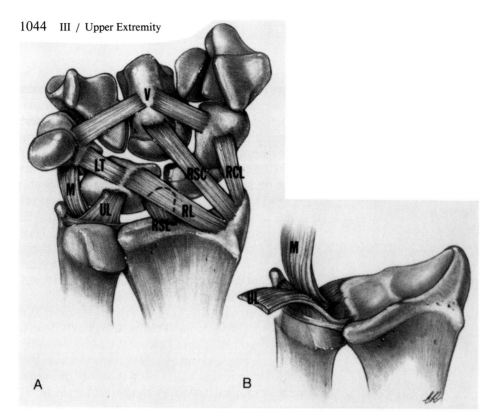

Figure 34–21

A, The extrinsic volar wrist ligaments; *B,* the ulnar carpal ligaments.   V = arcuate;   LT = lunate-triquetral; M = ulnar carpal meniscus homologue; UL = ulnolunate; RSL = radioscapholunate; RL = radiolunate;   RSC = radioscaphocapitate; RCL = radial collateral. (Illustration by Elizabeth Roselius, © 1985. Reprinted with permission from Taleisnik, J. The Wrist. Churchill Livingstone, New York 1985.)

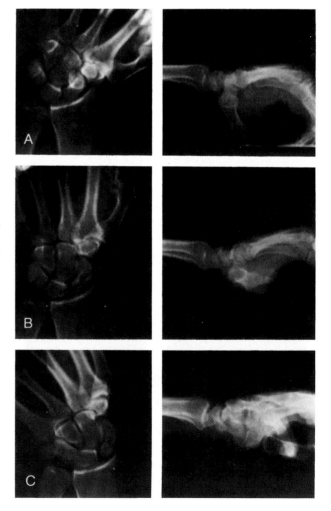

Figure 34–22

A, In radial deviation, the proximal carpal row deviates toward the radius, translates toward the ulna, and flexes as seen by visualizing the lunate on the lateral x-ray film. *B,* With the wrist in neutral, the capitate, lunate, and radius are nearly colinear. *C,* In ulnar deviation, the proximal row deviates toward the ulna, translates toward the radius, and extends as visualized by the lunate on the lateral x-ray film.

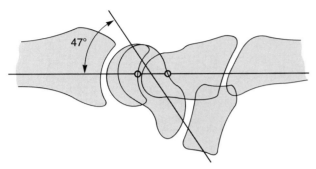

Figure 34-23

The normal scapholunate angle as represented in the original drawings from Linscheid and co-workers. (From Linscheid, R.L., et al. J Bone Joint Surg 54A:1612-1632, 1972.)

Because the primary wrist motors all insert into the metacarpals, all wrist motion is controlled by the bony configuration and ligamentous attachments of the carpals. The exact mechanism by which these displacements occur is not well established. Some authors feel that the triquetrohamate articulation exerts the major control,[145] while others feel that the scaphoid and its attachments are most important. At present, a descriptive analysis is the most that can be offered. In 1972 in a seminal article, Linscheid, and colleagues[79] described what was then known about carpal mechanics and emphasized the importance of the proximal row as an intercalated segment. They also pointed out some clinically useful radiographic measurements. In a true lateral radiograph of the normal wrist, the long axis of the scaphoid when measured against the long axis of the lunate was found to be 47° with a range of 30 to 60° (Fig. 34-23). Further, the radius, lunate, and capitate long axes are colinear or with slight volar flexion of the lunate. If the lunate is dorsiflexed with respect to the radius, dorsal intercalated segment instability (DISI) is said to exist (Fig. 34-24A). Conversely, if the lunate is palmar flexed with respect to the radius, then volar

intercalated segment instability (VISI) is said to be present (Fig. 34-24B). This nomenclature assumes that the lunate is representative of the proximal row and therefore the entire intercalated segment. These patterns (DISI and VISI) are commonly seen in clinically important wrist instabilities. Youm and Flatt[147] have defined carpal height as the distance between the base of the third metacarpal and the distal articular surface of the radius. They further defined the carpal height ratio as this distance divided by the length of the third metacarpal. A normal ratio is 0.54 ± 0.03 (Fig. 34-25). Thus, a wrist exhibiting longitudinal collapse DISI or VISI from whatever cause would have a decreased carpal height measurement and a decreased carpal height ratio.

Mechanism of Injury

Most clinically important carpal dislocations and fracture dislocations result from falls on the palm of the hand resulting in a hyperextension injury to the wrist. The exact amount of force and its direction of application as well as the strength and stiffness of the wrist structures will determine the precise nature of the injury. A very common pattern is one in which the distal row is displaced dorsal to the proximal row. For this to occur, there must be a failure of the connecting structures between the two rows, and this may be a scaphoid fracture or tear of the scapholunate and scaphoradial ligaments as occurs in a scapholunate disassociation. If the force is more extreme, a complete perilunate dislocation may occur wherein the energy of the injury is not dissipated until the capitolunate and triquetrohamate ligaments are torn as well.

An attempt to reproduce these mechanisms in vitro has been made by Mayfield and co-workers.[87] They loaded cadaver wrists to various degrees of destruction and demonstrated four stages of perilunate instability, which they termed progressive perilunate instability.

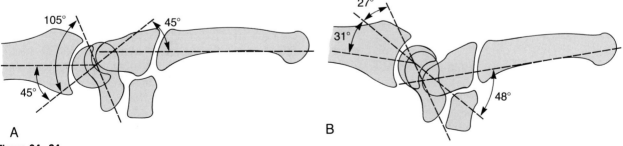

A   B

Figure 34-24

A, Dorsal intercalated segment instability. The scapholunate angle is high (105°), the capitolunate angle is high (45°), and the radiolunate angle is high (45°). The intercalated segment is represented by the lunate. *B,* Volar intercalated segment instability. The scapholunate angle is low (27°). (From Linscheid, R.L., et al. J Bone Joint Surg, 54A:1612-1632, 1972.)

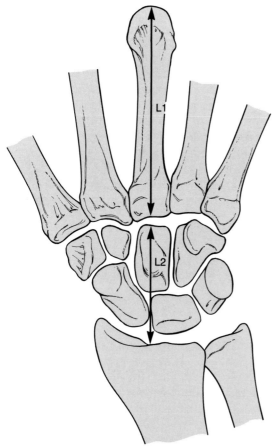

Figure 34-25

Measurement of the carpal height index: Distance (L2) from the radicarpal line to the base of the third metacarpal is divided by the length of the third metacarpal (L1). The normal index is 0.54 ± 0.3 mm. (Redrawn from Youm, Y; Flatt, A. Clin Orthop 149:21-32, 1980.)

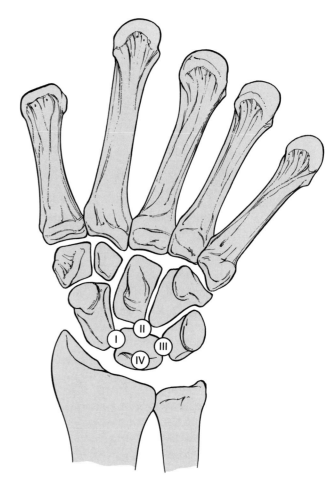

Figure 34-26

The pathomechanics and progressive perilunar instability pattern demonstrated by Mayfield and co-workers. I = scaphoid instability with respect to the lunate; II = scaphoid plus capitate instability with respect to the lunate; III = scaphoid plus capitate plus triquetrum instability with respect to the lunate; IV = lunate dislocation. (From Mayfield, J.R.; et al. J Hand Surg, 5:226-241, 1980.)

The mechanism of injury was extension, ulnar deviation, and intercarpal supination. Thus, Stage I is scapholunate instability caused by tearing of the scapholunate interosseous ligament and radioscapholunate ligaments; this corresponds clinically with scapholunate dissociation. Stage II includes lunate capitate subluxation caused by the injury propagating through the volar capitolunate capsule (space of Poirier). Stage III includes lunate triquetral subluxation caused by the injury continuing through the triquetrolunate interosseous ligament and the volar lunate triquetral ligament. Stage IV is lunate subluxation with respect to the scaphoid, capitate, triquetrum, and radius due to tearing of the dorsal radiolunate ligaments, which allows the lunate to rotate anteriorly into the carpal canal based on its intact volar radiolunate ligament (Fig. 34-26). Therefore, volar dislocation of the lunate is the ultimate in perilunate instability. It should be emphasized that these studies did not produce isolated ulnar side

instabilities, and the mechanisms for these remain unknown, although clinical experience suggests that some may be caused by rotational injury such as hyperpronation or hypersupination as when a drill bit on a power drill binds, twisting the hand.

Because of our incomplete knowledge regarding the etiology and diagnosis of carpal instability, especially the more subtle dynamic forms, a universally useful classification does not exist. Green and O'Brien[54] have nevertheless described a classification that aids in the recognition and treatment of the more common perilunate instabilities.

Diagnosis

The severe instabilities that are obvious on routine roentgenograms are relatively easy to diagnose; it is the

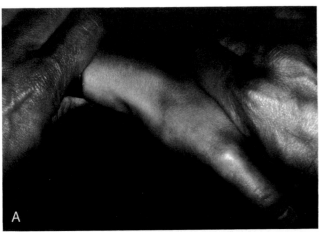 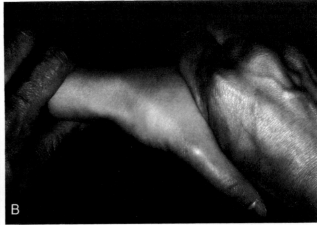

Figure 34–27

A, Volar shift test. The examiner stabilizes the distal forearm while simultaneously pushing the hand in the volar direction. Normally, a painless "shift" is felt by the examiner and patient. This generally represents midcarpal laxity and should be tested against the normal side. *B,* Dorsal shift test. The examiner stabilizes the distal forearm with one hand and simultaneously pushes the hand dorsally. Normally, very little motion is felt. In patients with dorsal intercalated segment instability, increased motion, pain, or both compared with the normal side is a positive finding.

subtle instabilities that may present as wrist pain with normal radiographs that are difficult. Approach these patients by keeping in mind that not all instabilities are painful and not all painful wrists are due to instability. In the history, one should look for an episode of trauma such as a fall on the outstretched hand. The patient should be asked about "clicks" or "clunks." The patient can sometimes localize the exact point of pain if any. The type of activity that worsens the symptoms is important. In the physical examination, palpate for tenderness of the first dorsal compartment (De Quervain's tenosynovitis), the anatomic snuffbox (scaphoid fracture), the first carpometacarpal joint (arthritis), the scapholunate interval (scapholunate ligament tear or ganglion), the triquetrolunate joint (triquetrolunate ligament tear), the radioulnar joint (instability), the extensor carpi ulnaris tendon (tendonitis or subluxation) and the extensor carpi ulnaris-flexor carpi ulnaris interval (ulnar impingement on the carpus, triangular fibrocartilage tear). Volarly, palpate the pisiform (fracture, arthritis), and hook of the hamate (fracture).

Several stress tests are useful. In the dorsal and volar shift test, the forearm is stabilized with one hand and the wrist translated dorsally and volarly with the other hand. It is normal to be able to subluxate the wrist volarly (midcarpal joint) but not dorsally, which may indicate scapholunate instability (Fig. 34–27A,B). A similar test may be applied to the ulnocarpal relationship: pushing the ulnar head down while pushing the ulnar carpus up often evokes pain in ulnar impingement syndromes (the ulna carpal shift test) (Fig. 34–28). There is also the triquetrolunate ballottement test[112] wherein the lunate is stabilized with one hand

and the triquetrum is passively shifted dorsally and palmarly with the other hand, which may elicit pain. Active and passive motion of the wrist should be recorded and one should note any dyssynchronous movements or "clunks." Measurement of grip strength on both wrists is also very important, as any significant wrist disease will usually reduce grip strength.

Routine Radiography

Routine Views. The mainstay of diagnosis remains radiography. Routine views should include posteroan-

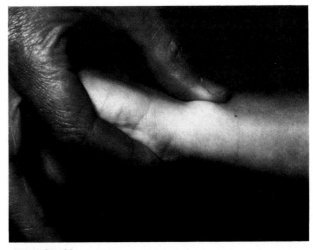

Figure 34–28

Ulnar carpal shift test. The examiner pushes down on the ulnar head and up on the pisiform. If the test is positive, pain is felt by the patient in the extensor carpi ulnaris and flexor carpi ulnaris interval. This may be found in cases of ulnar-carpal impingement.

terior (PA), true lateral with the wrist in neutral in all planes, and a 45° oblique with the wrist in 45° of pronation with respect to the cassette. Bellinghausen and colleagues[8] have pointed out that three smooth lines can be drawn on a normal PA view of the wrist. If these lines are broken, an instability can be suspected. The proximal line describes the proximal articular surfaces of the proximal row, the middle line describes the distal articular surfaces of the proximal row, and the distal line outlines the proximal articular surfaces of the distal row (Fig. 34–29). On the PA view, increased overlap of a carpal, especially the lunate, to the capitate should be sought. If the lunate presents a triangular as opposed to quadrilateral appearance, a perilunate instability may be suspected. The scaphoid normally appears elongated. If it appears foreshortened and demonstrates a "ring" bicortical density, this means it has become abnormally vertical with respect to the radius, as occurs in scapholunate dissociation and volar intercalated segment instability patterns. Check also for increased space in the scapholunate interval (>3 mm in scapholunate dissociation). Also assess carpal height.[147] On the lateral view, as has already been discussed, look for any disruption of the normal colinear relationship of the capitate, lunate, and radius.[46] Also measure the scapholunate angle to check for scapholunate dissociation (angle >60° or volar intercalated segment instability pattern (angle <30°). It must be emphasized that because of the normal flexion and extension of the proximal row in radial and ulnar deviation, all measurements must be made on radiographs in which the third metacarpal is aligned parallel to the long axis of the radius in all planes.

Other Views. If the routine radiographs are normal and the clinician suspects an instability, a stress or motion series may be helpful.[46] These views include a PA view in radial deviation, neutral, and ulnar deviation; anteroposterior view with fist (compression); and lateral views in radial deviation, neutral, and ulnar deviation. Look for the same malalignments as described for the static views.

Cineradiography

This can be helpful when the static films are normal or suspicious but not conclusive.[109] They are most useful when the radiologist has a clear idea of what is being sought or if the surgeon performs the studies with the radiologist in attendance. The wrist is actively or passively moved in radial and ulnar deviation and examined in the PA and lateral and oblique planes. Evidence of dyssynchronous motion is sometimes found.

Arthrography

There has been a good deal of experience with this modality, as reported by Kricun, Palmer, and Schwartz, among others.[68,103,118] The method allows identification of scapholunate and triquetrolunate interosseous ligament tears, triangular fibrocartilage tears, synovitis, occult ganglia, and large cartilage defects. However, it can be misleading, since in addition to false positives and negatives, the demonstration of a scapholunate interosseous or lunate-triquetrum interosseous ligament communication does not necessarily mean that the patient's symptoms are related to these findings. This is partly because the interosseous ligaments have a thin membranous central portion that probably does not contribute significantly to ligament function. After the age of 50, these tears become increasingly common[92] and the arthrogram becomes less useful. The study is most meaningful in the normal younger wrist, especially in patients under 20 years of age.

Bone Scan

This nonspecific but fairly sensitive test will be positive if there is a fracture or synovitis present. By itself it is not useful in diagnosing carpal instability but may furnish objective evidence of an abnormality. If negative, severe wrist disease is less likely.

Polytomography and Computerized Axial Tomography

At present, these tests may be useful in more clearly measuring subtle changes in the capitolunate and radiolunate angles on the lateral views.[80] They are very

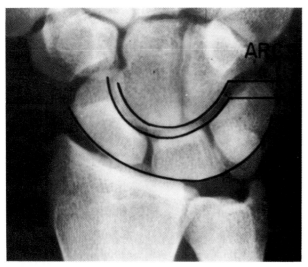

Figure 34–29

In the normal wrist, three smooth arcs can be drawn on the anteroposterior x-ray film. If there is a break in any of these three lines, an intracarpal malalignment should be strongly suspected. (From Bellinghausen, H.W., et al. J Bone Joint Surg 65A:999, 1983.)

useful in diagnosing fractures and malunited scaphoid fractures.

Magnetic Resonance Imaging

Attempts to visualize torn ligaments by magnetic resonance imaging have so far not proven successful. However, as image clarity improves with better technology, this may become a useful technique.

Arthroscopy

This newly applied technique has shown promise in diagnosing obscure wrist pain,[113] but its role in increasing our appreciation of carpal instability remains to be demonstrated. Some authors have also described treatment of wrist instabilities using the arthroscope; however this work is too preliminary to draw firm conclusions at present.

SPECIFIC DISLOCATIONS

Dorsal Perilunate/Volar Lunate Dislocation

This is the most common carpal dislocation[52,97] and as discussed previously, is the ultimate stage in perilunate instability (Mayfield Stage IV) (Fig. 34 – 30). All the soft tissue structures connecting the lunate to the rest of the carpus are torn while the volar radiolunate and ulnar lunate ligaments remain intact. The capitate and the rest of the carpus come to lie dorsal to the lunate. Depending on the degree of injury, the lunate either will be in its normal position with respect to the radius and the rest of the carpus dorsal (dorsal perilunate dislocation) or will be anteriorly displaced and rotated with the capitate and other carpal bones in more or less normal relationship to the radius (lunate dislocation). These dislocations are stages of the same injury; the only difference is that in lunate dislocation, the dorsal radiolunate ligaments are torn.

Treatment

If the injury is acute or occurred less than two weeks previously, closed reduction is often successful. However, even after reduction, these are very unstable injuries and it is usually necessary to internally fix the scaphoid, lunate, and capitate to each other. Percutaneous fixation has been advocated by some, but Green[52] and others are of the opinion that this is difficult to achieve and further that it is necessary to repair at least the anterior ligaments to properly treat the problem. Therefore, closed reduction is indicated immediately, especially if there is median nerve compression or associated injuries, but open fixation should be performed as soon as it is safe to do so. The end result is influenced by the timing of reduction, and earlier is

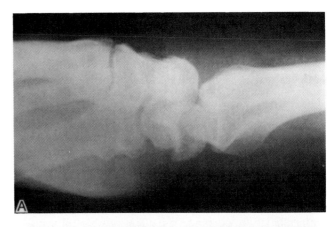

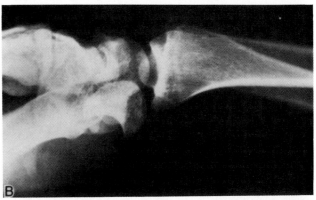

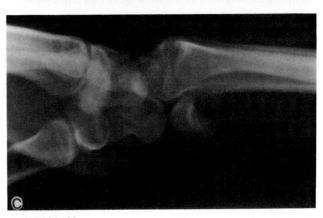

Figure 34–30

In a patient with a carpal dislocation the initial lateral radiograph may depict a configuration at any point in the spectrum of injury. *A,* Dorsal perilunate dislocation; *B,* an intermediate stage; *C,* volar lunate dislocation. (From Green, D.P. Operative Hand Surgery, Vol. 2. Churchill Livingstone. 1988, p. 885, by permission.)

better. Although successful results have been reported in isolated cases as late as four to five months postinjury,[53] the best results are seen when definitive treatment is performed within one to two weeks.

Technique. Closed reduction is best accomplished by longitudinal traction in finger traps with 10 to 15 lbs of counterweight on the upper arm.[52] We use the wrist

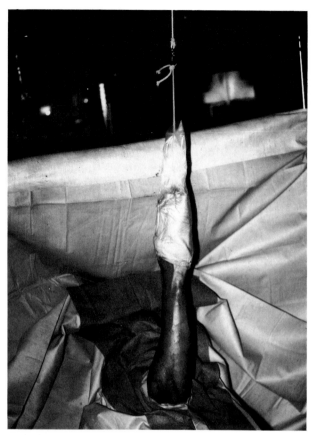

Figure 34–31

The patient is supine, with the upper arm taped to an arm board. The hand is suspended through finger traps to an overhead pulley system, and weight (2.25 to 3.15 kg) is applied.

arthroscopy set-up with 6 kg of weight applied to the thumb, index, and middle fingers by finger traps through the shoulder holder* (Fig. 34–31). The arm is strapped to an arm board to provide countertraction. Green[52] recommends a PA and lateral radiograph at this point to better delineate the extent of injury. After 10 minutes of traction has been applied, the finger traps are removed and the surgeon's thumb stabilizes the lunate volarly while the opposite hand is used to push the capitate over the dorsal pole of the lunate and reduce it into the lunate concavity. The arm is then placed in a short arm thumb spica cast with the wrist in slight palmar flexion. Repeat radiographs are then taken to assess the adequacy of reduction. It is important to be certain that the scapholunate angle is within normal range since dorsal intercalated segment instability is a very common consequence of this injury. If routine radiographs are difficult to interpret, lateral

* Dyonics Inc., 160 Dascomb Road, Andover, MA 01810.

polytomes or CT scans can be helpful. If alignment is anatomic, then cast immobilization can be continued for 12 weeks with repeat radiographs at 1 to 2 week intervals.

In our experience, treatment with cast alone is not usually successful. Occasionally, it is possible to fix these percutaneously, and this approach may be indicated in the multiple trauma patient when open fixation must be delayed. This is a difficult technique. Our method is to have an assistant stabilize the forearm while the surgeon holds the hand placing his or her thumb over the dorsum of the capitate. Then while exerting a volar translation force on the capitate, a single 0.054-in smooth Kirschner wire is driven from the capitate into the lunate distally to proximally. This stabilizes the capitolunate relationship. Image intensifier or routine radiographs are then taken to check reduction and wire position. If satisfactory, the proximal pole of the scaphoid is then pushed down (anteriorly from dorsally) while the surgeon drills a single 0.054-in wire through the snuffbox across the scaphoid into the capitate and a second 0.054-in wire from the scaphoid into the lunate. Again, the reduction and wire placement are checked radiologically. If satisfactory, the wires are cut just below the skin. A U-shaped above-elbow splint is applied for the first week until swelling subsides, followed by a short above-elbow thumb spica for six weeks and a below-elbow cast for six weeks for a total of twelve weeks of immobilization. The casts are changed every two to three weeks, otherwise they can become loose and the wires may also loosen. If closed reduction fails or percutaneous fixation is not successful, then open reduction and internal fixation is indicated. As mentioned above, we prefer this method as the initial treatment in most situations.

There has been controversy regarding the best surgical approach. Campbell and colleagues[19] reported a dorsal approach in nine patients and a volar approach in four patients, all without the complication of avascular necrosis. They preferred the dorsal approach because (1) it is usually necessary to remove scar tissue in the lunate space and (2) it is easier to visualize and align the carpal bones through a dorsal approach. Dobyns and co-workers[31] advocated a dorsal and volar approach to repair the volar ligaments. Green and O'Brien[53] and Taleisnik[131] also recommend a volar approach to effect ligament repair. Adkinson and Chapman[2] reported good results with a dorsal approach only, indicating that it is not necessary to suture the volar ligaments if bony reduction is achieved and maintained with Kirschner wires.

Our preference is to treat these injuries with open reduction and internal fixation with Kirschner wires through a dorsal approach. If the patient has a median neuropathy, we also perform a volar incision to release the flexor retinaculum, explore the nerve, and repair the volar wrist capsule. However, in our experience, the dorsal approach alone is adequate to reduce and fix the dislocation and suture repair of the volar ligaments is not absolutely necessary. Use the straight dorsal approach already described in the section on fracture treatment. After the extensor pollicis longus is retracted radially, the entire dorsal carpus is in view as the dorsal capsule has been torn and stripped off the radius by the injury. The proximal pole of the scaphoid and capitate are easily visualized and the lunate is hidden underneath. Reduction is obtained by traction on the hand and then pushing up on the lunate from anteriorly after clearing the lunate space of soft tissue. Reduction of the lunate can be facilitated by placing a blunt periosteal elevator between the capitate head and the lunate and levering the lunate up dorsally. Any small osteochondral fragments are removed and the capitolunate relationship aligned and stabilized by pushing the capitate volarly and driving a smooth 0.054-in Kirschner wire across the capitate into the lunate from distal to proximal. It is also helpful to radially deviate the capitate on the lunate approximately 10° before pinning. The scaphoid is then reduced to the lunate by pushing firmly down anteriorly on the proximal pole of the scaphoid and radially deviating the wrist. One 0.054-in Kirschner wire is then driven through the scaphoid into the capitate and a second wire through the scaphoid into the lunate. Radiographs are taken to assess reduction and pin placement. Closure is accomplished in routine fashion, although the dorsal capsule may be badly damaged and irreparable. A U-shaped above-elbow splint is applied with the wrist in neutral position and changed to a short above-elbow thumb spica cast at one week, which is left on for four weeks. A short arm cast is then applied for a further six to eight weeks. The pins are removed at ten to twelve weeks and prolonged therapy begun. Motion is emphasized initially, followed by strengthening exercises. It is important to examine these patients every two to three weeks to change the cast and inspect the pins to guard against loosening. Most patients will gain approximately 50% of normal motion, and some stiffness is the rule.[53]

Transscaphoid Perilunate Dislocation

This injury (Fig. 34–32) occurs by a mechanism very similar to that in dorsal perilunate dislocation except the energy is transmitted through the waist of the scaphoid instead of through its ligamentous attachments to the lunate. The indications and techniques of closed reduction are the same as for dorsal perilunate/volar lunate dislocation, including adequate anesthesia

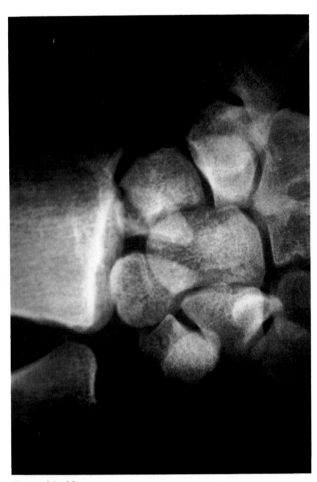

Figure 34–32

A transscaphoid perilunate dislocation with an associated radiostyloid fracture.

(axillary block or general anesthesia), 5 to 10 minutes of traction, and manipulation by stabilizing the lunate and proximal pole scaphoid fragment with one hand while maintaining traction and flexing the capitate and the distal row with the other hand until the capitate snaps over the dorsal pole of the lunate and rests in the scapholunate concavity. It is important to have adequate postreduction radiologic confirmation of exact reduction of the scaphoid, since any malalignment of this fracture will not only prejudice its healing but will also cause instability (usually dorsal intercalated segment) to persist. A U-shaped above-elbow splint is applied for one week with the wrist in slight flexion and radial deviation, followed by a short above-elbow thumb spica cast for six weeks, followed by a short arm cast for six weeks, or until the fracture is healed radiologically. The cast should be changed every two to three weeks to keep it snug. Since it is difficult to adequately visualize the fracture through plaster, lateral polytomes or lateral computerized tomographs are used to gauge both the initial reduction of the scaphoid, the capito-lunate relationship, and the healing of the scaphoid. Unfortunately, even with excellent initial reduction, the scaphoid usually angulates and the wrist collapses into DISI with the proximal row and proximal pole of the scaphoid angulated dorsally and the distal pole of the scaphoid and distal row angulated volarly.

Late correction is difficult and usually unsuccessful. Therefore, although closed reduction can be done as an emergency measure when a multiple trauma patient is being stabilized, this author, Green and O'Brien,[53] and others[19,20,93] advocate early open reduction and internal fixation as the treatment of choice. The technique is controversial. Some authors prefer a volar approach, some a dorsal approach, and some use both. We use a dorsal approach just as for the dorsal perilunate dislocation and for the same reasons. The disadvantage of this method is that if there is comminution of the volar cortex of the scaphoid, it is not possible to add a bone graft to maintain scaphoid alignment after reduction. Also, the volar ligaments cannot be repaired. Often, just as in a dorsal perilunate/volar lunate dislocation, the question becomes moot since a carpal tunnel release must be done to release the median nerve.

A straight dorsal incision is made centered a few millimeters ulnar to Lister's tubercle. The extensor pollicis longus is retracted radially, and the dorsal wrist capsule mobilized radially and ulnarly. (It will have been stripped off the carpus and distal radius by the injury.) The head of the capitate will come into view with the distal pole of the scaphoid. Any blood and fibrin are removed from the scapholunate fossa, and traction is applied to the hand. The lunate and the attached proximal pole of the scaphoid are pushed up (dorsal) while the capitate and distal scaphoid fragment are pushed down (volar) over the dorsal pole of the lunate. Again this maneuver can be facilitated with a blunt periosteal elevator placed in the fracture site and used as a lever. Reduction and stability are then checked clinically by radially and ulnarly deviating the wrist. Even though the reduction may appear stable, we routinely use internal fixation because of the high risk of later malalignment. Two methods are useful. The easiest method is with Kirschner wires. After reduction, two 0.054- or 0.045-in smooth Kirschner wires can be placed from the proximal pole of the scaphoid across the fracture site through the distal pole and then drawn distally until the ends are in the subchondral bone in the proximal pole so as not to project into the radioscaphoid joint. After radiographs confirm anatomic reduction of the fracture and proper placement of the wires, the wound is closed and a U-shaped above-elbow splint is applied for one week. This is followed by a short above-elbow thumb spica cast for six weeks and then a short arm thumb spica cast for a further six weeks or until the scaphoid is healed radiologically. The wires usually have to be removed by three months as they tend to become loose.

An alternative method of internal fixation is the Herbert screw, which has the advantages of providing better internal fixation without protruding wires and may obviate the need for long-term cast immobiliza-

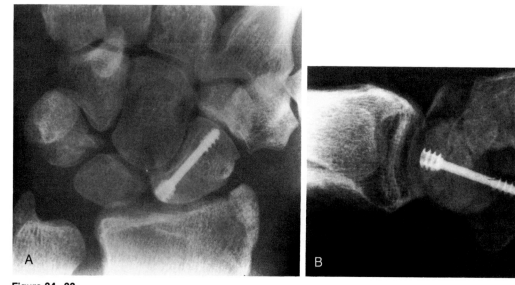

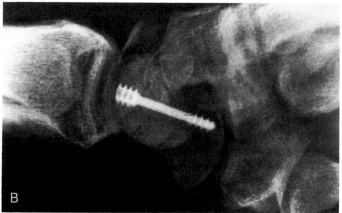

Figure 34–33

A and B, Anteroposterior and lateral postoperative radiographs demonstrating a Herbert screw used to fix the scaphoid fracture in a patient with a transscaphoid perilunate dislocation.

tion (Fig. 34–33). The only drawback is the exacting technique required, especially as the jig cannot be used with a dorsal approach. For the experienced operator, the screw may be the preferred method.

If the volar cortex of the scaphoid is comminuted or if the patient is seen two to three weeks after the injury with established DISI collapse, then an initial volar approach is preferable. A skin incision is made over the flexor carpi radialis tendon, which is exposed and retracted ulnarly. The radial artery is protected. The dorsal sheath of the flexor carpi radialis is incised longitudinally and pericapsular fat is divided. The anterior capsule of the wrist is divided and the proximal pole scaphoid and lunate are visualized. Fibrin and clot are removed from the fracture surface and dorsally as far as possible by placing traction on the hand. This should expose the distal fragment of the scaphoid and the head of the capitate. The proximal fragment is then pushed dorsally while the distal fragment is pulled volarly. If reduction is successful, then internal fixation and/or bone graft can be performed. We recommend bone graft if the volar cortex of the scaphoid is sufficiently comminuted to preclude anatomic reduction and adequate fixation. Since a volar approach does not allow good visualization of the critical scapholunate-capitate relationship, radiologic assessment or a dorsal incision will have to be made. Internal fixation is then performed either by driving two 0.045-in smooth Kirschner wires from distal pole to proximal pole or using the Herbert screw technique as already described in treatment of scaphoid fractures. Closure is routine and aftercare is as already described for the dorsal approach. Again, stiffness is a common sequel of these injuries and so vigorous and prolonged rehabilitation is necessary.

It is not rare to have an accompanying radial styloid fracture, in which case these injuries are termed transradial transscaphoid fracture-dislocations. If the radius fracture is large and in one piece, it should be treated by internal fixation since it may contribute to ligamentous and bony stability of the wrist. If small or comminuted, excision is a reasonable option.

Transtriquetral Perilunate Fracture-Dislocation

In some carpal dislocations, the plane of injury propagates ulnarly not between the lunate and triquetrum, but through the triquetrum. The proximal portion of the triquetrum stays with the lunate, and the distal fragment displaces dorsally with the capitate and distal row analogous to the transscaphoid perilunate dislocation. Treatment is the same as for the perilunate dislocation, and the triquetral fracture will be reduced automatically. We recommend internal fixation of the fracture and the carpus.

Capitate Hamate Diastasis

If a hand is severely crushed, a cleavage plane may be created between the capitate and hamate and third and fourth metacarpals (Fig. 34–34). This injury will propagate proximally through the triquetrum or between it and the hamate. The diagnosis is easy to overlook, and one should be suspicious in a patient with divergence between the middle and ring fingers where the hand has been flattened by considerable force. The injury is best visualized on a PA view. It is important to reduce and fix this diastasis as failure to do so will destroy the transverse arch of the hand and cause rotational malalignment of the fingers. Primiano and Reef[108] performed carpal tunnel release and internal fixation in their four patients. Garcia-Elias and co-authors[41] summarized all 13 cases reported in the literature up to 1985, including four of their own patients, and concluded that closed reduction produced good long-term results.

Scapholunate Dissociation

This entity may be defined as dyssynchronous movement of the scaphoid with respect to the lunate. Normally, although the scaphoid is the most mobile bone in the proximal row, its motions are similar in direction and amplitude to those of the lunate and triquetrum.[114]

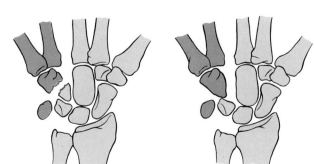
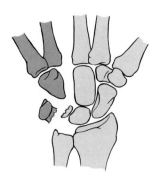

Figure 34–34

The three patterns of capitate-hamate diastasis described by Garcia-Elias and colleagues. (Redrawn from Garcia-Elias, M., et al. J Bone Joint Surg 67B:289, 1985.)

If this synchronous motion with respect to the lunate is lost, then scapholunate dissociation is said to exist. There is no general agreement as to which ligaments are the most important in stabilizing the scaphoid to the lunate, but evidence exists to support the idea that several structures are important in this regard, including the scapholunate interosseous ligament, the radiolunate triquetral ligament, and perhaps the dorsal radiolunate triquetral ligament. A history of dorsiflexion injury is sought although not always found. The patient will complain primarily of radial dorsal wrist pain, which may be localized on palpation to the scapholunate interval or dorsal rim of the radius. There will often be a positive dorsal shift test with increased pain at the capitate head as it subluxes dorsally out of the lunate concavity. When complete dissociation exists, the scaphoid rests in an abnormally vertical position relative to the radius, and the proximal pole may be subluxated dorsally out of the radial facet (Watson test[143]—see next section). Since the stabilizing link function of the scaphoid is lost, the midcarpal joint collapses into dorsal intercalated segment instability (DISI) with the lunate and triquetrum resting in dorsiflexion and the capitate and distal row migrating proximally and radially to lie against the dorsal aspect of the proximal row and in the gap between the scaphoid and lunate. On the posteroanterior radiograph, (1) the carpal height ratio is reduced (<0.54); (2) there is increased overlap of the lunate on the capitate with a more triangular shape of the lunate; (3) the triquetrum is also dorsiflexed, which gives it a wider posteroranterior appearance; (4) there is an increased gap between the scaphoid and lunate greater than 2 to 3 mm (so-called Terry Thomas sign); and (5) the scaphoid appears fore-

shortened (Fig. 34–35). Also, since the long axis of the bone is more nearly parallel with the x-ray beam, one sees the distal pole superimposed on the proximal pole, the so-called ring sign. On the lateral view, the scapholunate angle is greater than 60° and the lunate and triquetrum are dorsiflexed with respect to the radius and capitate (DISI).

Clinical Examination

Watson has described a test wherein the examiner pushes on the distal pole of the scaphoid volarly and tries to force the proximal pole of the scaphoid dorsally out of the radial facet. In the more subtle forms of this dissociation, the diagnosis is not easy to make and not all of the signs noted above will be present. For these patients, stress views in radial deviation, ulnar deviation, fist views, and cineradiography may be necessary. Arthrography can be helpful in the younger patient. Arthroscopy should prove to be a useful diagnostic tool since the scapholunate interosseous ligament, radioscapholunate ligament, radial lunate ligament, and scaphoid, lunate, and radial proximal articular surfaces can all be directly visualized.

Treatment

This issue is best considered in terms of early and late treatment as the methods and prognosis for each differ. It should also be pointed out that two of the most prominent authorities on the wrist, R.L. Linscheid and J.H. Dobyns, have stated that "treatment of this condition is seldom satisfactory."[78] Unfortunately, our own experience supports their conclusion.

Acute Scapholunate Dissociation. These injuries are often missed and in fact may be relatively asympto-

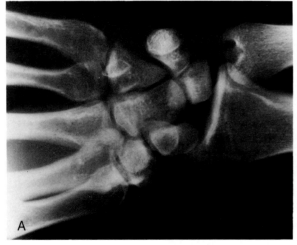 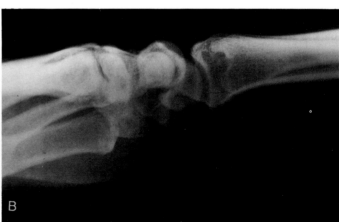

Figure 34–35

A and B, Anteroposterior and lateral x-ray films of scapholunate diastasis.

matic initially. If, however, one does see an acute injury, most authors, including this one, recommend open reduction and internal fixation. In our hands, closed reduction has never succeeded. The difficulty of closed reduction in this injury is probably due to the paradox of the scaphoid,[86] which can be described as follows. To close the scapholunate gap, radial deviation of the wrist, which compresses the scapholunate joint, should be done. However, this causes the scaphoid to assume a more vertical position, thereby increasing scapholunate angulation. Conversely, to align the scaphoid more horizontally, ulnar deviation of the wrist should be performed, which distracts the scapholunate joint, increasing the gap. Nonetheless, it may be possible to accomplish closed reduction with the maneuvers described below. Our preference is for open reduction and internal fixation with ligament repair. Other authors have recommended closed reduction and percutaneous fixation using the image intensifier or plain radiography to guide reduction and pin placement.

Technique. After adequate axillary block or general anesthesia, the capitolunate joint is reduced by volar translocation and radial deviation of the capitate on the lunate by pushing volarly and radially on the hand while stabilizing the forearm with the opposite hand. This is very similar to the volar shift test (see Fig. 34–27A). The assistant then drives a 0.054-in or 0.045-in smooth Kirschner wire across the capitolunate joint, and its position is checked by radiograph. Next, the scaphoid is reduced by 15 to 20° of radial deviation and simultaneous downward (anteriorly directed) pressure over the proximal pole of the scaphoid. A second 0.054-in or 0.045-in smooth Kirschner wire is then introduced across the scaphocapitate joint and a third wire across the scapholunate joint. Again, reduction and wire placement are checked radiologically. The wires are bent at right angles, and cut under the skin. After an initial one week of U-shaped thumb spica splinting, a solid short-arm thumb spica cast is applied and left in place for 10 weeks and changed at two to three week intervals. Alternative methods of wire placement have been described including two pins though the scaphoid to the capitate and two pins thorugh the scaphoid to the lunate.[97] Dobyns and Linscheid suggest one pin through the radius into the lunate and a second pin through the radius into the scaphoid.[31] Our preference is open reduction through a dorsal approach and pin placement as described previously for closed reduction and percutaneous pinning. Additionally, if there is significant scapholunate interosseous ligament to repair, 2-0 horizontal mattress sutures are placed if possible through bone to reconstruct the scapholunate interosseous ligament.[31] This tech-

nique is especially useful if the scapholunate interosseous ligament is avulsed from its attachment to the rim of the scaphoid or lunate. Aftercare is the same as for closed reduction and percutaneous fixation.

Chronic Scapholunate Dissociation. As noted previously, this is much more commonly seen than the acute form. Diagnosis rests on the same clinical and radiographic findings, although one must be aware that arthritis of the radioscaphoid joint and capitate head may also exist. Treatment of chronic scapholunate dissociation is controversial and difficult and the results are unpredictable. No single procedure has been uniformly successful in treating this problem.

Soft Tissue Methods. Since the dividing line between acute and chronic is not distinct but is arbitrarily drawn at three weeks by some[133] and three months by others,[75] the first option for treatment of chronic instability is the same as for acute instability; that is, open reduction through a dorsal approach, pinning of the three key carpals (i.e., capitate, lunate, and scaphoid), and repair of the scapholunate interosseous ligament, if possible.

Blatt[11] has described a soft tissue technique that does not rely on reconstruction of the scapholunate ligament and recreation of the scapholunate linkage that Linscheid recommends.[75] Rather, he creates a dorsal capsulodesis that horizontalizes the scaphoid (Fig. 34–

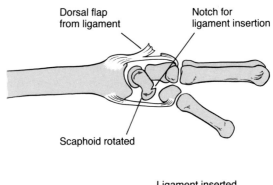

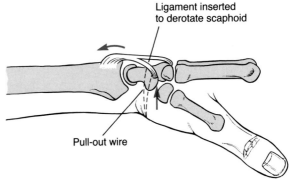

Figure 34–36

Blatt's technique of dorsal capsulodesis for chronic rotary subluxation of the scaphoid. (Redrawn from Blatt, G. Hand Clin 3:81–102, 1987.)

36). He exposes the wrist through a dorsal approach and dissects a 1-cm wide flap of dorsal capsule left attached to the dorsal rim of the radius. The scaphoid is then reduced and pinned to the capitate with a single 0.045-in Kirschner wire. A trough is created in the distal dorsal pole of the scaphoid and the flap attached with a pull-out wire led volarly. Motion is begun when the cast is removed at two months. The Kirschner wire is removed at three months. We have no experience with this technique.

The third type of soft tissue reconstruction that has been described is ligament reconstruction using tendon grafts. These are complicated, technically demanding procedures with unpredictable results. Dobyns and Linscheid[31,102] have described a method using drill holes in the scaphoid and lunate through which is passed a strip of extensor carpi radialis brevis or longus tendon in an attempt to reconstruct the scapholunate interosseous ligament and restore the scapholunate linkage. They emphasize several technical points: (1) careful drilling of the holes to avoid fractures; (2) passage of good quality tendon graft; (3) overreduction of the radiolunate-capitate and scaphoid joints and using three Kirschner wires to maintain reduction; and (4) postoperative immobilization with the Kirschner wires for six to eight weeks followed by part-time splinting for an additional six weeks. Rehabilitation after this procedure requires six to twelve months. Taleisnik[131] uses a combined dorsal and volar exposure and in addition reconstructs the scapholunate ligament. He prepares a strip of flexor carpi radialis, leaves it attached distally, and passes it through the lunate from volar to dorsal, then across to the scaphoid from dorsal to volar, then through the volar rim of the radius and sutures it to itself. He feels this technique is difficult, complex, and not totally reliable.

Intercarpal Arthrodesis. Because of the difficulty with and variable results of soft tissue procedures, some authors have proposed various limited intercarpal ararthrodeses to stabilize the wrist.

SCAPHOLUNATE ARTHRODESIS. This procedure appears to be a logical solution to the problem of chronic scapholunate dissociation since it addresses the key feature of this instability directly. Unfortunately, several surgeons who have had experience with it report low arthrodesis rates.[54] Nonetheless, clinical improvement and radiologic reduction can be achieved even in the face of nonunion. In common with all surgery for chronic scapholunate disassociation, no large series showing uniformly good results has been reported.

The technique is as follows. Expose the proximal half of the scaphoid, lunate, and capitate through a dorsal approach. Using a power burr or hand instrument, create cavities in the adjacent articular surfaces of the

scaphoid and lunate. Then reduce or overreduce the capitate to the lunate as described for reduction of acute dissociation. Pin this joint with a 0.054-in Kirschner wire from capitate to lunate. Then reduce the scaphoid to the lunate and pin this joint and the scaphocapitate joint with 0.054-in Kirschner wires. Follow this by tightly packing the scapholunate joint with cancellous bone graft harvested either from the distal radius or the iliac crest. Close in routine fashion and apply a U-shaped above-elbow splint for one week followed by a short arm cast for ten weeks changed at two to three week intervals. Then remove the wires and begin range of motion exercises followed by strengthening exercises. Total rehabilitation usually takes four to six months.

SCAPHOLUNATE-CAPITATE ARTHRODESIS. This technique improves the fusion rate and will solve the instability problem. However, there is at least a 50% loss of motion, and late changes may occur at the nonarthrodesed joints. Again, there is a paucity of data supporting this approach. In our hands, total intercarpal fusion including the scaphoid, lunate, capitate, triquetrum, and hamate has added nothing to the morbidity and has been predictable over the short term.

The technique is as follows: Expose the wrist through a dorsal subperiosteal approach as already described being careful not to expose the common digital extensor tendons. Remove cartilage and subchondral bone to expose cancellous bone at all the intercarpal joints. Reduce the wrist, taking care to preserve anatomic alignment of the proximal articular surface of the proximal row and preserve the external dimensions of the wrist. Stabilize all the intercarpal joints with 0.054-in or 0.042-in smooth Kirschner wires. Pack all the denuded surfaces tightly with cancellous bone harvested from the iliac crest. Close in layers over a drain. Place the wrist in a U-shaped above-elbow splint, which is changed at 48 hours. Apply a solid short arm cast at one week and change it every two to three weeks until three weeks or solid union has occurred by radiograph; then begin rehabilitation. It will require three to six months for the patient to return to heavy activity.

SCAPHOTRAPEZIAL TRAPEZOID ARTHRODESIS. This is a bony method to treat the vertical collapse pattern of the scaphoid. As with Blatt's technique, there is no attempt to restore scapholunate linkage. Watson[142] has popularized this arthrodesis, although it was first described by Peterson and Lipscomb in 1967 (Fig. 34–37).[106] Both Watson[142] and Kleinman[67] have described acceptable clinical results with this technique. Kleinman[66] has emphasized the change in wrist kinematics that occurs and has also reported 11 complications in his series of 41 patients. As with the Blatt dorsal capsulodesis procedure, the rationale is to prevent the

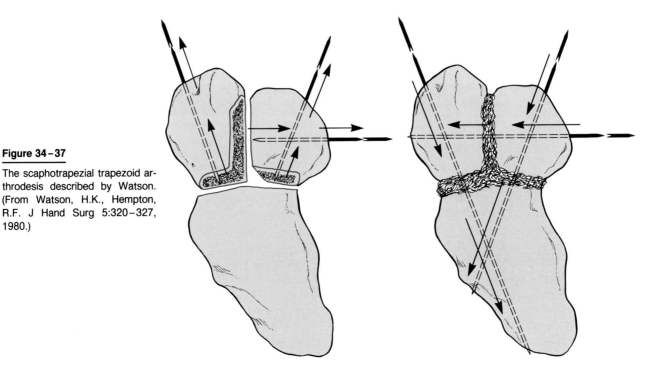

Figure 34-37

The scaphotrapezial trapezoid arthrodesis described by Watson. (From Watson, H.K., Hempton, R.F. J Hand Surg 5:320-327, 1980.)

scaphoid from assuming the vertical position that allows the proximal pole to sublux dorsally out of the radial facet with consequent arthritis and midcarpal collapse. More experience with this procedure is reported than with any of the other arthrodesis operations, but our personal experience has not been uniformly satisfactory and we no longer use it.

The Watson technique begins with a transverse incision made over the dorsoradial aspect of the wrist over the scaphoid. Nerves and tendons are retracted, and the scaphoid, trapezium, and trapezoid are exposed with a transverse incision through the wrist capsule. The articular surfaces of the distal scaphoid, proximal trapezium, proximal trapezoid, and trapezial trapezoid joints are denuded of cartilage. Bone graft is harvested from the distal radius through a second transverse incision between the first and second extensor compartments. The three bones are then aligned properly with the scaphoid at 45° to the long axis of the radius, and the normal external configuration at the three bones is preserved. At least three 0.045-in Kirschner wires are then prepositioned: one to cross each prepared articular surface and left protruding at the joint surface. To secure proper scaphoid position, two more Kirschner wires are driven across the scaphoid into the capitate after aligning the proximal pole to the lunate. Cancellous bone is packed into the joints, and the wires are driven across. Cortical bone is then added. Radiographs are taken to confirm proper alignment and wire placement. No pins should cross into the radius or ulna. The wires are cut under the skin and a bulky

dressing applied with a long arm splint. At 10 days, a long arm cast is applied including the index and middle fingers. Four weeks postoperatively, this is removed and a short arm cast applied. All fingers are allowed to be moved. At eight weeks, if radiographs demonstrate satisfactory healing, the pins are removed and a light volar splint applied. Range of motion of the wrist is begun. At nine weeks, all immobilization is stopped and full activity begun.

Author's Preferred Methods

For the patient with acute scapholunate instability, we prefer open reduction and soft tissue repair to attempt to restore the scapholunate linkage as described by Linscheid. For the chronic problem, we also attempt a soft tissue reconstruction of the scapholunate linkage using locally available ligament. This usually means placing drill holes in the scaphoid and threading 2-0 absorbable (Maxon) sutures in horizontal mattress fashion into the ligament remnant on the lunate. The capitolunate relationship is then reduced and pinned with a single 0.054-in or 0.062-in Kirschner wire. The scaphoid is reduced to the lunate and fixed with two pins: one from the scaphoid to the capitate and one from the scaphoid to the lunate. The sutures are then tied. A dorsal capsulodesis is performed by imbricating the dorsal radioscapulolunate triquetral ligament as part of the closure. The pins are cut off under the skin and left in place for three months. Protected radiocarpal motion is begun at six weeks and full motion is encouraged after the pins

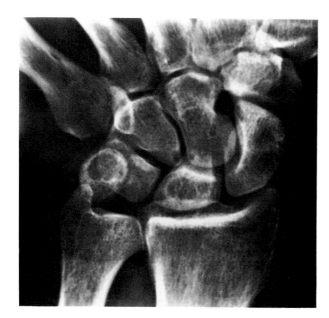

Figure 34–38

An x-ray film of a patient with triquetrolunate instability. Note the triquetrolunate step-off in ulnar deviation.

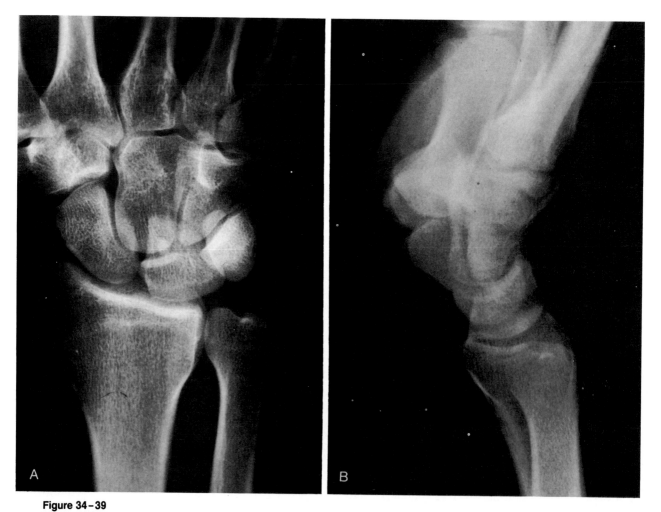

Figure 34–39

A and B, Volar intercalated segment instability, nondissociated (volar midcarpal instability), demonstrated on these radiographs.

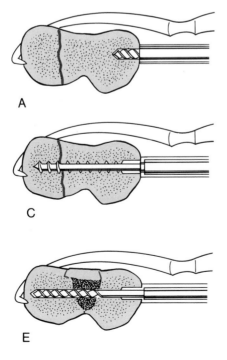

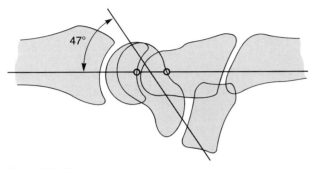

graphic changes denoting osteoarthritis, but only three had symptoms.[88] Overgaard and Solgaard in a seven-year follow-up found that 17 of 56 patients (30%) had radiographic evidence of osteophytes, and eight patients (14%) had advanced radiographic changes.[70] The occurrence of osteoarthritis in their series was related not to residual dorsal angulation or radial shortening but rather to the initial displacement and to advanced age at the time of injury. Frykman found a high rate (19%) of distal radioulnar joint arthritis, which was frequently symptomatic.[38]

Tendon complications include peritendinous adhesions involving both the extensor and flexor tendons, as well as tendon rupture. The tendon observed to rupture most frequently is the extensor pollicis longus.[17,30] This in particular may follow relatively undisplaced fractures, suggesting an ischemic cause rather than attritional rupture over a bony spike. In most cases, tendon transfer using the adjacent extensor indicis proprius provides a predictable reconstructive alternative.

Recognition of the role of anatomic restoration in functional recovery has led to greater interest in osteotomy of malunited distal radius fractures.[35,50,87,97] The techniques described by Fernandez should be referred to by any surgeon considering this complex reconstructive procedure.[35]

There are some additional complications that are less well known but merit some elaboration. In most cases these particular complications prove transient and do not require specific treatment. Occasionally, however, they can prove troublesome.

The first of these complications is cubital tunnel syndrome. Because of the altered mechanics of the upper extremity following a distal radius fracture, patients are more prone to lean on the elbow and maintain it in a flexed position. As a consequence, symptoms of cubital tunnel syndrome (parenthesias involving the little and ulnar half of the ring fingers) may develop. This particular problem can ordinarily be aborted by early recognition, elbow padding, and advice.

A second and unusual complication is "pseudo-Dupuytren's" nodules. A small nodule will often be seen to develop at the distal palmar crease, particularly overlying the ring metacarpal. It may be tender for weeks or even months. As a rule, it is not progressive and does not result in any contracture. The tenderness will generally subside spontaneously.

A third, unusual complication is piso-triquetral pain. Many fractures of the distal radius occur following a fall on the outstretched hand, and there may be a substantial amount of impact loading initially directed at the heel of the hand, delivering an injury to the piso-triquetral joint. Local tenderness on direct pressure and side-to-side movement detected on ballottement will be noted. On occasion, symptoms may persist for a substantial period of time, necessitating more aggressive treatment.

The final complication, which has not been well documented, is that of exacerbation of preexistent osteoarthritis of the carpometacarpal joint of the thumb. Because many of the patients with distal radius fractures are in the older age population, preexistent osteoarthritis involving the base of the thumb is not uncommon. It is important to recognize that this may exist when treating patients with plaster splints or casts. A cast that is applied too tightly or that constricts mobility of the carpometacarpal joint of the thumb can exacerbate an indolent problem and may ultimately cause more disability than the fracture itself.

Conclusion

Fractures of the distal radius are common injuries, particularly among the older age population. A favorable outcome, even in the presence of some residual deformity, can be anticipated in most, but not all, patients. However, the orthopedic surgeon cannot be complacent about the management of these injuries. As expressed by Edwards and Clayton in 1929, "What would be considered a good result in an old arthritic patient might be deplored as a comparative failure in a young working man."[32]

Treatment must be individualized based on the fracture pattern, energy of injury, associated problems, quality of bone, functional requirements of the patient, and patient compliance — far more factors than simply the chronologic age of the individual. The restoration and maintenance of anatomy will enhance the potential for a full functional outcome, but the various methods available to maintain fracture position are themselves associated with significant complications. Attention to detail and careful patient follow-up are critical, whether considering plaster immobilization, external skeletal fixation, or even an operative approach.

REFERENCES

1. Alffram, P.A.; Göran, C.H.B. Epidemiology of fractures of the forearm. J Bone Joint Surg 44A:105–114, 1962.
2. Altissimi, M.; Antenucci, R.; Fiacca, C.; Mancini, G.B. Long-term results of conservative treatment of fractures of the distal radius. Clin Orthop 206:202–210, 1986.
3. Anderson, R.; O'Neill, G. Comminuted fractures of the distal end of the radius. Surg Gynecol Obstet 78:434–440, 1944.
4. Aro, H.; Koirunen, J.; Katevuo, K.; et al. Late compression

neuropathies after Colles' fractures. Clin Orthop 233:217–225, 1988.

5. Atkins, R.M.; Duckworth, J.; Kanis, J.A. Algodystrophy following Colles' fracture. J Hand Surg 14B:161–164, 1989.

6. Axelrod, T.J.; McMurtry, R.Y. Open reduction and internal fixation of comminuted intraarticular fractures of the distal radius. J Hand Surg 15A:1–11, 1990.

7. Axelrod, T.; Paley, D.; Green, J.; McMurtry, R.Y. Limited open reduction of the lunate facet in comminuted intraarticular fractures of the distal radius. J Hand Surg 13A:372–377, 1988.

8. Bacorn, R.W.; Kurtzke, J.F. Colles' fracture: A study of 2,000 cases from the NY State Workmen's Compensation Board. J Bone Joint Surg 35A:643–658, 1953.

9. Bartosh, R.A.; Saldana, M.J. Intraarticular fractures of the distal radius: A cadaveric study to determine if ligamentotaxis restores radiopalmar tilt. J Hand Surg 15A:18–21, 1990.

10. Bell, M.J.; Hill, R.J.; McMurtry, R.Y. Ulnar impingement syndrome. J Bone Joint Surg 67B:126–129, 1985.

11. Bickerstaff, D.R.; Bell, M.J. Carpal malalignment in Colles' fractures. J Hand Surg 14B:155–160, 1989.

12. Böhler, L.B. Die funktionelle bewegungsbehandlung der "typischen radiusbrueche." Münch Medi Wochenschr 20:387, 1923.

13. Bower, W.H. The distal radioulnar joint. In: Green, D.P., ed. Operative Hand Surgery, Ed. 2. Philadelphia, J.B. Lippincott, 1988, pp. 939–989.

14. Bradway, J.; Amadio, P.C.; Cooney, W.P. Open reduction and internal fixation of displaced, comminuted intraarticular fractures of the distal end of the radius. J Bone Joint Surg 71A:839–847, 1989.

15. Brand, P.W.; Beach, R.B.; Thompson, D.E. Relative tension and potential excursion of muscles in the forearm and hand. J Hand Surg 3:209–219, 1981.

16. Carrozzella, J.; Stern, P.J. Treatment of comminuted distal radius fractures with pins and plaster. Hand Clin 4:391–397, 1988.

17. Cassebaum, W.H. Colles' fracture. A study of end results. JAMA 143:963–965, 1950.

18. Chapman, D.R.; Bennett, J.B.; Bryan, W.J.; Tullos, H.S. Complications of distal radius fractures: Pins and plaster treatment. J Hand Surg 7:509–512, 1982.

19. Clancey, G.J. Percutaneous Kirschner-wire fixation of Colles' fractures. J Bone Joint Surg 66A:1008–1014, 1984.

20. Clyburn, T.A. Dynamic external fixation for comminuted intraarticular fractures of the distal end of the radius. J Bone Joint Surg 69A:248–254, 1987.

21. Cole, J.M.; Obletz, B.E. Comminuted fractures of the distal end of the radius treated by skeletal transfixion in plaster cast: An end-result study of thirty-three cases. J Bone Joint Surg 48A:931–945, 1966.

22. Collert, S.; Isacson, J. Management of redislocated Colles' fractures. Clin Orthop 135:183–186, 1978.

23. Colles, A. On the fracture of the carpal extremity of the radius. Edinb Med Surg J 10:182–186, 1814.

24. Cooney, W.P. Management of Colles' fractures. Editorial. J Hand Surg 14B:137–139, 1989.

25. Cooney, W.P.; Dobyns, J.H.; Linscheid, R.L. Complications of Colles' fractures. J Bone Joint Surg 62A:613–619, 1980.

26. Cooney, W.P.; Linscheid, R.L.; Dobyns, J.H. External pin fixation for unstable Colles' fractures. J Bone Joint Surg 61A:840–845, 1979.

27. De Oliveira, J.C. Barton's fractures. J Bone Joint Surg 55A:586–594, 1973.

28. De Palma, A.F. Comminuted fractures of the distal end of the radius treated by ulnar pinning. J Bone Joint Surg 34A:651–662, 1952.

29. Dias, J.J.; Wray, C.C.; Jones, J.M.; Gregg, P.J. The value of early mobilization in the treatment of Colles' fractures. J Bone Joint Surg 69B:463–467, 1987.

30. Dobyns, J.H.; Linscheid, R.L. Complications of treatment of fractures and dislocations of the wrist. In: Epps, C.H., Jr., ed. Complications in Orthopaedic Surgery. Philadelphia, J.B. Lippincott, 1978, pp. 271–352.

31. Dowling, J.J.; Sawyer, B., Jr. Comminuted Colles' fractures. Evaluation of a method of treatment. J Bone Joint Surg 34A:651–662, 1952.

32. Edwards, H.; Clayton, E.B. Fractures of the lower end of the radius in adults. Br Med J 1:61–65, 1929.

33. Ekenstam, F.; Engkvist, O.; Wadin, K.; et al. Results from resection of the distal end of the ulna after fractures of the lower end of the radius. Scand J Plast Reconstr Surg 16:177–181, 1982.

34. Ellis, J. Smith's and Barton's fractures—a method of treatment. J Bone Joint Surg 47B:724–727, 1965.

35. Fernandez, D.L. Correction of post-traumatic wrist deformity in adults by osteotomy, bone grafting and internal fixation. J Bone Joint Surg 64A:1164–1178, 1982.

36. Fernandez, D.L. Avant-bras segment distal. In: Müeller, M.E.; Nazarian, S.; Koch, P., eds. Classification AO des Fractures. Les Os Longs. Berlin, Springer-Verlag, 1987, pp. 106–115.

37. Friberg, S.; Lindstrom, B. Radiographic measurements of the radiocarpal joint in normal adults. Acta Radiol (Stockh) 17:249, 1976.

38. Frykman, G. Fracture of the distal radius including sequelae—shoulder hand finger syndrome, disturbance in the distal radioulnar joint and impairment of nerve function. A clinical and experimental study. Acta Orthop Scand (Suppl.) 108:1–155, 1967.

39. Gartland, J.J. Jr.; Werley, C.W. Evaluation of healed Colles' fractures. J Bone Joint Surg 33:895–907, 1951.

40. Gelberman, R.H.; Szabo, R.M.; Mortensen, W.W. Carpal tunnel pressures and wrist position in patients with Colles' fractures. J Trauma 24:747–749, 1984.

41. Golden, G.N. Treatment and programs of Colles' fracture. Lancet 1:511–514, 1963.

42. Green, D.P. Pins and plaster treatment of comminuted fractures of the distal end of the radius. J Bone Joint Surg 57A:304–310, 1975.

43. Green, D.P.; O'Brien, E.T. Open reduction of carpal dislocation. Indications and operative techniques. J Hand Surg 3:250–265, 1978.

44. Hollingsworth, R.; Morris, J. The importance of the ulnar side of the wrist in fractures of the distal end of the radius. Injury 7:263–266, 1976.

45. Howard, P.W.; Stewart, H.D.; Hind, R.E.; Burke, F.D. External fixation or plaster for severely displaced comminuted Colles' fractures? J Bone Joint Surg 71B:68–73, 1989.

46. Jakob, R.P.; Fernandez, D.L. The treatment of wrist fractures with the small AO external fixation device. In: Uhthoff, H.K., ed. Current Concepts of External Fixation of Fractures. Berlin, Springer-Verlag, 1982, pp. 307–314.

47. Jenkins, N.H. The unstable Colles' fracture. J Hand Surg 14B:149–154, 1989.

48. Jenkins, N.H.; Jones, D.G.; Johnson, S.R.; Mintowt-Czyz, W.T. External fixation of Colles' fractures: An anatomical study. J Bone Joint Surg 69B:207–211, 1987.

49. Jones, R. Injuries of Joints. London, Henry Frowde and Hodder & Stoughton, 1915, p. 110.

50. Jupiter, J.B.; Masem, M. Reconstruction of post-traumatic deformity of the distal radius and ulna. Hand Clin 4:377–390, 1988.

51. Jupiter, J.B.; Lipton, H. Operative treatment of intraarticular fractures of the distal radius. Clin Orthop (in press).

52. Knirk, J.L.; Jupiter, J.B. Intraarticular fractures of the distal end of the radius in young adults. J Bone Joint Surg 68A:647–659, 1986.

53. Leung, K.S.; Tsang, H.K.; Chiu, K.H.; et al. An effective treatment of comminuted fractures of the distal radius. J Hand Surg 15A:11–17, 1990.

54. Lewis, M.H. Median nerve decompression after Colles' fracture. J Bone Joint Surg 60B:195–196, 1978.

55. Lidstrom, A. Fractures of the distal radius. A clinical and statistical study of end results. Acta Orthop Scand 41:1–118, 1959.

56. Linscheid, R.L. Kinematic considerations of the carpal joint. Clin Orthop 202:27–39, 1986.

57. Lucas, G.L.; Sachtjen, K.M. An analysis of hand function in patients with Colles' fractures treated by rush rod fixation. Clin Orthop 155:172–179, 1981.

58. Lynch, A.C.; Lipscomb, P.R. The carpal tunnel syndrome and Colles' fractures. JAMA 185:363–366, 1963.

59. McBride, E.D. Disability Evaluation, Ed. 4. Philadelphia, J.B. Lippincott, 1948.

60. McCarroll, H.R., Jr. Nerve injuries associated with wrist trauma. Orthop Clin North Am 15:279–287, 1984.

61. McMurtry, R.Y.; Jupiter, J.B. Fractures of the distal radius. In: Browner, B.; Jupiter, J.; Levine, A.; Trafton, P., eds. Skeletal Trauma. Philadelphia, W.B. Saunders, 1991.

62. McQueen, M.; Caspers, J. Colles fracture: Does the anatomic result affect the final function? J Bone Joint Surg 70B:649–651, 1988.

63. McQueen, M.M.; MacLaren, A.; Chalmers, J. The value of remanipulating Colles' fractures. J Bone Joint Surg 68B:232–233, 1986.

64. Melone, C.P., Jr. Articular fractures of the distal radius. Orthop Clin North Am 15:217–236, 1984.

65. Melone, C.P. Open treatment for displaced articular fractures of the distal radius. Clin Orthop 202:103–111, 1986.

66. Mohanti, R.C.; Kar, N. Study of triangular fibrocartilage of the wrist joint in Colles' fracture. Injury 11:321–324, 1980.

67. Müller, M.E.; Nazarian, S.; Koch, P., eds. Classification AO des Fractures. Les Os Longs. Berlin, Springer-Verlag, 1987.

68. Nakata, R.Y.; Chand, Y.; Matiko, J.D.; et al. External fixators for wrist fractures: A biomechanical and clinical study. J Hand Surg 10A:845–851, 1985.

69. Older, T.M.; Stabler, E.U.; Cassebaum, W.H. Colles' fracture: Evaluation of selection of therapy. J Trauma 5:469–476, 1965.

70. Overgaard, S.; Solgaard, S. Osteoarthritis after Colles' fracture. Orthopaedics 12:413–416, 1989.

71. Owen, R.A.; Melton, L.J.; Johnson, K.A.; et al. Incidence of a Colles' fracture in a North American community. Am J Public Health 72:605–613, 1982.

72. Palmer, A.K. Fractures of the distal radius. In: Green, D.P., ed. Operative Hand Surgery, Ed. 2. Philadelphia, J.B. Lippincott, 1988, pp. 991–1026.

73. Palmer, A.K. The distal radioulnar joint. Hand Clin 3:31–40, 1987.

74. Pattee, G.A.; Thompson, G.H. Anterior and posterior marginal fracture-dislocations of the distal radius. Clin Orthop 231:183–195, 1988.

75. Peltier, L.F. Fractures of the distal end of the radius. An historical account. Clin Orthop 187:18–22, 1984.

76. Pool, C. Colles's fracture. A prospective study of treatment. J Bone Joint Surg 55B:540, 1973.

77. Porter, M.L. Pilon fractures of the wrist: Displaced intraarticular fractures of the distal radius (in press).

78. Porter, M.; Stockley, I. Functional index: A numerical expression of post-traumatic wrist function. Injury 16:188–192, 1984.

79. Porter, M.; Stockley, I. Fractures of the distal radius. Intermediate and end results in relation to radiologic parameters. Clin Orthop 220:241–251, 1987.

80. Riis, J.; Fruensgaard, S. Treatment of unstable Colles' fractures by external fixation. J Hand Surg 14B:145–148, 1989.

81. Rubinovich, R.M.; Rennie, W.R. Colles' fracture: End results in relation to radiologic parameters. Can J Surg 26:361–363, 1983.

82. Saito, H.; Shibata, M. Classification of fractures at the distal end of the radius with reference to treatment of comminuted fractures. In: Boswick, J.A. Jr., ed. Current Concepts in Hand Surgery. Philadelphia, Lea & Febiger, 1983, pp. 129–145.

83. Sarmiento, A.; Pratt, G.W.; Berry, N.C.; Sinclair, W.F. Colles' fracture: Functional bracing in supination. J Bone Joint Surg 57A:311–317, 1975.

84. Sarmiento, A.; Zagorski, J.B.; Sinclair, W.F. Functional bracing of Colles' fractures: A prospective study of immobilization in supination vs. pronation. Clin Orthop 146:175–183, 1980.

85. Scheck, M. Long-term follow-up of treatment of comminuted fractures of the distal end of the radius by transfixation with Kirschner wires and cast. J Bone Joint Surg 44A:337–351, 1962.

86. Seitz, W.H. Jr.; Putnam, M.D.; Dick, H.M. Limited open surgical approach for external fixation of distal radius fractures. J Hand Surg 15A:288–293, 1990.

87. Short, W.H.; Palmer, A.K.; Werner, F.W.; Murphy, D.J. A biomechanical study of distal radial fractures. J Hand Surg 12A:529–534, 1987.

88. Smaill, G.B. Long-term follow-up of Colles' fracture. J Bone Joint Surg 47B:80–85, 1965.

89. Solgaard, S. Classification of distal radius fractures. Acta Orthop Scand 56(3):249–252, 1985.

90. Solgaard, S.; Binger, C.; Soelund, K. Displaced distal radius fractures. Arch Orthop Trauma Surg 109:34–38, 1989.

91. Sponsel, K.H.; Palm, E.T. Carpal tunnel syndrome following Colles' fracture. Surg Gynecol Obstet 121:1252–1256, 1965.

92. Stein, A.H. Jr.; Katz, S.F. Stabilization of comminuted fractures of the distal inch of the radius: Percutaneous pinning. Clin Orthop 108:174–181, 1975.

93. Stein, A.H. The relation of median nerve compression to Sudek's syndrome. Surg Gynecol Obstet 115:713–720, 1962.

94. Stewart, H.D.; Innes, A.R.; Burke, F.D. Factors affecting the outcome of Colles' fracture: An anatomical and functional study. Injury 16:289–295, 1985.

95. Stewart, H.D.; Innes, A.R.; Burke, F.D. The hand complications of Colles' fractures. J Hand Surg 10B:103–106, 1985.

96. Szabo, R.M.; Weber, S.C. Comminuted intraarticular fractures of the distal radius. Clin Orthop 230:39–48, 1988.

97. Taleisnik, J.; Watson, H.K. Midcarpal instability caused by malunited fractures of the distal radius. J Hand Surg 9A:350–357, 1984.

98. Thompson, G.H.; Grant, T.T. Barton's fractures—reverse Barton's fractures: Confusing eponyms. Clin Orthop 122:210–221, 1977.

99. van der Linden, W.; Ericson, R. Colles' fracture: How should its displacement be measured and how should it be immobilized? J Bone Joint Surg 63A:1285–1291, 1981.

100. Vaughn, P.A.; Lui, S.M.; Harrington, I.J.; Maistrelli, G.L. Treatment of unstable fractures of the distal radius by external fixation. J Bone Joint Surg 67B:385–389, 1985.

101. Villar, R.N.; Marsh, D.; Rushton, N.; Greatorex, R.A. Three years after Colles' fracture. J Bone Joint Surg 69B:635–638, 1987.

102. Weber, E.R. A rational approach for the recognition and treatment of Colles' fractures. Hand Clin 3:13–21, 1987.

103. Weber, S.C.; Szabo, R.M. Severely comminuted distal radial fracture as an unsolved problem: Complications associated with external fixation and pins and plaster techniques. J Hand Surg 11A:157–165, 1986.

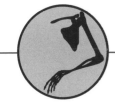

James F. Kellam, M.D.
Jesse B. Jupiter, M.D.

36

Diaphyseal Fractures of the Forearm

The supporting skeleton and articulations of the upper extremity serve to position its terminal unit, the hand, in space. In the adult, exacting management of diaphyseal fractures of the radius and ulna is necessary to assure forearm motion. These injuries can even be viewed as intraarticular fractures with the forearm "joint" providing supination and pronation. Unsatisfactory treatment can lead to loss of this motion as well as muscle imbalance and disability of hand function.[26,45,67]

The difficulties in forearm fracture management have long been recognized.[21,38,61,71] With the exception of a series by Evans,[26] most authors have been unable to achieve acceptable results in the adult forearm fracture with closed reduction and plaster cast immobilization. Even in Evans' series, there was greater than 50° loss of forearm rotation in nearly 30% of patients. Hughston[38] noted an exceptionally high rate of unsatisfactory results in isolated displaced radius (Galeazzi) fractures. Charnley,[16] writing in his classic book that advocated the nonoperative method of fracture care, recommended the operative treatment of adult forearm fractures.

Early operative efforts had disappointing outcomes that were as much the result of inadequate methods of internal fixation as any other reason. Knight and Purvis[40] reported on a high rate of nonunion with inadequate plate fixation despite additional plaster immobilization. Smith and Sage[69] developed a specific intramedullary nail for the radius and ulna. This still required open reduction and an above-the-elbow cast for three months, yet a nonunion rate close to 7% was described. Marek[43] modified the nailing approach, developing a square nail and changing the insertion point in the radius from the styloid to Lister's tubercle. An operative exposure and long-arm cast were required. Although union was described as 100%, a 22% unsatisfactory functional outcome was observed.

Perhaps in no other area of the appendicular skeleton has plate fixation had as dramatic an impact as in diaphyseal fractures of the adult forearm. Burwell and Charnley[12] in 1964 published a landmark paper reviewing 218 fractures in 150 patients treated with noncompressing Burns or Sherman plates. Even with these now-antiquated plates, the authors noted excellent results, provided the plates were at least 3.5 inches long and had six or more screws, and comminution did not exceed 50% or more of the cortical diameter. Plaster immobilization was infrequently used.

The advent of the compression plate originated by Danis in 1947 extended the percentage of predictable functional outcome with forearm plating.[19] In 1975, Anderson et al. published their experience using the principles of stable fixation of AO/ASIF[52] and noted union in 97.9% of radius fractures and 96.3% of ulnar fractures treated with compression plates.[2] Their results have subsequently been duplicated by a number of other investigators,[13,15,31,33,36,54,61,63,79] thus making compression plating of forearm fractures the standard by which all other treatments must be measured.

Goals of Treatment

To ensure maximal functional outcome, the goals of treatment of forearm fractures should be (1) anatomic reduction of the skeleton, restoring bony length, rotation, and the interosseous space; and (2) secure fixation of the skeleton to enable early soft tissue rehabilitation.

Classification of Diaphyseal Forearm Fractures

Currently, there is no universally accepted classification of diaphyseal fractures of the forearm. To be useful, a classification must document a number of factors, including the fracture location, pattern, soft tissue involvement, and proximal or distal radio-ulnar joint involvement.

Although based on relatively arbitrary factors, the forearm has been considered by many to be divided into thirds for surgical classifications (Fig. 36–1). The proximal third of the radius extends from the radial tuberosity to the beginning of the radial bow. The middle third includes the radial bow to the point at which the diaphysis begins to straighten. The distal third of the radius extends out to the metaphyseal flare.

The ulna, by contrast, is relatively straight, and can be divided into thirds based solely on linear dimensions (see Fig. 36–1).

The enveloping and interconnecting soft tissues must always be considered in identifying patterns of forearm injury.

In order to address the need for greater specification in forearm fracture classification, the Orthopaedic Trauma Association (Fig. 36–2) and the AO/ASIF (Fig. 36–3) have developed comprehensive classification systems of diaphyseal fractures that will become increasingly important as trauma centers compare results of treatment protocols.

Treatment

NONOPERATIVE

Indications

In the adult forearm fracture, the primary indication for nonoperative treatment is the isolated ulnar shaft fracture that has resulted from a direct blow ("nightstick fracture") (Fig. 36–4). Even if the fracture is displaced by 25% to 50% of the shaft width, the ulna can be effectively stabilized with a long-arm plaster cast for eight to ten weeks or a functional fracture brace. The latter has been reported by Sarmiento et al.[64,65] to successfully maintain the anatomic position of the bone when using a carefully made interosseous mold in the brace.

When located in the distal third of the ulna, displacement, particularly shortening, can result in deformity of the distal radio-ulnar joint articulation. If treating this fracture nonoperatively, this possibility must be carefully monitored.

With nondisplaced radial shaft fractures, nonoperative treatment may prove successful, provided the anatomic bow of the radius is maintained. The time to healing may be prolonged as the intact ulna prevents coaptation of the radius fracture.

OPERATIVE

Displaced fractures of the forearm diaphysis are best treated by operative means. To date, this has been most predictably accomplished with plate fixation and early functional rehabilitation. However, despite widespread acceptance of plate fixation, a number of issues continue to exist. These include timing, surgical technique, surgical approaches, fixation techniques, indications for ancillary bone graft, and postoperative management. With the exception of certain isolated ulnar fractures, all displaced fractures of the diaphysis of the radius and/or ulna are managed by open reduction and internal fixation. Despite widespread acceptance of plate fixation, a number of issues remain. These include timing, surgical technique, surgical approaches, fixation techniques, indications for ancillary bone graft, and postoperative management.

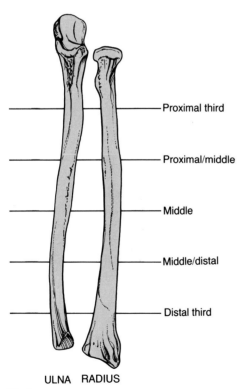

Proximal third

Proximal/middle

Middle

Middle/distal

Distal third

ULNA   RADIUS

Figure 36–1

Division of the forearm skeleton into thirds for surgical classification.

Shaft Fractures

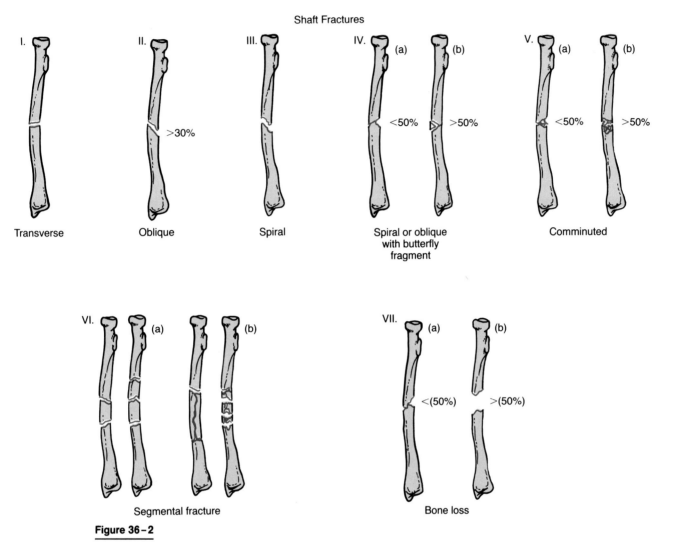

Figure 36–2

The classification for diaphyseal forearm fractures recommended by the Orthopaedic Trauma Association.

Timing

Although at one point it was suggested that operative intervention should be delayed to assure a higher rate of union,[69] this is no longer considered necessary. To the contrary, early operative treatment permits decompression of the fracture hematoma as well as ease of reduction of the fracture fragments, thus minimizing soft tissue trauma. Even many open forearm fractures have now been shown to be safely treated by immediate operative treatment (see section on open forearm fracture).[15,48] There are situations, however, such as polytrauma or a compromised soft tissue envelope, in which surgery is best delayed to allow either systemic or local conditions to improve.

Surgical Technique

The majority of fractures of the forearm can be readily approached with the patient supine and the forearm abducted onto a hand table. In this position, however, it is necessary to flex the elbow to gain access to the ulnar shaft. This factor has encouraged some surgeons to position the patient in the prone position. The ulna is approached with the forearm in pronation, and the radius is approached with the forearm supinated. However, this position may prove uncomfortable with regional block anesthesia and may increase the anesthetic risk in a medically compromised patient.

The use of a pneumatic tourniquet is advisable in most cases. The exception is in those situations in

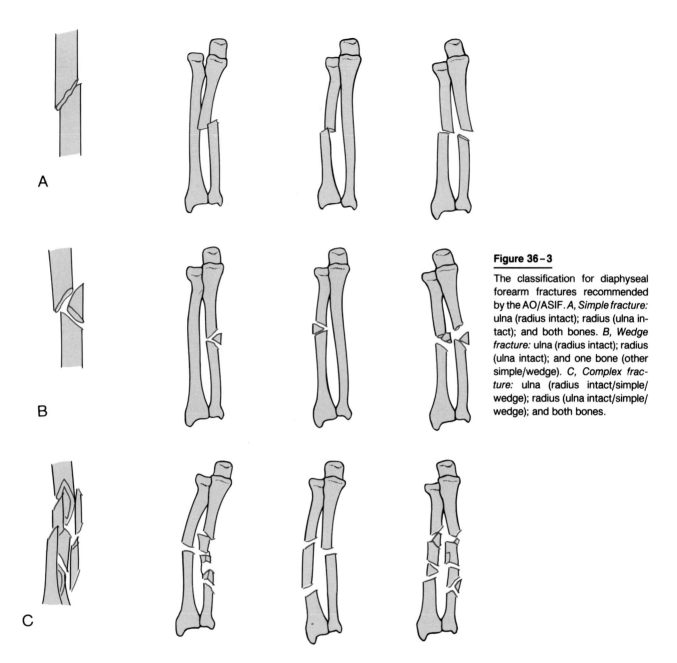

Figure 36-3

The classification for diaphyseal forearm fractures recommended by the AO/ASIF. *A, Simple fracture:* ulna (radius intact); radius (ulna intact); and both bones. *B, Wedge fracture:* ulna (radius intact); radius (ulna intact); and one bone (other simple/wedge). *C, Complex fracture:* ulna (radius intact/simple/wedge); radius (ulna intact/simple/wedge); and both bones.

which the soft tissue envelope is extremely traumatized (see section on open forearm fracture). Avoiding tourniquet-induced ischemia will aid the surgeon in assessing the viability of the compromised skeletal muscle during the surgical approach and debridement.

When a tourniquet is used, it is best left inflated for 90 to 120 minutes at most. The tourniquet should always be released prior to wound closure to assure control of bleeding.

Surgical Approaches

The wide variability of fracture patterns and soft tissue trauma make it vital that the surgeon become familiar with several surgical approaches to the forearm skeleton.[17]

Radius

Two general approaches have been advocated for the diaphysis of the radius: the anterior approach as described by Henry[35] and the dorsal approach of Thompson[78] (Table 36–1). The anterior approach is extensile, permitting ready extension across the elbow or onto the hand, presents a flat surface of the radius distally, and is ideal when fasciotomies are required. However, when the proximal radius is approached anteriorly, the surgeon is confronted with the major neu-

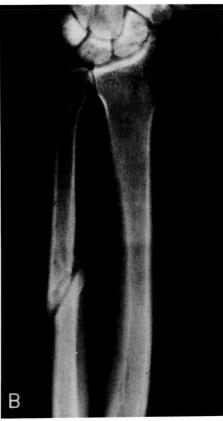
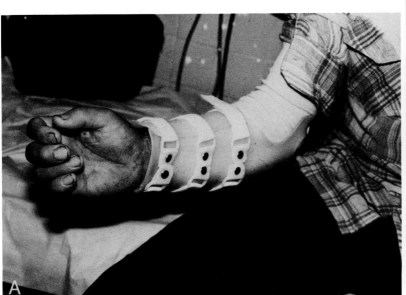

Figure 36-4

Minimally displaced nightstick fracture of the ulna treated effectively with a long-arm functional brace. Note the early callus.

rovascular structures of the forearm as they fan out anteriorly in front of the elbow.

The dorsal or Thompson approach is advantageous in that it is essentially subcutaneous for the distal half of its course. The proximal radius is readily approached as well, with only the common extensors covering the bone. Additionally, the plate can be applied along the dorsoradial cortex or "tension" side. The disadvantages include limited access to the anterior surface in the event a fasciotomy is required, the vulnerability of the posterior interosseous nerve to injury in the proximal third exposure, and the fact that it is not truly an extensile approach.

Anterior Approach. In the anterior approach, the patient is positioned supine with the arm abducted and forearm supinated. To approach the proximal radius, an incision is made starting at the lateral bicipital sulcus, extending across the elbow flexion crease, and distal to the midforearm. The brachioradialis muscle is identified and the fascia along the medial border incised (Fig. 36-5A). The lateral cutaneous nerve of the forearm is protected. The brachioradialis is retracted laterally and the biceps and brachialis tendons identified and retracted medially. The lacertus fibrosus must be divided. The radial nerve can be visualized at this juncture. The branches of the nerve can be identified,

Table 36-1.

Surgical Approaches to the Radius

Approach	Advantages	Disadvantages	Recommendation
Anterior (Henry)	Extensile; allows fasciotomy	Neurovascular structures proximally	Proximal third, distal third fractures
Posterior (Thompson)	Easy; plate on tension side	Not extensile	Middle third fractures

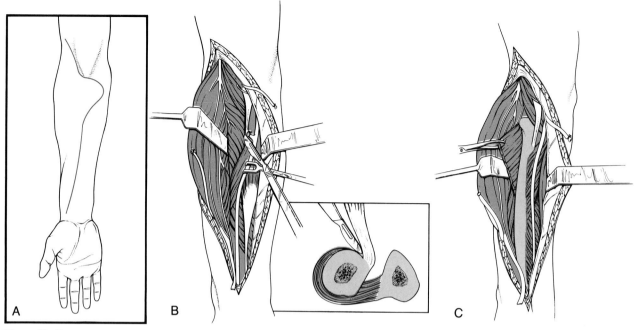

Figure 36–5

Anterior surgical approach to the radius. *A,* The surgical incision starts at the lateral bicipital sulcus, extending across the elbow flexion crease, and passes distally along the medial border of the brachioradialis. *B,* With the forearm maximally supinated, the supinator muscle is dissected off the proximal radius. The posterior interosseous nerve is protected within the two layers of the muscle. *C,* With the supinator detached, the brachioradialis and radial wrist extensors are readily mobilized to expose much of the radial diaphysis.

with the superficial sensory branch tracking over the supinator and passing distally into the forearm while the posterior interosseous nerve enters into the supinator muscle (Fig. 36–5*B*). With the forearm maximally supinated, the supinator muscle is dissected off the proximal radius with the posterior interosseous nerve protected within the two layers of the muscle. With the supinator detached, the brachioradialis and extensor carpi radialis longus and brevis can be mobilized radially to identify much of the radial shaft (Fig. 36–5*C*).

For more distal extension, the incision is carried distally one fingerbreadth lateral to the edge of the biceps to the radial styloid. The fascia is split longitudinally along the ulnar border of the brachioradialis. This muscle, as well as the remainder of the "mobile wad," can be taken radially. On the undersurface of the brachioradialis will be seen the superficial branch of the radial nerve. The radial artery will also be identified at this point lying on top of the flexor digitorum superficialis and across the pronator teres. The radius can be pronated, directing the surgeon to complete access to the dorsoradial surface (see Fig. 36–5*C*). If dissection is required to extend distally to the carpal tunnel, the palmaris longus will serve as a landmark in the identification of the median nerve, which lies between it and the flexor carpi radialis. The palmaris longus and median nerve can be retracted radially, with the superficial

and deep flexors taken ulnarly. This will reveal the pronator quadratus, which is elevated off the radius from its radial side. Complete access to the radius is gained from the distal articular margin into the forearm.

Closure of the anterior approach is straightforward. The only muscles that ordinarily require reattachment are the supinator proximally and the pronator quadratus distally. The remainder of the muscles will fall into place. The deep fascia is never closed. The subcutaneous tissue and skin are closed over a suction drain.

Dorsolateral or Thompson Approach. The dorsolateral approach is best suited to fractures of the proximal and middle thirds of the radius. The patient is positioned supine with the shoulder abducted and the arm resting on a hand table. The incision extends from the lateral epicondyle of the humerus along the dorsal border of the "mobile wad of Henry" (the extensor carpi radialis brevis and longus and brachioradialis muscles) down to the radial styloid. The length of incision is determined solely by the fracture. The fascia between the digital extensors and mobile wad is split. This interval is sometimes more apparent distally where the outcropping muscles of the thumb cross over the radius. Often a fibrous band can be identified between the extensor carpi radialis brevis and extensor digitorum communis. This "seam" is then developed

Figure 36-6

Dorsolateral approach to the radius. *A,* The surgical approach extends between the extensor carpi radialis brevis and extensor digitorum communis, exposing the supinator muscle in the proximal third of the forearm. *B,* The supinator muscle is elevated off the radius, providing access to the proximal and middle third of the radius.

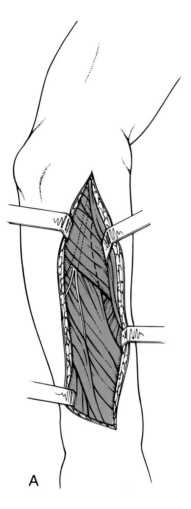

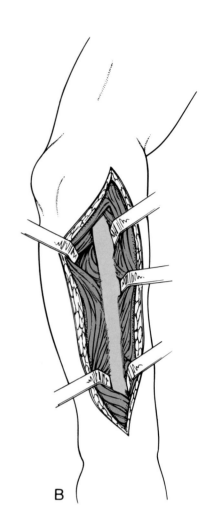

A

B

proximally in the direction of the lateral epicondyle. This will expose the supinator in the proximal third of the forearm (Fig. 36–6*A*).

At this point the posterior interosseous nerve has pierced the supinator anteriorly and is running at right angles to the muscle's fibers. The nerve can be identified by separating the fibers of the supinator at a level approximately three fingerbreadths distal to the radial head (Fig. 36–6*B*). The radius is next supinated to identify the insertion of the supinator muscle, which is elevated off the radius. The posterior interosseous nerve has entered the muscle more proximally and will be protected as the muscle is elevated. Ready access has now been gained to the proximal and middle third of the radius.

To expose the distal third, the surgeon must identify the exact location of the superficial radial nerve as it passes between the brachioradialis and digital extensors. The outcropping muscles of the thumb cross obliquely over the radius at this level. These are readily elevated to permit a plate to be placed beneath them.

The remainder of the radius distally is virtually subcutaneous.

Wound closure of the dorsal approach can be accomplished through closure of only the subcutaneous tissue and skin over a suction drain.

Ulna

The ulna lies in a subcutaneous position throughout its length in the forearm. The only structure of significance that crosses the ulna is the dorsal cutaneous branch of the ulnar nerve, which passes onto the dorsal surface of the flexor carpi ulnaris muscle approximately 6 to 8 cm proximal to the ulnar styloid. Consequently, when an incision is made along the distal third of the ulna, care must be taken to identify and protect this nerve.

To approach the ulnar shaft, an incision is made parallel and just slightly dorsal or volar to its palpable crest. The extensors are detached from the dorsal crest of the ulna. A plate can be applied either on the flexor or extensor surfaces, depending on the fracture configuration and the preoperative plan. This incision can be extended proximally to expose the olecranon or distal humerus. The ulnar nerve at this juncture must be identified and protected (Fig. 36–7).

Fixation Techniques

The forearm is a two-bone structure; thus reduction and fixation of one bone will present significant difficulty in obtaining reduction of the other bone. Consequently, it is advisable to expose both fractures and reduce the least comminuted fracture first, holding it provisionally with a plate and two clamps. This establishes length and facilitates reduction of the second fracture. Provisional fixation is applied to the second bone, and radiographs are obtained. When exposing an isolated diaphyseal fracture, assessment of the proximal and distal articulations is mandatory.

The fracture reduction can be controlled in a number of ways. The simplest way is to visualize the interdigitation of the fracture line and the contour of the diaphysis. This may not be easy with an extremely comminuted fracture. In this instance, following provisional fixation of both fractures, supination and pronation of the forearm is tested. If full forearm rotation has been restored, then the reduction should be considered acceptable, and a functional result can be anticipated. If forearm rotation is not complete, the fracture must be reduced again and rotation rechecked. Radiographic control of the reduction is mandatory.

Plate Application

The plate that has gained widespread acceptance is the 3.5-mm dynamic compression plate. In the vast majority of individuals, this plate, applied with appropriate technique and of adequate length, will be of sufficient strength to support functional loading while the fracture heals. In most cases, a minimum of eight cortices above and below the fracture will be required, the exception being a pure transverse fracture, which is effectively held with six cortices on each side (Fig. 36–8). In cases of comminution, 10- or 12-hole plates are recommended (Fig. 36–9).

Whenever possible, an interfragmentary screw is added either through the plate or in conjunction with the implant (Fig. 36–10). In pure transverse fractures, this will not be possible. In fractures with an oblique configuration, the plate is precontoured to sit slightly (1 mm) off the shaft over the fracture (Fig. 36–11A). The fracture is reduced and the plate applied by placing one screw in the fragment that has its obliquity facing away from the plate (Fig. 36–11B). This will allow the fragment, with its "spike" directly under the plate, to be pulled into the plate and fracture when compression is applied by the insertion of the load screw in the other fragment (Fig. 36–11C). Following this, a screw is placed as an interfragmentary lag screw through the plate across the oblique fracture line (Fig. 36–11D,E).

Spiral fractures are optimally fixed with the use of interfragmentary screw fixation over the length of the spiral. These screws serve as the primary means of achieving compression of the fracture. A plate is then applied as a "neutralization" plate spanning the fracture lines. The plate should be long enough to have screws in at least six cortices of cortical bone on either side of the fracture (see Fig. 36–10).

The management of comminuted fractures is more difficult. The first priority is to preserve the soft tissue attachments to the comminuted fragments. The approach to the skeleton should be extraperiosteal except at the fracture site. In the badly comminuted fracture, the surgeon should avoid attempting to reduce all the fragments and instead use the plate to maintain length and alignment; thus it functions as a "strut" plate. The more extensive the comminution, the greater will be the length of plate required to provide stable fracture fixation. The use of a distractor can prove invaluable in gaining length without extensive stripping of the bony fragments (Fig. 36–12).[44] Cancellous bone grafting should be performed at this time. As a general rule, if there exists a greater than one third loss of cortical contact opposite the plate or absolute stability cannot be assured, then cancellous bone grafting is indicated.

Segmental fractures can prove problematic. Two plates can be used if one plate is not long enough. When

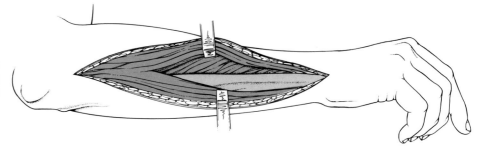

Figure 36–7

The surgical approach to the ulnar diaphysis is made parallel and just dorsal or volar to the palpable crest of the shaft.

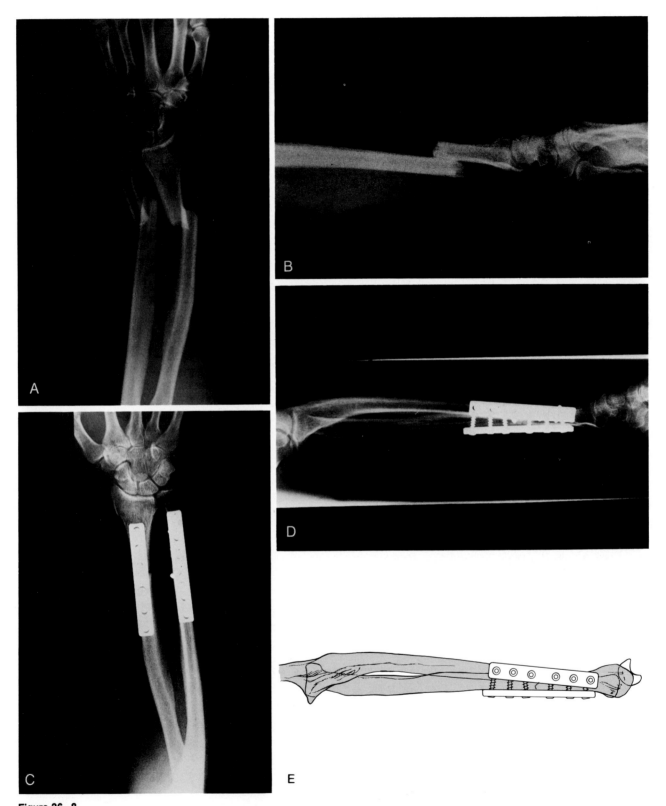

Figure 36–8

A 32-year-old construction worker sustained a transverse fracture of the distal third of both radius and ulna of his right dominant limb. *A* and *B*, Transverse fractures of both radius and ulna at the junction of mid to distal third of the forearm seen in AP and lateral radiographs. *C* and *D*, The fractures were each stabilized with six-hole 3.5-mm DC plates with an excellent functional outcome. *E*, Schematic of the internal fixation.

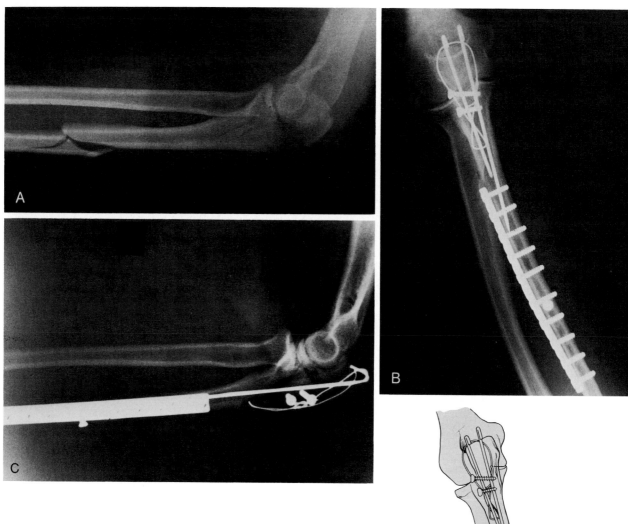

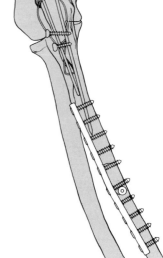

Figure 36–9

Complex ulna fracture including a large wedge fragment and a more proximal comminuted olecranon fracture. *A,* Lateral radiograph of a complex ulnar fracture including a large wedge fragment and a more proximal comminuted olecranon fracture. *B* and *C,* AP and lateral radiographs revealing stable internal fixation of the ulnar diaphysis with a ten-hole 3.5-mm DC plate neutralizing an interfragmentary lag screw, as well as a combination of interfragmentary screw and tension band fixation of the olecranon fracture. *D,* Schematic of the fixation.

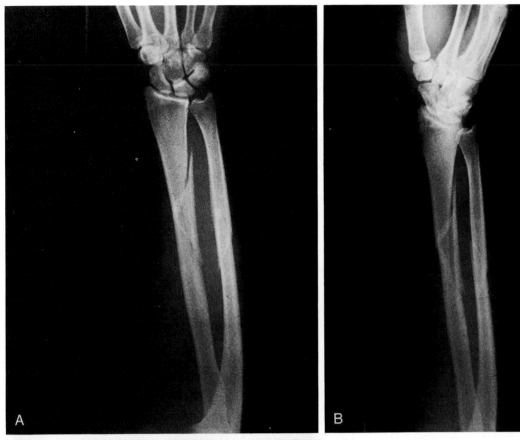

A

B

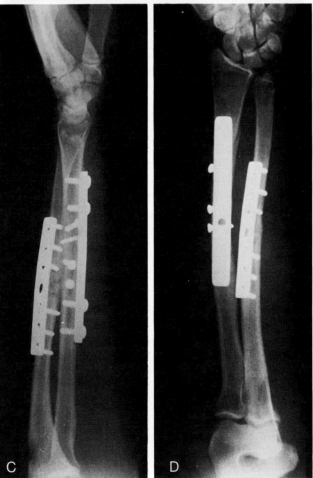

C   D   E

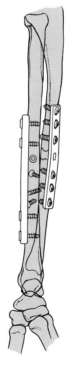

Figure 36–10

Spiral fracture of the radius treated with multiple interfragmentary lag screws and a plate. *A* and *B*, AP and lateral radiographs demonstrating a spiral fracture of the radius and transverse fracture of the ulnar diaphysis. *C* and *D*, AP and lateral radiographs revealing multiple interfragmentary screws providing compression across the spinal fracture. These screws are protected with a 3.5-mm DC plate. A six-hole DC plate securely stabilizes the transverse ulnar diaphysis fracture. *E*, Schematic demonstrating interfragmentary lag screws across the spiral fracture with a neutralization plate applied.

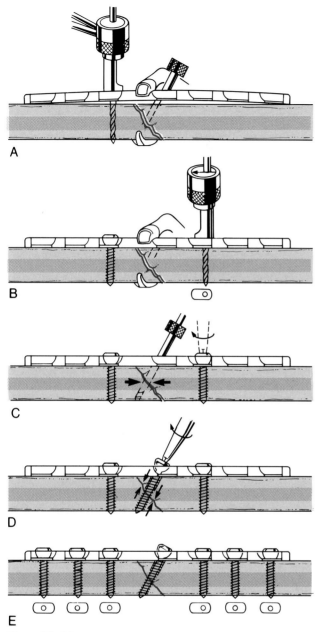

Figure 36–11

Schematic representation of the technique of applying a DC plate to an oblique forearm shaft fracture. *A,* The plate is precontoured to sit 1 mm off the shaft over the fracture site. The fracture is reduced, the plate is held with a clamp, and a screw is applied in a *neutral* mode in the fragment, which has its obliquity facing away from the plate. *B,* The gliding hole for an interfragmentary lag screw through the plate can next be drilled with a 3.5-mm drill bit. *C,* A screw is next applied in the "load" or compression position in the opposite fragment, which will allow this fragment to be "pulled into" the plate when compression is applied. *D* and *E,* The interfragmentary lag screw is then placed through the plate by drilling the far cortex with a 2.5-mm drill bit, tapping it with a 3.5-mm tap, and placing an appropriate length screw. *F,* The remainder of the screws are applied through the plate.

applying two plates to the bone, one should be at a right angle to the other (Fig. 36–13). The ulna, being a straight bone, is more amenable to intramedullary nailing to stabilize a segmental fracture.

The ulnar plate is most easily applied to the flat medial border, whereas the location of the plate on the radius will depend to a large degree on the surgical approach. For fractures of the proximal and middle thirds, the radial plate is ordinarily applied on the anterior or dorsolateral surface. The flat anterior surface of the distal radius is the preferred surface for fractures of the middle to distal third.

Indications for Ancillary Bone Graft

As a rule, cancellous bone grafting is recommended when comminution or bone loss has presented an anatomic reduction of the fracture fragments. The recommendation of Anderson et al. to use bone grafts if greater than one third of the diaphyseal cortex is deficient has become widely accepted.[2] In fact, the use of cancellous grafts in comminuted fractures has resulted in union rates comparable to those for closed, noncomminuted fractures.[15]

The anterior iliac crest is an excellent source for graft, although the distal radius or olecranon will provide adequate cancellous graft for most fractures. Great care must be taken to avoid placing graft across the interosseous space, especially with fractures of both forearm bones located at the same level, in order to prevent a synostosis from developing.

In the setting of high-energy trauma or gunshot wounds, significant bone loss may exist. Either acutely or once soft tissues have stabilized, a plate can be applied to ensure skeletal length and rotation and to maintain the interosseous space. In seven to ten days a cancellous graft can be used to span the defect. Rapid incorporation will generally ensue, given the well-vascularized environment in the forearm (Fig. 36–14).

Wound Closure

At the completion of internal fixation, the tourniquet is deflated and hemostasis assured. Wounds should never be closed under undue tension. Rather, it is advisable to leave the wound open and return to the operating room in 48 to 72 hours for either delayed closure or split-thickness skin grafts. In the interim, the wounds are covered with moist saline dressings.

With extensive soft tissue loss, flap coverage may be required. It has been our experience to treat skeletal injuries with internal rather than external fixation, as this best assures not only union but also maintenance of the functional anatomy.

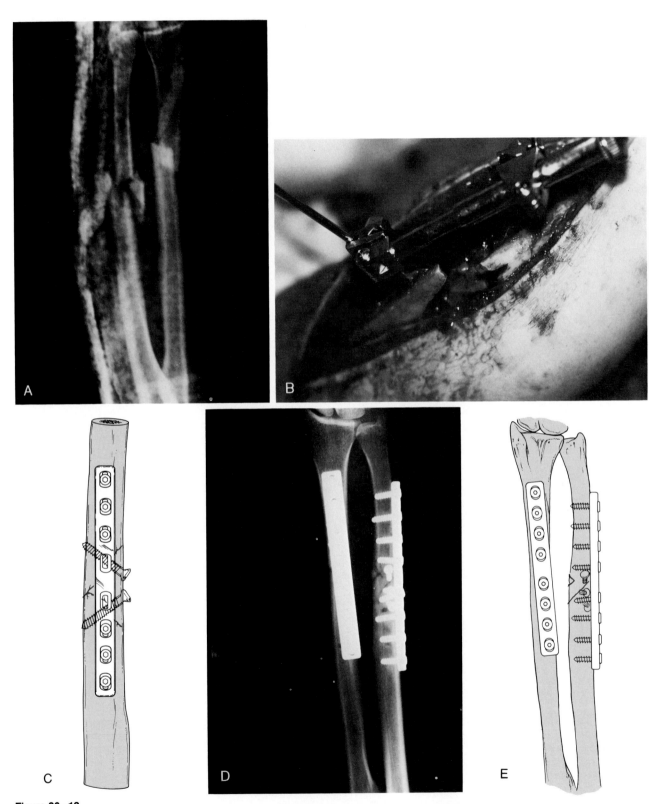

Figure 36–12

An open comminuted both-bone forearm fracture that occurred in a 27-year-old physician. *A,* AP radiograph demonstrating a comminuted ulnar and radial fracture. *B,* A minidistractor was applied to the ulnar shaft to distract the major fragments while the smaller fragments were teased into place. *C,* Schematic of the distractor in place. *D,* The fragments were fixed securely with interfragmentary lag screws, and eight-hole DC plates were applied to both ulnar and radial fractures. *E,* Schematic of plates in position.

Illustration continued on following page

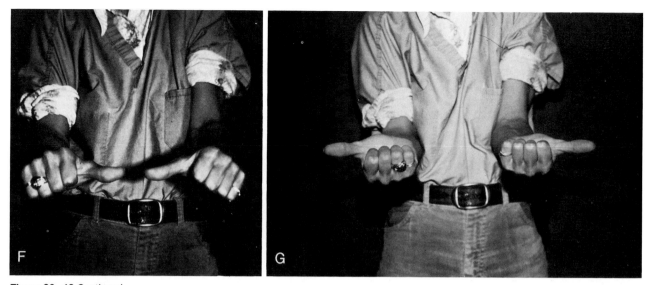

Figure 36-12 *Continued*

F and *G*, Normal function resulted.

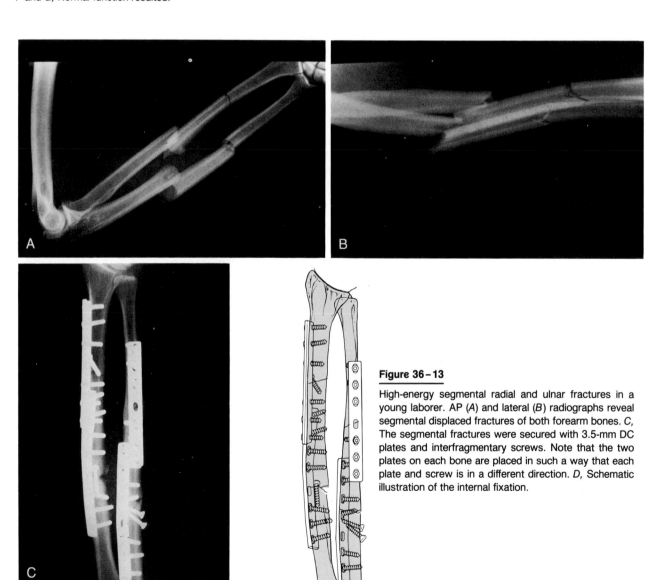

Figure 36-13

High-energy segmental radial and ulnar fractures in a young laborer. AP (*A*) and lateral (*B*) radiographs reveal segmental displaced fractures of both forearm bones. *C*, The segmental fractures were secured with 3.5-mm DC plates and interfragmentary screws. Note that the two plates on each bone are placed in such a way that each plate and screw is in a different direction. *D*, Schematic illustration of the internal fixation.

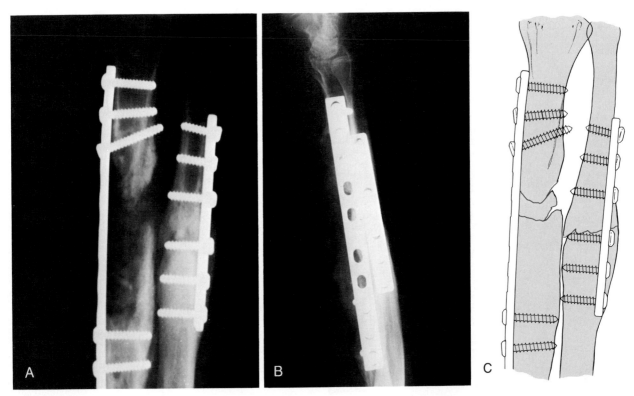

Figure 36–14

A 28-year-old man sustained a high-energy injury to his right forearm with extensive skeletal and soft tissue loss. Following extensive debridement, the ulna was stabilized with a six-hole DC plate. A groin flap was elevated and inset to cover the soft tissue defect. Ten days later, the radius was brought to length with a distractor and a "strut" plate was applied; the defect was filled with cancellous iliac crest graft. AP (*A*) and lateral (*B*) radiographs four weeks postoperatively demonstrate early incorporation of the cancellous graft. *C*, Schematic illustration of the internal fixation.

Postoperative Management

Closed, diaphyseal fractures treated with plate fixation are usually supported with a resting forearm plaster splint for patient comfort. Active digital and elbow motion is encouraged from the onset. Forearm rotation can be initiated once the patient is comfortable and wound healing has been assured, generally within three to five days postoperatively. If any question exists regarding the stability of the internal fixation or patient reliability, external functional bracing should be instituted in a manner such as that advocated by Sarmiento et al. (see Fig. 36–4*A,B*).[64] This provides excellent support of the forearm skeleton through a careful interosseous mold created in the splint, yet permits functional use of the extremity.

In general, most forearm fractures treated with plate fixation will heal within three to four months. During this period, the patient should be permitted to use the extremity for activities of daily living, avoiding only heavy lifting and sports. Once radiographic union has occurred, the patient may resume a normal life-style. Radiographic findings of callus, resorption at the frac-

ture site, or implant loosening should alert the treating physician to the possibility of instability of the internal fixation.

Open Fracture

The enhanced functional results achieved by anatomic skeletal restoration of forearm fractures have extended the application of plate fixation to the management of most open forearm fractures. Clinical studies by Moed et al.[48] and Chapman et al.[15] have documented a low rate of late infection: 1 of 79 fractures in 50 patients and 2 of 129 fractures in 87 patients, respectively. The results of these studies, as well as the experience of many other centers, have shown that infection and nonunion following internal fixation of open forearm fractures are uncommon.[12,21,22,31,36]

The management of the open forearm fracture demands meticulous attention to detail, both with the soft tissue as well as the skeleton. Cultures are obtained prior to debridement and are followed by broad-spectrum antibiotics and appropriate tetanus prophylaxis. A tourniquet is applied but not necessarily inflated in

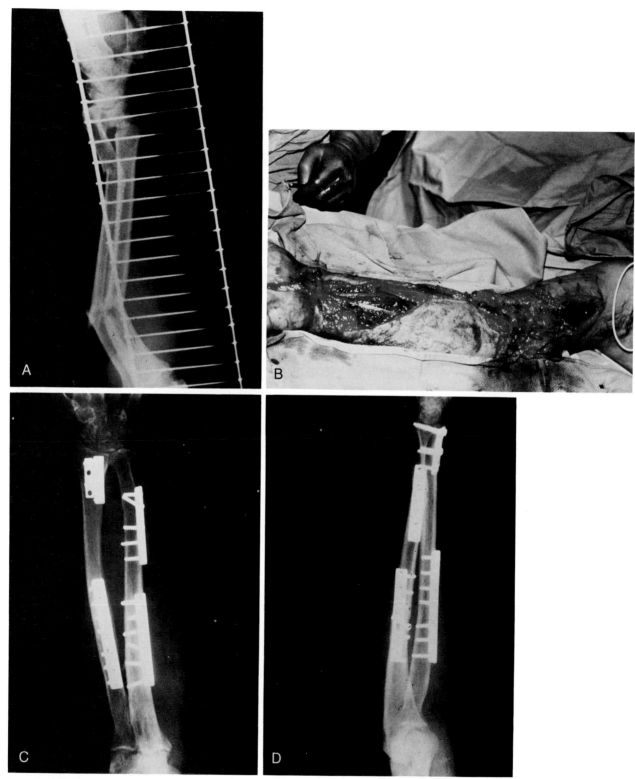

Figure 36–15

A 60-year-old laborer had his right (dominant) arm crushed in a press. *A,* Radiograph revealing segmental fractures of the radius and ulna, both of which were open. *B,* Extensive debridement and forearm decompression were achieved through an anterior approach. AP (*C*) and lateral (*D*) radiographs reveal segmental plating of the fractures. Excellent function resulted.

those wounds with extensive skeletal muscle trauma. Mechanical debridement, pulsed lavage, and direct debridement of the fracture ends through extensile exposures form the foundations of wound care. All devascularized tissue, including loose fragments of bone, should be excised. Anatomic reduction of the fractures is followed by plate fixation, with placement of the plates, whenever possible, under viable soft tissue coverage. The surgically created wounds can be closed, leaving the traumatic wounds open. Antibiotics are generally continued for two to five days postoperatively (Fig. 36–15).

Depending to some degree on the extent of the wound, nature of contamination, and associated injuries, a "second look" is recommended between 48 and 72 hours postoperatively. At that point, definitive wound closure can be considered. Delayed primary closure or split-thickness skin graft can be done in most Gustilo grade 1 or 2 wounds. In those wounds with extensive soft tissue loss or exposed plates, remote pedicled or microvascular flaps are required (see Chapter 15). At the time of definitive wound closure, cancellous iliac crest graft should be considered for those fractures with bone loss or comminution opposite the plate.[15,48]

In patients with extensive soft tissue loss, extreme contamination, or polytrauma, there may be occasions when internal fixation should be delayed. The application of external fixation or skeletal traction through a metacarpal pin will help to maintain skeletal length and alignment and soft tissue length until the patient is returned to the operating room for a repeat wound debridement. At that point, a judgment can be made to convert the internal fixation if the wound appears clean (Fig. 36–16). The combination of rigid skeletal fixation, meticulous soft tissue care, early wound closure, and liberal use of cancellous bone grafts has not only reduced the incidence of complications with these severe injuries, but has also maximized functional recovery.[15,48]

SPECIFIC LESIONS

Distal Third

Fractures involving the distal third of the forearm are deceptively difficult to treat. Situated at the junction of the diaphysis and metaphysis, these fractures prove unstable and offer a limited zone in which secure fixation can be achieved with plates and screws.

A particularly troublesome fracture is the short oblique fracture of the radius (Fig. 36–17). Often com-

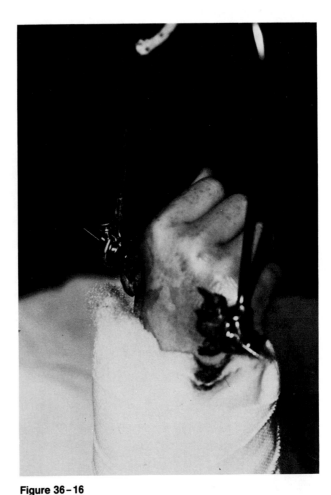

Figure 36-16

A heavily contaminated open forearm fracture that occurred in a horse stable and was treated with extensive debridement and temporary skeletal traction with a pin placed through the second and third metacarpal.

minuted, it is inherently unstable and not infrequently associated with disruption of the distal radioulnar joint. Viewed by some as just a metaphyseal fracture, external skeletal fixation spanning the fracture into pins in the metacarpals has been advocated. With this technique, the fixation must remain at least eight weeks to offset the likelihood of settling or displacement (Fig. 36–18). This is an even greater possibility when the fracture is comminuted. It has been our preference to advise open reduction and internal fixation with a plate acting as a buttress plate (Fig. 36–19). The management of associated distal radioulnar joint disruption is identical to that outlined with the Galeazzi fracture.

Fractures of the ulnar shaft at this level can also lead to functional limitations if allowed to shorten or angulate, thereby altering the mechanics of the distal radioulnar joint.

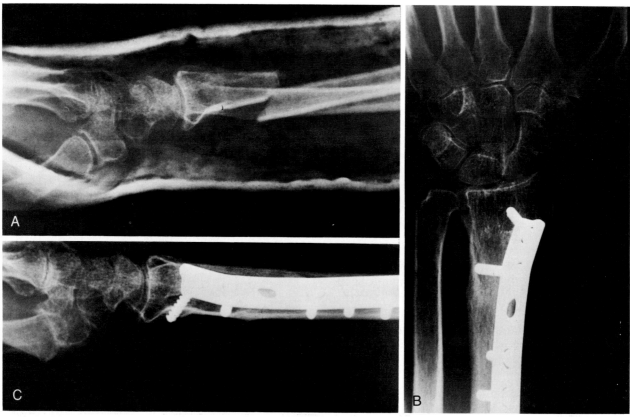

Figure 36–17

A short oblique fracture of the distal radius in a 56-year-old man. The fracture was initially treated with a cast. However, a follow-up radiograph (A) revealed an unsatisfactory alignment. AP (B) and lateral (C) radiographs one year following plate fixation with a 4.5-mm DC plate. Full function resulted.

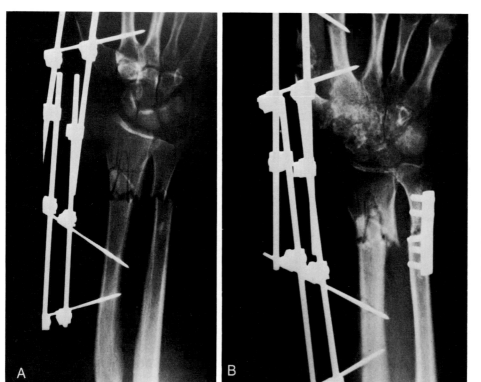

Figure 36–18

A comminuted fracture of the distal radius and ulna in a 50-year-old woman. A, The fracture was initially treated with skeletal fixation with the pins placed in the proximal radius and metacarpals. B, The ulna was fixed with a five-hole DC plate, but the radius was maintained in the external fixateur. Settling occurred at the fracture site with disruption of distal radioulnar joint function.

Figure 36-19

A 32-year-old woman with multiple injuries had this short oblique radius fracture treated in a splint for six weeks. *A,* AP radiograph demonstrating a short oblique distal radius fracture with shortening and disruption of the distal radioulnar joint. *B,* At surgery the extensor carpi ulnaris was found interposed between the ulnar head and distal radius. *C* and *D,* The fracture was taken down, lengthened, and secured with a 4.5-mm T plate. Residual disruption of the distal radioulnar joint remained, limiting the forearm rotation to 30% of normal.

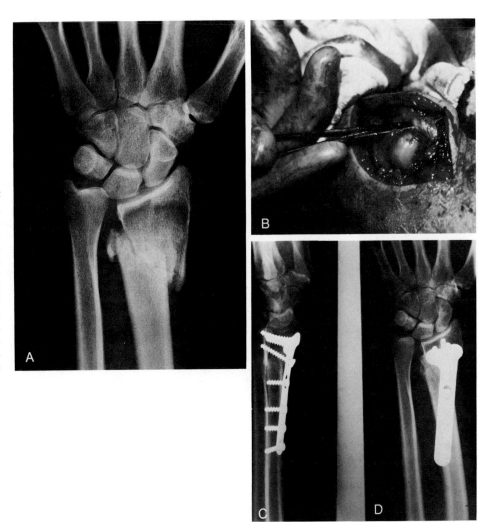

Galeazzi Fracture

Isolated fractures of the distal third of the radius can prove troublesome. Commonly referred to as the Galeazzi fracture,[28] they have also been called the reverse Monteggia fracture,[80] Piedmont,[38] or Darrach-Hughston-Milch[66] fracture. Whatever the eponym, its distinguishing feature is the associated subluxation or dislocation of the distal radioulnar joint (DRUJ).

The Galeazzi fracture is uncommon, with an incidence varying from 3%[84] to 6%[28,50,64] of all forearm fractures. Commonly thought to be the result of an axial load on a hyperpronated forearm,[47,81,84] the mechanism has never been reproduced in laboratory models.[27,51] More common in males,[21,47,50] its clinical features include pain and deformity at the distal radioulnar joint in association with a fracture of the radial shaft, most often at the juncture of the middle and distal thirds. The DRUJ disruption has also been observed to occur with isolated proximal or middle third

fractures of the radius.[47] As there may be substantial soft tissue swelling, the diagnosis must be confirmed radiographically. The radius fracture commonly has a short, oblique pattern, often angulated dorsally on the lateral view and shortened on the anteroposterior radiograph (Fig. 36-20).

The following radiographic findings suggest traumatic disruption of the DRUJ in the presence of an isolated fracture of the radial diaphysis[50]:

1. Fracture of the ulnar styloid at its base.

2. Widening of the distal radioulnar joint space as seen on the anteroposterior radiograph.

3. Dislocation of the radius relative to the ulna seen on a true lateral radiograph.

4. Shortening of the radius beyond 5 mm relative to the distal ulna.

Treatment

It is generally recognized that a Galeazzi fracture is best treated operatively. Campbell noted this in 1941, term-

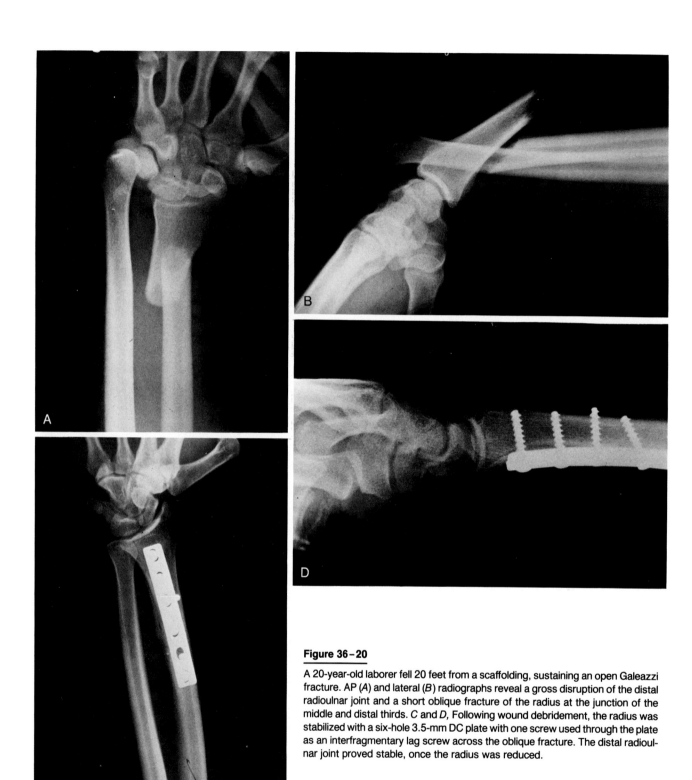

Figure 36–20

A 20-year-old laborer fell 20 feet from a scaffolding, sustaining an open Galeazzi fracture. AP (*A*) and lateral (*B*) radiographs reveal a gross disruption of the distal radioulnar joint and a short oblique fracture of the radius at the junction of the middle and distal thirds. *C* and *D*, Following wound debridement, the radius was stabilized with a six-hole 3.5-mm DC plate with one screw used through the plate as an interfragmentary lag screw across the oblique fracture. The distal radioulnar joint proved stable, once the radius was reduced.

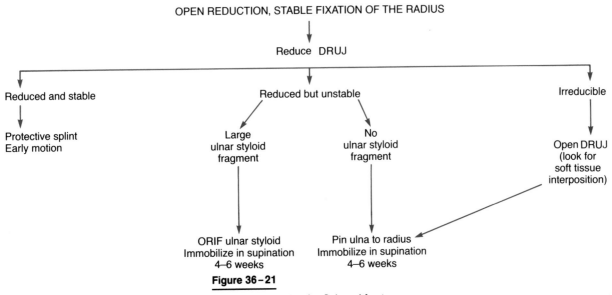

OPEN REDUCTION, STABLE FIXATION OF THE RADIUS

Reduce DRUJ

Reduced and stable → Protective splint / Early motion

Reduced but unstable → Large ulnar styloid fragment → ORIF ulnar styloid / Immobilize in supination / 4–6 weeks

Reduced but unstable → No ulnar styloid fragment → Pin ulna to radius / Immobilize in supination / 4–6 weeks

Irreducible → Open DRUJ (look for soft tissue interposition)

Figure 36–21

Treatment algorithm for Galeazzi fractures.

ing the Galeazzi fracture "a fracture of necessity."[76] The difficulties with nonoperative treatment were subsequently confirmed in 1957 by Hughston, who identified unsatisfactory results in thirty-five of the thirty-eight cases (92%) treated by closed reduction and plaster immobilization.[38] He identified several deforming forces that are not adequately controlled by plaster. These include the muscle pull of the brachioradialis, pronator quadratus, and thumb extensors as well as the weight of the hand. Although his criteria for a satisfactory result were strict (comprising union, anatomic alignment, no loss of length, no subluxation of the DRUJ, and no limitation of forearm rotation), succeeding clinical studies have supported his observations.[21,41,47,50,84]

The distal third of the radius is readily approached through the anterior (Henry) exposure. Stable internal fixation is most reliably achieved through compression plate fixation with a minimum of five and preferably six screws. Medullary nails or smaller plates may not control the deforming forces and have been associated with delayed union and nonunion.[21,50,75]

Once the anatomic reduction is secured and the plate provisionally applied with two screws, radiographs are obtained in both the anteroposterior and true lateral planes to control the DRUJ. If reduction has been achieved, then stability is tested clinically with rotation of the forearm (Fig. 36–21). If stable throughout full forearm rotation, there is no need for postoperative immobilization and early functional rehabilitation.

If reduction of the DRUJ can be achieved but proves unstable with forearm rotation, two options are available. In those cases in which there is an associated frac-

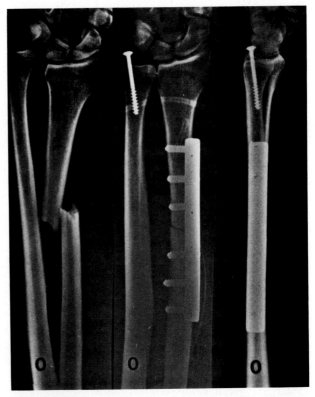

Figure 36–22

A Galeazzi fracture associated with continued instability of the distal radioulnar joint in spite of anatomic reduction and internal fixation of the radius. Once fixation of the large styloid fragment was achieved, the joint proved stable.

ture of the ulna styloid at its base, open reduction and fixation of the styloid with Kirschner wires or a small screw can effectively stabilize the DRUJ in some cases (Fig. 36–22).[47] If the reduction is stable clinically, the forearm should be immobilized in supination by an above-elbow cast brace for four to six weeks to allow for soft tissue healing. If no styloid fracture is present, the distal ulna can be transfixed to the radius with one or two 0.062-inch Kirschner wires left for four weeks. The forearm should also be immobilized in supination by an above-elbow cast brace during this time (Fig. 36–23).

In the unlikely event that DRUJ cannot be reduced, a soft tissue block should be suspected. The DRUJ can be approached through a dorsal incision and the source of the block identified and removed. In most reported cases, the extensor carpi ulnaris tendon has been the cause (see Fig. 36–19B) of the irreducible DRUJ. Instability of the DRUJ may also result from failure to recognize the injury, in part because of inadequate radiographs postoperatively or intraoperatively.

Complications

The complications of the Galeazzi fracture are not uncommon, with Moore et al. reporting a 39% incidence in 36 patients.[50] These include nonunion, malunion, infection, instability of the DRUJ, refracture following plate removal, and nerve injury associated with the operative treatment. Nonunion or malunion have been most commonly reported in association with plaster casts and inadequate internal fixation.[50,66,75] Instability of the DRUJ may be due to failure to recognize the injury, in part the result of inadequate x-rays films taken postoperatively or intraoperatively.

The radial nerve is the nerve most frequently injured. In Moore et al.'s series, six dorsal sensory and one pos-

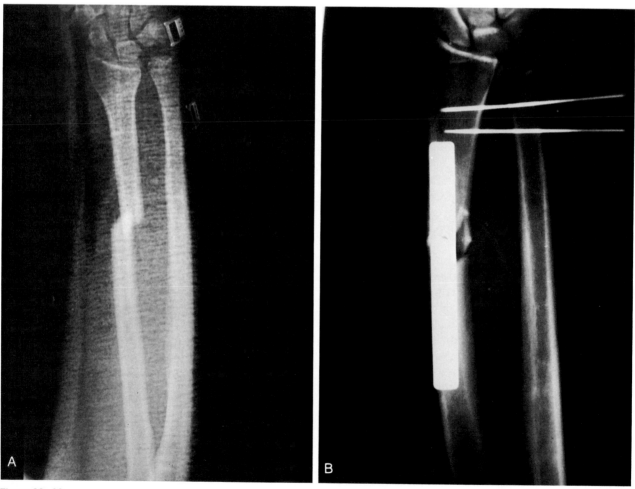

Figure 36–23

Despite stable fixation of the radius fracture, the distal ulna remained unstable even with the forearm supinated. Therefore the ulna was stabilized to the distal radius with two Kirschner wires for four weeks.

terior interosseous nerves were injured.[50] In the six dorsal sensory nerve injuries, three occurred with an anterior approach and three with a dorsal approach. In four of six cases, the nerve was not identified at the time of surgery.

Monteggia Lesion

Fracture of the proximal ulna with a dislocation of the radial head bears the eponym of Monteggia, who first described this association in Milan in 1814.[49] Bado

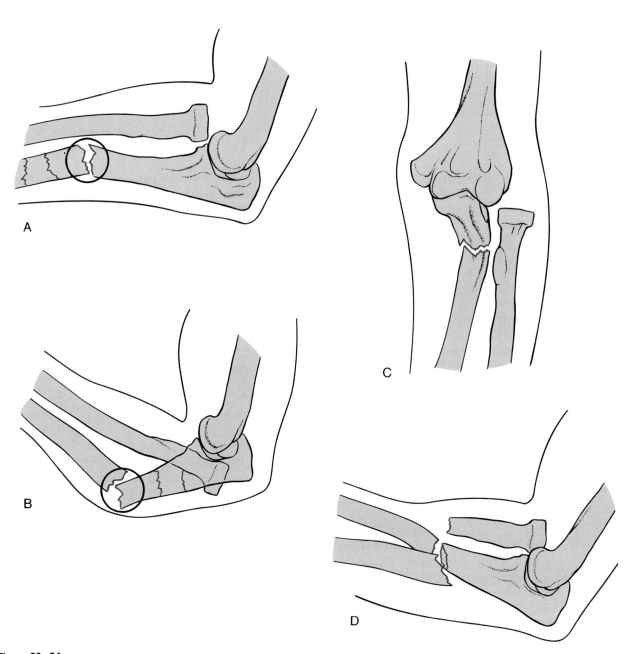

Figure 36–24

The classification of Monteggia lesions by Bado. *A,* Type I: anterior angulation of the ulnar fracture and anterior dislocation of the radial head. *B,* Type II: posterior angulation of the ulnar fracture and posterior dislocation of the radial head. *C,* Type III: fracture of the proximal ulna metaphysis and lateral dislocation of the radial head. *D,* Type IV: anterior dislocation of the radial head and fracture of the radial and ulnar shafts.

coined the term "Monteggia lesion" to encompass a number of traumatic lesions having in common disruption of the radio-humeral-ulnar joint in conjunction with a fracture of the ulna at any level.[5]

Although much has been published regarding the various presentations, treatment options, and complications, the Monteggia lesion remains a relatively uncommon injury, its incidence varying between 1% and 2% of all forearm fractures.[12,13,60,66] Problems arise in understanding these lesions in part because few individual surgeons have a wide experience. The literature can also be misleading, as a number of series combine adult and pediatric injuries.

It has become acceptable to categorize Monteggia fractures in terms of the direction of the dislocation of the head of the radius: anterior, posterior, or lateral. The ulnar fracture has characteristically been located at the junction of the proximal and middle thirds, although it is not unusual for it to occur proximal or distal to this. The apex of angulation of the ulnar fracture is in the same direction as the displacement of the radial head (Fig. 36–24). Bado expanded the categories to include a fourth group—anterior dislocation of the radial head with a fracture of both the ulna and radius at the proximal third of the forearm.[4]

The type I anterior lesion was long thought to be the result of a direct blow to the posterior aspect of the forearm, fracturing the ulna and forcing the radial head anteriorly.[70,72] Evans, however, in experiments on cadavers was able to create this lesion with a hyperpronation force on the forearm with the humerus held fixed in a vise.[25] He postulated that this injury was instead the result of a fall on the outstretched hand with the forearm fixed in maximal pronation. Rotation of the torso on this fixed pronated forearm results in fracture of the ulna; the radius is forced into hyperpronation and is levered anteriorly by the forearm of the fractured ulna.

The anterior dislocation (Bado type I) has been considered the most common type, comprising as much as 60% to 80% of all Monteggia lesions in some series (Fig. 36–24A).[7,72] The posterior and lateral dislocations have been considered to be less common. However, as these series tend to combine both adult and pediatric injuries, these published incidences may in fact not be universally the same in adult trauma centers.

In series by Penrose[56] and Pavel et al.,[55] the posterior presentation proved more common than previously recognized (Fig. 36–24B). The authors identified three distinct components to this injury. These include (1) a comminuted fracture of the proximal ulna near the coronoid, frequently including a triangular or quadrangular fragment; (2) posterior dislocation of the proximal radius; and (3) a triangular chip fracture of the anterior aspect of the radial head resulting from a shearing injury against the capitellum (Fig. 36–25A,B). Penrose[56] felt this lesion more closely resembled a variation of a posterior dislocation of the elbow, except in this case the ligamentous attachments of the elbow prove stronger than the ulnar shaft. To prove this theory, he placed cadaver humeri on a rigid support with the elbow at 60° of flexion and the forearm in moderate pronation. A direct blow was given across the wrist, resulting in posterior dislocation of the elbow. When the upper anterior surface of the ulna was notched, a similar force consistently produced the posterior Monteggia lesion he observed clinically. Unlike the anterior Monteggia lesion, which occurs frequently in the pediatric age group, this lesion is more likely to be seen in a middle-aged adult, typically resulting from a fall on the outstretched hand with the elbow flexed approximately 60° and the forearm pronated around 30°. At the Massachusetts General Hospital from 1981–1988, 20 adult Monteggia fractures had been treated surgically; 14 were this posterior variant.

The third type of Monteggia fracture, that with a lateral displacement of the radius, has been identified in both pediatric and adult patients. It has been attributed to be the result of a primary adduction force[58] or of both angulation and rotation.[53] This lesion has been associated with radial nerve trauma.[73] The clinical presentation of all Monteggia lesions is a painful elbow that resists attempts at elbow flexion, extension, or forearm rotation. The neurovascular status must be evaluated, as associated posterior interosseous, anterior interosseous, and ulnar nerve lesions have all been reported.[11,24,74]

The Monteggia lesion may be misdiagnosed on the initial examination. Whereas the ulnar fracture is readily apparent, the radius dislocation can be overlooked. Several factors account for this.[30] The injury is uncommon and thus is not always suspected. With associated soft tissue swelling or deformity about the elbow, the position of the radial head can be difficult to assess. In addition, the radial head may have been reduced when the ulna fracture was splinted. The radiographs may not be adequate if they are centered on the ulna fracture and miss the elbow.

In the presence of an isolated forearm diaphyseal fracture, the clinician must always anticipate the possibility of injury to the other bone. A line drawn through the radial shaft and head should contact the capitellum in any position of flexion or extension of the elbow if the radial head is correctly located.[46]

Closed treatment remains standard for most pediatric fractures. In the adult displaced Monteggia lesion, operative reduction and stable fixation are mandatory. The ulna fracture must be anatomically reduced and securely stabilized in order to assure an accurate repo-

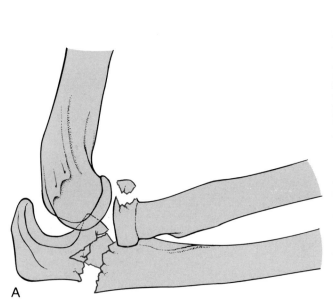

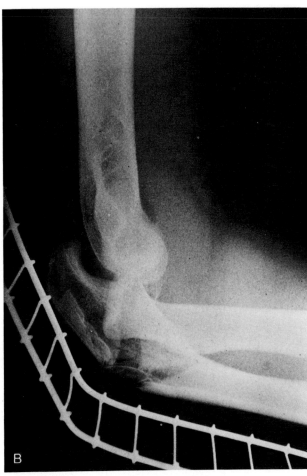

Figure 36–25

A, Schematic of a posterior Monteggia lesion. The features of this fracture dislocation include (1) comminuted fracture of the proximal ulna near the coronoid, (2) posterior dislocation of the proximal radius, and (3) triangular chip fracture of the radial head resulting from shearing against the capitellum. *B,* Lateral radiograph of a posterior Monteggia lesion in a 36-year-old man.

sition of the radial head. In most instances, this is best accomplished with a plate, although excellent results have sometimes been observed with intramedullary rods.

Once operative fixation is achieved, the surgeon must assure the stability of the radial head by fully flexing and extending the elbow and rotating the forearm, preferably under image intensification. Instability of the radial head or incomplete reduction usually suggests a malreduction of the ulnar fracture.[66] This is especially true with a posterior lesion. A comminuted metaphyseal ulna fracture, unless rigidly secured, tends to flex at the fracture site, levering the radial head posteriorly. In these fractures, a plate applied on the dorsal surface of the ulna better assures an anatomic reduction and functions mechanically as a tension band (Fig. 36–26).

If the radial head cannot be relocated despite an ana-

tomic reduction of the ulna (less than 10% of cases), the incision should be extended as a Boyd-Thompson approach, reflecting the anconeus, extensor carpi ulnaris, and supinator muscles from the ulna and exposing the radio-capitellar joint. Soft tissue interposition will likely prove to be the source of the inability to reduce the radial head and can be either the joint capsule, annular ligament, or, in some instances, the posterior interosseous nerve.

Boyd and Boals[8] described a procedure to stabilize the radial head by reconstructing a new annular ligament using a strip of forearm fascia elevated from distal to proximal. Our experience as well as that of others[61] has been that this is rarely, if ever, necessary and is fraught with the possibility of residual scarring and loss of forearm rotation.

In a radial head fracture, the fracture fragment may also serve to block reduction or elbow motion. A large,

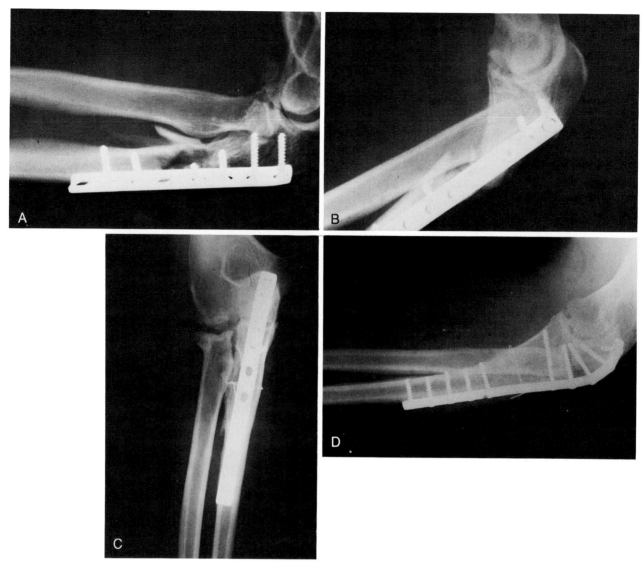

Figure 36-26

A 44-year-old male had a posterior Monteggia lesion treated with a plate applied to the lateral surface of the ulna. Incomplete reduction of the radial head was noted. *A,* Lateral radiograph showing inadequate skeletal fixation with the plate. Note the persistent posterior subluxation of the fractured radial head. *B,* The fracture displaced with the inadequate fixation. AP *(C)* and lateral *(D)* radiographs five months after revision surgery including placement of a 12-hole 3.5-mm DC plate on the tension side and radial head resection.

single fragment is best fixed internally, whereas a smaller fragment should be excised. A comminuted radial head represents one of the indications for a radial head Silastic arthroplasty.

Complications of Monteggia lesions are many and can be disabling. These include loss of motion, malunion, nonunion, and nerve palsy, which most often involves the posterior interosseous nerve. The prognosis is good, with recovery beginning within six to eight weeks after injury.[39] If, however, there is no evidence of nerve function by this period, then exploration is advisable. Tardy radial nerve palsy has been reported with longstanding radial head dislocation and responds well to nerve exploration and radial head excision.[3,42]

Malunion can follow failure to diagnose the radial head dislocation, inadequate reduction of the ulnar fracture, or unstable internal fixation. When recognized, consideration can be given to osteotomy of the ulna and plate fixation. In longstanding deformities, radial head resection may be necessary.

Nonunion of the ulna fracture almost always reflects inadequate skeletal fixation. In the absence of infection, union is readily achieved with a plate applied on the dorsal (tension) surface and, in some instances, supplemented by iliac crest bone graft.

Plate Removal and Refracture

Concern regarding "stress protection" of the bone under a plate, "stress concentration" at the end of the plate, and patient discomfort has led many in the past to recommend removal of forearm plates. The actual incidence of a fracture occurring beyond a plate is unknown but does pose a problem in the athlete involved in contact sports.

Plate removal, however, is not without complications. Refracture following forearm plate removal has been reported to be less than 4% in some series[15,21] and as high as 25% in others.[20,37] The basis for this wide variation of incidence is better understood when the number of factors that contribute to refracture in these series is analyzed. Premature plate removal (at times less than one year following injury), delayed union or nonunion, and inadequate technique were all identified by Deluca et al. and Hidaka and Gustilo as causes of refracture.[20,37]

Bone loss under a plate was long thought to be induced by a mechanical unloading of the bone ("stress protection") by the implant. It has now been demonstrated by Perren and co-workers that the initial porosis observed under a plate is the result of local circulatory disturbance and necrosis followed by bony remodeling.[57] According to these observations, plate removal should be considered only after the remodeling is complete and the cortex under the plate returned to a near normal condition.

Given these observations, should forearm plates be removed? It has become our policy to not recommend routine removal of the plates. If plates are to be removed, radiographic evidence of cortical remodeling under the plate should be present—often requiring two years after plating.

What, then, should be done for the high-demand athlete? Again, the plate is best left in place until cortical remodeling is evident. Following plate removal, the forearm should be protected with a functional forearm brace for six weeks. Return to activity should occur three to four months after removal.

If pain is the reason for plate removal, the surgeon must identify whether the pain is at the site of the original fracture. Should this be the case, adequate imaging, including radiographs and tomographs, should be considered to define the status of fracture healing.

Synostosis

Cross union between the forearm bones, first described by Gross in 1864,[32] has subsequently been identified in conjunction with nearly every form of forearm

trauma.[62,82,83] Although it is more commonly located in the middle and proximal third, the distal forearm is not entirely spared from this troublesome complication (Fig. 36–27).

The true incidence of cross union secondary to forearm fractures is difficult to accurately determine, as not all reported series address this issue. Vince and Miller reviewed 2381 reported forearm fractures in the literature and identified a combined incidence of approximately 2%.[82] The incidence may be higher with Monteggia fractures, particularly those involving both forearm bones along with dislocations of the radial head.[9,79]

A number of etiologic factors have been implicated in the formation of cross union, but the most likely causes include high-energy trauma involving open fractures,[10,59] infection,[13] multiple trauma involving head injuries,[29,82] and delayed (i.e., several weeks) internal fixation.[23,71,82] Less common but also possible factors include nonanatomic reduction with narrowing

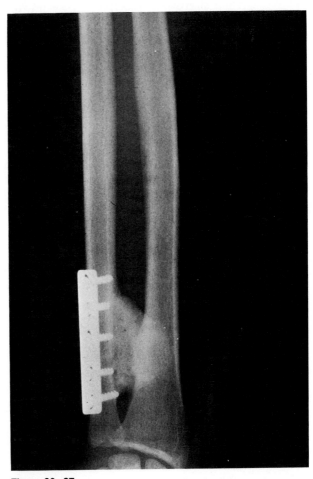

Figure 36–27

A large bony synostosis from a fracture of the distal ulna. This resulted in complete absence of forearm rotation.

of the interosseous space, onlay bone grafting, or the use of screws that are too long and cross the interosseous membrane.[6,18,40]

Although there have been no studies specifically identifying measures to prevent synostosis, it would appear that those fractures (open or closed) treated early with stable internal fixation and mobilized in the early postoperative period have little risk of developing cross union.[31,34,36]

The pessimism that surrounds the treatment of this problem should perhaps be reserved for synostosis in the proximal third of the forearm. In this area, there is a risk of neurovascular injury and a real chance of recurrence of the bony block, which may not at all be the case in the middle or distal third of the forearm.

Surgical excision with or without interposition of muscle,[10] fat,[85] or silicone[68] should be considered between one and two years following injury. Serial bone scans may assist in documenting the biologic activity of the synostosis. However surgery beyond two years after injury faces a compromised outcome because of muscle atrophy and fibrosis of the interosseous membrane.[82]

Assessment of Outcome

Normal function and skeletal union are the goals of treatment of adult forearm fractures. Therefore any assessment of outcome must address these criteria as well as associated complications. The assessment criteria of Anderson et al.[2] continue to function as a reliable means of identifying outcome and allow a more accurate comparison of the results of different studies (Table 36–2).

In their series of 330 acute fractures in 244 patients,

Anderson et al.[2] recorded 85% satisfactory or excellent results. Union rates for radius fractures were 97.9% within an average of 7.4 weeks and 96.3% within 7.3 weeks for ulnar fractures. Infection occurred in 2.9% of cases and nonunion in 2.9% of cases. In this series, 4.5-mm DC plates were used for the most part.

In a more recent series using the same grading system, Chapman et al.[15] evaluated 129 diaphyseal forearm fractures. They used primarily 3.5-mm DC plates; union was recorded in 98% of fractures, and 92% of patients achieved a satisfactory or excellent result. Infection was found in 2.3% of cases.

In other series reporting on the higher rates of complications associated with plate fixation of forearm fractures,[21,75] the authors emphasize that the source of most of the complications is lack of attention to detail, errors in judgment, or errors in technique.

Table 36–2.
Outcome Evaluation Scale

Excellent	Union with less than 10° loss of elbow or wrist flexion/extension
	Less than 25% loss of forearm rotation
Satisfactory	Union with less than 20° loss of elbow or wrist flexion/extension
	Less than 50% loss of forearm rotation
Unsatisfactory	Union with >30° loss of elbow or wrist flexion/extension and with >50% loss of forearm rotation
Failure	Malunion, nonunion, or unresolved chronic osteomyelitis

Source: Anderson, L.D., et al. J Bone Joint Surg 57A:287–297, 1975.

REFERENCES

1. Alexander, A.H.; Lichtman, D.M. Irreducible distal radio-ulnar joint occurring in a Galeazzi fracture. Case report. J Hand Surg 6:258–261,1981.
2. Anderson, L.D.; Sisk, T.D.; Tooms, R.E.; Park, W.I. III. Compression-plate fixation in acute diaphyseal fractures of the radius and ulna. J Bone Joint Surg 57A:287–297, 1975.
3. Austin, R. Tardy palsy of radial nerve from a Monteggia fracture. Injury 7:202, 1976.
4. Bado, J.L. The Monteggia lesion. Clin Orthop 50:71–76, 1967.
5. Bado, J.L. The Monteggia Lesion. Springfield, IL, Charles C Thomas, 1962.
6. Botting, T.D.J. Post-traumatic radio-ulnar cross-union. J Trauma 10:16–24, 1970.
7. Boyd, H.B.; Boals, J.C. The Monteggia lesion. Clin Orthop 66:94, 1969.
8. Boyd, H.B. Surgical exposure of the ulna and proximal third of the radius through one incision. Surg Gynecol Obstet 71:87, 1940.
9. Brady, L.P.; Jewett, E.L. A new treatment of radio-ulnar synostosis. South Med J, 53:507–512, 1960.
10. Breit, R. Post-traumatic radio-ulnar synostosis. Clin Orthop 174:149–152, 1983.
11. Bruce, H.E.; Harvey, J.P.; Wilson, J.C. Monteggia fractures. J Bone Joint Surg 56A:1563, 1974.
12. Burwell, H.N.; Charnley, A.D. Treatment of forearm fractures in adults with particular reference to plate fixation. J Bone Joint Surg 46B:404–424, 1964.
13. Caden, J.G. Internal fixation of fractures of the forearm. J Bone Joint Surg 43A:1115–1121, 1961.
14. Cetti, N.E. An unusual cause of blocked reduction of the Galeazzi injury. Injury 9:59–61, 1977.
15. Chapman, M.W.; Gordon, J.E.; Zissimos, A.G. Compression plate fixation of acute fractures of the diaphysis of the radius and ulna. J Bone Joint Surg 71A:159–169, 1989.
16. Charnley, J. The Closed Treatment of Fractures, Ed 3. New York, Churchill Livingstone, 1961.
17. Crenshaw, A.H. Campbell's Operative Orthopaedics, Ed. 7. St. Louis, C.V. Mosby, 1987, p. 94.
18. Crowie, R.J. Fractures of the forearm treated by open reduction and plating. Br J Surg 44:263–266, 1956.

19. Danis, R. Theorie et pratique de l'osteosyntheses. Paris, Mason, 1947.
20. Deluca, P.A.; Lindsey, R. W.; Rowe, P.A. Refracture of bones of the forearm after the removal of compression plates. J Bone Joint Surg 70A:1372–1376, 1988.
21. Dodge, H.S.; Cady, G.W. Treatment of fractures of the radius and ulna with compression plates. A retrospective study of one hundred and nineteen fractures in seventy-eight patients. J Bone Joint Surg 54A:1167–1176, 1972.
22. Elstram, J.A.; Pankovich, A.M.; Eqwele, R. Extra-articular low-velocity gunshot fracture of the radius and ulna. J Bone Joint Surg 60A:335–341, 1978.
23. Emery, M.A. The incidence of delayed union and non-union following fractures of both bones of the forearm in adults. Can J Surg 8:285–287, 1965.
24. Engber, W.D.; Keene, J.S. Anterior interosseous nerve palsy associated with a Monteggia fracture. Clin Orthop 174:133, 1983.
25. Evans, E.M. Pronation injuries of the forearm with special reference to anterior Monteggia fractures. J Bone Joint Surg 31B:579, 1949.
26. Evans, E.M. Rotational deformities in the treatment of fractures of both bones of the forearm. J Bone Joint Surg 27:373–379, 1945.
27. Frykman, G. Fracture of the distal radius including sequelae—shoulder hand finger syndrome, disturbance in the distal radio-ulnar joint and impairment of nerve function. A clinical and experimental study. Acta Orthop Scand 108(suppl):1–155, 1967.
28. Galeazzi, R. Ueber ein besonderes Syndrom bei Verletzungen im Bereich der Unterarmknocken. Arch Orthop Unfallchir 35:557–562, 1934.
29. Garland, D.E.; Dowling, V. Forearm fractures in the head-injured adult. Clin Orthop 176:190–196, 1983.
30. Giustra, P.E.; Killoran, P.J.; Furman, R.S.; Root, J.A. The missed Monteggia fracture. Radiology 10:45, 1974.
31. Grace, T.G.; Eversmann, W.W. Jr. Forearm fractures: Treatment by rigid fixation with early motion. J Bone Joint Surg 62A:433–438, 1980.
32. Gross, S.D. A System of Surgery, Ed. 3. Philadelphia, Blanchard and Lea, 1864, pp. 916–917.
33. Hadden, W.A.; Reschauer, R.; Seggl, W. Results of AO plate fixation of forearm shaft fractures in adults. Injury 15:44–52, 1983.
34. Hall, R.H.; Bugg, E.I.; Vitolo, R.E. Intramedullary fixation of fractures of the forearm. South Med J 45:814–818, 1982.
35. Henry, W.A. Extensile Exposures, Ed. 2. New York, Churchill Livingstone, 1973, p. 100.
36. Hicks, J.H. Fractures of the forearm treated by rigid fixation. J Bone Joint Surg 43B:680–687, 1961.
37. Hidaka, S.; Gustilo, R.B. Refracture of bones of the forearm after plate removal. J Bone Joint Surg 66A:1241, 1984.
38. Hughston, J.C. Fracture of the distal radius shaft. Mistakes in management. J Bone Joint Surg 39A:249–264, 1957.
39. Jessing, P. Monteggia lesions and their complicating nerve damage. Acta Orthop Scand 46:601, 1975.
40. Knight, R.A.; Purvis, G.D. Fractures of both bones of the forearm in adults. J Bone Joint Surg 31A:755–764, 1949.
41. Kraus, B.; Horne, G. Galeazzi fractures. J Trauma 25:1093–1095, 1985.
42. Lichter, R.L.; Jacobsen, T. Tardy palsy of the posterior interosseous nerve with a Monteggia fracture. J Bone Joint Surg 57A:124, 1975.
43. Marek, F.M. Axial fixation of forearm fractures. J Bone Joint Surg 43A:1099–1114, 1961.

44. Mast, J.; Jakob, R.; Ganz, R. Planning and Reduction Techniques in Fracture Surgery. New York, Springer-Verlag, 1989.
45. Matthews, L.S.; Kaufer, H.; Garver, D.F.; Sonstegard, D.A. The effect on supination-pronation of angular malalignment of fractures of both bones of the forearm. J Bone Joint Surg 64A:14–17, 1982.
46. McLaughlin, H.L. Trauma. Philadelphia, W.B. Saunders, 1959.
47. Mikic, Z.D. Galeazzi fracture-dislocations. J Bone Joint Surg 57A:1071–1080, 1975.
48. Moed, B.R.; Kellam, J.F.; Foster, J.R.; et al. Immediate internal fixation of open fractures of the diaphysis of the forearm. J Bone Joint Surg 68A:1008–1017, 1986.
49. Monteggia, G.B. Instituzione Chirugiche, Ed. 2. Milan, G. Maspero, 1813–1815.
50. Moore, T.M.; Klein, J.P.; Patzakis, M.J.; Harvey, J.P. Jr. Results of compression plating of closed Galeazzi fractures. J Bone Joint Surg 67A:1015–1021, 1985.
51. Moore, T.M.; Lester, D.K.; Sarmiento, A. The stabilizing effect of soft tissue constraints in artificial Galeazzi fractures. Clin Orthop 194:189–194, 1985.
52. Mueller, M.E.; Allgoewer, M.; Schneider, R.; Willenegger, H. Manual of Internal Fixation, Ed. 2. Berlin, Springer-Verlag, 1979.
53. Mullick, S. The lateral Monteggia fracture. J Bone Joint Surg 33A:543, 1977.
54. Naiman, P.T.; Schein, A.J.; Siffert, R.S. Use of ASIF compression plates in selected shaft fractures of the upper extremity. A preliminary report. Clin Orthop 71:208–216, 1970.
55. Pavel, A.; Pitman, J.M.; Lance, E.M.; Wade, P.A. The posterior Monteggia fracture. A clinical study. J Trauma 5:185, 1965.
56. Penrose, J.H. The Monteggia fracture with posterior dislocation of the radial head. J Bone Joint Surg 33B:65, 1951.
57. Perren, S.M.; Cordey, J.; Rahn, B.A.; et al. Early temporary porosis of bone induced by internal fixation implants. Clin Orthop 232:139–151, 1988.
58. Pollen, A.G. Fractures and Dislocation in Children. Edinburgh, Churchill Livingstone, 1973.
59. Razeman, J.P.; Decoulx, J.; Leclair, H.P. Les synostoses radio-cubitales post-traumatiques de l'adulte. Acta Orthop Belgica 31:5–23, 1965.
60. Reckling, F.W.; Cordell, L.D. Unstable fracture-dislocations of the forearm: The Monteggia and Galeazzi lesions. Arch Surg 96:999–1007, 1968.
61. Reckling, F.W. Unstable fracture-dislocation of the forearm (Monteggia and Galeazzi lesions). J Bone Joint Surg 64A:857–863, 1982.
62. Sage, F.P. Medullary fixation of fractures of the forearm: A study of the medullary canal of the radius and a report on 50 fractures of the radius treated with a pre-bent triangular nail. J Bone Joint Surg 41A:1489–1516, 1959.
63. Sargent, J.P.; Teipner, W.A. Treatment of forearm shaft fractures by double-plating. A preliminary report. J Bone Joint Surg 47A:1475–1490, 1965.
64. Sarmiento, A.; Cooper, J.S.; Sinclair, W.F. Forearm fractures. Early functional bracing—a preliminary report. J Bone Joint Surg 51A:297–304, 1975.
65. Sarmiento, A.; Latta, L.L. Closed Functional Treatment of Fractures. New York, Springer-Verlag, 1981.
66. Schatzker, J.; Tile, M. The Rationale of Operative Fracture Care. Berlin, Springer-Verlag, 1987.
67. Schemitsch, E.H.; Richards, R.R.; Kellam, J.F. The measurement of radial bow and its relationship to outcome following plate fixation of fractures of both bones of the adult forearm. Presented to the Canadian Orthopaedic Research Society, June, 1988.

68. Schneider, C.F.; Leyra, S. Siliconized Dacron interposition for traumatic radio-ulnar synostosis. Case report. J Med Assoc Ala 33:185–188, 1964.

69. Smith, H.; Sage, F.P. Medullary fixation of forearm fractures. J Bone Joint Surg 39A:91–98, 1957.

70. Smith, F.M. Monteggia fractures. An analysis of twenty-five consecutive fresh injuries. Surg Gynecol Obstet 85:630–640, 1947.

71. Smith, J.E.M. Internal fixation in the treatment of fractures of the shaft of the radius and ulna in adults. J Bone Joint Surg 41B:122–131, 1959.

72. Speed, J.S.; Boyd, H.B. Treatment of fracture of the ulna with dislocation of the head of the radius (Monteggia fracture). JAMA 115:1699, 1940.

73. Spinner, M.; Freundlich, B.D.; Teicher, J. Posterior interosseous nerve palsy as a complication of Monteggia fractures in children. Clin Orthop 58:141, 1968.

74. Stein, F.; Grabia, S.L.; Deiffer, P.A. Nerve injuries complicating Monteggia lesions. J Bone Joint Surg 53A:1432, 1971.

75. Stern, P.J.; Drury, W.J. Complications of plate fixation of forearm fractures. Clin Orthop 175:25–29, 1983.

76. Stewart, M. Discussion of paper. J Bone Joint Surg 39A:264, 1957.

77. Teipner, W.A.; Mast, J.W. Internal fixation of forearm diaphyseal fractures: Double plating versus single compression (tension band) plating. A comparative study. Orthop Clin North Am 11:381–391, 1980.

78. Thompson, J.E. Anatomical methods of approach in operations on the long bones of the extremities. Ann Surg 68:309–329, 1918.

79. Tile, M.; Petrie, D. Fractures of the radius and ulna. J Bone Joint Surg 51B:193, 1969.

80. Valande, M. Luxation en arriere du cubitus avec fracture de la diaphyse radiale. Bull et Membres de la Soc Nat de Chir 55:435–437, 1929.

81. Vesely, D.G. The distal radio-ulnar joint. Clin Orthop 51:75, 1967.

82. Vince, K.G.; Miller, J.E. Cross-union complicating fractures of the forearm. Part I—adults. J Bone Joint Surg 69A:640–653, 1987.

83. Watson, F.M. Jr.; Eaton, R.G. Post-traumatic radio-ulnar synostosis. J Trauma 18:467–468, 1978.

84. Wong, P.C.N. Galeazzi fracture-dislocation in Singapore 1960–1964. Incidence and results of treatment. Singapore Med J 8:186–193, 1967.

85. Yong-Hing, K.; Tchang, S.P.K. Traumatic radio-ulnar synostosis treated by excision and a free fat transplant. A report of two cases. J Bone Joint Surg 65B:433–435, 1983.

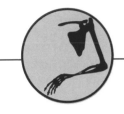

Jesse B. Jupiter, M.D.
David K. Mehne, M.D.

37

Trauma to the Adult Elbow and Fractures of the Distal Humerus

Part I   Trauma to the Adult Elbow

Jesse B. Jupiter, M.D.

The elbow represents the intermediate articulation of the upper extremity connecting the brachium to the forearm and hand. The joint is composed of three distinct articulations—the radiocapitellar, ulnotrochlear, and proximal radioulnar—all contained in one synovium-lined capsule. This cubital complex acts to position the forearm and hand in space and serves a vital load-carrying function.

Two degrees of freedom of motion exist: flexion and extension centered in the ulnotrochlear joint and pronation and supination through the radiocapitellar and proximal radioulnar articulations in conjunction with the distal radioulnar joint. This unique arrangement represents the evolutionary adaptation of the bipedal mammalian forelimb for the tasks of manipulation and prehension. A greater understanding of the functional anatomy of the elbow can be gained from even a brief evolutionary perspective.

As mammal-like reptiles evolved around 280 to 180 million years ago, the forelimb became drawn into the torso (Fig. 37–1). The distal humerus was composed of two large bulbous condyles separated by a shallow groove, whereas the proximal ulna developed a low longitudinal ridge to articulate between the condyles. This condylar arrangement reflected the greater weight-bearing requirement of the forelimb along with an increasing degree of flexion and extension. The straight medial margin of the radial head indicated there was limited axial rotation of the radius, whose major function was weight bearing (Fig. 37–2*B*).[44]

The ancestral prosimians (premonkeys) that existed 100 to 35 million years ago adopted a tree-living habitat, and one now can observe a greater specialization of the forelimbs for climbing.[15] The intercondylar groove of the distal humerus assumed more of a pulley shape. The proximal ulna developed a deepened greater sigmoid notch and anterior shelflike projection (a primitive coronoid process) (Fig. 37–2*D*). These changes reflected a shift in the burden of weight bearing and stability from the radius to the humeroulnar articulation. This functional transition, along with a more oval radial head, allowed for a slightly increased range of forearm rotation.[118] The hominoid apes (25 to 12 million years ago) represented a more advanced stage of primate evolution in which locomotion was characterized by a predominance of arm swinging, or brachiation. The trochlea became wider and deeper, creating a more congruent ulnotrochlear joint that became the major determinant of mediolateral stability. With the stabilizing and weight-bearing role of the radiocapitellar joint virtually eliminated, the circular radial head became capable of providing a full range of forearm rotation in any degree of elbow flexion or extension. The hand could now be placed into a vast number of positions during brachiation (Fig. 37–2*F*).[57,70]

The evolutionary split between the ancestral apes and early man likely occurred from 6 to 15 million years ago. As bipedalism evolved, the upper extremity came to be used primarily for prehension and manipulation. The architecture of the contemporary human

1125

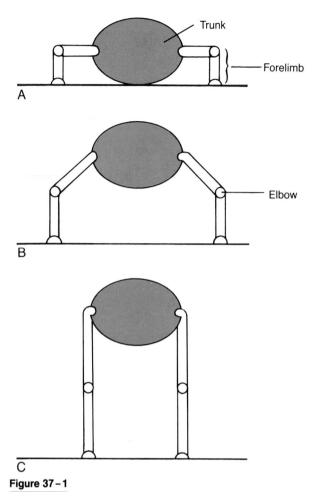

Figure 37–1

During the process of evolution, the forelimb became drawn into the torso.

elbow, however, differs from that of the ancient and modern apes only in small proportional measurements (see section on distal humerus).[36,100]

Radial Head Fractures

Fractures of the head of the radius are relatively common injuries and are involved in nearly 20% of all elbow trauma.[47,127] While much has been written regarding the management of these fractures, confusion and debate regarding optimal treatment continue. Support can be found for virtually every type of treatment, from prolonged immobilization to operative fixation and rapid functional loading. With a greater recognition of fracture patterns and associated soft tissue injuries as well as improved methods of fracture fixation, the simplistic universal approach of radial head excision has become subject to increasing scrutiny.[55]

Although loss of strength resulting from loss of the proximal part of the radius,[78] valgus instability,[79] and proximal migration of the radius leading to wrist pain[119] have all been observed clinically with radial head excision, the functional role of the radial head remains in question. Studies of static loading across the elbow have suggested that as much as 60% of force is transmitted across the radiocapitellar articulation,[3,4,37,126] although Morrey et al. found force transmission during physiologic muscle contracture to be considerably lower than that reported with static load-

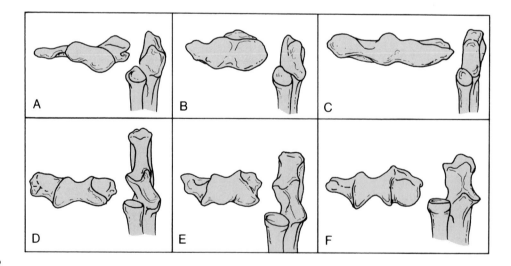

Figure 37–2

Major stages in the structural development of the elbow. The left drawing in each frame represents the distal end of the humerus (ventral surface facing interior); the right drawing is the corresponding radius and ulna rotated 180°. *A*, Primitive terrestrial quadruped elbow (345 to 230 million years ago). *B*, Early mammal-like reptiles (280 to 180 million years ago). *C*, First mammalian elbows (230 to 180 million years ago). *D*, The prosimian (premonkey) elbow (100 to 135 million years ago). *E*, Primitive anthropoid monkey elbow (35 to 25 million years ago). *F*, Hominoid ape elbow (25 to 12 million years ago). (Modified from Jenkins FA. Am J Anat 137:281–298, 1973.)

Table 37-1.

Scharplatz and Allgoewer Classification of Elbow Injuries

Fractures and fracture-dislocations 2° to axial forces

    Transverse olecranon fractures

    Comminuted olecranon fractures

    Transverse or comminuted olecranon fractures with anterior dislocation of radius and ulna

    Transverse or comminuted olecranon fractures with anterior dislocation of radial head (atypical Monteggia)

    Fractures of ulnar shaft with anterior dislocation of radial head (Monteggia)

    Fractures of coronoid process with posterior dislocation of olecranon

Fractures 2° to transverse and lateral forces

    Marginal fracture radial head

    Marginal fracture radial head with disruption of the distal radioulnar joint

Source: Modified from Scharplatz, D.; Allgöwer, M. Fracture-dislocation of the elbow. Injury 1976, 7:143–159, by permission of the publishers Butterworth-Heinemann Ltd ©.

ing.[77] Similarly, the extent of the radial head's role in resisting valgus stress has been disputed by a number of investigators.[42,79,81,89,108]

MECHANISM OF INJURY

The early experimental efforts of Thomas[121] and later of Oldeberg-Johnson[85] suggested that radial head fractures were the result of a fall on an outstretched hand with the forearm in pronation. The axial load can be of varying force and direction and can result in a variety of associated soft tissue and skeletal injuries. These include carpal fractures,[53] distal radioulnar joint, and interosseous membrane disruption,[22,26,28,69,119] Monteggia fracture-dislocations, capitellar fractures,[97] and soft tissue injury about the elbow.[7]

CLASSIFICATION

The classification of radial head fractures has undergone considerable evolution. Scharplatz and Allgoewer classified injuries about the elbow into two major groups on the basis of the direction of the force of the injury[104]: injuries resulting from pure axial forces and those secondary to forces leading to varus or valgus displacement (Table 37–1). The early classifications of radial head fractures by Carstam,[17] Bakalim (Fig. 37–3),[8] and Mason[66] (Fig. 37–4) were based solely on radiographs and failed to take into account associated injuries. Johnston added a fourth category to Mason's classification, identifying those fractures associated with an elbow dislocation.[47] This latter association has also been documented by a number of authors.[10,20,33,80]

As routine radiographs will project the radial head only in a two-dimensional profile, it is likely that some overlap exists within the arbitrary limits of these classifications. More recent interest in internal fixation of articular fractures has extended to the radial head, stimulating classification systems that will prove of value when comparing the results of series of operative treatments (Fig. 37–5).

DIAGNOSIS

Tenderness or swelling over the lateral surface of the elbow or limitation of active or passive elbow or forearm motion should alert the examiner to the possibility of a radial head fracture. Routine anteroposterior and lateral radiographs may not provide an accurate representation of the individual fracture pattern. The x-ray view described by Greenspan and Norman is recommended in those cases in which accurate identification of the fracture pattern will influence the method of treatment.[35] This so-called radiocapitellar view is accomplished by positioning the patient as for a lateral x-ray view, but angling the tube 45° toward the shoul-

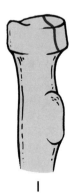 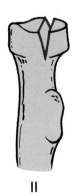 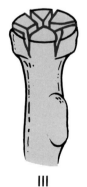 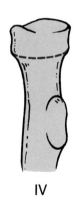 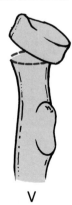

   I   II   III   IV   V

Figure 37-3

The classification system of Bakalim.

Type I

Type II

Type III

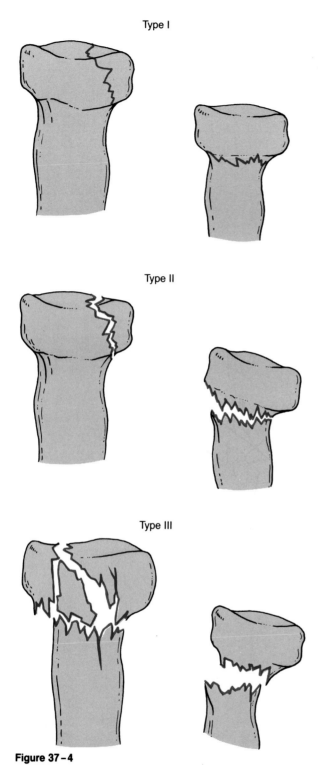

Figure 37–4

The modified Mason classification system for radial head fractures.

der. Palpation of the wrist and distal radioulnar joint should form a part of the examination of every case of suspected radial head fracture.

Aspiration of the radiocapitellar joint is of value not only in confirming the diagnosis of radial head fracture but also in reducing associated discomfort. It can prove invaluable in determining whether a bony block to forearm or elbow motion exists as a result of displacement of the fracture. For many, a block to motion represents an indication for surgery.[106] The technique, as described by Quigley, is performed under aseptic conditions. The forearm is pronated to minimize the possibility of trauma to the radial nerve, and the needle is introduced through the center of a triangle formed by the radial head, the tip of the olecranon, and the lateral epicondyle.[92] Aspiration of the hemarthrosis accompanied by instillation of a local anesthetic can be done through the same needle (Fig. 37–6). In one study by Fleetcroft, improved results were noted in nondisplaced or minimally displaced radial head fractures when the joint was aspirated and early mobilization encouraged versus early mobilization alone.[29]

TREATMENT

Although these fractures are considered by many to be a relatively benign injury, the outcome can be disappointing. This is a reflection not just of the treatment rendered but also (and more likely) of the nature of the original trauma and associated injuries. It is therefore of fundamental importance to define the presence or absence of other soft tissue or skeletal injury and to classify the fracture accordingly. The vast majority of fractures prove to be isolated events and can be effectively treated by conservative means.

RADIAL HEAD FRACTURE: NO OR MINIMAL DISPLACEMENT

Radial head fractures with no or minimal displacement consist of articular fractures with little or no separation or impaction (Fig. 37–7). The well-aligned, impacted radial neck fractures can also be included in this group.

Concern for residual loss of elbow motion has led many to recommend early mobilization of the forearm and elbow for these "stable" fractures.[1,41,65,128] Several studies, in fact, have suggested improved results, including shorter disability time and enhanced elbow mobility, with early functional motion following minimally displaced radial head fractures.[41,128] Early mobilization, however, should be considered cautiously when the fracture involves a large segment of the articular surface. In a series reported by Radin and Riseborough, displacement and resultant loss of mobility occurred in some instances of "stable" fractures involving more than one third of the articular surface that were permitted freedom of motion early following injury.[93]

Figure 37-5

The classification system of Schatzker and Tile for radial head fractures. *A*, Type I: wedge. May be displaced or nondisplaced. *B*, Type II: impaction. Part of the head and neck remain intact. The fracture is tilted and impacted. Comminution is variable. *C*, Type III: severely comminuted. No portion of the head and neck remains in continuity; comminution is severe.

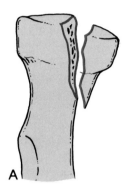
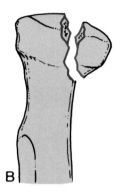
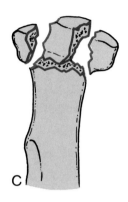

Treatment Recommendation

Early mobilization should be considered for those "stable" fractures that involve less than one third of the articular surface or in the elderly, low-demand individual. In the active individual, however, fractures involving more than one third of the articular surface should be treated with splint or sling support for a minimum of two weeks, followed by protected functional activities for an additional seven to ten days.

TWO-PART DISPLACED RADIAL HEAD FRACTURES

There is a diversity of opinions regarding the approach to management of two-part displaced radial head fractures. This is in part because of the fact that this fracture pattern can vary in the amount of articular surface involved, the extent of impaction of the fracture fragment, the presence or absence of comminution in the radial neck, and the associated soft tissue involvement (Fig. 37-8).

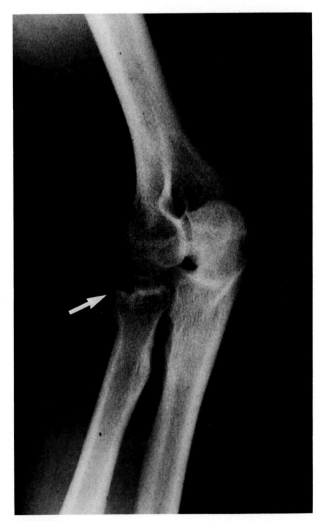

Figure 37-7

A minimally displaced radial head fracture can be treated with splinting provided there is no block to forearm or elbow motion.

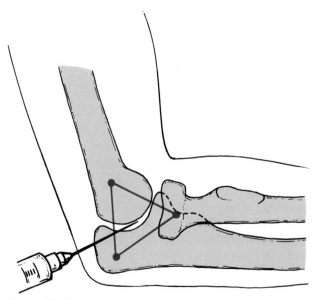

Figure 37-6

Aspiration of the radiocapitellar joint is performed with a needle introduced through the center of a triangle formed by the radial head, the tip of the olecranon, and the lateral epicondyle.

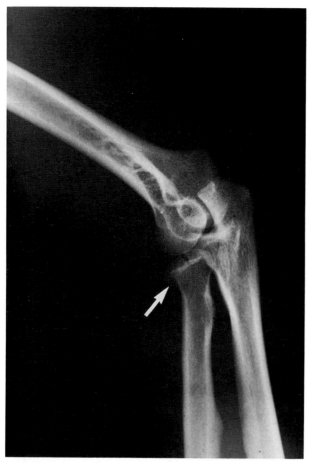

Figure 37-8

Two-part radial head fractures can vary widely in the extent of articular surface involved, amount of displacement, degree of radial neck involvement, and associated soft tissue injury.

Treatment Recommendation

It is of fundamental importance to assess the amount of forearm rotation and elbow flexion. When no block to motion exists and there is no palpable incongruity of the articular surface, conservative treatment with a splint will provide a good result.[76] If, however, a definable block to motion is demonstrated, operative intervention should be considered. At this point the presence of associated soft tissue or skeletal trauma becomes an essential factor in the decision-making process.

Displaced Two-Part Fractures Without Associated Injury

Displaced two-part fractures without associated injury are preferably treated by open reduction and internal fixation. Although good results have been reported following excision of the radial head for these fractures, some studies have noted proximal migration of the radius[69,112,119] and reduction of grip strength.[78]

Improvements in small implant design and application have made internal fixation of the radial head more reliable.[12,86,107,123] The surgical approach is through a standard lateral incision identifying the interval between the anconeus and extensor carpi ulnaris muscles. Through a longitudinal capsulotomy, the fracture hematoma is debrided, providing exposure to the fracture fragments. Most often the fracture will involve the anterolateral portion of the radial head, which makes it accessible to reduction and provisional fixation with Kirschner wires.[47] One or two 2.7-mm or 2.0-mm screws or self-compressing Herbert screws will afford sufficient stability to permit postoperative functional mobilization. The differential pitch of the threads of the Herbert screw provides a modest amount of interfragmentary compression, but a more important feature is the ability to sink the implant beneath the articular rim of the radial head (Fig. 37-9).

If the articular fragment is impacted and requires elevation for restoration of the articular surface, a small defect will be produced beneath the elevated fragment. This is best filled with cancellous bone graft, which is readily available from the lateral epicondyle of the humerus.

Displaced Fracture With Soft Tissue Injury

When the displaced two-part radial head fracture is associated with an elbow dislocation or distal radioulnar joint and interosseous membrane disruption, preservation of the radial head becomes a higher priority (Fig. 37-10). If internal fixation of the fracture is not feasible, several treatment options exist. If the fracture fragment involves less than one third of the surface of the head, excision of the fragment is one option.[17] Other options include replacement of the head with a silicone prosthesis and exploration and repair of the medial ligament complex of the elbow in conjunction with radial head resection.

Prosthetic replacement offers the advantages of more normal articular relationships, pain relief, intrinsic stability, and elimination of proximal migration of the radial shift.[38,114] Early implants were made of vitallium, stainless steel, and acrylic. The currently available design is made of silicone rubber, which has several unfortunate material properties. In the first place, studies by Carn et al. have suggested that the silicone rubber prosthesis is too flexible and thus is unable to transmit physiologic forces from the proximal radius to the capitellum; consequently it fails in its function as a static spacer.[16] A second problem can result from silicone prosthetic fracture and resultant particulate syno-

Figure 37–9

A 38-year-old female sustained a displaced two-part radial head fracture. On examination, a palpable block to forearm rotation was appreciated. *A,* An intraoperative photograph shows the extent of articular displacement. *B,* The fracture was secured with two Herbert screws. Full motion was regained within one week postoperatively.

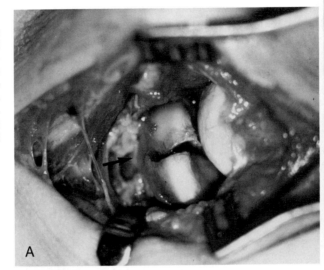
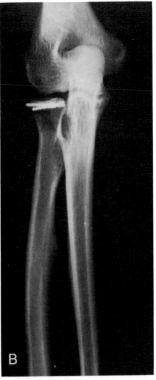

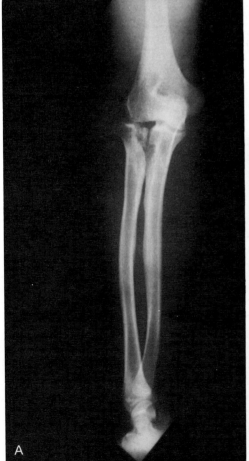
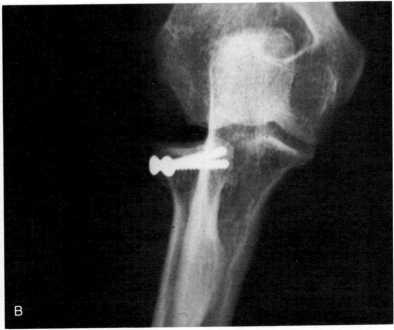

Figure 37–10

A 27-year-old male sustained a high-energy injury to his right dominant extremity. Pain was noted at his distal radioulnar joint, and a displaced two-part radial head fracture was seen on radiograph *(A). B,* Open reduction and internal fixation were performed using two 2.7-mm screws.

vitis, leading to local pain and further implant loosening.[34,131]

The technique of silicone radial head replacement bears mentioning, as attention to detail can offset prosthetic failure. As described by Swanson et al.,[116] the head is resected at the metaphyseal flare, preserving as much of the radial neck as possible. The cut edges are smoothed to keep bony spikes from cutting through the implant, and an implant as large as possible is used, centering the stem of the prosthesis over the center of the axis of rotation of the radius to minimize shearing on the implant.

Much has been said in the literature regarding the timing of surgery for radial head fractures. Some have felt that any surgery should be performed expeditiously to avoid heterotopic bone or myositis ossificans,[33,47,122] whereas others have recommended that surgery be considered within the first week after injury.[17,66] It is likely that the timing of the actual surgery is less important than the nature of both the original injury and the manner in which the surgery is executed.

COMMINUTED FRACTURES OF THE RADIAL HEAD

More commonly associated with higher energy trauma, comminuted fracture patterns are rarely amenable to stable internal fixation. Soft tissue swelling and ecchymosis suggest the likelihood of capsular, brachialis, or ligamentous injury, including a dislocation that has undergone spontaneous reduction.[46] Capitellar fractures, Monteggia fracture-dislocations, and wrist and forearm injuries may also accompany the comminuted radial head fracture. In view of the possibility of significant soft tissue trauma, the timing of surgery in this setting may be of more significance. Although this is uncommon, some patients have had satisfactory outcomes following early postinjury mobilization and delayed (beyond six weeks) radial head excision.[9]

Although radial head resection represents the most commonly performed procedure for comminuted fractures, it has been observed to be associated with instability and late posttraumatic arthritis when performed in the setting of medial collateral ligament or interosseous membrane disruption (Fig. 37–11).[22,26,28,48,69,74,119]

Treatment Recommendation

In the setting of a low-energy injury, an elderly patient, or a lack of physical findings suggestive of associated soft tissue disruption, resection of the radial head alone is a straightforward approach that in most instances

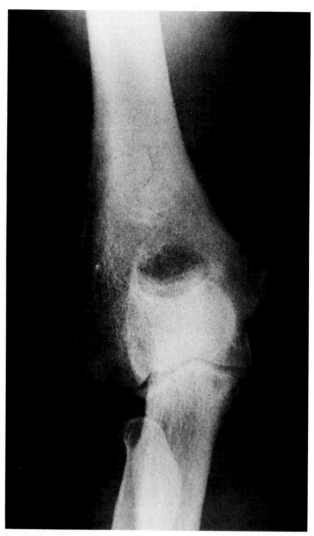

Figure 37–11

A 50-year-old male presented two years following fracture-dislocation of his elbow, treated initially with a closed reduction and radial head resection. Pain, instability, and symptoms of ulnar neuritis were observed. The radiograph demonstrates evidence of ulnohumeral arthritis.

will not be associated with long-term sequelae.[18] If, however, medial collateral ligament instability or disruption of the distal radioulnar joint is observed (the Essex-Lopresti lesion), then treatment should consist of either internal fixation of the radial head or silicone replacement (Fig. 37–12). Following radial head reconstruction or replacement, the elbow should be tested for valgus stability, and manual testing of the stability of the distal radioulnar joint should be carried out. Should valgus instability be observed, exploration and repair of the medial collateral ligament complex are recommended. Similarly, if distal ulnar instability is present, then it is best to pin the ulna to the radius

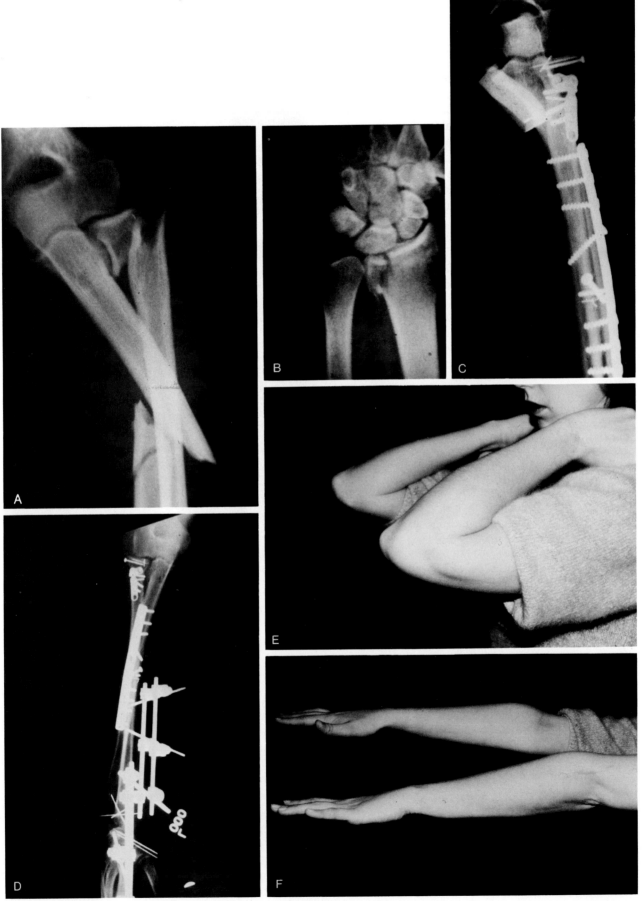

Figure 37-12

Illustration continued on following page; legend on following page.

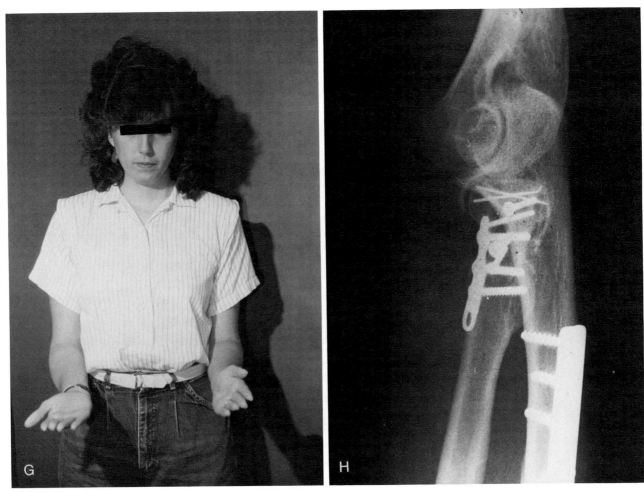

Figure 37-12 *Continued*

A 24-year-old woman was involved in a high-energy motorcycle accident. Multiple fractures were noted in her left dominant limb. *A*, The radiograph demonstrates complex radial head and neck fractures. *B*, Fractures were also noted to involve the ulnar shaft, distal radius, scaphoid, and capitate; disruption of the distal radioulnar joint was also present. *C*, Open reduction and internal fixation of the radial head and neck were performed with an interfragmentary 2.0-mm screw, two threaded 0.028-in Kirschner wires, and a minifragment T plate. *D*, The remainder of the forearm injuries were treated with internal and external fixation. *E* and *F*, Postoperatively the patient regained full elbow flexion and extension. *G*, Forearm supination was limited because of residual disruption of the distal radioulnar joint. *H*, Radiographs revealed excellent union with calcification noted in the pericapsular tissues. (From Jupiter, J.B. J Hand Surg 11A:279-282, 1986.)

with the forearm in supination. Elbow flexion and extension can then be started, with the Kirschner wire left in place for four to six weeks (Fig. 37-13).

COMPLICATIONS

Complications associated with radial head fractures can be divided into two major categories: those associated with the fracture and those following radial head excision.

For the most part, complications with nonoperative treatment are loss of motion and pain. These have generally been reported in association with the more complex comminuted radial head fractures and, rarely, with the minimally displaced variant.

Reported complications with radial head excision are well documented. These include loss of grip strength,[22,26,28,116,119] pain at the wrist,[69] valgus instability,[42,89,108] heterotopic bone,[122] and posttraumatic arthritis of the trochlear-olecranon articulation.[74,80]

Olecranon Fractures

The olecranon represents the proximal articulating unit of the ulna. Together with the coronoid process, the olecranon forms the greater sigmoid notch, which, in turn, articulates with the trochlea of the distal humerus. This articulation provides the flexion-extension movement of the elbow joint, and its intrinsic architec-

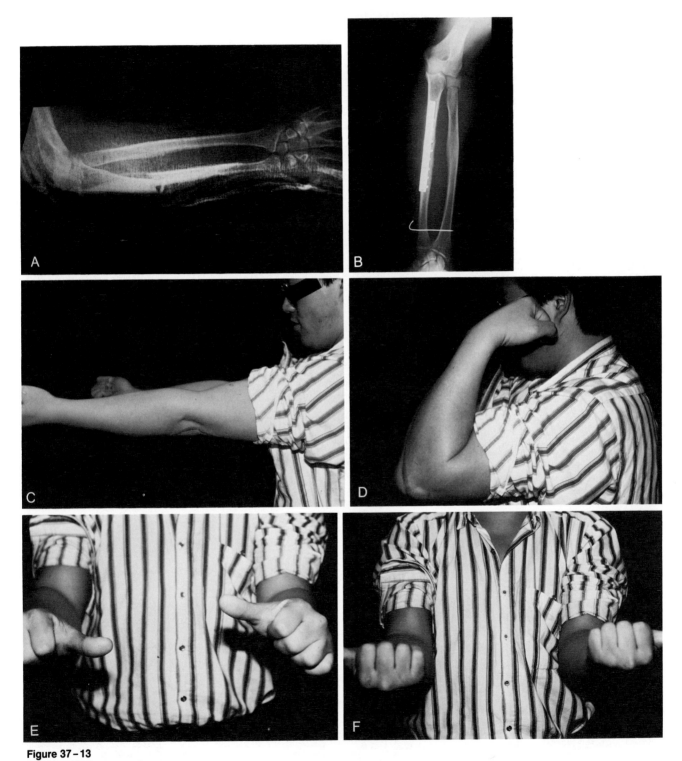

Figure 37–13

A 28-year-old man sustained a high-energy injury to his left upper extremity. *A,* The radiograph reveals a comminuted, displaced radial head fracture, ulnar shaft fracture, distal radius fracture, and disruption of the distal radioulnar joint. *B,* Following resection of the comminuted radial head fragments and plate fixation of the ulna, a silicone radial head prosthesis was placed. In addition, with the forearm in supination, the distal ulna was pinned to the radius. Full elbow motion *(C and D)* and nearly full forearm motion *(E and F)* resulted.

ture adds to the stability of the elbow. The triceps tendon inserts onto the olecranon with extension both medially and laterally to insert onto the periosteum of the proximal ulna as well as the fascial envelope of the proximal forearm. The ulnar nerve passes through the cubital tunnel beneath the medial epicondyle of the distal humerus to exit along the medial olecranon and enter the volar aspect of the forearm between the two heads of the flexor carpi ulnaris.

The subcutaneous position of the olecranon renders it vulnerable to direct trauma. Fracture patterns can be the result of a number of different mechanisms, including a direct blow, a fall on the outstretched hand with the elbow in flexion, or higher-energy trauma, which is associated with radial head fractures or elbow dislocation.[104,114,130]

Fractures of the olecranon represent intraarticular injuries and as such will often manifest as swelling, pain, and an effusion. The fracture itself may be palpa-

ble. A true lateral radiograph will be necessary to accurately identify the plane of the fracture, the number of fracture fragments, and the extent of articular disruption. A radiocapitellar view may be of help if there appears to be a concomitant injury or displacement of the radial head.

A number of classifications of olecranon fractures have been described, with only modest variation. The type of fracture is the single most important factor in determining the optimal type of treatment. Although surgeons have traditionally looked to apply one form of treatment for all olecranon fractures, it has become quite apparent that the mechanical characteristics of the various fracture patterns differ and that not all are amenable to one single method.

Colton classified olecranon fractures into two major groups: undisplaced (type I) and displaced (type II).[19] A type I undisplaced fracture is defined as having less than 2 mm of separation and no increase in displace-

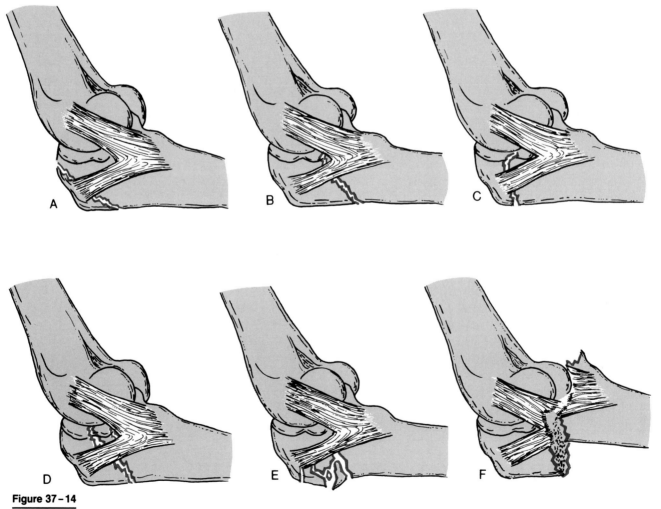

Figure 37-14

Colton's classification of olecranon fractures. *A*, Avulsion; *B*, oblique; *C*, transverse; *D*, oblique with comminution; *E*, comminuted; *F*, fracture-dislocation.

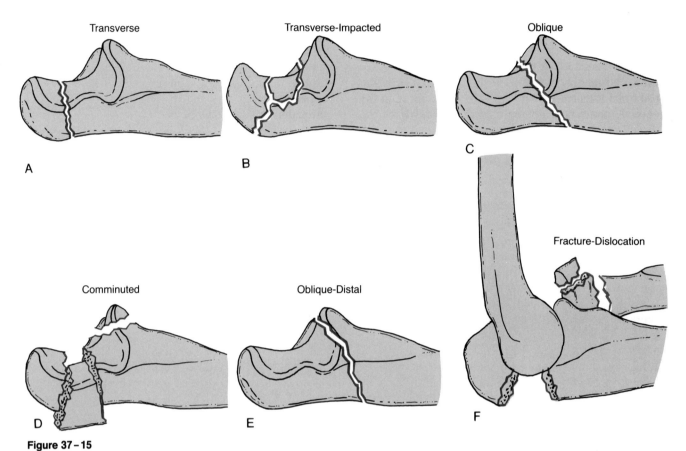

Figure 37–15

Schatzker's classification system of olecranon fractures. *A*, Transverse; *B*, transverse impacted; *C*, oblique; *D*, comminuted; *E*, oblique distal; *F*, fracture-dislocation.

ment with flexion to 90°, with the patient able to extend the elbow against gravity (Fig. 37–14). Colton further subdivided the displaced fractures into type IIA, avulsion; IIB, oblique and transverse; IIC, comminuted; and IID, fracture-dislocations.

Schatzker addressed the mechanical considerations of fractures with specific reference to the requirements placed on the internal fixations.[105] He considered transverse fractures (occurring at the deepest point of the trochlear notch) to be either simple (two fragments) or complex (involving comminution or depression of the articular surface). A separate group includes the oblique fractures, which extend distally from the midpoint of the trochlear notch. These prove less stable with tension band wiring alone. His final group consists of comminuted fractures. These may include (1) fractures of the coronoid process, (2) fractures extending distally beyond the midpoint of the trochlear notch, and (3) fractures or dislocations of the radial head (Fig. 37–15).

The goals of treatment of olecranon fractures should include the following features[14]: articular restoration, preservation of motor power of extension, stability,

avoidance of stiffness, and limitation of possible associated complications. Nondisplaced fractures, although uncommon, can be effectively treated by immobilization of the limb in a long-arm splint or cast with the elbow flexed at 90° for four weeks. A radiograph should be obtained in seven to ten days to ensure that displacement of the fracture has not occurred.

DISPLACED FRACTURES

Treatment Recommendation

Displaced fractures require operative treatment. Avulsion fractures of the proximal olecranon, although in reality extraarticular fractures, should be treated operatively, as they disrupt the insertion of the triceps mechanism. These fractures are more common in the elderly, and operative treatment consists of suturing the triceps back to the proximal ulna using strong nonabsorbable suture placed through drill holes.[101,125] A tension band wire can be used to reinforce the repair.

Two types of treatment exist for the displaced intraarticular olecranon fractures: open reduction and internal fixation or fragment excision and triceps reconstruction. The evolution of these very divergent approaches can be more clearly understood by reviewing the history of olecranon fracture treatment. Interest in operative treatment was generated by the poor results of immobilization, initially recommended with the elbow in extension, which led to loss of motion. This was then followed by immobilization in flexion, resulting in displacement of the fragments and weak extension.[23] This led innovative surgeons, starting with Lister in 1883, to use a variety of techniques and materials to securely stabilize the olecranon to permit functional motion and avoid displacement.[61,68,82,124,129,132] Although each technique was advocated enthusiastically, none proved satisfactory for each type of fracture pattern. This in part stimulated the concept of fragment excision and triceps reattachment.[25] Popularized by McKeever and Buck, this technique has gained acceptance by some authors, particularly for the elderly patient.[2,32,71,101]

In determining treatment for a displaced olecranon fracture, the classification system of Schatzker is of great help. Despite some authors' enthusiasm for olecranon excision, there are certain fractures for which this method is not advisable. These include fractures associated with elbow instability, avulsion of the coronoid, or comminution extending toward the distal aspect of the olecranon and fractures in younger individuals with high functional demands. An et al., in a biomechanical model, confirmed the important stabilizing function of the olecranon and noted that the proximal portion of the olecranon has a greater effect on joint constraint than had been generally appreciated.[5]

TRANSVERSE FRACTURES

Treatment Recommendation

The transverse fracture, whether simple or involving comminution or depression of the articular surface, is amenable to the mechanically effective tension band fixation technique. This technique is based on the placement of a wire loop dorsal to the midaxis of the ulna. In this position, the tensile or distraction forces at the fracture site are transformed into compressive forces. Two Kirschner wires are used to act as an internal splint offsetting rotational and angular displacement forces. The Kirschner wires are placed in parallel extending proximal dorsal to distal anterior to just catch the anterior cortex of the ulna distal to the fracture line (Fig. 37–16). This technique will offset some of the reported difficulties of the Kirschner wires backing out and causing discomfort and limitation of motion.[45,64,83]

The placement of the wire loop is fundamental to the effectiveness of the technique. A hole is drilled with a 2.0-mm drill bit dorsal to the midaxis of the ulna and at least 2.5 to 3 cm distal to the fracture for the placement of the tension band wire. As a rule, the distance spanned by the wire from the fracture should be at least equal to the distance from the fracture to the tip of the

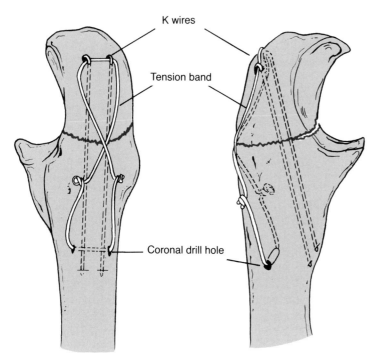

K wires

Tension band

Coronal drill hole

Figure 37–16

A transverse olecranon fracture is optimally treated by a tension band wire technique. Note the placement of the two parallel Kirschner wires from dorsal proximal to anterior distal to engage in the anterior cortex. This minimizes the problem of Kirschner wire migration.

olecranon. The tension band wire is passed deep to the triceps tendon and held in place by the two parallel Kirschner wires, which will be bent around the tension wire as they are impacted into the proximal ulna (Fig. 37–16). The tension wire is carefully tightened with the elbow in extension. This will result in a slight overre-

duction of the fracture at the articular surface that will disappear as the elbow actively flexes.

A transverse fracture with depression of the articular surface should have the articular surface elevated and, if possible, secured with an interfragmentary screw. At times, cancellous bone will be needed to support the

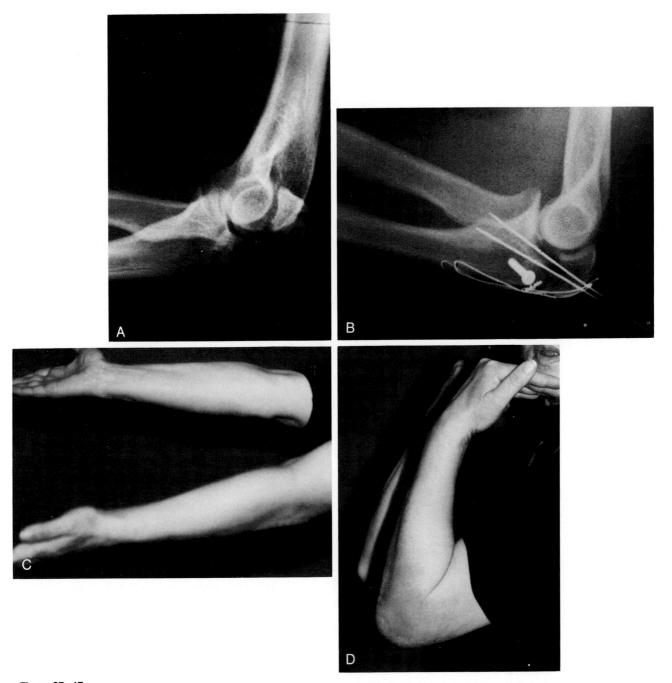

Figure 37–17

A 38-year-old female sustained an impacted transverse olecranon fracture. *A,* The lateral radiograph reveals an impacted transverse olecranon fracture. *B,* Following elevation of the major articular fragment, an interfragmentary lag screw was placed. A double tension band loop secured the comminuted dorsal ulnar cortex. Note the oblique position of the Kirschner wires just prior to bending the wires. *C* and *D,* Full flexion and extension were achieved within three weeks after injury.

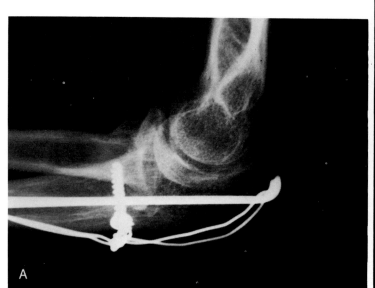

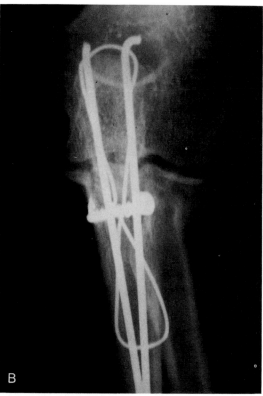

Figure 37–18

An oblique olecranon fracture was fixed with an interfragmentary lag screw and a tension band wire and two Kirschner wires.

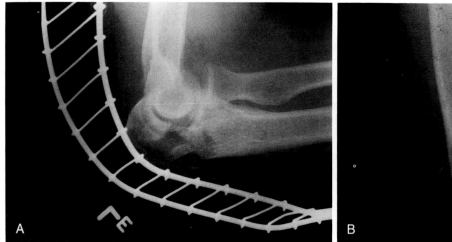

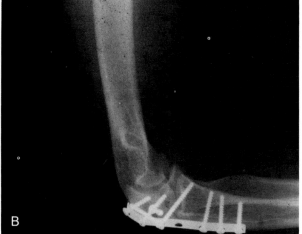

Figure 37–19

A 55-year-old female fell 10 feet off a ladder, landing directly on her left elbow. *A,* The lateral radiograph reveals an extensively comminuted olecranon fracture extending to the very distal aspect of the semilunar notch. *B,* The fragments were carefully teased into place and held with interfragmentary screws and a contoured 3.5-mm third tubular plate. Note how the plate conforms to the shape of the proximal olecranon and the screws are directed at various angles.

articular restoration. This is readily available from the lateral epicondylar area of the distal humerus. A tension band will effectively protect the articular elevation and permit early active functional aftercare (Fig. 37–17).

Oblique fractures should have, whenever possible, an interfragmentary lag screw placed across the fracture line. This compression screw can be neutralized against rotational or translational forces either by a tension band wire or by a dorsally applied plate (Fig. 37–18).

Displaced comminuted fractures that extend to and include the coronoid process present the most difficult of all olecranon fractures to treat with internal fixation. At times, as a result of high-energy trauma, these can be associated with instability of the elbow. Tension band wiring will not be effective for these fractures. Plate fixation applied on the dorsal surface is necessary. The plate, a 3.5-mm dynamic compression (DC), reconstruction, or third tubular, can be contoured to project proximally around the tip of the olecranon. This will enhance the hold of the screws in the cancellous bone, as they will now be directed in two directions. Cancellous bone graft should be used both to help support the articular reconstruction and to fill in any defects in the cortex opposite the plate (Fig. 37–19). Difficulty in maintaining secure fixation of olecranon fractures, particularly comminuted fractures in the elderly, has led some to continue to advocate olecranon excision and triceps reattachment.[21,32] In a low-demand elbow, this technique has proved effective even with as much as two thirds of the olecranon excised, provided no instability is present. Studies by Gartsman et al.[32] using functional and mechanical strength evaluations suggested that elbow strength following excision and reattachment is equal to that with internally fixed olecranon fractures. Strength was significantly less, however, following both procedures when compared with the contralateral uninjured control elbow. Yet in the series of Gartsman et al., the technique of internal fixation varied, and the elbow was immobilized, thus delaying the functional aftercare of the patient. It remains to be demonstrated whether excision and triceps reattachment is functionally as effective as properly executed internal fixation combined with early postoperative rehabilitation.

COMPLICATIONS

Complications specific to fractures of the olecranon include loss of elbow flexion and extension, malunion, nonunion, and posttraumatic arthritis. Lack of extension is not uncommon to all traumatic injuries about the elbow, although it has not generally been a major factor with olecranon fractures.[27]

Nonunion has been reported in a number of series of olecranon fractures, although it, too, is uncommon. More often than not, treatment will be successful with a plate applied dorsally to function as a tension band.

Posttraumatic arthritis can be problematic, as the sigmoid notch–trochlea articulation is important in providing intrinsic stability to the elbow. Fortunately, it is not a common occurrence.

Dislocation of the Elbow

Dislocation of the elbow accounts for 20% of all dislocations, second only to glenohumeral and finger joints. Elbow dislocations occur most commonly in the younger individual, with the peak ages between 5 and 25 years. Along with disruption of the joint capsule and restraining ligaments, accessory injuries are not uncommon. These include skeletal injuries such as radial head or neck fractures (see section on radial head fractures), capitellum injury, avulsion of the coronoid process of the ulna,[95,110] and avulsion of the medial or lateral epicondyles in the younger individuals. Associated soft tissue injuries can involve vascular compromise[60,62,115] or neurologic trauma,[30,67,90,94,111,113] with the latter usually involving stretch injury to the median or ulnar nerve.

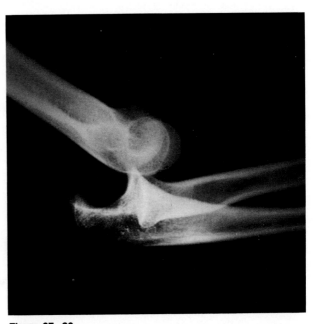

Figure 37–20

A 26-year-old female who was six months pregnant fell on her outstretched left arm. Radiographs were not obtained at the time of injury because of her pregnancy. Because of persistent pain and swelling about her left elbow, she sought medical attention one week after injury. Radiographs revealed a complete posterolateral dislocation of her elbow, which had remained dislocated for one week.

Although elbow dislocation may be diagnosed clinically, swelling often obscures the bony landmarks about the elbow (Fig. 37–20). Supracondylar distal humerus or associated fractures must be considered, making radiographic examination essential.

The radiographic studies will define the type of dislocation. Dislocation of both the radius and ulna together is by far the most common type and can be posterior, medial, lateral, or anterior to the distal humerus. The radius and ulna can also be in divergent directions. Dislocation of either the radius or ulna alone has been reported but is exceptionally uncommon (Fig. 37–21).

The posterior or posterolateral dislocation is found in more than 80% of all elbow dislocations.[56,60,99] Two theories have been promoted to explain the mechanism of this injury. The hyperextension theory suggests that force is taken on the hand with the elbow extended.[39,59] The olecranon thus impinges on the olecranon fossa, with further energy levering the ulna

and radius from their capsular constraints. The brachialis muscle may be torn or the coronoid process avulsed. Continued extension force results in the tearing of the epicondylar attachments of the capsule and ligaments, and in some instances an abduction force results in injury to the radial head or capitellum.

The second theory suggests that the dislocation occurs with the elbow slightly flexed and subject to axial compressive loading.[87] The radial collateral ligament and lateral capsule tear, with resulting posterior dislocation of the forearm on the humerus.

Whatever the mechanism, in the posterior or posterolateral elbow dislocation the distal humerus drives through the anterior capsule and brachialis, with the final position of the forearm dependent to some degree on the direction of the force. True lateral or anterior dislocations are extremely rare. In the anterior dislocation, the soft tissue injury may be severe, as this may be the result of a violent blow to the olecranon. This is also

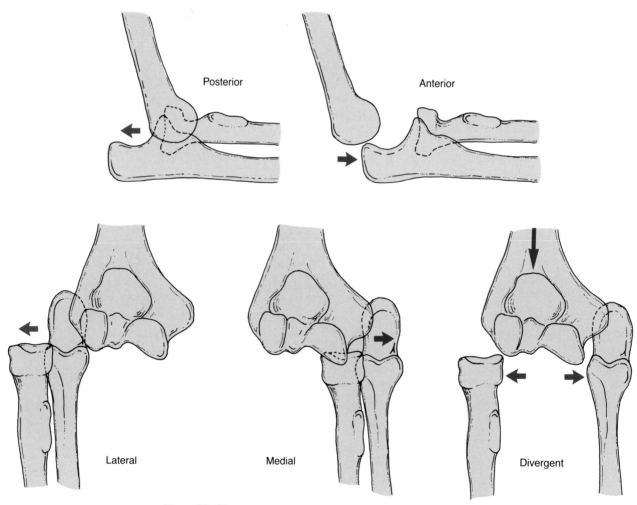

Figure 37–21

An elbow dislocation is defined by the direction of the forearm bones.

often the case with divergent dislocations in which the radius is displaced from the ulna and both are dislocated from the humerus.

TREATMENT

The goal of treatment of any elbow dislocation is the restoration of articular alignment performed as expeditiously and atraumatically as possible. Prior to any reduction must come a careful neurovascular assessment documenting any sensory or motor deficit. Although an elbow dislocation can often be reduced without any anesthetic, especially before soft tissue swelling has advanced, it is preferable to do this under regional or general anesthesia to minimize the required force.

Several methods have been described for reduction of the common posterior dislocation.[58,59,73,84,88] Perhaps the most predictable is that of gentle traction applied to the forearm with countertraction on the brachium. Residual medial or lateral displacement of the elbow joint can be corrected, followed by gentle flexion of the forearm. The reduction is often appreciated by a palpable and occasionally audible "clunk." Undue force is counterproductive, and care should also be taken not to hyperextend the forearm too vigorously in

order to minimize additional trauma to the brachialis muscle. Following manipulation, the reduction is confirmed by both radiograph and examination. The elbow should be ranged from full extension to full flexion to ensure that no block to motion exists and to document any instability in the plane of motion. In addition, the elbow is subjected to varus and valgus stress both in full extension and in moderate flexion. For the more unusual medial or lateral dislocations, more sustained traction and countertraction will be required. Rotation of the forearm may also aid in reducing the translational displacement (Fig. 37–22).

POSTREDUCTION MANAGEMENT

With the elbow held at 90°, a well-padded splint is applied. Adequate access to the hand and wrist is mandatory to permit careful monitoring of the neurovascular status. In the event of signs or symptoms suggesting vascular compromise or neurologic dysfunction, forearm compartment pressure measurements should be performed at once at the bedside (see Chapter 13). Arterial inflow can also be documented at the bedside using digital cuff impedance plethysmography or formal arteriography.[11]

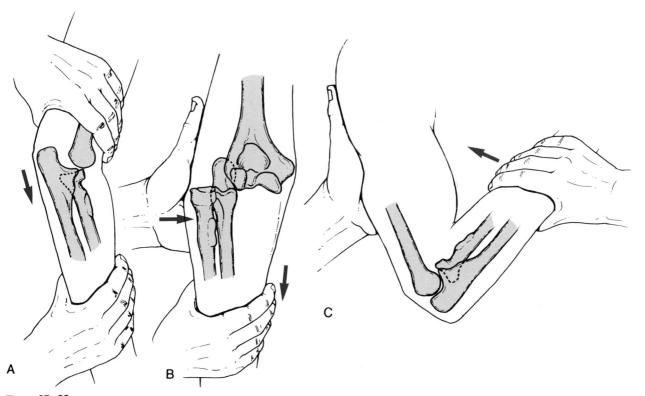

Figure 37–22

Reduction of a posterior elbow dislocation consists of (A) longitudinal traction, (B) correction of lateral or medial displacement, and (C) flexion of the elbow.

In those cases in which no instability was noted following reduction, immobilization need be for only seven to ten days, followed by a program of active exercises out of a removable splint. For those elbows with a tendency toward redislocation during stress in the operating room, it is advisable to continue immobilization for two to three weeks. Control radiographs are necessary within three to five days after reduction to make certain the joint remains congruent.[52] Immobilization beyond three weeks will have significant adverse effects, particularly residual loss of motion and elbow flexion contractures.[49,50]

Open reduction of simple (without fracture) elbow dislocations is rarely indicated. In fact, a prospective study by Josefsson et al. demonstrated no significant difference between the results of operative and those of nonoperative treatment of simple dislocations.[52] However, studies of surgical treatment have revealed the extent of soft tissue injury, even with uncomplicated dislocations.[21,24,43,63] Complete rupture of the medial collateral ligament has been described in nearly all cases and disruption of the lateral collateral ligaments in most. In addition, extensive injury to the anterior capsule and brachialis muscle is common. This supports the biomechanical studies of Morrey and co-workers, who demonstrated that as much as 50% of elbow stability is provided by the congruent articulations of the trochlea and olecranon.[78,79]

A number of investigations have suggested favorable long-term outcome from simple elbow dislocations.[49,51,52,60,72,84,91] Josefsson et al., in a review of 52 patients seen on average 24 years after injury, found that more than 50% had no residual symptoms.[49] There were no complaints referable to instability, although 19 patients had some loss of motion, and follow-up radiographs revealed no loss of the articular space, although periarticular calcification was seen in 76%.

Favorable results are not as common with elbow dislocations associated with fractures of the radial head, olecranon, or coronoid process. Radial head fracture has been observed to occur in 5% to 10% of all elbow dislocations,[59] and the outcome of these fractures is considerably worse than that of simple radial head fractures.[1,20,47,80,122] Complications have included loss of motion, posttraumatic arthritis, instability, and ulnar neuritis. Myositis ossificans has been noted in some studies.[122] When faced with a radial head fracture associated with humeroulnar dislocation, efforts should be made to maintain the radial head either through open reduction and internal fixation or with a silicone rubber prosthesis. Should this not prove possible and instability to valgus stress is obvious in the operating room following radial head excision, a me-

dial incision and repair of the medial collateral ligaments is advisable.

Dislocations associated with olecranon fracture can be exceptionally complex injuries and may be the result of high-energy trauma with extensive soft tissue injury. In this setting, myositis may be more likely to occur. As with any complex intraarticular fracture, joint reconstruction and early mobilization should be the goals of treatment, although these may not always be possible when soft tissue reconstruction is necessary (Fig. 37–23). Additionally, posterior radiocapitellar dislocations can occur with fracture of the olecranon, and these, too, can prove surgically challenging (see Chapter 36, on forearm posterior Monteggia lesions).

Fracture of the coronoid process has been identified in as many as 10% to 15% of elbow dislocations.[95,110] Along with acting as the anterior buttress of the greater sigmoid notch of the olecranon, the coronoid provides attachment for both the anterior bundle of the medial collateral ligament and the middle part of the anterior capsule.[95] Regan and Morrey classified these fractures into the following three types (Fig. 37–24)[95]:

I: Avulsion of the tip.
II: A single or comminuted fracture involving 50% or less of the coronoid.
III: A single or comminuted fracture involving more than 50% of the coronoid.

They, as others, identified more instability and complications with elbow dislocations associated with displaced, major coronoid process fractures. Despite this,

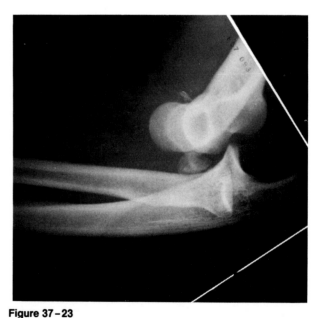

Figure 37–23

A posterior fracture-dislocation of the elbow with displacement of the tip of the coronoid process.

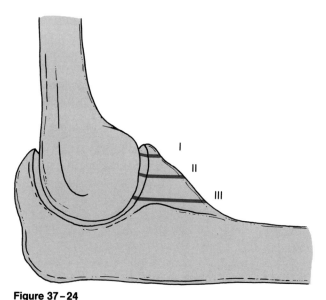

Figure 37–24

The coronoid fracture has been classified into three types by Regan and Morrey.

rarely have open reduction and internal fixation of coronoid process fractures been required to assure stability following closed reduction of the dislocation.[59,110] In the past it has been recommended in these situations that a longer duration of immobilization (three to four weeks) in greater flexion is preferable to surgery. This may well result in a loss of full mobility and a permanent elbow flexion contracture, yet this must be weighed against the possibility of myositis ossificans developing as a result of surgical dissection within the brachialis. Our preference in these unusual situations is to consider surgical stabilization of the displaced coronoid fracture performed at the time of the initial treatment, followed by protected mobilization for five to seven days postoperatively. A hinged orthosis may protect against varus-valgus instability during the early phase of ligament healing.

The displaced coronoid fracture, which presents a block to full elbow motion, is perhaps the one definitive indication for operative reduction and surgical stabilization of these injuries.

Considerably more uncommon are the medial, lateral, divergent, and pure radial head dislocations. A clinical presentation of a distorted elbow despite normal length of the brachium and forearm should raise the suspicion of a medial or lateral elbow dislocation.[91] The radiograph will show the distal humerus to be completely uncovered from its normal articulation with the greater sigmoid notch. The method of reduction has already been described (see treatment section under Elbow Dislocation).

The divergent dislocation, which is exceptionally

uncommon, is usually associated with more violent trauma. In this injury, the ulna is dislocated posteriorly, and the radial head and radius are dislocated anteriorly. A closed, manipulative reduction should be attempted, but repositioning of the radius may prove problematic and require open reduction. A careful pre- and postoperative assessment of neurovascular status is mandatory with this complex injury.

Traumatic radial head dislocation without concomitant ulnar fracture is extremely rare in the adult; isolated anterior and posterior dislocations have been described.[13,40,102,103] Closed reduction by means of longitudinal traction with the elbow in extension followed by forearm supination while maintaining direct pressure over the radial head has been recommended,[13] although open reduction may be necessary.

COMPLICATIONS

The complications of elbow dislocations can be disabling and include recurrent instability, stiffness, myositis ossificans, heterotopic calcification, and neurovascular dysfunction.[31,56,94,98]

Recurrent or "habitual" dislocation is uncommon but can be exceptionally difficult to treat. A number of causes have been postulated to account for this chronic instability, including attenuation of the collateral ligaments, residual articular defects in the trochlear or semilunar notch, nonunion of a large coronoid fracture, and failure of the anterior capsule to heal.[117] Osborne and Cotterill postulated the cause to be located on the lateral side and devised a repair based on this.[87]

Given the fact that the pathology of elbow dislocations has never clearly been defined, it is no small wonder that a number of surgical procedures have been devised for the treatment of this problem. Milch placed a tibial bone block into the tip of the coronoid,[75] whereas Reichenheim described transfer of the biceps tendon into the region of the coronoid, through a drill hole, and out the dorsal aspect of the ulna.[96] Kapel described creating a "cruciate" ligament using a strip of the triceps aponeurosis left attached distally and a similar strip of the biceps tendon brought through the brachialis into a hole drilled into the olecranon fossa.[54] Arafiles described a similar concept using a strip of free tendon graft.[6] Osborne and Cotterill recommended reattaching what they believed to be a deficient posterolateral capsule and lateral collateral ligament to a roughened area along the lateral distal humerus,[87] whereas Schwab et al. focused their attention more on the role of the medial collateral ligament, advising either surgical reattachment or reconstruction with a free tendon graft.[108]

Part II   Fractures of the Distal Humerus

David K. Mehne, M.D. • *Jesse B. Jupiter, M.D.*

The Distal Humerus

FUNCTIONAL ANATOMY

The elbow can be characterized as a hinge joint in that it has only a single axis of rotation.[164] By definition, this represents a constrained joint. In the case of the elbow, the ulna rotates with respect to the humerus around a transverse axis. The cylindrical part of the elbow, consisting of the semilunar notch of the proximal ulna, articulates around the trochlea of the distal humerus, which represents the central axis of this joint (Fig. 37–25).

The term "trochlea" is derived from the Greek word meaning "pulley," although to the modern eye it appears more like a spool. The trochlea functions effectively as the articulating axis of the joint by virtue of its being held between two bony columns, much like the ends of a spool of thread that are held between the thumb and index finger (Fig. 37–26). The end of the skeleton of the humerus splits in a wishbone fashion to form the two columns that support the trochlea. By interconnecting with these divergent columns, the terminal part of the elbow joint most resembles a triangle. This factor is fundamental in the understanding of the proper mechanics of intraarticular distal humerus fractures. With disruption of any one of the three arms of this triangle, the entire construct is weakened more

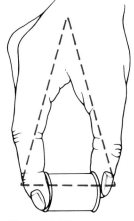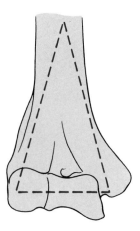

Figure 37–26

The trochlea functions as the articulating axis of the distal humerus. It is held between two bony columns much like the ends of a spool of thread held between the thumb and index finger.

than might be expected.[169] This is an important issue and helps to explain why instability will result after internal fixation of fractures unless all three arms of this triangle are effectively stabilized.

However, defining the distal humeral articulation as a triangle based on the trochlea ignores the capitellum. There are reasons to consider the capitellum and its articulation with the radius as a joint separate from the elbow (i.e., the trochlea-ulna joint). Mechanically, the radiocapitellar joint contributes to the function of forearm rotation and is independent of elbow flexion and extension. In short, it is possible to have an arthrodesis of the elbow joint and yet have full forearm rotation. Furthermore, if this joint is eliminated (e.g., with removal of the radial head), elbow flexion and extension should not be affected.

On viewing the distal humerus from a posterior aspect, the trochlea and its articular surface are readily appreciated to be centrally located between the lateral and medial distal humerus columns from which the trochlea is suspended. On the other hand, the capitellum is not seen, and only on viewing the distal humerus from the anterior surface does it become apparent that the capitellum represents the cartilage-covered anterior surface of the lateral column. It may well be best to view it as such rather than as an integral articular part of the distal humerus and elbow joint. It can be removed from the distal humerus traumatically or surgically and not

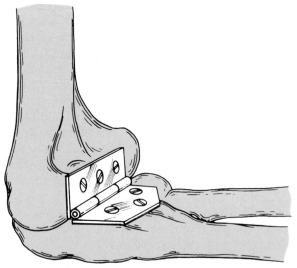

Figure 37–25

The elbow represents a true hinge joint with a single axis of rotation.

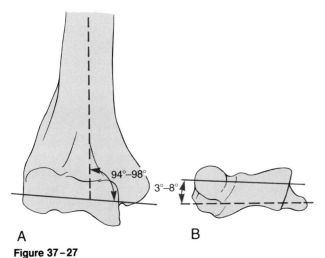

Figure 37-27

The axis of the trochlea is in valgus with respect to the longitudinal axis of the distal humerus (A) and in internal rotation with respect to the transverse axis (B).

in any way interfere with the structural integrity of the "distal humeral triangle."

Although the ulnotrochlear joint behaves as a hinge joint with a single axis of rotation, the motion of the elbow appears more complex clinically. This may be a result in part of the fact that the trochlear axis is not parallel to any ordinate body axis, and the consequent forearm projection of elbow extension-flexion actually traverses several sagittal planes. In fact, the forearm always remains within a single plane, which is oblique to the sagittal and coronal planes of the body. The trochlear axis with respect to the longitudinal axis of the humerus is approximately 94° in valgus in males and 98° in females (Fig. 37-27). In addition, the trochlear axis is externally rotated between 3° and 8° with respect to a line connecting the medial and lateral epicondyles.[164] This therefore places the forearm in external rotation when the elbow is in 90° of flexion (see Fig. 37-27).

This normal valgus position of the elbow is commonly referred to as the "carrying angle" of the elbow. Functionally, it allows the positioning of objects away from the body when they are held with the elbow in extension. When this is considered in depth, it becomes clear that with the elbow in full extension, an object is truly suspended rather than carried. This puts the shoulder girdle musculature at a mechanical disadvantage, as the lever arm of the upper extremity is located at a substantial distance. Any attempt to hold an object away from the body leads to fatigue of the shoulder abductors within a few seconds.

A second source of confusion with the common rationale for a "carrying angle" is the fact that if a heavy object is handheld with the elbow in extension, then the laws of physics dictate that the center of gravity of the object must be precisely below the center of rotation of the shoulder. The positioning of the "pendulum" that is holding this object really has very little to do with the ultimate position of what the pendulum is suspending (Fig. 37-28). Thus one generally sees the trunk of the body tilted, which is functionally more efficient than it would be if the elbow had a greater "carrying angle." A final argument against the stated purpose of the "carry-

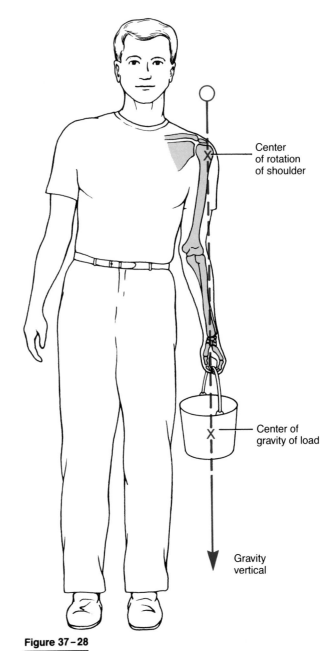

Figure 37-28

With the elbow in full extension, an object held is truly suspended rather than carried.

ing angle" is that in functional activities of the upper extremity, the angle is really manifested only in the anatomic position (i.e., with the humerus in neutral rotation and the forearm in full supination). In fact this position is rarely assumed in the activities of daily living. The most common upper extremity posturing for carrying objects is with the humerus in 45° of internal rotation and the forearm in 45° of supination, leaving the limb in position with the palm facing the thigh. Little, if any, elbow angulation is apparent in this position.

SURGICAL ANATOMY

When viewed from a posterior approach, which is the standard surgical view, the humeral shaft divides into longitudinal medial and lateral columns. These columns terminate distally where the transversely oriented trochlea connects between. The medial column ends approximately 1 cm proximal to the distal end of the trochlea, whereas the lateral column extends to the distal aspect of the trochlea (Fig. 37–29).

Bounded by the triangular structure of the distal humerus is a similarly triangular-shaped depression, the olecranon fossa. This fossa accommodates the proximal tip of the olecranon in full elbow extension. A layer of fatty tissue, the posterior fat pad, is normally contained within the fossa. This fat pad is sandwiched between two layers of the posterior joint capsule (i.e., the fibrous layer, which is superficial to the fat pad, and the synovial layer, which is deep).[168] With the presence of an intraarticular effusion, the fat pad is displaced posteriorly and will become visible on the lateral radiograph with the so-called "posterior fat pad sign" (Fig. 37–30). In normal elbow extension, the fat pad displaces to

permit room for the tip of the olecranon. This displacement, which is posterior as well as superior, is also visible if a lateral radiograph is obtained of the extended elbow. Following trauma or surgery, this posterior fat pad will at times become adherent to the olecranon fossa and undoubtedly contributes to the commonly noted loss of full elbow extension following major trauma to the elbow.

The medial and lateral columns are not as apparent from an anterior perspective (see Fig. 37–29). This is primarily because there is no counterpart to the deep olecranon fossa to put the columns in relief. There are, however, a small coronoid fossa just proximal to the trochlea and an even smaller radial fossa just proximal to the capitellum. These two fossae are separated by a longitudinal ridge of bone that continues distally with the lateral lip of the trochlea. This longitudinal ridge and the lateral trochlear lip form the anatomic division between the lateral and medial columns. The coronoid fossa and trochlea are situated between the two columns and form a symmetric intercolumnar arch (see Fig. 37–29). The medial column begins at the medial border of this arch.

The medial column of the distal humerus diverges from the humeral shaft at an approximately 45° angle. The proximal two thirds of this column is cortical bone. The distal one third of the column represents the medial epicondyle,[170] which is composed of cancellous bone and is ovoid in cross section. The medial and superior surfaces of the medial epicondyle serve as the origins of the flexor muscle mass of the forearm. The medial epicondyle additionally serves as the origin for the anterior and posterior bundles of the ulnar (medial) collateral ligament.[151,154,174,175,191]

It is of surgical importance to recognize that the infe-

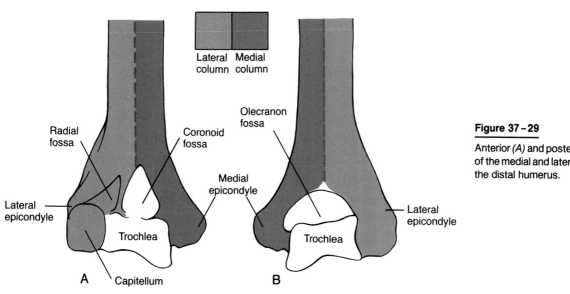

Figure 37–29

Anterior *(A)* and posterior *(B)* views of the medial and lateral columns of the distal humerus.

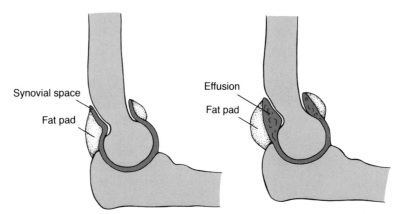

Figure 37-30

With an intraarticular effusion, the fat pads will be displaced and become visible on radiograph.

Synovial space

Fat pad

Effusion

Fat pad

rior surface of the medial epicondyle is available for the placement of internal fixation. The ulnar nerve, which runs in the cubital tunnel below this, can be transferred anteriorly, and the entire posterior medial column can be utilized for the placement of internal fixation. As there are no articulations on the anterior aspect of the medial column, screws can penetrate anteriorly and not interfere with articular function. The triangular shape of this medial column should be kept in mind, as it affords an excellent purchase for screws; these should be directed somewhat medially to obtain purchase on the anteromedial cortex, which is more substantial.

The lateral column of the distal humerus diverges from the humeral shaft at the same level as the medial column but subtends at approximately a 20° angle with reference to the humeral shaft axis. The proximal half of this column is cortical bone, with the posterior aspect being broad and flat and ideal for accepting a plate. The distal half of the lateral column is cancellous bone that is somewhat more complex from both an anatomic and a surgical point of view. From the posterior view, this part of the lateral column begins at the level of the middle of the olecranon fossa. As it extends distally, it begins to gradually curve anteriorly. The anconeus muscle covers the lateral column as it follows the curvature of the adjacent trochlea. At the most distal point of this curve, the capitellar cartilage begins. This represents the distal limit that would allow internal fixation posteriorly. The concept of the columnar structure of the distal humerus is important when considering the placement of internal fixation, because the anterior aspect of the lateral column cannot be seen directly from the posterior view. One must bear in mind that the trochlea lies *between* the two columns, whereas the capitellum is *part* of the lateral column. It therefore follows that the olecranon and coronoid fossae associated with the trochlea are intercolumnar, whereas the radial fossa associated with the capitellum is part of the lateral column. The radial fossa is vulnera-

ble to screw penetration when applying internal fixation on the posterior aspect of the lateral column.

When viewed from the anterior surface, a rough ridge of bone is seen projecting laterally farther along the lateral column from its proximal tubular portion. This is the lateral supracondylar ridge. The brachioradialis and extensor carpi radialis longus muscles originate from this ridge, which ultimately blends distally with the lateral epicondyle. The lateral epicondyle, although smaller than its counterpart on the medial side, represents the point of origin of the radial collateral ligament[154] of the elbow. The common extensor muscle origin comes off the lateral tip of the epicondyle posterior to the radial collateral ligament (Fig. 37-31).

Medially and anteriorly, the lateral column is bounded by the longitudinal ridge. Proceeding distally, the column indents to form the shallow radial fossa. Just below this the capitellum juts out anteriorly as a hyaline cartilage-covered incomplete hemisphere. The midpoint of this hemisphere is directly anterior and is an arc of only 180° in the sagittal plane. This must be compared with an articular arc of 270° for the trochlea. The rotational center of the capitellum is displaced between 12 and 15 mm forward of the humeral shaft axis and is aligned with the trochlear axis. Thus the ulna and radius flex and extend coaxially.

The trochlea is the intercolumnar "tie-rod." It has the form of a spool and is comprised of medial and lateral lips with an intervening sulcus. The sulcus articulates with the semilunar notch of the proximal ulna, and the adjacent lips offer medial and lateral stability to this simple articulation. The anterior and distal aspects of the lateral trochlear lip are of a different radius of curvature than the medial lip, thus changing the symmetry of the trochlea. This asymmetry gives the impression that the trochlea is mechanically complex. Although many have felt that this asymmetric shape positions the ulna in a different axis from flexion to extension,[191] London has shown that it is part of a pure

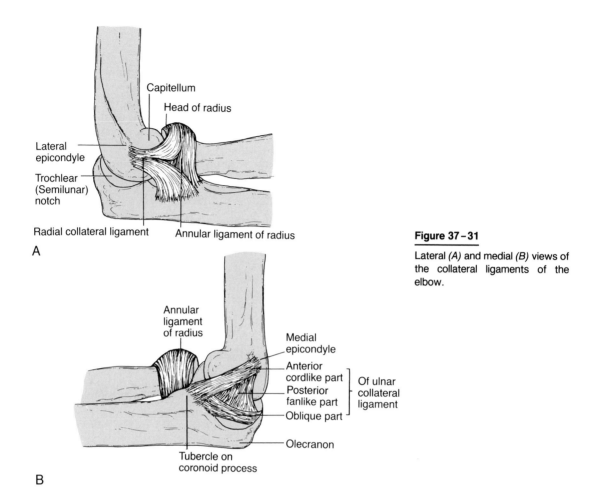

Figure 37–31

Lateral *(A)* and medial *(B)* views of the collateral ligaments of the elbow.

and simple hinge joint.[164] As depicted in Figure 37–32, when the trochlea is viewed end on and the "missing" anterolateral and posteromedial lips are "filled in," it can be seen to be a symmetric spool.

The anatomic division of "condyle" has been absent in this description. Although entrenched in the anatomic and orthopedic literature, this term may well represent a pathologic description rather than a true anatomic division. The word "condyle" comes from the Greek word *kondylos,* which means "knuckle," and can be defined in general as "a rounded projection

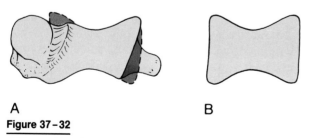

Figure 37–32

A, The trochlea viewed end on. *B,* The anterolateral and posteromedial lips "filled in" so that the trochlea resembles a symmetric spool.

of bone."[145] Although this term accurately describes the distal femur or head of the metacarpals, there are really no obvious structures that lend themselves anatomically to this term in the distal humerus. For this reason we have chosen not to define this as part of the delineated anatomic divisions of the distal humerus; instead we will use it to describe skeletal disruption of the distal humerus.

GENERAL CLASSIFICATION

Traditional classifications of fractures of the distal humerus have centered on the anatomic concept of the terminal end of the humerus structured as condyles (hence the terms "condylar," "transcondylar," and "bicondylar" fractures). As discussed, the distal humerus is more precisely described and understood as two diverging columns supporting an intercalary articular surface (i.e., the trochlea). By changing the term "condyle" to "column," the general fracture categories will be maintained and the fractures more accurately described (Table 37–2).

Table 37–2.

Classification of Distal Humeral Fractures

I. Intraarticular fractures
   A. Single-column fractures
      1. Medial
         a. High
         b. Low
      2. Lateral
         a. High
         b. Low
   B. Bicolumn fractures
      1. T pattern
         a. High
         b. Low
      2. Y pattern
      3. H pattern
      4. Lambda pattern
         a. Medial
         b. Lateral
   C. Capitellum fractures
   D. Trochlear fractures
II. Extraarticular intracapsular fractures
   A. Transcolumn fractures
      1. High
         a. Extension
         b. Flexion
         c. Abduction
         d. Adduction
      2. Low
         a. Extension
         b. Flexion
III. Extracapsular fractures
   A. Medial epicondyle
   B. Lateral epicondyle

Single-Column Fractures

Single-column fractures are rare, making up only 3% to 4% of fractures of the distal humerus.[162,174] Lateral column fractures are more common than medial.[170,174,176] These fractures traverse either the medial or lateral column, extending distally through the intercolumnar portion of the distal humerus. The separated fragment represents the distal portion of the fractured column along with the adjacent part of the trochlea. In fact, the extent of the trochlea that separates with the columnar fragment is directly related to how high proximally or low distally the columnar fracture is. The higher the fracture, the larger the trochlear fragment that separates with the column (Fig. 37–33).

Classification

Single-column fractures have traditionally been considered condylar fractures, with the classification of Milch considered standard.[170,174,176,180] Milch divided the fractures into two types, based on whether the "lateral wall of the trochlea" remained attached to the main mass of the humerus (type 1) or fractured away from it (type 2). He considered the type 2 pattern as a "fracture-dislocation" because of the radius and ulna displacing along with the fracture fragment. On the basis of this, he suggested that type 1 injuries may be treated nonoperatively, whereas type 2 injuries fared better with operative intervention.[170]

It has been our impression that displacement has less to do with the fracture involving the lateral trochlear ridge than with which fragment has the greater capsular

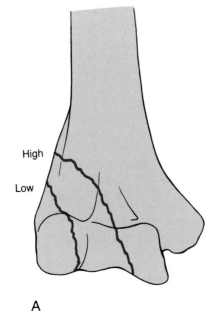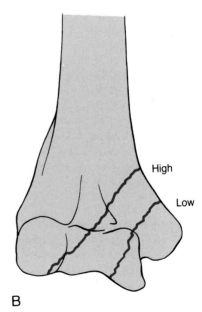

Figure 37–33

Single-column fractures of the distal humerus. A "high" fracture involves the majority of the trochlea and is unstable, as the ulna displaces with the fracture fragment. "Low" fractures are inherently stable.

A

B

attachment and if either of the collateral ligaments is ruptured.[174]

The present classification is based on our columnar concept of the distal humerus. There are two basic categories of single column fractures, depending on which column is dissociated from the remainder of the humerus. The level of the fracture (proximal or distal) represents, in reality, a continuum, but it is useful to categorize these injuries as high or low.

High fractures share the following characteristics:

1. The fractured column includes the majority of the trochlea.

2. The ulna and radius follow the displacement of the fractured column.

3. Internal fixation is reliable and technically straightforward, as there is sufficient skeleton for the placement of internal fixation devices in the distal fragment.

Low fractures, on the other hand, have opposite characteristics.

History and Physical Examination

The mechanism of fracture has been well delineated in past studies. Milch suggested that these fractures may be caused by an abduction or adduction force,[170] but this has never been definitively supported. The fracture may be the result of a motor vehicle accident,[139] a direct blow to the elbow, or a fall on an outstretched hand. The elbow manifests with swelling, pain, and restricted movement. High fractures are clinically more unstable than low fractures and may occur as apparent varus or valgus deformity.[186] A collateral ligament injury may be associated with the fracture[180] but may not be apparent until after internal fixation of the fracture. The neurovascular status of the distal extremity must be evaluated and documented with both high and low single-column fractures.

Standard anteroposterior (AP) and lateral radiographs of the elbow are often sufficient to diagnose a single-column fracture. A radial head–capitellum view may be necessary to differentiate a lateral column fracture from a capitellum fracture.[153] This view may also undercover an occult radial head fracture. Tomography or computed tomography may be of additional value in precisely defining the skeletal and articular injury.

Management

Although these injuries, both high and low, represent intraarticular fractures, some authors continue to advocate closed reduction for the low fractures.[174] There are certain disadvantages of closed treatment of any intraarticular elbow fracture, including prolonged im-

mobilization, the potential for early or late displacement, and residual incongruity of the articular surface leading to instability and posttraumatic arthritis.

It is our opinion that displaced single-column fractures are best treated by open reduction and internal fixation followed by early mobilization of the elbow, but there are certain situations in which internal fixation may not be advisable. These include, for example, the polytraumatized patient in whom extensive peripheral surgery may not be indicated at the time of initial stabilization and long-bone skeletal management. In these cases, a closed reduction can be considered with splinting of the fracture in 90° of elbow flexion. With fractures of the lateral column, the forearm should be maintained in supination, whereas with fractures of the medial column, the forearm should be maintained in pronation.[174,180] In the event that reduction cannot be achieved, overhead traction can be considered.

When considering a surgical approach, the surgical planning, technique, and postoperative regimen are similar to those described for bicolumn fractures, with only a few exceptions. These include the fact that the ulnar nerve generally does not need anterior transposition with lateral column fractures. In the restoration of the mechanical integrity of the distal humeral triangle, a single plate is generally needed in addition to the distal transtrochlear screw fixation.

Postoperative care and rehabilitation are essentially the same as for bicolumn fractures, and the reader is referred to that section.

Bicolumn Fractures

Bicolumn fractures are the most common type of fracture of the distal humerus and the most difficult to treat. The fracture disrupts each component of the distal humeral triangle (see section on functional anatomy), resulting in a dissociation of each column from the other and from the proximal humeral shaft.

Incidence

Statistics regarding the incidence of bicolumn fractures vary widely in the literature, from a low of 5% of all distal humeral fractures[161] to a high of 62%.[165] In terms of overall incidence of skeletal fractures, they are uncommon. Of 4536 consecutive fractures treated at the Massachusetts General Hospital in one clinical study, only 14 (0.31%) were bicolumn fractures.[165]

Mechanism of Injury

Although many have considered the bicolumn fracture to be the result of a "wedging" apart of the distal humerus by the olecranon,[140,149,187] this has not been duplicated in mechanical studies. In cadaver studies per-

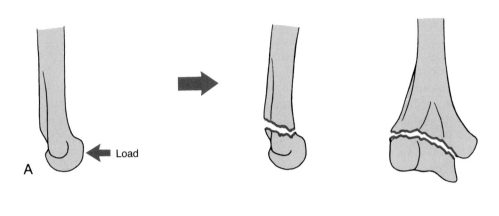

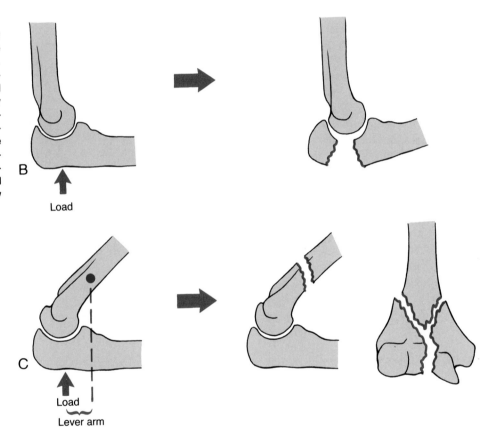

Figure 37-34

Fracture patterns about the elbow commonly reflect the magnitude and direction of the force of injury. *A,* A transcolumn fracture will result from an axial load directed through the forearm with the elbow flexed at 90°. *B,* An olecranon fracture often represents a direct impact on the olecranon with the elbow flexed at 90°. *C,* An intercondylar fracture of the distal humerus will occur with an axial load on the olecranon with the elbow flexed 90°.

formed at the University of Southern California biomechanical laboratories, a direct force applied to the olecranon with the elbow flexed at 90° repeatedly resulted in transverse olecranon fractures. Only with the elbow flexed beyond 90° were bicolumn fractures produced (Fig. 37-34).

Associated Injury

Although sporadic reports exist of associated neurologic or vascular injury with closed bicolumn fractures, these are exceptionally uncommon.[134,140] However, open bicolumn fractures are not uncommon, with in-

cidence varying from 20% to as much as 50% in some series.[150,160,169]

Classification

Considerable modifications in the classification of bicolumn fractures have developed since Reich's original description in 1936 of T and Y classifications.[177] Riseborough and Radin in 1969 subdivided these into four categories based on separation, rotation, and comminution of the distal articular fragments.[179] With increased interest in the surgical approach to these fractures has come a realization that these classifications do not accurately reflect the extent of the injury or help in surgical planning. The AO classification has expanded the definition of the intraarticular components, but it, too, is lacking in identifying the anatomy of the columnar involvement.

The following classification system addresses the specific characteristics of the various types of bicolumn fractures in order to help in the preoperative planning of internal fixation:

1. *High T fracture.* A transverse fracture line divides both columns proximal to or at the upper limits of the olecranon fossa (see Fig. 37–43A).

2. *Low T fracture.* This fracture is among the most common and the most difficult to treat. A transverse line crosses the olecranon fossa usually just proximal to the trochlea, leaving relatively small distal fragments (see Fig. 37–44A).

3. *Y fracture.* In this pattern, oblique fracture lines cross each column, joining in the olecranon fossa to form a distal vertical line. The oblique fracture lines and the large fragments with broad fracture surfaces make this a relatively straightforward fracture to treat with internal fixation (see Fig. 37–45A).

4. *H fracture.* In this pattern, the medial column is fractured above and below the medial epicondyle. The lateral column is fractured in a T or Y configuration. The trochlea is thus rendered a free fragment and is also at risk for avascular necrosis. This may be the most difficult fracture pattern to treat (see Fig. 37–46A).

5. *Medial lambda fracture.* The most proximal fracture line exits medially with the lateral fracture line distal to the lateral epicondyle, leaving a small zone for internal fixation on the lateral side (see Fig. 37–47A).

6. *The lateral lambda fracture.* This fracture pattern is similar to an H fracture without the lateral column fracture. Although technically not a true bicolumn fracture (as the medial column remains intact), it still requires fixation approaches similar to those for bicolumn fractures (see Fig. 37–48A).

Clinical Presentation

Commonly the elbow is swollen and may be deformed. The arm may also appear shortened because of proximal migration of the distal fragment and arm.[174] The neurovascular status must be carefully checked. Additionally, the posterior soft tissue envelope should be inspected carefully and examined for the possibility of an open wound, which will be present in more than one third of cases.[138,150,160,169,186]

Standard AP and lateral radiographs will generally provide an adequate projection of the fracture pattern. Additionally, in the operating room an AP view with traction on the arm can further define the intraarticular aspect of these fractures.

Treatment

Until the 1970s, the vast majority of studies dealing with this fracture tended to approach these injuries in one of two ways: conservative or operative. The conservative approach ranged from no treatment to traction methods and casting.[138,161,173,177] The operative approaches were based on surgical exposure and limited internal fixation. The results of these treatment methods are difficult to analyze, as the rating systems used were quite different and frequently quite broad. For example, an excellent result could include, in

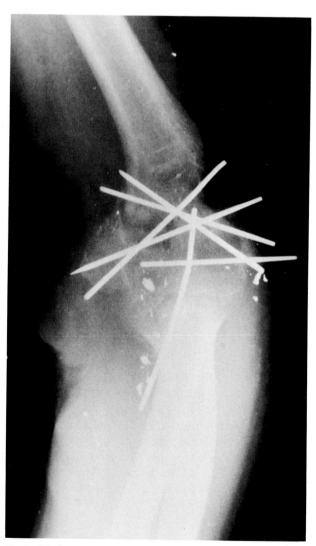

Figure 37–35

Flexible wire fixation of complex distal humeral fractures does not provide sufficient stability to allow early mobilization and can result in loss of reduction and limited motion.

some, a 60° flexion contracture.[141] Riseborough and Radin expressed the general consensus well in their review published in 1969 when they stated, "Open reduction and adequate internal fixation is not easy, and seemed to offer little chance of a good outcome" (Fig. 37–35).[179] The technical difficulties with the operative treatment of these fractures have been confirmed by other authors as well.[149,161,165,172,173,185–187]

In 1985, Jupiter et al. reported on 39 fractures treated in one AO center in Switzerland with open reduction and internal fixation (ORIF).[160] Thirteen patients had excellent results, and 14 had good results, with the conclusion being that ORIF can provide a predictable outcome and offer a chance at a functional restoration, even in the elderly patient. These results have been subsequently confirmed in other studies.[150,169] All of these authors have identified the need to provide stable fixation of both columns using plates and screws.

Preoperative Planning

Ideally surgery should be performed as soon as possible, preferably within two to three days of the fracture. Special considerations are required for the polytraumatized patient. A molded posterior splint or overhead traction can be used to stabilize these injured limbs while the more serious systemic injuries are treated.

The surgical tactic is planned preoperatively based on the fracture type as determined by good-quality radiographs. A full complement of instrumentation, including plates and screws of differing sizes, should be available when contemplating the surgical stabilization of these fractures. A sterile arm tourniquet, fine dissecting instruments, and a sharp osteotome complete the surgical armamentarium necessary for these procedures.

General anesthesia is preferred, as these surgical procedures can prove lengthy, and iliac crest bone graft may be required. The lateral decubitus position is a versatile one, allowing exposure of the iliac crest and the entire arm[169] without the potential problems incurred with the patient in a prone position (Fig. 37–36).[158] With the patient placed in the lateral position and the sterile tourniquet high on the arm, an 8- to 10-in roll of folded drapes can be tucked between the arm and the chest wall, suspending the arm for ease of access.

Operative Technique

A longitudinal incision is made over the posterior aspect of the arm beginning 15 to 20 cm proximal to the tip of the olecranon, curving slightly medially at the elbow to skirt the olecranon, and returning to the midline and extending approximately 5 cm distal to the tip of the olecranon (Fig. 37–37). The ulnar nerve is dissected free for a distance of approximately 6 to 8 cm proximal to the cubital tunnel and 5 cm distal to the cubital tunnel. If it appears that internal fixation will be necessary in the vicinity of the cubital tunnel and medial epicondyle, then the ulnar nerve is transposed anteriorly to the medial epicondyle. The fascia over the flexor carpi ulnaris is split, and the muscle is split to allow the nerve to rest without tension in its new position.

At this point, the triceps insertion is isolated and the

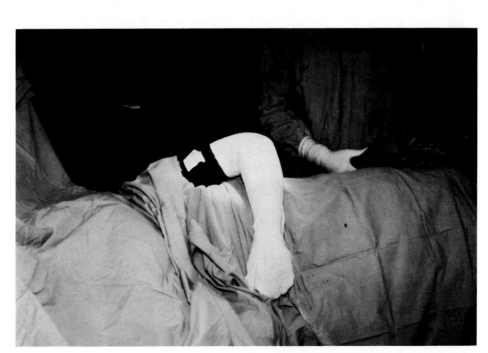

Figure 37–36

The lateral decubitus position provides a versatile approach to fractures about the elbow. Exposure of the entire arm as well as the iliac crest is facilitated.

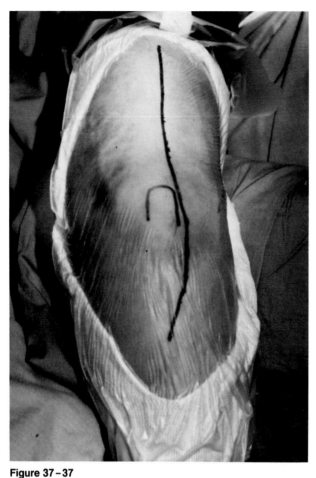

Figure 37–37

The skin incision for fractures of the distal humerus is extensile, skirting just around the olecranon tip.

distal triceps separated from adjacent soft tissues. The joint capsule is freed up from both sides of the olecranon, leaving only the attachment of the triceps tendon. Gauze is passed through the trochlear notch of the ulna to act as a suspensory sling and provide countertraction during the course of the olecranon osteotomy. The osteotomy can be performed using either a fine-bladed saw or a sharpened, thin osteotome. If a saw is chosen, the osteotomy should be completed with an osteotome, which will produce a more irregular surface for later reduction and fixation. The osteotomy is directed either perpendicular to the long axis of the shaft of the ulna in a transverse manner or in a chevron fashion with the apex pointing distally. The advantages of the latter are the ease of repositioning following completion of the distal humeral fixation and the broader surface of cancellous bone for more rapid union. Predrilling of the olecranon can be considered if the surgeon chooses to use a large screw such as 6.5-mm cancellous screw (Fig. 37–38).

Once osteotomized, the olecranon and triceps are wrapped in moist gauze and retracted proximally, exposing the fracture. The fracture surfaces and small fracture fragments are gently debrided of hematoma and irrigated using pulsed lavage to help clear the hematoma atraumatically. At this point consideration is given to the approach to reduction and internal skeletal fixation.

The principle of fixation of these fractures is to anatomically reconstruct and stably secure each side of the distal humeral triangle. It must be borne in mind that these fractures prove difficult to securely fix for a number of anatomic reasons, including the following:

1. The distal fragments are small and limit the number of screws that can be placed.

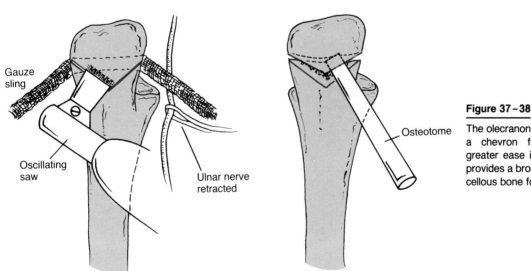

Gauze sling

Oscillating saw

Ulnar nerve retracted

Osteotome

Figure 37–38

The olecranon osteotomy made in a chevron fashion allows for greater ease in repositioning and provides a broader surface of cancellous bone for healing.

2. The distal fragments are cancellous bone, which also presents a problem in gaining stable purchase with screws.

3. The hardware must avoid the articular surfaces and three fossae to maintain full motion.

4. The complex skeletal and articular geometry in this area make plate contouring difficult.

Although modifications must be made depending on the specific fracture patterns, the principles of internal fixation apply to all fracture types. A standard fixation is illustrated in Figure 37–39. Fractures of the trochlea can be secured with an interfragmentary compression screw. The "tie-rod" is then reconstructed back onto the medial and lateral columns using plates. The reconstruction plate offers distinct advantages in the dis-

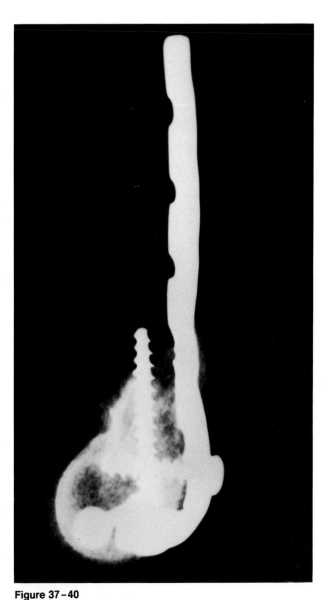

Figure 37–40

The medial epicondyle can be "cradled" by a 90° bend in the plate. The two distal screws will be perpendicular to each other, providing a mechanical interlocking construct.

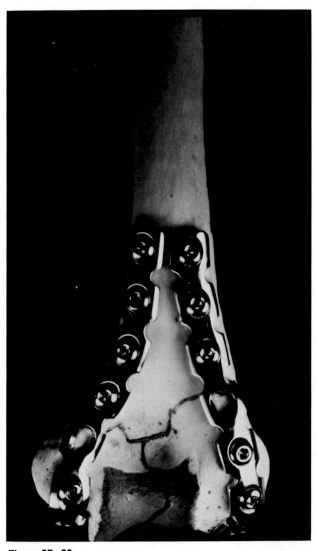

Figure 37–39

Two-column fixation of the distal radius with contoured 3.5-mm reconstruction plates.

tal humerus, as it can be bent in three dimensions to match the complex geometry of the distal humeral columns. The medial epicondyle can be "cradled" by a 90° bend in the distal part of the plate (Fig. 37–40). This bend is achieved by placing two instruments in the adjacent holes at the distal part of the plate and applying a torque (Fig. 37–41). Thus the two distal screws will be perpendicular, providing a mechanical interlocking construct, the strength of which exceeds the combined pullout strengths of each of the screw threads.

The lateral plate is applied as distally as possible until it almost abuts the posterior border of the capitellar

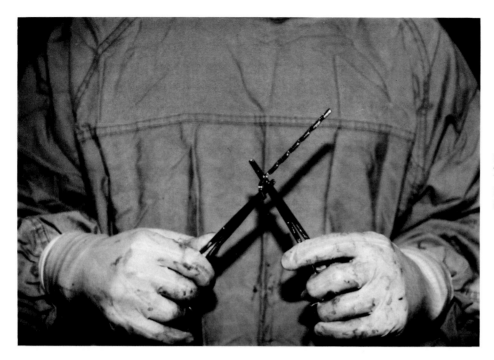

Figure 37–41

The reconstruction plate can be bent by placing two Kocher clamps in the distal two holes.

cartilage. The most distal screw is directed proximally to avoid the capitellum and to provide a mechanical interlocking construct (Fig. 37–42).

The order of fixation will vary and must be tailored to the individual fracture pattern. At times it may be advisable to fix the longer fracture planes first, which ordinarily involves one of the columns. One other basic principle that should be maintained is to contour the plates and fix them from a distal-to-proximal direction, as the distal plate position is the most critical to maximize the distal screw purchase.

Fixation of Specific Fracture Types

High T Fracture. The high T fracture proves to be the simplest fracture to securely fix, because the distal fragments are relatively large. In view of the fact that the

Figure 37–42

The plate on the posterior aspect of the lateral column can extend distally onto the posterior aspect of the distal column.

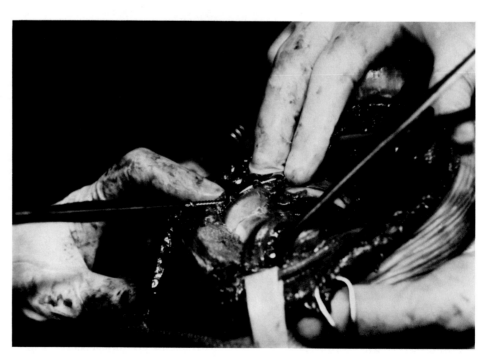

vertical fracture line is the longest, it is generally fixed first with a transverse lag screw (Fig. 37–43).

Low T Fracture. The low T fracture is the most common fracture, and the particular problem is often the fixation of the lateral fragment. For this reason, the medial column is ordinarily fixed first, as this proves to be the most straightforward fixation. The medial column can be secured to the lateral column by a long malleolar screw placed through the distal plate hole, achieving purchase more proximally in the lateral column. The lateral column can be secured using a plate that is twisted sagittally around the lateral column (Fig. 37–44).

Y Fracture. The oblique fracture planes permit interfragmentary compression screws. In the Y fracture, plates only have to function as neutralization plates (Fig. 37–45).

H Fracture. In principle, the trochlear fragment must be realigned onto the distal columns. The three distal fragments are reduced with a pointed reduction forceps onto the two upper columns. A temporary transverse Kirschner wire is helpful in stabilizing the trochlea and preventing displacement of the fragments when the interfragmentary 4.0- or 6.5-mm screw is introduced. The medial and lateral columns are secured in the previously described manner (Fig. 37–46).

Medial Lambda Fracture. The difficulty with the medial lambda fracture is the minimal purchase area available in the lateral fragment. Additionally, the medial trochlear fragment is too small for screw purchase, such as can be done with the low T fracture. The lateral column can be secured with two 4.0-mm screws, bringing the capitellum to the medial column and accomplishing distal transverse fixation. Two lateral 4.0-mm screws then secure the same fragment to the lateral plate to provide fixation of the entire lateral column. The medial column is secured with a standard 3.5-mm reconstruction plate (Fig. 37–47).

Lateral Lambda Fracture. In lateral lambda fractures the trochlea is a free fragment, as in the H fracture, but the medial column is intact; therefore efforts can be directed primarily toward securing the trochlear fragment onto the medial column. Standard plate fixation may be utilized on the medial column. The two distal holes of the plate are overdrilled with a 3.5-mm drill bit to allow passage of 4.0-mm cancellous screws. The distal plate can be twisted sagittally, placing the two distal screw holes onto the medial trochlea. The two 4.0-mm screws are then directed transversely through the plate holes and into the trochlea and the capitellum. Both screws secure the plate and lag the distal fragments together. The proximal portion of this plate is then

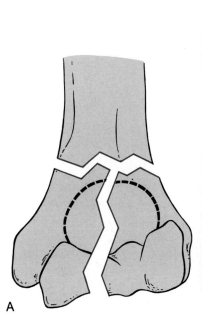
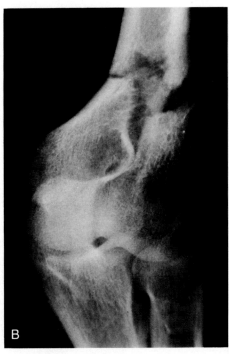
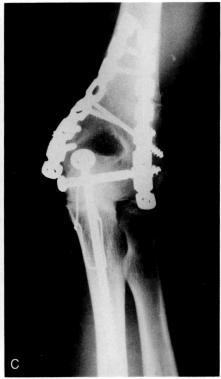

Figure 37–43

A to *C*, The high T fracture is the most straightforward bicolumn fracture to secure with internal fixation, because the distal fragments are large.

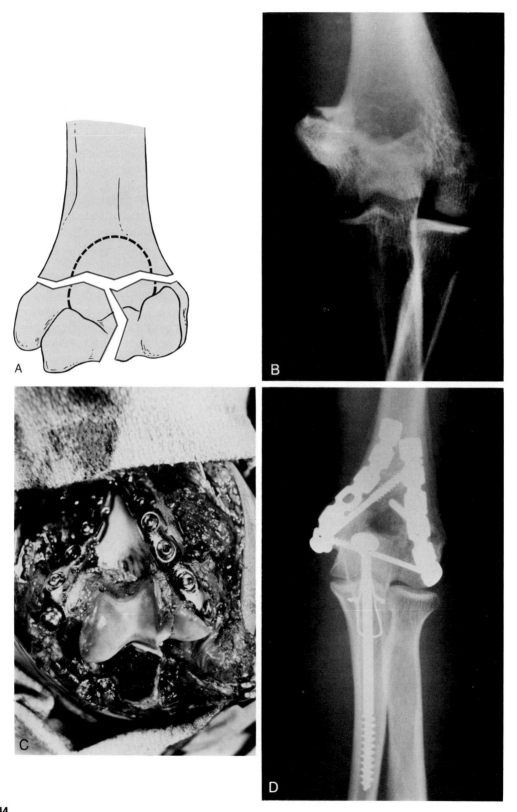

Figure 37–44

A and *B*, The low T bicolumn fracture. *C*, Intraoperative view of internal fixation of low T fracture. Note that both plates extend distally along the columns of the distal humerus. *D*, Radiograph of internal fixation of low T bicolumn fracture.

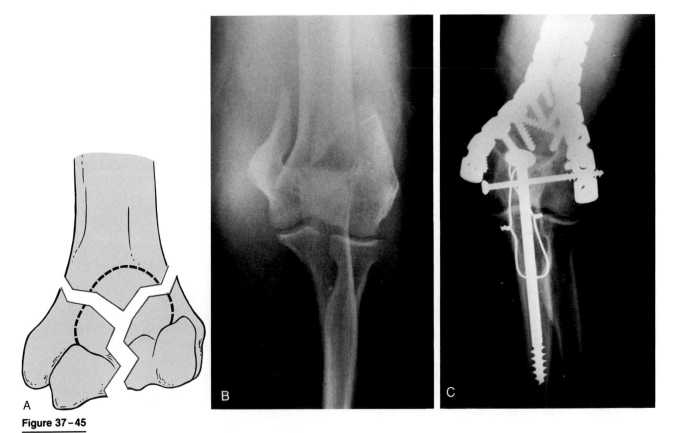

Figure 37-45

A and *B,* The Y bicolumn fracture has oblique fracture planes that permit intrafragmentary compression of screws across the fracture line. *C,* Stable fixation of a Y bicolumn fracture.

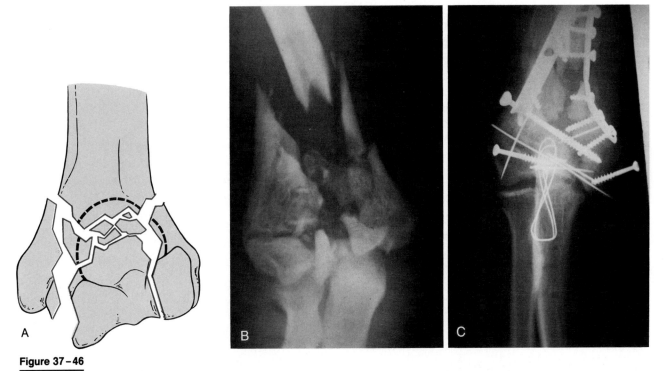

Figure 37-46

A and *B,* The H fracture is the most complex of the bicolumn fractures. *C,* Stability was achieved with internal fixation. Elbow motion of 125° flexion and −40° extension resulted.

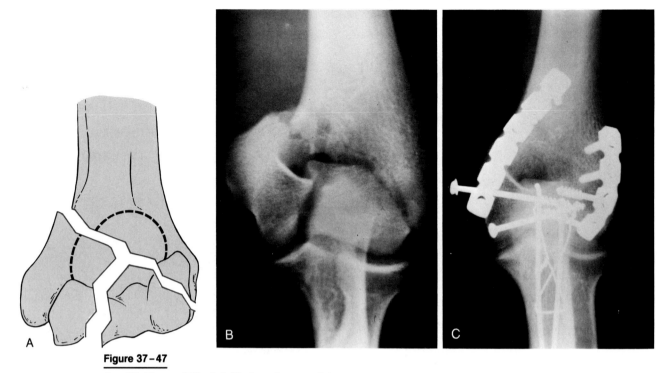

Figure 37-47

A and *B,* The medial lambda bicolumn fracture. *C,* Internal fixation of a medial lambda bicolumn fracture.

secured to the medial column in a standard fashion. Lateral column fractures of this type can be readily fixed with a standard plate technique (Fig. 37–48).

Reattachment of the Olecranon Osteotomy

The olecranon osteotomy can be secured either with a 6.5-mm screw placed over a washer (see section on olecranon fractures), also incorporating a tension band wire, or with two Kirschner wires. The surgeon should be able to put the elbow through a full range of motion without obstruction by hardware or demonstration of fracture instability (Fig. 37–49). A small suction drain is placed in the depths of the wound, and the wound is closed in layers. A sterile, bulky, soft dressing and a posterior molded splint are applied. The drain can be removed 24 hours postoperatively, and the patient can be started on a program of active exercises as soon as the wound appears stable. Immobilization should be considered for comfort only. A sling can provide sufficient stabilization and avoid the potential postoperative stiffness that may come from prolonged immobilization. The patient can rest the elbow on a padded tabletop and concentrate on relaxing the biceps muscle, letting the elbow extend over a period of 15 to 20 seconds. Extension is alternated with active flexion, also exerted over a 15- to 20-second period.

As the radiographs demonstrate bone healing, usually within four to six weeks, the patient is permitted to perform active extension exercises and to slowly add resistance to active flexion and extension exercises. Passive exercises by the patient in both extension and flexion can be started, but the patient is instructed to stretch only to the point of discomfort, not to the point of pain.

Evaluation of Outcome

The commonly accepted parameters of elbow function include the following[175]:

1. Range of motion:
    a. Elbow extension (normal, 0°)
    b. Elbow flexion (normal, 140° to 150°)
    c. Forearm supination (normal, 85°)
    d. Forearm pronation (normal, 75°)
2. Strength:
    a. Elbow flexion
    b. Elbow extension
    c. Grip

Most activities of daily living can be performed in a range of motion of 30° to 130°.[169] Lack of extension is more easily compensated for than loss of flexion.

Anticipated Results

In predicting final range of motion, it is often not the fracture pattern that determines the ultimate outcome, but the energy absorbed by the elbow in the initial

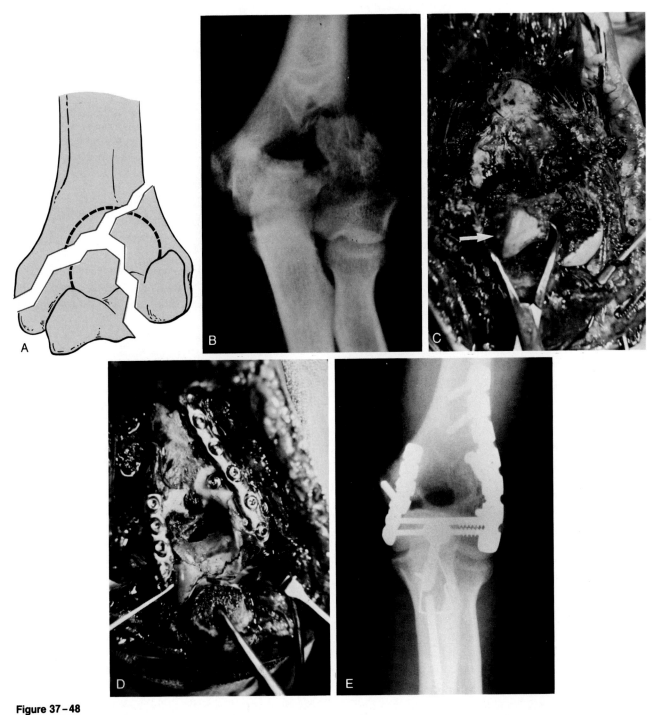

Figure 37–48

A and B, The lateral lambda bicolumn fracture. C, Intraoperative view of the trochlea (arrow) held with pointed clamp. It is completely devoid of soft tissue attachment. D, Intraoperative view of lateral lambda fracture after reassembling trochlear fragments and securing construct back to humeral column. E, Radiograph of internal fixation of lateral lambda fracture.

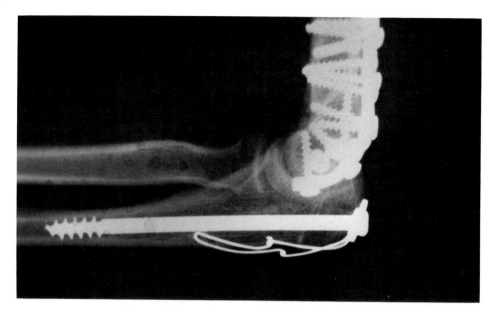

Figure 37–49

The olecranon osteotomy can be secured either with a 6.5-mm screw placed over a washer or with a tension band wire technique.

trauma.[160,169] High-energy injuries such as sideswipe injuries, falls from a height, motor vehicle trauma, and gunshot wounds all result in greater soft tissue trauma leading to scarring and diminished range of motion. A successful result in a patient with a low-energy lesion is generally considered to be a 15° to 140° range of motion.[150,160,169] Flexion generally returns first, usually within two months. Extension returns more slowly, and final outcome may not be reached until four to six months.[150,169] Supination and pronation are essentially unaffected by bicolumn fractures, particularly when the fracture is mobilized early.[134,138,141,148,157,173,177]

Exertional pain may be expected in about 25% of patients. This does not appear to be related to the energy of trauma, the range of motion, or radiographic arthrosis.[160,169]

Complications

Failure of Fixation. Failure of fixation most often results from a lack of secure fixation of the plates and screws at the time of surgery. This is usually seen at the junction of the distal articular fracture patterns and the humeral shaft. Clinically, fixation failures are accompanied by pain, decreased range of motion, and radiographic evidence of implant loosening or breakage. If the elbow is left as it is, nonunion can be anticipated.[160] If the internal fixation breaks or pulls out from the bone or if the fracture fragments displace into a position that is not acceptable for ultimate function, early reoperation should be considered. If, however, the loosening is noted at an early stage without complete disruption of the reconstruction, cast immobilization can be considered. This offers the possibility of obtaining union, but

at the expense of a loss of mobility and ultimate elbow stiffness.

Nonunion. Although uncommon, nonunion can be disabling.[133,140,160,169] It is more likely to occur with fractures resulting from high-energy trauma or as a result of fixation failure. Treatment is based on the patient's symptoms, but reoperation and secure fixation of the nonunion with compression plates are generally required. In a nonunion at the supracondylar level, dual plate fixation in a manner similar to that described for primary fractures has been shown to be effective.[133] Bone grafting is necessary in atrophic or synovial nonunions but may not be necessary with compression fixation of hypertrophic or fibrous nonunions (Fig. 37–50; see Chapter 20).

Nonunion of an Olecranon Osteotomy. Nonunion of an olecranon osteotomy has been recognized by a number of authors.[133,160,169] Fixation failure has been associated with the use of a number of different types of techniques. This is in part because the osteotomy, with its smooth "fracture" planes, is intrinsically less stable. The use of a chevron-shaped osteotomy should diminish the incidence of this. Nonunions are treated by a repeat osteosynthesis; a plate applied along the subcutaneous border of the ulna is preferable. If the initial osteotomy involved only the proximal olecranon and the nonunion fragment was relatively small, then excision of the fragment and reattachment of the triceps tendon can also be considered.

Infection. Considering the fact that a substantial number of these fractures are open and the surgery is long and complicated, infections are uncommon. Infection rates in the literature range from 0% to

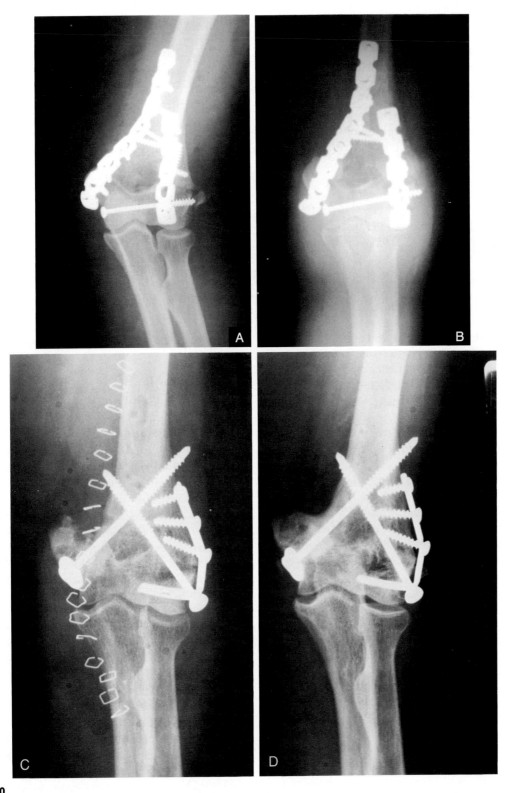

Figure 37–50

A, A bicolumn fracture was internally fixed with two plates and an interfragmentary screw. *B*, Five months postoperatively instability of the fixation and nonunion were noted. *C*, Stable fixation of the nonunion with a contoured plate along the lateral column. *D*, Radiograph 12 months after fixation of the nonunion.

6%.[134,137,138,140,150,160,169] They have been described more commonly in grade III open wounds but have not been associated with one type of treatment more than another.

Tardy Ulnar Palsy. Tardy ulnar palsy has been described in as many as 15% of cases in one series.[160] It may be preventable by transferring the ulnar nerve at the time of surgery, particularly if screws or plates extend in the vicinity of the cubital tunnel.

Capitellum Fractures

Capitellum fractures are extremely rare. It is estimated that they account for 1% of all elbow fractures and about 6% of all distal humeral fractures.[174] Although there are slight variations in fracture patterns, these injuries are essentially a shear fracture in a coronal plane displacing the capitellum from the lateral column of the distal humerus. This fracture has been described as occurring more frequently in females than in males.[143,152] Capitellum fractures may be associated with radial head fractures as well as posterior elbow dislocations.[163,174]

Most capitellum fractures are "complete" fractures as originally described by Hahn[155] and Steinthal[183a] in the nineteenth century. This fracture has been called the Hahn-Steinthal fracture in subsequent literature.[135,147,181] A second, less common type involves only the shell of the anterior cartilage of the capitellum with a thin layer of subcondylar bone. This lesion has been called the Kocher-Lorenz fracture.[135,147,152,163,181]

A more contemporary and more useful classification is that proposed by Bryan and Morrey.[174] Type I fractures are complete fractures of the capitellum; type II, the more superficial lesions of Kocher-Lorenz; and type III, comminuted capitellar fractures (Fig. 37–51).

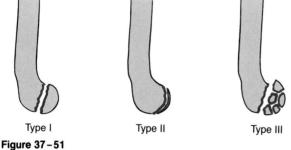

| Type I | Type II | Type III |

Figure 37–51

Fractures of the capitellum can be divided into type I, complete capitellum fracture; type II, the more superficial lesion of Kocher-Lorenz; and type III, comminuted capitellar fracture.

Clinical Presentation

Historically this is an injury of middle-aged or elderly patients. The presentation is like that of a radial head fracture, with swelling and tenderness localized along the lateral aspect of the elbow. Pain will be noted with forearm rotation.

Standard AP and lateral radiographs will demonstrate the fracture in most cases. At times this fracture may be confused with a displaced lateral epicondyle fracture. Type II fractures are more difficult to diagnose, as the extent of subcondylar bone involvement may be minimal. A radial head–capitellum view will be helpful in these cases.[153]

As with all elbow trauma, careful examination of the wrist and shoulder is mandatory.

Treatment

Because this fracture is uncommon, it would be unusual for any individual to have had a large clinical experience. The literature reflects a wide variety of recommendations, extending from closed treatment[142,147,152,178] to surgical excision[135,166] to open reduction and internal fixation.[143,146,163,165] Although closed reduction has been described, if the fracture is displaced, successful reduction and maintenance of reduction are unpredictable. Some have advocated excision of the fracture fragment,[147] although one study of 11 fractures treated by excision and followed for an average of five years noted that results were unsatisfactory.[152] With the evolution in small-fragment fixation methodology, open reduction and internal fixation of these fractures have gained favor.[139,158,163,165]

Type I. Consideration should be given to a closed reduction with this fracture pattern. However, the timing of surgery is critical if closed reduction is contemplated. It should be done as soon as possible, with general or regional anesthesia affording complete muscle relaxation. With the patient in the supine position, traction is applied by an assistant to the supinated forearm with the elbow held at 90° of flexion. Downward pressure by the surgeon's thumb is applied to the capitellar fragment.[142] If a successful anatomic reduction is achieved, the elbow should be immobilized in a well-molded posterior splint or long-arm cast for a minimum of three to four weeks, following which active assisted range-of-motion exercises can be initiated. Success with closed treatment is contingent on achieving an anatomic or near-anatomic reduction.

If the closed reduction proves unsuccessful or there is a delay of several days from the time of fracture, open reduction and internal fixation should be considered (Fig. 37–52). A lateral approach is recommended, with

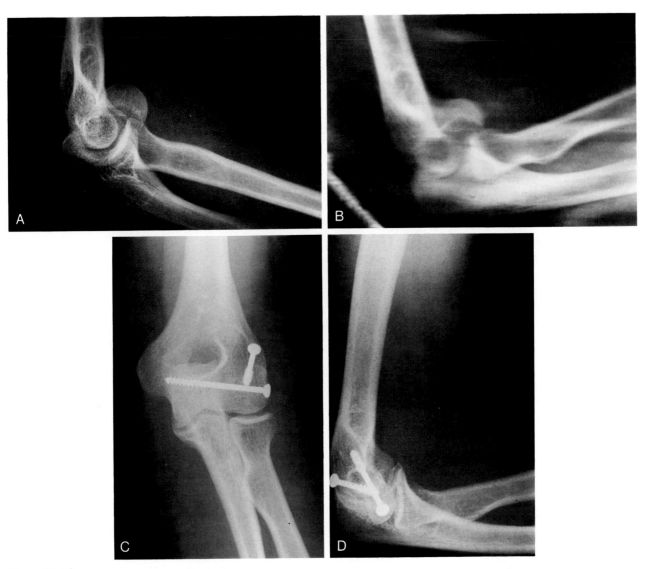

Figure 37-52

A displaced type I capitellar fracture in a 28-year-old female. *A*, The lateral radiograph demonstrates the rotational displacement of the capitellum. *B*, Lateral tomography provides an excellent picture of the extent of displacement. *C* and *D*, Through a lateral approach, anatomic repositioning and stable fixation were achieved with two screws. Full motion was regained.

the incision begun 2 cm proximal to the lateral epicondyle and extending 3 to 4 cm distal to the radial head. The common extensor origin is detached with a sharp osteotome and reflected distally to expose the lateral elbow joint. The capitellar fragment is reduced, temporarily held in place with a sharp reduction forceps, and provisionally secured with a Kirschner wire. Internal fixation can be achieved with 2.0-mm miniscrews used in a lag fashion or 4.0-mm cancellous screws placed from posterior to anterior. The Herbert screw is also applicable in these cases, its advantage being that it can be buried underneath the cartilage in the subcondylar bone.

Care is taken to avoid damage to the radial nerve, which lies between the brachioradialis and brachialis muscles. The most likely cause of damage is excessive soft tissue retraction while gaining the exposure.

Should the fixation prove secure, postoperative mobilization can be initiated as soon as tolerated. Should the fixation not prove rigid, it is then necessary to support the elbow for three to four weeks in a posterior splint or cast.

Type II and Type III Fractures. Internal fixation of shear fractures or comminuted fractures is not easily accomplished. In most cases, excision of the fragments is advisable. The surgical approach is the same as for type I fractures, and the techniques of exposure and resection are straightforward. Again, it is advisable to consider surgery as early as possible following the injury. The results of excision can be expected to be good in the short term,[135,147] but long-term results have been less favorable, revealing loss of motion or instability.[143,147,152]

Complications

The principal complication to be expected from a capitellar fracture is loss of elbow motion.[143,152] This has been associated more with fragment excision than with open reduction and internal fixation.

A less common complication is avascular necrosis of the capitellar fragment.[135,174] It is likely that avascular necrosis of capitellar fractures is more common than generally appreciated but may not become apparent clinically or radiologically because of a rapid revascularization of the small fragment. In the event that this does occur and becomes symptomatic, delayed excision is indicated.[152]

Finally, an additional complication is a nonunion of the capitellar fragment. Should this prove to be painful or associated with significant loss of elbow motion, capitellar fragment excision along with a soft tissue elbow release through a lateral approach can improve overall function.

Extraarticular Intracapsular Fractures: Transcolumn Fractures

Pathologic Anatomy

Transcolumn fractures traverse both columns of the distal humerus without violating the articular surface. Although the fracture line may be above the olecranon fossa, it is usually somewhat lower and may in fact represent an intracapsular fracture. These fractures occur in four basic patterns: high, low, abduction, and adduction.

The high and low fractures can be further subdivided into extension and flexion patterns. We have characterized these fractures into the following subgroups (Fig. 37–53).

High extension fractures. The fracture line is oblique, extending from a posterior proximal position to a low anterior position with posterior displacement.

High flexion fracture. The fracture line is oblique, beginning proximally anteriorly and extending distally with anterior displacement.

Low extension fracture. The fracture is slightly oblique or transverse with posterior displacement.

Low flexion fracture. The fracture line is slightly oblique or transverse with anterior displacement.

Abduction fracture. The fracture line is oblique with a lateral proximal–to–distal medial direction. There is lateral displacement.

Adduction fracture. The fracture line is oblique, with the line extending from proximal medial to distal lateral with a medial displacement.

Incidence

These fractures are more common in the pediatric patient, and are exceptionally rare in adults. Figure 37–54, which represents a compilation of statistics from several references,[159,174,180,182] illustrates that transcolumn fractures are exceptionally uncommon. High extension fractures are the most common of the transcolumn fractures.

Diagnosis

Transcolumn fractures most often are the result of a fall. The extension fractures have been believed to be associated with a fall on the outstretched hand with a posteriorly directed force on the distal humerus.[139] The flexion fractures, on the other hand, have been thought to result from an anteriorly directed force on the posterior distal humerus.[184] Adduction and abduction fractures result from axial loading on the distal humerus with an additional varus or valgus component. The patient with the flexion pattern may also give a history of direct trauma over the posterior distal humerus, usually with the elbow flexed.[173,180,183]

The transcolumn fracture is manifested as noticeable swelling in the elbow area, and deformity may be appreciated if the fracture is displaced. Posterior displacement may be apparent with extension fractures, and anterior displacement with flexion fractures.

The vascular supply of the extremity must be checked expeditiously. Although uncommon, brachial artery injury may occur with any of these fracture patterns and particularly with the extension pattern. In the presence of excessive swelling at the fracture site with diminished or absent distal pulses, arteriography should be considered. An assessment must also be made of the compartments in the forearm.[189] Finally, neurologic status must be checked, as injury to all of the three major nerves has been documented. The radial and median nerves have been more commonly associated with extension injuries, whereas the ulnar nerve has been associated with flexion fractures.

Routine AP and lateral radiographs are generally adequate to define a transcolumn fracture. The AP radiograph alone will differentiate a low or high fracture pattern, even in the presence of an oblique fracture line. However, it may not be able to differentiate between a transcolumn fracture and a bicolumn injury. This is particularly important, as the bicolumn fracture is a

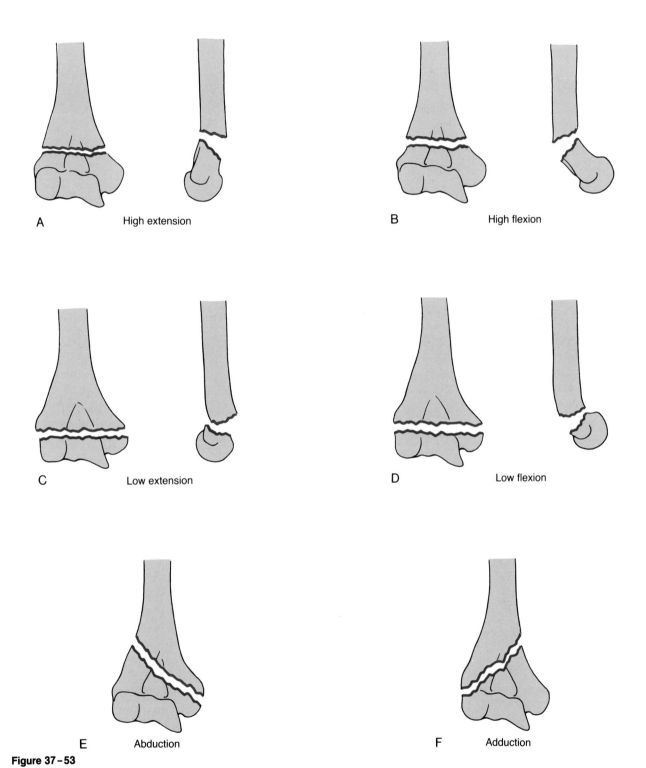

Figure 37–53

A to F, Transcolumn fractures. These fractures occur in four basic patterns: high, low, abduction, and adduction. The high and low fractures can be further subdivided into extension and flexion patterns. When compared with other fractures of the distal humerus, transcolumn fractures are uncommon.

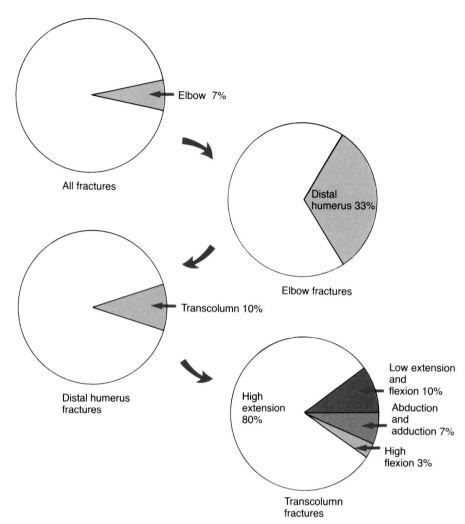

Figure 37-54

The relative incidence of various fractures of the distal humerus is depicted in this diagram. Note the rarity of transcolumn fractures.

much more common injury. The lateral radiograph will distinguish a flexion pattern from an extension pattern and will also identify the extent of the obliquity of the fracture plane. More advanced imaging techniques such as tomography and computed tomography (CT) scanning may be helpful but are usually not necessary.

Management

The literature is relatively limited with regard to studies specifically dealing with these fractures. For the most part, they have been included in papers related to adult bicolumn fractures[141,149,160,173,191] or in papers describing general elbow trauma.[137,144,156,184] In the past, most authors advocated closed reduction and plaster immobilization of these fractures.[146,159,165,171,189] However, current indications for closed reduction of an adult transcolumn fracture are limited and include the poor surgical risk patient or those fractures associated with pathologic conditions that limit stable internal fixation.

The techniques of closed reduction are the same as for any fracture. With extension fractures, the extended position of the distal fracture fragment should be maintained while traction is applied to the humerus and countertraction applied to the distal arm. The surgeon uses both thumbs in pushing the distal fragment distally and anteriorly. Reduction is checked either with fluoroscopy or with AP and lateral radiographs. If a satisfactory reduction is achieved, the elbow is extended between 10° and 20° of maximum flexion and placed in a well-padded but well-molded splint.

Flexion fractures are more difficult to maintain in a reduced position with a posterior molded splint. In these cases, the cylindrical casting technique described by Sultanpur may be more effective.[184] This technique is designed to maintain a posterior force on the distal humeral fragment with the forearm flexed. This is achieved by having a well-molded forearm cast "shoving backward" on the forearm with a counterforce provided by the posterior portion of a cylindrical arm cast. The arm cylinder portion is initially applied while traction is maintained directly on the humeral epicondyle. The elbow, at this juncture, is in flexion. When the cast hardens, the surgeon then places one hand posteriorly to support the cast while pushing the patient's forearm posteriorly with the other hand to reduce the fracture. The forearm plaster is then applied to complete a circumferential long-arm cast. Complications associated with the closed reduction of these fractures include damage to the brachial artery, which can be the result of hyperflexion, particularly in the setting of significant soft tissue swelling. Should this occur, the elbow must be extended until distal pulses can be appreciated. If there is any suspicion that arterial damage has oc-

curred, an intraoperative arteriogram is recommended.

In the event that closed manipulation fails to achieve or maintain a reduction, a number of authors have advocated olecranon traction, either overhead[172] or sidearm.[174] Percutaneous pin fixation, although very successful in the pediatric age group, has not gained widespread application in the adult. Because fixation is not stable using this technique, the fracture must be immobilized for a period of between four and six weeks, which may result in prolonged or permanent elbow stiffness.

Percutaneous Fixation. The indications for percuta-

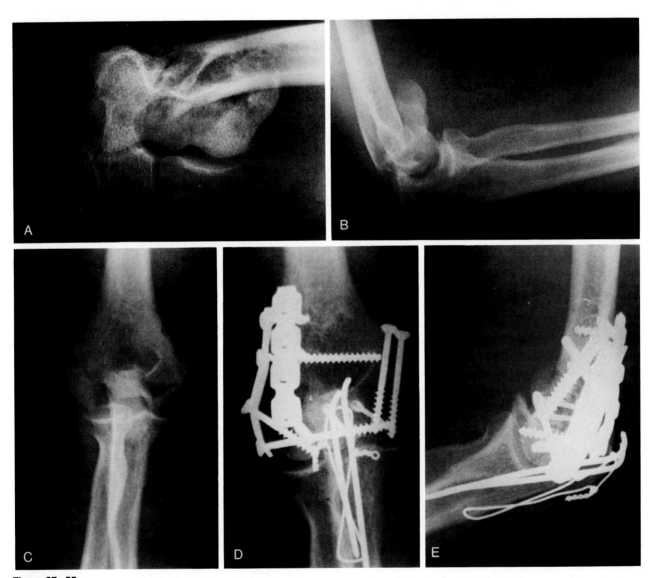

Figure 37–55

A 50-year-old female fell while hiking and landed on her elbow. AP *(A)* and lateral *(B)* radiographs demonstrate the displaced transcolumn fracture. *C,* An AP radiograph with traction applied to the forearm provides a clearer picture of the fracture pattern. *D* and *E,* Through an olecranon osteotomy, the articular fragments were secured with screws and plates, providing fixation secure enough to permit postoperative mobilization.

neous fixation include a low transcolumn fracture with osteoporotic bone or any other transcolumn fracture in which reduction cannot be attained and the patient's condition or the clinical situation is not appropriate for open reduction and internal fixation. With the patient in the supine position, the fracture is reduced as previously described. Image intensification is of tremendous help in both the reduction and the pin placement. With the elbow maintained in 90° of flexion, smooth pins are placed from each epicondyle across the fracture line into the opposite cortex. The pins are directed at a 35° to 45° angle through the longitudinal axis of the humeral shaft. A right-handed surgeon will find it easier to insert the lateral pin first in a right distal humeral fracture and the medial pin first in a left distal humeral fracture.[159] If radiographs confirm a satisfactory fracture reduction and pin placement, the pins are cut off, protruding just outside the skin. Any skin tension around the pins must be liberally released. Skin edges compressed by a pin are prone to develop a localized cellulitis. The pin tract wounds are covered with antibiotic ointment, and a well-molded posterior splint is applied with the elbow in 90° of flexion and the forearm held in neutral rotation.

Potential complications with this approach especially involve damage to the ulnar nerve. This can be avoided either by identifying the nerve directly or by using smooth pins introduced from the anterosuperior medial epicondyle, thus avoiding the cubital tunnel.

Once the postoperative swelling has diminished, conversion from a posterior splint to a long-arm cast is done. The pins can be removed without any anesthesia in the office between four and five weeks postoperatively. Depending on the fracture stability and radiographic appearance of union, the extremity may be further immobilized in a cast or, if it appears stable, protected in a sling.

Open Reduction and Internal Fixation. For the most part, a well-planned and executed internal fixation will offer the patient the most favorable chance of union as well as function. It is our belief that this treatment should be considered in all adult displaced transcolumnar fractures, unless the patient's general condition contraindicates surgery or the surgeon does not feel that a stable fixation can be achieved. The timing, technique, and postoperative care of transcolumnar fractures are identical to those of bicolumn fractures, with one exception: the two columns do not have to be fixed to each other distally. This in fact facilitates the internal fixation (Fig. 37–55).

Postoperative care with stable internal fixation of transcolumnar fractures is identical to that for bicolumn fractures. Controlled mobilization, under the supervision of a therapist, is an integral part of the overall treatment program.

REFERENCES

Trauma to the Adult Elbow

1. Adler, J.B.; Shafton, G.W. Radial head fractures. Is excision necessary? J Trauma 4:115–136, 1964.
2. Adler, S.; Fay, G.F.; MacAusland, W.R., Jr. Treatment of olecranon fractures. Indications for excision of the olecranon fragment and repair of the triceps tendon. J Trauma 2:597–602, 1962.
3. Amis, A.A.; Dowson, D.; Wright, V. Elbow joint force predictions for some strenuous isometric actions. J Biomech 8:765–775, 1980.
4. Amis, A.A.; Dowson, D.; Wright, V.; Miller, J.H. The derivation of elbow joint forces and their relation to prosthesis design. J Med Eng Technol 3:229, 1979.
5. An, K.N.; Morrey, B.F.; Chao, E.Y.S. The effect of partial removal of proximal ulna on elbow constraint. Clin Orthop 209:270–279, 1986.
6. Arafiles, R.P. Neglected posterior dislocation of the elbow: A reconstruction operation. J Bone Joint Surg 69B:199–203, 1987.
7. Arvidson, H.; Johansson, O. Arthrography of the elbow joint. Acta Radiol 43:445, 1955.
8. Bakalim, C. Fractures of radial head and their treatment. Acta Orthop Scand 41:320, 1970.
9. Broberg, M.A.; Morrey, B.F. Results of delayed excision of the radial head after fracture. J Bone Joint Surg 68A:669–674, 1986.
10. Broberg, M.A.; Morrey, B.F. Results of treatment of fracture-dislocation of the elbow. Clin Orthop 216:109–119, 1987.
11. Broudy, A.; Jupiter, J.; May, J.W. Jr. Management of supracondylar fracture with brachial artery thrombosis in a child: A case report and literature review. J Trauma 19:540–543, 1979.
12. Bunker, T.D.; Newman, J.H. The Herbert differential pitch bone screw in displaced radial head fracture. Injury 16:621–624, 1985.
13. Burgess, R.C.; Sprague, H.H. Posttraumatic posterior radial head subluxation. Clin Orthop 186:192–194, 1984.
14. Cabanela, M. Olecranon fractures. In: Morrey, B.F., ed. The Elbow and Its Disorders. Philadelphia, W.B. Saunders, 1987.
15. Campbell, B.G. Human Evolution: An Introduction to Man's Adaptations, Ed. 2. Chicago, Aldine, 1974.
16. Carn, R.M.; Medige, J.; Curtain, D.; Koenig, A. Silicone rubber replacement of the severely fractured radial head. Clin Orthop 209:259–269, 1986.
17. Carstam, N. Operative treatment of fractures of the upper end of the radius. Acta Orthop Scand 19:502–526, 1950.
18. Coleman, D.A.; Blair, W.F.; Shurr, D. Resection of the radial head for fracture of the radial head. J Bone Joint Surg 69A:385–392, 1987.
19. Colton, C.L. Fractures of the olecranon in adults: Classification and management. Injury 5:121–129, 1973–1974.
20. Conn, J., Jr.; Wade, P.A. Injuries of the elbow: A ten-year review. J Trauma 1:248–268, 1961.
21. Copf, F.; Holz, V.; Schauwecker, H.H. Biomechanische probleme bei ellenbogenluxationen mit frakturen am processus coronoideus und radius koepfchen. Langenbeck's Arch Chir 350:249–254, 1980.

22. Curr, J.; Coe, W. Dislocation of the inferior radio-ulnar joint. Br J Surg 34:74–77, 1946.

23. DeLee, J.C.; Green, D.P.; Wilkins, K.E. Fractures and dislocations of the elbow. In: Rockwood, C.; Green, D.P., eds. Fractures and Dislocations. Philadelphia, J.B. Lippincott, 1985, pp. 559–652.

24. Duerig, M.; Mueller, W.; Ruedi, T.P.; Gauer, E.F. The operative treatment of elbow dislocation in the adult. J Bone Joint Surg 61A:239–244, 1979.

25. Dunn, N. Operation for fracture of the olecranon. Br Med J 1:214–215, 1939.

26. Edwards, G.; Jupiter, J.B. The Essex-Lopresti lesion revisited. Clin Orthop 234:61–69, 1988.

27. Ericksson, E.; Sahlen, O.; Sahdahl, V. Late results of conservative and surgical treatment of fracture of the olecranon. Acta Chir Scand 113:153–166, 1957.

28. Essex-Lopresti, P. Fractures of the radial head with distal radioulnar dislocation. J Bone Joint Surg 33B:244–247, 1951.

29. Fleetcroft, J.P. Fractures of the radial head: Early aspiration and mobilization. J Bone Joint Surg 66B:141–142, 1984.

30. Galbraith, K.A.; McCullough, C.J. Acute nerve injury as a complication of closed fractures or dislocations about the elbow. Injury 11:159–164, 1979.

31. Garland, D.E.; O'Halloren, R.M. Fractures and dislocations about the elbow in the head injured adult. Clin Orthop 168:38–41, 1982.

32. Gartsman, G.M.; Sculco, T.P.; Otis, J.C. Operative treatment of olecranon fractures—excision or open reduction with internal fixation. J Bone Joint Surg 63A:718–721, 1981.

33. Gaston, S.R.; Smith, F.M.; Baab, D.D. Adult injuries of the radial head and neck: Importance of time element in treatment. Am J Surg 78:631–635, 1949.

34. Gordon, M.; Bullough, P.G. Synovial and osseous inflammation in failed silicone-rubber prostheses. J Bone Joint Surg 64A:574–580, 1982.

35. Greenspan, A.; Norman, A. The radial head capitellar view. Useful technique in elbow trauma. AJR 8:1186–1190, 1982.

36. Gregory, G.K. The humerus from fish to man. Am Mus Novit 1400:1–54, 1949.

37. Halls, A.A.; Travill, A. Transmission of pressures across the elbow joint. Anat Rec 150:243–248, 1964.

38. Harrington, I.J.; Tountas, A.A. Replacement of the radial head in the treatment of unstable elbow fractures. Injury 12:405–409, 1981.

39. Hassman, G.C.; Brunn, F.; Neer, C.S. Recurrent dislocation of the elbow. J Bone Joint Surg 57A:1080–1084, 1975.

40. Heidt, R.S. Jr.; Stern, P.J. Isolated posterior dislocation of radial head. Clin Orthop 168:136–138, 1982.

41. Holdsworth, B.J.; Clement, D.A.; Rothwell, P.N. Fractures of the radial head—the benefit of aspiration: A prospective controlled trial. Injury 18:44–47, 1987.

42. Hotchkiss, R.N.; Weiland, A.J. Valgus stability of the elbow. Orthop Trans 10:224, 1986.

43. Jacobs, R.L. Recurrent dislocation of the elbow joint. A case report and review of the literature. Clin Orthop 74:151–154, 1971.

44. Jenkins, F.A. The functional anatomy and evolution of the mammalian humero-ulnar articulation. Am J Anat 137:281–298, 1973.

45. Jensen, C.M.; Olsen, B.B. Drawbacks of traction-absorbing wiring (TAW) in displaced fractures of the olecranon. Injury 17:174–175, 1986.

46. Johansson, O. Capsular and ligament injuries of the elbow joint. Acta Chir Scand Suppl 287, 1962.

47. Johnston, G.W. Follow-up of one hundred cases fracture of head of the radius with a review of the literature. Ulster Med J 31:51–56, 1962.

48. Josefsson, P.O.; Gentz, C.F.; Johnell, O.; Wendenberg, B. Dislocation of the elbow and intraarticular fractures. Clin Orthop 246:126–130, 1988.

49. Josefsson, P.O.; Johnell, O.; Gentz, C.F. Long-term sequelae of simple dislocation of the elbow. J Bone Joint Surg 66A:927–930, 1984.

50. Josefsson, P.O.; Gentz, C.F.; Johnell, O.; Wendeberg, B. Dislocation of the elbow and intraarticular fractures. Clin Orthop 246:126–130, 1989.

51. Josefsson, P.O.; Johnell, O.; Wendeberg, B. Ligamentous injuries in dislocations of the elbow joint. Clin Orthop 222:221–225, 1987.

52. Josefsson, P.O.; Gentz, C.F.; Johnell, O.; Wendeberg, B. Surgical versus non-surgical treatment of ligamentous injuries following dislocations of the elbow joint. J Bone Joint Surg 69A:605–608, 1987.

53. Jupiter, J.B. The management of fractures in one upper extremity. J Hand Surg 11A:279–282, 1986.

54. Kapel, O. Operation for habitual dislocation of the elbow. J Bone Joint Surg 33A:707–714, 1951.

55. Keon-Cohen, B.T. Fractures at the elbow. J Bone Joint Surg 48B:1623–1639, 1966.

56. Kini, M.G. Dislocation of the elbow and its complications. J Bone Joint Surg 22:107–117, 1940.

57. Kluge, A.G. Chordate Structure and Function, Ed. 2. New York, Macmillan, 1977, pp. 179–269.

58. Lavine, L. A simple method of reducing dislocations of the elbow joint. J Bone Joint Surg 35A:785–786, 1953.

59. Linscheid, R.L. Elbow dislocations. In: Morrey, B.F., ed. The Elbow and Its Disorders. Philadelphia, W.B. Saunders, 1985, pp. 414–432.

60. Linscheid, R.L.; Wheeler, D.K. Elbow dislocations. JAMA 194:1171–1176, 1965.

61. Lister, J. An address on the treatment of fracture of the patella. Br Med J 2:855, 1883.

62. Louis, D.S.; Ricciardi, J.E.; Spengler, D.M. Arterial injury: A complication of posterior elbow dislocation. A clinical and anatomical study. J Bone Joint Surg 56A:1631–1636, 1974.

63. Mackay, I.; Fitzgerald, B.; Miller, J.H. Silastic replacement of the head of the radius in trauma. J Bone Joint Surg 61B:494, 1979.

64. Maeko, D.; Szabo, R.M. Complications of tension-band wiring of olecranon fractures. J Bone Joint Surg 67A:1396–1401, 1985.

65. Mason, J.A.; Shutkin, N.M. Immediate active motion in the treatment of fractures of the head and neck of the radius. Surg Gynecol Obstet 76:731–737, 1943.

66. Mason, M. Some observations on fractures of the head of the radius with a review of one hundred cases. Br J Surg 42:123–132, 1954.

67. Mateo, I. A radiological sign of entrapment of the median nerve in the elbow joint after posterior dislocation. A report of two cases. J Bone Joint Surg 58B:353–355, 1976.

68. McAusland, W.R. The treatment of fractures of the olecranon by longitudinal screw or nail fixation. Ann Surg 116:293–296, 1942.

69. McDougall, A.; White, J. Subluxation of the interior radio-

ulnar joint complicating fracture of the radial head. J Bone Joint Surg 39B:278–287, 1957.

70. McHenry, H.M.; Corruccini, R.S. Distal humerus in hominoid evolution. Folia Primatol 23:227–244, 1975.

71. McKeever, F.M.; Buck, R.M. Fractures of the olecranon process of the ulna. JAMA 135:1–5, 1947.

72. Mehlhoff, T.L.; Noble, P.C.; Bennett, J.B.; Tullos, H.S. Simple dislocation of the elbow in the adult. Results after closed treatment. J Bone Joint Surg 70A:244–249, 1988.

73. Meyn, M.A.; Quigley, T.B. Reduction of posterior dislocation of the elbow by traction on the dangling arm. Clin Orthop 103:106–108, 1974.

74. Mikic, Z.D.; Vukadinovic, S.M. Late results in fractures of the radial head treated by excision. Clin Orthop 181:220–228, 1983.

75. Milch, H. Bilateral recurrent dislocation of the ulna at the elbow. J Bone Joint Surg 18:777–780, 1936.

76. Miller, G.K.; Drennan, D.B.; Maylahn, D.J. Treatment of displaced segmental radial head fractures. Long term follow-up. J Bone Joint Surg 63A:712–717, 1981.

77. Morrey, B.F.; An, K.N.; Stormont, T.J. Force transmission through the radial head. J Bone Joint Surg 70A:250–256, 1988.

78. Morrey, B.F.; Chao, E.Y.; Hui, F.C. Biomechanical study of the elbow following excision of the radial head. J Bone Joint Surg 61A:63–68, 1979.

79. Morrey, B.F.; An, K.N. Articular and ligamentous contributions to the stability of the elbow joint. Am J Sports Med 11:315–319, 1983.

80. Morrey, B.F. Radial head fracture. In: Morrey, B.F., ed. The Elbow and Its Disorders. Philadelphia, W.B. Saunders, 1985.

81. Morrey, B.F.; An, K.N. Functional anatomy of the ligaments of the elbow. Clin Orthop 201:84–90, 1985.

82. Mueller, M.E.; Allgoewer, M.; Schneider, R.; Willenegger, H. Manual of Internal Fixation, Ed. 2. New York, Springer-Verlag, 1979.

83. Murphy, D.F.; Greene, W.B.; Dameron, T.B. Displaced olecranon fractures in adults. Clin Orthop 224:215–223, 1987.

84. Nevasier, J.S.; Wickstrom, J.K. Dislocation of the elbow: A retrospective study of 115 patients. South Med J 70:172–173, 1977.

85. Odeberg-Johnson, G. On fractures of the proximal portion of the radius and their causes. Acta Radiol 3:45, 1924.

86. Odenheimer, K.; Harvey, J.P. Jr. Internal fixation of fractures of the head of the radius. J Bone Joint Surg 61A:785–787, 1979.

87. Osborne, G.; Cotterill, P. Recurrent dislocation of the elbow. J Bone Joint Surg 48B:340–346, 1966.

88. Parrin, R.W. Closed reduction of common shoulder and elbow dislocations without anaesthesia. Arch Surg 75:972–975, 1957.

89. Pribyl, C.R.; Kester, M.A.; Cook, S.D.; et al. The effect of the radial head and prosthetic radial head replacement on resisting valgus stress at the elbow. Orthopaedics 9:723–726, 1986.

90. Pritchard, D.J.; Linscheid, R.L.; Svien, H.J. Intraarticular median nerve entrapment with dislocation of the elbow. Clin Orthop 90:100–103, 1973.

91. Protzman, R.R. Dislocation of the elbow joint. J Bone Joint Surg 60A:539–541, 1978.

92. Quigley, T.B. Aspiration of the elbow joint in treatment of fractures of the head and neck of the radius. New Engl J Med 240:915–916, 1949.

93. Radin, E.L.; Riseborough, E.J. Fractures of the radial head. J Bone Joint Surg 48A:1055–1064, 1966.

94. Rana, N.A.; Kenwright, J.; Taylor, R.G.; Rushworth, G. Complete lesion of the median nerve associated with dislocation of the elbow joint. Acta Orthop Scand 45:365, 1974.

95. Regan, W.; Morrey, B. Fractures of the coronoid process of the ulna. J Bone Joint Surg 71A:1348–1354, 1989.

96. Reichenheim, P.P. Transplantation of the biceps tendon as a treatment for recurrent dislocation of the elbow. Br J Surg 35:201, 1947.

97. Reith, P.L. Fractures of the radial head associated with chip fractures of the capitellum in adults; surgical considerations. South Surgeon 14:154, 1948.

98. Roberts, J.B. The surgical treatment of heterotopic ossification of the elbow following long-term coma. J Bone Joint Surg 61A:760–763, 1979.

99. Roberts, P.H. Dislocation of the elbow. Br J Surg 56:806–815, 1969.

100. Romer, A.S.; Parsons, T.S. The Vertebrate Body, Ed. 6. Philadelphia, Saunders College Publishing, 1986.

101. Rowe, C. The management of fractures in elderly patients is different. J Bone Joint Surg 47A:1043–1059, 1965.

102. Ryu, J.; Pascal, P.E.; Levine, J. Posterior dislocation of the radial head without fracture of the ulna. A case report. Clin Orthop 168:136–138, 1982.

103. Salama, R.; Wientroub, S.; Weissman, S.C. Recurrent dislocation of the head of the radius. Clin Orthop 125:156, 1977.

104. Scharplatz, D.; Allgoewer, M. Fracture-dislocation of the elbow. Injury 7:143–159, 1976.

105. Schatzker, J. Olecranon fractures. In: Schatzker, J.; Tile, M., eds. The Rational Basis of Operative Fracture Care. New York, Springer-Verlag, 1987.

106. Schatzker, J. Fractures of the radial head. In: Schatzker, J.; Tile, M., eds. The Rational Basis of Operative Fracture Care. New York, Springer-Verlag, 1987.

107. Schmueli, G.; Herold, H.Z. Compression screwing of displaced fractures of the head of the radius. J Bone Joint Surg 63B:535–538, 1981.

108. Schwab, G.H.; Bennett, J.B.; Woods, G.W.; Tulles, H.S. Biomechanics of elbow instability. The role of the medial collateral ligament. Clin Orthop 146:42–52, 1980.

109. Schwartz, R.P.; Young, F. Treatment of fractures of the head and neck of the radius and slipped radial epiphysis in children. Surg Gynecol Obstet 57:528–537, 1933.

110. Selesnick, F.H.; Dolitsky, B.; Haskell, S.S. Fracture of the coronoid process requiring open reduction with internal fixation. Case report. J Bone Joint Surg 66A:1304–1306, 1984.

111. Sharma, R.K.; Covell, N.A.G. An unusual ulnar nerve injury associated with dislocation of the elbow. Injury 8:145–147, 1976.

112. Stephen, I.B.M. Excision of the radial head for closed fracture. Acta Orthop Scand 52:409, 1981.

113. Strange, F.G. St. C. Entrapment of the median nerve after dislocation of the elbow. J Bone Joint Surg 64B:224–225, 1982.

114. Stugh, L.H. Anterior dislocation of the elbow with fracture of the olecranon. Am J Surg 75:700–703, 1948.

115. Sturm, J.T.; Rothenberger, D.A.; Strate, R.G. Brachial artery disruption following closed elbow dislocation. J Trauma 18:364–366, 1978.

116. Swanson, A.B.; Jaeger, S.H.; LaRochelle, D. Comminuted fractures of the radial head. The role of silicone implant replacement arthroplasty. J Bone Joint Surg 63A:1039–1049, 1981.

117. Symeonides, P.P.; Paschaloglov, C.; Stavrov, Z.; Pangalides, T. Recurrent dislocation of the elbow. Report of three cases. J Bone Joint Surg 57A:1084–1086, 1975.

118. Szaly, F.S.; Dagosto, M. Locomotor adaptations as reflected on the humerus of paleogene primates. Folia Primatol 34:1–45, 1980.
119. Taylor, T.K.F.; O'Connor, B.T. The effect upon the inferior radio-ulnar joint and excision of the head of the radius in adults. J Bone Joint Surg 46B:83–84, 1964.
120. Thomas, T.T. A contribution to the mechanism of fractures and dislocations in the elbow region. Ann Surg 89:108, 1929.
121. Thomas, T.T. Fractures of the head and the radius. An experimental study and recent report of cases. Univ Penn Med Bull 18:184–197;221–234, 1905.
122. Thompson, H.C. III; Garcia, A. Myositis ossificans: Aftermath of elbow injuries. Clin Orthop 50:129, 1967.
123. Vierhout, R.J.; Oostvogel, H.J.M.; Van Vroonhoven, J.M.V. Internal fixation of the head of the radius. Neth J Surg 35:13–16, 1983.
124. Wadsworth, T.G. Screw fixation of the olecranon after fracture or osteotomy. Clin Orthop 119:197–201, 1976.
125. Wainwright, D. Fractures of the olecranon process. Br J Surg 29:403–406, 1941–1943.
126. Walker, P.S. Human Joints and Their Artificial Replacements. Springfield, IL, Charles C Thomas, 1978, pp. 182–183.
127. Watson-Jones, R. Fractures and Other Bone and Joint Injuries, Ed. 2. Baltimore, Williams and Wilkins, 1941.
128. Weseley, M.S.; Barenfeld, P.A.; Eisenstein, A.L. Closed treatment of isolated radial head fractures. J Trauma 23A:36–39, 1983.
129. Willenegger, H. Problems and results in the treatment of comminuted fractures of the elbow. Reconstr Surg Traumatol 11:118–127, 1969.
130. Wolfgang, G.; Burke, F.; Bush, D.; et al. Surgical treatment of displaced olecranon fractures by tension band wiring technique. Clin Orthop 224:192–204, 1987.
131. Worsing, R.A.; Engber, W.D.; Lange, T.A. Reactive synovitis from particulate Silastic. J Bone Joint Surg 64A:581–585, 1982.
132. Zuelzer, W.A. Fixation of small but important bone fragments with a hook plate. J Bone Joint Surg 33A:430–436, 1951.

Fractures of the Distal Humerus

133. Ackerman, G.; Jupiter, J. Nonunion of fractures of the distal end of the humerus. J Bone Joint Surg 70A:75–83, 1988.
134. Aitken, G.K.; Rorabeck, C.H. Distal humeral fractures in the adult. Clin Orthop 207:191–197, 1986.
135. Alvarez, E.; Patel, M.; Nimberg, P.; et al. Fractures of the capitellum humeri. J Bone Joint Surg 57A:1093–1096, 1975.
136. Anson, B.J.; Maddock, W.G., eds. Callander's Surgical Anatomy. Philadelphia, W.B. Saunders, 1958.
137. Boehler, L. The Treatment of Fractures, Vol. I, Ed. 5. New York, Grune and Stratton, 1956.
138. Brown, R.F.; Morgan, R.G. Intercondylar T-shaped fractures of the humerus. Results in ten cases treated by early mobilization. J Bone Joint Surg 53B:425–428, 1971.
139. Bryan, R.S. Fractures about the elbow in adults. AAOS Instr Course Lect 30:200–223, 1981.
140. Bryan, R.S.; Bickel, W.H. "T" condylar fractures of the distal humerus. J Trauma 11:830–835, 1971.
141. Cassebaum, W.H. Open reduction of T and Y fractures of the lower end of the humerus. J Trauma 9:915–925, 1969.
142. Christopher, F.; Bushnell, L. Conservative treatment of fractures of the capitellum. J Bone Joint Surg 17:489–492, 1935.
143. Collert, S. Surgical management of fractures of the capitellum humerus. Acta Orthop Scand 48:603–606, 1977.
144. Conwell, H.E.; Reynolds, F.C., eds. Key and Conwell's Management of Fractures, Dislocations, and Sprains, Ed. 7. St. Louis, C.V. Mosby, 1961.
145. Dorland's Illustrated Medical Dictionary, Ed. 24. Philadelphia, W.B. Saunders, 1965.
146. DePalma, A.F. The Management of Fractures and Dislocations, Vol. II. Philadelphia, W.B. Saunders, 1970.
147. Dusuttle, R.; Coyle, M.; Zawalsky, J.; Bloom, H. Fractures of the capitellum. J Trauma 25:317–321, 1985.
148. Eastwood, W.J. The T-shaped fracture of the lower end of the humerus. J Bone Joint Surg 19:364–369, 1937.
149. Evans, E.M. Supracondylar Y fractures of the humerus. J Bone Joint Surg 35B:381–385, 1953.
150. Gabel, G.T.; Hanson, G.; Bennett, J.B.; et al. Intraarticular fractures of the distal humerus in the adult. Clin Orthop 216:99–107, 1987.
151. Grant, J.C.B. Grant's Atlas of Anatomy, Ed. 6. Baltimore, Williams and Wilkins, 1972.
152. Grantham, S.A.; Norris, T.R.; Bush, D.C. Isolated fracture of the humeral capitellum. Clin Orthop 161:262–269, 1981.
153. Greenspan, A.; Norman, A. Radial head-capitellar view: An expanded imaging approach to elbow injuries. AJR 8:1186, 1982.
154. Guyot, J. Atlas of Human Limb Joints. Berlin, Springer-Verlag, 1981.
155. Hahn, N.F. Fall von einer besonderes varietaet der frakturen des ellenbogens. Zeitsch Wund Geburt 6:185, 1853.
156. Hamilton, F.H. A Practical Treatise on Fractures and Dislocations, Ed. 8. Philadelphia, Lea Brothers and Co., 1891.
157. Hasner, E.; Husky, J. Fractures of the epicondyle and condyle of the humerus. Acta Chir Scand 101:195, 1951.
158. Heim, V.; Pfeiffer, K.M. Small Fragment Set Manual. Berlin, Springer-Verlag, 1982.
159. Jones, K.G. Percutaneous fixation of fractures of the lower end of the humerus. Clin Orthop 50:53–69, 1967.
160. Jupiter, J.B.; Neff, U.; Holzach, P.; Allgoewer, M. Intercondylar fracture of the humerus. J Bone Joint Surg 67A:226–239, 1985.
161. Keon-Cohen, B.T. Fractures at the elbow. J Bone Joint Surg 48A:1623–1639, 1966.
162. Knight, R.A. Fractures of the humeral condyle in adults. South Med J 48:1165–1173, 1955.
163. Lansinger, O.; More, K. Fractures of the capitellum humeri. Acta Orthop Scand 52:39–44, 1981.
164. London, J.T. Kinematics of the elbow. J Bone Joint Surg 63A:529–536, 1981.
165. MacAusland, W.R.; Wyman, E.T. Fractures of the adult elbow. AAOS Instr Course Lect 24:165–181, 1975.
166. Mazel, M.S. Fracture of the capitellum. J Bone Joint Surg 17:483–488, 1935.
167. McLaughlin, H.L. Some fractures with a time limit. Surg Clin North Am 35:555, 1955.
168. McVay, C.B. Surgical Anatomy, Vol. II, Ed. 5. Philadelphia, W.B. Saunders, 1971.
169. Mehne, D.K.; Matta, J. Bicolumn fractures of the adult humerus. Presented at the 53rd Annual Meeting of the American Academy of Orthopaedic Surgeons, New Orleans, LA, 1986.
170. Milch, H. Fractures and fracture-dislocations of the humeral condyles. J Trauma 4:592–607, 1964.
171. Milch, H. Fracture Surgery. A Textbook of Common Fractures. New York, Hoeber, 1959.
172. Miller, O.L. Blind nailing of the T fracture of the lower end of the humerus which involves the joint. J Bone Joint Surg 21:933–938, 1939.

173. Miller, W.E. Comminuted fractures of the distal end of the humerus. J Bone Joint Surg 46A:644–656, 1964.

174. Bryan, R.S.; Morrey, B.F. Fractures of the distal humerus. In: Morrey, B.F., ed. The Elbow and Its Disorders. Philadelphia, W.B. Saunders, 1985, pp. 302–339.

175. Morrey, B.F.; An, K. Functional anatomy of the ligaments of the elbow. Clin Orthop 201:84–89, 1985.

176. Niemann, M. Condyle fracture of the distal adult humerus. South Med J 70:915, 1977.

177. Reich, R.S. Treatment of intercondylar fractures of the elbow by means of traction. J Bone Joint Surg 18:997–1004, 1936.

178. Rhodin, R. Treatment of fractures of the capitellum. Acta Chir Scand 86:475, 1942.

179. Riseborough, E.J.; Radin, E.L. Intercondylar T fractures of the humerus in the adult. A comparison of operative and nonoperative treatment in twenty-nine cases. J Bone Joint Surg 51A:130–141, 1969.

180. DeLee, J.C.; Green, D.P.; Wilkins, K.E. Fractures and dislocations of the elbow. In: Rockwood, C.A. Jr.; Green, D.P., eds. Fractures, Ed. 2 Philadelphia, J.B. Lippincott, 1984.

181. Simpson, L.A.; Richards, R.R. Internal fixation of a capitellar fracture using Herbert screws. Clin Orthop 209:166–169, 1986.

182. Siris, I.E. Supracondylar fractures of the humerus. Surg Gynecol Obstet 68:201–222, 1939.

183. Smith, F.M. Surgery of the Elbow, Ed. 2. Philadelphia, W.B. Saunders, 1972.

183a. Steinthal, D. Die isolirte Fraktur der eminentia Capetala in Ellenbogengelenk. Zentralb Chir 15:17, 1898.

184. Sultanpur, A. Anterior supracondylar fracture of the humerus (flexion type): A simple technique for closed reduction and fixation in adults and the aged. J Bone Joint Surg 60B:383–386, 1978.

185. Speed, J.S. Surgical treatment of condylar fractures of the humerus. AAOS Instr Course Lect 7:187–194, 1950.

186. Suman, R.K.; Miller, J.H. Intercondylar fractures of the distal humerus. J R Coll Surg Edinb 27:276–281, 1982.

187. VanGorder, G. Surgical approach in supracondylar "T" fractures of the humerus requiring open reduction. J Bone Joint Surg 22:278–292, 1940.

188. Watson-Jones, R. Fractures and Joint Injuries, Vol. II, Ed. 4. Baltimore, Williams and Wilkins, 1955.

189. Whitesides, T.E., Jr.; Hanley, T.C.; Morimoto, K.; Harada, H. Tissue pressure measurements as a determinant for the need of fasciotomy. Clin Orthop 113:443, 1975.

190. Wickstrom, J.; Meyer, P.R. Fractures of the distal humerus in adults. Clin Orthop 50:43–51, 1967.

191. Warwick, R.; Williams, P.C., eds.: Gray's Anatomy, Ed. 36. Philadelphia, W.B. Saunders, 1980.

192. Zagorski, J.B.; Jennings, J.J.; Burkhalter, W.E. et al. Comminuted intraarticular fractures of the distal humeral condyles: Surgical vs. non-surgical treatment. Clin Orthop 202:197–204, 1986.

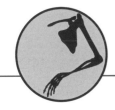

E. Frazier Ward, M.D.
Felix H. Savoie, M.D.
James L. Hughes, M.D.

38

Fractures of the Diaphyseal Humerus

*F*ractures of the humeral diaphysis account for approximately 3% of all fractures.[2,21,25,28,32,36] A variety of options are available in the management of these injuries.* Although satisfactory results have been reported for both operative and nonoperative methods of management, the character of the fracture and the needs of the patient will usually mandate a particular treatment option. In order to appreciate the diverse management requirements of these fractures, a knowledge of basic anatomy and function is essential.*

Anatomy

The shaft of the humerus extends from the upper border of the insertion of the pectoralis major to the supracondylar ridge distally. The cylindrical proximal humerus assumes a more triangular shape in its distal one third. Three borders divide the humeral shaft into three surfaces (Fig. 38–1): the anterior border, extending from the greater tuberosity proximally to the coronoid fossa; the medial border, extending from the lesser tuberosity to the medial supracondylar ridge; and the lateral border, extending from the posterior aspect of the greater tuberosity to the lateral supracondylar ridge. The anterolateral surface presents the deltoid tuberosity and the sulcus for the radial nerve and profunda brachii artery. The anteromedial surface forms the floor of the intertubercular groove. The anterolateral and anteromedial surfaces blend distally, at which point they provide the origin for the brachialis muscle.

The posterior surface contains the spiral groove for the radial nerve and the origin of the medial and lateral heads of the triceps (Fig. 38–1).[20,45,55,57,72]

The medial and lateral intermuscular septa divide the arm into anterior and posterior compartments. The biceps brachii, coracobrachialis, brachialis, and anconeus muscles, the brachial artery and vein, and the median, musculocutaneous, and ulnar nerves are contained in the anterior compartment. The triceps brachii and the radial nerve constitute the posterior compartment (Fig. 38–2).

The blood supply to the humeral diaphysis arises from branches of the brachial artery. One or more nutrient vessels may emanate from this artery, the profunda brachii artery, or the posterior humeral circumflex artery, to course distally and provide the intramedullary circulation. The periosteal circulation likewise depends on these vessels, multiple small muscular branches, and the arterial anastomosis about the elbow. Care must be taken to avoid disruption both of the intramedullary and of the periosteal circulation during operative fracture management.[20,45,55,57,72]

General Considerations

An analysis of fractures of the humeral diaphysis reveals the effect of the muscular forces acting on the shaft at varying levels (Fig. 38–3). In fractures occurring above the insertion of the pectoralis major, the proximal fragment is displaced into abduction and external rotation owing to the action of the rotator cuff musculature (Fig. 38–3*A*). Fractures occurring in the interval between the insertion of the pectoralis major

---

* References 1–19, 21–33, 36, 38–46, 51–54, 56, 58–63, 65–71, 72, 74, 76–79, 81–85, 87, 88, 91, 92, 95–102, 104–109.

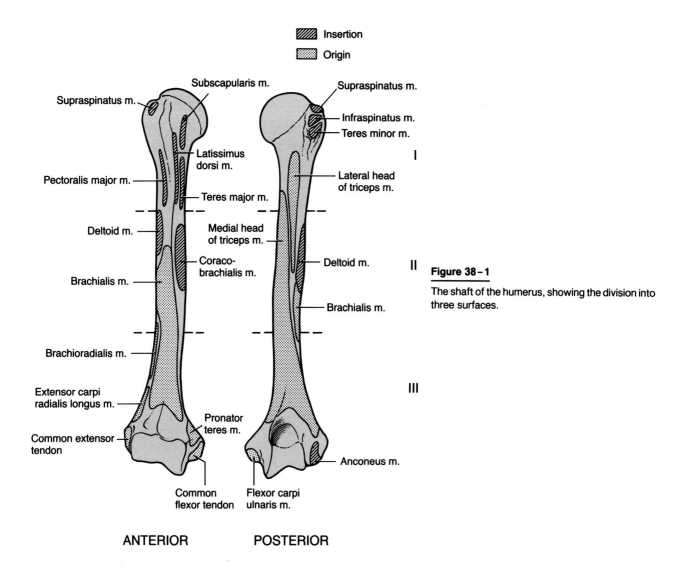

Insertion
Origin

Supraspinatus m.
Subscapularis m.
Supraspinatus m.
Infraspinatus m.
Teres minor m.
Latissimus dorsi m.
Pectoralis major m.
Lateral head of triceps m.
Teres major m.
Deltoid m.
Medial head of triceps m.
Coraco-brachialis m.
Deltoid m.
Brachialis m.
Brachialis m.
Brachioradialis m.
Extensor carpi radialis longus m.
Common extensor tendon
Pronator teres m.
Anconeus m.
Common flexor tendon
Flexor carpi ulnaris m.

I

II

III

ANTERIOR   POSTERIOR

Figure 38–1

The shaft of the humerus, showing the division into three surfaces.

proximally and the deltoid insertion distally result in adduction of the proximal fragment and proximal and lateral displacement of the distal fragment (Fig. 38–3B). Fractures distal to the insertion of the deltoid muscle result in abduction of the upper fragment and proximal displacement of the distal fragment by unopposed muscle contraction (Fig. 38–3C).[36]

The energy absorbed by the humerus during the fracture is an important determinant of the amount of displacement. Low-energy fractures may be held in position by the internal splinting effect of the intermuscular septa. The weight of the arm aids in preserving alignment and length in these low-velocity injuries. High-energy fractures result in comminution of the bone and disruption of the soft tissues, with loss of this internal splinting effect.

A consideration other than the location of the fracture and the amount of energy absorbed and/or dissipated in the injury is the mobility of the shoulder and the elbow joints, which tend to minimize the effect of posttraumatic angulation and rotational deformities. Klenerman has shown experimentally that the musculature around the humerus will accommodate 20° of anterior angulation and 30° of varus angulation without compromising function or appearance.[67] The normal mobility in the shoulder and elbow joints will compensate for this degree of deformity.

Classification

A classification system for humeral shaft fractures should include the following factors influencing the selection of the management program (Table 38–1): the anatomic location of the fracture, its "personality" or character, the condition of the surrounding soft tissues, and disease intrinsic to the bone itself that may affect the eventual outcome. The management plans of

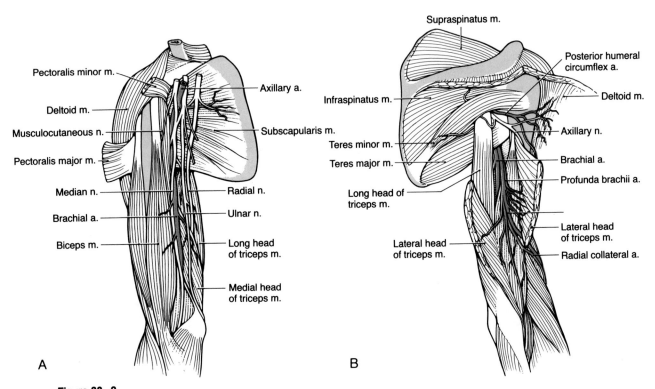

Figure 38-2

The muscular and neurovascular structures of the upper arm are divided into anterior (*A*) and posterior (*B*) compartments.

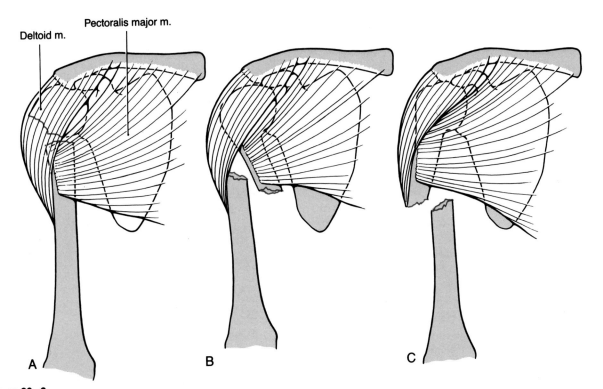

Figure 38-3

The muscular attachments to the shaft of the humerus cause different degrees of displacement, depending on the level of the fracture: *A*, The proximal fragment is abducted and externally rotated by the rotator cuff musculature in fractures occurring above the insertion of the pectoralis major. *B*, The deltoid muscle displaces the distal fragment proximally and laterally in fractures occurring proximally, between its insertion and that of the pectoralis major. *C*, Fractures distal to the insertion of the deltoid muscle result in abduction of the proximal fragment.

Table 38-1.

Classification of Humeral Shaft Fractures

Anatomic Location
  Above the pectoralis major insertion
  Below the pectoralis major insertion, above the deltoid insertion
  Below the deltoid insertion

Fracture Personality (Direction and Character of the Fracture
  Transverse
  Oblique
  Spiral
  Segmental
  Comminuted

Associated Soft Tissue Injury (Gustilo)
  Open
    Grade 1
    Grade 2
    Grade 3
  Periarticular injury
    Glenohumeral
    Elbow joint
  Nerve injury
    Radial nerve
    Median nerve
    Ulnar nerve
  Vascular injury
    Brachial artery
    Brachial vein

Intrinsic Conditions of the Bone
  Normal
  Pathologic
    Metabolic
    Metastatic
    Infectious
  Incomplete fractures

Epps and of Bone have been combined and modified to provide a useful system.[9,36]

In addition to anatomic location, the personality of the fracture is important in the selection of the treatment modality. Transverse fractures that are not internally splinted by the intramuscular septa may be difficult to control, while oblique fractures usually unite without difficulty. Spiral fractures in the distal one third (Holstein-Lewis fracture) may produce a radial nerve injury.[56] Segmental injuries are also difficult to control and delayed union of one or both fracture sites is common. Comminuted fractures, which often involve soft tissue injury, are difficult to manage by internal fixation but unite well with nonoperative fracture management.

Associated soft tissue injuries may dictate the mode of treatment.[49,50] Gustilo grade I (low energy, less than 1 cm wound) and grade II (moderate energy and soft tissue damage, wound greater than 1 cm) open fractures respond well to stable internal fixation and soft tissue care, while grade III (high energy, wound greater than 10 cm) injuries may require external fixation.[9,13,48,49,50,63] Open injuries with associated nerve or vascular damage may require stabilization to protect the repair of these structures.[27,80,90,93,94]

Conditions intrinsic to the bone itself may make certain options untenable, as in the case of a severely osteoporotic individual who is best managed by fracture bracing or intramedullary stabilization rather than plate osteosynthesis.[106]

Diagnosis

HISTORY AND PHYSICAL EXAMINATION

In most cases the patient sustaining a humeral shaft fracture will recall the specific traumatic event that produced the fracture. Falls on the arm, twisting injuries, industrial accidents, penetrating injuries, and motor vehicle accidents are the most common causes of these injuries. The individual will present with all the cardinal signs of a fracture: pain, swelling, deformity, and crepitation. Shortening of the upper arm and mobility of the fracture site may also be observed.

After a general baseline physical examination, attention is focused on the injured upper extremity. The neurovascular status of the entire limb should be evaluated at multiple levels. The soft tissue compartments of the arm and forearm should be examined, and the possibility of a compartment syndrome considered. The proximal and distal articulations should also be carefully evaluated. Abrasions, lacerations, or puncture wounds may indicate an open injury, necessitating emergent management.

RADIOGRAPHIC EXAMINATION

The standard radiographic evaluation of the humerus should include two views taken at 90° to one another. The shoulder and elbow joints should both be included on each view. These films should be obtained by moving the patient, rather than simply rotating the injured extremity at the fracture site.

In pathologic lesions, staging studies (e.g., technetium bone scan, computerized tomography, and magnetic resonance imaging) may be necessary to delineate the extent of the disease before treatment can be instituted.

Management

The numerous methods available for the management of humeral shaft fractures allow a wide latitude in the selection of a specific technique.* Historically, closed treatment has been associated with a certain rate of delayed union and nonunion.[36] However, recent advances in fracture bracing have alleviated many of these problems and have made this method the treatment of choice for the nonoperatively managed fracture of the humeral diaphysis.[4,79,97] Similar advances in fracture stabilization over the last two decades have made operative fracture management a viable alternative in these patients, with rapid recovery of normal function.[66,83,84,107,108]

As mentioned, Klenerman has shown that 20° of anterior angulation and 30° of varus angulation are well tolerated by the musculature around the humerus. The humerus can tolerate up to 3 cm of shortening as a result of overriding fracture fragments with little functional deficit.[67] However, greater deformity indicates a need for open reduction and operative stabilization. The algorithm presented in Figure 38–4 represents our approach to these injuries. In all cases, fracture management is combined with early motion and rehabilitation of the injured extremity to limit the problems associated with fracture disease.

CLOSED TREATMENT MODALITIES

Most humeral shaft fractures can be managed nonoperatively, with an expected union rate of 90 to 100%. Close supervision and frequent review are necessary to obtain a satisfactory result. The pattern of the fracture, mechanism of injury and amount of energy involved, associated swelling and soft tissue injuries, body habitus, functional level, and compliance of the patient should all be considered in the selection of a management option. Although many different alternatives are available, functional fracture bracing has replaced all other modalities as the treatment of choice for these injuries. Initial management is directed toward reduction and immobilization of the fracture. In most cases a coaptation splint or hanging arm cast is used until the immediate postfracture pain has subsided, usually in three to seven days. A functional fracture brace is then applied. Union rates of 90 to 100% have been reported with this device. Other methods of nonoperative management include the Velpeau dressing, sling and swathe, abduction splint, shoulder spica cast, and skeletal traction.

* References 1–19, 21–33, 36, 38–46, 48, 51–54, 56, 58–63, 65–71, 72, 74, 76–79, 81–85, 87, 88, 91, 92, 95–102, 104–109.

Hanging Arm Casts

The hanging arm cast technique, introduced by Caldwell in 1933, remains a standard management technique for humeral shaft fractures.[16,17,59,72,92] It is most often used to obtain reduction in shortened oblique, spiral, and transverse fractures. Once reduction is adequate, an alternative method of treatment may be utilized or the hanging arm cast continued. If continuation of the hanging arm cast is elected, the fracture must be closely monitored for distraction and nonunion.

Specific principles should be followed when utilizing the hanging arm cast technique. A lightweight cast, extending from 2 cm proximal to the fracture across the elbow joint to the wrist with the elbow at 90° and the forearm in neutral rotation, is placed by standard techniques. The cast must be secured at the wrist by wire or plaster loops.[16,17,36,59,72,92] The anterior/posterior and varus/valgus alignment at the fracture site is controlled by the attachment of the suspension strap to these loops (Fig. 38–5). The patient should be instructed to remain in an erect or semierect posture at all times so that the arm is always in a dependent position. Frequent reevaluation is necessary. Weekly radiographic examination is essential during the initial three to four weeks of treatment. Active assisted shoulder and hand exercises should be instituted as pain permits, and these maneuvers should be combined with isometric exercises for the remainder of the arm.

Limitations in the use of the hanging arm cast to manage a diaphyseal fracture of the humerus include resultant shortening, angulation and rotational deformities, and delayed union and nonunion. These complications are more common in obese and noncompliant patients. However, most authors have reported a union rate of 93 to 96% with this technique.[16,17,59,66,72,92] Adherence to proper techniques by the physician, proper patient selection, and patient cooperation are necessary to obtain these success rates.

Currently, a hanging arm cast may be used initially to obtain reduction of the fracture and a fracture brace substituted once satisfactory alignment has been achieved, but this is not necessary when there is an acceptable initial reduction. These patients are better managed by immediate fracture bracing or by immobilization with a coaptation splint until the acute fracture pain has subsided and a functional brace can be applied.

Velpeau Dressing

Gilchrist has described an inexpensive, easily applied device for immobilization of the shoulder and humerus (Fig. 38–6B).[44] A similar but more restrictive device is

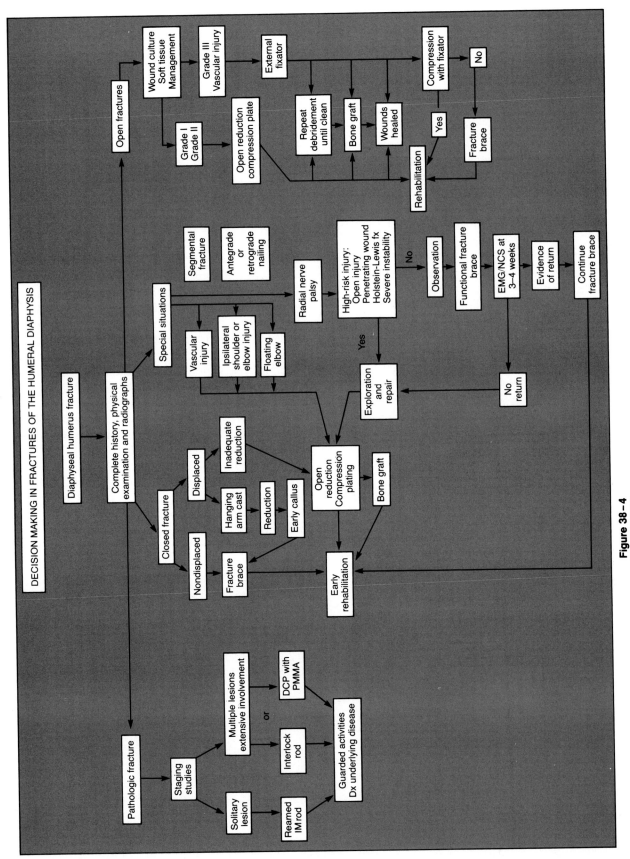

Figure 38–4

Algorithm for management of humeral shaft fractures.

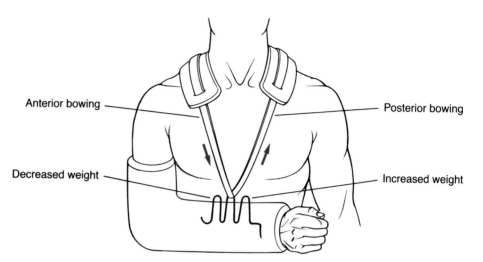

Figure 38-5

The hanging arm cast is used both to obtain reduction of the fracture and to allow union in this reduced position.

the sling and swathe dressing (Fig. 38–6A), which is most useful in nondisplaced or minimally displaced fractures in children under eight years of age or in elderly patients who are unable to tolerate other methods of management. Pads composed of various materials can be placed in the axilla to control the angulation of the fracture site. Although a Velpeau dressing is seldom utilized except in situations as described above, a functional fracture brace should be substituted as soon as possible without compromising the patient.

Coaptation Splint

The sugar tong or U splint, supplemented by collar and cuff, has been utilized in acute humeral shaft fractures (Fig. 38–7).[8,23,32] The plaster extends from the axilla around the elbow and over the deltoid. Stockinette, held in place by benzoin and supplemented by pad-

ding, is applied to the arm prior to the application of the plaster of Paris splints.

This technique has the advantage of allowing motion of the hand, wrist, and (to a limited extent) elbow. Disadvantages include axillary irritation, shortening of the fracture, angular union and displacement, patient discomfort, and the bulkiness of the immobilization device.

Indications for the use of a coaptation splint include the initial management of a nondisplaced or minimally displaced fracture and inability to tolerate a hanging arm cast. A functional fracture brace is substituted as soon as possible.

Abduction Splint — Shoulder Spica Cast

Although used infrequently, a plaster or orthoplast splint supporting the arm in abduction has been advo-

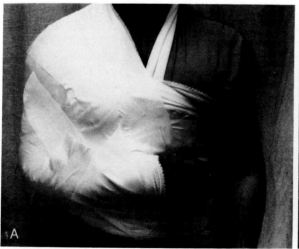

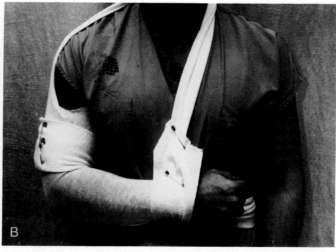

Figure 38-6

A Velpeau dressing (A) and a Jacksonville sling (B) are most often used in patients who are unable to tolerate a hanging arm cast.

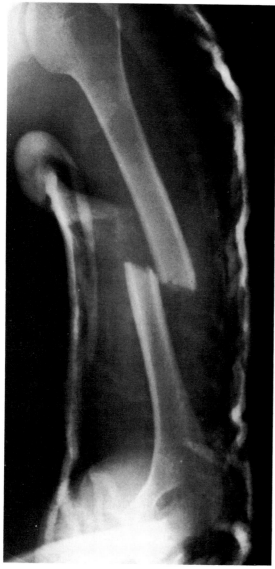

Figure 38-7

The coaptation splint, applied using U-shaped plaster from the axilla around the upper arm to the shoulder, is useful for acute fractures.

cated for certain humeral shaft fractures (Fig. 38-8).[54,102] Disadvantages that limit the effectiveness of these devices include the unusual and awkward position of the arm, immobilization of the shoulder, and the pressure on the rotator cuff.

Skeletal Traction

Skeletal traction may be applied via a transolecranon Kirschner wire or a wing nut. Provisional stabilization of a comminuted fracture may be attained with skeletal traction in certain instances in which other modalities are contraindicated, but it is rarely necessary. If utilized, care should be taken to protect the ulnar nerve during insertion of the traction device by utilizing blunt dissection to the cortical bone and pin insertion from the medial side.[36]

Functional Bracing

Sarmiento pioneered the concept of functional bracing of humeral fractures in 1977.[97] An orthoplast or polypropylene sleeve utilizes the hydraulic forces within the arm combined with the force of gravity acting through an extended elbow to maintain fracture alignment while allowing mobilization of the entire upper extremity. Although initially designed as a wraparound sleeve, current braces utilize an anterior shell with a contour for the biceps tendon and a posterior shell with a triceps contour to ensure adequate compression and support for the fracture. One of the shells is designed to fit inside the other, and Velcro straps hold the brace in proper position. These modifications have minimized the angular deformities that occurred in the initial series. Current devices may be custom-made or prefabricated (Fig. 38-9).

This technique represents an advance in nonoperative fracture management and should be considered the treatment of choice in all nonoperatively managed diaphyseal humerus fractures. The fractures are usually stabilized initially by one of the previously mentioned methods until the acute pain and swelling have subsided. The patient is then placed in the functional fracture brace and rehabilitation begun. The patient should be instructed to remain erect as much as possible and to use the injured extremity as tolerated. Motion of the shoulder and elbow joints are encouraged. Abduction is limited to 60 to 70° until evidence of fracture healing is present. Although a sling may be used in conjunction with the fracture brace, it leads to varus and internal rotation deformity and should be discontinued as soon as patient comfort allows. The brace is worn for a minimum of eight weeks postfracture. It can be removed once the patient has regained a minimum of 90° of pain-free abduction. Union rates of 96 to 100% have been reported with these devices.[4,79,97]

Complications include angular deformities and skin maceration. Obesity, especially in female patients with large, pendulous breasts, may increase angular deformity. However, this same obesity will often minimize the cosmetic defect associated with the angulation. Normal daily hygiene will prevent skin maceration.

Although an extension over the shoulder is available, it is seldom necessary. This extension restricts motion of the shoulder girdle while providing little additional support. It is most often used in comminuted fractures and in those involving the proximal one third of the humerus. However, these injury patterns are difficult

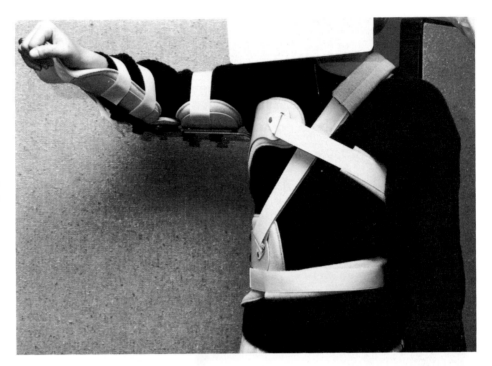

Figure 38-8

The abduction splint, or shoulder spica cast, has been advocated for certain humeral shaft fractures.

to manage by this technique, and alternative treatment methods should be considered.

External Fixation

External fixation has been utilized effectively in certain humeral fractures (Fig. 38-10). The major indications

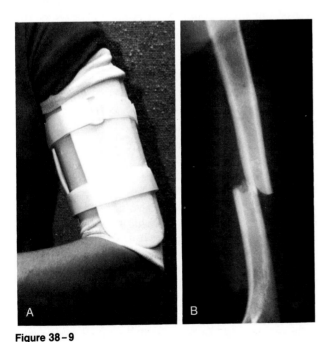

Figure 38-9

The humeral fracture brace (A), uses hydraulic forces to maintain fracture alignment, while allowing mobilization of the entire upper extremity.

for external fixation include open fracture with extensive soft tissue and bone defects; extensively comminuted fractures in patients requiring mobilization; burn patients in whom easy repetitive access to the affected areas of the skin is required; and possibly patients with ipsilateral fractures of the humerus, radius, and ulna (the floating elbow).[13,47,62]

Both Brooker and Green have outlined placement techniques for external fixation of humeral shaft fractures (Fig. 38-11).[13,47] Two pins are placed above and below the fracture with radiographic control of the alignment. Each pin should be inserted under direct visualization to prevent soft tissue injuries. Recently, the advent of radiolucent carbon fiber rods has allowed the fracture to be evaluated properly with a fixator in place. Any malalignment can be corrected by adjustment of the fixator under radiographic control. A major complication during fracture manipulation and placement of the fixator is neurovascular injury. In order to avoid this, external fixator pins must be inserted under direct visualization in the middle third and especially the distal third of the humerus. Kamhin and associates reported radial nerve injuries during manipulation of the fracture.[63] If this occurs, immediate exploration is indicated. Other problems encountered in the use of external fixation include pin tract infection, muscle and tendon impalement, and nonunion of the fracture.[47] These sequelae can be avoided by meticulous pin care by the patient, adherence to proper technique, and adjustment of the fixator to provide compression when indicated.

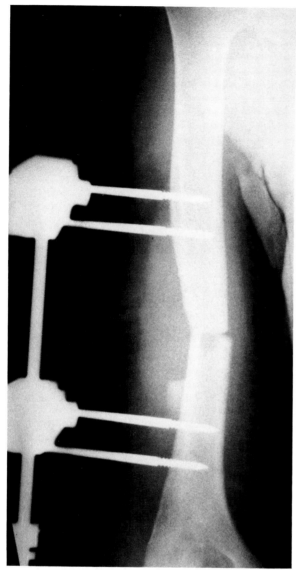

Figure 38-10

The external fixator can be used effectively to maintain reduction of humeral shaft fractures while allowing adequate management of soft tissue injuries.

The major advantage of external fixation is that of allowing management of associated soft tissue injuries. When these problems have been remedied, the fixator should be removed and a functional brace substituted.

OPERATIVE MANAGEMENT OF HUMERAL SHAFT FRACTURES

Traditionally surgeons have been taught to manage humeral shaft fractures nonoperatively owing to the high union rate and infrequent complications.[36] However, operative osteosynthesis may be preferable in certain situations. Failure of closed reduction, associated articular injuries, vascular or nerve injuries, associated ipsilateral forearm fractures, segmental fractures, and pathologic fractures are indications for operative stabilization of humeral shaft fractures (Table 38-2). The polytrauma patient with multiple extremity or multisystem injuries should also be considered for acute operative stabilization of a diaphyseal humerus fracture. A relative indication may be the transverse or short oblique fracture in an active individual, as these are more prone to delayed union.[98] Operative stabilization may be accomplished by the placement of an intramedullary rod or by the use of plates and screws.

Surgical Approach to the Humerus

There are three basic approaches to the shaft of the humerus.[20,55,57] Of these, the anterolateral and posterior approaches are most often used for operative stabilization of fractures of the humerus.[57] The anteromedial approach is seldom used owing to the potential for significant neurovascular injury.

Anterolateral Approach. The anterolateral approach is most often utilized for fractures of the proximal and middle thirds of the humeral shaft (Fig. 38-12). The patient is placed supine with a light padding under the shoulder to support the scapula. The forearm is placed in a supinated position while the shoulder is abducted 60°. The skin incision may begin as proximal as 5 cm distal to the coracoid process, passing along the anterior border of the deltoid muscle and the lateral bicipital sulcus. The incision may be continued in line with the lateral border of the biceps to within 7.5 cm of the elbow joint. The superficial and deep fascia are divided, with care being taken to protect the cephalic vein. The humerus is approached between the deltoid and pectoralis major muscles proximally, and through the brachialis muscle more distally. The innervation of the brachialis muscle is preserved during this approach, as its lateral portion is supplied by the radial nerve and the medial portion by the musculocutaneous nerve. Distal retraction of the brachialis muscle is facilitated by flexion of the elbow joint. The radial nerve as it winds around the humeral shaft is protected by the lateral half of the brachialis muscle. In its most distal extent, the approach continues between the biceps brachii medially and the brachioradialis laterally. Plate osteosynthesis of the humeral shaft through this approach is facilitated by partial detachment of the deltoid insertion and subperiosteal dissection of the origin of the brachialis. The hazards of this approach are the proximity of the radial nerve laterally and the lateral antebrachial cutaneous nerve medially.[57]

Posterior Approach. The posterior approach splits the triceps to expose the posterior humeral shaft in its

Figure 38–11

Technique for placement of the external fixator: two 1-cm incisions are made in the skin approximately 7 cm proximal and 7 cm distal to the fracture site. Utilizing blunt dissection, the underlying soft tissues are spread until the bony aspect of the humerus is uncovered. The soft tissue guide is then placed to protect these tissues. Both cortices of the humeral shaft are drilled and two transfixing pins are inserted, one proximal and one distal to the fracture site. The fracture is then reduced, either under direct vision or with fluoroscopic control. A single connecting rod is then placed in universal clamps attached to the two pins. Utilizing the same technique, two more transfixing pins are inserted, one proximal and one distal to the fracture site, to complete the stabilization procedure. The connecting rod is then attached to all four pins approximately 1 to 2 inches from the skin edge. A second connecting rod can be used to secure rigidity of the frame. Radiographic confirmation of pin placement and fracture reduction is then obtained. The possible areas of pin placement for stabilization are illustrated.

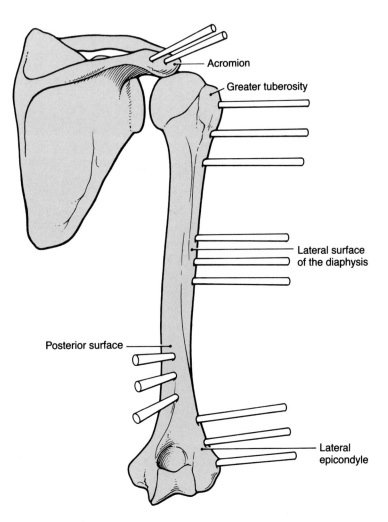

middle two thirds (Fig. 38–13). This approach is indicated in those procedures in which the humeral shaft fracture involves the middle or distal thirds, or when revision or repair of radial nerve injury is necessary.

The patient is placed in the prone or lateral position with the arm abducted 90° over an elbow rest. The

Table 38–2.

Operative Indications For Humeral Shaft Fractures

Failure to maintain or control reduction by closed technique
Concomitant articular fractures
Neurovascular injuries
Associated ipsilateral forearm fractures
Segmental fractures
Impending potential fractures in pathologic bone
Polytrauma with multiple extremity fractures
Transverse or short oblique fracture in an active individual

elbow and shoulder joints are draped free in the operative field. The skin is incised along the posterior surface of the arm, following a line joining the posterior edge of the acromion with the olecranon. This incision begins at the free border of the deltoid and ends 4 cm proximal to the tip of the olecranon. During deep dissection the posterior border of the deltoid is identified and the fascia divided. The lateral brachial cutaneous nerve should be preserved. Blunt dissection develops the interval between the long and lateral heads of the triceps, and the radial nerve and profunda brachii vessels are noted and protected. Sharp dissection is necessary to extend the incision distally to the olecranon. The medial head of the triceps is then divided and the humeral shaft exposed proximally and distally. Proximal dissection is limited by the axillary nerve and posterior humeral circumflex vessels. One disadvantage to this approach is that the radial nerve and profunda brachii vessels are directly involved in the incision. If future surgery is contemplated, extreme care must be taken to identify and protect these structures during this approach to prevent their injury.[57]

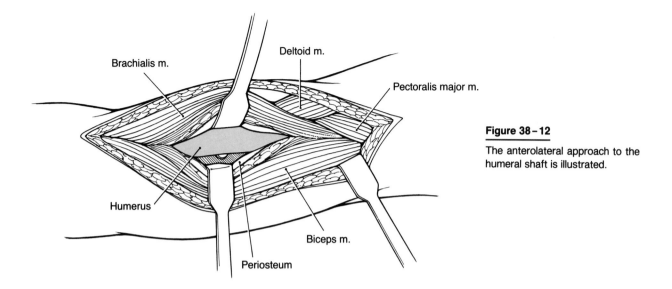

Figure 38-12

The anterolateral approach to the humeral shaft is illustrated.

Anteromedial Approach. The anteromedial surface of the humeral shaft can be approached posterior to the intermuscular septum along a line extending proximally from the medial epicondyle (Fig. 38-14). The ulnar nerve must be freed from the triceps muscle and retracted medially. The triceps is then separated from the posterior surface of the medial intermuscular septum and adjacent humeral shaft. The median nerve and brachial artery are at risk during the exposure. This approach is seldom used in fracture stabilization.

Figure 38-13

The posterior approach to the humeral shaft is demonstrated.

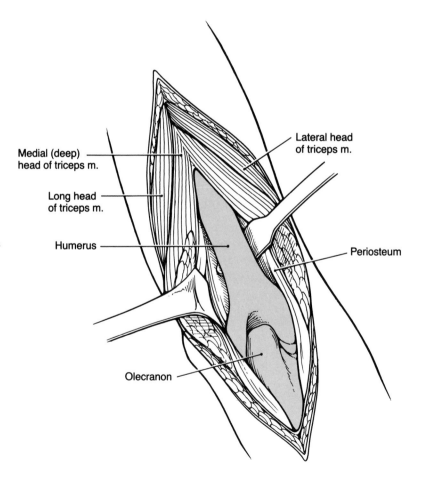

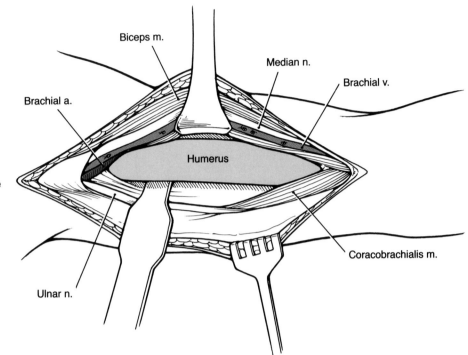

Figure 38–14

The anteromedial approach to the humeral shaft is illustrated.

Technique of Plate Osteosynthesis

Preoperative evaluation of the fracture should dictate the proper approach and method of fixation. The fracture is exposed, evaluated, debrided of hematoma, and anatomically reduced. If there are multiple fragments, the humerus is reconstructed in stepwise fashion by reducing one piece to another until the shaft is reconstructed. Provisional stabilization via reduction clamps or Kirschner wires may facilitate this process. Whenever possible, lag screw fixation should be included as part of the overall fracture plan. If during the preoperative evaluation, it was determined that lag screw fixation outside of the plate was indicated, it is inserted at this time by standard AO technique. A broad 4.5-mm dynamic compression plate contoured to adequately fit the shaft is then applied. In a transverse fracture, the plate is applied in compressive mode. In all other fractures, it is applied to neutralize the rotational and bending forces around the fracture and thereby protect the lag screw fixation. In all operative stabilizations of the humeral shaft, it is essential that a minimum of six, and preferably eight cortices (minimum three to four screws), be obtained both above and below the fracture site for adequate fixation (Fig. 38–15A,B). Radiographic confirmation of the reduction should be obtained both in the provisional stabilization phase and prior to skin closure.[9,52,77,83–85,106]

Specific problems associated with plate osteosynthesis include infection, radial nerve palsy, and failure

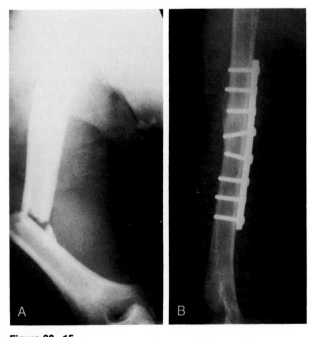

Figure 38–15

A, The humeral shaft fracture has been inadequately reduced. B, Open reduction and internal fixation with a dynamic compression plate was accomplished.

of fixation. Adequate preoperative planning to reduce operative time, prophylactic antibiotics, and meticulous soft tissue techniques will reduce the incidence of infection. Adequate exposure and gentle handling of the soft tissues will decrease the risk of radial nerve palsy.[44,82,106]

Failure of fixation may be a result of poor technique or of patient disease. As mentioned, a minimum of six to eight cortices should be obtained both proximal and distal to the fracture site in each case. The use of dual plates results in excessive destruction of soft tissues and stress shielding of the bone and is not recommended. Cancellous bone graft should be used to reconstitute all bony defects. A functional fracture brace may be used to protect the fixation in patients with poor bone quality. Each of these factors should be considered preoperatively in determining whether or not fixation is indicated, and specific solutions devised for each problem prior to undertaking surgical intervention.

Intramedullary Nailing

Intramedullary fixation of the humeral shaft is gaining in popularity, due in part to the successful management of fractures of the femur and tibia by this method. Indications for closed intramedullary nailing of the humerus include the inability to achieve satisfactory alignment of a diaphyseal fracture by closed techniques, fractures in the midportion of the humerus, segmental fractures, delayed nonunion, osteopenic bone, pathologic or impending pathologic fractures, displaced midshaft transverse, short oblique, or spiral fractures, and any diaphyseal humerus fracture in a polytraumatized patient. Contraindications to closed intramedullary nailing include humeral fractures associated with neurologic deficit, open Gustilo grade 3 fractures, and established atrophic nonunions. In these patients, an open intramedullary nailing technique should be utilized if this treatment option is selected.

Two types of nails may be used for intramedullary nailing. The basic straight Küntscher cloverleaf nail may be inserted either antegrade or retrograde into the humerus. The tibial nail, with its angulated proximal end, provides better rotational control and is most often used in antegrade nailing. The retrograde approach with the tibial nail is technically more demanding. Each of these nails may be easily drilled to create an interlocking nail, or a commercially available interlocking tibial nail may be used when this type of fixation is required. The present interlocking tibial nail insertion handles allow rapid interlocking in the proximal humerus. A distal interlocking screw is inserted under image intensification control.

Technique

Proximal Approach. This approach is used for middle and distal third fractures (Fig. 38–16). The patient is placed in a lawn chair or similar reclining support with the arm draped free in the sterile field. A 4-cm incision is made lateral to the acromion, and the greater tuberosity is exposed. The supraspinatus tendon is incised in line with its fibers, and the arm is adducted and flexed across the chest. The standard intramedullary awl is introduced through the greater tuberosity under fluoroscopic control. The ball tip guide wire is then passed across the fracture site to the distal fragment. The position of the guide wire in both the proximal and distal fragments is checked in two planes by fluoroscopy. Once adequate positioning is obtained, sequential reaming is accomplished until a satisfactory purchase is obtained above and below the fracture site. The guide wire is exchanged for the driving guide wire and the intramedullary nail is inserted (Fig. 38–17A, B). If purchase cannot be obtained or rotational control is poor, interlocking fixation can be utilized. In pathologic bone, polymethyl methacrylate can improve fixation but should be utilized only when interlocking fixation is not possible.

The interlocked screws are placed through the rod under image intensification control. A 3.2-mm drill bit is inserted across the bone, through the interlocking hole in the nail. The depth of the screw hole is measured, tapped using a 4.5-mm tap, and the appropriate length screw inserted.[9,22,68-71,106-109]

Distal Approach (Fig. 38–18). Fractures involving the diaphysis and proximal one third of the humerus are best managed by retrograde intramedullary nailing. A triceps splitting incision 1 cm proximal to the olecra-

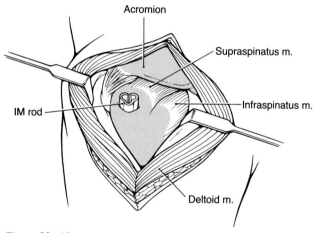

Figure 38–16

The proximal approach for intramedullary nailing of the humeral shaft fractures is demonstrated.

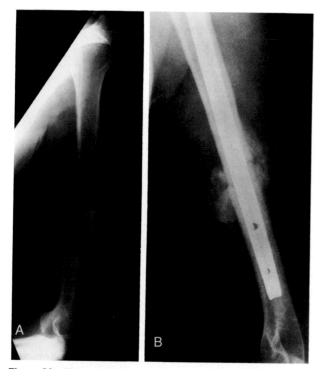

Figure 38–17

Fracture of the diaphyseal humerus in a polytrauma patient (*A*) is stabilized using a proximally inserted, reamed intramedullary rod (*B*).

non fossa but well distal to the spiral groove and radial nerve is utilized in this technique. The medullary canal is entered with a 4.5-mm drill bit through the posterior cortex of the humerus 2 cm above the olecranon fossa (Fig. 38–18*B*). This hole is enlarged with a high speed router (Fig. 38–18*C*). The entrance hole is then over-reamed in a decreasing angular fashion until the reamer can be inserted in line with the humeral shaft. This allows proper orientation for both reamer and rod insertion. A ball tip guide is passed retrograde across the fracture site into the proximal fragment and its position checked in two planes by fluoroscopy. Sequential reaming is then accomplished until satisfactory purchase is obtained. In this case, the reamer should extend across the fracture site for a distance of approximately 1 to 2 cm and not fully into the proximal fragment. Full reaming may result in loss of proximal fixation or in damage to the proximal articular surface of the humerus. The guide wire is then exchanged and the intramedullary rod passed into the shaft of the humerus, stopping 1 to 1.5 cm from the humeral head (Fig. 38–18*D*). It is essential in this technique that a 3.5-mm screw be utilized to block the rod in its distal portion in order to prevent its dislodging or backing out (Fig. 38–19*B*).[9,69–71,106,107]

If purchase is inadequate during intramedullary rod fixation, an interlock rod may be substituted utilizing the same technique.[106] The screws are then inserted under fluoroscopic control proximally and distally to provide stable fixation and rotational control (Fig. 38–20).[107]

Fractures involving the area of the radial sulcus with displacement have the potential for disruption of the radial nerve by either the reamer or the intramedullary device. In these cases, a small incision at the fracture site is recommended for identification and protection of the radial nerve prior to reaming and rod placement.

Intramedullary stabilization is an effective alternative to plate osteosynthesis in the polytraumatized patient in whom crutch walking will be necessary, and in fractures resulting from intrinsic bone abnormalities. It is the authors' opinion that closed nailing of diaphyseal humerus fractures will become a standard method of management in the near future.

The senior author has reported a series of 35 patients with diaphyseal humerus fractures managed by intramedullary Küntscher nailing.[107,108] Seventeen fractures were located in the proximal third of the humerus and eighteen in the middle third. The average time to fixation was 12 days. Fourteen of these injuries involved pathologic fractures. Thirty of these fractures were approached proximally, while five were stabilized by the distal approach. The nail lengths ranged from 22 to 26 cm and the widths from 9 to 14 mm. All distally inserted nails were supplemented by 3.5-mm blocking screws inserted at the distal incision. Thirty-four fractures in 33 patients united primarily. Two patients have persistent nonunion of the fracture site, one of which was a pathologic fracture in which a noninterlocked intramedullary nail was used.

Two patients sustained nondisplaced split supracondylar fractures during intramedullary rod insertion via a proximal approach. Each of these required open cerclage wiring and united uneventfully. No other complications were noted in this series.

Eight patients, six women and two men, managed by interlocked intramedullary fixation have also been reported by the senior author.[108] The primary indication for modified interlocked Küntscher nailing of the humerus was an established nonunion in osteopenic bone. Five of the eight fractures had failed to respond to both conservative and previous surgical management. Seven of the eight patients regained normal function of the arm after interlock stabilization.

Although currently a technically demanding procedure, the rapid return of normal function and the satisfactory results achieved by intramedullary stabilization of diaphyseal humerus fractures will make this method

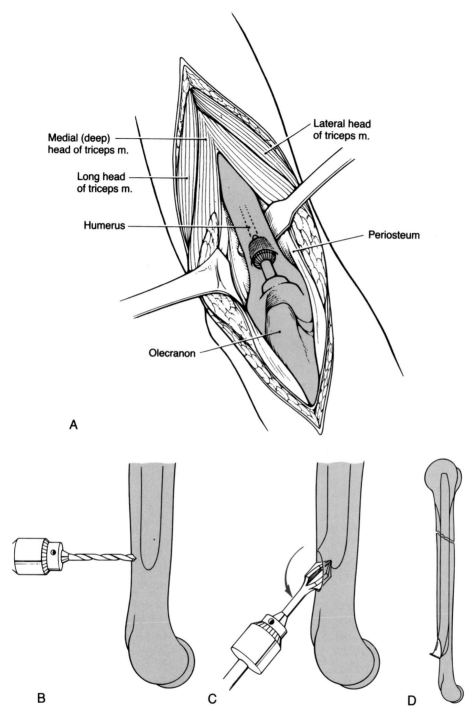

Medial (deep) head of triceps m.

Long head of triceps m.

Humerus

Olecranon

Lateral head of triceps m.

Periosteum

A

B

C

D

Figure 38–18

The distal approach and steps in retrograde intramedullary rod fixation of a fracture of the diaphyseal humerus: *A*, Surgical approach. *B*, The posterior cortex is entered 2 cm proximal to the olecranon fossa with a 4.5 mm drill bit. *C*, The 4.5-mm hole is enlarged in an oblique direction with a high-speed router to allow the reamer access to the intramedullary canal. The access hole is then enlarged by the reamer until it can be inserted in line with the axis of the humeral shaft. The fracture is then reduced, and the ball-tip guide is placed across the fracture site. *D*, The canal is then reamed to no more than 1 to 2 cm across the fracture site; (see text) with the flexible intramedullary reamer, the guide rods are exchanged, and the rod is inserted. A 3.5-mm screw is inserted through the hole in the distal end of the rod to prevent its extrusion.

of management the treatment of choice for these injuries.

FLEXIBLE INTRAMEDULLARY DEVICES

Flexible intramedullary devices, such as Ender pins, Hackenthal nails, and Rush rods, have been utilized in the management of humeral shaft fractures (Fig. 38–21). Multiple rods should be placed in order to obtain adequate stability of the fracture site. Advantages include ease of insertion and minimal associated morbidity. Disadvantages include less than adequate stabilization of the fracture with poor rotational control. These implants may be indicated for pathologic fractures and in certain open humerus fractures. A functional brace should be utilized in conjunction with these devices to prevent fracture displacement (Fig. 38–21).[14,31,36,51,87,88,91,97]

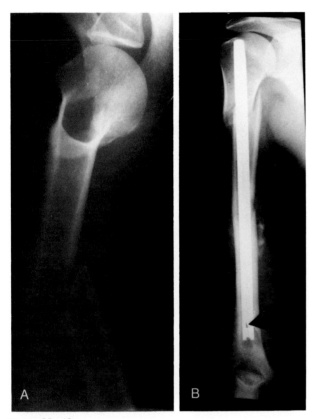

Figure 38–19

This segmental fracture of the diaphyseal humerus (*A*) was stabilized using a retrograde reamed intramedullary rod (*B*). Note the 3.5-mm block screw placed to prevent a loss of fixation *(arrow)*.

SPECIAL CONSIDERATIONS

Open Fractures

Open fractures constitute an orthopedic emergency.[49,50] It is imperative that they receive acute operative debridement and stabilization.[37,49,50] A sterile dressing should be draped over the wound and the humerus splinted until the patient reaches the operating room. Tetanus toxoid or antitoxin, as indicated, should be given in the emergency room.[34]

The open wound should be irrigated thoroughly and debrided, as described by Gustilo and colleagues.[49,50] Aerobic, anaerobic, and fungal cultures should be taken both before and after debridement.

Plate osteosynthesis may be elected in grade 1 and grade 2 fractures. In grade 3 injuries, external fixation is usually considered the treatment of choice. In each case, the wounds are left open initially and the patient is returned to the operating room every 48 hours until the wounds are determined to be clean and closure is accomplished, either by skin closure or the use of grafts. If indicated, cancellous bone grafting may be utilized at the final debridement to augment fracture healing.

Operative stabilization of open humeral shaft fractures not only provides stability to the fracture but also allows management of the soft tissue injuries. When proper fracture and soft tissue techniques are employed, osteosynthesis of open humeral shaft fractures does not increase the risk of infection and allows immediate rehabilitation of the entire upper extremity.

Pathologic Fractures

When pathologic conditions affect the humeral shaft, the strength of the cortical bone is decreased.[24,43,74] The

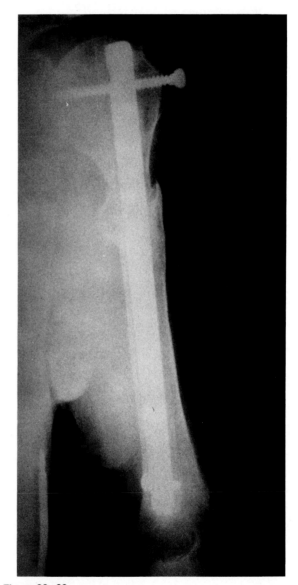

Figure 38–20

In fractures that remain rotationally unstable despite intramedullary rod fixation, the intramedullary rod can be interlocked by using proximal and distal screws to provide stable fixation and rotational control.

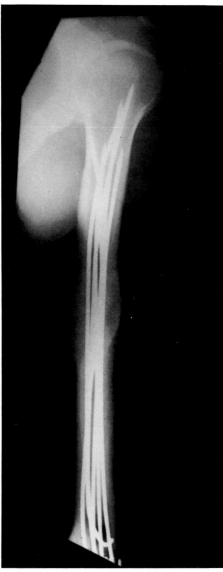

Figure 38-21

A flexible intramedullary device can be used as an internal splint in pathologic fractures and in certain open humeral fractures.

etiology of the underlying disease (e.g., metastatic tumor) may compromise the union of the fracture, resulting in delayed or nonunion if nonoperative methods of management are utilized.[75,89] Internal fixation is often necessary to decrease the associated morbidity and to obtain union. Single and dual plates have the disadvantage of relying on the screw-bone interface for stability. Unreamed intramedullary devices, such as Rush rods or Ender pins, provide poor rotational control and do not prevent distraction of the fracture fragments but may act as an internal splint of sufficient strength to obtain union.[22,60,96,109] A reamed intramedullary rod, with or without interlocked fixation, usually

provides the best stabilization of these injuries.[107] Once the fracture is stabilized, treatment of the underlying pathologic condition can be accomplished (Fig. 38-22).[43,67,74]

The Polytrauma Patient

In the patient with multisystem injuries, acute operative stabilization of diaphyseal humerus fractures should be considered imperative. Stabilization of long bone injuries in the acute period results in decreased

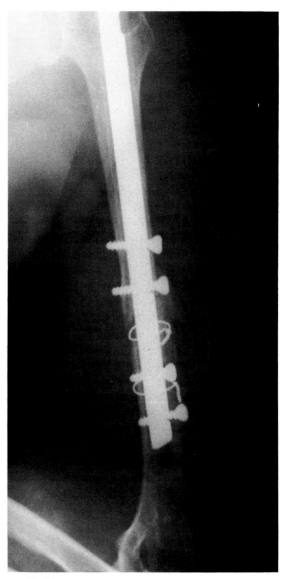

Figure 38-22

A pathologic fracture may require a special fixation. The humeral interlocked rod or a custom modification most often provides satisfactory stabilization in these patients.

systemic complications and earlier, more functional recovery in these patients. Operative stabilization of a diaphyseal humerus fracture in these cases also benefits the patient by allowing immediate use of the extremity so that he can assist in his own care.

In a polytraumatized patient who will be using crutches, intramedullary rod stabilization is indicated. Immediate "weight bearing" is well tolerated by the intramedullary device and may actually speed healing of the humeral shaft fracture.[107] Plate osteosynthesis in this particular situation requires four to six weeks before crutch walking can be instituted.

Radial Nerve Palsy

Radial nerve palsy may occur in up to 18% of closed humeral shaft fractures.[35,43,64,77,90,109] Of these, more than 90% will constitute a neurapraxia, and the patient will recover spontaneously within three to four months of the injury.[90] It is important to note whether the nerve became nonfunctional during the injury or after the initial or emergent management of the fracture. Occurrence during initial fracture management may represent a laceration of the nerve by the bone fragments during manipulation, and operative exploration should then be considered mandatory.[43,90]

In the complete absence of clinical evidence of return of function, radial nerve dysfunction should be evaluated six weeks postinjury by electromyography and nerve conduction studies. The search for objective evidence of return should be directed toward motor response, primarily in the brachioradialis and extensor carpi radialis longus and brevis muscles. If action potentials are present, conservative management can be continued. However, if denervation fibrillation or complete denervation is noted on these tests, surgical exploration and repair, with or without cable grafts, is indicated.

Neurapraxic radial nerve injury is most often associated with transverse fractures of the humeral shaft. In the authors' experience, 95% of these patients recover within four months of injury. Special situations requiring primary operative exploration of the nonfunctional radial nerve include open fracture, fractures associated with penetrating injuries, and the spiral oblique fracture of the middistal third of the humerus (Holstein-Lewis fracture).[35,43,56,64,77,90,109] A primary repair of the injured nerve and an open reduction and stable fixation of the humeral fracture should be carried out at the time of exploration. Muscle should be interposed between the fracture site and the nerve repair to prevent the repaired nerve's incorporation into the bone healing response.

Postoperative Management and Rehabilitation

In the presence of stable fixation, motion of the elbow and shoulder joints can be instituted immediately. Elbow motion should be stressed and attained within two weeks of operative intervention. Lightweight strengthening exercises should be begun when tolerated, but heavy resistance training should be delayed until evidence of fracture union is present, usually by six weeks postoperatively.

Complications

The primary complications resulting from the management of humeral shaft fractures are malunion, nonunion, infection, and radial nerve deficit.[36] Epps has described several factors affecting the prognosis of fractures of the humeral shaft:

1. Spiral-oblique and comminuted fractures unite more quickly than transverse, segmental, or open fractures.

2. Fractures in proximity to or associated with joint injuries have less satisfactory results.

3. In closed fractures with marked displacement, the interposition of soft tissues may make reduction impossible.

4. Neurovascular damage results in a decreased functional outcome.

5. Patient compliance will affect the final result. These factors should be considered initially and should aid in the selection of the proper treatment for the injured patient (see Fig. 38–4).[36]

MALUNION

An angular malunion of 20 to 30° or shortening of 2 to 3 cm rarely presents a problem. The wide range of motion of the shoulder joint may also minimize the effect of rotational malunion of up to 15°, and even greater deformity may be tolerated with minimal functional impairment. Cosmesis should seldom be considered an indication for operative intervention, and one should be cautious in considering or recommending skeletal surgery in such cases. However, if surgery is indicated, osteotomy with stable internal fixation may provide a satisfactory method of reconstruction.

NONUNION

Nonunion of humeral shaft fractures develops in 2 to 5% of nonoperatively managed injuries and in up to

25% of fractures managed by primary open reduction and internal fixation.* Nonunion occurs more frequently in open fractures, high-velocity injuries, segmental fractures, poorly reduced fractures, and fractures with inadequate operative stabilization. Preexisting conditions, such as shoulder or elbow stiffness, result in increased stress on the fracture site and predispose the patient toward the development of a nonunion. Other causative factors include poor soft tissue coverage, severe obesity, metastatic carcinoma, alcoholism with resulting osteoporosis, corticosteroid treatment, and polytrauma.[12,36,39,40,109]

Physiologic considerations, including vascularity of the fracture site, nutritional status of the patient, and the presence of systemic disease should be evaluated prior to treatment of the nonunion. When these factors have been considered, a management plan can be formulated. The objective should be reduction with stable internal fixation, supplemented by the liberal use of cancellous bone graft. Intramedullary nail stabilization is preferred in patients with osteopenic or pathologic bone, while compression plate stabilization is recommended for those patients with adequate bone stock.

If plate osteosynthesis is planned, the plate and screw fixation must be stable enough to withstand disruptive stress until union occurs. At least eight cortices (minimum of four screws) should be obtained both proximal and distal to the nonunion site. This usually will require the use of a minimum ten-hole broad dynamic compression plate to achieve adequate stability (Fig. 38–23). In selected cases, a narrow dynamic compression plate may be substituted when the humeral diameter will not accommodate the larger plate. Supplemental external support with a fracture brace is recommended to allow immediate rehabilitation of the extremity. The use of corticocancellous onlay grafts opposite the plate may increase the rigidity of fixation and aid in screw purchase near the nonunion site.

Intramedullary rod stabilization is also an acceptable method of managing diaphyseal nonunions (Fig. 38–24), and it is especially appropriate for fractures of the proximal and distal one third. Stabilization with plate and screws in these fractures will result in inadequate fixation on one side of the nonunion. Three to 5 cm of cortical contact to the rod should be obtained above and below the fracture site. Interlocked fixation to provide additional rotational stability and maintain length may be necessary and should be available if adequate cortical contact cannot be obtained intraoperatively.

All established nonunions are managed by supplemental bone grafts and either intramedullary nailing or

---

* References. 7,9,10–12,18,19,29,39,40,77,82.

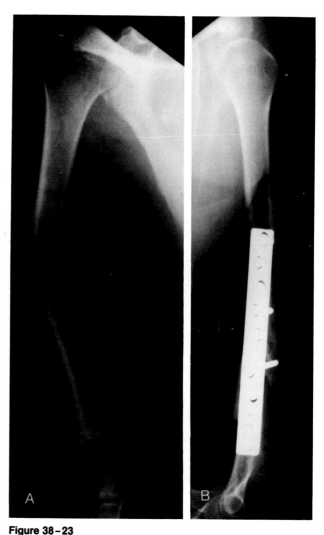

Figure 38–23

A humeral nonunion often responds to stabilization with a technically adequate dynamic compression plate. This nonunion (A) was managed with dynamic compression plate stabilization (B), with resultant union.

fixation with a broad dynamic compression plate. An intramedullary nail is preferred if the bone is osteopenic. Closed intramedullary rodding can be performed for delayed union or nonunion in the absence of interposed fibrous scar tissue. If closed intramedullary nailing is utilized, a thoracotomy tube can deliver bone graft to the site of the nonunion. Closed or open intramedullary fixation is the treatment of choice in patients using ambulatory support, such as crutches, a walker, or a cane.

Satisfactory results can be obtained with a stable fixation of humeral nonunion. Boyd, Campbell, Müller, Savoie and Culpepper, and Küntschner have reported union in approximately 90% of cases.[10–12,19,69–71,77,82]

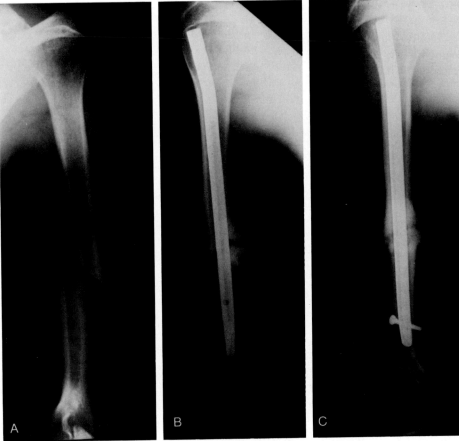

Figure 38–24

Intramedullary rod stabilization, with or without the addition of interlocked screw fixation, can be used in the management of humeral nonunions: *A*, nonunion; *B*, intramedullary rod stabilization; *C*, fracture union.

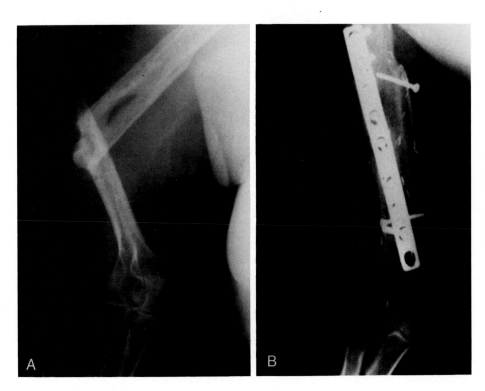

Figure 38–25

Humeral nonunion with a bone deficit (*A*) should be considered to require reconstruction. Vascularized autogenous fibula graft (*B*) can provide satisfactory union with restoration of function.

Infected Nonunion

A direct correlation has been shown between instability and infection.[10,12] Stabilization of the nonunion with *complete* debridement of infected nonviable tissue including bone, irrigation of the wound, and systemic antibiotics will lead to union in the majority of cases. The use of antibiotic-impregnated methylmethacrylate or a local antibiotic infusion pump may be necessary to eradicate the infection. Intramedullary stabilization or plate and screw fixation is often contraindicated in infected cases but may be utilized when the infection has been eradicated.

Rarely is amputation necessary for prolonged infected nonunion of the humeral diaphysis. Amputation should be considered for life-threatening infections, in situations in which the limb is so severely diseased that function would be better with a prosthesis, and in cases in which the infection cannot be controlled by local and systemic treatment.

Nonunion with Bone Loss

A nonunion with a bone deficit of 5 cm or more should be considered a reconstructive case. Methods of reconstituting this deficit include full-thickness corticocancellous autografts, vascularized bone transfer, and humeral allograft.[1,98] Techniques for each method include excision of all nonviable tissue, including the bone ends, reestablishment of the medullary canal on each side, and interposition of the graft with stable fixation.[1,58] Supplemental cancellous autograft should be utilized at both ends of the interpositional graft. Jupiter has reported a series of problem upper extremity injuries managed by vascularized fibula transfer with excellent results (Fig. 38–25).[1,62]

NEUROLOGIC COMPLICATIONS

Radial nerve injury is the most common neurologic complication associated with humeral fractures. Transient, neurapraxic injuries are most commonly noted following transverse or short oblique fractures of the humerus. Transection of the radial nerve has been noted most commonly with open fractures, fractures associated with penetrating injuries, and historically with the spiral oblique fracture of the distal humerus (Holstein-Lewis fracture).[35,43,56,77,90,108] The management of this complication has been discussed previously.

Transient palsy of the anterior interosseous, median, and ulnar nerves is rare. If present, spontaneous recovery usually occurs within 10 weeks of injury. Median nerve palsy associated with a supracondylar process may require release of the associated fibrous band in order to obtain return of normal function.

VASCULAR COMPLICATIONS

Vascular injuries associated with humeral shaft fractures are rare and most often occur in open fractures or with penetrating injuries.[27,80,93] If arterial injury is suspected or in high-risk injuries as detailed earlier, arteriography should be used to determine the site of injury and to accomplish vascular repair. Vascular reconstruction should be considered an absolute indication for stable fixation of the fracture, either with plate and screw stabilization or by external fixation. In most cases, bone stabilization should precede arterial reconstruction. Fasciotomy of the arm, forearm, and hand may be necessary when flow has been reestablished.

Conclusion

Primary union can be obtained in humeral shaft fractures in more than 90% of cases if proper techniques are utilized. Closed management by functional fracture bracing allows early rehabilitation and union and should be considered the nonoperative method of choice. With meticulous preoperative planning, precise technique, and careful attention to possible complications, results equal to those of nonoperative management, with the added advantages of decreased morbidity and earlier return to function, can be obtained with operative fracture management.

REFERENCES

1. Ackerman, G.; Jupiter, J.B. Nonunion of fractures of the distal end of the humerus. J Bone Joint Surg 70A:75–83, 1988.
2. Adams, J.C. Outline of Fractures. Edinburgh, E. & S. Livingstone, 1968.
3. Baker, D.M. Fractures of the humeral shaft associated with ipsilateral fracture dislocation of the shoulder: Report of a case. J Trauma 11:532, 1971.
4. Balfour, G.W.; Mooney, V.; Ashby, M. Diaphyseal fractures of the humerus treated with a ready-made fracture brace. J Bone Joint Surg 64A:11–13, 1982.
5. Banks, S.W.; Laufman, H. An Atlas of Surgical Exposures of the Extremities. Philadelphia, W.B. Saunders, 1964, pp. 63–97.
6. Bell, M.J.; Beauchamp, C.G.; Kellam, J.K.; McMurtry, R.Y. The results of plating humeral shaft fractures in patients with multiple injuries. J Bone Joint Surg 67B:293–296, 1985.
7. Bennett, G.E. Fractures of the humerus with particular reference to nonunion and its treatment. Ann Surg 103:994, 1936.
8. Bohler, L. The Treatment of Fractures. Supplementary Volume. New York, Grune & Stratton, 1966.
9. Bone, L. Fractures of the shaft of the humerus. In: Chapman, M.W., ed. Operative Orthopedics, Vol. 1. Philadelphia, J.B. Lippincott, 1988, pp. 221–234.

10. Boyd, H.B.: Symposium: Treatment of ununited fractures of the long bones. J Bone Joint Surg 47A:167, 1965.

11. Boyd, H.B.; Anderson, L.D.; Johnston, D.S.: Changing concepts in the treatment of nonunions. Clin Orthop 43:37, 1965.

12. Boyd, H.B.; Lipinski, S.W.; Wiley, J.H. Observation on nonunion of the shaft of the long bones with a statistical analysis of 842 patients. J Bone Joint Surg 43A:159, 1961.

13. Brooker, A.F.; Edwards, C.C. External Fixation—The Current State of the Art. Baltimore, Williams & Wilkins, 1979.

14. Brumbeck, R.J.; Bosse, M.J.; Poka, A.; Burgess, A.R. Intramedullary stabilization of humeral shaft fractures in patients with multiple trauma. J Bone Joint Surg 68A:960–969, 1986.

15. Burney, F.; Demolder, V.; Hinsen Kamp, M.; Posquin, C. The treatment of fractures of the humeral shaft with external fixation. Proceedings of Seventh International Symposium on External Fixation, Avignon, France, 1980.

16. Caldwell, J.A. Treatment of fractures in the Cincinnati General Hospital. Ann Surg 97:161, 1933.

17. Caldwell, J.A. Treatment of fractures of the shaft of the humerus by hanging cast. Surg Gynecol Obstet 70:421, 1940.

18. Cameron, B.M. Shaft Fractures and Pseudarthroses. Springfield, IL, Charles C Thomas, 1966.

19. Campbell, W.C. Ununited fractures of the shaft of the humerus. Ann Surg 105:135, 1937.

20. Carroll, S.E. A Study of the nutrient foramina of the humeral diaphysis. J Bone Joint Surg 45B:176–181, 1963.

21. Cave, E.A. Fractures and Other Injuries. Chicago, Year Book, 1958.

22. Chapman, M.W. Closed intramedullary nailing of the humerus. Instr. Course Lect, Vol. 31, 1982.

23. Charnley, J. The Closed Treatment of Common Fractures. Baltimore, Williams & Wilkins, 1961.

24. Cheng, D.S.; Seitz, C.B.; Eyre, H.J. Nonoperative management of femoral, humeral, and acetabular metastases in patients with breast carcinoma. Cancer 45:1533–1537, 1980.

25. Christensen, S. Humeral shaft fractures: operative and conservative treatment. Acta Chir Scand 133:455, 1967.

26. Comfort, T.H. The sugar tong splint in humeral shaft fractures. Minn Med 56:363–366, 1973.

27. Connolly, J. Management of fractures associated with arterial injuries. Am J Surg 120:331, 1970.

28. Conwell, H.E.; Reynolds, F.C. Management of Fractures, Dislocations and Sprains, 7th ed. St. Louis, C.V. Mosby, 1961.

29. Coventry, M.B.; Laurnen, E.L. Ununited fractures of the middle and upper humerus: Special problems in treatment. Clin Orthop 69:192, 1970.

30. Dameron, T.B.; Grubb, S.A. Humeral shaft fractures in adults. South Med J 74:1461–1467, 1981.

31. DeGeeter, L. Treatment of diaphyseal humeral fractures by percutaneous pinning. Acta Chir Belg 69:198, 1970.

32. DePalma, A.F. The Management of Fractures and Dislocations. Philadelphia, W.B. Saunders, 1970.

33. Doran, F.S.A. The problems and principles of the restoration of limb function following injury as demonstrated by humeral shaft fractures. Br J Surg 31:351, 1944.

34. Doty, D.B.; et al. Prevention of gangrene due to fractures. Surg Gynecol Obstet 125:284, 1967.

35. Duthie, H.L. Radial nerve in osseous tunnel at humeral fracture site diagnosed radiographically. J Bone Joint Surg 39B:746, 1957.

36. Epps, C.H., Jr. Fractures of the shaft of the humerus. In: Rockwood, C.A., Jr.; Green, D.P., eds. Fractures in Adults, Vol. 1. Philadelphia, J.B. Lippincott, 1984, p. 653.

37. Epps, C.H., Jr.; Adams, J.P. Wound management in open fractures. Am Surg 27:766, 1961.

38. Fenyo, G. On fractures of the shaft of the humerus. Acta Chir Scand 137:221, 1971.

39. Fisher, D.E. Nonunions of the humeral shaft. Minn Med, pp. 395–403, 1972.

40. Foster, R.J.; Dixon, G.L.; Bach, A.W.; et al. Internal fixation of fractures and non-unions of the humeral shaft. J Bone Joint Surg 67A:857–864, 1985.

41. Friedman, R.J.; Smith, R.J. Radial nerve laceration twenty-six years after screw fixation of a humeral fracture. J Bone Joint Surg 66A:959–960, 1984.

42. Gallagher, J.E.; Black, J.R. Humeral intramedullary nailing—a new implant. Injury 16:374–376, 1985.

43. Garcia, A. Jr.; Maeck, B.H. Radial nerve injuries in fractures of the shaft of the humerus. Am J Surg 99:625–627, 1960.

44. Gilchrist, D.K. A stockinette Velpeau for immobilization of the shoulder girdle. J Bone Joint Surg 49A:750–751, 1967.

45. Goss, C.M., ed. Gray's Anatomy, 25th ed. Philadelphia, Lea & Febiger, 1950.

46. Granz, R.; Isler, B.; Mast, J.W., Jr. Internal fixation technique in pathological fractures of the extremities. Arch Orthop Traumat Surg 103:73–80, 1984.

47. Green, S.A. Complications of external skeletal fixation. In: Uhthoft, H.K., ed. Current Concepts of External Fixation. Heidelberg, Springer-Verlag, 1982, pp. 43–52.

48. Gregersen, H.N. Fractures of the humerus from muscular violence. Acta Orthop Scand 42:506, 1971.

49. Gustilo, R.B.; Anderson, J.T. Prevention of infection in the treatment of 1025 open fractures of the long bones. Retrospective and prospective analysis. J Bone Joint Surg 58A:453–458, 1976.

50. Gustilo, R.B.; Simpson, L.; Nixon, R.; Ruiz, A. Analyses of 511 open fractures. Clin Orthop 66:148–154, 1969.

51. Hall, R.F.; Pankovich, A.M. Ender nailing of acute fractures of the humerus. J Bone Joint Surg 69A:558–567, 1987.

52. Hampton, O.P., Jr.; Fitts, W.T., Jr. Open Reduction of Common Fractures. New York, Grune & Stratton, 1959.

53. Harris, W.H.; Jones, W.N.; Aufranc, O.E.: Fracture Problems. New York, Grune & Stratton, 1959.

54. Holm, C.L. Management of humeral shaft fractures. Fundamental nonoperative technics. Clin Orthop 91:132–139, 1970.

55. Hollinshead, W.H. Anatomy for Surgeons, Vol. 3. New York, Hoeber-Harper, 1958.

56. Holstein, A.; Lewis, G.B. Fractures of the humerus with radial nerve paralysis. J Bone Joint Surg 45A:1382–1388, 1963.

57. Hoppenfeld, S.; De Boer, P. Exposures in Orthopedics. Philadelphia, J.B. Lippincott, 1984, pp. 47–75.

58. Huckstep, R.L. Fibula replacement of humerus. J Bone Joint Surg 65B:101, 1983.

59. Hudson, R.T. The use of the hanging cast in treatment of fractures of the humerus. South Surg 10:132, 1941.

60. Hunter, S.G. The closed treatment of fractures of the humeral shaft. Clin Orthop 164:192–198, 1962.

61. Junkin, H.D. The Topography of Pins, Precision Pinning of Fractures. Bloomington, IN, American Fracture Association, 1971.

62. Jupiter, J.B. The treatment of complex nonunions of the humeral shaft with a combination of surgical techniques. J Bone Joint Surg. 72A:701–707, 1990.

63. Kamhin, M.; Michaelson, M.; Waisbrod, H. The use of external skeletal fixation in the treatment of fractures of the humeral shaft. Injury 9:245–248, 1977.

64. Kettlekamp, D.B.; Alexander, H. Clinical review of radial nerve injury. J Trauma 7:424, 1967.

65. Key, J.A.; Conwell, H.E. Fractures, Dislocations and Sprains. St. Louis, C.V. Mosby, 1956.

66. Klenerman, L. Fractures of the shaft of the humerus. J Bone Joint Surg 48B:105–111, 1966.
67. Klenerman, L. Experimental fractures of the adult humerus. Med Biol Eng 7:357, 1969.
68. Kunec, J.R.; Lewis, R.J. Closed intramedullary rodding of pathologic fractures with supplemental cement. Clin Orthop 188:183–186, 1984.
69. Küntscher, G. The Küntscher method of intramedullary fixation. J Bone Joint Surg 40A:17, 1958.
70. Küntscher, G. Intramedullary surgical technique and its place in orthopaedic surgery: My present concept. J Bone Joint Surg 47A:809, 1965.
71. Küntscher, G. Practice of Intramedullary Nailing. Springfield, IL, Charles C Thomas, 1967.
72. LaFerte, A.D.; Nutter, P.D. The treatment of fractures of the humerus by means of hanging plaster cast—"hanging cast." Ann Surg 114:919, 1941.
73. Laing, P.G. The arterial supply of the adult humerus. J Bone Joint Surg 38A:1–105, 1956.
74. Lancaster, J.M.; Koman, A.L.; Gristina, A.G.; et al. Treatment of pathologic fractures of the humerus. South Med J 81:52–55, 1988.
75. MacAusland, W.R., Jr.; Wyman, E.T. Management of metastatic pathological fractures. Clin Orthop 73:39–51, 1970.
76. Mann, R.; Neal, E.G. Fractures of the shaft of the humerus in adults. South Med J 58:264–268, 1965.
77. Mast, J.W.; Spiegel, P.G.; Harvey, J.P.; Harrison, C. Fractures of the humeral shaft. Clin Orthop 12:254–262, 1975.
78. Mazet, R., Jr. A Manual of Closed Reduction of Fractures and Dislocations. Springfield, IL, Charles C Thomas, 1967.
79. McMaster, W.C.; Tivnon, M.C.; Waugh, T.R. Cast brace for the upper extremity. Clin Orthop 109:126–129, 1975.
80. McNamara, J.J.; Brief, D.K.; Stremple, J.F.; Wright, J.K. Management of fractures with associated arterial injury in combat casualties. J Trauma 13:17, 1973.
81. Mears, D.C.; Maxwell, G.P.; Vidal, J.; et al. Clinical techniques in the upper extremity. In: Mears, D.C., ed. External Skeletal Fixation. Baltimore, Williams & Wilkins, 1983, pp. 458–520.
82. Müller, M.E. Treatment of nonunions by compression. Clin Orthop 43:83, 1965.
83. Müller, M.E.; Allgower, M.; Willenegger, H. Technique of Internal Fixation of Fractures. New York, Springer-Verlag, 1965.
84. Müller, M.E.; Allgower, M.; Schneider, R.; Willenegger, H. Manual of Internal Fixation. New York, Springer-Verlag, 1970.
85. Naiman, P.T.; Schein, A.J.; Siffert, R.S. Use of ASIF compression plates in selected shaft fractures of the upper extremity. A preliminary report. Clin Orthop 71:208–216, 1970.
86. Newman, A. The supracondylar process and its fracture. Am J Roentgenol Radium Ther Nucl Med 105:844, 1969.
87. Nummi, P. Supramid pin in medullary fixation. Acta Chir Scand 137:67, 1971.
88. Nummi, P. Intramedullary fixation with compression for the treatment of fracture in the shaft of the humerus. Acta Chir Scand 137:71, 1971.
89. Parrish, F.F.; Murray, J.A. Surgical treatment for secondary neoplastic fractures—a retrospective study of 96 patients. J Bone Joint Surg 52A:665–686, 1970.
90. Pollock, F.H.; Drake, D.; Bovill, E.G.; et al. Treatment of radial neuropathy associated with fractures of the humerus. J Bone Joint Surg 63A:239–243, 1981.
91. Pritchett, J.W. Delayed union of humeral shaft fractures treated by closed flexible intramedullary nailing. J Bone Joint Surg 67B:715–718, 1985.
92. Raney, R.B. The treatment of fractures of the humerus with the hanging cast. North Carolina Med J 6:88, 1945.
93. Rich, N.M.; Baugh, J.H.; Hughes, C.W. Acute arterial injuries in Vietnam, 1000 cases. J Trauma 10:359, 1970.
94. Rich, N.M.; Metz, C.W.; Hutton, J.E.; et al. Internal versus external fixation of fractures with concomitant vascular injuries in Vietnam. J Trauma 11:463–473, 1971.
95. Rüedi, T.; von Hochsetter, A.H.C.; Schlumpf, R. Surgical Approaches for Internal Fixation. Heidelberg, Springer-Verlag, 1984, pp. 15–41.
96. Rush, L.V.; Rush, H.L. Intramedullary fixation of fractures of the humerus by the longitudinal pin. Surgery 27:268, 1950.
97. Sarmiento, A,; Kinman, P.B.; Calvin, E.G.; et al. Functional bracing of fractures of the shaft of the humerus. J Bone Joint Surg 59A:596–601, 1977.
98. Savoie, F.H.; Culpepper, D. Humeral nonunion: A comparative study of internal fixation techniques. In press.
99. Sisk, D.T. Fractures and fracture dislocations of the shoulder and humerus. In: Gossling, H.R.; Pillsbury, S.L., eds. Complications of Fracture Management. Philadelphia, J.B. Lippincott, 1984, pp. 301–306.
100. Spak, I. Humeral shaft fractures—treatment with a simple hand sling. Acta Orthop Scand 49:234–239, 1978.
101. Stern, P.J.; Mattingly, D.A.; Pomeroy, D.L.; et al. Intramedullary fixation of humeral shaft fractures. J Bone Joint Surg 66A:639–646, 1984.
102. Stewart, M.J.; Hundley, J.M. Fractures of the humerus. A comparative study in methods of treatment. J Bone Joint Surg 37A:681–692, 1955.
103. Stewart, M.J. Fractures of the Humeral Shaft. In: Adams, J.P., ed. Current Practice in Orthopaedic Surgery. St. Louis, C.V. Mosby, 1964.
104. Terry, R.J. A study of the supracondyloid process in the living. Am J Phys Anthropol 4:129, 1921.
105. Thompson, R.G.; Compere, E.L.; Schnute, W.J.; et al. The treatment of humeral shaft fractures by the hanging cast method. J Int Coll Surg 43:52–60, 1965.
106. Vander Griend, R.A.; Tomasin, J.; Ward, E.F. Open reduction and internal fixation of humeral shaft fractures. J Bone Joint Surg 68A:430–433, 1986.
107. Vander Griend, R.A.; Ward, E.F.; Tomasin, J. Closed Küntscher nailing of humeral shaft fractures. J Trauma 25:1167–1169, 1985.
108. Ward, E.F.; White, J. Interlocked intramedullary nailing of the humerus. Orthopedics 12:135–141, 1989.
109. White, R.R.; Ward, E.F. Küntscher nailing of the humerus. In: Seligson, D., ed. Concepts in Intramedullary Nailing. New York, Grune & Stratton, 1985, pp. 219–233.

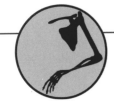

Tom R. Norris, M.D.

39

Fractures of the Proximal Humerus and Dislocations of the Shoulder

Pathology

Fractures of the proximal humerus have gained more attention recently with many advances in the field. The diagnosis has been facilitated with adaptation of three right-angle trauma series roentgenograms in the acute setting. Supplemental diagnostic imaging techniques have improved with the advent of computerized tomography (CT) for more accurate assessment of bony displacement and wear. Magnetic resonance imaging (MRI) offers the possibility of cartilage evaluation in epiphyseal injuries and in soft tissue, rotator cuff, and labrum attachment injuries in patients of all ages. Recently, with the more standard use of a four-segment classification system for fracture and fracture-dislocations, comparisons of the diagnosis, management, and long-term outcome of similar injuries are becoming possible. There have been improvements in fixation techniques during open reductions and in the understanding of the role of prosthetic replacement to maximize anatomic restoration while minimizing immobilization time during which stiffness develops. The elderly no longer need be denied effective surgical treatment,[33,34,241] especially at a time in life when the shoulders are often needed for ambulation with canes or crutches. Maintenance of good shoulder function may make the difference in whether these patients can remain independent of nursing home care.[241]

Although a few excellent articles* have been written on the treatment of proximal humeral fractures, there have not been many long-term studies on the more rare three- and four-part lesions, nor have adequate rating

*References 33, 84, 179, 180, 198, 249.

systems been adopted for general use. Often, with each new article produced, authors have reported different methods for evaluating these complex injuries. In much of the older literature the history and analyzable care of these fractures are unavailable. It has been difficult to compare the many overlapping and confusing terminologies that assign different weights to anatomic restoration, pain relief, motion, strength, stability, function, and complications.[33,179]

Fractures in the adult proximal humerus tend to occur along the lines of the old epiphyseal plate scar, with patterns involving four important segments (Fig. 39–1).[31,179] These include the articular surface; the lesser tuberosity with subscapularis attached; the greater tuberosity with the supraspinatus, infraspinatus, and teres minor attached at their respective facets; and the shaft of the humerus. To understand the pathologic changes caused by fractures and fracture-dislocations of the proximal humerus, it is important to understand the developmental and normal adult anatomy of the glenohumeral joint.

Relevant Anatomy and Biomechanics

In the infant, the proximal humeral epiphysis is spherical, and the epiphyseal plate is convex inferiorly with its apex posterior and medial to its center.[42] There are three centers of ossification. The central or major center of ossification appears within four to six months of birth in the humeral head.[93a] The greater tuberosity appears at approximately three years and the lesser tuberosity by five years. These coalesce between four and six years and close between 18 and 20 years (Fig. 39–2).

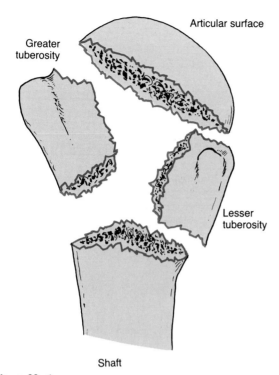

Figure 39–1

Codman's four-segment proximal humerus fracture classification.

The glenohumeral joint has the greatest range of motion of any joint in the body. The loose ligaments that allow this motion provide a passive restraint against instability. The most important of these is the inferior glenohumeral ligament complex, with anterior and posterior bands and an axillary pouch in between. The anterior band travels from the humeral neck inferiorly up along the anterior glenoid rim. It becomes confluent with the anterior glenoid labrum. When taut in abduction and external rotation, it is the prime shoulder stabilizer, but is more relaxed when the arm is at the side. The less well developed posterior band travels superiorly from the humeral neck to the posterior glenoid rim to join the posterior glenoid labrum. This composite tissue superiorly becomes confluent with the origin of the long head of the biceps at the supraglenoid tubercle (Fig. 39–3).

Normally, the humeral head is retroverted 35° to 40° to articulate with the scapula. The shoulder joint is not located in the sagittal or coronal plane of the body; its axis of motion begins on the curved chest wall, 35° to 40° away from the sagittal plane of the body. This has important implications in imaging and in reconstruction.

The average adult humeral head has a 44-mm radius of curvature. It is located slightly higher than the greater tuberosity and lateralizes the rotator cuff attachments. This architecture has important biome-

chanical implications for overhead elevation. Minor alterations accompanying head collapse or superior malunion of the greater tuberosity lead to major disruptions in motion, particularly elevation.

The small, flat glenoid cavity provides minimal bony support to the large humeral head. Only 25% to 30% of the humeral head articulates with the glenoid at any one time. The labral and ligamentous attachments accommodate this shallow, relatively flat surface to the more rounded curve of the humeral head. The intact humeral head is the fulcrum through which the rotator cuff and the long head of the biceps act as a force coupled with the deltoid to provide elevation of the arm while fixing the head within the glenoid cavity. The active power of the rotator cuff serves to protect the passive ligamentous stabilizers from overstretching or tearing. Rotation and elevation are lost if the head fulcrum is destroyed by fracture, dislocation, avascular necrosis, or surgical resection.

There is a rich periosteal network of blood supply to the humeral head. The majority of the direct blood supply to the humeral head derives from the arcuate artery of Laing supplied by the anterior and posterior circumflex humeral arteries, which derive from the third division of the axillary artery just above the teres major muscle (Fig. 39–4). These anastomose at the lower border of the biceps groove. These arcuate ascending branches travel with the biceps superiorly. They enter the cortex in the biceps groove or arborize to enter the tuberosities to provide the major blood supply to the articular surface of the humeral head. The consistent terminal artery passes up the lateral biceps to enter the medial portion of the greater tuberosity.[68] The anterior circumflex humeral artery provides the predominant supply to the arcuate artery. The posterior circumflex artery also sends a branch to the greater tuberosity posteromedially, but this supply is less significant.[85,132] To an even lesser extent, blood supply is provided through the tendon insertions on the tuberosities. Injury to the axillary artery or to the ascending branches by fracture or surgery is associated with an increased incidence of osteonecrosis.

Approximately two thirds of full overhead motion occurs through the glenohumeral joint and one third through the scapulothoracic articulation.[96,101,215] The humeral head fulcrum is lost if the articulation is destroyed or the articular surface is discarded. With loss of this fulcrum, rotation is lost as well as abduction. For full overhead elevation, external rotation with an intact humeral head fulcrum is necessary.[178]

The shoulder requires power and strength for normal function. Although it has been described as a non–weight-bearing joint when compared with hips and knees, it is load bearing, with significant forces across

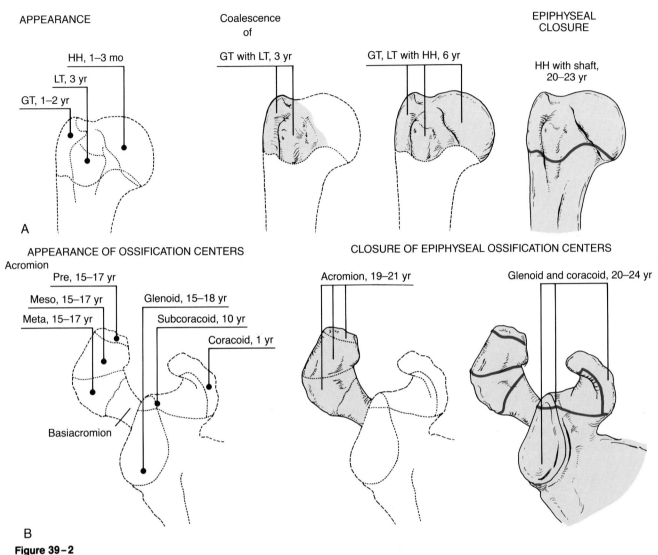

Figure 39-2

Appearance and closure of shoulder ossification centers. *A*, Proximal humerus. *B*, Outer scapula and glenoid. Basiacromion—present at birth; GT = greater tuberosity; HH = humeral head articular surface; LT = lesser tuberosity; Meso = mesoacromion; Meta = metaacromion; Pre = preacromial epiphysis. (Redrawn from Hodges, P.C. AJR 30:809, 1933.)

the glenohumeral articulation. When the arm is held in 90° of abduction, the joint reaction force equals 90% of body weight. These forces understandably increase with overhead lifting, with throwing, when weight is added to the hand, and when lifting is done away from the body.

The rotator cuff and deltoid each provide approximately 50% of the power needed for overhead lifting. These, combined with the scapula stabilizers, allow positioning of the arm in space with power and precision. During elevation the humeral head is stabilized in the glenoid primarily by the supraspinatus and secondarily by the subscapularis, infraspinatus, and long head of the biceps (Fig. 39-5).

Disruption of any of these intricate mechanisms can result in pain and loss of function, coordination, stability, and strength. Tearing of the rotator cuff, either from impingement or with a displaced greater tuberosity avulsion, destabilizes the shoulder and allows superior subluxation to occur with attempted elevation. There is a loss of the lever arm and a loss of active power, even if the passive motion is still present. Long-standing loss may result in fixed superior displacement of the humeral head and, eventually, cuff tear arthropathy.[189] The subacromial and subdeltoid bursae can no longer lubricate the normal gliding motions of the shoulder. Minor tuberosity displacements and varus malunions of surgical neck fractures compromise free motion in the subacromial space. Scarring with fracture or surgery may further restrict motion. Formation

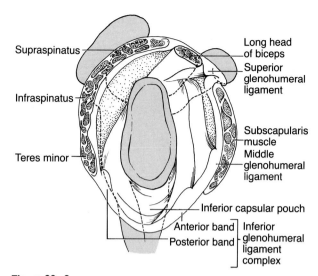

Figure 39–3

Glenoid cavity: relationship of glenohumeral ligaments, rotator cuff, and long head of biceps origins. (Redrawn from Hodges, P.C. AJR 30:809, 1933.)

of adhesions during the repair process, combined with long periods of immobility, obliterates the normal capsular recesses. A painful shoulder results from stiffness, even if the other factors are no longer contributory.

Minor losses of humeral length between the head and deltoid insertion can alter seriously the deltoid length–tension ratios on Starling's curve.[190,266] The effective deltoid contraction may be spent reducing an inferior humeral head subluxation, with little contraction left for elevation power (Fig. 39–6).

Between 47% and 80% of proximal humerus fractures are nondisplaced.[105] The rotator cuff, periosteum, and long head of the biceps hold many fractures together. Nondisplaced and minimally displaced fractures generally do not disrupt the rotator cuff or interfere with the blood supply to the humeral head and therefore seldom require surgery. These can be treated closed with early gentle motion as soon as pain subsides and security of the fracture fragments is assured. However, with displaced fractures and fracture-dislocations of the proximal humerus, severe disability may occur. Avulsion of the greater tuberosity is pathognomonic of a concomitant rotator cuff tear.[31,56,84,180,218] Pain, poor motion, and loss of strength and endurance are common in the treatment of proximal humerus fractures.[118,198–200,235] Results are seldom satisfactory when near-normal anatomy cannot be restored.

Epiphyseal Fractures

Three percent of epiphyseal fractures occur through the proximal humerus. Fractures through the proximal

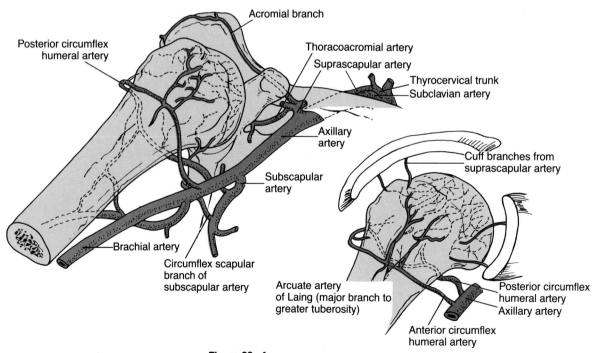

Figure 39–4

Vascular supply to the shoulder region.

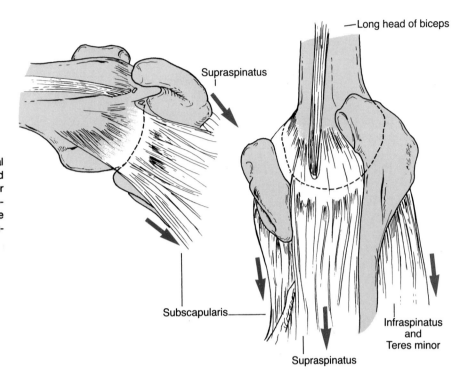

Figure 39–5

Rotator cuff forces to the proximal humerus serve to center the head in the glenoid, prevent superior ascent, and rotate the arm. The rotator cuff provides 50% of the power for elevation as a force coupled with the deltoid.

humeral epiphyseal plate occur most frequently in patients who are between the ages of 10 years and 16 years,[61,186] but they can occur anytime between birth and epiphyseal closure at approximately 18 years.[20,42]

No injuries separating the three secondary centers of ossification have been reported in children.[42]

Injuries at birth usually are fractures through the epiphyseal plate between the humeral diaphysis and

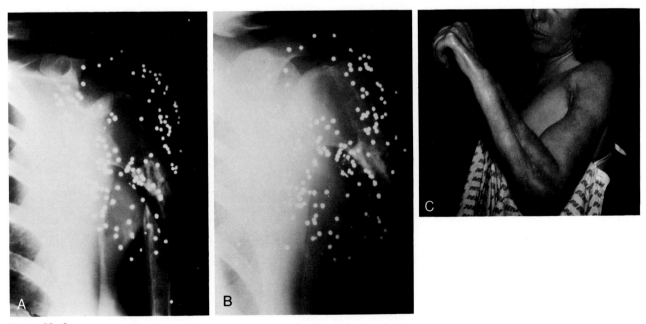

Figure 39–6

Inferior instability from bone loss in proximal humerus. *A*, Five-centimeter bone loss between the deltoid origin and insertion following a shotgun blast. *B*, Effective deltoid muscle contracture is spent on reduction of humeral head with little left for arm elevation. *C*, Volkmann's ischemic contracture resulted from axillary artery injury with failure of the first of two saphenous vein grafts.

the proximal epiphysis rather than dislocations of the shoulder. The epiphysis cannot be seen roentgenographically, but with reduction, abundant fracture callus is seen by two to three weeks (Fig. 39–7). Fluoroscopy, arthrography, and ultrasound have confirmed that the head remains located within the glenoid cavity with this displaced birth fracture.[20,48] In a study of 12 stillborn infants, Dameron and Reibel[42] demonstrated that it was extremely difficult to displace the metaphysis posteriorly at the epiphyseal plate. However, with the humerus extended and abducted, the metaphysis could be displaced anteriorly quite easily. This was explained by the asymmetric dome of the metaphysis with the high point posterior and medial through the center and with the much stronger, thicker attachment of the posterior periosteum along the posterior surface of the humerus (Fig. 39–8A).

The anterior periosteum is relatively weaker and thinner. As in adult fractures, the pectoralis major displaces the shaft anterior and medial to the proximal fragment. In the stillborn infants, the periosteal envelope was stripped distally yet still connected the proximal epiphysis to the shaft even when the metaphysis protruded through the periosteum. Eighty percent of humeral growth occurs from the proximal epiphysis, and even untreated displaced fractures remodel without loss of humeral length in children younger than 11 years.[186]

The rotator cuff muscles attach proximally to the epiphysis at the lesser and greater tuberosities. These hold the proximal fracture fragment in normal position. The pectoralis major attaches to the metaphysis at the junction with the epiphyseal plate. In the stillborn infants, no triangular fragment of bone accompanied the fracture at the epiphyseal plate through the zone of hypertrophied cartilage cells and adjacent to the zone of provisional calcification (Fig. 39–8B).[42]

The weakest link in the ossification chain is the zone of degenerating cartilage cells and osteoid tissue. Thus, in the infant, the zone of resting cells is not involved. Growth disturbances do not occur unless there is axial compression or crushing, as in Salter-Harris type V fracture (see below).

Aitken classified fractures of the proximal humerus into three types (Fig. 39–9). Salter and Harris expanded this classification of epiphyseal injuries to five types. Their types I and II account for most proximal humeral epiphyseal injuries (Fig. 39–10). Aitken's type I fracture, the only type he had actually seen, correlates with the Salter-Harris type II injury.

In stillborn infants Dameron and Reibel[42] were only able to produce the Salter-Harris type I fracture through the hypertrophied cartilage zone adjacent to the zone of provisional calcification. This is similar to fractures produced in experimental animals.[16,225]

In infants and young children, Salter type I epiphyseal injuries occur with the greatest frequency, whereas in older children and adolescents, Salter type II (Aitken type I) injuries predominate following coalescence of the ossification centers.

The increased incidence of epiphyseal fractures in children aged 10 to 16 years relates primarily to an

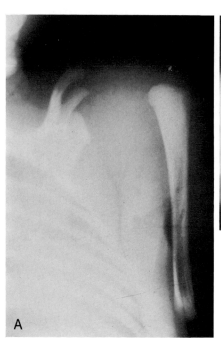

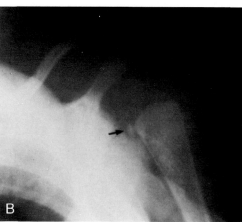

Figure 39–7

Obstetric proximal humeral epiphyseal fracture. *A*, At birth with complete displacement. *B*, At three weeks with callus, demonstrating that this is a fracture rather than a dislocation.

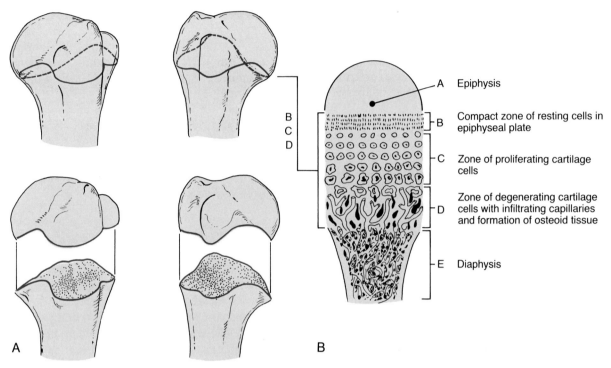

Figure 39-8

Proximal humeral epiphyseal plate. *A*, The epiphyseal plate is located on an asymmetric posteromedial dome at the proximal humerus metaphysis. *B*, The proximal humeral epiphyseal plate below the three epiphyseal centers of ossification. Most fractures occur through zone D without damaging the epiphysis or subsequent growth. (Modified from Aitken, A.P. Surg Clin North Am 43(6):1575–1580, 1963.)

increase in contact sports or to falls from heights onto an adducted and extended arm. In the United States, boys predominate with 55% of the fractures, whereas in Scandinavia, girls sustain 62%. This predominance for girls occurred between the ages of 9 and 14 years, and 50% of the fractures occurred during horseback riding.[209]

These lesions clinically involve Salter-Harris type I or II fractures. No Salter-Harris type III, IV, or V fractures have been identified in patients younger than 17 years.[42,236] Up to 20% of angulation will correct, and metaphyseal translation will correct in the absence of rotation, but rotatory deformities will not correct.[29,42,252]

In addition to classifying epiphyseal fractures by type, Neer and Horwitz[186] classified proximal humeral fractures into four grades of displacement: grade I (up to 5 mm); grade II (up to one third shaft diameter); grade III (up to two thirds shaft diameter); and grade IV (greater than two thirds shaft diameter, which includes

Figure 39-9

Aitken classification of fractures of the proximal humeral epiphysis.

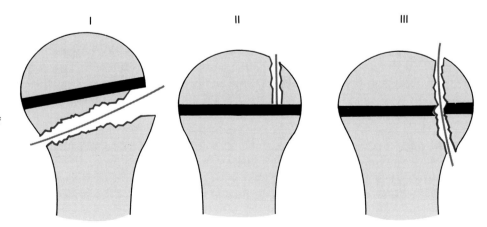

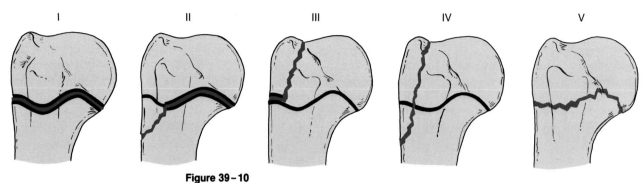

Figure 39–10

Salter-Harris classification, modified for the proximal humerus.

complete separation). In the younger patient, there is greater potential for correction by epiphyseal growth. In this extensive study, no growth inequities were noted with proximal humerus epiphyseal fractures in children younger than 11 years of age.[186]

The multiplanar glenohumeral joint compensates for minor discrepancies better than do other joints. Moderate shortening and angular deformities, not infrequent in children 12 years and older, are seldom objectionable. After age 11, 1- to 3-cm permanent growth discrepancies occur in children with minor grades I and II displacement (11%), and with grade IV displacement (33%). Aggressive treatment is usually not indicated because of the extensive remodeling that can occur from the proximal epiphysis. With persistent displacement, closed reduction is indicated to obtain greater than 50% overlap of the fragments.[186] Soft tissue interposition precluded a closed reduction in 9 of Fraser et al.'s 43 patients (21%).[61] The biceps was involved in three and the periosteum or deltoid muscle in six. If the fracture is unstable or irreducible, open reduction with smooth K wire pinning is advocated in older children.[121] Other methods of holding closed reductions have included "Statue of Liberty" casts, hanging arm casts, and olecranon pin traction. Each of these has had its complications, including gross angulation, nonunion, and malunion with hanging arm casts, ulnar nerve parasthesias with olecranon pin placement, and transient brachial paresis and/or physis destruction with the overhead Statue of Liberty position in a cast.[252] In one instance, permanent contracture from abduction cast positioning required an open release. This resulted in an epiphysiolysis with a 4-cm shortening.[252]

In Clement et al.'s[29] review of 148 epiphyseal fractures, 17 of 25 malunions were acceptable and eight were not. Twenty-one patients with multiple trauma underwent surgery following failed closed reduction, neglected fractures, or secondary displacement in plas-

ter. In older children, the fractures were treated the same as for those in adults.

The proximal humeral epiphysis closes between ages 18 and 20 years. The scar of the epiphyseal plate persists. In young adults, the ligamentous glenohumeral attachment is relatively weaker when compared with the bone. Dislocations predominate. In middle age, the rotator cuff attachments, especially the supraspinatus, replace the ligaments as the structure most susceptible to injury. First-time dislocations occurring in individuals older than 40 years have a 50% to 80% chance of occurring from tearing of the rotator cuff rather than from detachment of the glenoid labrum.[3,157,160,192] An anterior mechanism involves avulsion of the subscapularis,[192] whereas a posterior mechanism involves rupture of the supraspinatus, infraspinatus, and teres minor.[37,157,160] With advancing age, the greater tuberosity cavitates, and the shaft is devoid of cancellous bone, yet the scar of the epiphyseal plate persists. The cortical bone is thin at the lower part of the greater tuberosity and humeral head, where fractures most commonly occur; it is thickest at the supraspinatus attachment.[79] If the rotator cuff attachments are attached to the tuberosities, they may rupture with avulsion of the tuberosities through the weakened, senile bone.

Incidence

Proximal humeral fractures account for 4% to 5% of all fractures.[243] They may occur in any age group, with the earliest noted at the time of birth. Three percent of epiphyseal injuries are to the proximal humerus, most commonly in patients aged 10 to 16 years and secondary to hard falls and contact sports.[186,220] There is an increased frequency in the older middle-aged and elderly groups.[95,220] This increased frequency is attributable to advanced osteoporosis.[79,125]

In a Rochester, Minnesota, study,[220] 586 fractures of

the humerus occurred in 564 of the city's 53,000 residents during a ten-year period. Fractures of the proximal humerus comprised 45% of the initial fractures and 69% of recurrent fractures. In adults, the incidence rate was lowest in the third decade. From there it began to rise with similar incidence rates for both sexes until age 50. Thereafter the rate rose for both sexes, but the female:male ratio was 4:1. The greatest number of fractures in adult males appeared during the active ages between 30 and 60, whereas in women there was a dramatic exponential increase after menopause. Fractures in women in the upper age group were 37 times more frequent than in those in their fourth decade. In Kristiansen et al.'s study[125] of 565 proximal humeral fractures in 500,000 people, 77% of the fractures in all age groups involved were in women. Again this was thought to be a result of advanced osteoporosis.

Jensen et al.[107] demonstrated that the frequency of osteoporotic fractures varied inversely with bone mineral content. Other causative factors, in addition to lack of hormone replacement after menopause, include alcoholism and gastric resection for peptic ulcer disease.[95] Proximal humeral fractures more reliably correlate with bone fragility than do fractures of the spine, upper femur, pelvis, or distal radius.[95,107] Thus with advancing age, less trauma is required to sustain a fracture of the proximal humerus. In patients younger than 50 years, the most common causes of humeral fractures involve violent trauma, such as falls from heights, motor vehicle accidents, and contact sports. In patients older than 50 years, a fracture can result from minimal to moderate trauma, such as a fall from the standing position or less.[107] Seventy-six percent of the fractures involving the surgical neck of the humerus, the most likely area for fracture, occurred in individuals older than 65 years.[259]

Mechanisms of Injury

When the history of the shoulder injury can be recalled, it often reveals one or a combination of mechanisms occurring to produce a fracture of the proximal humerus. A direct blow to the anterior, lateral, or posterolateral aspect of the humerus can result in fracture. In younger patients, this might occur in a motor vehicle or skiing accident, whereas in the older individual, this may occur simply from a fall from standing height or less.

An axial load transmitted to the humerus through the elbow or extended hand and forearm when the elbow is locked in extension can also result in fracture. The displacement of the distal fragment depends on the position of the hand and elbow at the time that the axial load is applied. This has been documented in epiphyseal injuries when the metaphysis and diaphysis of the humerus displace anteriorly or posteriorly depending on whether the elbow was in front or behind the coronal plane of the body at the time of the fall.[263] Indirect focuses are brought into play in a fall on an outstretched abducted arm with the forearm pronated. The greater tuberosity is unable to clear the acromion, and the humeral neck levers against the acromion to produce fracture, fracture-dislocation, or dislocation depending on the relative strengths of the bone and surrounding ligaments.[183] Combinations of rotational forces and forward, backward, or lateral positioning of the arm have been deduced by the history given or by the resultant position of the fracture fragments in an effort to understand what forces could be applied to obtain closed reductions.[1,13,39,242,263,264]

Violent muscle contractures are produced in grand mal seizures and strong electric shock. The large internal rotators and adductors of the arm easily overpower the external rotators, resulting in a locked posterior fracture-dislocation.[17,72,201,205] During electroconvulsive therapy, the least current necessary to produce a major convulsion is 100 V for a duration of 0.3 s. During a ten-year study of 2200 patients undergoing electroconvulsive therapy, 37,000 convulsions were induced that resulted in 53 fractures; 16 of these were to the shoulder region.[116] Elsewhere the fracture rate with this therapy has been reported to be between 0.9% and 2.8%[122,162,226] Fractures to the shoulder in Kelly's review occurred four times for each 10,000 convulsions induced, or 6.8 fractures per 1000 patients treated.[116]

Convulsive seizures are thought to be the most common cause of bilateral posterior fracture-dislocations of the shoulder. These may occur either as locked head impression fractures or as four-part fractures.[51,142,144]

Pathologic fractures have occurred from local tumor, such as multiple myeloma, metastic tumor, or metabolic disorders.[133,140,270] Lancaster et al. reviewed their treatment of 57 lesions (40 pathologic fractures and 17 impending pathologic fractures) with various types of intramedullary fixation, including prosthetic replacement.[133,134] Zych and Montane described a successful treatment using humeral head replacement for a pathologic fracture superimposed on a chronic posterior fracture-dislocation following a seizure.[270] Li et al. reviewed the cortical irregularities in the medial aspect of the proximal humeral metaphysis leading to pathologic fractures in Gaucher's disease and have compared these with an infiltrative lesion seen in 60% of leukemia patients. The mechanism for fracture in these patients is closely related to the destruction of cortical bone.

Identification prior to fracture and prophylactic treatment are most efficacious.

It is important to determine the amount of trauma involved in fractures of the proximal humerus. Motor vehicle accidents, falls from heights, falls resulting from high speed (e.g., as in skiing), and injuries resulting from high-velocity gunshot wounds often have greater implications as to their associated injuries than do less traumatic injuries. However, those patients in whom the bone is weakened, either because of osteoporosis from aging, menopause, a premature hysterectomy, alcoholism, or gastric resection or because of osteomalacia that commonly follows phenytoin therapy, are predisposed to more serious injuries from only minimal trauma.

Consequences of Injury

The majority of proximal humeral fractures are non-displaced. These are treated expectantly with immobilization until pain subsides and then with gradual resumption of motion with pendulum and other passive exercises for nondisplaced or minimally displaced fractures to maintain the gliding planes. Rigorous passive stretching or active motion is avoided until healing is assured. This requires the understanding and cooperation of the patient to maximize the result for these simple injuries. Even so, sympathetic dystrophy, which occasionally occurs, can prolong the recovery period. The early postmenopausal female seems most prone to this complication.

Displaced fractures and fracture-dislocations result in pain, weakness, stiffness, and loss of function, which can be very disabling. In the adolescent and young adult, it interferes with all activities but is most noticeable in sports. Growth disturbances are rare injuries occurring in patients in the first decade but may be involved in 20% of the epiphyseal injuries occurring in patients in the second decade.[239] No cases of traumatic arthritis or osteonecrosis resulting from fractures alone have been reported in patients in the first two decades.

In the active middle-aged group, these fractures may interfere with livelihood, sports, and daily living. Loss of humeral length, with secondary deltoid weakening, traumatic arthritis, acute or chronic dislocations, rotator cuff tears with tuberosity displacement, nerve injuries, and (less frequently) axillary vessel injuries add to the fracture complications.[190,241] Fixed retraction of the tuberosities occurs as a result of a muscle pull with associated rotator cuff tears. Often, adequate radiographs in three right-angle planes have not been obtained. Soft tissue injuries may be easily missed, as they may be masked by pain, swelling, or instability caused

by fracture.[4] Because of scarring in the subacromial space with contracture of the joint capsule, fixed retractions of the tuberosities resulting from muscle pull are associated with stiffness and rotator cuff tearing. As little as a 2-mm greater tuberosity superior displacement has been associated with postfracture impingement and tearing of the rotator cuff.[115] This occurs especially in three- and four-part fractures treated with closed reduction; in these, persistent pain, shoulder stiffness, and functional disability are usual.[30,118,179,241] A number of reconstructive procedures have been described for treatment of displaced proximal humeral fractures. For three- and especially four-part fractures that retain the humeral head, the failure rate is high when the head is retained either because of stiffness that occurs while awaiting secure healing or because of late osteonecrosis that occurs during the ensuing two years.[118,132,137,179,180,221] Reattachment of the rotator cuff to the shaft with head removal likewise has had poor results because of the loss of an adequate fulcrum and subsequent pain, stiffness, and weakness.[111,118,175,176] Prosthetic humeral head replacement has gained increasing acceptance as shoulder reconstruction techniques have improved.[187,190,241,249]

Although only 20% of proximal humeral fractures have generally been considered to be displaced or minimally displaced,[183,220] Jakob, reporting for the AO group,[105] described 53% of these fractures as displaced. Thus, the more serious or displaced fractures may be more common than previously thought. The major anatomic concerns involve tearing of the rotator cuff with resultant weakness; loss of blood supply to the articular surface, leading to late collapse; soft tissue interposition that precludes closed reduction; and bone malunions or nonunions, which mechanically preclude motion. Pain, stiffness, weakness, and function disabilities result from any of these.

Adequate radiographs are essential to avoid misdiagnosis. Between 50% and 80% of the posterior fracture-dislocations are missed by the first examining physician.[53,82,86,201] Patients with multiple trauma resulting from motor vehicle accidents frequently have chest, abdominal, and cervical spine injuries. Often shoulder fractures, fracture-dislocations, and articular fractures of the glenoid are missed or neglected until more serious life-threatening cranial, thoracic, and abdominal injuries have been treated. Ironically, the shoulder lesions may be the most debilitating residual injury after all others have healed.[3,100,155]

Commonly Associated Injuries

The most common injury associated with wide separation of the tuberosities in the proximal humerus is a rotator cuff tear. The muscles attaching to the tuberosities are the deforming forces. A longitudinal tear at the rotator interval between the supraspinatus and subscapularis occurs with displacement of either tuberosity (Fig. 39–11B).

In 10% to 25% of anterior shoulder dislocations there is an avulsion of the greater tuberosity.[156,169,222,258] Two mechanisms can account for the two-part greater tuberosity fractures, in which the tuberosity remains behind in a normal position relative to the glenoid as the humerus dislocates anteriorly. In one, the tuberosity fragment is imbedded in the empty capsular sleeve from which the humerus has dislocated.[156] On reduction, the tuberosity fragment assumes anatomic position. In these situations, a rotator cuff interval tear may not have occurred, and the reduction reapproximates any capsular stripping (Fig. 39–11A–E).

The second mechanism in which the tuberosity remains in its premorbid position involves a massive rotator cuff avulsion without detachment from the tuber-

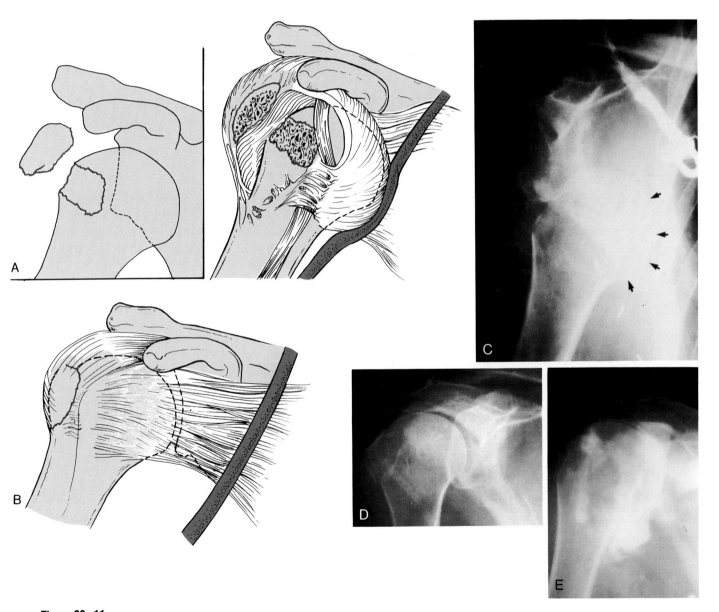

Figure 39–11

Variations of pathology in two-part greater tuberosity fractures associated with anterior shoulder dislocations. A through E: capsular stripping without rotator cuff tear. A, Diagram of anterior dislocation with greater tuberosity displacement allowed by capsular stripping in the absence of a rotator cuff tear. B, Anatomic reduction of tuberosity with reduction of shoulder dislocation and closure of capsular envelope. C,D, Clinical examples of pathologic conditions depicted in A and B with (E) no cuff tear on arthrography.

Illustration continued on following page

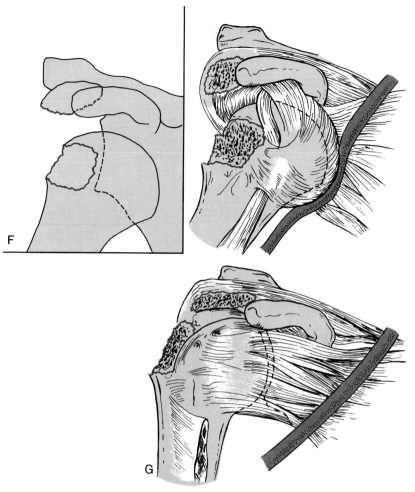

Figure 39–11 *Continued*

F through *H*: greater tuberosity avulsion associated with longitudinal rotator interval tear between subscapularis and supraspinatus. *F*, anterior dislocation and greater tuberosity fracture with longitudinal tear of rotator cuff at rotator interval between supraspinatus and subscapularis. *G*, Persistent greater tuberosity retraction superiorly with supraspinatus tear following closed reduction.

osity. There is an obligatory rotator interval tear (Fig. 39-11*F* and *G*). On reduction it displaces superiorly if the supraspinatus alone is involved (Fig. 39-11*H*) or posteriorly into the spinoglenoid notch if the supraspinatus, infraspinatus, and teres minor are involved. Early reduction and rotator cuff repair are essential if useful shoulder function is to be obtained (Fig. 39–11*F* through *H*).[156]

A rare third mechanism involves a greater tuberosity fracture that does not stay in an anatomic position but accompanies the anterior dislocation of the humeral head. On reduction of the dislocation, the tuberosity is not accurately reduced. (Fig. 39-11*I*). This raises a distinct possibility of an additional rotator cuff tear from the tuberosity, which is associated with a painful, prolonged postreduction course. Diagnostic tests to evaluate the status of the rotator cuff and early treatment are worthwhile (Fig. 39–11*J*).[156]

A fourth mechanism involves a large tuberosity fragment that may involve the groove of the long head of the biceps. If the biceps tendon slips posteriorly from the groove, it may occupy a position behind the dislocated head and prevent reduction or result in immediate redislocation if reduction is temporarily obtained (Fig. 39–11*K*).[72,106,156] Repeated closed reductions are contraindicated due to the increased chances of additional nerve injuries or myositis ossificans. Open reduction is necessary to remove the interposed long head of the biceps prior to reduction of the fracture-dislocation.

In severe trauma, multiple fractures of the ipsilateral extremity may occur in addition to the proximal humeral fracture. Pierce and Hodurski[214] reported that in 21 patients who sustained ipsilateral radial and ulnar fractures, more than 50% experienced residual nerve injury, which included the brachial plexus, radial, and ulnar nerves. These fractures of the proximal third of the humerus were associated with poor results. Shaft and more distal humeral fractures may have an unsuspected associated proximal humeral fracture or fracture-dislocation (Fig. 39–12).[113] These were often missed in victims of motor vehicle accidents because of

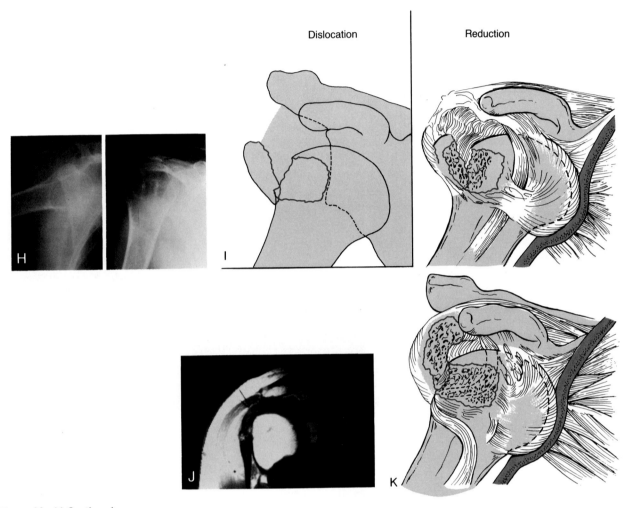

Figure 39–11 *Continued*

H, Clinical roentgenogram of *F* and *G*. *I*, Incomplete tuberosity displacement with cuff detached from tuberosity leading to persistent tear on reduction. *J*, MRI documentation of persistent cuff avulsion from anatomically reduced greater tuberosity. *K*, Greater tuberosity fracture or tear of the transverse humeral ligament or both permits interposition of the biceps long head, which precludes a closed reduction.

associated cervical spine injuries, brachial plexus injuries, thoracic cage injuries with rib fractures and subsequent pneumothoraces, abdominal injuries, and scapular injuries, as well as unsuspected glenoid fractures.

NERVE INJURIES

The neurovascular bundle is anteromedial to the glenohumeral joint and is subject to injury with anterior glenohumeral dislocations, fracture-dislocations, and fractures involving the surgical neck of the humerus. Injury may occur either from direct contact with the fracture fragments or from traction injuries.[32,268]

Nerve injuries are more common when humeral head dislocation accompanies fracture of the proximal humerus. In this instance, a greater tuberosity fracture is most frequently accompanied by an isolated axillary nerve injury.[232] Traumatic brachial plexus injuries can be classified as either infraclavicular or supraclavicular.[2,32,173,245] In a review of 420 operative cases for brachial plexus palsies, 25% of the injuries were infra- or retroclavicular, and 75% were supraclavicular. Fifteen per cent of the 420 operative cases were at double levels.[2] Ninety per cent of the injuries occurred in patients aged 15 to 30 years and were the result of automobile or motorcycle accidents. Anterior or inferior shoulder dislocations cause most isolated axillary nerve and posterior cord lesions. In Alnot's series,[2] 80% of the isolated axillary nerve lesions were neurapraxias that recovered in four to six months. However, in Seddon's[232] series, 44% had complete recovery, 12% had incomplete recovery, and 44% had no recovery. Vio-

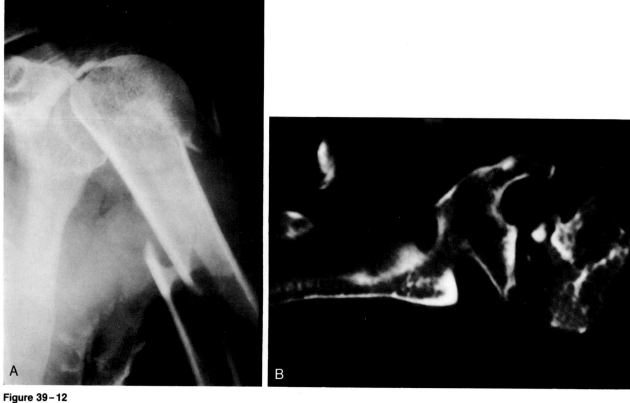

Figure 39–12

A, Three-part greater tuberosity proximal humeral fracture combined with midshaft diaphyseal fracture. *B,* Treatment of the diaphyseal fracture alone resulted in severe glenohumeral arthritis that later required replacement.

lent downward and backward movement of the shoulder causes brachial plexus stretch injuries, and multiple trauma involving fractures of the clavicle, scapula, or upper humerus causes diffuse lesions of the secondary trunks and terminal branches, which are often accompanied by vascular damage. Atraumatic downward and backward movement of the shoulder is associated with axillary and suprascapular or musculocutaneous nerve stretching or tearing. Ruptures of the axillary nerve in the quadrilateral space, of the suprascapular nerve at the suprascapular notch adjacent to the coracoid, and of the musculocutaneous nerve avulsion from its entry point into the coracobrachialis are the most frequent injuries.

When diagnosed by electromyography (EMG), the incidence of axillary and other types of nerve lesions in glenohumeral dislocations and humeral neck fractures is 20% to 30%. In patients older than 50 years, it is as high as 50%.[11,54,211]

Nerve injuries can be easily overlooked, as pain and immobilization make it difficult to diagnose palsy in the early posttraumatic period. Sensory loss does not routinely accompany an axillary nerve lesion.[8,11] Fortunately, most of the palsies resolve within a few weeks.

Although persistent deltoid palsy caused by an axillary nerve lesion is rare, a long delay in reinnervation will be disadvantageous if the nerve has been severed or ruptured. Muscle transfers for deltoid paralysis as late salvage procedures have had poor results. For this reason Narakas[174] and others[22,32,232] advocate exploring infraclavicular nerve lesions early after very severe trauma.

In four-part fractures of the proximal humerus, Stableforth reported brachial plexus injuries in 6.1%, of which only one third made complete recovery.[241]

VASCULAR INJURIES

Vascular injuries with rupture of the axillary artery have been reported in approximately 5% of four-part fractures of the proximal humerus.[241] Treatment has included above-elbow amputation for gangrene after rupture of the axillary artery, ligation of third and fourth intercostal vessels to control hypovolemic shock from a displaced head fragment entering the pleural cavity, and repair or ligation of atherosclerotic axillary artery ruptures. Swelling and collateral circulation may mask the extent of the vascular injury. Abduction for evaluation of the axillary artery may be difficult as a result of pain and muscle spasm. The peripheral pulses, including the radial artery, should be palpated, but collateral circulation may provide a peripheral pulse even with an axillary artery injury. Other signs include parasthesias, pallor or cyanosis depending on whether it is an arterial or venous injury, and an expanding hematoma. Parasthesias may be secondary to poor distal circulation and suggest a vascular injury. The key to successful treatment is early diagnosis and repair.[87,230,269]

Fractures through the surgical neck of the humerus, with or without additional accompanying dislocation, have resulted in rupture, thrombus formation, and pseudoaneurysms of the axillary artery.[32,89,136,145,161,240,250,261,268] If a vascular injury is suspected, Doppler and arteriographic studies are recommended. If reconstruction is indicated, a fracture must be internally fixed to prevent fracture displacement, which could compromise the vascular repair. Serial Doppler examinations postoperatively are then necessary to detect thrombus formation[268]; otherwise thrombosis and severe ischemia, accompanied by Volkmann's contracture, may result (Fig. 39–6C).

Another complication of vascular injury is late osteonecrosis of the articular surface. The blood supply through the anterior and posterior circumflex humeral arteries and the ascending arcuate artery to the articular surface can be damaged by fractures or by surgical procedures with extensive mobilization that disrupt these vessels,[244] especially if the terminal arcuate arterial supply to the articular segment is involved.[68,132] Thus even two-part fractures through the surgical neck are occasionally associated with osteonecrosis, although it is more common in three-part fractures and most common in four-part fractures and fracture-dislocations. Displacement at the anatomic neck carries the greatest risk for osteonecrosis with disruption of the blood supply to the articular surface.

Chest wall damage[241] has been reported in 2.5% of four-part fracture and fracture-dislocation injuries. Intrathoracic dislocations of the humeral head combined with surgical neck fractures of the humerus, pneumothorax, and pneumohemothorax have been reported with fractures of the proximal humerus.[69,81,179,212]

Evolution of Classification

It has been very difficult to compare the many overlapping and confusing terminologies used to evaluate proximal humeral fractures and fracture-dislocations. They have been categorized by the anatomic level of fracture,[12,119] but this classification cannot identify all lesions and cannot differentiate between the more serious displaced lesions and nondisplaced fractures.

Classification according to the mechanism of injury, proposed by Dehne,[45] has undergone many modifications.[46,63,91,257] Neer[179] points out that adduction and abduction fractures of the proximal humerus can both be diagnosed in the same injury depending on whether the radiograph is taken with the arm in internal or external rotation. Thus the usefulness of this classification is limited.[179] The anatomy and mechanisms of fracture are not fully addressed, and the natural history and clinical management are not apparent from a mechanistic classification alone.[118] Unfortunately, with the many different classifications, the more serious fractures are often combined with the nondisplaced fractures. Thus much of the history and analyzable care of appropriate treatment for these fractures is unavailable, since the results of nondisplaced and displaced fractures are quite different.

For epiphyseal injuries, both the Aitken and Salter-Harris classifications, which are based on the anatomic components, are useful. In older reports using the Aitken system, neither disruption of blood supply to the articular surface nor tears of the rotator cuff have been reported. The more complete Salter-Harris classification proposes every possible type of epiphyseal injury. Prior to the use of MRI, identification of injuries within the cartilage of the proximal humerus was extremely difficult. However, with newer diagnostic techniques, injuries previously undescribed may be appreciated. Epiphyseal crushing may be correlated with shortening caused by up to 20% of the displaced fractures occurring in those older than 10 years.[239]

Neer and Horwitz[186] introduced the concept of displacement in differentiating epiphyseal injuries. Given that no type III, IV, or V epiphyseal fractures have been described in the proximal humerus and that these fractures through the epiphyseal plate do not affect longitudinal growth unless there is some crushing of the plate, then the nondisplaced and minimally displaced fractures in the Neer and Horwitz classification may be grouped as one type, with the completely displaced, significantly angulated, or rotated fractures grouped as a second category, regardless of the direction of displacement or rotation.

Codman[31] and deAnquin and deAnquin[44] emphasized vascular considerations and their importance to fractures involving the articular segment of the proximal humerus. Neer,[179] realizing this, made Codman's four-segment classification clinically useful by basing it on the degree of displacement or angulation of an anatomic segment. He combined the advantages of the three classifications using the anatomic level of the fracture and differentiated between the less serious nondisplaced fractures and the more serious displaced lesions. From this classification, one would hope to predict the integrity of the blood supply to the articular surface and whether rotator cuff tear has occurred.

Neer's classification system is based on imaging studies of the three original epiphyseal centers of ossification and the shaft segment. The first segment is the articular surface. A fracture may displace it through the anatomic neck level, split the head segment, or both. The second segment is the greater tuberosity with its muscle and tendon units, consisting of the supraspinatus, infraspinatus, and teres minor, attached. These muscles serve to abduct and externally rotate the head. This segment is often comminuted, and there may be

differences in sizes, location, and number of rotator cuff muscles involved with the fracture fragments. Generally, however, displacement of any portion of the greater tuberosity is significant. The number of comminuted nondisplaced fracture fissures that may occur are not thought to alter either the blood supply to the articular surface or the ability to differentiate whether rotator cuff integrity is still present.

The third segment consists of the lesser tuberosity with its attached subscapularis, which internally rotates the humeral head. This muscle opposes or balances the forces of those attached to the greater tuberosity.

The fourth segment is the shaft at the subtuberous or surgical neck level. When this classification was origi-

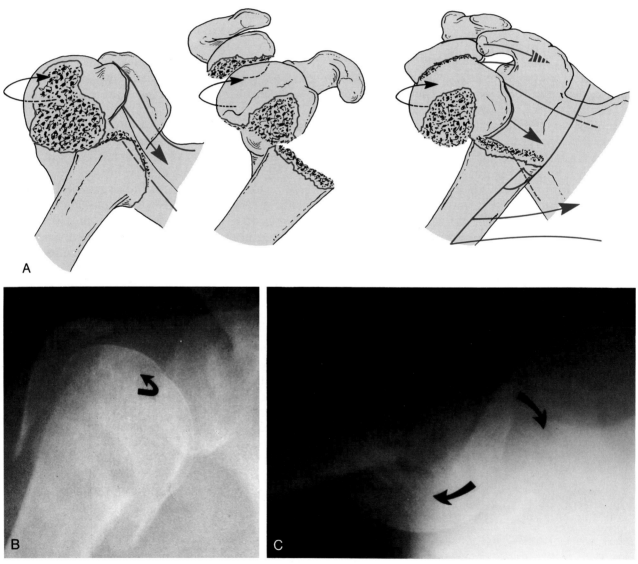

Figure 39-13

Three-part greater tuberosity fracture. The pectoralis displaces the unimpacted shaft anteriorly and medially. The greater tuberosity is retracted by the spinati and teres minor. The articular surface is rotated posteriorly by the intact subscapularis. There is a rotator interval tear.

nally presented in 1970, it stressed that with accurate imaging studies, fractures of the proximal humerus could be classified as displaced or nondisplaced. A fracture is considered displaced if any major segment is displaced 1 cm or more or angulated greater than 45°. Empirically, multiple fracture fissures without displacement of 1 cm are less likely to disrupt the blood supply to the articular surface. These are referred to as one-part fractures or minimally displaced fractures in which the periosteum, joint capsule and rotator cuff attachments hold the fracture fragments together.[31] The stable fractures are grouped together for treatment purposes (i.e., for early functional exercises to avoid stiffness), whereas displaced fractures are considered for closed reductions, open reductions, or prosthetic replacement.

Two-part fractures involve displacement of one segment from the remaining group. The isolated greater tuberosity avulsion and surgical neck two-part fractures are more common. Two-part lesser tuberosity avulsion and isolated anatomic neck fractures are very rare. An isolated two-part fracture involving a tuberosity often accompanies a dislocation of the shoulder away from the tuberosity attachment. The innocent-appearing isolated greater tuberosity avulsion may accompany an anterior shoulder dislocation in which the dislocation has spontaneously reduced prior to the radiograph. If the tuberosity is in anatomic position, the fracture would be classified as a one-part fracture in this classification. If it displaced, it would be a two-part fracture. When isolated two-part lesser tuberosity fractures occur, a posterior dislocation should be taken for granted until accurate imaging studies can disprove it. The axillary view roentgenogram or CT scan are diagnostic.

Three-part fractures involve displacement of three major segments: the head, the shaft at the surgical neck, and one tuberosity. The muscle pull through the remaining intact tuberosity is unopposed, and the unimpacted articular surface rotates to face the avulsed tuberosity. For example, in a three-part greater tuberosity displaced fracture, the intact lesser tuberosity will rotate the head posteriorly. These fractures can be best visualized in the axillary or lateral scapular views, in which the articular surface faces posteriorly and the shaft is disengaged (Fig. 39–13). In the three-part lesser tuberosity displaced fracture, the intact greater tuberosity rotates the articular surface until it faces anteriorly. A rotator cuff tear usually occurs between the subscapularis and supraspinatus (Fig. 39–14). There are few reports of this relatively rare series of fractures, and unfortunately the cases are often mixed with cases involving other two-, three-, and four-part fracture patterns.[5,30,84,179,180,209,216,246]

In four-part displaced fractures, each major segment is displaced. The articular surface may be impacted on the upper shaft, displaced laterally, or dislocated anteriorly or posteriorly. The external rotators retract the greater tuberosity posteriorly and superiorly, or their combined force may retract the greater tuberosity posteriorly to the spinoglenoid notch at the base of the spine of the scapula. The lesser tuberosity is retracted anteromedially. The primary shaft-deforming force is the pectoralis major, which retracts the shaft medially.

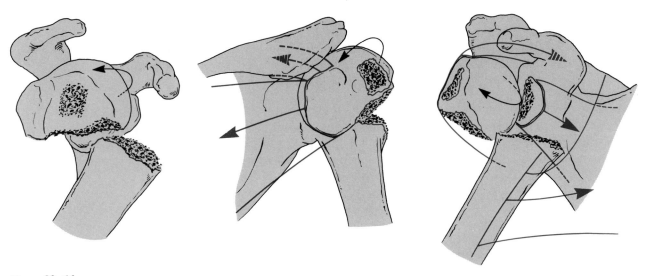

Figure 39–14

Three-part lesser tuberosity fracture. The intact spinati and teres minor attaching to the greater tuberosity rotate the articular segment anteriorly. The avulsed lesser tuberosity and displaced shaft no longer balance the head in neutral rotation. There is a rotator interval tear.

The rotator cuff tears at the interval between the supraspinatus and subscapularis (Fig. 39–15).

Thus the terminology is based on the fate of the major segments rather than on the number of fracture lines or mechanism of injury, with the exception of the articular surface. Articular impression fractures and head-splitting fractures are considered separately.

Fracture-dislocations refer to a loss of contact of the humeral head with the glenoid in association with articular surface impression fractures. Displaced two-, three-, or four-part fractures may accompany an anterior, posterior, or lateral dislocation of the articular surface. When the articular surface is a free fragment, manipulation of the arm can change it from any one of the positions to another. The significance of having separate categories for fractures and fracture-dislocations is that the latter generally involve more extensive damage outside the joint and have a greater potential for neurovascular injury.[32,159] The axillary artery and the brachial plexus cords and branches travel anteromedial to the glenohumeral joint. The axillary nerve passes immediately inferior to the glenohumeral joint capsule.

Posterior articular impression fractures, referred to as Hill-Sachs lesions,[92] occur with anterior glenohumeral dislocations. The posterior articular surface is crushed on the anterior glenoid rim. Similarly, anterior articular surface impression fractures, sometimes referred to as reverse Hill-Sachs lesions, result from the posterior glenoid rim compressing the anterior articular surface with a posterior, locked fracture-dislocation.

Head-splitting fractures may occur in the absence of a dislocation. The double articular contour seen on imaging studies is indicative of a more serious articular incongruence (Fig. 39–16).

Studies involving malunion of the greater tuberosity and malposition of the tuberosity from a varus surgical neck malunion indicate a need to more carefully evaluate these lesions.[105,199,200,202] The limit of 1-cm displacement or 45° angulation may be too generous for classifying the lesion as nondisplaced, especially when the tuberosity assumes a position superior to the articular surface when the arm is resting at the side. On elevation, the normally small clearance in the subacromial space, if compromised, leads to impingement and tearing of the rotator cuff. McLaughlin considered a 0.5-cm superior displacement of the greater tuberosity a significant lesion worthy of an open reduction.[159,160]

POTENTIAL DEFICIENCIES OF THE NEER CLASSIFICATION

In Neer's original classification,[179] group I fractures were categorized as nondisplaced and group II–VI fractures as displaced. Group II involved displacement of the anatomic neck, group III involved variations of the surgical neck fracture, group IV involved fractures of the greater tuberosity, group V those of the lesser tuberosity, and group VI involved fractures associated with dislocations. This classification combines two-, three-, and (potentially) four-part greater tuberosity fractures in group IV; similarly, in group V, the two-,

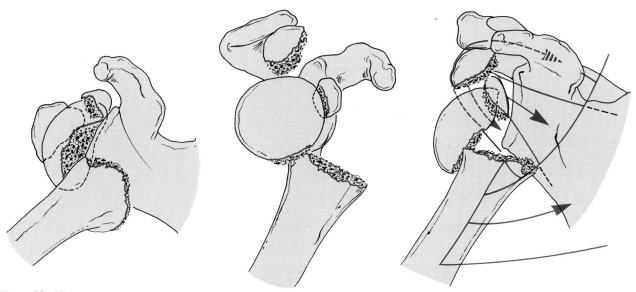

Figure 39–15

Four-part fracture. The shaft and tuberosities are displaced by their muscle attachments. The articular surface can be dislocated or subluxated in an anterior, posterior, inferior, or lateral direction, or it may be impacted on the upper shaft. Vascular supply to the articular surface is disrupted. A longitudinal tear is present between the subscapularis and supraspinatus.

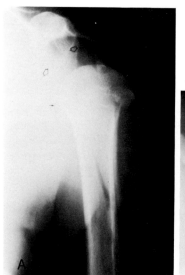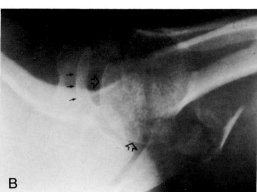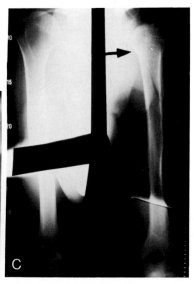

Figure 39-16

Head-splitting fracture. *A*, Anteroposterior roentgenogram. *B*, Axillary roentgenogram. The double articular contour is indicative of a displaced split of the humeral head. *C*, Scanograms permit determination of how much above a fixed point on the upper shaft the articular surface should rest in order to restore humeral length with proper deltoid tension.

three- and (potentially) four-part lesser tuberosity fractures are combined. In group VI, all fracture-dislocations, whether they are two-, three- or four-part and are associated with anterior or posterior dislocations, are combined. This would not be a problem if each of the segment classifications were noted when comparing results, but unfortunately many subsequent articles discussed results in terms of the overall groupings. For example, two-, three- and four-part fractures involving the greater tuberosity might all be discussed as group IV injuries.[30]

In subsequent revisions of the classification, Neer dropped the group I through VI listings that allowed authors to inappropriately combine two-, three-, and four-part fractures as one in their analyses.[183]

Jakob et al.[105] criticized the Neer classification for not having adequate subgroupings for detailed analysis and documentations. They argued that the displacement classification had not been established clinically or experimentally. For example, they were concerned that a valgus, impacted four-part fracture might have continued articular surface viability or acceptable function despite avascular necrosis. It did not have a separate category. Also, the classification of the displaced anatomic neck fracture did not emphasize the seriousness of the anticipated and almost universally disastrous complication of avascular necrosis. They proposed a fracture classification in keeping with the AO system used for other joints. In this classification there are 25 variables in nine groups that consider undisplaced fissure lines as significant components and

separate fractures into extracapsular or two segments (group A), partially intracapsular or three segments (group B), and intracapsular or four segments (group C). Each group includes a scaled subclassification from less to more serious lesions. While this new proposal would allow detailed study of many fractures and their variables, when compared with the Neer classification, it has not solved the issues raised. It is more confusing and difficult to use for the shoulder than the Neer system, which is presently the most logical classification as supported by the literature.

Bigliani[10] has expanded the Neer classification to include head-splitting and head impression fractures (Fig. 39-17). Outcome results of fracture treatment should be analyzed for each group separately; this will enable more meaningful comparison modalities.

Diagnosis

HISTORY

A detailed history should include items related to the patient's health and expectations and details of the injury. History of the former begins with the patient's age, sex, handedness, and occupation and how the injured extremity is used in daily life. A good understanding of the patient's general health (i.e., whether he or she has osteoporosis or any other metabolic disorder that might interfere with wound or fracture healing) is of critical importance. For example, in uremic bone disease from chronic renal dialysis, patients may develop

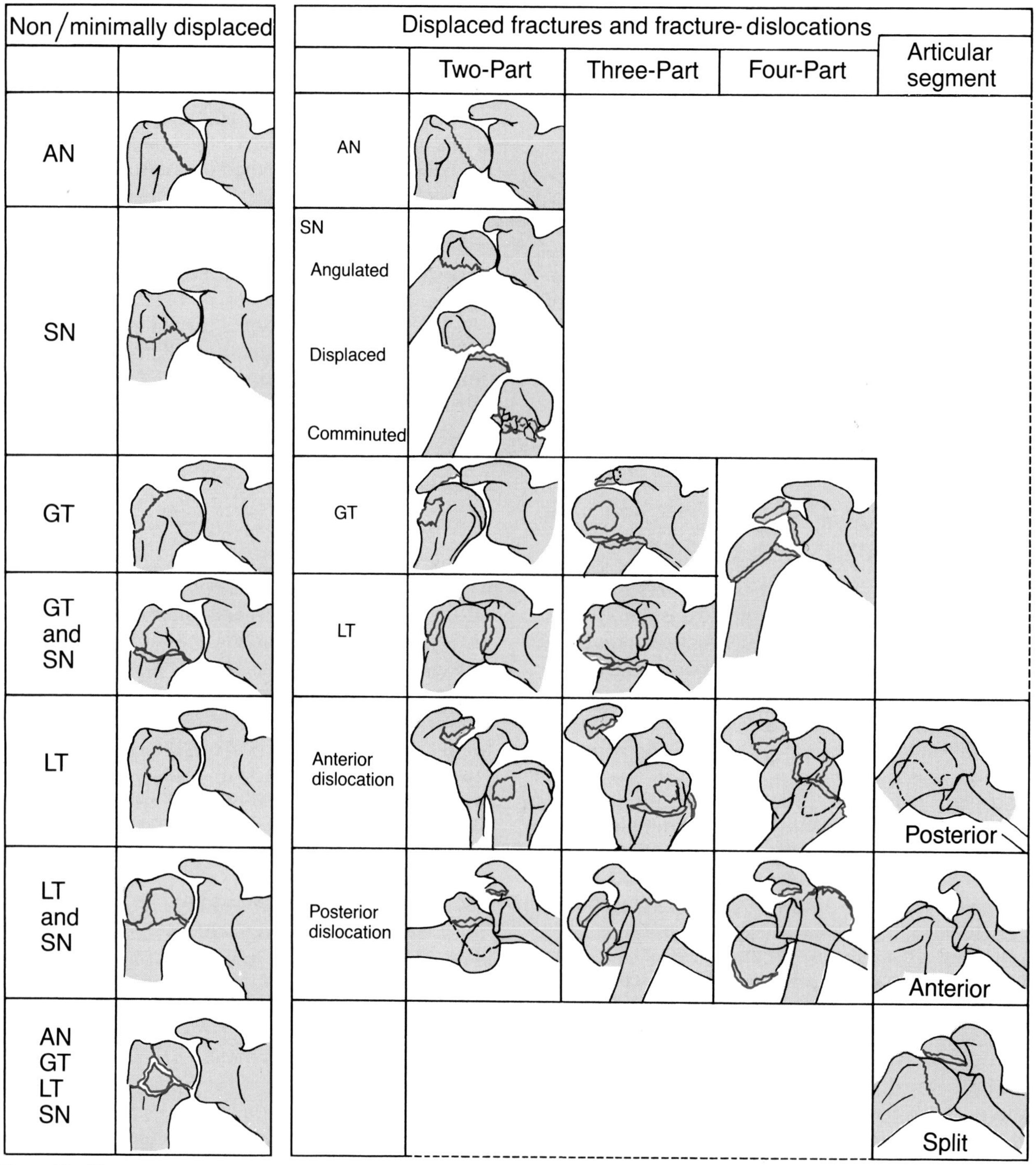

Non/minimally displaced		Displaced fractures and fracture-dislocations			
		Two-Part	Three-Part	Four-Part	Articular segment
AN		AN			
SN		SN Angulated Displaced Comminuted			
GT		GT			
GT and SN		LT			
LT		Anterior dislocation			Posterior
LT and SN		Posterior dislocation			Anterior
AN GT LT SN					Split

Figure 39-17

Four-part classification for fractures and fracture-dislocations. AN = anatomic neck; GT = greater tuberosity; LT = lesser tuberosity; SN = surgical neck.

aluminum intoxication, osteomalacia, and secondary hypoparathyroidism.[103] Those patients with seizure disorders who are on phenytoin commonly will have osteomalacia with more brittle, easily fragmented cortical bone at the time of fracture or internal fixation.

Such patients are more likely to have unilateral or even bilateral posterior fracture-dislocations of the shoulders, with or without other accompanying fractures. In addition, after age 50, osteoporosis increases in an exponential manner in women. This has serious implications in terms of whether screws or plates will hold in the softer, senile bone. Expectations regarding postoperative activities may also directly influence the type of treatment chosen.

An assessment of the psychologic well-being of the patient and his or her ability to understand and follow postoperative directions during a long and complicated rehabilitation, and an assessment of his or her motivation (specifically, the potential for self-destructive behavior, either consciously or unconsciously) are important to obtain at the initial setting.[205] If alterations to these assessments are necessary later in the course of treatment, then modifications as to the type of mobilization, supervised therapy, and necessary explicitness of directions required can be made.

In some patients, a previous shoulder injury may have occurred. A prior history of recurrent dislocations or chronic rotator cuff tear would complicate any new acute injury.

The mechanism of injury (i.e., whether the trauma was mild, moderate, or violent) is an important factor to combine with the physiologic status of the patient and the roentgenographic findings. The extent of vascular and neurologic compromise and the time of onset of these potentially rapidly deteriorating symptoms are essential to monitor frequently; otherwise, ischemia or a compartment syndrome may develop.

PHYSICAL EXAMINATION

To obtain a meticulous evaluation of all injured anatomic parts, they must be adequately visualized. A gown is placed above the breasts and below the shoulders for women; men are disrobed from the waist up. An examining table in the middle of the room permits evaluation of a seated patient from the front, the side, or behind. In the supine position, other muscles can be relaxed, and the patient can be made more comfortable during this portion of the evaluation.

In proximal humeral fractures, the deltoid and soft tissue may mask significant fracture displacement or dislocation. Swelling and ecchymosis will develop with time. By approximately 48 hours following injury, ecchymosis may extend down the chest wall or to the elbow in proximal fractures.

Other areas are evaluated prior to addressing the proximal humerus fracture. The cervical spine is assessed for any tenderness. If there is any question, cervical spine radiographs are obtained prior to any movement of this area. Direct tenderness over fresh or healing fractures has always been a useful clinical sign for the ribs, clavicle, acromion, and humerus and will often indicate the area of concern. Pain or tenderness

may be elicited indirectly with motion or with longitudinal compression or distraction.

The length of the arm from the posterior acromion to the olecranon tip is measured and compared with the opposite side. Any shortening is important to note both at this time and at the time of treatment. Scanograms provide an additional method of assessing shortening. Shortening between the deltoid origin and insertion is especially important to note. Maintenance of the length of the deltoid is essential if it is to function adequately along Starling's curve following fracture healing.

Neurovascular evaluation is carried out for all components of the upper extremity. Gentle motion and isometric contractures generally are sufficient to allow palpation of the muscle group contractions as a screening test for muscle integrity and nerve supply. In the absence of ipsilateral forearm and hand injuries, radial, median, and ulnar nerve function can be assessed without disturbance of the proximal humerus fracture.

An attempt is then made to evaluate the biceps, the triceps, the three divisions of the deltoid, the spinati, the pectoralis, the latissimus dorsi, and the trapezius muscles. Dermatomal sensory patterns are recorded, but unfortunately, the presence of sensibility in the axillary distribution in the lateral arm is not a reliable test for concomitant axillary motor function.[11]

Complicated injuries involving open fractures are splinted, and much of the evaluation that does not require the patient's subjective input or attempt to demonstrate muscle function can be delayed until the patient is taken to the operating room, where more complete evaluation is undertaken at the time of debridement.

It is important to remember that neurovascular injuries occur in 5% to 30% of complex fractures of the proximal humerus. Several helpful clinical signs in the evaluation of closed fractures include estimation of the stability of the fracture and whether there is a dislocation. With gentle longitudinal traction, damage to the neurovascular structures would not be anticipated. When the humerus is grasped at the elbow and the arm gently rotated, an assessment can be made as to whether the humeral head rotates with the shaft. With careful manipulation and longitudinal traction, crepitus is a common finding with a displaced or unstable fracture unless there is soft tissue muscle interposition. The lack of crepitus with a displaced fracture and the inability to obtain an accurate closed reduction suggest soft tissue interposition.

Dislocations of the shoulder are associated with visible or palpable depressions in the skin. With an anterior dislocation the head is anterior, medial, and inferior. A sulcus is palpable posteriorly and laterally beneath the

AP in scapular plane.

Arm supported in sling.

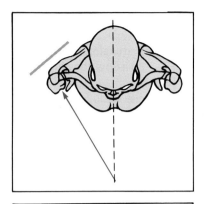

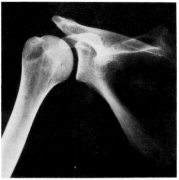

No overlap of head and glenoid.

Lateral in scapular plane.

Arm supported in sling.

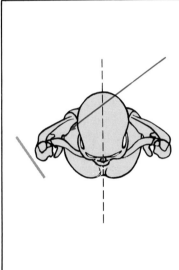

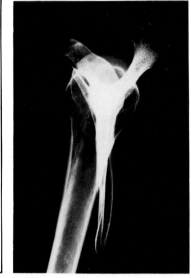

90° to AP.

Head in center of

Identify anterior and posterior displacement.

Identify greater tuberosity displacement.

Evaluate shape of acromion for etiology of impingement or cuff tears.

Emergency axillary.

Arm is gently abducted.

Tube at the hip.

Involved shoulder supported on pad.

Arm holds IV pole or is supported by assistant.

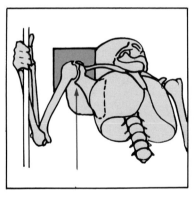

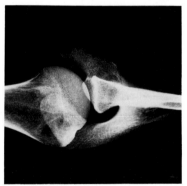

Evaluate glenoid for uneven wear or rim fractures.

Identify anterior and posterior dislocation.

Identify displaced tuberosities.

Identify unfused acromial epiphysis.

Figure 39–18

Trauma series views. (From Norris, T.R. In: Chapman, M.W.; Madison, M., eds. Operative Orthopaedics. Philadelphia, JB Lippincott, 1988, pp. 203–220.)

acromion. With posterior dislocations, the coracoid becomes prominent, and an anterior sulcus is present. The arm is usually held in adduction and internal rotation unless there is a concomitant fracture of the surgical neck or shaft. In the rare subspinus posterior dislocation, the arm is held in abduction.

In the standard posterior dislocation, there is fre-

quently a loss of forearm supination and an inability to externally rotate the arm. The axis of the humerus is directed posteriorly. There is a loss of rotation at 90° (or at maximal abduction if this is less than 90°).

Fracture-dislocations are less striking than the true dislocations. Any flattening or loss of contour is less than in true dislocations. The arm may hang in a more normal position at the side, but the head does not rotate with the remaining shaft of the humerus.

Early muscle atony with inferior subluxation of the humeral head is common and must be distinguished from an axillary nerve injury. EMG and nerve conduction studies at the time of injury may exclude prior injury and give a baseline for comparison two to three weeks later when the information used to assess the extent of nerve involvement is available.[11] Although sometimes difficult at the time of fracture, it is useful to evaluate both spinati, the three divisions of the deltoid, the musculocutaneous nerve, and the more distal radial, median, and ulnar nerves to determine whether deficits are the result of local nerve injury or of injury at the level of the brachial plexus.

Vascular evaluation is undertaken if vessel injury is suspected. An axillary artery injury is more rare than nerve injuries. Collateral circulation may mask arterial laceration or thrombosis,[33,34] and distal pulses may be intact. Clinical ischemia may be absent initially,[145] but an expanding hematoma suggests a vascular injury.

IMAGING

The glenohumeral articulation lies between the sagittal and coronal planes of the body. Five views are standardly used to evaluate this joint. These include three right-angle trauma series views in the plane of the scapula and anteroposterior (AP) views in internal and external rotation. Computerized tomography, three-dimensional reconstructions, additional plain radiographic imaging, arthrography, ultrasonography, and MRI all allow the shoulder injuries to be more fully defined.

Precise radiographs are critical to establishing an accurate diagnosis in shoulder trauma.[248] All too often injuries are missed with radiographs obtained in the plane of the body rather than in the plane of the scapula centered on the glenohumeral joint. Overlapping structures preclude full definition of the injuries. With advances in the understanding of the four-part classification system and what the orthopedist seeks for purposes of treatment, radiologists now seldom include the transthoracic lateral view.

Five Screening Roentgenographic Views

Trauma Series (Three Views)

The humeral articular surface relative to the glenoid and the relationship of the four segments to each other are defined in three-dimensional space with three right-angle trauma series views (Fig. 39–18).[183,198] These views are taken in the sagittal, coronal, and axial scapular planes rather than in the sagittal plane of the body. The scapular AP view centered on the glenohumeral joint is a 30° posterior oblique view. The joint space is defined clearly without overlap of the head and glenoid in the absence of subluxation or dislocation.

Figure 39–19

Examples of pathologic findings seen with rotational anteroposterior views following an anterior dislocation and reduction. *A*, Internal rotation; Hill-Sachs posterolateral humeral head impression fracture. *B*, External rotation; the greater tuberosity is missing from its normal location on the humerus following a displaced two-part greater tuberosity fracture and anterior dislocation.

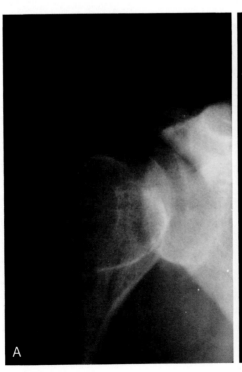
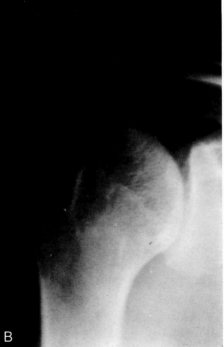

This is in contradistinction to the AP rotational views taken in the sagittal plane of the body. Alternate views for posterior head displacement are taken between 30° and 45° posterior oblique, with a 45° to 60° caudal angulation.[65,123,255]

Rotational AP Views (Two Views)

When the head moves with the shaft, particularly in late cases of nonunion or malunion, the internal and external rotational views in the anteroposterior plane supplement the three-view trauma series to comprise the five standard screening views recommended for routine shoulder evaluations (Fig. 39–19). The AP in internal rotation and the Stryker notch[78] are the two projections most likely to demonstrate a posterolateral humeral head impression fracture.

In the external rotation view the greater tuberosity is normally seen. When it is absent, the axillary view is mandatory to locate the large avulsions that are retracted by both spinati toward the base of the scapular spine. This fragment may be difficult to appreciate on the AP because of superimposition with the humeral head.

Overpenetrated rotational AP and lateral scapular views will locate calcium deposits. Occasionally a rotator cuff avulsion with a small fragment of tuberosity can be confused with a calcium deposit (Fig. 39–20).

Anteroposterior views in the sagittal plane of the body do not adequately demonstrate posteromedial displacement, and a posterior fracture-dislocation is

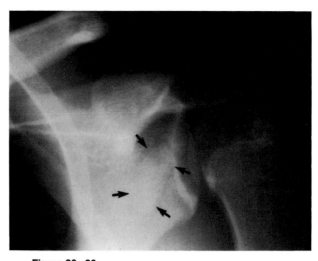

Figure 39-20

Isolated lesser tuberosity fracture with medial retraction.

frequently missed.[38,53,71,86] Overlap of the head and glenoid is expected in the AP view taken in the sagittal plane of the body, but it is indicative of a posterior dislocation or fracture-dislocation in the view taken in the sagittal plane of the scapula (Fig. 39–21). All variations of either AP view adequately demonstrate an anterior dislocation and anterior shaft displacement, but the tuberosity positions may not be as well defined.

The lateral scapular view is taken at right angles to the scapular AP view; thus at a 60° anterior oblique angle, the view parallels the scapular spine. The head

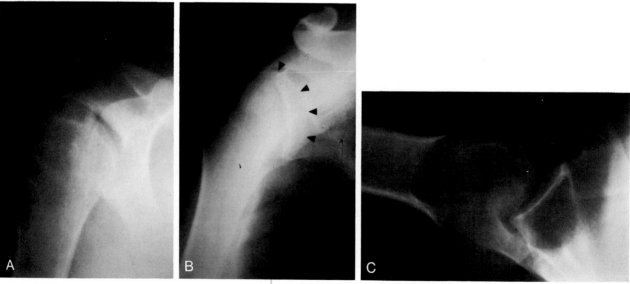

Figure 39-21

Anteroposterior roentgenograms. *A*, In sagittal plane of the body (missed posterior dislocation). *B*, In sagittal plane of the scapula, overlap of the head and glenoid indicates a dislocation. *C*, Axillary or CT views are the best views with which to diagnose a posterior dislocation or fracture-dislocation.

overlaps the glenoid evenly and entirely to sit in the center of the Y formed by the scapular spine and coracoid superiorly and the scapular body inferiorly in the normal view (Fig. 39–22). In this projection, an anterior dislocation is easily appreciated. More information is added as to tuberosity and shaft displacement. The larger avulsed greater tuberosity fragments that overlap the head in the AP views are usually distinguishable posteriorly. Slight scapular malpositioning leads to confusion when defining the status of the humeral head. Use of fluoroscopy in positioning the patient enables an inexperienced technician to superimpose the axillary and vertebral borders of the scapula. Once superimposed, the head will be centered on the glenoid in a normal shoulder. Posterior prominence suggests a posterior fracture-dislocation.

In three-part fractures involving the surgical neck and one tuberosity, the head will point to the side of the avulsed tuberosity. This can be distinguished on the lateral scapular and axillary views but not as well on the AP view.

The axillary roentgenograph is the most useful in assessing the humeral head and glenoid relationships. Although anterior dislocations can easily be distinguished in the AP and lateral scapular views, subluxations, fracture-dislocations, and dislocations in the posterior direction are more subtle. The axial view is more

difficult to obtain[60] but will avoid missing less common but equally debilitating injuries.

The axillary view and specific modifications are the best views with which to evaluate the articular surface of the humeral head and glenoid. Cystic defects in the humeral head and glenoid[234] and fractures of the coracoid base, distal clavicle, and acromion are also well visualized in the axial projections. In acute trauma, an assisted axillary view is obtained with gentle longitudinal traction applied at the elbow and abduction between 25° and 50° in the coronal plane of the scapula. The radiographic plate is placed at the top of the shoulder to the neck and often is steadied by the patient's opposite hand. The tube at the hip is directed cephalad and medial, with enough scapula visualized to determine accurate glenoid version, to adequately depict humeral head articular and glenoid rim fractures, and to appreciate any subluxations or dislocations. The patient can be supine and hold an intravenous (IV) pole[71,198] or can be positioned on the opposite, uninjured side (see Figs. 39–18 and 39–21C).[131,219]

Other axillary modifications include the West Point axillary view to visualize the anteroinferior glenoid rim and the Bloom-Obata[10a] apical axillary view for posterior head displacement (Fig. 39–23). Anterior rim fractures or ectopic calcification in many anteroinferior labral detachments with instability can be delin-

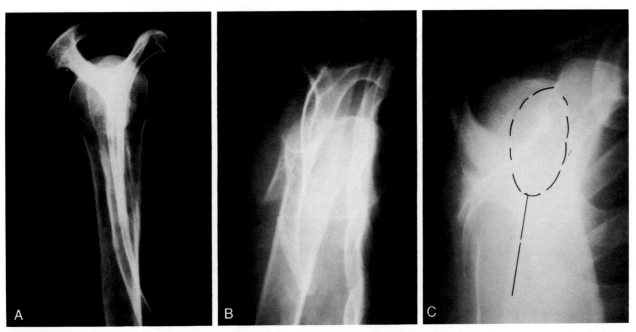

Figure 39–22

A, Lateral or scapular Y views. The humeral head is centered on the glenoid located at the junction of the coracoid process, scapular spine, and scapular body. *B*, In an anterior dislocation with two-part surgical neck fracture and axillary nerve palsy, the humeral head is anterior to the glenoid in a subcoracoid position. *C*, In a posterior fracture-dislocation, more of the head is posterior to the glenoid at the center of the scapular Y formed by the coracoid process and the body and spine of the scapula. Slight scapular rotation makes diagnosis by this view alone difficult.

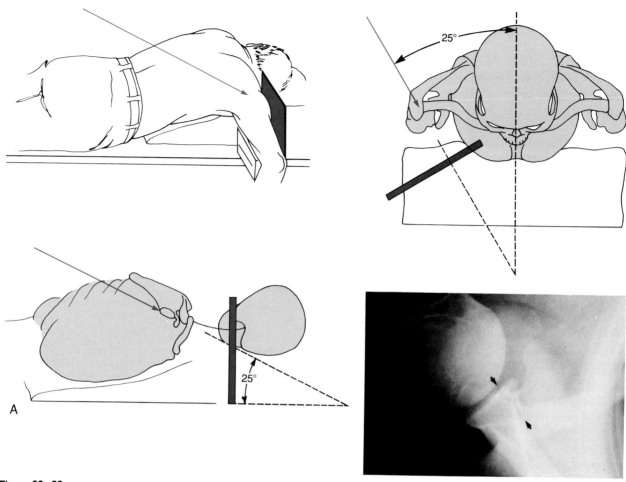

Figure 39–23

West Point axillary view to visualize the anteroinferior glenoid rim for evidence of a labral detachment of rim fracture. *A,* Roentgenographic evaluation. *B,* Anteroinferior rim fracture following anterior dislocation.

eated with the West Point axillary view or, alternatively, the Cuello supine axillary view with the arm in external rotation.[195,219]

The Bloom-Obata apical oblique view is specifically for defining whether there is a posterior dislocation or fracture-dislocation. No manipulation of the arm is necessary, but an elderly patient often has trouble leaning backward over the x-ray table and cassette during the positioning.

Low-dose CT scans now offer the most accurate method for evaluation of complex proximal humeral fractures. When CT scans and standard radiographs were compared, CT scans were superior in assessing the location of fracture lines, displacement of fracture fragments relative to their normal position, rotation of the humeral articular surface, and fractures of both the glenoid and the humeral head.[27,168,195,198,205] In Castagno et al.'s study, CT findings altered the treatment method in 15 of 17 patients.[27] Nine showed no significant displacement and therefore were treated by closed

means when by plain radiographs the fractures were judged to be displaced or intermediate.[27] In six of the remaining eight patients undergoing surgery, unsuspected abnormalities guided the type of surgical treatment. In their study, the craniocaudal displacement was not as well demonstrated as the horizontal displacement when these views were reconstructed in the axial plane. CT is superior to MRI in depicting bony detail (Table 39–1).

CT with contrast is more comprehensive than regular arthrotomography. It is ideal for evaluating Hill-Sachs defects[50] and labral detachments at the glenoid rim.[166]

OTHER STUDIES

Three-Dimensional Reconstruction

Three-dimensional (3D) reconstruction from CT scans is now available in many hospitals. This allows the radiologist and orthopedist to rotate the fractures in

Table 39–1.

Common Uses for CT

Nondisplaced fracture
Greater or lesser tuberosity displacement
Four-part fracture
Posterior fracture-dislocation
Avascular necrosis with collapse
Tuberosity malunion
Glenoid version evaluation
Loose bodies

any direction and review in real time the position and displacement of any fractures or fracture-dislocations. If clarification is desired, nonessential structures such as the ribs or scapula can be eliminated from the screen. This technique gives the treating surgeon an unparalleled opportunity to make an accurate diagnosis and plan for reconstruction.

The uncompressed CT tape can also be used to generate three-dimensional plastic models with the assistance of a numerically controlled milling machine (Cemax). These models are of more use in reconstructive cases where there is fracture malunion or abnormal and eccentric wear of the glenoid (Fig. 39–24).[196–198,203,204]

Evaluation of Concomitant Rotator Cuff Tears

If there is wide displacement of one tuberosity from the other, then a rotator interval cuff tear is assumed to have occurred. With dislocations of the shoulder in patients older than 40 years, avulsion of either the subscapularis or external rotators is most common. 3D imaging studies to evaluate these injuries include ultrasonography, arthrography, and MRI. Ultrasonography is presently the least expensive; no radiation is employed, and the other shoulder can still be compared. However, it is still a test that is operator dependent, with a steep learning curve for the ultrasonographer. It and magnetic resonance imaging may both miss the smaller cuff tears less than 1 cm in size.

Arthrography is still the gold standard with which to determine whether there is a full-thickness cuff tear or an incomplete tear on the articular side. It is not as helpful as the clinical examination or MRI in evaluating the size of the tear.

In trauma care, MRI is used in the evaluation of soft tissue lesions of the rotator cuff and of neurovascular injuries involving the brachial plexus and axillary artery and in the assessment of osteonecrosis following trauma, with or without open reduction and internal fixation. Osteonecrosis may not be appreciated on plain films for up to two to four years, but with MRI it

Figure 39–24

Three-part fracture with malunion of the greater tuberosity and loss of humeral length by scanograms. *A*, Anteroposterior roentgenogram showing varus malunion. *B*, Three-dimensional reconstruction confirms varus malunion through the upper shaft, inferior subluxation of the humeral head, and poor position of the greater tuberosity directly over the humeral shaft. Late prosthetic reconstruction required bipolar osteotomy of the greater tuberosity and repositioning lower than the articular surface and more laterally in a more normal location. See Reference No. 203.

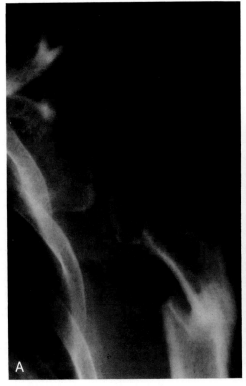

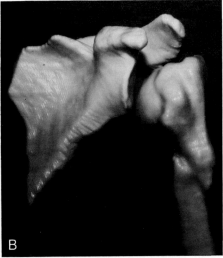

can be seen prior to any changes visualized on the plain roentgenograms. (How much earlier these changes are visible on MRI is not known.)

One advantage of MRI over other studies is that there is no ionizing radiation. Disadvantages include the expense and the fact that bone imaging for fractures is not as clear. Patients who are claustrophobic will have difficulty with MRI and CT examinations. In most settings, premedications can relieve the anxiety associated with the process. Patients who weigh 300 pounds or more may not fit in the scanners.

Fluoroscopy

Fluoroscopy is rarely used but has distinct advantages in positioning the patient for roentgenograms, in determining motion at a delayed union or nonunion site, and in evaluating stability in those cases where the degree of stability is the determining factor for open reduction and internal fixation.

Arteriography and Venography

Arteriography and venography are performed in those patients in whom serious arterial or venous injury is suspected. It is especially helpful in evaluating a nonunion at the surgical neck secondary to a pseudoaneurysm of the axillary artery with dissolution of the medial cortex at the fracture site.[261]

EMG and Nerve Conduction Studies

EMG and nerve conduction studies are appropriate to distinguish old injuries from fresh injuries. They also supplement the clinical examination when pain and fracture instability may preclude an adequate evaluation. The incidence of nerve injury related to proximal humeral fractures and dislocations is much higher than clinically appreciable, although many of these resolve in the early postinjury period.

Essential Studies to Rule Out Other Injuries

Additional studies depend on the clinical presentation of the injury and the ability to diagnose it with the clinical examination and the original imaging studies. There is great variation among observers when interpreting plain roentgenograms of proximal humeral fractures.[128] Suspected injuries include neurovascular and soft tissue injuries and tendon disruptions in the shoulder region. The invasive and noninvasive studies available for these structures have been outlined previously. Other injuries may occur to the head, cervical spine, thorax, or abdomen, especially following severe trauma such as motor vehicle accidents. Scapular fractures, with or without proximal humeral fractures, are frequently associated with other more central and much more serious injuries. A multidisciplined approach in the evaluation of each of these areas is necessary when any additional injuries are suspected. For example, after a serious fall or motor vehicle accident, a patient with neck pain or suspected neurologic injury should have screening lateral cervical spine and swimmer's view films performed to ensure that there is no unstable fracture-dislocation in this region.

DIFFERENTIAL DIAGNOSIS

Differential diagnosis of proximal humeral fractures includes muscle contusion or sprain, rupture of the rotator cuff, dislocation of the shoulder in the absence of fracture, brachial plexus injury, infection, disruption of the axillary artery, and thrombosis of the axillary vein. Imaging studies combined with the history and physical examination enable differentiation of these injuries.

Management

There has been an evolution in the management of fractures of the proximal humerus. One must define the structural changes, perform an adequate neurologic and vascular evaluation, rule out occult infection or tumor, and assess the patient's overall medical and psychological status (i.e., the ability to undergo treatment and rehabilitation procedures that are appropriate for the injury).

The realization that a poor initial result is very difficult to later reconstruct makes the comminuted fracture of the proximal humerus a potentially difficult fracture to treat.[34] Bony and soft tissue anatomy must be restored early for unstable or displaced fractures and rotator cuff tears.

Options for treatment include a sling with early motion; closed reduction; humeral head excision with or without rotator cuff repair[110,111,185]; primary arthrodesis; external fixation; closed pinning; open reduction and internal fixation with sutures, intramedullary devices, plates, screws, staples, or pins; and prosthetic arthroplasty. In general, closed reduction is possible for two-part fractures at the surgical neck unless soft tissue interposition precludes it. Open reduction and internal fixation are used for two- and three-part fractures, and prosthetic replacement is used for four-part fractures and for three-part fractures in osteoporotic patients.

Fifty percent to eighty percent of proximal humeral fractures are nondisplaced or minimally displaced and stable.[105,179,180] These fractures are held together with the periosteum and rotator cuff and are splinted by the long head of the biceps tendon. Adequate imaging studies should be obtained to ensure that a minimally displaced fracture is not an occult fracture-dislocation, that the greater tuberosity displacement is less than 0.5 cm, and that the articular surface is intact. Given these circumstances, treatment consists of a sling to support these fractures and assist in supporting any transient inferior subluxation that often occurs. Early range of motion to prevent adhesions and stiffness resulting from scarring of tendons, joint capsule, and bursa is begun as pain and stability allow.[21,31,46,64]

Unimpacted fractures at the surgical neck are not held together by the rotator cuff. These are protected with a sling with the arm at the side to relax the deforming force of the pectoralis major until the head and shaft rotate in unison. Then gentle pendulum exercises may be added until there is sufficient strength in the union to allow progressive exercises. These fractures are at special risk for further displacement and disabling nonunions when treated with distraction, when exercises forcing rotation are begun too early, or when manipulations are used to treat an anticipated frozen shoulder.

Displaced fractures block motion, result in weakness, and may cause persistent disabling pain.[182] Displaced fractures at the surgical neck may be adequately treated with closed reduction, assuming there is no interposition of soft tissue and the reduction can be maintained. Fractures at the tuberosity level treated closed have had disappointing results.[66,165,246] Abduction casts and splints to bring the distal fragment to the proximal one are not recommended. The intact rotator cuff does not abduct the head. The subscapularis anteriorly and the infraspinatus and teres minor posteriorly prevent head abduction unless the distal shaft eccentrically engages the head. These theoretic understandings fail to take into account the more important pectoralis major and latissimus dorsi, which pull the shaft anteriorly and medially. This deforming force is increased with abduction (Fig. 39–25).[26,183] Furthermore, abduction casts can be heavy, uncomfortable, and prevent early assisted motion. Additional deforming forces are added as the arm extends posteriorly when the patient is supine.[46,56,99,191]

The weight of the arm alone provides 10 to 15 pounds of distraction force, which can be supported by a sling or collar and cuff to reduce and maintain the fracture position.[46] A hanging arm cast giving additional distraction has been successfully used by several physicians.[23,24,97,99,257] Unfortunately, this requires some fine tuning. In many patients the heavy hanging arm cast has overly distracted the fracture sight and

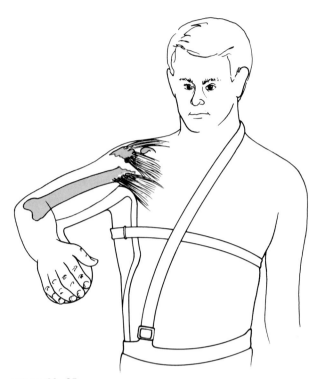

Figure 39–25

Deforming forces of the pectoralis with arm in abduction. The pectoralis pulls the humeral shaft toward the chest while displacing the fracture at the surgical neck.

given an increased lever arm at the apex of the fracture, thus increasing the likelihood of malunion or nonunion.[90,183] At this level the arm is difficult to immobilize with casts coming up only to the fracture site.

Traction, overhead or at the side, with olecranon pin fixation for surgical neck fractures[24,117] is reserved for comminuted upper shaft fractures in which patients are confined to bed with multiple other injuries. Neviaser[191] preferred adduction and flexion of the arm, whereas Callahan[25,26] proposed keeping the arm at the side for epiphyseal fractures; abduction was specifically avoided.[179]

With improvements in instrumentation and fracture care, olecranon pin traction has largely been abandoned and replaced with external fixators,[125,126,130] closed pinning,[126,141,153] open external fixation,[239] or intramedullary rods placed antegrade using open techniques or retrograde using semiclosed means.[80,210]

Open reduction and internal fixation has been advocated for displaced fractures or fracture-dislocations in which closed reductions have not been stable or successful. Many internal fixation techniques have been employed, including nonabsorbable sutures, wire loops, simple screws, staples, blade plates, AO buttress plates, Kirschner wires, Steinmann pins, Mouridian rods, Rush rods, Ender rods, and combinations of these.[52,70,77,84,90,99,110,111,118,120,124,135,163,164,171,172,179,180,185,194,198-200,229,241,244] Some series present a high risk of complications, with unacceptable reductions as high as 16%; residual hardware impingement, 15.6%; infection, 12.5%; avascular necrosis, 12.5%; and hardware loosening requiring removal, 6%.[124] In Kristiansen's study,[124] only 45% of the patients followed for two to seven years had an excellent or satisfactory result, whereas 55% had an unsatisfactory or poor result. Unfortunately, many studies comparing the results of treatment combine all levels of fractures, thereby precluding meaningful interpretation as to how well a particular type of fracture responded to a certain treatment.

Fracture type and bone quality may dictate the type of treatment because of the higher incidence of avascular necrosis following the extensive stripping and dissection necessary with the use of AO buttress plates and the poor ability of osteoporotic bone to hold screws. Sturzenegger et al.[244] have suggested "minimal osteosynthesis" with simple screws and tension bands in an effort to avoid the extensive stripping needed for plate fixation and the attendant risks to the remaining blood supply. Avascular necrosis occurred in 34% of their patients in whom plate fixation was used for three- and four-part fractures. With fracture reduction and fixation, all efforts are taken to preserve the arcuate artery ascending the lateral aspect of the biceps groove from the anterior circumflex artery.[68,132]

Complications of open reduction and internal fixation include malunion, nonunion, and avascular necrosis[199,200] leading to a painful, stiff shoulder. Other complications include arthritis secondary to screw penetration of the joint, varus surgical neck nonunion with greater tuberosity entrapment, valgus malunion secondary to an overly tight tension band, and a refracture after manipulation under anesthesia for residual stiffness. Neer[179,180] reported a 75% incidence of avascular necrosis in four-part fractures treated with open reduction and internal fixation. Hagg and Lundberg[77] reported only 35% good or excellent results following open reduction and internal fixation of three- and four-part fractures. Both closed and open reductions resulted in poor motion. Avascular necrosis is noted to occur up to three-and-a-half years following the injury, thus indicating that long-term follow-up is necessary.[137]

Isolated reports have indicated that open reduction and internal fixation of four-part fractures are a predictable means of treating these injuries without avascular necrosis. In reviewing these reports, however, either the preoperative radiographs demonstrated that a tuberosity was still attached,[33] or the postoperative report did not include ranges of motion, an estimation of

pain, or an assessment of return of function.[137] These will be considered further in the section on complications. The goal of any open reduction and internal fixation is to restore enough stability so that the fracture can heal; to allow early motion; and to avoid stiffness, hardware complications, and late avascular necrosis.

The value of prosthetic replacement is increasingly recognized for establishing early stability for the more comminuted or complicated proximal humeral fractures.[55,129,175-178,182,185,187,198,203,217,237,249,253,254]

CURRENT ALGORITHM

Between 50% and 80% of fractures of the proximal humerus are nondisplaced or minimally displaced. No reduction is necessary. A sling for support is used early, and gentle pendulum exercises are begun as tolerated by the patient. Special care is taken to avoid strong passive exercises that might displace a fracture that would otherwise go on to uncomplicated healing. Some stiffness is anticipated, and therefore the balance between mobilization and protection should be kept in mind.

An algorithm for displaced fractures requires that individual decisions be based on the medical health of the patient, the quality of the bone and its ability to hold fixation if internal fixation is anticipated, and the overall ability of the patient to cooperate with the necessary postoperative rehabilitation. Some patients will respond to specific instructions, whereas others need immobilization that cannot be removed in the early healing periods if compliance is a serious issue.[205]

In general, fractures that can be treated with closed reduction do not include large tears of the rotator cuff or greater tuberosity avulsions. Fractures that can be treated with open reduction require assessment and then protection of any remaining blood supply to the humeral head. Prosthetic replacement is preferred for three-part fractures in osteoporotic patients, for all four-part fractures, and for head-splitting fractures. Fractures with dislocations are indicative of additional soft tissue and, possibly, neurovascular injury (Fig. 39–26).

SPECIAL CONSIDERATIONS FOR POLYTRAUMA PATIENTS

Fractures of the proximal humerus may be associated with other multiple joint injuries, combined injuries of the shaft and proximal humerus, neurovascular injuries, or more central injuries to the body. Those associated with forearm fractures have a higher incidence of nerve injury within that extremity than do isolated

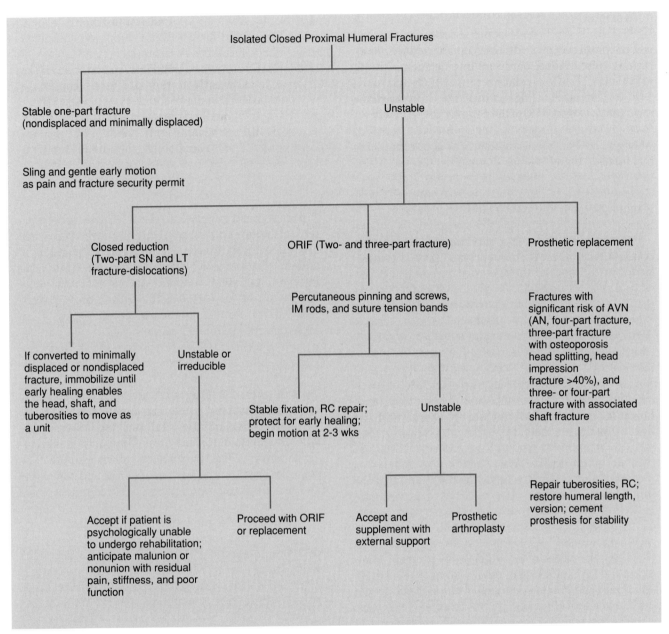

Figure 39–26

Algorithm for isolated closed proximal humeral fractures. AN = anatomic neck; AVN = avascular necrosis; IM = intramedullary; LT = lesser tuberosity; ORIF = open reduction and internal fixation; RC = rotator cuff; SN = surgical neck.

proximal humerus fractures alone. Proximal humeral fractures resulting from falls from a height or from motor vehicle accidents not infrequently have associated head, cervical spine, chest, or abdominal injuries.

Proximal humeral fractures may be splinted during evaluation of other injuries to prevent additional injury. Chest injuries involving rib fractures associated with a pneumothorax and abdominal injuries involving ruptures of the spleen take priority in definitive treatment. Injuries of the cervical spine, if unstable, should be treated operatively or placed in protective halo traction.

Head injuries are associated with an increased incidence of myositis ossificans in the region of the extremity fracture. These regions should be stabilized and any additional bleeding into the soft tissues prevented to lessen this incidence. Heterotopic ossification may be asymptomatic or associated with mild pain and decreased range of motion.[15]

When there are associated nerve or vascular injuries, reduction of any dislocations and operative stabilization of unstable fractures permit early repair of the neurovascular structures. Fractures should be stabilized first. The management of fractures associated with nerve injuries is still controversial. An adequate screening examination of any neurologic deficit is important prior to fracture manipulation for a closed reduction. If the fracture is open, then the nerve can be explored at the time of wound debridement and fracture stabilization. With multiple injuries to the same extremity, to both humeri, or to other areas, stabilization of proximal humeral fractures simplifies the care and permits earlier mobilization. It would be difficult to splint the arm to the chest wall in a patient with a flail chest, as such splinting would interfere with ventilation and care of the chest injury.

The AO/ASIF group has advocated stable internal fixation for displaced intraarticular fractures.[229] Although the necessity for immaculate repair of these fractures is seldom questioned, an attitude of benign neglect still abounds with regard to major fractures of the glenohumeral joint.[34] In high-energy fractures of the proximal humerus associated with other serious injuries, the proximal humerus is often overlooked or neglected.[231] These fractures do not do well with this form of care.[7,33,34,152,224,231,241,249] Open reduction and internal fixation are recommended for open fractures with nerve injuries, any fractures with vascular injuries, bilateral injuries, and fractures into the joint. Proximal humeral fractures are often overlooked or confused with brachial plexus injuries; therefore imaging procedures should be undertaken and should be of sufficient quality to obtain the information desired concerning fractures and dislocations. Alternative forms of treatment for the multiple trauma patient include external fixation,[238] temporary external fixation prior to delayed open reduction and internal fixation,[93] and prosthetic replacement. Excision of the humeral head, with or without repair of the rotator cuff, and primary arthrodesis of the shoulder have little role in acute fracture care.

There are three levels of priorities in the treatment of polytrauma patients:

1. Acute care: airway, head, chest, abdomen, spine stabilization.

2. Proximal extremity fixation: open reduction and internal fixation of shaft and proximal humerus fractures with brachial plexus injury.[19]

3. Distal fractures: joint reconstruction may benefit from complex imaging studies prior to surgery.

Open fractures have been classified by Gustilo et al.[75,76] as follows:

Type I: Wound <1 cm long, clean.
Type II: Wound >1 cm, no extensive soft tissue damage, flaps, or avulsion.
Type III: Open segmental fracture, extensive soft tissue damage, traumatic amputations.
   IIIA: Adequate soft tissue coverage despite high-energy open fracture.
   IIIB: Extensive soft tissue stripping and wound contamination, high-velocity gunshot wound or farming accident.
   IIIC: Open fracture with vascular injury requiring repair.

Management begins with debridement, prophylactic antibiotics, temporary external fixation (when soft tissue injury precludes initial internal fixation)[238] and delayed soft tissue closure. When soft tissue healing permits, then internal fixation is undertaken. Bone grafting in the proximal humerus is recommended for delayed union or nonunion at 10 to 16 weeks.[75,76,238]

INDIVIDUAL TREATMENT PROCEDURES

Treatment for fractures of the proximal humerus may be broadly grouped in the categories listed in Table 39–2. There are many general considerations as to the type of treatment deemed most effective for a particular patient and the "personality" of the fracture. The activities, health, and wishes of the patient, the risks and benefits of treatment, and the effectiveness of the

Table 39–2.
Treatment Options for Fractures of the Proximal Humerus

Sling
Closed reduction and sling
   Coaptation splints
   Hanging arm cast
Percutaneous pinning
External fixation
Open reduction and internal fixation
   Sutures or wires — simple repair or tension band fixation
   Intramedullary rods
      Rush
      Ender
      Mouridian nail
      Humeral locking nail
   Tension band and intramedullary Ender rods
   Screws
   Plates and screws
Prosthetic arthroplasty

possible treatment methods are important considerations. The surgeon should be familiar with the specialized techniques of shoulder surgery and its prolonged aftercare. Some fractures are difficult to treat in the acute setting with operative reconstruction using either fixation or prosthetic arthroplasty. However, they are much more difficult to treat with subsequent surgery because of subacromial, capsular, and muscular scarring; fixed retractions of the tuberosities and rotator cuff; fracture malunion, malrotation, or angulation; osteonecrosis of the humeral head, often associated with progressive rotator cuff contracture; and possible damage to the brachial plexus. An early reduction without repeated manipulations is preferable to avoid heterotopic ossification. A surgery that has a high incidence of failure should not be used when a safer or more predictable procedure can be done acutely.

Any vascular compromise requires immediate evaluation and treatment with fracture stabilization. Vascular repair or grafting can then proceed expeditiously without risk of disruption by an unstable fracture.

Preoperative planning and preparation require an assessment of the patient's health, a neurovascular examination, and a definition of the potentially injured structures. This neurovascular evaluation may be supplemented with EMG and nerve conduction studies, Doppler sonograms, or arteriograms. Imaging studies should be made in at least three planes to determine fracture classification, fracture stability, and potential tears of the rotator cuff. CT or MRI scans supplementing the routine studies add more clarification to the diagnosis, thereby assisting in the decision of whether to operate and in planning for a repair.[168] The type of repair required will depend on whether there is an open or closed fracture and the type of fracture. A full assortment of plates, screws, intramedullary rods, and prostheses should be available in the operating room, as the type of treatment may change intraoperatively (e.g., when internal fixation is not secure or when additional fractures are displaced during the operation). For most cases, general anesthesia is preferred. However, a closed reduction can be undertaken using midazolam hydrochloride and intravenously or intramuscularly administered pain medication. If general anesthesia is precluded for health reasons in an elderly patient, the operation can be done with an intrascalene block.[18,35] However, this is contraindicated when a patient has a suspected neurologic injury preoperatively. It is also more difficult for the surgeon to test the patient's neurologic status in the early postoperative period following regional anesthesia. Good muscle relaxation by block or general anesthesia is especially important in a patient with a dislocation combined with a nondis-

placed fracture. Full muscle relaxation with an open technique lessens the likelihood of displacement of the fracture with the manipulation required for reduction of the dislocation.

Contraindications to surgery include poor patient health, patient wishes, or the surgeon's unfamiliarity with both the procedures required and the treatment of their complications.

General Considerations and Operative Approaches

Open fractures require immediate debridement and, if possible, fixation. If these are delayed for reasons of extensive contamination, then treatment for infection and secondary wound closure may be necessary. This does not preclude intramedullary internal fixation prior to wound closure.[247]

There are reports of an increase in the incidence of myositis ossificans with delay in treatment. Schatzker and Tile advised avoiding surgery on the third to seventh day following injury.[229] Neer noted an increased incidence after three weeks following fracture. However, in practice, the specific observations are only estimates of an increased incidence of myositis. The risks of myositis are present following any displaced fracture or dislocation. Adequate stabilization diminishes further soft tissue injury. The fractures should be stabilized as soon as the patient is medically clear and a surgeon with experience in treating these fractures is available.

A Gelfoam mattress is placed on the operating table. The patient is positioned supine in a semi-fowler's or beach chair position unless only a posterior surgical approach is anticipated. Then the lateral decubitus position is selected, and the McConnell body positioning frame is employed. The upper section of the table is replaced with a McConnell gel-padded headrest (Fig. 39–27) that is adjusted to protect the cervical spine in slight flexion and approximately 10° of deviation to the opposite side. This gives more exposure superiorly in the region of the neck. The patient is positioned to the side of the table to enable the arm to be extended off the edge. The scapula is padded forward with a gel bolster. Potential pressure points to the skin and nerves are padded. Eye cups or a narrow gel pad are placed over the taped eyes. A towel is then wrapped around the head to exclude the hair and anesthesia tubes from the operative field. Additional gel pads are wrapped around the opposite elbow and both heels and placed under the opposite wrist as the opposite arm is tucked into the side. If there is a possibility that bone grafts in addition to what is available in the local field of surgery

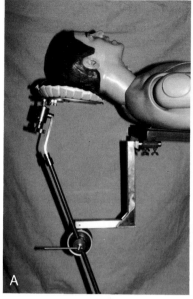

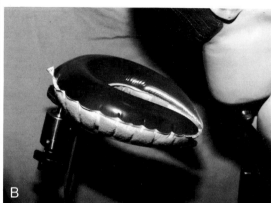

Figure 39-27

A, McConnell headrest. The headrest is adjusted and can be positioned through a series of universal joints to protect the cervical spine. *B*, The gel pads provide secure fixation with minimal, evenly distributed pressure holding the head and neck.

may be necessary, then the two potential donor sites are the ribs and the iliac crest. All areas for potential surgery are degreased with alcohol and a skin degreaser, Freon (made by Miller-Stephenson). Adherent Steri-drapes seal the head and neck to the headrest and a U-shaped Steri-drape beginning under the axilla with the tails upward permits full exposure from the base of the neck as far anterior, posterior, and inferior as necessary. If bone graft from a rib is anticipated, the U-shaped Steri-drape is lowered in a male or a separate area is prepped for a concealed inframammary incision in a female. Grafts obtained from the iliac crest frequently require a bolster under the opposite hip to permit exposure of the crest. The opposite hip is chosen to enable simultaneous shoulder surgery and harvesting of an iliac crest bone graft.

The arm is then prepped with 1% iodine solution, suspended from the wrist with the McConnell arm holder, and then reprepped while the surgical team scrubs. The arm is placed in sterile towels and an impervious stockinette and secured with sterile Coban. Prophylactic antibiotics are given prior to the skin incision and every four to six hours thereafter for 48 hours. The cell saver is routinely employed for these procedures.[14] The skin incision is marked with methylene blue. The largest Ioban-adherent Steri-drape then covers the skin, and a second piece is used for the axilla. The arm remains freely moveable. The arm is positioned using the McConnell arm holder (Fig. 39-28).

There are four utility approaches utilized in fracture care. The most common is the deltopectoral approach for any fractures involving the surgical neck or lesser

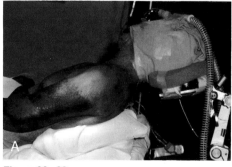

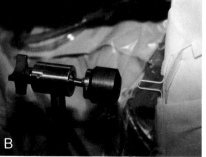

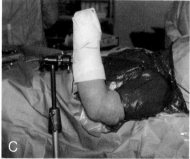

Figure 39-28

Semi-Fowler's beach chair position for anterior and superior approaches to the shoulder. *A*, The cervical spine is protected in slight flexion. The headrest permits superior exposure of the shoulder girdle without obstruction by the operator. *B*, The McConnell arm positioner attached to the forearm enabling (*C*) the arm to be positioned in any rotation or elevation.

tuberosity. With isolated greater tuberosity fractures, a superior approach with a lateral deltoid split may be sufficient. Alternatively, an anterior acromioplasty or superior approach permits decompression of the subacromial space without the need for transacromial osteotomy or Cubbins detachment of the entire deltoid.[40,181] Occasionally a posterior approach is necessary for posterior and inferior glenoid fractures, but this approach is seldom necessary for isolated proximal humeral fractures or for prosthetic replacement.

Deltopectoral Approach

A 15-cm deltopectoral incision begins at the clavicle, passes over the coracoid, and extends to the deltoid insertion (Fig. 39–29). The cephalic vein is preserved with either the deltoid or pectoralis major. The clavipectoral fascia is incised. Richardson retractors or an abdominal Balfour retractor are used to retract the deltoid laterally and cephalad and the intact coracoid muscles medially. Abduction of the arm and release of the anterior 1 cm of the deltoid insertion and the upper half of the pectoralis provide more wound relaxation if necessary. The key landmark is the long head of the biceps. If the rotator cuff and tuberosities are intact at the biceps groove, then the fracture type will determine the type of glenohumeral arthrotomy.

For a two-part surgical neck fracture, the joint rarely needs to be open. For a posterior dislocation in which the articular deficit in the head is less than 20%, an opening through the subscapularis is used, but if the deficit is between 20% and 40%, then an osteotomy of the lesser tuberosity enables transfer into the humeral head deficit.

In three-part fractures, the joint is already exposed by avulsion of one of the two tuberosities. The longitudinal tear of the rotator cuff at the interval between the subscapularis and supraspinatus can be extended proximally.

In four-part fractures, both tuberosities are usually separated, but in the rare instance in which they are still intact at the biceps groove, the groove is osteotomized, and the cuff is opened through the rotator interval. Heavy traction sutures using no. 5 nonabsorbable nylon are placed through the rotator cuff insertion at the tuberosity level. This is the one predictable area of firm cortical bone where sutures will not pull through, but through the midportion of the tuberosity in an elderly patient, the sutures may cut through the soft bone like a Gigli saw.

Superior Approach Without Anterior Acromioplasty (Fig. 39–30A)

An incision is made over the lateral border of the acromion along Langer's skin lines. The skin is undermined, and a point is selected just posterior to the anterolateral corner of the acromion to split the deltoid.

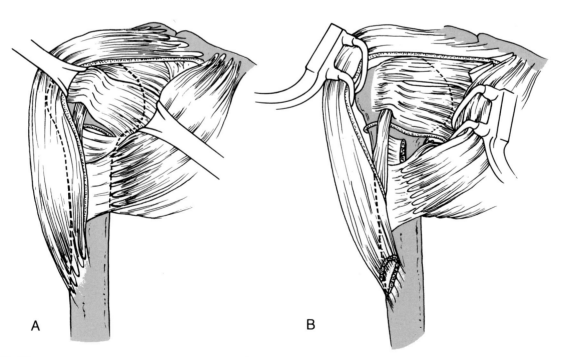

A   B

Figure 39–29

The deltopectoral approach preserves the cephalic vein. The coracoid is left intact to protect the brachial plexus. Richardson retractors (A) or self-retaining Balfour retractors (B) maintain exposure to the proximal humerus.

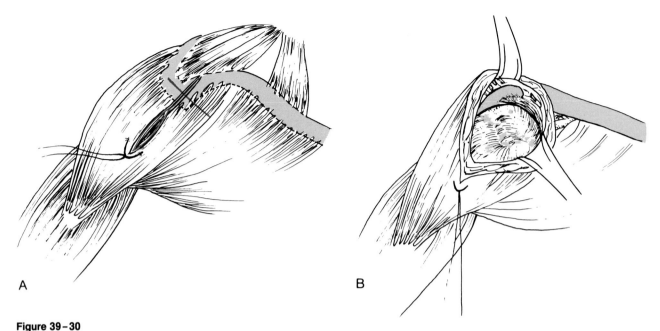

Figure 39-30

A, Superior approach without anterior acromioplasty with a deltoid split. *B,* Anterior acromioplasty approach. The skin incision is along Langer's skin lines and perpendicular to the deltoid split or detachment.

The acromial branch of the thyroacromial artery is co-agulated. Small Richardson retractors are placed to retract the deltoid. Any underlying hemorrhagic bursa is excised. A stay suture is placed at the distal portion of the deltoid split 5 cm below the acromion to prevent injury to the axillary nerve. This operative approach is commonly used for greater tuberosity avulsions.

Superior Approach With Anterior Acromioplasty

An incision is made over the midportion of the acromion along Langer's skin lines paralleling the antero-posterior direction of the acromion (Fig. 39-30B). This is carried from the posterior acromion down beyond the anterior edge of the acromion, midway to the coracoid. After undermining circumferentially, a split is made in the deltotrapezius fascia over the anterior acromion 1 cm posterior to the anterior acromial margin. It is continued down the deltoid similar to the deltoid-splitting incision. The acromial branch of the thoracoacromial artery is coagulated. The anterior deltoid is dissected off the anterior acromion, preserving Sharpey's fibers with the deltoid for later attachment. The coracoacromial ligament is resected.

The McConnell arm holder is utilized to provide longitudinal traction to the arm to enable better visualization of the subacromial space. Visualization may also be aided with a flat Darrach elevator in the subacromial space to push inferiorly on the humeral head.

A 1-in osteotome at the top margin of the acromion is directed posteriorly to bevel any anterior beaking of the acromion. The undersurface of the anterior third of the acromion is removed. The inferior surface of the remaining acromion is parallel to the posterior two thirds of the acromion. With a combination of rongeurs and rasps, the undersurface of the acromion is reshaped, with care taken to remove any rim of bone that may project inferiorly at the deltoid origin laterally or the acromioclavicular (AC) joint medially. If arthritic, the outer clavicle is excised to enable adduction of the arm without contact between the clavicle and the medial acromion. Alternatively, a modified arthroplasty is performed with removal of any inferiorly projecting spurs. Scar and adhesions in the subacromial bursa are released to provide access to the rotator cuff and tuberosities.

Posterior Approach (Fig. 39-31)

In the posterior approach, the patient is placed in the lateral decubitus position on the Gelfoam mattress, and all pressure points are padded. The gel bolster in the shape of an intravenous (IV) bag is placed underneath the opposite chest wall to protect both the brachial plexus and the opposite shoulder. The head is sealed to a Mayfield or McConnell neurosurgical headrest padded with gel bolsters. The arm is positioned with a McConnell arm holder from the opposite side of the table.

An incision is made parallel to the scapular spine or perpendicular to this over the glenohumeral joint level.

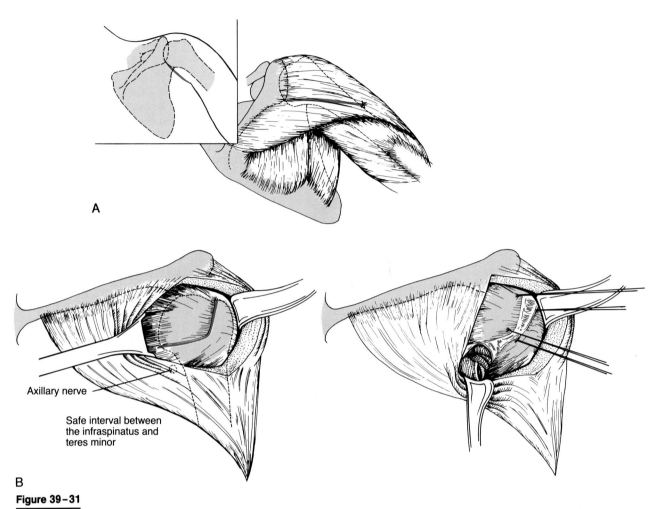

Figure 39-31

A, Posterior approach, longitudinal incision. The posterior deltoid is split up to 8 cm from the acromion to expose the infraspinatus and teres minor. *B*, Vertical infraspinatus arthrotomy with any horizontal component at the "safe interval" between the infraspinatus and teres minor.

After undermining, the deltoid is split between 6 and 8 cm from the level of the posterior spine of the scapula, care being taken not to injure the axillary nerve. Alternatively, the arm can be abducted and the inferior border of the deltoid retracted in a cephalad manner. The latter provides exposure to the posterior scapula but is more difficult with posterior capsule repairs. The critical point in the exposure is the location and protection of the axillary nerve with its branches along the undersurface of the deltoid and to the teres minor.

In general, the goal of fixation or prosthetic replacement is to maintain the length of the deltoid myofascial sleeve by reconstructing the full length of the humerus. The version of the head segment or the replacement is maintained at approximately 35° of retroversion unless it is altered for longstanding instability and in order to prevent recurrent instability. If both tuberosities and the surgical neck are involved, then the metaphyseal bone used for support of the prosthetic replacement is often not sufficient to prevent the prosthesis from loosening, spinning, or subsiding. Methylmethacrylate fixation within the shaft permits fixation in proper version with restoration of humeral length.

Proximal humeral fractures associated with glenoid rim fractures may be approached either anteriorly or posteriorly. There is a high incidence of late instability if glenoid rim fractures are not treated. The bony rim with its capsular attachments or the capsular attachments alone are repaired.

Tuberosity fixation is best accomplished with nonabsorbable sutures in both vertical repairs to the shaft and horizontal repairs to the prosthesis and other tuberosity. If the surgical neck is involved, intramedullary fixation with rods or prosthetic replacement should be considered. Although wire gives more secure fixation in the acute fracture setting, complications include late breakage and migration.[188,269]

Intraoperative Complications

Intraoperative complications include fractures of the humeral shaft from forceful manipulation, displacement of previously nondisplaced fractures, poor holding of sutures in the tuberosities, damage to the deltoid with retraction, and damage to the axillary nerve or brachial plexus. These occur in all surgeons' practices, but awareness will lessen their frequency.

An intraoperative shaft fracture may be avoided by gentle manipulation and avoidance of strong rotational torques. If a closed reduction is not possible, avoid repeated attempts and proceed early with open treatment. Nerve injuries have been reported with closed fracture manipulation, with repeated attempts at closed reduction, and with use of the foot in the axilla for countertraction with reductions of dislocations.

Once a shaft fracture has occurred, intramedullary fixation with rods or a long-stemmed prosthesis is preferred. Alternatively, a shaft fracture can be stabilized with AO plates and screws if a prosthesis is not needed or if other forms of intramedullary fixation are not deemed sufficient.[19]

Problems with secure fixation of the tuberosities are best approached by repairing the tuberosities at the junction of the rotator cuff with the tuberosity. Here the bone is the hardest. Suture through the rotator cuff at this junction, then loop around the tuberosity to repair it both to the adjacent tuberosity and to the shaft.

If additional relaxation is necessary, the deltoid is protected by abducting the arm and releasing the anterior portion of the deltoid insertion rather than the origin. The axillary nerve can be identified on the undersurface of the deltoid through a deltopectoral approach. The brachial plexus is most easily protected by leaving the coracoid muscles intact to avoid a traction injury.

Late rotator cuff dehiscence can occur with a tension band repair when the tension band circles around the undersurface of the rotator cuff (Fig. 39–32A). A vertical tension band repair pulls on the hard tuberosity, whereas the horizontal portion of the tension band in the absence of intramedullary fixation can erode through the rotator cuff (Fig. 39–32).

Essential Aftercare

In general, these procedures are performed to give maximal stability to the fracture fragments. Rehabilitation is custom tailored to the patient and the fracture and is easier, more comfortable, and more assured with firm internal fixation[208] with or without prosthetic replacement. External support using a sling, abduction splint or pillow, or shoulder spica cast is an alternate method of postoperative immobilization. Hanging arm casts are avoided. Any potential benefit is lost if the patient becomes supine. Physical therapy is preferred to assist with early passive range of motion, but it should be delayed if there are tissue deficits or a lack of secure fixation or if patient understanding and compliance are not assured. A large number of problems involving healing of the tuberosities or rotator cuff have been reported with the use of physical therapy in the first three weeks following complicated fractures of the proximal humerus.[249]

Hardware removal is considered if there is impingement, pain, or a late need for lysis of scar and adhesions. Forceful manipulation should be avoided to avoid fracture or cuff tear.

One-Part Fractures

One-part fractures are nondisplaced or only minimally displaced (less than 0.5 cm when the fracture involves the greater tuberosity or 1 cm between any other segments) (Fig. 39–33). They are angulated less than 45°. Their incidence ranges between 47% and 85% of all proximal humeral fractures.[30,79,105,149,179,180,220] The rotator cuff and periosteum and long head of the biceps splint these fractures in position.

Treatment

The arm is placed in a sling for comfort with support. Early gentle, passive range of motion, beginning with pendulum exercises, is begun as tolerated and advanced as fracture healing is assured.[218]

Indications

Indications are the same as for stable fractures involving the head, the tuberosities, and the shaft, all of which move as a unit, regardless of the number of fracture fragments.

Contraindications

Early motion is not started as soon for those fractures that have been recently converted to nondisplaced or minimally displaced fractures that are not stable. If the fracture does not move as a unit, then early passive motion may result in a nonunion or malunion.

Aftercare

The exercises are advanced as the security of the fracture permits. A sling is worn to support the arm. This, along with early deltoid isometrics, provides upward support in an effort to prevent inferior humeral head subluxation and promote fracture healing. Phase I passive exercises usually can be begun four to five days after the fracture. Pulley and supine external rotation may be instituted by seven to eight days. Additional isometrics are added by three weeks. Active exercises

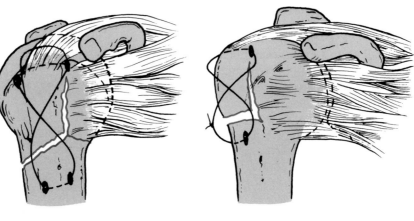

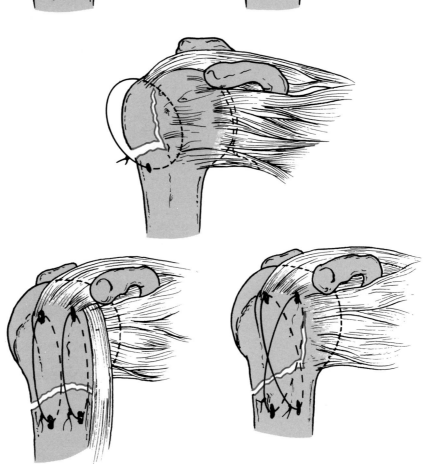

Figure 39–32

A and *B*, This suture does not include the tuberosity. It is passed through the soft tissue (rotator cuff), differentiated in *B*, in which the bone and cuff are included. In *A*, the suture may erode the cuff. *C*, Suture passage that includes the cuff insertion and tuberosity for good proximal holding power. The rotator interval is closed between the supraspinatus and the subscapularis. *D*, Simple vertical or crossed sutures (shown in *E*) are satisfactory as long as the cuff is included. *E*, Suture through the tuberosity without including the hard bone at the cuff insertion may cut through the bone.

commence at approximately six to eight weeks if healing permits.

Frequent clinical and roentgenographic evaluations are important to assess progress and ensure that no displacement has occurred.

One-Part Fracture With Dislocation

When dislocations are associated with nondisplaced or minimally displaced one-part fractures, additional care must be taken with reduction if displacement of the fracture is to be avoided. General anesthesia provides more adequate relaxation for reduction, but the reduc-

tion may also be gently performed using open techniques.

Displaced Fractures and Fracture-Dislocations of the Proximal Humerus

Two-Part Fractures and Fracture-Dislocations

Anatomic Neck. One seldom has the opportunity to treat isolated anatomic neck fractures of the proximal humerus. They are not seen in childhood[42] and are quite rare in adults,[183] constituting only 0.54% of proximal humeral fractures.[105] Indications for treatment of

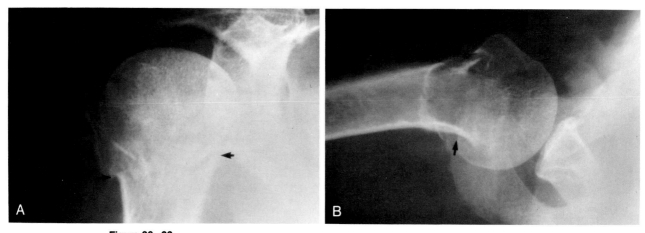

Figure 39-33

One-part nondisplaced surgical neck fracture (*arrows*). *A*, Anteroposterior view. *B*, Axillary view.

these fractures are displacement or dislocation. Closed reduction alone with postulated disruption of the blood supply to the articular surface has resulted in malunion and collapse.[183] There are no reported cases of successful closed reduction or closed pinning for isolated, displaced, or dislocated anatomic neck fractures with long-term follow-up. The preferred treatment is an early prosthetic replacement to avoid the malunion and collapse that is almost certain to occur when the blood supply to the articular surface has been disrupted. Alternatively, open reduction and pinning may be considered in the younger patient. It is preferred to treat this fracture early, obtain an accurate reduction, and then begin early rehabilitation and regain range of motion as soon as fracture security permits.

As with all fractures considered for operative treatment, preoperative planning requires a general evaluation of the patient's medical condition and wishes and adequate imaging studies. In surgery, the patient is positioned for a deltopectoral approach. The coracoid muscles are left intact to protect the brachial plexus. An opening in the subscapularis and anterior capsule 1 cm from their insertion on the lesser tuberosity allows full visualization of the humeral head and, if necessary, the glenoid. The humeral head is positioned anatomically under direct vision. Screws, K wires, or Steinmann pins are inserted through the tuberosities up into the head. Under direct vision the arm can then be externally rotated to ensure that the articular cartilage has not been violated (Fig. 39-34).

If the head is found to be dislocated on opening the subscapularis, then a bone hook can be used to pull laterally on the upper humeral shaft, with the arm in some flexion and abduction to relax the deltoid. This will give sufficient room to retrieve the displaced or dislocated articular surface. Once it has been anatomically positioned, it can be fixed with Steinmann pins, K wires, or screws. Any wires or pins should be watched carefully and removed if they break or begin to migrate or when healing permits, usually by six weeks.[148] Intraoperative complications to avoid include fragmentation of the head and penetration of the fixation through the articular surface. If secure fixation is not achieved or there is fragmentation of the articular surface, this procedure should be abandoned and converted to a humeral head replacement (Fig. 39-35).

The long deltopectoral approach without deltoid detachment is ideal for a humeral head replacement. The fracture occurs along the scar of the old epiphyseal line. If there is any bony deficiency, the humeral head is used as additional bone graft; the metaphyseal bone is still present for support and rotatory control of the prosthesis. The subscapularis is opened 1 to 2 cm medial to its insertion on the lesser tuberosity. The elbow is lowered off the operative table and the shaft pushed upward in the deltopectoral interval. Suture retraction on the supraspinatus and subscapularis permits trial replacement of humeral prostheses with the thin stem. To preserve the normal 30° to 40° of retroversion, the fin of the humeral head prosthesis is placed just posterior to the groove of the long head of the biceps tendon.

The prosthetic stem size can be determined by radiographs in two right-angle planes. Templates are available if needed. The T-handled humeral reamers for each stem size can be passed down the length of the humerus. My preference is to judge the stem size by radiograph, use the thin stem for a trial, and then use a medium or large stem if the canal permits. One passage enables a press fit in those fractures with an intact calcar and metaphyseal bone that prevent rotation. The prosthesis is cemented if it pistons easily upward or subsides

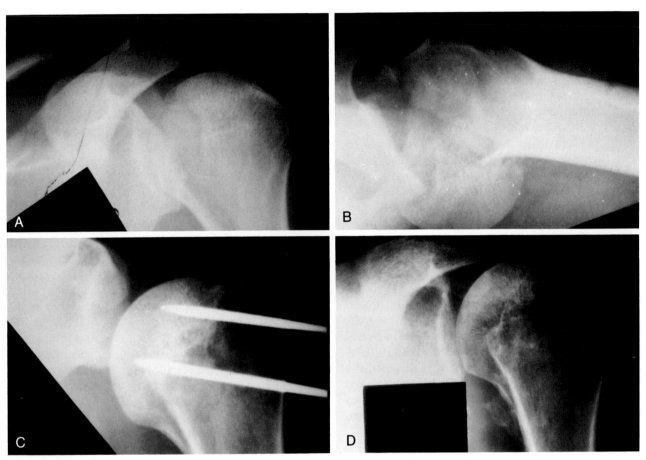

Figure 39-34

Posterior dislocation—two-part anatomic neck posterior fracture-dislocation. *A*, The anteroposterior view was not diagnostic for the first three orthopedic surgeons assessing this fracture-dislocation. *B*, The axillary view demonstrating the posterior head displacement enabled the diagnosis to be established. *C*, Open reduction and internal fixation with two Steinmann pins. *D*, Four-month follow-up with pin removal at six weeks shows good early healing of articular surface. A longer follow-up will be needed to ensure that late collapse with avascular necrosis does not occur. (Courtesy of Charles A. Rockwood, Jr., M.D.)

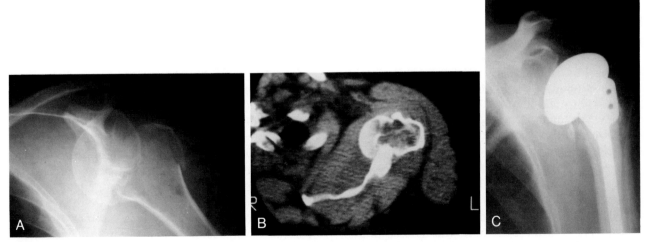

Figure 39-35

Two-part anatomic neck fracture/anterior dislocation. *A*, Anteroposterior view with anatomic neck fracture and nondisplacement of greater tuberosity fracture. *B*, CT scan demonstrating anterior dislocation of articular surface. *C*, Postoperative prosthetic replacement.

with the articular surface below the greater tuberosity level. If the bone is soft or fragmented, the prosthesis is cemented to avoid late subsidence.

A trial reduction is then performed. Tension is estimated in planning for cuff closure. The trial component is removed, and sutures are placed to close the rotator cuff prior to the final placement of the prosthesis and are then retracted out of the way. Once the prosthesis has been press fit into the shaft, these replaced sutures are tied. A drain is placed through the upper portion of the deltoid and out through the skin posteriorly. The deltopectoral interval and rotator cuff are closed with nonabsorbable sutures. The nonabsorbable sutures in the deltopectoral interval mark the interval in the event that reoperation is necessary later. The cephalic vein is preserved with either the deltoid or pectoralis.

Several absorbable subcutaneous sutures are placed. The skin is reapproximated with a deep subcuticular 2-0 Prolene layer, and the skin edges are further reapproximated with Steri-strips. The patient is transferred to the recovery room, still on the prophylactic antibiotics that will be continued for the first 48 hours following surgery. The arm is protected with a sling and swathe as long as the patient experiences any nausea from anesthesia. A continuous passive motion apparatus may be used on an intermittent basis to rotate the arm from the sling position on the abdomen out to a neutral position and elevate it in the first 30° to 40° of flexion range. Elevation beyond this is not necessary in the acute postoperative setting, but elevation up to this point does assist in decreasing pain and the need for postoperative medications in most patients. A patient-controlled anesthesia machine is generally employed for the first 24 hours postoperatively. Pendulum exercises are begun on the following day and continued through the early healing phases. Sutures are removed between 10 and 14 days following surgery, and the gentle passive exercises are advanced as tolerated.

If long pins have been placed, they can be removed at six to eight weeks. Screws are left in place permanently unless the humeral head begins to collapse. If screw penetration through the articular surface is discovered, the patient is returned to surgery early. The screw can be replaced with a shorter screw or removed, or the internal fixation can be converted to a humeral head replacement. Resurfacing of the humeral and glenoid side will likely be necessary with longstanding collapse or screw penetration through the surface.

Follow-up care and rehabilitation begin with early pendulum exercises to preserve glenohumeral motion. These are advanced in a routine fashion as the security of the repair permit.

Surgical Neck — General Considerations. Displaced fractures of the surgical neck are the most common fracture of the proximal humerus. These subtuberous fractures comprise a large percentage of the proximal humerus epiphyseal fractures and between 60% and 65% of all proximal humeral fractures in adults.[105] In the adult the shaft fracture may be impacted, angulated greater than 45°, displaced anteriorly and medially by the pull of the pectoralis, comminuted, occur with or without extension into the tuberosities, or be associated with an anterior dislocation of the shoulder. These fractures are often associated with infraclavicular brachial plexus lesions, but fortunately most patients recover.

Frequently these fractions are unstable after closed reduction because of the fracture configuration or secondary to interposition of the long head of the biceps, subscapularis, or deltoid muscles. The common prior practice of using an abduction cast to meet a slightly abducted proximal fragment usually exacerbates the displacement either by the shaft catching the medial cortex of the proximal fragment to increase the varus angulation or by the increased pectoralis pull with attempted abduction, which displaces the shaft anteriorly and medially. Similarly, a hanging arm cast increases the anterior angulation, resulting in a high incidence of malunion or nonunion.[190,199,200] Although the hanging arm cast may give distraction early on at the fracture site, as the muscles fatigue it may overpull. Furthermore, when the patient lies down, any potential benefit it may have had is lost.

The treatment of these fractures varies depending on the architecture of the fracture, the amount of comminution, and whether a stable closed reduction can be maintained. Fractures in polytrauma patients benefit from open reduction and internal fixation to permit ease of care.

The epiphyseal fractures in the young are managed differently from the three types of surgical neck fractures in the adult. The treatment will vary depending upon the patient's age and fracture architecture.

Epiphyseal Fractures. In the very young, epiphyseal fractures simulate an anterior dislocation of the shoulder prior to the appearance of the proximal physis. Even if unreduced, the intact posterior periosteum will fill in with bone, and the proximal humerus will remodel without apparent deformity. Beyond the age of 9 years, up to 30% of patients may show a growth disturbance.[42,186]

The indication for reduction is complete displacement or angulation greater than 45°. Under general anesthesia and with radiographic or, preferably, fluoroscopic control, these fractures are reduced in adduction, full forward flexion, and neutral rotation. With slight traction on the arm in this overhead position, the anterior angulated shaft is reduced with a posterior force on the upper shaft. This utilizes the intact posterior periosteum as a stabilizing hinge. The fragments lock together without crushing the physeal plate. The arm is lowered and immobilized across the chest to relax the pectoralis. Rarely, these have been treated with the arm positioned near the salute position in an abduction cast, using Saha's[224a] assumption that the zero position will relax all the deforming muscles about the shoulder. This is not an entirely benign treatment, as brachial plexus stretch injuries have occurred with prolonged overhead positioning. A safer position is 90° forward flexion held by a cast or overhead olecranon pin traction if the fracture redisplaces with the arm at the side.

Fractures that are reducible but unstable in an adolescent 16 years or older may be treated with minimal internal fixation using percutaneous pinning[77,141] or with an open reduction through a deltopectoral approach and fixation with two Steinmann pins. These pins should be buried deep enough that they do not irritate the skin and yet not too deep to be retrievable through incisions made under a local anesthetic at three to six weeks, or they should extend sufficiently beyond the skin to minimize additional skin irritation that may result in a secondary infection. Relaxing incisions should be made if skin tenting occurs, and daily pin care should be administered to decrease the likelihood of pin complications (Fig. 39–36).

After pin removal, pendulum exercises can be started. Active motion is begun when the fracture is secure, but resistive exercises should be avoided if there

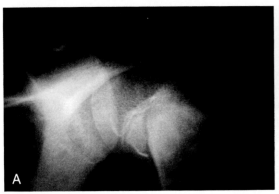

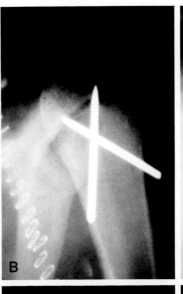

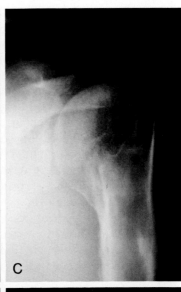

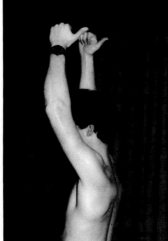

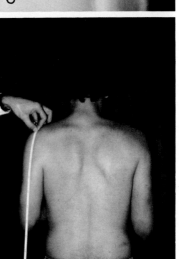

Figure 39–36

Two-part surgical neck epiphyseal fracture. *A*, Film showing a two-part surgical neck fracture in a 15-year-old male with polytrauma. *B*, Open reduction and stabilization with two crossed Steinmann pins. *C*, Remodeling and healing three years later. *D*, Mild limitation of elevation. *E*, Three-centimeter shortening of proximal humerus at three years.

is any suggestion of motion at the fracture site or, in general, if there is still tenderness at the epiphyseal line. Before advancing in treatment stages, new roentgenograms should document fracture position and healing, and all pins should be removed. Alternate forms of reduction include olecranon pin traction with the arm at the side[26] or in adduction and flexion.[191]

Two-Part Surgical Neck Fractures in the Adult

IMPACTED AND ANGULATED. Impacted surgical neck fractures are angulated with the apex anteriorly. The posterior periosteal hinge is intact. Although impacted fractures were not considered in the AO classification, in the absence of a tuberosity avulsion,[105] they form one of the three important types described by Neer for displaced two-part surgical neck fractures. Angulated fractures comprise approximately 26% of displaced proximal humerus fractures, and a small percentage of them occur with fissure lines extending up into one or both tuberosities.[105] If these are stable, consideration should be given to accepting the deformity, with the understanding that elevation will be lost in direct proportion to the fracture angulation. A varus malunion with the greater tuberosity rotated up into the subacromial space will not be tolerated well by an active patient or by one who needs overhead elevation.[109,183,184]

At the time of closed reduction, the surgeon should be prepared for the possibility of an open reduction. These fractures may be reduced following the administration of intramuscular (IM) or IV pain medication and muscle relaxants or, preferably, under general anesthesia (which results in better muscle relaxation) and fluoroscopic control. Varus angulation is corrected with longitudinal traction and gentle arm pressure from lateral to medial at the fracture site and with forward flexion and adduction of the arm to relax the pectoralis and latissimus dorsi. Once the fracture is disimpacted and realigned, an upward compression at the elbow may reimpact the fracture for a stable closed reduction. The arm is lowered to the side and immobilized in a sling and swathe with the elbow across the abdomen. If the fracture cannot be maintained in a reduced position, then some form of fixation should be employed, either closed pinning at the deltopectoral interval or an open reduction.

Once this fracture has been rendered stable by closed reduction, the essential aftercare includes sling support for two to three weeks followed by gentle pendulum exercises and continued support until four to six weeks, when fracture healing is far enough advanced that additional gentle passive exercises can be added. No exercises are begun unless the head and shaft rotate in unison. Manipulation of the arm with strong passive motion prior to completion of fracture healing is to be avoided. Although the surgeon, the patient, and the treating therapist are understandably eager to reestablish glenohumeral motion to avoid long-term stiffness, early aggressive physical therapy has been a frequent cause of proximal humeral nonunion at the surgical neck. This leads to prolonged disability with the necessity of open treatment (Fig. 39–37).[199]

The patient can graduate to gentle stretching and

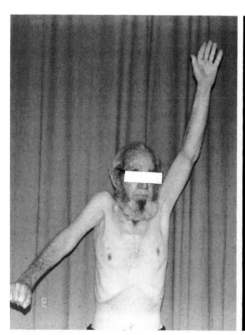
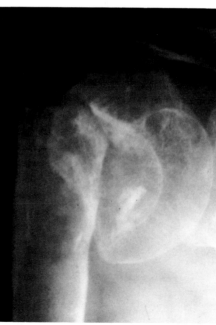

Figure 39–37

Two-part surgical neck nonunion following chiropractic manipulation prior to healing. Poor motion and poor pain relief resulted prior to reconstruction.

active resistive exercises by approximately six weeks. It may take 9 to 12 months to regain full range of shoulder motion, strength, and endurance.

DISPLACED. Approximately 22% of proximal humeral fractures are displaced through the surgical neck.[105] Most are stable once they are reduced by longitudinal traction in flexion and adduction while applying a posterior force on the upper humerus. They are immobilized in adduction with a sling and swathe for three to six weeks, at which point gentle pendulum exercises may be begun if the head and shaft rotate in unison. Eighty percent of these fractures will heal more or less in approximately six weeks,[109] and then gentle passive stretching exercises may be added. Light resistive exercises may begin at approximately 10 to 12 weeks and advanced as tolerated.

Indications for open reduction include unstable fractures or polytrauma, where stabilization of proximal fractures permits easier care, earlier relief, and earlier rehabilitation.

A small number of these fractures are irreducible secondary to interposition of the long head of the biceps, subscapularis, or deltoid muscles (Fig. 39–38).

Occasionally these fractures are reducible but redisplace as soon as the surgeon releases the tension to hold the fracture. At this point options for treatment include closed pinning,[77,127,141] external fixators,[127,128] and open reduction and internal fixation.[5,9,41,198] Preoperative imaging studies are obtained to assess osteoporosis, rule out a dislocation, and identify any additional fracture fissures in preparation for surgery. Care is taken not to displace otherwise minimally displaced or undisplaced fragments preoperatively or intraoperatively. In fractures that are irreducible or appear to be reducible but are unstable with no bony crepitus, interposed tissue is usually found at the fracture site during open reduction.

The techniques for open reduction and internal fixation include figure-of-8 wiring with a tension band or a nonabsorbable heavy nylon suture, intramedullary rod fixation placed antegrade or retrograde, a combination of tension band and intramedullary rod fixation, Mouridian nail fixation, and fixation with plates and screws. My preferred technique combines the stability of intramedullary fixation and figure-of-8 suture with nonabsorbable no. 5 nylon (Teudec) suture. This

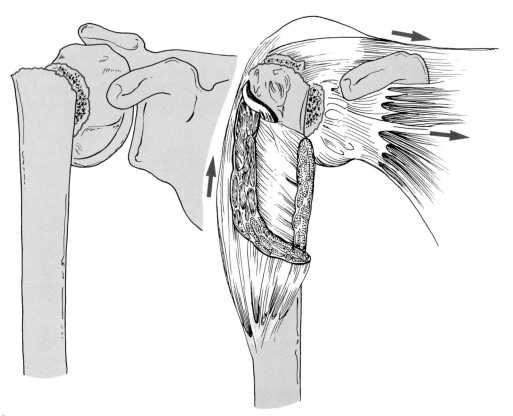

Figure 39–38

Interposition of long head of biceps in surgical neck fracture precludes stable reduction. Unless the long head is removed, a nonunion will result at the fracture site.

avoids the additional stripping involved with placement of plates and the propensity of screws to pull out of the soft metaphyseal bone in the head, as additional dissection is required, and it may compromise the long head of the biceps and the arcuate artery, which supplies blood to the articular surface, as a result of the placement of the proximal plate. The screws often do not hold well in the cancellous humeral head. This technique is exponentially more difficult in the elderly patient with osteoporosis. Plates, when secure, provide fixation for early rehabilitation but are not recommended in those with osteoporosis (Fig. 39–39). The three most common postoperative complications include impingement of the hardware on the acromion, loosening, and a significantly increased incidence of avascular necrosis. Occasionally, avascular necrosis occurs in closed two-part fractures as a result of extensive soft tissue and periosteal stripping, especially if the fracture fragments have injured the axillary artery or, more distally, the terminal arcuate artery supply to the articular segment.

The preferred operative technique combines intramedullary rod fixation with tension band compression at the fracture site. This avoids the extra dissection for plate fixation and the propensity for screws to pull out of the humeral head that can occur with the Mouridian nail or plate and screws. This is performed under general anesthesia or scalene block with the patient in the beach chair position. The patient is positioned high on the operative table and to the side, where the arm can be lowered over the edge for placement of the intramedullary rod through a deltopectoral approach. This is similar to the position used for prosthetic replacement. At surgery, a closed reduction is attempted with adduction and forward flexion to relax the pectoralis muscle pull.

Saha's zero or full overhead position, with the use of fluoroscopic guidance, may allow reduction when soft tissue otherwise precludes this in other positions. This is especially helpful when there is an associated anterior dislocation.

Open reduction is accomplished through a deltopectoral approach. Resection of the coracoacromial ligament provides more room superiorly. Interposed soft tissue is removed from the fracture site. This may consist of the deltoid, when the distal fragment has passed through it on the initial displacement, or the subscapularis or long head of the biceps (see Fig. 39–38). Holes for the modified Ender rods are made at the articular junction with the greater tuberosity. Alternatively, Rush rods as modified by Watson,[256a] with a suture hole through the top hook, can be used (Figure 39–40A, B). The placement of these rods and of the accompanying tension band sutures is technically demanding but provides intramedullary fixation, tension band compression over the fracture site, and sutures to keep the rods from migrating proximally.

Preliminary drill holes are made at the marginal junction of the articular surface in the greater tuberosity for two intramedullary rods that will later be passed for intramedullary fixation (Fig. 39–40C). Using an AO or Deschamp suture passer, a no. 5 nonabsorbable nylon suture is passed down one intramedullary entrance point and out the adjacent one proximally. This serves as the top portion of the figure-of-8 tension band repair. The two free ends are passed though the top smooth, rounded holes of the modified Ender or Rush rods.

A second set of drill holes is made in the shaft at a distance from the fracture site equal to that of the entrance point of the intramedullary rods. The figure-of-8

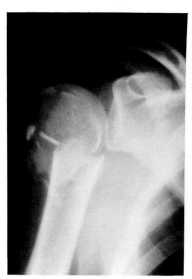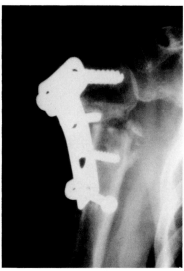

Figure 39–39

Two-part surgical neck fracture with nondisplaced greater tuberosity fragment. Plates and screws pulled out of soft bone on the two operative attempts for open reduction and internal fixation.

suture then crosses the fracture site for maximal tension band compression. One of the sutures is passed through the distal two drill holes in the shaft, which will later permit suture tying distal to the fracture site. The next two sutures are passed through one of the distal drill holes and up the intramedullary portion of the shaft beyond the fracture site. Then one suture is passed through each of the proximal intramedullary rod entrance holes, through the eyelet of the Ender rod, and back down through the same intramedullary hole to be used for that rod. Both sutures then exit distal to the fracture site through the opposite transverse hole drilled for the inferior portion of the tension band suture.

The intramedullary rods are then passed down through their proximal entrance holes beyond the fracture site and into the intramedullary cavity of the distal fragment. The fracture is anatomically reduced, and the rods are inserted just beneath the cortical entrance point proximally. The sutures through each rod are then tied distally to prevent the rod from later being pulled in a superior direction by the tension band suture (Fig. 39–40D). This ensures that there will be no

hardware impingement, thus eliminating the need for later hardware removal. The tension band suture is tied tightly to provide secure fixation, with the compression across the fracture site to permit early motion.

Fracture security is tested prior to closing the wound. The patient is placed in a sling and swathe and begun on pendulum exercises the first postoperative day. With secure fixation, Hemovac drainage and a modified version of the continuous passive motion apparatus may be started in the early postoperative period, as discussed in the section on rehabilitation (Fig. 39–40E, F).

Alternative techniques for intramedullary rod fixation include the use of retrograde Ender nails passed retrograde from the distal humerus. These are less likely to maintain an anatomic reduction, especially if there is fracture collapse. Any soft tissue interposition is more easily removed by a direct or antegrade approach. Advocated procedures using tension band techniques that grasp only the rotator cuff[143] without tuberosity support[143] risk rupture of the cuff (see Fig. 39–32A).

Alternate proximal approaches include the use of a Mouridian nail or an AO buttress T plate. Either of

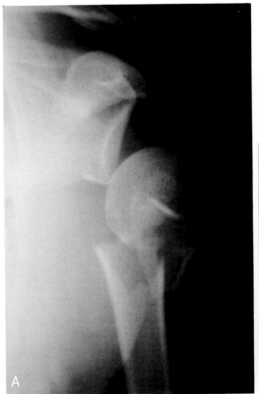
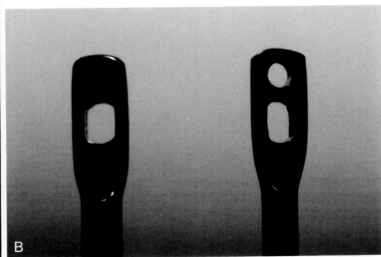

Figure 39–40

Technique of Ender intramedullary fixation combined with a tension band for two-part surgical neck fracture. *A,* Unstable two-part surgical neck fracture with inferior humeral head subluxation. *B,* Modification of Ender rod with small superior hole for no. 5 nonabsorbable nylon suture.

Illustration continued on following page

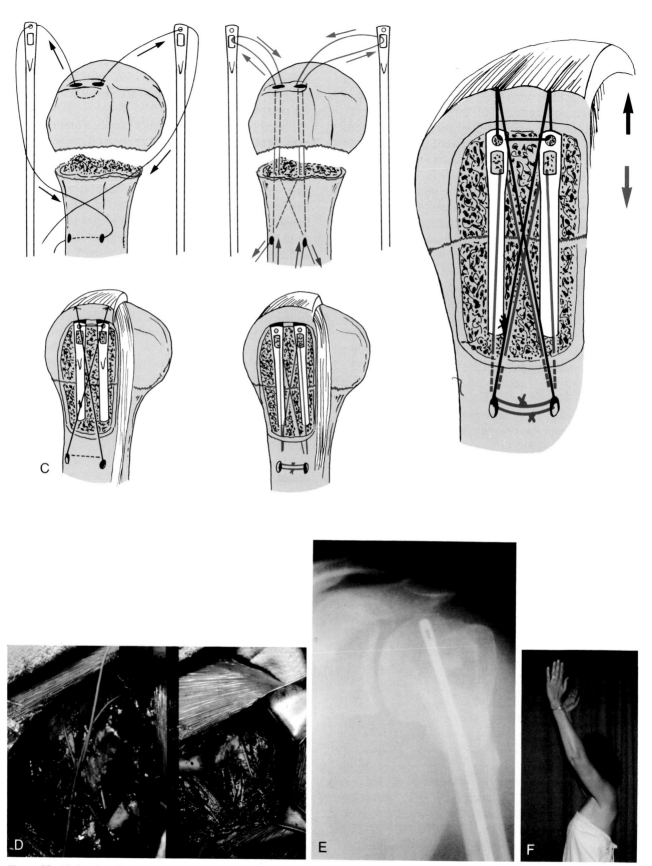

Figure 39-40 *Continued*

C, Technique of open reduction and internal fixation of two- and three-part surgical neck fractures with modified Ender rods. The superior hole is used for the figure-of-8 tension band. Additional sutures through the rods and secured through drill holes beyond the fracture site preclude the rods from migrating into the subacromial space. *D*, Conversion of unstable two-part surgical neck fracture to a stable one-part fracture that permits early motion. *E*, Satisfactory fracture healing six months postoperatively. *F*, Near-normal motion for elevation.

these may be satisfactory in young patients with good bone stock, but the previously described limitations of impingement or loosening still apply (see Fig. 39–38).

If closed pinning is chosen, two stiff Steinmann pins are placed from below in an upward direction. Care must be taken with this technique and with those involving external fixators to avoid the path of the axillary nerve passing 5 cm below the acromion in the region of the anterior and middle deltoid; thus the deltopectoral interval is the safest interval for pin placement. These external methods of fixation are recommended for temporary use prior to definitive treatment.[238] The open technique is recommended in polytrauma patients to avoid the complications of pin migration, breakage, pin tract infection, or loss of fixation in a patient who must be rolled from side to side in bed or mobilized out of bed. In other fractures (e.g., grade II open fractures of the tibia), open rodding has provided better fracture control with no increase in complications when compared with external fixation techniques.[247]

For olecranon pin traction, the arm is flexed and adducted to relax the deforming muscle forces of the pectoralis major. This technique has disadvantages in that the patient is confined to bed with more awkward positioning and greater postoperative care, and the potential overpull of the fracture encourages nonunion.

In special cases, humeral head prosthetic replacement will be beneficial for two-part surgical neck nonunion in which there is a small osteoporotic head in an elderly patient. Through the deltopectoral approach, a four-part fracture is created by splitting the tuberosities at the biceps groove. The articular surface is removed and saved for possible bone graft. The humeral component is cemented in normal retroversion at the proper height to preserve the length of the deltoid. The remaining technique is described in the section on four-part fractures.

METAPHYSEAL COMMINUTION. Surgical neck fractures with metaphyseal comminution denote a greater degree of trauma and are more difficult to manage. The comminution extends down the shaft from 1 to 5 cm. The intact rotator cuff holds the head in neutral rotation, while the pectoralis may pull one segment of the shaft in a medial direction. If placed in internal rotation in a Valpeau position, the fragments twist and collapse with shortening, the head may be pushed into a varus position by the upper shaft, and an undesirable malunion or nonunion is likely to result.

Neer[184] recommends reduction with muscle relaxation in overhead pin traction with the arm in a neutral position. Care must be taken to avoid overdistraction. Alternatively, and more simply, the fracture may be realigned and then maintained with immobilization in a plaster cast in forward flexion and adduction to relax the pectoralis muscle pull.[184]

Closed pinning is not usually possible, and traction risks nonunion. The hanging arm cast has a tendency to lever anteriorly at the fracture site, leading to nonunion or malunion. A posterior plaster slab beginning over the top of the shoulder and extending to the hand has less tendency to angulate the fracture than the hanging cast. Coaptation splints at a right angle to this from the axilla, around the proximal radius and ulna, and up to the lateral shoulder provide additional rotational control.

In polytrauma patients, these fractures are even more difficult to manage by closed means. My preference is to obtain an early anatomic reduction secured by internal fixation rather than risk malrotation, shortening with collapse, nonunion, or malunion, followed by a more difficult secondary reconstruction in a stiff, painful shoulder.

Three operative approaches for stabilization can be considered. My preference is any antegrade intramedullary rod fixation combined with tension band sutures. Heavy absorbable cerclage sutures secure the intermediate fragments with the attached pectoralis major and latissimus dorsi. The fracture fragments can be manipulated to ensure that the cerclage sutures do not include the neurovascular structures. Standard Rush rods are no longer used, as they have a propensity to migrate cephalad prior to fracture healing.

Alternate internal fixation techniques include the Mouridian intramedullary rod with screw fixation into the head,[171] the AO cloverleaf or buttress plate and screws,[88] and retrograde passage of Ender rods.[80,210]

Once the fracture is stabilized, aftercare is as described for other two-part surgical neck fractures treated with open reduction. Progress may be somewhat slower if there is concern that the fragments lack stability.

Possible neurovascular injury is evaluated pre- and intraoperatively. It is usually easier to stabilize the fracture prior to the more delicate nerve or artery repair.

Surgical Neck Fracture With Combined Glenohumeral Dislocation. Glenohumeral dislocations with surgical neck fractures increase the likelihood of an axillary or brachial plexus injury compared with isolated surgical neck fractures alone. The additional dislocation in a fracture is indicative of a greater extracapsular injury. Nerve status must be carefully assessed and documented prior to reduction.

Closed reduction can be accomplished with full overhead traction in flexion and adduction. In most of these dislocations, the head is anterior. It can be gently reduced with fingertip pressure. Any maneuvers that compress the brachial plexus (i.e., a socked foot in the axilla for countertraction) should be avoided.

Open reduction and internal fixation are appropriate if there is a nerve deficit or if a closed reduction is difficult in an individual without a concomitant nerve injury (Fig. 39–41). The operative approach is similar to that for two-part surgical neck fractures without an accompanying dislocation. The deltopectoral interval is opened, and the clavipectoral fascia is split. The intact coracoid muscles are retracted with a lateral Richardson retractor. An anteriorly dislocated head may require dissection off the brachial plexus. A bone hook is used to retract the humeral shaft laterally with the arm in forward flexion. The head is then gently manipulated off the brachial plexus and from the glenoid rim back into the joint.

Rarely, a posterior dislocation occurs within a non-displaced surgical neck fracture. This is an indication for an open reduction using the deltopectoral approach to avoid stronger closed manipulation, which risks displacing the surgical neck fracture.

As with any dislocation in individuals older than 40 years, there is a significant chance of a subscapularis avulsion anteriorly or rupture of the supraspinatus and infraspinatus superiorly and posteriorly. If found, the ruptured tendons are repaired back to their bony inser-

tion through drill holes in bone with nonabsorbable interrupted sutures. The rest of the procedure is described in the section on displaced two-part fractures of the surgical neck without dislocation.

Postoperatively the arm is supported in a lightweight fiberglass or orthoplast cast in neutral rotation and slight abduction or in a sling and swathe. Once adequate fixation has been achieved with the combined tension band and intramedullary rod technique, the arm can be positioned in neutral rotation to enable the patient to better overcome stiffness without the pectoralis displacing the shaft. The top half of the arm cast is removed when pendulum exercises are started (Fig. 39–42).

Deltoid atony from trauma is more likely when a fracture is combined with a dislocation. The arm is supported with a cast or sling to reduce any inferior subluxation. If the fracture-dislocation has been reduced closed, persistent inferior subluxation requires evaluation for nerve injury and cuff tear (Fig. 39–43).

Rehabilitation for these fractures is prolonged and often underestimated. The emphasis is placed on gentle passive motion early, followed by progressive active stretching and strengthening after the fractures have healed between 8 and 16 weeks. Prolonged stiffness and pain may occur. Manipulation under anesthesia is not recommended. Open release at 6 to 12 months follow-

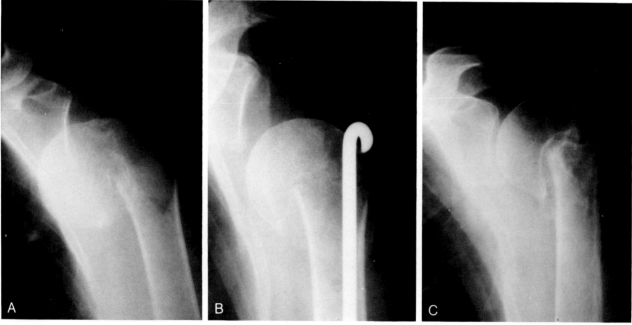

Figure 39–41

Two-part surgical neck fracture and anterior dislocation with associated axillary paralysis noted after prior attempts at a closed reduction. *A*, Injury film. *B*, Following open reduction and internal fixation with intramedullary rod and a nylon figure-of-8 tension band. Initially there was inferior humeral head subluxation, which resolved (*C*) as the axillary nerve returned.

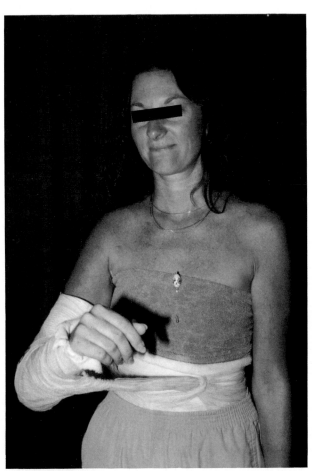

Figure 39-42

Postoperative position for two-part surgical neck fracture.

ing surgery, combined with removal of any prominent hardware, has proven to be gentle and effective when necessary.

Two-Part Greater Tuberosity Fractures. Two-part greater tuberosity fractures comprise 14% of displaced proximal humeral fractures with or without anterior dislocation.[105] It is the most common isolated fracture occurring in skiers.[258] Codman[31] described it as one of the worst proximal humeral fractures, because the supraspinatus is pulled off with the fracture. Anatomically, there are separate facets for the supraspinatus, infraspinatus, and teres minor insertions. Significant displacement of any or all of these facets is pathognomonic of a longitudinal tear of the rotator cuff. The more common displacement in the elderly is a small fragment that retracts into the subacromial space with a supraspinatus tear. In a young patient, both spinati and the teres minor retract the entire tuberosity posteriorly into the spinoglenoid notch. This fragment may be difficult to see on an anteroposterior roentgenogram, but in external rotation, the greater tuberosity will appear to be missing. Lateral scapular and axillary views demonstrate the retracted tuberosity. Additional elevation to determine the degree of displacement with CT is indicated if closed treatment is considered. CT more accurately depicts tuberosity displacement.

Indications for treatment include displacement greater than 5 mm.[158,256] Although treatment might be considered for even less superior displacement, it might later impinge. Other authors have arbitrarily used 1 cm as an indication for open reduction.[6,28,46,47,159,170,179,180,182,183,223,257]

Figure 39-43

A, Inferior glenohumeral subluxation frequently is associated with an acute fracture, bone loss, deltoid paresis, or a massive cuff tear. Two-and-a-half months following fracture, the persistent subluxation was secondary to muscle atony and a supraspinatus cuff avulsion demonstrated by MRI. The EMG was normal. Scanograms demonstrated only 1-cm loss of humeral length through the fracture site. B, MRI scan showing rotator cuff tear.

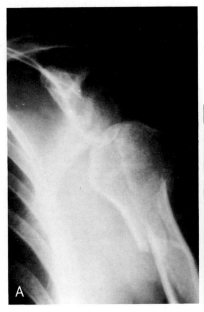

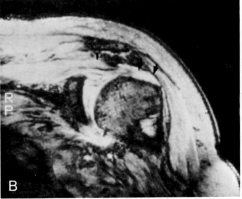

Contraindications to open treatment include severe medical problems that preclude anesthesia and medical or psychiatric problems that prevent the patient from cooperating with the early postoperative rehabilitation.

Early surgery is preferred to avoid fixed retraction of the muscles. A neglected displaced tuberosity may heal to the articular surface and thereby block elevation, resulting in a stiff, weak, and painful shoulder. With time, the articular segment softens, and with late treatment, a humeral head or total shoulder replacement combined with an anterior acromioplasty may be necessary.

For fresh fractures, the patient is placed in the beach chair position with the arm draped free. A 6-cm skin incision along Langer's skin lines is carried through the skin and subcutaneous tissue over the anterolateral aspect of the acromion for the superior approach. The deltoid is split distally from the acromion 5 cm. A stay suture distally protects the axillary nerve below. Richardson retractors are used to expose the underlying bursa and tuberosity fragment. The hemorrhagic bursa is excised. Two large skin hooks in the rotator cuff serve as handles for lateral traction. Nonabsorbable no. 2 or

no. 5 nylon sutures are placed through the rotator cuff at its attachment in the greater tuberosity to replace the skin hooks. The humerus is rotated and abducted to allow anatomic repositioning of the fragment.

Drill holes are made in the shaft distal to the fracture using a Hall drill to penetrate the cortex, followed by Rowe curved awls to connect with the fracture site.

In planning for the closure, the fracture architecture and its relationship to late impingement should be considered. Minimal upward displacement often results in late stiffness or secondary erosion of the cuff insertion. The tuberosity is trimmed to inset the fragment below the level of the humeral articular surface and is then secured with sutures (Figs. 39–44 and 39–45).

Alternatively, screws may be placed in the tuberosity with or without a washer,[88] but I prefer fixation using the hard bone at the cuff insertion to avoid the risk of screw loosening in soft cancellous bone or of intraarticular screw penetration.

Intraoperative complications to avoid include displacement of a nondisplaced or minimally displaced fracture at the surgical neck. Gentle manipulation, support of the humerus, and minimal rotatory torque protect the surgical neck. The suture repair can con-

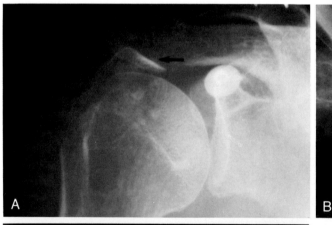

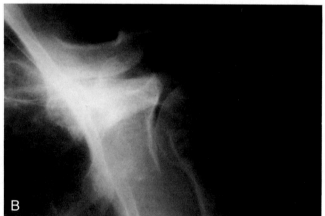

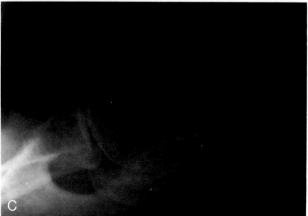

Figure 39–44

Two-part greater tuberosity fracture with rotator cuff tear. *A*, Two-part greater tuberosity avulsion involving the supraspinatus with superior tuberosity retraction. AP (*B*) and axillary (*C*) views of neglected two-part greater tuberosity avulsion leading to traumatic arthritis with posterior retraction of greater tuberosity.

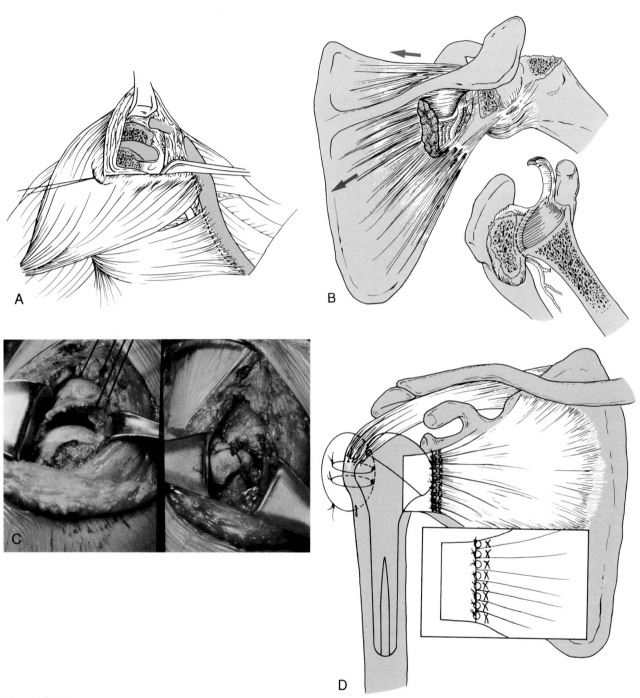

Figure 39-45

Two-part greater tuberosity fracture: operative approach. *A*, The operative approach for a retracted greater tuberosity fragment in a two-part fracture necessitates splitting the deltoid at the junction of the anterior and middle deltoid. For chronic or massive tuberosity avulsions, the anterior acromioplasty approach is added for decompression and exposure. *B*, The greater tuberosity is then mobilized by release of bursa and scar superficially and the posterior and superior capsule at the glenoid margin. The suprascapular nerve at the base of the spine of the scapula is 1.0 to 1.5 cm posterior to the glenoid margin and can be injured with blunt or sharp dissection. *C*, Traction sutures are passed around the tuberosity through the rotator cuff for mobilization and late repair as the tuberosity is replaced on the upper humerus. *D*, The technique of prosthetic replacement for traumatic arthritis using the deltopectoral approach includes subscapularis lengthening with coronal plane Z-plasty, mobilization of the retracted greater tuberosity with cuff attachments, vertical suture repair of the cuff and tuberosity to the shaft, and horizontal tuberosity fixation through the holes in the fin of the cemented prosthesis. A small-head prosthesis is usually required because of the difficulty in immobilizing the cuff with a retracted tuberosity.

tinue below the shaft fracture level. If displacement occurs at the surgical neck, then operative repair as for three-part greater tuberosity fractures is indicated.[198]

Aftercare is similar to that for one-part fractures, beginning with sling immobilization and early pendulum exercises, with advancing exercises at four to six weeks as tuberosity union progresses.

For late treatment of greater tuberosity avulsion fractures, the cuff may be more difficult to mobilize. There are two choices for operative approach: the deltopectoral and the superior or anterior acromioplasty approach. If no arthritis or need for replacement is anticipated, then the anterior acromioplasty approach is used, as it creates more room for the tuberosity while giving more exposure than the deltoid-splitting approach used for fresh fractures. The retracted greater tuberosity and its cuff attachments are freed superficial to the cuff from the acromion, deltoid, and trapezius. On the deep surface the capsule is released from the glenoid without disturbing the origin of the long head of the biceps. The coracoacromial and coracohumeral ligaments are released at the coracoid base. Skin hooks, traction sutures around the tuberosity, and persistence are necessary to bring the cuff laterally and cephalad for

repair to the avulsion site. The rotator interval is closed between the subscapularis and supraspinatus (see Figs. 39–44 and 39–45).

Postoperative treatment is similar to that for other two-part greater tuberosity avulsions. An abduction brace is sometimes used to relax the repair for the first four weeks. A prosthesis may be required for late treatment when the tuberosity has healed to the articular surface. If this can be determined preoperatively, then the head can be removed and the tuberosity osteotomized using the deltopectoral approach.

If an internal rotation contracture is present, the subscapularis is lengthened with a coronal plane Z-plasty (Fig. 39–46). Once the head has been removed, the greater tuberosity and retracted rotator cuff are mobilized in a manner similar to that used for the anterior acromioplasty approach (i.e., from anterior and below rather than from the superior approach). A short-head prosthesis is selected if the retracted cuff cannot be mobilized adequately to fit the tuberosity below the larger size articular surface (Fig. 39–47).

Two-Part Greater Tuberosity Fractures Associated With Anterior Dislocation. Greater tuberosity fractures may occur in up to one third of anterior shoulder

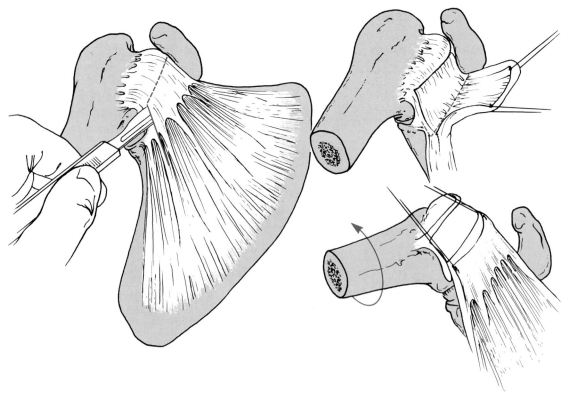

Figure 39–46

Coronal plane Z-plasty of the subscapularis and capsule. (From Norris, T.R. In: Watson, M., ed. Surgical Disorders of the Shoulder. London, Churchill Livingstone, 1991, p 496, by permission.)

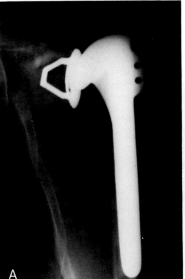
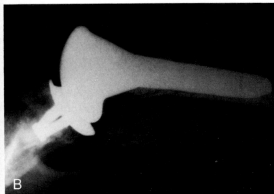

Figure 39–47

Two-part greater tuberosity fracture nonunion with traumatic arthritis treated with total shoulder replacement using a short-head prosthesis to permit tuberosity reapproximation. *A,* Anteroposterior view. *B,* Axillary view.

dislocations.[222] The glenohumeral joint frequently has reduced spontaneously prior to emergency treatment and imaging documentation.

There is a high incidence of nerve injury with luxatio erecta combined with a greater tuberosity fracture. The shoulder is reduced closed with elbow flexion, arm elevation in the plane of the scapula, and upward traction. Once reduced, the arm is lowered[62] and then evaluated for the amount of tuberosity displacement, as described in the previous section.

Closed reductions of subcoracoid anterior dislocations require longitudinal traction in mild abduction with pressure over the back of the greater tuberosity. Excessive abduction or rotation with reduction increases the likelihood of trapping the greater tuberosity displaced under the acromion. When this occurs, open

treatment is used.[207] Operative and postoperative management is described in the previous section.

Two-Part Lesser Tuberosity Fracture. Isolated lesser tuberosity avulsions are rare, comprising only 0.27% of all proximal humeral fractures and 0.5% of displaced fractures.[105] The fracture may be confused with a calcium deposit (Fig. 39–48). Although it is not usually clinically significant in the absence of a posterior dislocation,[183] it may be associated with late stiffness.

Similarly, if a portion of the articular surface accompanies the lesser tuberosity, then a malunion with a block to internal rotation may occur. Open reduction and internal fixation are recommended (Fig. 39–49). In the absence of an associated posterior dislocation, treatment consists of early sling protection, followed by early gentle motion to prevent stiffness. With displace-

Figure 39–48

Two-part lesser tuberosity fracture resulting in late stiffness. *A,* Lesser tuberosity avulsion (*arrow*) could be confused with a calcium deposit. *B,* Restricted elevation nine months following closed fracture treatment.

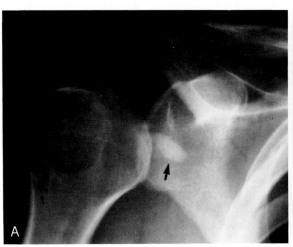
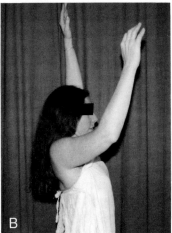

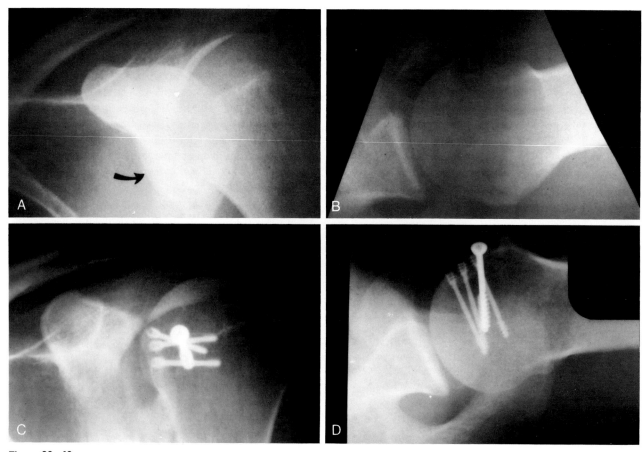

Figure 39–49

Herbert screw fixation of head-splitting fracture. *A,B,* AP and axillary radiographs of a 25-year-old patient following a motor vehicle accident with multiple injuries; grade II open femur fracture, closed with rods at ten days, and displaced lesser tuberosity fracture with 1.5- × 2.0-cm anteroinferior articular fragment attached to the capsule lesser tuberosity. A separate fragment of the lesser tuberosity formed the upper medial biceps groove. *C,D,* AP and axillary radiographs taken seven months postoperatively. Utilizing a deltopectoral approach, the subscapularis was elevated from the capsule. The articular surface was anatomically reduced, temporarily fixed with K wires, then permanently fixed with three Herbert screws 1 to 2 mm below the articular surface (one medially for compression and one each in the superior and inferior capsule reflection). The 4.0-mm cancellous screw was placed extraarticularly to restore the lesser tuberosity and biceps groove. Seven months later, full painless range of motion was restored without avascular necrosis or hardware loosening. (From Lange, R.H.; Engber, W.D.; Clancy, W.G. Orthopedics 9(10):1393–1398, 1986.)

ment of more than 1 to 1.5 cm, suture repair may be considered.

Preoperative planning, aside from caring for other associated injuries, requires adequate imaging studies to evaluate tuberosity displacement, articular surface involvement, and possible associated nondisplaced fractures at the surgical neck or missed posterior dislocations.

The surgical approach for repair using screw fixation is shown in Figure 39–49. If the articular surface is not significantly involved, then screw fixation, or suture fixation where screw fixation is not adequate, is used for young patients. With suture fixation, the subscapularis and capsule need not be separated. Utilizing the deltopectoral approach, the coracoid muscles are left intact. Special care is taken to preserve the anterior

circumflex humeral vessels at the inferior border of the subscapularis and, more importantly, the arcuate artery as it ascends the lateral biceps groove. Sutures are placed through the subscapularis insertion around the lesser tuberosity. The deep sutures are passed through drill holes connecting the avulsion site with the humeral shaft and greater tuberosity. If necessary, the lesser tuberosity is pared to permit a secure inset into the cancellous bed. The sutures are tied and tested for security. The rotator interval is closed, and then the glenohumeral joint is evaluated for stability prior to a layered closure (Fig. 39–50).

Postoperatively a sling is worn for four to five weeks. Pendulum exercises are started the first postoperative day, advancing to supine assisted elevation and pulley exercises for the first three weeks. Careful clinical and

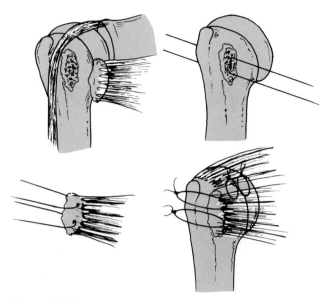

Figure 39-50

Screw or suture fixation of lesser tuberosity fracture. *A*, With head defect less than 20%, the tuberosity is repaired in its anatomic position. *B*, With head defect between 20% and 40%, the tuberosity is transferred into the head defect. Postoperatively, the arm is immobilized at the side in 15° external rotation to allow the posterior capsule to heal.

roentgenogram follow-up is necessary. Exercises are discontinued or diminished if there is any evidence of fracture displacement. By three to four weeks, gentle assisted external rotation is started. Active exercises commence at six to eight weeks when the tuberosity has healed.

Two-Part Lesser Tuberosity Fracture With Posterior Dislocation. Posterior dislocation is associated with a lesser tuberosity fracture in 1.3% of all displaced proximal humeral fractures[105]; thus it is more frequent than the isolated lesser tuberosity fracture. Unfortunately, unless adequate imaging studies in the axial plane are obtained, the dislocation may be missed. As will all dislocations, the incidence of nerve injury is higher than with fractures alone.

Preoperative planning includes careful documentation of neurovascular status and axillary views or CT scans to assess the amount of articular surface involvement. These fractures may also be associated with a nondisplaced fracture of the surgical neck.

General or scalene block anesthesia is recommended to lessen the chance of displacing other fractures. If there is no surgical neck fracture, then a closed reduction is attempted. Using image intensification, the arm is brought into forward flexion and adduction. With longitudinal traction and pressure on the humeral head from behind, the posterior dislocation is reduced while lowering the arm.

Once reduced, closed treatment presents a challenge. Better apposition of the lesser tuberosity is expected if the arm is internally rotated, but the shoulder may redislocate. The more important lesion to treat is the dislocation. Immobilization in 15° external rotation and 15° extension with the arm at the side allows the posterior capsule to heal. If the tuberosity displacement is significant, then either it can be ignored, with symptomatic treatment later if necessary, or an open reduction with fixation can be performed primarily. There is little published clinical experience clearly favoring either approach.[105,183,184]

If there is a surgical neck fracture, the arm cannot be levered across the glenoid to disengage the head safely, and an open reduction is necessary. With the patient in the beach chair position and under general anesthesia, the lesser tuberosity is identified through the deltopectoral approach. I prefer suspending the arm with the McConnell arm holder to avoid adding rotational torque that could displace the surgical neck fracture. Traction sutures are passed around the lesser tuberosity, and a Darrach or Fukuda retractor is placed across the glenoid to gently lever the humeral head back into the joint. Gentle external rotation allows placement of a flat elevator under the head. Once reduced, the lesser tuberosity is repaired, and the arm is supported with a light fiberglass or plastic cast at the side in 15° of extension and 40° external rotation for four to six weeks to allow the posterior capsule to heal.

Variations in operative findings may require alternative treatment. If there is an anterior articular impression fracture of up to 40% of the entire humeral articular surface, two options are available. The first is to transfer the lesser tuberosity into the defect and fix it with a screw (Fig. 39-51).[183,184] Alternatively, Gerber has fashioned articular graft harvested from the femoral head in fresh fractures treated with replacement.[67] Large head defects greater than 40% are treated with primary arthroplasty.

The timing of surgery influences the treatment. In late cases, scar precludes safe closed reduction. Joint changes after 6 to 12 weeks favor humeral replacement or possibly total shoulder replacement if the glenoid is involved. Active rather than passive range-of-motion exercises immediately following cast removal enable earlier rehabilitation. Forceful rotation is avoided. As with any posterior dislocation, upright elevation using a pulley is preferable to supine elevation in early rehabilitation. The latter stresses the posterior capsule more than is desired in the first three months after reduction.

Three-Part Fractures

In three-part fractures, the shaft and one tuberosity are displaced. The incidence varies in reported series from

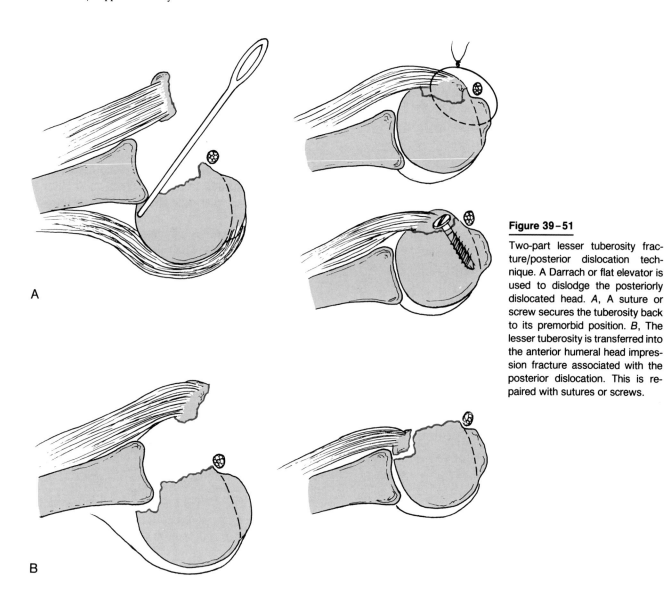

A

B

Figure 39–51

Two-part lesser tuberosity fracture/posterior dislocation technique. A Darrach or flat elevator is used to dislodge the posteriorly dislocated head. *A,* A suture or screw secures the tuberosity back to its premorbid position. *B,* The lesser tuberosity is transferred into the anterior humeral head impression fracture associated with the posterior dislocation. This is repaired with sutures or screws.

3% to 29% of displaced proximal humeral fractures without a dislocation.[105,179,183]

Treatment options include closed or no reduction followed by early motion and pain medications,[90] closed reduction and immobilization for three to four weeks,[83] open reduction and internal fixation,[5,30,73,74,77,83,84,124,179,180,198,209,216,228,244,246] and prosthetic replacement.[33,34,183,198,203,249]

Closed treatment is indicated for those patients for whom an anesthetic is deemed unsafe or for those with alcoholism or a similar disorder in which a modicum of postoperative cooperation is precluded. The likelihood of satisfactory results with closed treatment is less than 50%.[33]

Open treatment is indicated in an otherwise healthy patient to restore anatomy and repair the rotator cuff. Tuberosity displacement is pathognomonic of a longitudinal cuff tear. The tuberosity that remains intact with the head rotates the articular surface to face the side of tuberosity avulsion; the head is disimpacted from the shaft. For example, with a three-part greater tuberosity displaced fracture, the articular surface faces posteriorly. This is best visualized on axillary and lateral scapula projections. These fractures are poorly reduced using closed measures, and there is a risk of neurovascular injury with strong or repeated manipulations.

Contraindications to open reduction and internal fixation include osteoporosis or an inability to obtain satisfactory fixation.

Three-Part Greater Tuberosity Fractures. Surgery is performed when the patient can be scheduled by a surgeon experienced in shoulder reconstructive techniques. The patient is advised that a later lysis of scar and adhesions may be necessary. With flimsy tissue or soft bone, a prosthesis may be chosen. All necessary fixation devices and prostheses should be in the operating room prior to anesthetizing the patient.

The standard beach chair position with the supine patient high on the operative table and over to the side permits lowering the arm off the side. The head is protected in slight flexion with the McConnell headrest. A 15-cm deltopectoral incision from the clavicle to the deltoid insertion preserves the cephalic vein. The coracoid muscles are left intact to protect the brachial plexus. For ease of exposure, the upper half of the pectoralis and anterior 1 cm of the deltoid insertion may be released. The long head of the biceps serves as a guide to the shoulder joint. The displaced tuberosity (the greater tuberosity in most instances) is retrieved with skin hooks. Nonabsorbable sutures are placed through the rotator cuff insertion on the tuberosity for manipulation and reduction of the fracture relative to the humeral head, other tuberosity, and shaft. The surgeon has the choice of several forms of fixation, including suture or wire,[84] with or without intramedullary support, and plates and screws.

The technique for suture or wire fixation requires fracture reduction first between the tuberosities and head. Two 14-gauge colpotomy needles with stylets in place are passed through the subscapularis and lesser tuberosity, through the head, and out through the greater tuberosity and supraspinatus tendon. The malrotation of the head on the shaft is reduced. Two holes are drilled through the anterior humeral shaft below the greater tuberosity and lesser tuberosity and deep to the biceps. Two 20-gauge wires or no. 5 nonabsorbable nylon sutures are used. The first is passed through the shaft, crossing the fracture in a figure-of-8 centered on the surgical neck fracture with one end through the colpotomy needle. This needle is then removed, and the suture is tied securely. The process is then repeated with a second figure-of-8 through the second colpotomy needle, thereby converting this to a stable one-part fracture. The rotator interval tear is repaired. Stability is checked as the shoulder is passed through a full range of motion (Fig. 39–52A).

Intraoperative difficulties may include a poor rotator cuff that requires mobilization and repair and less-than-adequate holding power in the soft bone. Supple-

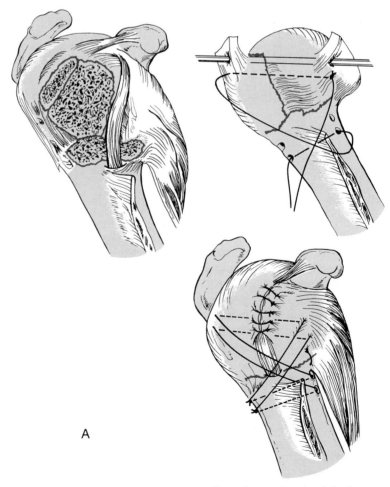

Figure 39–52

Techniques of three-part fracture fixation. A, Tension band fixation.

A

Illustration continued on following page

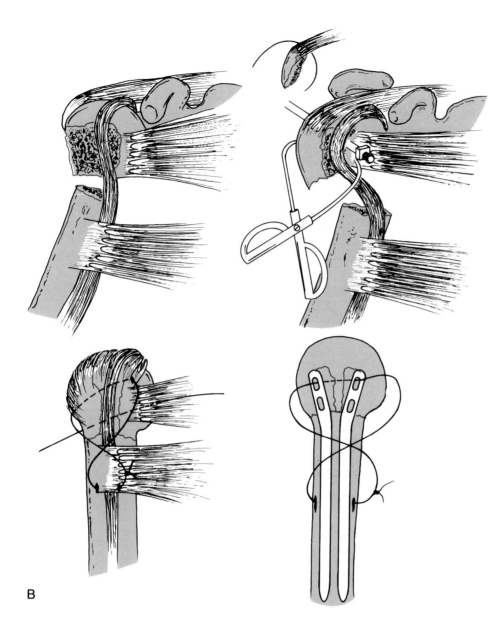

Figure 39–52 *Continued*

B, Tension band combined with intramedullary rods. (Modified from Hawkins, R.J., et al. J Bone Joint Surg 68A:1410–1414, 1986.)

B

mental intramedullary rods with tension band closure between both tuberosities adds additional stability with vertical fixation to the shaft and horizontal fixation to the intact tuberosity (Fig. 39–52*B*).

Wire can be tied more securely than no. 5 nylon, but it has a propensity to break with motion or tuberosity collapse; then migration of the pieces poses a significant problem.[148,183] My preference is to use nonabsorbable sutures with one figure-of-8 tension band and intramedullary rods with the second tension band to supplement the fixation.

AO cloverleaf plates provide another option in the younger patient. However, the possibility of postoperative impingement and the additional surgical exposure with the resultant increased incidence of avascular necrosis make this less desirable.[77,244] With an average patient age of 61 years for these fractures,[84] osteoporo-

sis is common. Plates and screws hold poorly in the upper humerus in this setting (Fig. 39–53).[84,198,229]

Prosthetic replacement is preferred when more secure fixation can be obtained, and exercises are started earlier to prevent disabling stiffness. Secondary procedures, although worthwhile, are still more difficult and have less favorable outcomes than the best procedure done primarily. Frequently second procedures are necessary in an older patient with soft bone or to revise a failed internal fixation. In malunions and nonunions, the glenoid is resurfaced if it is significantly involved and the rotator cuff can be reconstructed. The technique for humeral head replacement is reviewed in the section on four-part fractures.

Three-Part Lesser Tuberosity Fractures. Three-part fractures with lesser tuberosity displacement are much less frequent than those with greater tuberosity dis-

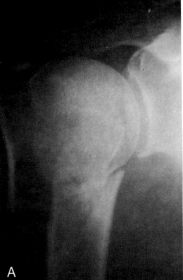

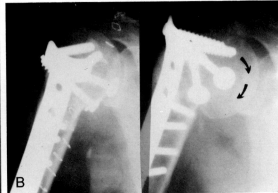

Figure 39–53

Poor screw and plate holding power in elderly patients with osteoporotic bone. *A,* Injury film showing three-part greater tuberosity fracture. *B,* Postoperative radiographs immediately and at four weeks with loss of fixation in the proximal humerus.

placement. The articular surface is rotated anteriorly by the intact external rotators.

Indications for and principles of surgery are the same as those for a three-part greater tuberosity and surgical neck fracture. In older individuals, prosthetic arthroplasty allows more secure fixation, thereby permitting earlier motion to lessen stiffness. For the combined three-part fracture and midshaft fracture, operative treatment using a long-stem prosthesis and employing the resected head as bone graft simplifies surgery and postoperative care. It also eliminates the risk of avascular necrosis, the need for hardware removal, and the risk of loosening or hardware impingement that is more common with plates and screws.[33,84,184,198,203,249]

The security of repair for three-part fractures treated with internal fixation or with prosthetic replacement and tuberosity fixation is determined at surgery. A 45° abduction brace with motion upward from the brace is used for four to six weeks if tension needs to be taken off the tuberosity repair. Otherwise the arm is placed in a sling at the side, and early pendulum motion is begun shortly after surgery. More aggressive stretching is avoided for the first three weeks; otherwise tuberosity and rotator cuff dehiscence is more likely.[249]

Active range of motion begins at six to eight weeks, with light resistive exercises begun at 12 weeks. Six to twelve months of daily stretching and long-term therapy will be necessary for individuals to gain elevation above 90°.

Hardware is removed if breakage, loosening, migration, or impingement occurs. Prosthetic replacement is undertaken for painful nonunion, malunion, or late arthritis.

Three-Part Fracture-Dislocations. Three-part displaced surgical neck shaft fracture-dislocations occur in two common patterns: an anterior head dislocation with a greater tuberosity fracture and a posterior head dislocation with a lesser tuberosity fracture. These dislocations have a greater chance of neurovascular injury with extensive capsular disruption and late avascular necrosis following closed or open fixation (Fig. 39–54).

With a three-part greater tuberosity displaced fracture–anterior dislocation, the subscapularis and anterior capsule may still provide some blood supply to the articular surface. The arcuate artery enters the lateral biceps groove as the terminal arterial supply, thus jeopardizing assured circulation to the head. Open reduction and internal fixation are more gentle and accurate than closed techniques.

Three-part lesser tuberosity fracture–posterior dislocations are often not well appreciated. An axillary view or CT scan may be necessary to diagnose the tuberosity displacement as well as the posterior dislocation. Closed reduction is possible in forward flexion and gentle abduction, but an open reduction through a deltopectoral approach is more gentle and allows for accurate tuberosity repair, cuff closure, and derotation of the head relative to the shaft.

The surgical techniques and aftercare have been described in the section on two-part fractures.

Four-Part Fractures and Fracture-Dislocations

In four-part fractures, the articular surface is detached from its blood supply. The small segment of articular surface may be dislocated anteriorly, posteriorly, laterally, or inferiorly or crushed. Both tuberosities are separated from the head and shaft and from each other. A longitudinal rotator cuff tear is present. In rare instances, the tuberosities are still joined at the biceps groove, but these are still treated as four-part fractures

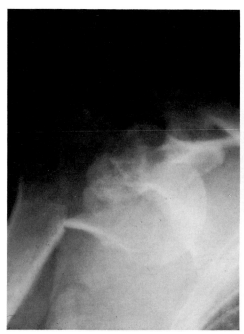
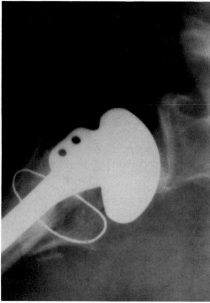

Figure 39-54

Three-part fracture with anterior dislocation of the articular surface also had comminution of the upper shaft. Tuberosity reconstruction around a cemented humeral head replacement out to proper length enabled earlier motion with less risk of the tuberosity avulsion encountered with other measures of open reduction and internal fixation.

(Fig. 39-55), more specifically through a deltopectoral approach without coracoid muscle detachment. The lesser tuberosity is isolated and controlled by two no. 5 nonabsorbable Tevdek sutures. The head is reduced, and the holding power of the head and greater tuberosity is assessed. In a young individual with good quality bone stock, an open reduction is undertaken, using a figure-of-8 suture technique with repair of the tuberosities to each other and to the shaft similar to that demonstrated for three-part greater tuberosity fractures (Fig. 39-52A). Additional stability can be obtained with intramedullary fixation demonstrated in Figure 39-52B.

Surgery is indicated to restore the anatomy securely so that motion can be instituted early to avoid stiffness. Open reductions and internal fixations are frequently discussed but seldom practiced.[33,34] Less secure fixation, hardware complications, avascular necrosis, and nonunion contribute to the poor results with efforts to save the small amount of articular cartilage.[33,34,77,187,188,244,249]

Prosthetic arthroplasty is the preferred treatment of all types of four-part fractures, head-splitting fractures, articular impression fractures of greater than 40% of the articular surface, selected malunions, nonunions, and osteoporotic three-part fractures. Earlier surgery is preferred to lessen the likelihood of heterotopic bone formation. Contraindications to replacement include active sepsis or widespread neurologic loss in which both the deltoid and the rotator cuff are not expected to recover. Infection requires debridement and control,

whereas irreversible neurologic deficits are corrected with an arthrodesis.

Early reports suggested that surgery be done in the first 48 hours,[178] but the safe time interval has been extended.[187] In general, surgery is performed as soon as it can be scheduled; it should not be delayed for late reconstruction, as pericapsular bone may form.

Preoperative planning should include a careful assessment of neurovascular status, medical condition, and fracture architecture. When swelling and pain make it difficult to clinically assess nerve status, EMG and nerve conduction studies can be obtained. Ninety percent of patients are medically cleared by an internist or cardiologist.

Scanograms are now routinely obtained preoperatively to determine how far above an identifiable point on the upper shaft the prosthesis should rest. Final adjustments can be made in surgery based on the tension in the long head of the biceps and rotator cuff.

The 15-cm deltopectoral incision begins at the clavicle, passes over the coracoid, and is carried down to the deltoid insertion. The cephalic vein is preserved. The clavipectoral fascia is incised. Richardson retractors or a self-retaining abdominal Balfour retract the deltoid laterally and cephalad and the intact coracoid muscles medially. Abduction of the arm and release of the anterior 1 cm of the deltoid insertion and the upper half of the pectoralis provide more exposure if necessary without detachment of the deltoid origin (Fig. 39-56).

The key landmark is the long head of the biceps. The rotator cuff and tuberosities, if they are intact at the

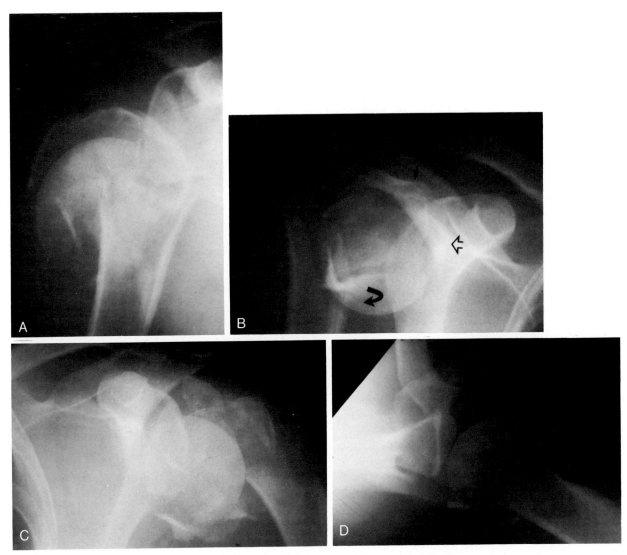

Figure 39–55

Four-part fracture. *A,* Lateral dislocation of the head and a surgical neck fracture, with the tuberosities still joined at the biceps groove (*open arrow*) without attachment to articular surface. *B,* There is a posterior dislocation of the head, the lesser tuberosity is an isolated fragment, and the greater tuberosity fracture has included the biceps groove. *C,* Anterior dislocation with head resting on brachial plexus. *D,* Axillary view following open reduction without tuberosity repair prior to prosthetic replacement.

biceps groove, are split along the interval joining the subscapularis and supraspinatus. The coracohumeral and coracoacromial ligaments are released. Two no. 5 traction sutures are placed through the rotator cuff near each tuberosity insertion; these will hold better than drill holes in the bone. The articular segment is then retrieved to save as potential bone graft to the tuberosities and shaft.

The McConnell arm holder can be used for gentle distraction for subacromial visualization as well as release of the coracoacromial ligament. If there is a prominent beak to the anterior acromion or inferior spurring at the acromioclavicular joint, then these are removed

with an osteotome or ronguer prior to humeral head replacement. These areas are visualized with relaxation of the deltoid in abduction. The deltoid is subperiosteally elevated with sharp dissection in preparation for the acromioplasty. If the deltoid is inadvertently released, then repair is accomplished after the acromioplasty with sutures through the remaining acromion.

The humeral shaft is delivered into the deltopectoral interval by extending the arm off the table and pushing upward at the elbow. The narrow humeral reamer is passed down the canal, and then a small- or large-head trial prosthesis with a narrow stem replaces the reamer. The ridge of the biceps groove on the shaft is located,

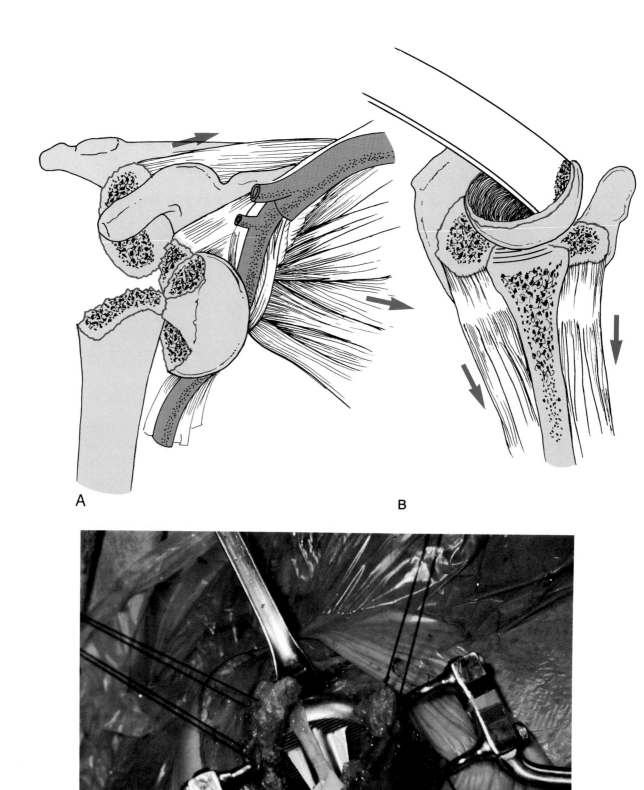

Figure 39-56

Technique of prosthetic replacement for four-part fractures. *A*, The articular surface is avascular and may rest on the brachial plexus. Rotator cuff muscles displace the tuberosities. The pectoralis, deltoid, and gravity displace the shaft. *B*, The axial view demonstrates the medial retraction of the tuberosities by their respective muscle attachments. In this illustration, the displaced head has been reduced. *C*, Operative photograph demonstrates biceps identification, tuberosity and cuff mobilization, and trial humeral head reduction, which preserves humeral length.

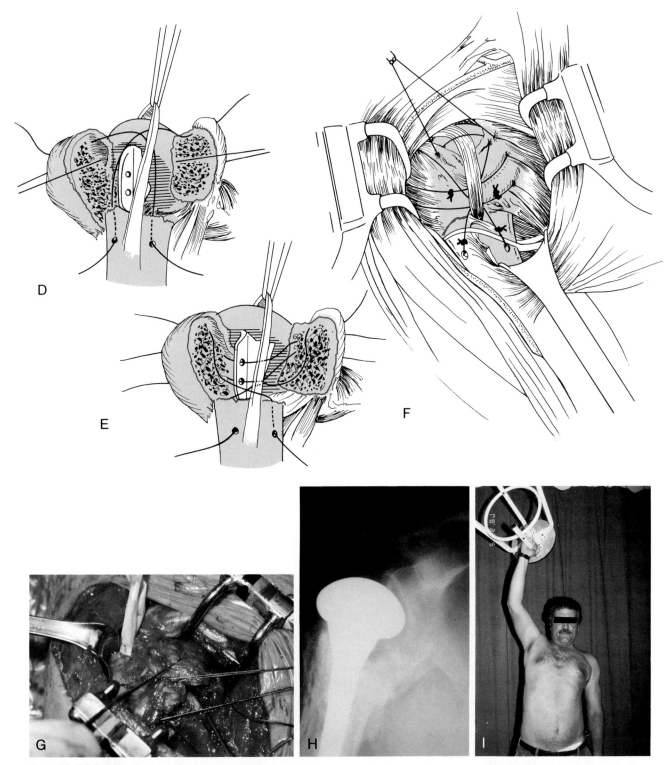

Figure 39–56 *Continued*

D, The long head of the biceps at the rotator interval is a key structure in identifying the lesser and greater tuberosity with displacement. Four-part fracture traction sutures are placed through the rotator cuff at their insertion on each tuberosity both for horizontal repair of the tuberosity to the shaft and to each fracture segment and for vertical repair through drill holes in the shaft. A trial reduction with a small-stem prosthesis enables the surgeon to assess the proper height with the aid of preoperative scanograms, the tension in the long head of the biceps tendon, and the ability to close the rotator cuff around the prosthesis. Note that the tuberosities make up a significant portion of the upper shaft. *E*, Once the prosthesis has been cemented in proper version and height, the tuberosities are approximated under the articular surface and above the diaphyseal shaft with vertical and horizontal fixation. *F*, Sutures preplaced in rotator interval are then tied. *G*, Reapproximation of tuberosities in the operative setting. *H*, Mild ectopic bone formation did not preclude a satisfactory result. *I*, Four-year clinical follow-up with good strength and mild restriction of motion.

and a notch for the fin is made with a ronguer just posterior to the biceps groove. This ensures proper version.

Common errors to avoid include removing too much bone and resting the prosthesis on the shaft without leaving room for the tuberosities. Otherwise the head subluxates inferiorly, as the deltoid myofascial sleeve is rendered too long. Unless the prosthesis restores the humeral length, it will be unstable with the functionally weakened deltoid. Too much retroversion will make it difficult to reposition the greater tuberosity, whereas less than the normal 30° to 35° of retroversion fosters anterior instability.[33]

Spinning of the prosthesis without normal metaphyseal bone support is more likely with both tuberosities displaced. Methylmethacrylate fixation is preferred with the prosthesis extended to length once the proper stem size has been selected. Prior to fixing the humeral component, vertical sutures are passed through drill holes in the shaft to provide tuberosity fixation.

A trial reduction is then performed. The mobilized tuberosities with cuff attachments are fitted below the level of the articular surface. This avoids greater tuberosity impingement and adds length to the upper shaft. The tuberosities can be held together with a towel clamp while determining proper head height.

With the trial prosthesis out, sutures to repair the longitudinal tear in the rotator cuff are placed but not tied. During the cementing of the prosthesis, the tuberosities are not forced over the humeral head; otherwise their pressure could cause the humeral component to subside prior to cement hardening. During methylmethacrylate curing, extra cement is removed from above the shaft level. The space between the cemented prosthesis and the shaft is filled in by the tuberosities. The traction sutures around each tuberosity are passed through the holes in the prosthetic fin. The vertical sutures in the shaft secure each tuberosity. Because of the stress riser effect of the prosthetic fin, wire sutures are avoided, as late breakage is often a problem.

The preplaced sutures for the rotator interval are closed, and the repair security is evaluated. Limits of motion determined intraoperatively are used to guide the postoperative rehabilitation.

The deltopectoral interval is closed over two Hemovac drains that exit posteriorly and superiorly. Following subcutaneous and a subcuticular skin closure, the arm is placed in a sling unless additional relaxation of the greater tuberosity repair is desirable. For these patients, a 45° abduction pillow, brace, or cast is used.

Essential aftercare includes ample postoperative support with early physician-guided passive range of motion beginning by one week. Active-assistive range of motion begins with early healing by six weeks. Isometric exercises are added at six weeks and isotonic exercises at twelve weeks.

Head-Splitting Fracture. Head-splitting fractures may occur with or without dislocation; often they are associated with other fractures (Figs. 39–16 and 39–49). Prosthetic replacement is the preferred treatment in order to avoid avascular necrosis, obtain secure fixation, and begin early motion.

Articular Defects With Dislocation

Posterior Head Defect (Hill-Sachs) and Anterior Dislocation. Impression fractures of the articular surface frequently occur with traumatic or recurrent dislocations. These are associated with labral detachments at the anteroinferior glenoid margin. A closed reduction is indicated. Repair of the labral detachment is performed in special circumstances primarily and routinely with recurrent instability. It provides stability without the need for infraspinatus or tuberosity transfer into the defect. Glenoid rim fractures with dislocations are associated with an 80% recurrent dislocation rate with closed treatment. Early fracture repair or late ligament advancement to the remaining glenoid margin effectively restores stability in the absence of more complicated bone blocks. Impression fractures of less than 30% to 40% would not be expected to cause recurrent dislocations alone.

For impression fractures greater than 50%, humeral head replacement and capsular repair are preferred early rather than waiting for the development of more advanced traumatic arthritis, which requires glenoid replacement. In individuals older than 40 years, imaging studies are important to rule out a rotator cuff tear. A poor result is anticipated with both a neglected large humeral head defect and cuff tear.

Glenoid bone grafting with replacement is considered for deficient glenoids secondary to eccentric wear or loss of more than 25% of the anterior glenoid in late reconstruction for traumatic arthritis.[204] With acute fractures involving 25% or more of the glenoid, an early open reduction with internal fixation is preferred. When treatment is delayed, with loss of contact and motion between the head and glenoid, then replacement for bone loss and articular surface changes may be necessary.

Essential aftercare is directed to the ligamentous stability of the shoulder repair rather than the impression fracture. Immobilization of the arm in internal rotation with a sling for three to five weeks with early pendulum exercises protects the ligament repair while decreasing stiffness. Exercises are advanced after five weeks (Fig. 39–57).

Anterior Head Impression Fracture (Reverse Hill-Sachs) and Posterior Dislocation. Humeral head defects of less than 20% are treated early with closed re-

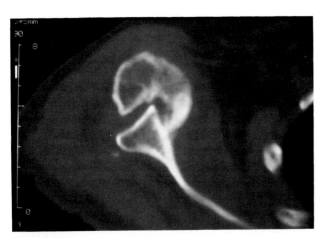

Figure 39-57

Anterior dislocation with large posterior humeral head impression fracture. In this case the articular surface was soft. Humeral head replacement was performed without the need for glenoid resurfacing.

duction under general anesthesia. The arm is flexed forward, internally rotated, and adducted to disengage the head from the posterior glenoid rim. With longitudinal traction and anterior pressure on the head from behind, the head is gently reduced. The arm is externally rotated and lowered to the side and is then immobilized in 15° extension and external rotation for five to six weeks in a light fiberglass cast.

Contraindications for closed reduction are a fixed dislocation that is not easily reducible or an undisplaced fracture at the surgical neck or tuberosity.

With head impression fractures between 20% and 40%, a closed reduction may be attempted with similar treatment as for the smaller impression fractures (Fig. 39-58).

Alternatively, Neer's modification, using the lesser

tuberosity,[183,184,193] of McLaughlin's subscapularis transfer[102,158] to the anteromedial head defect is effective in preventing recurrent posterior dislocations.[86] The lesser tuberosity is osteotomized to convert this to a two-part lesser tuberosity fracture in acute cases (Fig. 39-59). The operative technique and rehabilitation are as described for two-part lesser tuberosity fractures. Results of the tuberosity transfer have been superior to those for the subscapularis transfer alone.[85]

In chronic cases, it is more likely that a replacement will be necessary. Rather than osteotomizing the lesser tuberosity, a subscapularis coronal plane Z-plasty preserves the tuberosity while giving the option for lengthening a contracted subscapularis (see Figs. 39-46 and 39-59B).

Preoperative discussion prior to a closed or open reduction of a posterior fracture-dislocation should review the risks of redislocation, intraoperative fracture, and nerve injury and the possible need for a humeral head replacement at the time of surgery or later, as necessary. Displacement of previously nondisplaced fractures changes the treatment indications to those for the new type of displaced fracture encountered.

Intraoperative complications include the inability to reduce the fracture using closed treatment, enlargement of the head defect, shaft fracture, and continued gross instability following reduction.

During open reduction, the head may be discovered to have more comminution and fragmentation than previously appreciated or to have a generalized arthritis. Humeral head or total shoulder replacement with rotator cuff balancing and reconstruction are then considered. Should the shaft fracture with closed or open reduction, a long-stem prosthesis is recommended if humeral head replacement is indicated; otherwise intramedullary or ASIF plate fixation, rather than closed

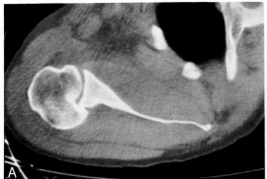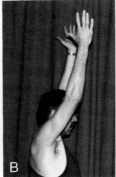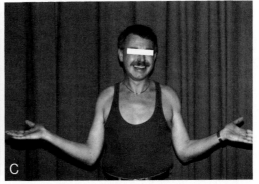

Figure 39-58

Posterior fracture-dislocation of the humeral head. *A*, This responded to a closed reduction and became stable when immobilized in a lightweight fiberglass waistband cast with the arm in 15° extension, 10° abduction, and 15° external rotation for five weeks. *B,C*, Three months following fracture, the shoulder is stable with good return of elevation and rotation.

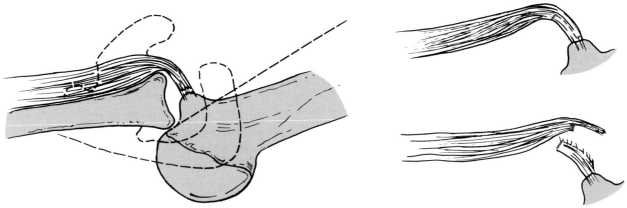

Figure 39–59

A, Lesser tuberosity osteotomy permits transfer of the tuberosity into an anterior head defect. *B,* Alternatively, a subscapularis lengthening permits latitude at the time of closure for adjusting the tension and reestablishing external rotation. With a subscapularis and capsule contracture, each centimeter of lengthening permits an additional 20° of external rotation.

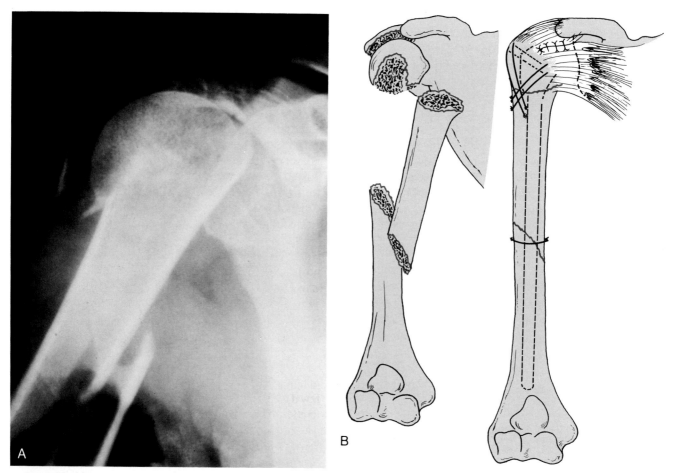

Figure 39–60

Long-stem prosthesis. *A,* Three-part fracture of the proximal humerus with diaphyseal midshaft fracture. *B,* Reconstruction of cuff and tuberosities and fixation of shaft fracture with long-stem prosthesis. (*B* Redrawn from Norris, T.R.; McElheney, E.: Seminars in Arthroplasty 1(2):138–150, 1990. W.B. Saunders.)

Table 39–3.

Preferred Treatment for Fractures and Fracture-Dislocations of the Proximal Humerus

Approximate incidence of fracture type	Type	Closed reduction	ORIF	Indications for prosthetic replacement
50%–80%	One-part nondisplaced			
10%	Two-part	LT, shaft	AN in child, GT irreducible or unstable shaft nonunion, symptomatic	AN in adult, AVN, SN nonunion with osteoporotic head, AVN, some MU, TA
3%	Three-part	Rare	LT, GT	LT or GT with osteoporosis or unstable after ORIF, MU, or NU
4%	Four-part			Repair tuberosities to shaft, rotator cuff, cement prosthesis
	Fracture-dislocation	Two-part A and P in absence of RCT	Two-part with cuff tear, three-part A or P (some)	Some three-part A or P, all four-part
	Head-splitting		Rare	Preferred
	Head impression	<20%, early	20%–40% with tuberosity transfer into defect	>40% chronic dislocations

Displaced fractures are those with >1 cm displacement and >45° angulation. Greater tuberosity fractures with greater than 0.5 cm displacement superiorly are now considered displaced.

Abbreviations: A = anterior dislocation; AN = anatomic neck, articular surface free segment; AVN = avascular necrosis; GT = greater tuberosity, shaft displaced at surgical neck; LT = lesser tuberosity; MU = malunion; NU = nonunion; ORIF = open reduction and internal fixation; P = posterior dislocation; RCT = rotator cuff tear; SN = surgical neck; TA = traumatic arthritis.

treatment, is recommended for shaft stabilization (Fig. 39–60).[206]

When good stability is restored with prosthetic replacement, pendulum exercises begin early. The posterior capsule is not stressed early. Active exercises commence at four to six weeks postoperatively and advance to isotonic strengthening at three months. It may take 9 to 12 months for maximal range of motion and strength to develop (Tables 39–3 and 39–4).

Pathologic Fractures

Lancaster et al.[134] reported on 57 humeral fractures or impending humeral fractures in patients with inoperable cancer. Fractures of the proximal humerus have been treated with cemented intramedullary fixation or prosthetic replacement with satisfactory results. Healing occurs by four months.[134,171] For sensitive tumors, local irradiation is used postoperatively.

Follow-up Care and Rehabilitation

IMMOBILIZATION

Following fractures of the proximal humerus, the arm is routinely protected in a sling between times of exercise. Adequate support is required for bone and fibrous healing. A 45° abduction brace or cast will relax the greater tuberosity repair in patients in whom fragile bone or soft tissue would benefit from additional support for the first four to five weeks. Avoiding early stress to the cuff and tuberosity repairs for three weeks has decreased the incidence of tuberosity and cuff dehiscence for the more complicated fractures.[33,249]

In fractures associated with posterior dislocation where postoperative instability is a concern, the arm is protected in a fiberglass or light plastic orthosis with the arm at the side in 15° extension and external rotation for four to six weeks to allow the posterior capsule to heal.

MOBILIZATION

When possible, early joint motion is begun in the first few days following surgery. With very secure internally fixed fractures, a continuous passive motion apparatus is used to externally rotate the arm to neutral and forward flex the arm up to 30°. There is a risk of splitting open the repair in disoriented or nauseated patients; thus its use has been limited to selected patients, in whom it is used for 2 hours and alternated with sling support for 2 hours to allow the patients to ambulate.

Table 39-4.

Common Pitfalls in Prosthetic Replacement for Fractures

Problem	Potential result	Solution
Prosthesis too low	Functionally weakens deltoid; inferior subluxation	Place tuberosities between shaft and head or bone graft to full humeral height
Prosthesis stem too narrow	Pistoning or spinning	Larger stem or methylmethacrylate fixation
Uncemented prosthesis without metaphyseal bone support	Loosening prior to tuberosity healing; subsidence	Larger stem or methylmethacrylate fixation
Prosthesis in varus	Greater tuberosity prominent; impingement shaft penetration	Redirect prosthesis at proper height and version
Subsidence	Greater tuberosity prominent; with impingement shaft penetration	Cement at proper height; bone graft PRN
Too much retroversion	Difficult GT attachment; posterior instability	Correct version; cement PRN
Too much anteversion	Anterior instability	Correct version; cement PRN
Tuberosity avulsion	Cuff retear; weakness; loss of elevation	Delay rehabilitation; trim tuberosity for fit; vertical and horizontal repair; bone graft
Intraoperative shaft fracture below prosthesis stem	Unstable fracture	Long-stem prosthesis with or without cement
Cerclage wiring of upper shaft fracture	Bone necrosis or wire breakage	Wire removal, bone graft

Abbreviations: GT = greater tuberosity; PRN = as necessary.

At surgery, the surgeon determines the safe range of motion, which then guides the early postoperative exercises. Frequently some passive rotation or elevation is possible from an abduction brace upward.

Exercises and mobilization are slow. Unfortunately, exercises cannot exceed the weakest combined suture and tissue strength. Mason et al. demonstrated that tendon repair strength is less at 10 to 12 days following surgery than on the day of repair. By three weeks, the repair is again as strong as when the sutures were first placed.[150,151]

PHYSICAL THERAPY

Determination of the length of immobilization, the amount of mobilization, and the appropriate exercises is made by the surgeon. With earlier passive motion, results in complex fracture care have improved.[184,187,188] Physician-directed exercises have been conveniently divided into three phases.[98]

Phase I Exercises

Phase I begins with passive assisted stretching exercises to avoid capsular contracture and adhesions in the subacromial, subdeltoid, and scapulothoracic gliding planes (Fig. 39-61). Early application of ice following surgery decreases swelling and pain. Later, moist heat precedes exercises prior to stretching. Ideally, exercises for short periods several times daily are preferred to extended exercises that invite more swelling and pain. The latter may actually retard progress.

In this first phase, the surgeon, a therapist, or family member assists the patient in stretching for elevation and rotation. Later the patient can do these alone. Early abduction and lateral wall climbing are avoided. During external rotational stretching with the elbow kept at a right angle, the forearm serves as a fulcrum for shoulder rotation. Arm extension behind the back is combined with internal rotation up the back.

Gentle isometrics (Fig. 39-62) to preserve muscle tone begin early following injury and are advanced by six weeks.

Phase II Exercises

In phase II exercises (Fig. 39-63), early active and advancing stretching is encouraged. The combination of passive assistance with elimination of gravity using a pulley or the opposite arm is important so as not to overly stress the healing fracture and cuff. The greatest forces across the joint are at 90° of abduction; therefore through this midrange, assisted motion is beneficial. Methods of gradually transferring the load in the operated arm without overstressing the early healing process are demonstrated in Figure 39-64. Muscle exercises using light resistance begin in phase II with the aid of rubber dam, but true isotonic strengthening is reserved for phase III. With complex fractures of the proximal humerus, isotonic strengthening is delayed

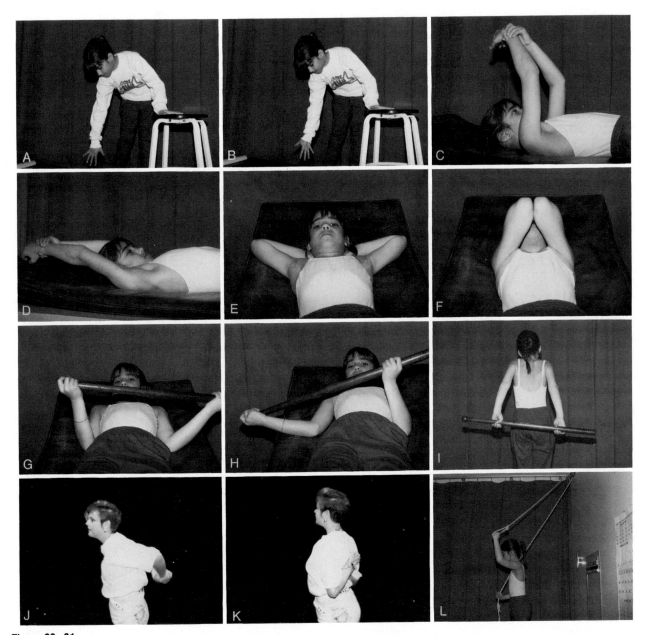

Figure 39-61

Phase I rehabilitation exercises include passive assisted exercises to maintain range of motion by preventing strong bursal and capsular adhesions. These are done several times a day for short periods to avoid unnecessary fatigue and soreness. *A,B,* Pendulum is begun with gravity-assisted elevation, supporting the body with the unoperated hand on a stable stool or counter. The arm is gently rotated in external rotation with the palm facing backward and in internal rotation with the palm facing upward. It can be moved downward in a clockwise or counterclockwise manner and supports active use of muscle and the muscle repairs. *C,D,* Supine passive elevation is performed with the assistance of the unoperated arm (or by the therapist or the physician) with slight distraction at the shoulder joint. *E,F,* When 120° of passive elevation are obtained, then external and internal rotation stretching can be started with the hands locked behind the neck. *G,H,* Supine passive external rotation with a stick or cane is performed with the elbow at a right angle to permit the forearm to serve as a fulcrum for shoulder rotation. This is performed with a slow, steady stretch, deep breaths with an open mouth for relaxation, and additional stretching within the security of the repair and the pain tolerance. *I–K,* Internal rotation is begun first by shoulder extension behind the back with the aid of a stick. The hands are moved closer on the stick until the unoperated hand can grab the wrist of the operated arm. Then the stick is discontinued and the arms are extended, followed by a flexion of the arms bringing the "hitch-hiking thumb" up the back for maximal internal rotation. *L,* Assisted passive elevation with a pulley permits gentle flexion once active-assisted motion is permitted. Then the arm is elevated to its maximal degree, and the unoperated arm then allows the operated arm to share the load as the arm is lowered. The overhead arm provides partial support as a means of early strengthening.

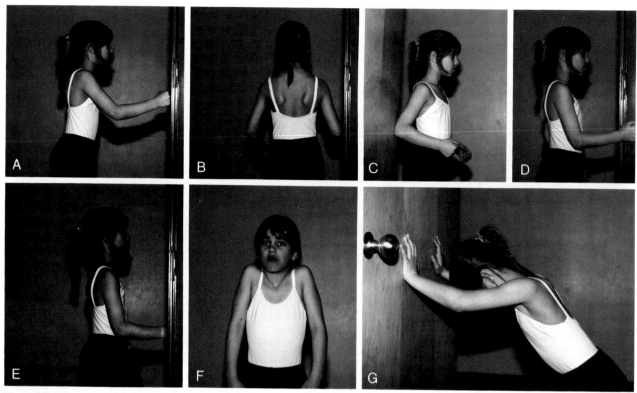

Figure 39-62

Isometric exercises for triphasic deltoid strengthening. *A*, anterior deltoid. *B*, Middle deltoid. *C*, Posterior deltoid. Internal rotation (*D*) and external rotation (*E*) are started at the end of phase I exercises to prevent loss of muscle bulk. Scapular stabilization exercises are used for the trapezius (*F*), and pushups for the rhomboids and serratus (*G*) are added.

for at least three months.[33,249] In general, two principles are followed: stretching is better accomplished with heat and relaxation, and distraction is less painful than compression for joint mobilization.

Overhead stretching exercises are advanced from ones that use a pulley to ones in which the individual can use his or her own weight to guide how much stretch is applied. All too often an individual may tighten to protect against a hard stretch applied by the surgeon or therapist. Overhead stretching can be done from a stable door or from a device such as a yachting cleat mounted on the wall. Just as in sit-ups, where knee flexion flattens and protects the lower back, overhead stretching requires the back to be rounded with the hips forward. Otherwise back pain results from apparent shoulder motion that is actually obtained by arching the lower spine.

Phase III Exercises

Phase III exercises (Fig. 39-65) involve heavier resistors and the use of Cybex and Nautilus equipment to build strength and endurance. Terminal stretching to obtain the last 15° of motion and to stretch a tightened posterior capsule often provides a surprising decrease

in the residual aching so commonly present following shoulder injuries.

EXPECTED DURATION OF DISABILITY

The duration of disability following proximal humeral fractures is often grossly underestimated.[30,184] Many authors feel that there are no significant improvements in function after six months.[57,118,138,147,167,267]

One-part fractures may recover motion early, but realistically, 6 to 12 months are necessary for maximum recovery of comfort, mobility, and strength following these[33] and more complex fractures.[84,184] Endurance is the last element of strength to recover. A weather-related ache and stiffness pain may persist. Among the many potential complications in operative and nonoperative management of displaced humeral fractures that may occur, pain, stiffness, and shoulder dysfunction may be permanent.[241]

APPROPRIATE ASSISTANCE AND LIVING ARRANGEMENTS

Individuals with isolated fractures at the proximal humerus will require some assistance in daily care. For an

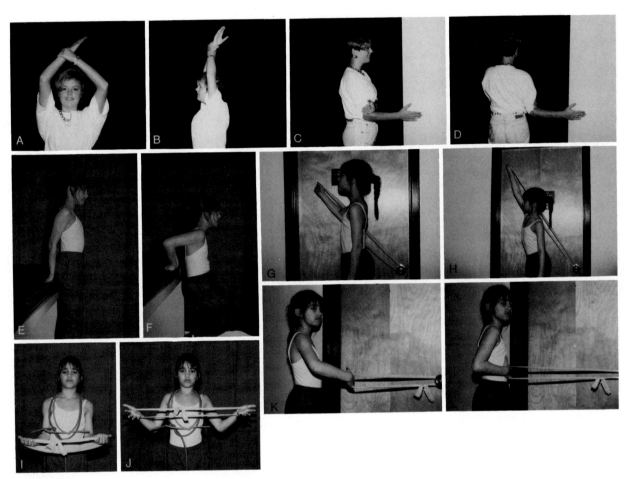

Figure 39–63

Phase II exercises include early active and assisted passive elevation and external and internal stretching. *A,B,* Phase II stretching in early strengthening for elevation. *C,D,* External rotation in a doorway. *E,F,* Internal rotation with the hands behind the back as the patient does deep knee bends. All of these are intended to provide more forceful stretching in these three directions. Active exercises for elevation using rubber resistors on a door for anterior deltoid (*G,H*), external rotation (*I,J*), and internal rotation (*K,L*) can be done with different strength resistors or wall weights for a pulley. The anterior deltoid strengthening exercises in a forward plane avoid impingement that might occur in abduction with residual stiffness. With the external rotation strengthening exercises, the hands are pushed apart equally and are farther apart then the elbows for maximum effect. If the elbow is kept forward for internal rotation strengthening, then the pectoralis and internal rotators are exercised, whereas if the elbow is brought backward, the posterior deltoid shares more of the load.

elderly individual who may normally require the assistance of canes or crutches for ambulation, residence in an extended-care facility, in a nursing home, or with relatives should be considered. Paraplegic individuals with cuff tears require six months of assistance with transfers to protect the cuff repair.

Assessment of Results

Documentation and assessment of results following proximal humeral fractures and fracture-dislocations present a unique challenge. Rating systems throughout the literature vary widely among authors. There has been considerable confusion, because types of fractures are often grouped together for evaluation of individual or combined treatments. Nondisplaced fractures are not always separated from displaced fractures. Little of the older literature is usable, as fracture types and treatments are not separated for analysis. Unfortunately, many contemporary authors still cannot agree on how to measure motion (i.e., elevation may be described as abduction in the coronal plane of the body, coronal plane of the scapula, or a flexion in the sagittal plane of the body; external rotation is reported by some with the arm at the side and by others in 90° of abduction). Functional results that are shown are often passive, with individuals leaning against a wall for elevation or holding their hands together behind the neck for external rotation.[229]

The factors that enable us to define the natural history of a specific fracture type as well as the response to

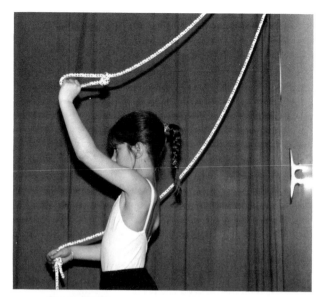

Figure 39–64

Combined active and assisted pulley strengthening.

nonoperative or operative management begin with an adequate fracture classification based on careful imaging and operative findings. Newer imaging techniques have improved diagnostic accuracy. Parameters evaluated during and following treatment include pain, range of motion, strength, stability, function, patient satisfaction, roentgenographic documentation of fracture healing, anatomic restoration, the need for additional operative procedures, and economic factors.

Numeric rating scales have been assigned to many of these factors, yet different authors weight categories differently.[179,180,187,188,190,227] For example, Sante[227] did not describe how much elevation was required for a satisfactory result; Knight and Mayne[118] chose 60°; Neer and McIlveen considered less than 90° to be unsatisfactory.[187,188]

Neer proposed a 100-point rating system in 1970 (Table 39–5),[179,180] and the American Academy of Orthopaedic Surgeons has adopted Neer's rating scale for evaluating total shoulder arthroplasty for fractures.[187,188] An excellent result occurs when the patient is enthusiastic about the operation, has full use, active elevation to within 35° of the normal side and rotation to within 90% of the normal side, and no significant pain. A satisfactory result occurs when the patient is satisfied, has no more than occasional pain or weather-related aches, and has good function for daily use and active elevation above the horizontal and within 50% of normal rotation. An unsatisfactory result is anything less than a satisfactory result. In a report prior to this, Neer et al.[190] included a limited goals category for pa-

tients with massive cuff, bone or neurologic deficits and in whom reconstruction was felt to be appropriate for pain relief but rehabilitation was directed more to stability than motion.[190] This type of category may be more beneficial in fracture analysis than consideration of these more difficult cases with the overall group. Otherwise there is a tendency to view all failures as being in a "limited goals" category.

Unlike the hip, which seems well adapted for a numeric rating, the shoulder has many unique functions that are not easily reduced to an overall number. It is now more informative to break out the results by categories when describing the effectiveness of fracture treatment.

Shoulder evaluation sheets popularized by Neer et al.[190] were computerized and expanded by Cofield[32a] (for shoulder arthroplasty), Norris,[203,205] Matsen and McLean,[154] and Johnson.[108] Through the American Shoulder and Elbow Surgeons research committee and its committee in the American Academy of Orthopaedic Surgeons, progress continues in efforts to standardize the reporting of data to facilitate comparison of results among colleagues (Fig. 39–66).[154] The Matsen-McLean program at the University of Washington in Seattle uses a menu-driven McIntosh system to rate only the involved shoulder. Data from examinations can be entered into a database using a Fourth Dimension structure. From these, standardized reports and more complex statistical analyses can be generated. Not shown are the history, diagnostic categories, and surgical portions of the evaluation. A program using the Norris shoulder evaluation system was developed by Omni MicroSystems, runs on an IBM-compatible computer, and has the capacity to compare both shoulders. This enables data presentation on both as required by the California Industrial Commission for shoulder evaluations.

Table 39–5. Neer 100-Point Rating System		
Category	**Points**	**Rating**
Pain	35	90–100: Excellent
Function	30	80–89: Satisfactory
Motion	25	70–79: Unsatisfactory
Anatomy	10	<70: Failure

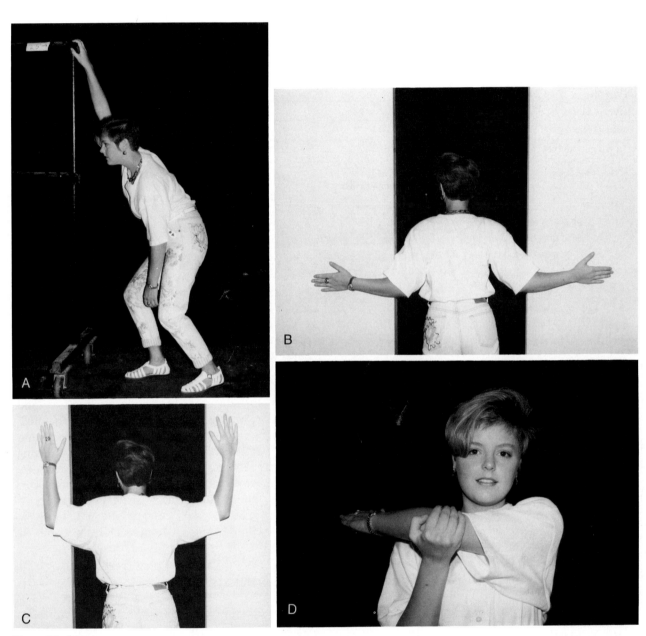

Figure 39–65

Phase III exercises. More advanced stretching with the arm on the end of a door is accomplished by leaning forward at the waist, rounding the back, and then providing a distraction force through the glenohumeral joint by lowering the body as the axilla moves forward and downward. Overhead elevation by arching the lower back is avoided to protect the lumbar spine (A). B,C, External rotation with the arms at the side and abduction and external rotation with the arms overhead can be accomplished by leaning through a doorway. D, Adduction with stretching of the arm across the chest stretches the posterior capsule, which relieves a form of secondary impingement and also improves the patient's ability to sleep on the operated shoulder. The phase III active strengthening exercises use increasing resistance with surgical tubing, wall weights over pulley, free weights, and Nautilus and Cibex equipment in the same four basic directions for strengthening and stretching (i.e., elevation, external and internal rotation, abduction). Heat applied prior to exercise assists in relieving stiffness. Ice applied prior to exercise assists in relieving pain, decreases swelling, and acts as a local anesthetic.

SHOULDER EXAMINATION DATA FORM
BASIC EVALUATION

| Name: | Chart # | Examination date |

List findings as (R/L) or (L/R) • Dominance (L) (R) • Bilateral? (Yes) (NO) • # Steroid injections ____

Diagnosis:

Previous Surgery:

Medications:

I. PAIN

5	4	3	2	1	0
No Pain	Slight	Moderate with activity	Moderate at rest	Marked	Completely disabling pain

II. MOTION

A. Patient sitting: (Enter motion or "NA" if not measured)

1. Active total elevation of arm: ____/____ degrees

2. Active external rotation with arm at side: ____/____ degrees

3. Active external rotation at 90° abduction: ____/____ degrees
(Enter NA if patient cannot achieve 90° of abduction)

4. Passive internal rotation: ____/____ degrees
(Circle segment of posterior anatomy reached by thumb, or circle "NA" if reach restricted by limited elbow flexion.)

1 = Less than trochanter	8 = L2	15 = T7	NA = Reach restricted
2 = Trochanter	9 = L1	16 = T6	by elbow flexion
3 = Gluteal	10 = T12	17 = T5	
4 = Sacrum	11 = T11	18 = T4	
5 = L5	12 = T10	19 = T3	
6 = L4	13 = T9	20 = T2	
7 = L3	14 = T8	21 = T1	

B. Patient supine:

1. Passive total elevation of arm: ____/____ degrees*
*Total elevation of the arm is measured by viewing the patient from the side and using a gromiometer to determine the angle between the arm and the thorax.

2. Passive external rotation with arm at side: ____/____ degrees

3. Passive rotation in 90° abduction:
   A. External: ____/____ degrees
   B. Internal: ____/____ degrees

4. Assisted horizontal cross-body adduction: ____/____ cm
(Measure from antecubital fossa to anterior tip of acromion.)

III. PAINFUL MOTION DIFFERENTIAL DIAGNOSIS
(Answer: Yes or No)

1. Painful arc of elevation
   A. Impingement   ____/____
   B. Stiffness   ____/____
   C. Arthritic   ____/____
   D. Instability   ____/____
2. Relieved by lidocaine ____/____
3. Crepitus
   A. Subacromial   ____/____
   B. Glenohumeral   ____/____

IV. DYNAMOMETER EXAM (Measure in kg.):
(Isometric contraction against resistance, arm in neutral position)

A. Forward flexion   ____/____
B. Abduction   ____/____
C. Extension   ____/____
D. External rotation   ____/____
E. Internal rotation   ____/____

Figure 39–66

Shoulder data forms.

R/L	**SHOULDER EXAMINATION DATA FORM: BASIC EVALUATION**	Page 2
L/R	Name:	Chart#:	Date:

V. STRENGTH: (5=normal, 4=good, 3=fair, 2=poor, 1=trace, 0=paralysis, NA=Not Available)

A. Anterior deltoid   ____/____   F. Triceps   ____/____   **Supraspinatus in
B. Middle deltoid   ____/____   G. Biceps   ____/____   90° coronal abduction
C. External rotation   ____/____   H. Supraspinatus** ____/____   with extended arm in
D. Internal rotation   ____/____   I. Serratus   ____/____   internal rotation
E. Trapezius   ____/____

VI. STABILITY: (5=normal, 4=apprehension, 3=rare subluxation, 2=recurrent subluxation,
            1=recurrent dislocation, 0=fixed dislocation, NA=Not Available)

A. Anterior   ____/____   *Usually related to cuff or tuberosity dehiscence.
B. Posterior   ____/____
C. Inferior   ____/____
D. Anterosuperior* ____/____

VII. FUNCTION: (4=normal, 3=mild compromise, 2=with difficulty, 1=with aid, 0=unable, NA=Not Available)

R/L
L/R
(Circle one)

____/____   A. Use back pocket?
____/____   B. Rectal hygiene?
____/____   C. Wash opposite underarm?
____/____   D. Eat with utensil?
____/____   E. Comb hair?
____/____   F. Use hand with arm at shoulder level?
____/____   G. Carry 10-15 lbs with arm at side?
____/____   H. Dress?
____/____   I. Sleep on shoulder?
____/____   J. Pulling?
____/____   K. Use hand overhead?
____/____   L. Throwing?
____/____   M. Lifting?
____/____   N. Do usual work?
____/____   O. Do usual sport?

VIII. ECONOMICS: (Mark box if "Yes")

❑ Receiving physical therapy?   ❑ Earning power same as before injury?
❑ Receiving home help?   ❑ Vocational rehabilitation in progress?
❑ Working light duty?   ❑ Legal claim settled?

IX. PATIENT RESPONSE: (mark anywhere on scale below)

Worse (0)   Same (1)   Better (2)   Much better (3)

Figure 39–66 *Continued*

EXPECTED RESULTS

In general, closed treatment has yielded satisfactory results in 90% of undisplaced fractures, 75% to 85% of reducible two-part surgical neck fractures, 50% of fractures involving the greater tuberosity, and less than 10% of four-part fractures and fracture-dislocations.[30,33,56,246] Longer immobilization times for undis-placed fractures result in longer physical therapy and disability times.[30]

Closed treatment of displaced fractures has yielded disappointing results.[66,165,246] Displaced fragments block movement, result in weakness, and cause permanent, disabling pain.[182]

Caution is suggested in accepting short-term follow-up. Although satisfactory radiographic appearance may be observed at one year,[213] the humeral head may collapse over the ensuing three years[143] with a poor final result.[124,139,180,241,244]

Open reduction and internal fixation using plates in preference to pin, suture, or wire repair have a significantly higher rate of avascular necrosis,[138,244,260] hardware loosening,[88,184,198,209] and subacromial impingement.[124,209] Regardless of technique, unrecognized screw or pin penetration through the humeral head can lead to poor results.[146,148,209,244]

ACTUAL RESULTS

Results can be analyzed according to treatment of specific fracture types. For nondisplaced fractures, lingering stiffness and a weather-related ache may continue; some permanent stiffness is found.[30,255]

Epiphyseal fractures in the growing child seldom cause a problem, even with gross displacement. Occasionally there is neurovascular injury, and in children older than nine or ten years, there may be some shortening. Otherwise these fractures remodel well despite displacement. Rotational deformities will not correct with remodeling.

In the adult, closed reduction has been associated with a high neurovascular injury rate and treatment by traction with a high nonunion rate.[109] In Jones' series, 9 of 13 fractures (69%) were reducible closed, but only 5 of 13 (38%) healed.[109] Two of his cases healed with reduction and closed pinning, but closed reductions were associated with nerve injury, further fracture displacement, and conversion to more unstable fractures with two or more components. An approximately 75% incidence of satisfactory results was noted with closed treatment by other authors.[30,139,241,246] Savoie et al.[228] quoted satisfactory results in all 12 patients treated who had three-part fractures. Eleven of twelve underwent open reduction and internal fixation. Nine of twelve had a 2-year follow-up. A slightly better range of motion was noted in the 5 of 12 in which an anterior acromioplasty was combined with the open reduction of the fractures. This small group (5 of 12) averaged 130° of elevation and 35° of external rotation.

In the absence of a dislocation, two-part greater tuberosity fractures had good results in only 46% of patients when treated by closed technique; 100% of fracture-dislocations had poor results with closed treatment.[30] Depending on the author's experience, displacement of the greater tuberosity has been associated with poor results if the tuberosity remained displaced between 0.5 cm and 1.5 cm or more.[115,165,180] Those with greater displacement were associated with fair to poor results.

Closed treatment of three-part fractures is associated with minimal to moderate pain and poor motion in those who were not acceptable operative candidates.[109] Open reduction and internal fixation were associated with good to excellent results, assuming the tuberosities could be accurately reduced and maintained without complications of healing, in more than 80% of the cases.[84,115,180] Average total elevation ranged from 120° to 130° with external rotation of 30°; abduction was only 81°.[84] The reoperations in Hawkins et al.'s series included prosthetic replacement following avascular necrosis, removal of broken and prominent wires, and revision of failed fixation when an AO plate and screw fixation pulled out early.[84] The last case was converted satisfactorily using open reduction with the tension band technique.

Prosthetic replacement for three-part fractures has been used by several authors.[184,198–200,202,203,249] Radiographs taken following open reduction and internal fixation of three-part fractures show significant humeral head deformities, avascular necrosis,[84] and malunions and nonunions in cases treated with plates and screws.[199,200,202] Avascular necrosis occurs in approximately 14% of three-part fractures following closed treatment and in up to 25% following open treatment.[244] Minimal internal fixation with the open pinning and tension band technique is associated with a fivefold decrease in the avascular necrosis rate when compared with open reduction and internal fixation with plates and screws.[244]

In the treatment of four-part fractures and fracture-dislocations, less than 10% good or excellent results are obtained with either closed reduction or open reduction and internal fixation.[30,104,180] Isolated reports of revascularization of the humeral head following open reduction and internal fixation indicate satisfactory healing.[120,213] Unfortunately, many of the cases referenced in the literature often have not been true four-part fractures with isolation of the articular fragment, and follow-up is not sufficient to rule out long-term osteonecrosis.[33,34,143]

Hagg and Lundberg[77] noted a 74% avascular necrosis rate when open reduction and internal fixation were used for these fractures. Prior to prosthetic replacement, late treatment of these injuries, with or without head excision, yielded poor results.[94,191,264] All authors agree that pain relief has been greater than 90% with prosthetic replacement, but there have been varying results with regard to function, motion, and strength.[262] Kraulis and Hunter[123a] reported satisfactory results in only 2 of 11 prosthetic replacements, whereas Neer and McIlveen have reported nearly 90% excellent results with an improved technique utilizing the long deltopectoral approach and better rehabilitation.[187] This has become the preferred technique of most surgeons.[10,44,49,114,149,198,203,216,241,249]

In summary, closed manipulation has not been satisfactory for four-part fractures and fracture-dislocations. It results in stiffness, persistent pain, and functional disability.[30,118,179,180] Reconstructive procedures in which the humeral head is retained often fail, particularly when the head collapses later from avascular necrosis.[118,135,221,241] Those treated with prosthetic replacement have consistently better pain relief and improved function, strength, and range of motion when compared with those treated nonoperatively or operatively with humeral head excision or open reduction and internal fixation. Although many argue that a second procedure can be performed to replace the humeral head if avascular necrosis occurs, it is much more difficult to obtain a satisfactory result following collapse of the humeral head and fixed retraction of the tuberosities following a prior failed surgery. My preferred method is to treat four-part fractures and fracture-dislocations with a prosthesis primarily to allow more normal reconstruction of the anatomy rather than await collapse with osteonecrosis, malunion, nonunion, or fixed scar with retraction of tuberosities. It is more difficult to obtain a satisfactory result with multiple operations. Contributing factors to the improved results with early prosthetic replacement,[187] as compared with a prior series,[176,180] include the following: the deltoid is not detached; the long head of the biceps is left intact; normal length of the shaft is restored for stability and muscle strength; the retroversion of 30° to 40° with proper length for the head provides stability; the prosthesis is made more secure with a good press fit or cement technique; the tuberosities and the cuff are repaired with nonabsorbable sutures below the articular surface; and gentle passive motion is started early, whereas active motion is delayed until the tuberosities have healed.

Complications

Complications following fractures of the proximal humerus are not uncommon, as these are difficult fractures to manage with any form of treatment. It is critical to make an accurate diagnosis, use safe and simple treatment techniques when possible, and be aware of the likelihood of complications following specific forms of treatment for a given fracture or fracture-dislocation.

NONUNION

Nonunion following surgical neck fractures is more common than previously thought.[190] It is promoted by traction at the fracture site, inadequate immobilization or fixation, and early range of motion prior to secure fracture healing (Fig. 39–37). Soft tissue interposition that precludes adequate reduction and the inability to maintain a reduction are additional causes (Fig. 39–39).[199] Following three- and four-part fracture fixation, nonunion may result from collapse following avascular necrosis or hardware or suture failure, with loss of fixation of one or more of the proximal humeral segments (Figs. 39–53 and 39–67).

Treatment of the nonunion will depend on the segments involved and whether traumatic arthritis has developed. With a greater tuberosity nonunion, mobilization and advancement laterally to its normal insertion requires freeing the capsule from the rotator cuff inferiorly and from scar superficially. The tuberosity is often trimmed for a better fit but should not be excised. With longstanding neglected cases combined with cuff

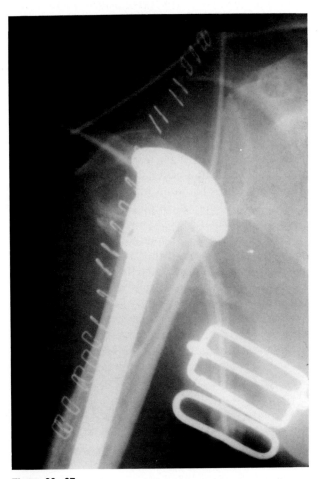

Figure 39–67

Four-part fracture with early tuberosity dehiscence. The technical error was in seating the prosthetic keel on the upper shaft without restoring humeral length. This results in inferior instability and promotes tuberosity dehiscence.

tear arthropathy, return of the tuberosity to its normal position may not be possible.

Surgical neck nonunions are ideally treated with open reduction and internal fixation as described for the original acute fractures; however, supplemental bone graft is usually desirable. Protection with a lightweight plastic orthosis or fiberglass cast is desirable until early healing has been obtained.

At times, the head is excavated from longstanding nonunion. Purchase in the osteoporotic bone is poor at best. For these, cemented humeral head replacement with excision of the remaining articular fragment provides solid intramedullary support. The excised humeral head is packed as bone graft for the nonunion site at the tuberosity and surgical neck levels (Fig. 39–37).[194,199] Nonunions following failed three- or four-part fracture treatment are more difficult to treat than the original acute fractures. The most frequently successful treatment has included a prosthetic replacement cemented out to length and reconstruction of the rotator cuff and tuberosities. Replacement of the glenoid is considered if it is also involved and a good cuff closure can be obtained.

MALUNION

Malunion in proximal humerus fractures is more common at the tuberosity level. It can occur from inadequate closed reductions, from tuberosity fractures missed as a result of inadequate roentgenograms, or from loss of reduction secondary to inadequate fixation. This is most common with the use of plate and screws in an osteoporotic head fragment.

Malunions are problematic because of stiffness, blocked range of motion, traumatic arthritis, and loss of length with collapse at the fracture site. In the absence of traumatic arthritis, the surgical treatment of a malunited greater tuberosity often requires a biplanar osteotomy with repositioning at a more anatomic level below the articular surface. Adhesions must be released superficial and deep to the tuberosity and muscles with release of the capsule. If the greater tuberosity is adherent to the articular surface, then a humeral head or total shoulder replacement may be necessary. Postoperatively, abduction splinting in approximately 45° for the first three to four weeks protects the tuberosity fixation while allowing for early bone and fibrous healing.

Osteotomy for a surgical neck malunion is technically difficult. The axillary nerve must be dissected free and protected. A closing or opening wedge osteotomy, mobilization of anatomic planes, fixation out to proper length, and adequate fixation to permit early motion may all be necessary for a satisfactory result. If traumatic arthritis has occurred, consideration is given to accepting the malunion as is, with loss of elevation, or replacing the humeral head. The latter simplifies adjustment of head height and early fixation in preparation for rehabilitation.

Some surgical neck malunions with anterior angulation of the shaft or prominent greater tuberosities result in greater tuberosity entrapment. The rotator cuff may secondarily erode from the superiorly malunited tuberosity (Fig. 39–68). Valgus malunions secondary to tight tension band repair and collapse in the absence of a combined intramedullary fixation have also been reported.[244]

AVASCULAR NECROSIS

Avascular necrosis occasionally occurs following some two-part fractures with injury to the axillary artery but is more frequent following three- and four-part fractures treated by closed or open means.[59,66,77,118,124,137,139,171,179,180,198,209,244,246] Extensive open reduction and internal fixation with stripping of the soft tissue invites avascular necrosis in the fixa-

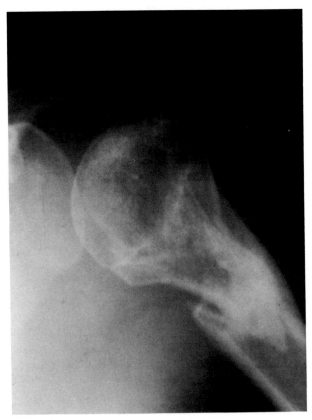

Figure 39–68

Varus malunion at the surgical neck rotates the greater tuberosity superiorly. The prominent tuberosity blocks elevation and concomitantly exposes the supraspinatus to more impingement wear.

tion of the more complicated three- and four-part fractures. The incidence of avascular necrosis was five times greater with plate and screw fixation techniques than with the more simple pinning and tension band techniques.[244] There are isolated reports[120] of treatment of four-part fractures without avascular necrosis. However, in one report, published radiographs demonstrated that the greater tuberosity was still attached,[120] and in another, a roentgenographic follow-up was reported without the benefit of clinical assessment of range of motion, pain, strength, or function. Follow-up of longer than two years is suggested, as Lee and Hansen noted an intact humeral head at two years that later collapsed at 3.5 years following treatment.[137]

In Sturzenegger et al.'s series,[244] three cases of sympathetic dystrophy were associated with avascular necrosis following open reduction and internal fixation of three- and four-part fractures. These progressed to moderate to marked traumatic arthritis with a poor function. With collapse, screw penetration into the joint may hasten traumatic arthritis.[146,198,244] Some patients with avascular necrosis and collapse of the humeral head have only mild to moderate symptoms, but the majority have disabling pain. Collapse may be so severe that the humeral head serves as a cavity that surrounds the glenoid or dislocates to catch on one edge of the glenoid.

There are advantages to replacing the humeral head early rather than waiting until the collapse is severe (Fig. 39–69). Prior to screw penetration through a collapsing head or severe muscle and capsular contraction with earlier replacement, one might not need to lengthen the subscapularis or replace the glenoid. However, longstanding avascular necrosis will likely require both, as the tissue is less elastic and the surgery is more difficult (Fig. 39–70).

Nerve injury may occur at the time of fracture, with closed reduction (particularly if there are several unsuccessful closed reductions), or with an open repair. Brachial plexus injury requires careful and repeated clinical and EMG and nerve conduction studies for assessment. The most common isolated nerve injured is the axillary nerve. Injuries to the musculocutaneous and suprascapular nerves are less common. If recovery does not begin by three months, then exploration is warranted. If the nerve is severed or ruptured, then both anterior and posterior approaches are necessary. Sural nerve grafting is the treatment of choice.

For longstanding suprascapular nerve injuries, latissimus dorsi transfer for external rotation power may be indicated. Tendon transfers for complete loss of the axillary nerve have been only minimally rewarding, whereas for isolated loss of the anterior deltoid alone, reapproximation of the pectoralis and middle deltoid has proven valuable.

Modification of the Clark transfer using the pectoralis major for restoration of elbow flexion following longstanding musculocutaneous nerve palsy has given superior results to transfers using the latissimus dorsi.

VASCULAR INJURY

Successful management of serious vascular injury requires early diagnosis and treatment. Clinical signs and

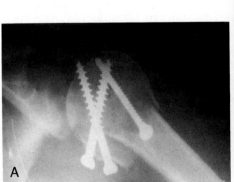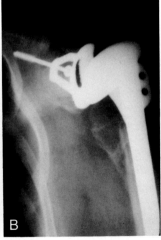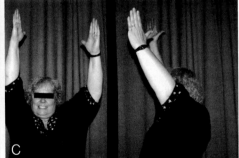

Figure 39–69

Complications of open reduction with screw fixation. *A,* Open reduction and internal fixation of three-part fracture with intraarticular screw. *B,* Advanced glenoid erosion was treated with a glenoid bone graft from the humeral head at the time of prosthetic replacement with (*C*) restoration of function and relief of pain.

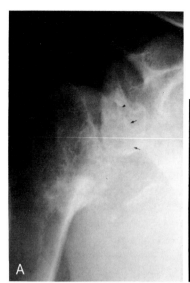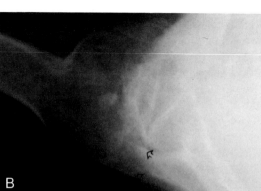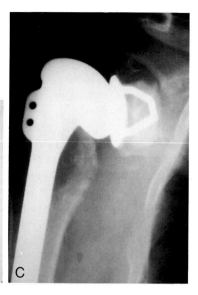

Figure 39–70

Late results of closed treatment of a head-splitting fracture at 10 years with disabling pain and only scapulothoracic motion. *A,B,* The enlarged humeral head cavity captures the glenoid and locks on the posterior rim. *C,* With an intact rotator cuff, prosthetic replacement provides the needed fulcrum for motion with pain relief.

diagnostic tests have been discussed previously. With advancing age, arteriosclerosis increases the risk of vascular injury from minor trauma. Complications in the treatment of vascular injury include Volkmann's contracture and gangrene (Fig. 39–6C).

JOINT STIFFNESS AND ADHESIVE CAPSULITIS

Muscle contractures and joint stiffness occur with prolonged immobilization. Unfortunately, satisfactory radiographic evidence of healing may accompany a poor functional result if mobilization has been delayed. There are scar and adhesions in the bursal and capsular structures. Once fracture stability has been obtained, then stretching exercises are the mainstay of treatment for three to six months. If hardware removal is considered, then open lysis of adhesions with release of scar and contracture, release of coracohumeral ligament and inferior glenohumeral capsule, and a gentle open manipulation under anesthesia followed by an intensive physical therapy program are the goals. If no hardware removal is required, then therapy might be considered for six to nine months prior to an open release.

There are significant risks with manipulations under anesthesia by closed techniques, including redisplacement of prior fractures or dehiscence of the rotator cuff.[244]

ROTATOR CUFF DEHISCENCE

Rerupture of a rotator cuff is seen with early unprotected active motion or aggressive passive motion prior to healing. It can also occur with manipulation under anesthesia and with prominent greater tuberosity malunions that chronically impinge under the acromion.

A deltoid split with longitudinal arthrotomy through the rotator cuff is protected for three weeks. Cuff repairs perpendicular to the direction of their fibers are protected for five weeks prior to active motion. For larger tears with extensive mobilization or transfers, motion at the shoulder level is assisted for several months.

DELTOID DEHISCENCE

Deltoid dehiscence or other problems with the deltoid origin occur following anterior acromioplasty, lateral acromionectomy, or a transacromial approach to the shoulder. With an anterior acromioplasty approach, the deltoid is repaired with nonabsorbable sutures and protected for three to five weeks. Lateral acromionectomy has been discarded as an operative approach. The transacromial approach for fracture repair has yielded more complications with malunions and nonunions following acromial fixation than would be expected with removing the deltoid from the anterior acromion and repairing it through an anterior acromioplasty approach.

INFERIOR SUBLUXATION OF THE GLENOHUMERAL JOINT

Inferior subluxation of the humeral head is not uncommon following trauma of the proximal humerus, fractures of the glenoid, tears of the capsule or ligament, dislocation of the shoulder with nerve injury, isolated brachial plexus injury, and postoperatively when adequate sling support is not provided.[266] Nontraumatic causes include stroke or hemaplegia, poliomyelitis, ligamentous laxity, apical lung tumor involving the brachial plexus, septic arthritis, neuralgic amyotrophy, hemophilic hemarthrosis, rheumatoid arthritis, and, in rare instances, the aging process.[43,266] Complete recovery is anticipated in the majority of cases. The humerus is supported with a sling to reduce the inferior subluxation. Isometric exercises for the deltoid and rotator cuff muscles are begun early. EMG studies may be considered for those thought to have nerve injuries. Inferior subluxation following a fracture of the proximal humerus occurs in 10% to 20% of patients.[58,251] Following open reduction and internal fixation, inferior subluxation is anticipated initially in all patients;[180] in the absence of nerve injury, diminished muscle tone because of fatigue is the most commonly recognized cause.[36,58,112] Intraoperative causes for inferior subluxation include axillary nerve injury and failure to restore full humeral length between the deltoid origin and insertion (Fig. 39–67).

HETEROTOPIC OSSIFICATION

Unwanted or pericapsular bone formation follows fractures with soft tissue injury outside of the joint. It is reported in up to 10% of proximal humerus fractures. It is more common in fracture-dislocations, but repeated unsuccessful closed reductions or a delay in treatment may also contribute.[179] Heterotopic bone can be a significant problem following head injury. Removal of the heterotopic ossification should only be considered if the ossification is mature (i.e., with sharp cortical margins) rather than active (i.e., with a fluffy roentgenographic appearance). This rarely occurs before six to nine months. Low-dose radiation treatment at the time of removal is considered for selective cases.

RECURRENT DISLOCATIONS

Recurrent shoulder instability may be expected with persistent labral or glenoid rim avulsions.[3,198,205] Treatment involves repair of the capsule back to the glenoid. Loss of humeral length, use of a prosthetic head that is too small, malunion of a humeral head, or malrotation of a prosthetic replacement can each result in recurrent shoulder dislocations.

Dehiscence of the rotator cuff superiorly and posteriorly presents as anterosuperior subluxation with attempted elevation, anterior dislocation, or, rarely, with inferior subluxation. Avulsion of the subscapularis

may be associated with either recurrent fixed anterior dislocation or recurrent posterior instability. Nerve injuries or muscle atony may produce an inferior subluxation. These are usually not associated with medial migration of the humeral head. Identification of the etiology of shoulder instability is essential in formulating the correct reconstructive plan.

ADDITIONAL FRACTURES

Additional unanticipated fractures may result from conversion of a nondisplaced fracture to a displaced fracture at the time of closed or open treatment or may occur at the shaft level with intraoperative reduction. The newly created fractures alter the course of treatment. If an intraoperative shaft fracture occurs at the time of open reduction and internal fixation, then AO plating of the shaft fracture, intramedullary fixation, or fixation with a long-stem humeral component are potential treatment options.[206] The long-stem humeral component is preferred for patients with three- or four-part fractures, as both levels can be clearly fixed without the extensive dissection that might be required with the application of plates and screws (Fig. 39–8).

Fractures occurring postoperatively about the tip of a prosthesis are difficult to control by closed means. Some angulation is anticipated with the fractures braces that are available. Nonunions at this level have not been easily treated with AO plating around the prosthesis. Two proposed techniques include an exchange prosthesis using a long stem with cerclage fixation and the technique advocated by Murnaghan (personal communication, 1990). In his operative technique, a fracture about the stem of a prosthesis was fixed with an AO plate distally through bone and proximally through Midas Rex drill holes in the prosthetic stem using screws bolted to the opposite cortex.

COMPLICATIONS OF PROSTHETIC REPLACEMENT

Use of a prosthesis with a large head provides better leverage. A small head allows easier closure of a contracted rotator cuff. If the head is too large, then cuff closure may not be possible, whereas if the head is too small, then with the lax capsule and rotator cuff, the shoulder may be unstable. The proper stem diameter is important, as a loose stem may result in pain and pistoning of the prosthesis. Late subsidence may be more common in the absence of cement fixation or intact calcar.

The prosthesis may be placed too low at the time of treatment if the length of the humerus has not been restored (Fig. 39–67). Important techniques used in assessing the prosthetic height include preoperative scanograms and assessment of the tension in the intact long head of the biceps and rotator cuff at the time of closure.

Improper version of a prosthesis can occur by placement in malrotation or by postoperative spinning following inadequate stem fixation. Placement of a prosthesis in a varus position is not uncommon when the prosthesis is placed on top of the shaft without restoring height; this is done by replacing the tuberosities above the shaft fracture and below the articular surface of the humeral head. Low head placement relative to the greater tuberosity results in impingement with loss of motion. Revision of a prosthesis is one of the most difficult orthopedic procedures to perform, as it involves inelastic tissue with retracted muscles, nerve injuries, and scar. In rare cases where the prosthesis has been placed in a varus position or where the greater tuberosity has healed over the center of the humeral shaft, there is a danger of placing a new prosthesis in a varus position with the stem through the shaft. Revision of a failed prosthesis can be exceedingly difficult if the prosthesis has been cemented in poor position. Neither single-piece Neer prosthetic components nor modular components fare well when the prosthesis is cemented either in a varus position or too low. Unfortunately, just changing a modular head does not solve the poor placement of the cemented stem; removal and repositioning of the stem are necessary. In revising one-piece humeral components, a shorter or more narrow stem can be recemented out to proper height for correction of version, but if there is an angular deformity, then removal of the cement column enables more accurate placement of the new prosthetic component. Difficulties with removal of the cement column, including fracture of the humerus, are compounded when the component stem has been cemented in a varus position. There is a risk of the high-speed bur engaging with the cement column and then easily bouncing through the opposite cortex.

In a preliminary report on the development of a new cement extraction technique, Wuh and Chin[265] have provided a simple and effective technique for cement extraction during revision of total hip arthroplasty that is applicable to the proximal humerus. Using their technique, the common complications of incomplete cement removal, cortical perforation, and shaft fracture can be avoided. It takes advantage of the mechanical properties of the bone-cement interface and bonding characteristics between new and aged methylmethacrylate. Once the prosthetic component has been removed, the old cement mantle is dried; new cement is chilled and then injected into the canal in a retrograde fashion up to the level of the existing cement mantle. A

Table 39–6.
Complications of Humeral Head Prosthetic Replacement

Loosening with subsidence, spinning, or pistoning
Malposition
    Version: anteverted with anterior instability; retroverted with posterior instability
    Too low, with instability
    Too high, with impingement
    Varus: head low, stem out shaft; narrow stem in large shaft
Soft tissue and bone:
    Dehiscence of tuberosities, rotator cuff, or deltoid
    Dislocation or subluxation
    Infection
    Heterotopic bone
    Nerve injury
    Humeral shaft bone defects with loss of length
    Tuberosity by excision
    Tuberosity malunion
    Contractures
    Intra- or postoperative humeral shaft fracture at distal prosthetic stem
    Inadequate aftercare

distally tapered, threaded extraction rod is placed down the central axis until seated in the floor of the cement mantle. After the new bone cement has hardened, a slap hammer is attached to the cement extraction rod and both the new cement and old cement are extracted as a unit. This technique may prove valuable in avoiding many potential complications.[265]

For satisfactory outcome, revision requires attention to all potential deficits. The prosthesis should be at the proper height and version with secure rotator cuff reconstruction. Bone deficits require grafting. Ample postoperative protection and support are necessary until sufficient healing has occurred to begin motion. Complications of prosthetic replacement are summarized in Table 39–6.

Summary

In summary, fractures of the proximal humerus may be extremely demanding. There are many pitfalls for the unwary patient and surgeon to avoid during the course of treatment. Emphasis is placed on complete and accurate diagnosis and the formulation of safe and simple techniques for restoration of stability, fracture healing, cuff integrity, motion, and function. Suture techniques and intramedullary fixation are well adapted for the proximal humerus. Prosthetic arthroplasty has proven to be of considerable value in the treatment of the more serious comminuted proximal humeral fractures and in the late reconstruction of malunions, nonunions, and traumatic arthritis.

REFERENCES

1. Aitken, A.P. Fractures of the proximal humeral epiphysis. Surg Clin North Am 43(6):1573–1580, 1963.
2. Alnot, J.Y. Traumatic brachial plexus palsy in the adult. Retro- and infraclavicular lesions. Clin Orthop 237:9–16, 1988.
3. Aston, J.W.; Gregory, C.F. Dislocation of the shoulder with significant fracture of the glenoid. J Bone Joint Surg 55A:1531–1533, 1973.
4. Baker, D.M.; Leach, R.E. Fracture-dislocation of the shoulder: Report of three unusual cases with rotator cuff avulsion. J Trauma 5:659–664, 1965.
5. Bandi, W. Zur operativen therapie der humeruskopf-und-hals-frakturen. Unfallheilkunde 196:38–45, 1976.
6. Bateman, J.E. The Shoulder and the Neck. Philadelphia, W.B. Saunders, 1972.
7. Bell, M.J.; Beauchamp, C.G.; Kellam, J.D.; McMurtry, R.Y. The results of plating humeral shaft fractures in patients with multiple injuries. J Bone Joint Surg 67B(2):293–296, 1985.
8. Berry, H.; Bril, V. Axillary nerve palsy following blunt trauma to the shoulder region: A clinical and electrophysiological review. J Neurol Neurosurg Psychiatry 45:1027–1032, 1982.
9. Bigliani, L.U. Treatment of two and three part fractures of the proximal humerus. American Academy Orthopaedic Surgeons Instructional Course Lecture. AAOS 38:231–244.
10. Bigliani, L.U. Fractures of the proximal humerus. In: Rockwood, C.A. Jr.; Matsen, F.A. III, eds. The Shoulder. Philadelphia, W.B. Saunders, 1990, pp. 278–334.
10a. Bloom, M.H.; Obata, W.G. Diagnosis of posterior dislocation of the shoulder with use of Velpeau axillary and angle-up roentgenographic views. J Bone Joint Surg 49A:943–949, 1967.
11. Blom, S.; Dahlback, L.O. Nerve injuries in dislocations of the shoulder joint and fractures of the neck of the humerus. A clinical and electromyographic study. Acta Chir Scand 136:461, 1970.
12. Bohler, L. Die behandlung von verrenkungsbruchen der schulter. Dtsch Z Chir 219:238–245, 1929.
13. Bourdillon, J.F. Fracture-separation of the proximal epiphysis of the humerus. J Bone Joint Surg 32B:35–37, 1950.
14. Boville, D.F.; Norris, T.R. The efficacy of intraoperative autologous transfusion in major shoulder surgery. Clin Orthop 240:137–140, 1989.
15. Bradway, J.K.; Kavanaugh, B.F.; and Cofield, R.H. Open reduction and internal fixation of displaced intra-articular fractures of the glenoid. Presented at the American Shoulder and Elbow Surgeons Sixth Open Meeting, New Orleans, Louisiana, February 11, 1990.
16. Brashear, H.R. Jr. Epiphyseal fractures. A microscopic study of the healing process in rats. J Bone Joint Surg 41A:1055–1064, 1959.
17. Breederveld, R.S.; Patka, P.; Dwars, B.J.; VanMourik, J.C. Shoulder injury caused by electric shock. Neth J Surg 39(5):147–148, 1987.
18. Brems, J.J.; Yoon, H.J.; Tetzlaff, J. Interscalene block anaesthesia and shoulder surgery. Presented at the American Shoulder and Elbow Surgeons Sixth Open Meeting, New Orleans, Louisiana, February 11, 1990.
19. Brien, W.; Downey, C.A.; Gellman, H.; et al. Management of humerus fractures in patients with brachial plexus injury. Presented at the American Shoulder and Elbow Surgeons Sixth Open Meeting, New Orleans, Louisiana, February 11, 1990.
20. Broker, F.H.L.; Burbach, T. Ultrasonic diagnosis of separation of the proximal humeral epiphysis in the newborn. J Bone Joint Surg 72A:187–191, 1990.
21. Brostrom, F. Early mobilization of fractures of the upper end of the humerus. Arch Surg 46:614, 1943.
22. Burge, P.; Rushworth, G.; Watson, N. Patterns of injury of the terminal branches of the brachial plexus. J Bone Joint Surg 67B:630–634, 1985.
23. Caldwell, J.A. Treatment of fractures in the Cincinnati General Hospital. Ann Surg 97:174–177, 1933.
24. Caldwell, J.A.; Smith, J. Treatment of unimpacted fractures of the surgical neck of the humerus. Am J Surg 31:141–144, 1936.
25. Callahan, D.J. Closed reduction of fractures of the proximal humerus: Anatomical considerations. Orthop Trans 7(3):425, 1983.
26. Callahan, D.J. Anatomic considerations. Closed reduction of proximal humeral fractures. Orthop Rev 13(3):79–85, 1984.
27. Castagno, A.A.; Shuman, W.P.; Kilcoyne, R.F.; et al. Complex fractures of the proximal humerus: Role of CT in treatment. Radiology 165(3):759–762, 1987.
28. Cave, E.A. Fractures and Other Injuries. Chicago, Year Book Medical, 1958.
29. Clement, J.L.; Cahuzac, J.P.; Gaubert, J.; et al. Fractures and epiphyseal separations of the upper end of the humerus. A critical analysis of 148 cases. Orthop Trans 12(2):299, 1988.
30. Clifford, P.C. Fractures of the neck of the humerus: A review of the late results. Injury 12:91–95, 1981.
31. Codman, E.A. The Shoulder. Boston, T. Todd, 1934.
32. Coene, L.N.; Narakas, A.O. Surgical management of axillary nerve lesions, isolated or combined with other infraclavicular nerve lesions. Periph Nerve Repair Regen 3:47–65, 1986.
32a. Cofield, R.H. Total shoulder arthroplasty with the Neer prosthesis. J Bone Joint Surg 66A:899–906, 1984.
33. Cofield, R.H. Comminuted fractures of the proximal humerus. Clin Orthop 230:49–57, 1988.
34. Cofield, R.H. The future of shoulder surgery. Orthopedics 11(1):179–181, 1988.
35. Conn, R.A.; Cofield, R.H.; Byer, D.E.; et al. Interscalene block anaesthesia for shoulder surgery. Clin Orthop 216:94–98, 1987.
36. Cotton, F.J. Subluxation of the shoulder—downward. Boston Med Surg J 185:405–407, 1921.
37. Craig, E.V. The posterior mechanisms of acute anterior shoulder dislocation. Clin Orthop 190:212–216, 1984.
38. Craig, E.V. Importance of proper radiography in acute shoulder trauma. Minn Med 68(2):109–112, 1985.
39. Crenshaw, A.H. Surgical approaches. In: Crenshaw, A.H., ed. Campbell's Operative Orthopaedics, Ed. 7. St. Louis, C.V. Mosby, 1987.
40. Cubbins, W.R.; Callahan, J.J.; Scuderi, C.S. The reduction of old or irreducible dislocations of the shoulder joint. Surg Gynecol Obstet 58(2):129–135, 1934.
41. Cuomo, F.; Flatow, E.L.; Miller, S.R.; et al. Open reduction and internal fixation of two- and three-part proximal humerus fractures. Presented at the American Academy of Orthopaedic Surgeons 57th Annual Meeting, New Orleans, Louisiana, February 10, 1990.
42. Dameron, T.B.; Reibel, D.B. Fractures involving the proximal humeral epiphyseal plate. J Bone Joint Surg 51A(2):289–297, 1969.
43. Dameron, T.B. Jr. Complications of the treatment of injuries to the shoulder. In: Epps, C.H., ed. Complications in Orthopaedic

Surgery, Vol. 1, Ed. 2. Philadelphia, J.B. Lippincott, 1986, pp. 273–274.

44. deAnquin, C.L.; deAnquin, A. Prosthetic replacement in the treatment of serious fractures of the proximal humerus. In: Baley, I.; Kessel, L., eds. Shoulder Injury. Berlin, Springer-Verlag, 1965, pp. 206–217.

45. Dehne, E. Fractures of the upper end of the humerus: A classification based on the etiology of trauma. Surg Clin North Am 25:28–47, 1945.

46. DePalma, A.F.; Cantilli, R.A. Fractures of the upper end of the humerus. Clin Orthop 20:73–93, 1961.

47. DePalma, A.F. Surgery of the Shoulder, Ed. 2. Philadelphia, J.B. Lippincott, 1973.

48. DeSimone, D.P.; Morwessel, R.M. Diagnostic arthrogram of a Salter I fracture of the proximal humerus in a newborn. Orthop Rev 17(8):782–785, 1988.

49. DesMarchais, J.E.; Morais, G. Treatment of complex fractures of the proximal humerus by Neer hemiarthroplasty. In: Bateman, J.E.; Welsh, R.P.. eds. Surgery of the Shoulder. Philadelphia, B.C. Decker, 1984.

50. Deutsch, A.L.; Resnick, D.; Mink, J.H. Computed tomography of the glenohumeral and sternoclavicular joints. Orthop Clin North Am 16(3):497–511, 1985.

51. Din, K.M.; Meggitt, B.F. Bilateral four-part fractures with posterior dislocation of the shoulder. J Bone Joint Surg 65B(2):176–178, 1983.

52. Dingley, A.; Denham, R. Fracture-dislocation of the humeral head: A method of reduction. J Bone Joint Surg 55A:1299–1300, 1973.

53. Dorgan, J.A. Posterior dislocation of the shoulder. Am J Surg 89:890–900, 1955.

54. Ebel, R. Uber die ursachen der axillaris parese bei schulterluxation. Msche Unfallheilk 76:445–449, 1973.

55. Edelman, G. Immediate therapy of complex fractures of the upper end of the humerus by means of acrylic prosthesis. Presse Med 59:1777–1778, 1951.

56. Einarsson, F. Fractures of the upper end of the humerus: Discussion based on follow-up of 302 cases. Acta Orthop Scand [Suppl] 32:10–209, 1958.

57. Ekstrom, T.; Lagergren, C.; von Schreeb, T. Procaine injections and early mobilisation for fractures of the neck of the humerus. Acta Chir Scand 130:18–24, 1965.

58. Fairbank, T.J. Fracture-subluxation of the shoulder. J Bone Joint Surg 30B(3):454–460, 1948.

59. Fellander, M. Fracture-dislocation of the shoulder joint. Acta Chir Scand 107:138–145, 1954.

60. Flinn, R.M.; MacMillan, C.L. Jr.; Campbell, D.R.; Fraser, D.B. Optimal radiography of the acutely injured shoulder. J Can Assoc Radiol 34(2):128–132, 1983.

61. Fraser, R.L.; Haliburton, R.A.; Barber, J.R. Displaced epiphyseal fractures of the proximal humerus. Can J Surg 10:427–430, 1967.

62. Freundlich, B.D. Luxatio erecta. J Trauma 23(5):434–436, 1983.

63. Funsten, R.V.; Kinser, P. Fractures and dislocations about the shoulder. J Bone Joint Surg 18:191–198, 1936.

64. Garceau, G.J.; Coglang, S. Early physical therapy in the treatment of fractures of the surgical neck of the humerus. J Indiana Med Assoc 34:293–295, 1941.

65. Garth, W.P.; Leberte, M.A.; Cool, T.A. Recurrent fractures of the humerus in a baseball pitcher. J Bone Joint Surg 70A(2):305–306, 1988.

66. Geneste, R.; et al. Closed treatment of fracture dislocations of the shoulder joint. Rev Chir Orthop 66:383–386, 1980.

67. Gerber, C. Femoral head allografts in the treatment of posterior fracture-dislocations with head impression fractures. Presented at the American Shoulder and Elbow Surgeons Closed Meeting, Santa Fe, New Mexico, November, 1988.

68. Gerber, C.; Schneeberger, A.; Vinh, T.S. The arterial vascularization of the humeral head. An anatomic study. Presented at the American Shoulder and Elbow Surgeons Sixth Open Meeting, New Orleans, Louisiana, February 11, 1990.

69. Glessner, J.R. Intrathorax dislocation of the humeral head. J Bone Joint Surg 43A:428–430, 1961.

70. Gold, A.M. Fractured neck of the humerus with separation and dislocation of the humeral head. Bull Hosp Joint Dis 32:87–99, 1971.

71. Golding, F.C. The Shoulder. The forgotten joint. Br J Radiol 35:149–158, 1962.

72. Goldman, A.; Sherman, O.; Price, A.; Minkoff, J. Posterior fracture dislocation of the shoulder with biceps tendon interposition. J Trauma 27(9):1083–1086, 1987.

73. Goss, T.P. Proximal humeral fractures revisited. Orthop Rev 16(11):17–24, 1987.

74. Gristina, A.G. Symposium: Management of displaced fractures of the proximal humerus. Contemp Orthop 15(1):61–93, 1987.

75. Gustilo, R.B.; Anderson, J.T. Prevention of infection in the treatment of 1025 open fractures of the long bones: Retrospective and prospective analysis. J Bone Joint Surg 58A:453–458, 1976.

76. Gustilo, R.B.; Mendoza, R.M.; Williams, D.N. Problems in the management of type III (severe) open fractures: A new classification of type III open fractures. J Trauma 24:742–746, 1984.

77. Hagg, O.; Lundberg, B.J. Aspects of prognostic factors in comminuted and dislocated proximal humeral fractures. In: Bateman, J.E.; Welsh, R.P., eds. Surgery of the Shoulder. Philadelphia, B.C. Decker, 1984.

78. Hall, R.H.; Isaac, F.; Booth, C.R. Dislocations of the shoulder with special reference to accompanying small fractures. J Bone Joint Surg 41A:489–494, 1959.

79. Hall, M.C.; Rosser, M. The structure of the upper end of the humerus with reference to osteoporotic changes in senescence leading to fracture. Can Med Assoc J 88:290, 1963.

80. Hall, R.F. Jr.; Pankovich, A.M. Ender nailing of acute fractures of the humerus. J Bone Joint Surg 69A(4):558–567, 1987.

81. Hardcastle, P.H.; Fisher, T.R. Intrathorax displacement of the humeral head with fracture of the surgical neck. Injury 12:313–315, 1981.

82. Hawkins, R.J.; Neer, C.S. II. Missed posterior dislocations of the shoulder. In: Bateman, J.E.; Welsh, R.P., eds. Surgery of the Shoulder. Philadelphia, B.C. Decker, 1984.

83. Hawkins, R.J.; Gurr, K. A review of 3-part displaced proximal humeral fractures: Operative vs. non-operative management. Orthop Trans 8(1):87, 1984.

84. Hawkins, R.J.; Bell, R.H.; Gurr, K. The three-part fracture of the proximal part of the humerus. J Bone Joint Surg 68A:1410–1414, 1986.

85. Hawkins, R.J.; Angelo, R.L. Displaced proximal humeral fractures. Selecting treatment, avoiding pitfalls. Orthop Clin North Am 18(3):421–431, 1987.

86. Hawkins, R.J.; Neer, C.S. II; Pianta, R.M.; Mendoza, F.X. Locked posterior dislocation of the shoulder. J Bone Joint Surg 69A(1):9–18, 1987.

87. Hayes, M.J.; Van Winkle, N. Axillary artery injury with minimally displaced fracture of the neck of humerus. J Trauma 23:431–433, 1983.

88. Heim, U.; Pfeiffer, K.M. Internal Fixation of Small Fractures. Technique Recommended by the AO-ASIF Group. New York, Springer-Verlag, 1987, pp. 85–106.

89. Henson, G.F. Vascular complications of shoulder injuries: A report of two cases. J Bone Joint Surg 38B:528–531, 1956.

90. Heppenstall, R.B. Fractures of the proximal humerus. Orthop Clin North Am 6(2):467–475, 1975.

91. Hermann, O.J. Fractures of the shoulder joint with special reference to the correction of defects. AAOS Instr Course Lect 2:359–370, 1944.

92. Hill, H.A.; Sachs, M.D. The grooved defect in the humeral head. A frequently unrecognized complication of dislocations of the shoulder joint. Radiology 35:690–700, 1940.

93. Hinsenkamp, M.; Burny F.; Andrianne, Y.; et al. External fixation of the fractures of the humerus. A review of 164 cases. Orthopedics 7(8):1309–1314, 1984.

93a. Hodges, P.C. Development of the human skeleton. AJR 30:809, 1933.

94. Honner, R. Bilateral posterior dislocations of the shoulder. Aust NZ J Surg 38:269–272, 1969.

95. Horak J.; Nilsson, B.E. Epidemiology of fracture of the upper end of the humerus. Clin Orthop 112:250, 1975.

96. Howell, S.M.; Imobersteg, A.M.; Seger, D.H.; Marone, P.J. Clarification of the role of the supraspinatus muscle in shoulder function. J Bone Joint Surg 68A(3):398–404, 1986.

97. Hudson, R.T. The use of the hanging cast in treatment of fractures of the humerus. South Surg 10:132–134, 1941.

98. Hughes, M.; Neer, C.S. II. Glenohumeral joint replacement and postoperative rehabilitation. Phys Ther 55:850, 1975.

99. Hundley, J.M.; Stewart, M.J. Fractures of the humerus: A comparative study in methods of treatment. J Bone Joint Surg 37A:681–692, 1955.

100. Imatani, R.J. Fractures of the scapula: A review of fractures. J Trauma 15:473–478, 1975.

101. Inman, V.; Saunders, M.; Abbot, C. Observations on the function of the shoulder joint. J Bone Joint Surg 26A:1–30, 1944.

102. Jackson, H.C. Treatment of fractures of the proximal humerus with missed posterior dislocation of the humeral head. Orthop Trans 9(2):201, 1985.

103. Jacobs, S.J.; Gilbert, M.S.; Einhorn, T.A. The treatment of fractures in uremic bone disease: Causes of failure and optimization of healing. Contemp Orthop 18(1):23–25, 1989.

104. Jager, M.; Wirth, C.J. Luxationstrummerfrakturen des humeruskopfes—resektion oder refixation der kopffragemente? Unfallheilkunde 84:26–32, 1981.

105. Jakob, R.P.; Kristiansen, T.; Mayo, K.; et al. Classification and aspects of treatment of fractures of the proximal humerus. In: Bateman, J.E.; Welsh, R.P., eds. Surgery of the Shoulder. Philadelphia, B.C. Decker, 1984.

106. Janecki, C.J.; Barnett, D.C. Fracture-dislocation of the shoulder with biceps tendon interposition. J Bone Joint Surg 61A(1):142–143, 1979.

107. Jensen, G.F.; Christiansen, C.; Boesen, J.; et al. Relationship between bone mineral content and frequency of postmenopausal fractures. Acta Med Scand 213(1):61–63, 1983.

108. Johnson, L. Patient information questionnaire. Okemos, MI, Instrument Makar, Inc., 1987.

109. Jones, A.R.; Brashear, H.R.; Dameron, T. B. Surgical neck fracture of the humerus with severe displacement: Factors related to union. Orthop Trans 11(3):457, 1987.

110. Jones, L. Reconstruction operation for non-reducible fractures of the head of the humerus. Ann Surg 97:217–225, 1933.

111. Jones, L. The shoulder joint—observations on the anatomy and physiology with analysis of reconstructive operation following extensive injury. Surg Gynecol Obstet 75:433–444, 1942.

112. Kapandji, I.A. The Physiology of Joints. New York, Churchill Livingstone, 1970, pp. 40–41.

113. Kavanaugh, J.H. Posterior shoulder dislocation with ipsilateral humeral shaft fracture. Clin Orthop 131:168–171, 1978.

114. Kay, S.P.; Amstutz, H.C. Shoulder hemiarthroplasty at UCLA. Clin Orthop 228:42–48, 1988.

115. Keene, J.S.; Huizenga, R.E.; Engber, W.D.; Rogers, S.C. Proximal humerus fractures: A correlation of residual deformity with long-term function. Orthopedics 6:173–178, 1983.

116. Kelly, J.P. Fractures complicating electroconvulsive therapy and chronic epilepsy. J Bone Joint Surg 36B:70–79, 1954.

117. Key, J.A.; Conwell, H.E. Fractures, Dislocations, and Sprains, Ed. 5. St. Louis, C.V. Mosby, 1951.

118. Knight, R.A.; Mayne, J.A. Comminuted fractures and fracture-dislocations involving the articular surface of the humeral head. J Bone Joint Surg 39A:1343–1355, 1957.

119. Kocher, T. Beitrage zur kenntnis einiger praktisch wichtiger fracturenformen. Basel, Carl Sallman Verlag, 1896.

120. Kofoed, H. Revascularization of the humeral head. A report of two cases of fracture-dislocation of the shoulder. Clin Orthop 179:175–178, 1983.

121. Kohler, R.; Trilland, J.M. Fracture and fracture separation of the proximal humerus in children: Report of 136 cases. J Pediatr Orthop 3(3):326–332, 1983.

122. Kolb, L.; Vogel, V.H. The use of shock therapy in 305 mental hospitals. Am J Psychiatry 99:90, 1942.

123. Kornguth, P.J.; Salazar, A.M. The apical oblique view of the shoulder: Its usefulness in acute trauma. AJR 149(1):113–116, 1987.

123a. Kraulis J.; Hunter, G. The results of prosthetic replacement in fracture-dislocations of the upper end of the humerus. Injury 8:129–131, 1976.

124. Kristiansen, B.; Christensen, S.W. Plate fixation of proximal humeral fractures. Acta Orthop Scand 57(4):320–333, 1986.

125. Kristiansen, B.; Barfod, G.; Bredesen, J.; et al. Epidemiology of proximal humeral fractures. Acta Orthop Scand 58(1):75–77, 1987.

126. Kristiansen, B.; Kofoed, H. External fixation of displaced fractures of the proximal humerus. J Bone Joint Surg 69B(4):643–646, 1987.

127. Kristiansen, B.; Kofoed, H. Transcutaneous reduction and external fixation of displaced fractures of the proximal humerus. J Bone Joint Surg 70B(5):821–824, 1988.

128. Kristiansen, B.; Andersen, U.L.S.; Olsen, C.A.; Varmarken, J.E. The Neer classification of fractures of the proximal humerus. Skeletal Radiol 17:420–422, 1988.

129. Krueger, F.T. Vitallim replica arthroplasty of shoulder: Care of aseptic necrosis of proximal end of humerus. Surgery 30:1005–1011, 1951.

130. Kyle, R.F.; Conner, T.N. External fixation of the proximal humerus. Orthopedics 11(1):163–168, 1988.

131. Lahde, S.; Putkonen, M. Positioning of the painful patient for the axial view of the glenohumeral joint. Rontgenblatter 38(12):380–382, 1985.

132. Laing, P.G. The arterial supply to the adult humerus. J Bone Joint Surg 38A:1105–1116, 1956.

133. Lancaster, J.M.; Koman, L.A.; Gristina, A.G.; et al. Pathologic fractures of the humerus. Orthop Trans 7(3):408, 1983.

134. Lancaster, J.M.; Koman, L.A.; Gristina, A.G.; et al. Pathologic fractures of the humerus. South Med J 81:52, 1988.

135. Lange, R.H.; Engber, W.D.; Clancy, W.G. Expanding applications of the Herbert scaphoid screw. Orthopedics 9(10):1393–1398, 1986.

136. LeBorgne, J.; LeNeel, J.C.; Mitland, D. Les lesions de l'artere axillaire et de ses branches consecutives a un traumatisme ferme de l'epaule. Ann Chir 27:587, 1973.

137. Lee, C.K.; Hansen, H.R. Post-traumatic avascular necrosis of

the humeral head in displaced proximal humeral fractures. J Trauma 21(9):788–791, 1981.

138. Lentz, W.; Meuser, P. Treatment of fractures of the proximal humerus. Arch Orthop Trauma Surg 96:283–285, 1980.

139. Leyshon, R. Closed treatment of fractures of the proximal humerus. Acta Orthop Scand 55:48–51, 1984.

140. Li, J.K.W.; Birch, P.D.; Davies, A.M. Proximal humeral defects in Gaucher's disease. Br J Radiol 61:579–583, 1988.

141. Li, X.R.; Wang, C.W.; Tao, P.X. Internal fixation by percutaneous pinning for the treatment of fracture of surgical neck of humerus. Acta Acad Med Wuhan 4(4):236–240, 1984.

142. Liebergall, M.; Mosheiff, R.; Lilling, M. Simultaneous bilateral fractures of the femoral necks and the proximal humeral heads during convulsion. Orthop Rev 17(8):819–820, 1988.

143. Lim, E.V.A.; Day, L.J. Thrombosis of the axillary artery complicating proximal humeral fractures. J Bone Joint Surg 69A(5):778–780, 1987.

144. Lindholm, T.S.; Elmstedt, E. Bilateral posterior dislocation of the shoulder combined with fracture of the proximal humerus. Acta Orthop Scand 51:485–488, 1980.

145. Linson, M.A. Axillary artery thrombosis after fracture of the humerus. A case report. J Bone Joint Surg 62A:1214, 1980.

146. Lower, R.F.; McNiesh, L.M.; Callahan, J.J. Complications of intraarticular hardware penetration. Complications Orthop May/June:89–93, 1989.

147. Lundberg, B.J.; Svenungson-Hartwig, E.; Wikmark, R. Independent exercises vs. physiotherapy in nondisplaced proximal humerus fractures. Scand J Rehab Med 11:133–136, 1979.

148. Lyons, F.R.; Rockwood, C.A. Perils of pins: Migration of pins used in shoulder surgery. Presented at American Shoulder and Elbow Surgeons Sixth Open Meeting, New Orleans, Louisiana, February 11, 1990.

149. Marotte, J.H.; Lord, G.; Bancel, P. L'arthroplastie de Neer dans les fractures et fractures-luxations complexes de l'epaule: A propos de 12 cas. Chirurgie 104:816, 1978.

150. Mason, M.D.; Shearon, C.G. The process of tendon repair. An experimental study of tendon suture and tendon graft. Arch Surg 25(4):615, 1932.

151. Mason, M.L.; Allen, H.S. The rate of healing of tendons. An experimental study of tensile strength. Ann Surg 113:424, 1941.

152. Mast, J.W.; Spiegel, P.G.; Harvey, J.P. Jr.; Harrison, C. Fractures of the humeral shaft: A retrospective study of 240 adult fractures. Clin Orthop 112:254–262, 1975.

153. Matsen, F. M. III. In: Sledge, C., ed. Proximal Humeral Fractures. Orthopaedic Update, Lifetime Medical Television (Sledge is Orthopaedic Host), 1989.

154. Matsen, F.M. III; McLean, D. The shoulder database—University of Washington shoulder and elbow service. American Shoulder and Elbow Surgeons Committee to the American Academy of Orthopaedic Surgeons, February, 1990.

155. McGahan, J.P.; Rab, G.T.; Dublin, A. Fractures of the scapula. J Trauma 20:880–883, 1980.

156. McLaughlin, H. Common shoulder injuries. Am J Surg 3:282–295, 1947.

157. McLaughlin, H.L.; Cavallaro, W.V. Primary anterior dislocation of the shoulder. Am J Surg 80:615, 1950.

158. McLaughlin, H.L. Posterior dislocation of the shoulder. J Bone Joint Surg 34A:584–590, 1952.

159. McLaughlin, H. Trauma. Philadelphia, W.B. Saunders, 1959.

160. McLaughlin, H.L.; MacLean, D.I. Recurrent anterior dislocations of the shoulder II. A comparative study. J Trauma 7:191. 1967.

161. McQuillan, W.M.; Nolan, B. Ischemia complicating injury. J Bone Joint Surg 50B:1090, 1970.

162. Meduna, L., von; Friedman, E. The convulsive-irritative therapy of the psychoses. JAMA 112:501, 1939.

163. Michaelis, L.S. Comminuted fracture-dislocation of the shoulder. J Bone Joint Surg 26:363–365, 1944.

164. Milch, H. The treatment of recent dislocations and fracture-dislocations of the shoulder. J Bone Joint Surg 31A:173–180, 1949.

165. Mills, H.J.; Horne, G. Fractures of the proximal humerus in adults. J Trauma 25(8):801–805, 1985.

166. Mink, J.H.; Harris, E.; Rappaport, M. Rotator cuff tears: Evaluation using double-contrast shoulder arthrography. Radiology 157:621–623, 1985.

167. Moriber, L.A.; Patterson, R.L. Jr. Fractures of the proximal end of the humerus. J Bone Joint Surg 49A:1018, 1967.

168. Morris, M.E.; Kilcoyne, R.F.; Shuman, W.; Matsen, F. III. Humeral tuberosity fractures: Evaluation by CT scan and management of malunion. Orthop Trans 11(2):242, 1987.

169. Moseley, H.F. Athletic injuries to the shoulder region. Am J Surg 98:401–422, 1959.

170. Moseley, H.F. Shoulder Lesions, Ed. 3. Edinburgh, E. and S. Livingstone, 1969.

171. Mouradian, W.H. Displaced proximal humeral fractures. Seven years' experience with a modified Zickel supracondylar device. Clin Orthop 212:209–218, 1986.

172. Muller, M.E.; Allgower, M.; Willenegger, H. The Technique of Internal Fixation of Fractures. Segmuller, G., translator. New York, Springer, 1965.

173. Narakas, A. Surgical treatment of traction injuries of the brachial plexus. Clin Orthop 133:71, 1978.

174. Narakas, A. Brachial plexus surgery. Orthop Clin North Am 12(2):303–323, 1981.

175. Neer, C.S. II. Articular replacement for the humeral head. J Bone Joint Surg 37A:215–228, 1955.

176. Neer, C.S. II. Indications for replacement of the proximal humeral articulations. Am J Surg 89:901–907, 1955.

177. Neer, C.S. II. Degenerative lesions of the proximal humeral articular surface. Clin Orthop 20:116–124, 1961.

178. Neer, C.S. II. Prosthetic replacement of the humeral head—indications and operative techniques. Surg Clin North Am 43:1077–1089, 1970.

179. Neer, C.S. II. Displaced proximal humeral fractures: Part I. Classification and evaluation. J Bone Joint Surg 52A:1077–1089, 1970.

180. Neer, C.S. II. Displaced proximal humeral fractures: Part II: Treatment of three-part and four-part displacement. J Bone Joint Surg 52A:1090–1103, 1970.

181. Neer, C.S. II. Anterior acromioplasty for the chronic impingement syndrome in the shoulder: A preliminary report. J Bone Joint Surg 54(1):41–50, 1972.

182. Neer, C.S. II. Four-segment classification of displaced proximal humeral fractures. AAOS Instr Course Lect 24:160–168, 1975.

183. Neer, C.S. II. Fractures about the shoulder. In: Rockwood, C.A.; Greene, D.P., eds. Fractures in Adults. Philadelphia, J.B. Lippincott, 1984.

184. Neer, C.S. II. Shoulder Reconstruction. Philadelphia, W.B. Saunders, 1990.

185. Neer, C.S. II; Brown, T.H.; McLaughlin, H. Fracture of the neck of the humerus with dislocation of the head fragment. Am J Surg 85:252–258, 1953.

186. Neer, C.S. II; Horwitz, B.S. Fractures of the proximal humeral epiphyseal plate. Clin Orthop 41:24–31, 1965.

187. Neer, C. S. II; McIlveen, S.J. Recent results and technique of prosthetic replacement for four part proximal humerus fractures. Orthop Trans Fall 10(3), 1986.

188. Neer, C.S. II; McIlveen, S.J. Humeral head replacement with

tuberosity and cuff reconstruction for 4 part displacement. Current results and technique. Rev Chir Orthop 74(suppl II):31, 1988.

189. Neer, C.S. II; Craig, E.V.; Fukuda, H. Cuff tear arthropathy. J Bone Joint Surg 65A(9):1232–1242, 1983.

190. Neer, C.S. II; Watson, K.C.; Stanton, F.J. Recent experience in total shoulder replacement. J Bone Joint Surg 64A:319–336, 1982.

191. Neviaser, J.S. Complicated fractures and dislocations about the shoulder joint. AAOS Instr Course Lect 44A:984–998, 1962.

192. Neviaser, R.J.; Neviaser, T.J.; Neviaser, J.S. The relationship of rotator cuff tears to primary and recurrent anterior shoulder dislocation in the older patient. Orthop Trans 11(2):247, 1987.

193. Nicola, F.G.; Ellman, H.; Eckardt, J.; Finerman, G. Bilateral posterior fracture-dislocation of the shoulder treated with a modification of the McLaughlin procedure. J Bone Joint Surg 63A(7):1175–1177, 1981.

194. Norris, T.R.; Turner, J.A. Surgical treatment of nonunions of the upper humerus shaft in the elderly. Orthop Trans 9:44, 1985.

195. Norris, T.R. Diagnostic techniques for shoulder instability. In: Stauffer, E.S., ed. American Academy of Orthopaedic Surgeons Instructional Course Lectures, Vol. 34. St. Louis, C.V. Mosby, 1985, pp. 239–257.

196. Norris, T.R. Bone grafts for glenoid deficiency in total shoulder replacements. In: The Shoulder. Proceedings of the Third International Conference on Surgery of the Shoulder. Tokyo, Professional Postgraduate Services, 1987, pp. 373–376.

197. Norris, T.R. 3D (CEMAX) reformation in the evaluation of complex glenoid wear of fracture. Presented at the American Shoulder and Elbow Surgeons Sixth Annual Meeting, Orlando, Florida, November, 1987.

198. Norris, T.R. Fractures and dislocation of the glenohumeral complex. In: Chapman, M.W.; Madison, M., eds. Operative Orthopaedics. Philadelphia, J.B. Lippincott, 1988, pp. 203–220.

199. Norris, T.R.; Boville, D.F.; Turner, J.A. A review of 28 proximal humerus fractures leading to nonunion. In: Post, M.; Hawkins R.J.; Morrey, B.F., eds. Surgery of the shoulder. St. Louis, C.V. Mosby, 1990, pp. 63–67.

200. Norris, T.R.; Boville, D.F.; Turner, J.A. Common problems with proximal humerus fractures leading to malunion: A review of 27 cases. Presented at the American Shoulder and Elbow Surgeons Fifth Open Meeting, Las Vegas, Nevada, February 12, 1989.

201. Norris, T.R. Recurrent posterior subluxations. Hosp Med April 1990, pp. 45–63.

202. Norris, T.R. Nonunions of the proximal humerus. Presented at the Fourth International Conference on Surgery of the Shoulder, New York, October 4–7, 1989.

203. Norris, T.R. Unconstrained prosthetic shoulder replacement. In: Watson, M., ed. Surgical Disorders of the Shoulder. London, Churchill Livingstone, 1991, pp 473–510.

204. Norris, T.R.; Hulsey, R.E. Bone grafts for glenoid deficiency in total shoulder replacements. Presented at the American Shoulder and Elbow Surgeons Sixth Open Meeting, New Orleans, Louisiana, February 11, 1990.

205. Norris, T.R. History and physical examination of the shoulder. In: Nicholas, J.A.; Hershman, E.B., eds. The Upper Extremity in Sports Medicine. St. Louis, C.V. Mosby, 1990.

206. Norris, T.R.; McElheney, E. The role of the long-stemmed humeral head prosthesis in treatment of complex humeral fractures and in revision arthroplasty. Semin Arthroplasty 1(2):138–150, 1990 (W.B. Saunders Co.).

207. Oni, O.O. Irreducible acute anterior dislocation of the shoulder due to a loose fragment from an associated fracture of the greater tuberosity. Injury 15(2):138, 1983.

208. Oster, A. Fracture-dislocations of the shoulder joint. Four cases treated with Vitallium prosthesis. Acta Chir Scand 135:499, 1969.

209. Paavolainen, P.; Bjorkenheim, J.M.; Slatis, P.; Paukku, P. Operative treatment of severe proximal humeral fracture. Acta Orthop Scand 54:374, 1983.

210. Pankovich, A.M. Update 1987—flexible intramedullary nailing of long bone fracture: A review. J Orthop Trauma 1(1):78–95, 1987.

211. Pasila, M.; Faroma, H.; Kiviluoto, O.; Sundholm, A. Early complications of primary shoulder dislocations. Acta Orthop Scand 49:260–263, 1978.

212. Patel, M.R.; Pardee, M.L.; Singerman, R.C. Intrathoracic dislocation of the head of the humerus. J Bone Joint Surg 45A:1712–1714, 1963.

213. Pettine, K.A. Open reduction and internal fixation of four-part fractures of the proximal humerus. Contemp Orthop 19(1):49–54, 1989.

214. Pierce, R.O.; Hodurski, D.F. Fractures of the humerus, radius, and ulna in the same extremity. J Trauma 19(3):182–185, 1979.

215. Poppen, N.K.; Walker, P.S. Forces at the glenohumeral joint in abduction. Clin Orthop 135:165–170, 1978.

216. Post, M. Fractures of the upper humerus. Orthop Clin North Am 11(2):289–252, 1980.

217. Richard, A.; Judet, R.; Rene, L. Acrylic prosthetic construction of the upper end of the humerus for fracture-subluxations. J Chir 68:537–547, 1952.

218. Roberts, S.M. Fractures of the upper end of the humerus: An end result study which shows the advantage of early active motion. JAMA 98:367–373, 1932.

219. Rokous, J.R.; Feagin, J.A.; Abbott, H.G. Modified axillary roentgenogram. A useful adjunct in the diagnosis of recurrent instability of the shoulder. Clin Orthop 82:84–86, 1972.

220. Rose, S.H.; Melton, L.J. III; Morrey, B.F.; et al. Epidemiologic features of humeral fractures. Clin Orthop 168:24, 1982.

221. Rosen, H. Tension band wiring for fracture dislocations of the shoulder. Chirurgie orthopedique et traumatologie: 12 eme congres de SICOT. Amsterdam, Excerpta Medica, 1973, pp. 939–941.

222. Rowe, C.R. Prognosis in dislocations of the shoulder. J Bone Joint Surg 38A(5):957–977, 1956.

223. Rowe, C.R.; Marble, H. Shoulder girdle injuries. In: Cave, E.F., ed. Fractures and Other Injuries. Chicago, Year Book Medical, 1958.

224. Ruedi, T.; Moshfegha, A.; Pfeiller, K.M.; Allgower, A. Fresh fractures of the shaft of the humerus: Conservative or operative treatment? Reconstr Surg Traumatol 14:65–74, 1975.

224a. Saha, A.K. "Zero-position" of the glenohumeral joints. Its recognition and clinical importance. Ann R Coll Surg Engl 22:223, 1958.

225. Salter, R.B.; Harris, W.R. Injuries involving the epiphyseal plate. J Bone Joint Surg 45A:587–622, 1963.

226. Samuel, E. Some complications arising during electrical convulsive therapy. J Ment Sci 89:81, 1943.

227. Sante, H.E. Fractures about the upper end of the humerus. Ann Surg 80:103–114, 1924.

228. Savoie, F.H.; Geissler, W.B.; Vander Griend, R.A. Open reduction and internal fixation of three-part fractures of the proximal humerus. Orthopedics 12(1):65–70, 1989.

229. Schatzker, J.; Tile, M. The Rationale of Operative Fracture Care. New York, Springer-Verlag, 1987, pp. 31–70.

230. Schuhl, J.F. Fracture-Dislocations of the Proximal Humerus. Lyon, These Medicine, 1973.
231. Scott, A.C.; Buckle, R.; Browner, B.D.; Hildreth, D.H. High energy proximal humerus fractures: Fracture patterns and results of treatment. Orthop Trans 13(1):42, 1989.
232. Seddon, H.J. Nerve lesions complicating certain closed bone injuries. JAMA 135(11):11–15, 1947.
233. Sedel, L. Results of surgical repair of brachial plexus injuries. J Bone Joint Surg 64B:54–66, 1982.
234. Seltzer, S.E.; Weissman, B.N. CT findings in normal and dislocating shoulders. J Can Assoc Radiol 36(1):41–46, 1985.
235. Sever, J.W. Fracture of the head of the humerus: Treatment and results. New Engl J Med 216:1100–1107, 1937.
236. Sherk, H.H.; Probst, C. Fractures of the proximal humeral epiphysis. Orthop Clin North Am 6(2):401–413, 1975.
237. Sisk, T.D. Campbell's Operative Orthopaedics, Ed. 6. St. Louis, C.V. Mosby, 1980, pp. 662–670.
238. Smith, D.K.; Cooney, W.P. External fixation of high energy upper extremity injuries. J Orthop Trauma 4(1):7–18, 1990.
239. Smith, F.M. Fracture-separation of the proximal humeral epiphysis. Am J Surg 91:627–635, 1956.
240. Smyth, E.H.J. Major arterial injury in closed fracture of the neck of the humerus: Report of a case. J Bone Joint Surg 51A:508, 1969.
241. Stableforth, P.G. Four-part fractures of the neck of the humerus. J Bone Joint Surg 66B:104–108, 1984.
242. Stewart, M.J.; Hudley, J.M. Fractures of the humerus: A comparative study in methods of treatment. J Bone Joint Surg 37A:681–692, 1955.
243. Stimson, B.B. A Manual of Fractures and Dislocations, Ed. 2. Philadelphia, Lea and Febiger, 1947.
244. Sturzenegger, M.; Fornaro, E.; Jakob, R.P. Results of surgical treatment of multi-fragmented fractures of the humeral head. Arch Orthop Trauma Surg 100:249, 1982.
245. Sunderland, S. Nerves and Nerve Injuries, Ed. 2. New York, Churchill Livingstone, 1978.
246. Svend-Hansen, H. Displaced proximal humeral fractures. A review of 49 patients. Acta Orthop Scand 45:359, 1974.
247. Swanson, T.V.; Sutherland, T.B.; Spiegel, J.D.; et al. A prospective Comparative study of the Lottes nail versus external fixation in 100 open tibia fractures. Presented at the Western Orthopaedic Association Northern California Chapter Spring Meeting, March 15–18, 1990.
248. Szalay, E.A.; Rockwood, C.A. Jr. Injuries of the shoulder and arm. Emerg Med Clin North Am 2(2):279–294, 1984.
249. Tanner, M.W.; Cofield, R.H. Prosthetic arthroplasty for fracture and fracture-dislocations of the proximal humerus. Clin Orthop 179:116–128, 1982.
250. Theodorides, T.; Dekeizer, G. Injuries of the axillary artery caused by fractures of the neck of the humerus. Injury 8:120, 1976.
251. Thompson, F.R.; Winant, E.M. Comminuted fracture of the humeral head with subluxation. Clin Orthop 20:94–97, 1961.
252. Tosovsky, V.; Stryhal, F. The conservative treatment of the fractures and dislocation of the extremities in children. Acta Univ Carol 111:1–145, 1986.
253. Valls, J. Acrylic prosthesis in a case with fracture of the head of the humerus. Bal Soc Orthop Trauma 17:61, 1952.
254. VanderGhirst, M.; Houssa, R. Acrylic prosthesis in fractures of the head of the humerus. Acta Chir Belg 50:31, 1951.
255. Wallace, W.A.; Hellier, M. Improving radiographs of the injured shoulder. Radiography 49(586):229–233, 1983.
256. Warren R. In: Gristina, A.G., ed. Symposium: Management of Displaced Fractures of the Proximal Humerus. Contemp Orthop 15(1):61–93, 1987.
256a. Watson, K.C. Modification of Rush pin fixation for fractures of the proximal humerus. Presented at the American Shoulder and Elbow Surgeons Annual Meeting, Santa Fe, New Mexico, November 3–5, 1988.
257. Watson-Jones, R. Fractures and Joint Injuries, Ed. 5, Vol. 2. Baltimore, Williams and Wilkins, 1955.
258. Weaver, J.K. Skiing-related injuries to the shoulder. Clin Orthop 216:24–28, 1987.
259. Wentworth, E.T. Fractures involving the shoulder joint. NY J Med 40:1282, 1940.
260. Weseley, M.S.; Barenfeld, P.A.; Eisenstein, A.L. Rush pin intramedullary fixation for fracture of the proximal humerus. J Trauma 17(1):29–37, 1977.
261. White, E.M.; Kattapuram, S.V.; Jupiter, J.B. Case report 241. Skeletal Radiol 10:178–182, 1983.
262. Willems, W.J.; Lin, T.E. Neer arthroplasty for humeral fracture. Acta Orthop Scand 56(5):394–395, 1985.
263. Williams, D.J. The mechanism producing fracture-separation of the proximal humeral epiphysis. J Bone Joint Surg 63B(1):102–107, 1981.
264. Wilson, J.C.; McKeever, F.M. Traumatic posterior (retroglenoid) dislocation of the humerus. J Bone Joint Surg 31A(1):160–172, 1949.
265. Wuh, H.C.K.; Chin, A.K. A preliminary report on the development of a new cement extraction technique. Presented at the Western Orthopaedic Association Northern California Chapter Spring Meeting, March 15–18, 1990.
266. Yosipovitch, Z.; Tikkva, P.; Goldberg, I. Inferior subluxation of the humeral head after injury to the shoulder. J Bone Joint Surg 71A(5):751–753, 1989.
267. Young, T.B.; Wallace, W.A. Conservative treatment of fractures and fracture-dislocations of the upper end of the humerus. J Bone Joint Surg 67B(3):373–377, 1985.
268. Zuckerman, J.D.; Flugstad, D.L.; Teitz, C.C.; King, H.A. Axillary artery injury as a complication of proximal humeral fractures: Two case reports and a view of the literature. Clin Orthop 189:234–237, 1984.
269. Zuckerman, J.D.; Matsen, F.A. Complications about the glenohumeral joint related to the use of the screws and staples. J Bone Joint Surg 66A(2):175–180, 1984.
270. Zych, G.A.; Montane, I. Acute fracture of the proximal humerus superimposed on a chronic posterior dislocation of the humeral head. South Med J 80(10):1307–1308, 1987.

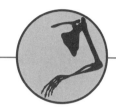

Michael E. Miller, M.D.
Jesse R. Ada, M.D.

40

Injuries to the Shoulder Girdle

*T*he shoulder joint owes its unique axial and rotational mobility to the unconstrained structure of its articulations. In addition to the sternoclavicular joint, only the muscular supports of the scapula and clavicle link the shoulder girdle to the axial skeleton. Codman[13] observed shoulder motion as a composite of movements at the scapulothoracic, sternoclavicular, acromioclavicular, and glenohumeral joints. He also recognized a rotational component of clavicular motion.

Teleologically, the skeletal and articular units of the shoulder girdle have evolved to provide a mobile platform for the musculature surrounding the proximal humerus. The most important part of this muscular array inserts as a unit around the head of the humerus and forms the rotator cuff. Treatment of injuries to the shoulder girdle should focus on preservation of rotator cuff function.

Scapular Fractures and Dislocations

Humans and other primates enjoy an unusual combination of strength and agility in the upper extremity. This is in part a product of the complex web of 18 muscle origins and insertions that suspend the scapula from the spine and thorax and the humerus from the scapula (Table 40–1).

The earliest treatise on scapular fractures is probably that of Desault[15] in 1805. Since then, a small number of studies have been published, all of which note the rarity of these fractures and the high incidence of associated injuries.[4,21,27,33,40–42,46,54,62,69,72,73]

Closed management has been the rule for the vast majority of these fractures. This is based on a belief that the results of nonoperative treatment are functionally and symptomatically good. However, results of more recent studies have raised questions regarding these observations.

FRACTURE PATTERNS AND CLASSIFICATION

Scapular fractures are best classified on a simple anatomic basis. We have evolved a classification system based on a series of 146 fractures in 116 scapulae (Fig. 40–1). The distribution of fracture types in our series is similar to that in many others reported (Table 40–2).

The most common fracture type occurs in the body of the scapula and seldom requires more than symptomatic treatment. Fractures of the scapular neck are second in frequency, with injuries of the scapular spine, glenoid, and acromion all of about equal occurrence. As will be noted from the presence of 148 fractures in 116 scapulae, complex multiple fracture patterns were common.

DIAGNOSIS

The diagnosis of these injuries is often made as an incidental finding seen on chest radiographs of the multiple trauma patient. Any patient with polytrauma and complaints of shoulder pain, especially in the presence of rib or pulmonary injury, should be examined closely for fractures of the scapula.

Anteroposterior tomography may suffice for most cases (Figs. 40–2 and 40–3), but in complex fractures, computed tomography (CT) scanning may be useful for defining displacements in the transverse plane

Table 40–1.

Muscle Origins and Insertions of the Scapula

Trapezius
Deltoid
Supraspinatus
Infraspinatus
Teres minor
Subscapularis
Teres major
Rhomboideus major
Rhomboideus minor
Levator scapulae
Long head of biceps
Short head of biceps
Coracobrachialis
Pectoralis minor
Serratus anterior
Long head of triceps
Latissimus dorsi
Inferior belly of omohyoid

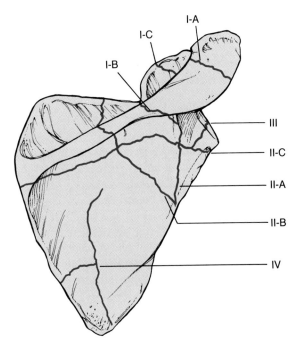

I-A: Acromion
I-B: Base of acromion, spine
I-C: Coracoid

II-A: Neck lateral to base of acromion—spine
II-B: Neck, extending to base of acromion or spine
II-C: Neck, transverse type

 III: Glenoid, intraarticular

 IV: Body

Figure 40–1

Classification of scapular fractures. Types I-A, I-B, II-A, II-B, II-C, and III most often require operative treatment.

Table 40–2.

Distribution of Fracture Types

Fracture Type	No.	%
I-A, acromion	18	12
I-B, spine	17	11
I-C, coracoid	7	5
II-A, II-B, II-C, neck	39	27
III, glenoid	15	10
IV, body	52	35
Total	148	100

(Figs. 40–4 and 40–5). CT imaging is also a valuable educational tool, providing the surgeon with a three-dimensional understanding of the fracture patterns.

MANAGEMENT

We have reviewed 148 fractures in 116 scapulae in 113 patients.[1] Included in this retrospective study were 24 patients with displaced scapular neck, spine, and intra-articular fractures. Follow-up ranged from two to eight years, with an average of 36 months. Patients averaged 25.9 years old, younger than in some series[55] but more in agreement with the usual age of multiple blunt trauma patients today. Ninety-six percent of these patients had associated injuries, with upper thoracic rib fractures being most common. This is to be expected, as most scapular fractures occur in high-energy multi-

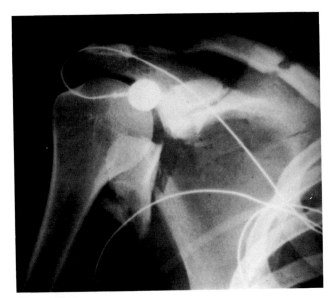

Figure 40–2

Complex intraarticular fracture of the scapula. (Radiograph courtesy of Roy Sanders, M.D.)

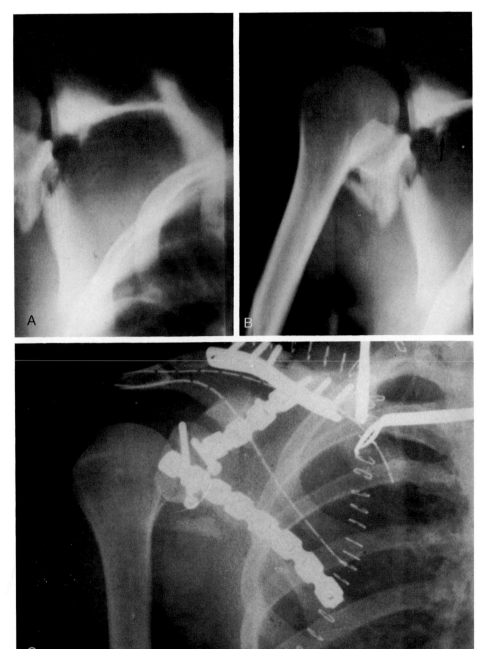

Figure 40–3

A and *B*, Tomography shows extension of fracture through the scapular spine (*arrow*) isolating the upper glenoid fragment and coracoid. *C*, Complex fixation required for stabilization as a result of clavicle fracture and intraarticular displacement. (Radiographs courtesy of Roy Sanders. M.D.)

ple trauma accidents as a result of direct impact over the scapular region. Pulmonary injuries were also frequent, with a 37% incidence overall, including a 29% incidence of hemopneumothorax and an 8% incidence of pulmonary contusion. Thirty-four percent had head injuries, with an 8% incidence of skull fractures. Ipsilateral clavicle fractures occurred in 25%, and 12% of patients had cervical spine injuries, with four permanent cord injuries overall (two quadriplegic, one paraplegic, and one Brown-Séquard lesion). Three of four

associated brachial plexus injuries recovered spontaneously.

The problems caused by scapular fractures depend on the location of the fracture, presence of comminution, and displacement. Union is rarely a problem; in our series, only one fracture failed to unite. The majority of problems were related to pain and loss of function following closed treatment.

Fractures of the body of the scapula (type IV) do well with closed treatment. Even in the presence of severe

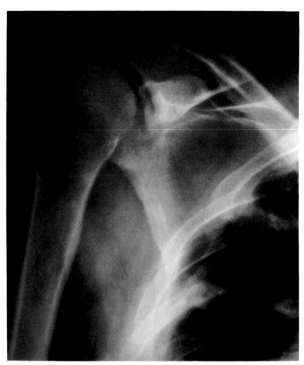

Figure 40–4

Intraarticular fracture of the glenoid.

displacement, patients in our study had neither pain nor loss of motion. Some patients did note painless "popping" or grating with motion at the scapulothoracic interface, but there were no functional deficits.

Displaced scapular neck fractures frequently caused abduction weakness and subacromial pain. The latter may be especially pronounced when patients lie on the affected side for sleep.

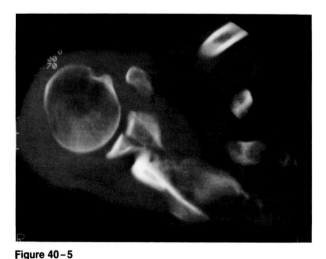

Figure 40–5

CT scan of same fracture seen in Figure 40–4 showing articular step-off.

Of the six acromioclavicular sprains that occurred, five were ipsilateral to the scapular fracture, and all were grade I or II. Four of these acromioclavicular injuries were associated with coracoid process fractures, a finding reported in the past with isolated acromioclavicular injuries.[36]

The only indirect injury was an avulsion fracture of the acromion that occurred in a patient with renal osteodystrophy.

The results in our 24 cases with displaced fractures of the neck and spine of the scapula demonstrated a high rate of associated disability. Patients with displaced neck fractures noted weakness of shoulder abduction. All patients with displaced glenoid fractures had decreased range of motion, and four of the six had pain with motion (one moderate and three severe). Of ten patients with comminuted scapular spine fractures, five complained of weakness with abduction activities. Fifty-seven percent of these patients had night pain, mostly in the subacromial area. These findings are summarized in Table 40–3.

Many of these posttraumatic complaints are probably explained by rotator cuff dysfunction following scapular fractures.

ROTATOR CUFF DYSFUNCTION FOLLOWING SCAPULAR FRACTURE

At less than 90° of abduction, the glenoid reactive force of the deltoid results in a shear vector.[13] The transverse orientation of the rotator cuff muscles in the scapula creates a normalizing or compressive force across the glenoid that neutralizes this destabilizing tendency (Fig. 40–6).[57] It has been our observation that angular or translational change from the normal position of the glenoid caused by fracture displacement affects the lever arm of the rotator cuff muscles and the generation of these compressive forces. As the tilt of the glenoid increases, some of the compressive forces of the rotator cuff are converted to a shear or sliding force. Because this conversion to shear forces approximates the tangent of the tilt angle, the situation worsens markedly at about 45° of glenoid tilt.

Fractures of the spine of the scapula also cause rotator cuff dysfunction, with patients complaining of pain and weakness with abduction and night pain.

When found in combination with scapular neck and body fractures, these scapular spine injuries can produce the so-called "Z" deformity (Fig. 40–7) and collapse of the scapula. In such a situation, a degree of direct injury to the rotator cuff musculature, proportional to the displacement and comminution evident on radiography, must be assumed. Nevaiser[46] described a problem of "pseudorupture" of the rotator

Table 40–3.

Follow-up Study of 24 Patients

Fracture Type	No.	Decreased Range of Motion	Pain	Weakness With Exertion	Pain With Exertion	Popping
Displaced Neck Fractures	16	3 (20%)	8 (50%) (Night 6, 75%)	6 (40%)	7 (46%)	4 (25%)
Intra-articular	6	6 (100%)	6 (100%)	4 (66%)	4 (66%)	4 (66%)
Comminuted spine	11	5 (45%)	7 (63%) (Night 4, 57%)	5 (45%)	2 (20%)	3 (30%)

cuff in patients with scapular fractures and thought this was a result of hemorrhage into the cuff musculature with resulting paralysis. We suggest that chronic problems also occur as a result of such hemorrhage as well as from direct muscle trauma.

Management of scapular fractures, then, should aim at restoring and preserving rotator cuff function.

Based on our review of available studies and on our own patient group, we feel that surgical management has a place in the treatment of some displaced fractures of the scapula. In addition to the obvious cases of intra-articular derangement caused by displaced glenoid (type III) fractures, fractures for which surgery is suited include scapular neck fractures with more than 40° angulation in either the transverse or coronal plane and fractures of the scapular neck with 1 cm or more displacement. Scapular spine fractures at the base of the acromion and those with more than 5 mm of displace-

ment may be at risk for the development of nonunion and thus should also be considered for surgical treatment. These findings are summarized in Table 40–4.

Operative management of scapular fractures has been reported almost exclusively by European surgeons,[19,20,23,24,28] with isolated cases seen in North America.[5] The series of Hardegger and Simpson[24] is among the largest surgical experiences reported, with 79% of their 37 patients having good to excellent results.

SURGICAL APPROACHES AND TECHNIQUES

Accurate radiographic assessment and preoperative planning are essential in surgical treatment of scapular fractures. A true anteroposterior radiogram and a lateral "Y" view to assess displacement of the glenoid in the coronal plane (Fig. 40–8) are essential minimum studies. In those cases with obvious or suspected fractures of the glenoid (type III), CT scanning provides needed information as to the best surgical approach (Fig. 40–9). Glenoid fractures with an anterior fragment, for example, should be treated through an anterior dissection, whereas any fracture involving the body or spine or a displaced posterior fragment must be approached from the dorsal route.

Anterior glenoid fragments can be easily seen through the standard Bankart dissection using a deltopectoral incision. In addition, the articular surface of the glenoid is more clearly seen from the anterior approach because of the anteversion of the scapula and glenoid face on the thorax. In large or muscular patients, the coracoid process or the conjoint tendon of the short head of the biceps-coracobrachialis must be taken down to afford satisfactory visualization of the medial extent of the neck of the glenoid. Fixation may generally be obtained using 3.5-mm AO cortical screws, although in some instances it may also require small plates.

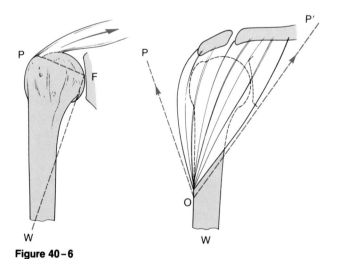

Figure 40–6

The pull of the rotator cuff (P) results in a normalizing force of the humeral head against the glenoid. The action of the deltoid, if not modified by the rotator cuff, produces a combination of shear force vectors. (From Codman, E.A. The Shoulder. Boston, T. Todd and Co., 1934, pp. 32–64.)

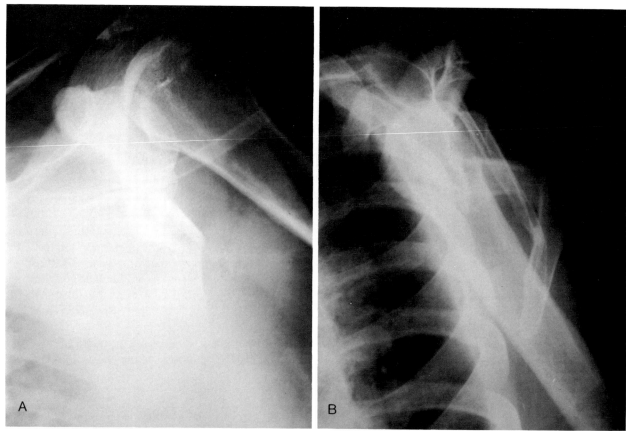

Figure 40-7

Complex type II-B scapular fracture, which on lateral view shows a Z pattern collapse.

The majority of injuries must be viewed and treated from a posterior approach, as they are often complex fracture patterns involving more than one area of the scapula. Most frequently, displaced fractures of the scapular neck and glenoid are associated with fractures of the scapular spine and body. Limited surgical exposures[11] will prove frustrating; thus we recommend the extensile exposure of the so-called Judet incision (Fig. 40-10) for almost all complex fractures. The robust

Table 40-4.
Indications for Operative Treatment of Scapular Fractures

Fracture Type	Displacement
I-A, I-B	More than 5-8 mm
II-A, II-B, II-C	More than 40° angular displacement in transverse or coronal plane; 1 cm or more displacement of glenoid surface.
III	3-5 mm step-off of joint surfaces

blood supply to the scapula (Fig. 40-11) aids in fracture healing, even in the presence of extensive soft tissue dissection. With reasonable care, the two major vascular structures, the suprascapular and circumflex scapular arteries, can be avoided.

Posterior Surgical Approach

The patient is positioned semiprone with the extremity draped free in the operative field for manipulation during fracture reduction. The incision is made from the base of the acromion along the inferior margin of the scapular spine to the medial scapular border, then curved inferiorly along the medial border to the inferior angle. The tough dorsal fascia is incised along the lower edge of the scapular spine and the medial scapular margin, revealing the medial edge of the infraspinatus and the scapular spine. The posteromedial edge of the deltoid is sharply dissected away from the spine and base of the acromion. This is very important in muscular patients, or visualization of the lateral scapular margin and neck of the scapula will be limited. The deltoid is reattached by closure of the fascia adherent to its origin.

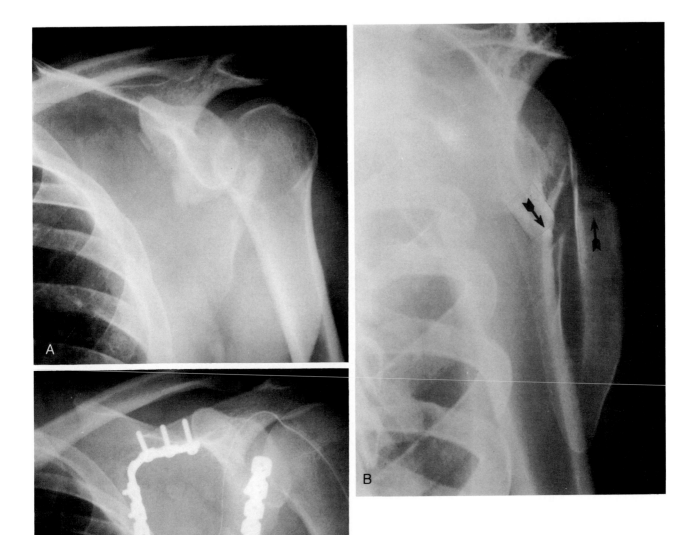

Figure 40–8

A, Type II-C scapular neck fracture. The fracture exits the medial scapular border beneath the scapular spine (*arrow*). *B,* Lateral view showing complete displacement of the fracture margins (*arrows*) of the lateral scapular border. *C,* Anatomic reduction of the fracture with fixation in two planes using 3.5-mm reconstruction plates.

The entire infraspinatus is then cut away from the medial scapular border and spine. Starting with sharp dissection, this can be continued along the infraspinatus fossa with a sharp periosteal elevator, eventually revealing the lateral scapular border and the neck of the scapula by reflecting the entire muscle flap laterally on its neurovascular pedicle (Fig. 40–12). The inferior face of the scapular spine, base of acromion, lateral scapular border, and neck can now be seen. If desired,

the posterior part of the glenoid may be seen through a small arthrotomy.

Reduction maneuvers and fixation patterns vary with fracture types, but a few useful points should be considered. It is very helpful to have two assistants for these demanding cases. Purchase on scapular spine fragments is easily gained with a bone-holding clamp inserted through small keyhole incisions along the superior border of the scapular spine. Because of the

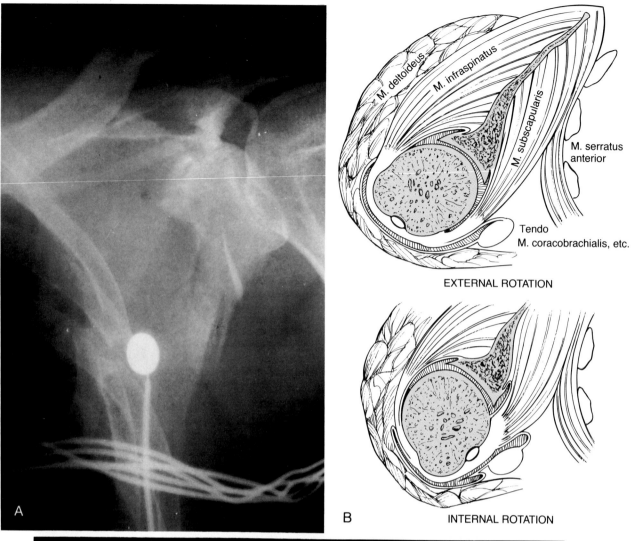

M. deltoideus

M. infraspinatus

M. subscapularis

M. serratus anterior

Tendo
M. coracobrachialis, etc.

EXTERNAL ROTATION

INTERNAL ROTATION

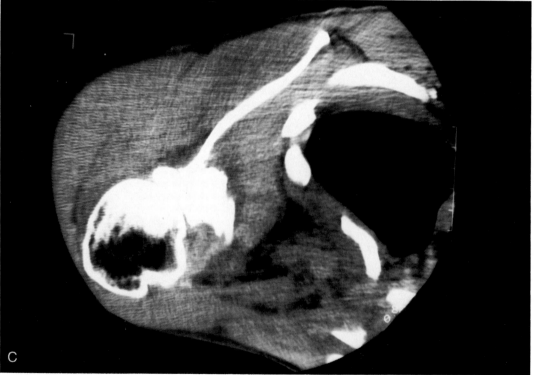

Figure 40–9

See legend on opposite page

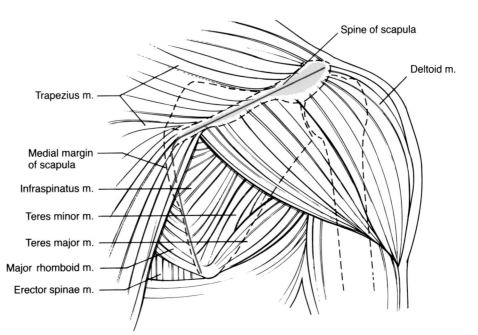

Figure 40-10

Judet posterior approach to the scapula. (From von Torklus, D.; Nicola, T. Atlas of Orthopaedic Exposures. Baltimore, Urban & Schwarzenberg, 1986.)

Spine of scapula

Deltoid m.

Trapezius m.

Medial margin of scapula

Infraspinatus m.

Teres minor m.

Teres major m.

Major rhomboid m.

Erector spinae m.

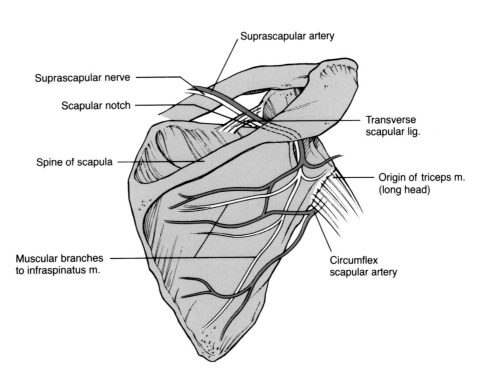

Figure 40-11

Extensive blood supply to the scapula. (From von Torklus, D.; Nicola, T. Atlas of Orthopaedic Exposures. Baltimore, Urban & Schwarzenberg, 1986.)

Suprascapular artery

Suprascapular nerve

Scapular notch

Spine of scapula

Transverse scapular lig.

Origin of triceps m. (long head)

Muscular branches to infraspinatus m.

Circumflex scapular artery

Figure 40-9

A, Fracture of the neck of the glenoid, with inferomedial displacement. *B*, Normal relationship of the rotator cuff musculature with the neck of the scapula. *C*, CT scan of this fracture shows the subscapularis to be impaled on the rotated fragment of scapular neck (*arrow*). (*B* from Codman, E.A. The Shoulder. Boston, T. Todd and Co., 1934.)

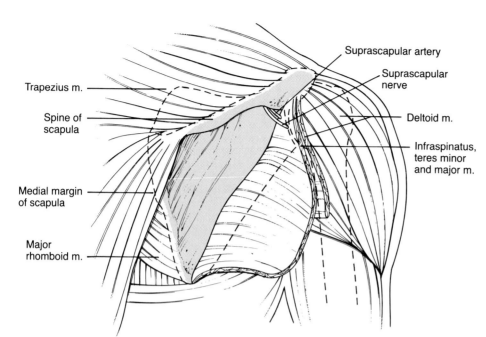

Trapezius m.

Spine of
scapula

Medial margin
of scapula

Major
rhomboid m.

Suprascapular artery

Suprascapular
nerve

Deltoid m.

Infraspinatus,
teres minor
and major m.

Figure 40-12

The entire infraspinatus may be reflected on its neurovascular pedicle. (From von Torklus, D.; Nicola, T. Atlas of Orthopaedic Exposures. Baltimore, Urban & Schwarzenberg, 1986.)

complex web of muscle attachments on the scapula, reduction of displaced fragments must be done with patience and with the aid of complete muscle relaxation by the anesthetist. Small Hohmann retractors and a dental pick can be used to good advantage for realigning fracture margins.

Fixation of simple scapular neck fractures, even those that are widely displaced, can be accomplished with one plate along the lateral scapular margin (Fig. 40-13). The AO 3.5-mm compression plates or reconstruction plates should be used, along with 3.5-mm cortical bone screws. The $\frac{1}{3}$ tubular plates, although

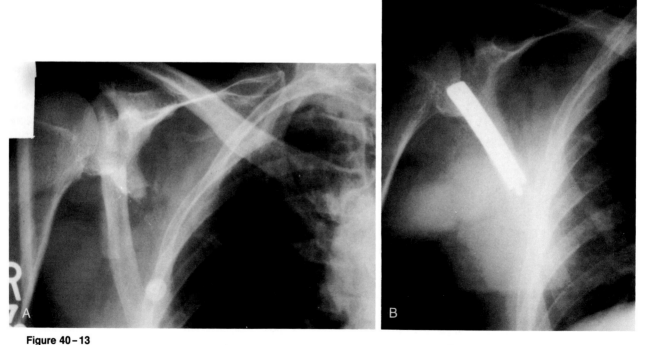

Figure 40-13

Displaced type II-B scapular neck fracture. Fixation with a single 3.5-mm compression plate successfully restores the lateral border.

somewhat easier to contour, are too weak to withstand the large muscle forces and bending movements generated in the shoulder and may break with exercise.

The lateral scapular margin, although only 10- to 14-mm thick, is very dense cortical bone that provides surprisingly strong purchase for the newer AO 3.5-mm cortical screws. More complex fractures may require bidirectional fixation with two plates (see Fig. 40–8C).

Fixation of scapular spine fractures should be done from the inferior surface of the spine so as not to endanger the suprascapular neurovascular bundle or impinge on the relatively tight confines of the supraspinatus muscle itself.

Extremely complex fractures, which include fractures of the glenoid, neck and spine of the scapula, and the clavicle, may require fixation of the clavicle. The intact coracoclavicular ligaments may displace fragments contiguous with the coracoid, making reduction and maintenance of fixation more difficult (see Fig. 40–3C). Such fractures may require a combined anterior and posterior approach, but the majority of even the most complex fractures of the scapula can be treated through the posterior dissection alone.

The incision is closed with a small suction drain left in the infraspinatus fossa, and the dorsal fascia is reapproximated with no. 0 interrupted absorbable suture, followed by routine skin closure. Full, active range of motion is encouraged as soon as tolerated, but Codman's exercises should be started on the second or third postoperative day. These exercises allow the shoulder to come to a fully abducted position with the patient bent over at the waist and gravity as the passive force. A complete program of rotator cuff strengthening therapy, using resistive strengthening exercises after the third postoperative week, is mandatory for a good result.

With reasonable care, good results should be expected in most cases. Our own series of ten patients has thus far been satisfactory; all patients have regained a minimum of 80 to 85° of glenohumeral abduction, none have night pain or rest pain, and there have been no neurovascular complications or infections.

Scapulothoracic Dislocations

The scapula is usually dislocated by high-energy trauma, and patients with these injuries have exceedingly complex multisystem problems. Dislocations may be characterized as intrathoracic or lateral. These injuries are rare.

Intrathoracic dislocation, in which the inferior scapular angle is traumatically inserted between two ribs, is managed by abduction of the arm and direct manipulation of the scapula, with immobilization for three to six weeks.

More ominous is the lateral scapulothoracic dislocation. As described by Oreck et al.[49] and later by Rubenstein et al.,[56] this injury is the harbinger of a major neurovascular disruption of the forequarter and can be thought of as a partial, closed amputation. Diagnosis is based on lateral displacement of the scapula seen on a well-centered plain radiograph of the chest. Arteriography and immediate vascular repair are recommended by both Oreck et al. and Rubenstein et al.[49,56]

Sternoclavicular Dislocations

Sternoclavicular dislocation, an uncommon injury, is of two general types: anterior and posterior. In addition, patients younger than 25 years may suffer this injury as a growth plate fracture-dislocation.

The mechanism of injury is usually a direct force or blow on the point of the shoulder or on the clavicle itself. At least one case of sternoclavicular dislocation has also been reported as a sequela of seizure activity.[14]

ANTERIOR STERNOCLAVICULAR DISLOCATION

The patient usually complains of pain localized to the joint with abduction/external rotation, and the joint is usually quite tender. Neer,[44] in his review of sternoclavicular injuries, described the difficulty in some cases of discerning whether a dislocation is anterior or posterior. The patient must be given a thorough neurovascular examination, although few anterior dislocations have any major associated injuries.

Radiography using apical lordotic views may be helpful, but only computed tomography is accurate enough to fully characterize these lesions.[16,38] In patients aged 25 years or younger, these injuries may constitute a Salter type I or II physeal injury, a finding difficult to substantiate with any study other than tomography or CT scanning (Fig. 40–14).

Treatment

In anterior dislocation of the sternoclavicular joint, the joint is very unstable when reduced. The major considerations in treatment of acute, chronic, or recurrent anterior sternoclavicular joint dislocations are symptomatic and cosmetic, as they generally have little long-term functional impact. The clavicle itself is pinioned by powerful muscular insertions of the pectoralis major, sternocleidomastoid, and trapezius. Loss of stability at its least mobile end is thus minimized. Further-

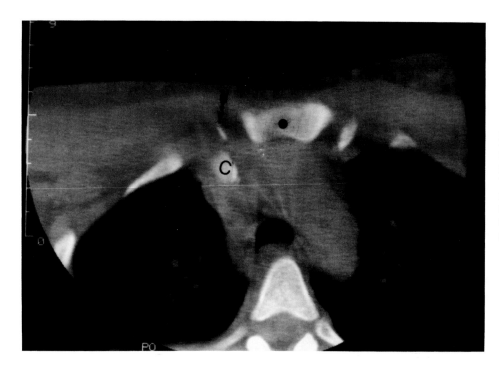

Figure 40–14

CT scan of posterior sternoclavicular joint dislocation in a young adult. The sternum (*dot*) and the medial clavicular epiphysis (*arrow*) maintain their normal relationship, while the clavicle (C) is displaced posteriorly.

more, the contribution of the clavicle for most daily activities is minimal; complete claviculectomy may result in little functional limitation of the forequarter.[70]

Closed Reduction

Despite the inherent instability of anterior dislocations, a closed reduction should be attempted, particularly in view of the functionally benign nature of these injuries. (Surgical procedures are discussed in the section on posterior sternoclavicular dislocation.)

The reduction maneuver consists of abduction of the affected shoulder using a sandbag or a rolled towel under the patient's thoracic spine as a fulcrum. For patient comfort, as well as muscle relaxation, general anesthesia should be used. If the reduction is stable, the limb should be held with a Velpeau bandage for a period of six weeks, with elbow exercises and glenohumeral rotation begun at three weeks during daily furloughs from the bandage. If posteriorly directed distraction force on the shoulder girdle is required to maintain reduction, a plaster jacket or figure-of-8 bandage may be tried. Commercially available soft figure-of-8 bandages exert insufficient force for the management of clavicle fractures in adults[3] and are just as ineffectual for sternoclavicular dislocations.

In the probable event that the anterior dislocation cannot be held reduced by closed means, three alternatives must be considered: acceptance of the deformity, with the small likelihood of a functional deficit; resection of the medial end of the clavicle; and (least preferable) surgical stabilization of the medial end of the clavicle.

POSTERIOR STERNOCLAVICULAR DISLOCATION

Treatment

Posterior dislocations of the sternoclavicular joint are produced by the same mechanisms of injury as the more benign anterior type: a blow on the point of the shoulder or direct trauma to the clavicle. However, because of the subjacent mediastinal and cervical structures, these injuries are potentially more serious and require more aggressive diagnosis and management.

Diagnosis is based on physical and radiographic findings similar to those described for anterior dislocations, with some important differences. In addition to pain, the patient may complain of dysphagia or dyspnea as a result of compression of the esophagus or trachea. Major vascular structures are also at risk for compression (Fig. 40–15), and thus a careful neurovascular assessment is required.

Closed Reduction

Posterior dislocations of the sternoclavicular joint are reduced by a maneuver similar to that described for anterior dislocations. Often a towel clip or pointed bone-holding forceps must be used percutaneously to gain enough purchase to coax the clavicle back to its desired position. In the majority of cases, these injuries are stable when reduced, and the patient can then be managed with a sling and swathe for approximately three weeks before active exercises are begun. We

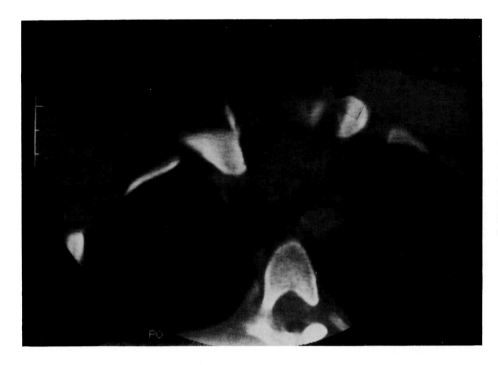

Figure 40–15

CT scan of posterior sternoclavicular dislocation. The clavicle (C) is compressing the underlying brachiocephalic vein. The sternoclavicular joint space on the uninjured and injured sides (*arrows*) are demonstrated well.

prefer to wait at least 12 to 16 weeks before allowing full activities and contact sports after these injuries.

Surgical Management

Surgical stabilization of acute or chronically dislocated sternoclavicular joints can be justified only in the presence of posterior dislocations that cannot be managed with closed techniques. Although primary open treatment of anterior dislocations has its advocates,[17] open management should be reserved for those patients who have intractable pain or in whom the lesion appears to be amenable to soft tissue repair for stabilization. Because of the widely reported complications of Kirschner wire fixations of the sternoclavicular joint, such procedures are to be condemned.[48] One author, in his report of intrathoracic dislocation of Kirschner wires after fixation of these injuries, suggested that this problem ". . . requires treatment by a surgeon with good experience in thoracic surgery."[!][30]

In their review of fixation methods, Booth and Roper[9] described fixation of the medial end of the clavicle with the manubriosternal end of the sternocleidomastoid. The tenodesis transfer of the subclavius described by Burrows,[12] which appears to be physiologically sound, carries the same risks shared by other methods of fixation: potentially hazardous results because of vital structures apposed to the operative field and possible disfigurement created by scar tissue replacing the medial prominence of the clavicle. Although Burrows reported excellent results, there have been too few of these repairs reported by other surgeons to know whether such soft tissue procedures are efficacious in other hands. In cases undertaken for cosmetic reasons, Booth and Roper have warned that "the scar looks worse than the lump."[9]

If an excision of the medial end of the clavicle is chosen because of persistent pain, care must be taken to avoid removal of too much of the clavicle, with resultant ablation of the costoclavicular ligament. Not more than 1 to 1.5 cm of the medial end of the clavicle should be resected. The situation is analogous to the removal of the distal end of the clavicle for treatment of a painful acromioclavicular joint, in which resection of bone sufficient to disturb the intact coracoclavicular ligaments may unnecessarily destabilize the clavicle.

Because the medial clavicular growth plate is among the last to close at the end of growth, any patient younger than 25 years with a sternoclavicular dislocation should be suspected of having a growth plate separation, and in younger patients extensive bone remodeling can be expected.[37]

Fractures of the Clavicle

Clavicle fractures in adults, like those in children, will heal with minimal treatment in the vast majority of cases. Nonunion rates have been reported to be between 0.1% and 5%,[43,71] but for reasons discussed later, the occurrence in adults is probably underestimated.

Although a fall on the outstretched hand is often cited as the common mechanism of injury, Stanley et al.[59] found that direct trauma was the more likely cause in the majority of cases in adults. In either case, when the sternoclavicular joint remains intact, a posteriorly directed force on the entire shoulder or the scapula itself may bend and break the clavicle over the fulcrum of the first rib.

In their study of healing problems in 140 clavicle fractures in adults, White et al.,[67] using several criteria to analyze their patients, found a much higher incidence of delayed union and nonunion (23%) than had previously been reported. They found significantly higher rates of delayed union and nonunion in high-energy injuries but did not find a significant effect of displacement or comminution within the high- or low-energy groups. They did not recommend initial surgical care even in their high-energy group, because the results of delayed surgery have generally been excellent. We agree with their conclusions in most cases.

White et al.[67] found a higher rate of delayed healing for patients treated with slings than for those treated with a figure-of-8 brace, but had only a small group on which to base this observation. Andersen et al.[3] compared plain sling treatment to figure-of-8 bracing and found no difference in adults. We feel that a sling and swathe is best for adults with clavicle fractures.

Most series of acute fixation of clavicle fractures have been from western Europe and typically report complication rates in excess of 10%.[51]

INDICATIONS FOR ACUTE SURGICAL TREATMENT

Injuries to the underlying vascular structures associated with clavicle fractures require exploration and stabilization as a logical part of the vascular repair and protection of the vessels after surgery. Restraint should be exercised in patients with brachial plexus injury, since as many as two thirds of these patients will recover spontaneously.[60]

Depending on the degree of surrounding soft tissue trauma, open fractures of the clavicle may also require stabilization. In these cases, as well as in some cases of established nonunion, external fixation has been successfully employed by at least one group.[58] In patients with head injuries or seizures, tenting of the skin by sharp bone fragments becomes worrisome. It is our opinion that in neurologically normal patients, the major skin injury takes place at the time of initial trauma and is not likely to progress. In those patients lacking normal proprioception or pain inhibition, fixation of clavicle fractures that are tenting the skin may be indicated. Depending on the nursing needs of the patient, a shoulder spica cast may suffice if a good closed reduction is obtained. An exceptional case is seen in Figure 40–16.

Clavicle Fractures That Fail to Unite

For reasons reviewed by Jupiter and Leffert,[29] most nonunited clavicle fractures are in the middle third of the bone; here the medial and lateral compound "S" curves unite in a region almost totally devoid of cancellous bone and muscle coverage and subject to the most pronounced bending and rotational stresses in the entire bone. Indications for surgical intervention in chronic cases are relatively simple. Most surgical candidates have a painful nonunion that limits function and range of motion. Also, patients with brachial plexus compression and thoracic outlet syndrome have been reported.[6] Wilkins and Johnston[68] have observed that most painful nonunions are of the hypertrophic type and that atrophic nonunions are frequently asymptomatic. For reasons described previously in the section on sternoclavicular joint injuries, surgery for cosmetic reasons alone is likely to be disappointing and should be avoided.

Recent reviews of surgery for chronic nonunion or pseudarthrosis are in general agreement as to indications for surgery and method of treatment: pain, loss of function, and brachial plexus compression.[18,29,39,58,68]

Although intramedullary pin fixation has had its proponents,[47] most authors agree that plate fixation is far better and more likely to produce a satisfactory outcome. Because resection of the nonunion is necessary in many cases, the observation made by Eskola et al.[18] becomes more important; all four of their patients with shortening of the clavicle averaging 17 mm or more complained of abduction weakness. This weakness may be attributed to restriction of the scapula in an adducted position by the shortened clavicle. The technique of sculptured bicortical interposition bone graft described by Jupiter and Leffert[29] should thus be considered in patients with resection gaps of more than 10 mm. The AO 3.5-mm compression or reconstruction plates should be used for most patients. The implants must be carefully shaped because of the complex curves and twists of the clavicular surface. After fixation, motion should be restricted for not more than three to four weeks unless bone quality or tenuous fixation indicates a need for more prolonged support.

The fixation of nonunited clavicle fractures should be undertaken with caution, and the patient should have a clear conception of the risks of continued nonunion, loss of fixation, and infection. A hypertrophic scar may result in spite of the care exercised in wound planning and closure. Despite these risks, however, the series cited previously reported an 85% to 95% rate of good to excellent results overall, and a careful surgeon with a reasonably compliant patient should expect to match these favorable outcomes.

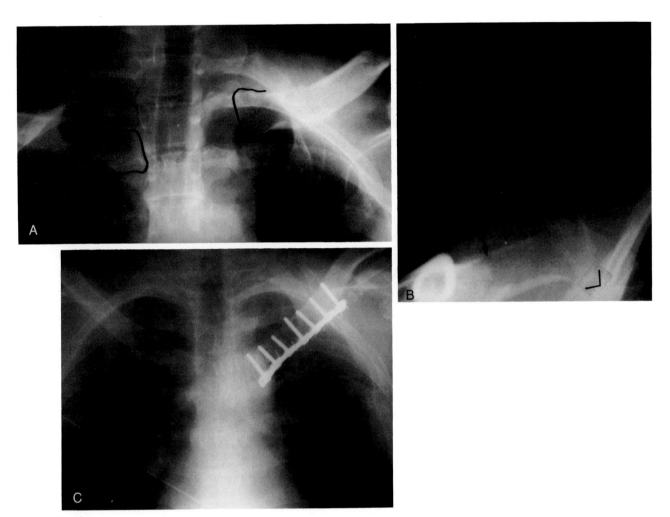

Figure 40–16

A, Anterior dislocation of the sternoclavicular joint with accompanying fracture of the clavicle in mentally retarded seizure patient. The fracture was tenting the skin as a result of severe anterior angulation. *B*, Posterior oblique radiographic view shows the displaced medial end of the clavicle (*brackets*) and the clavicle fracture (*arrow*). *C*, Sternoclavicular joint reduction and clavicle fracture fixation in place. With the clavicle reduced and fixed, the sternoclavicular joint was stable with a simple soft tissue repair.

Acromioclavicular Dislocations and Fractures of the Lateral End of the Distal Clavicle

Since the 1940s, the treatment of acute acromioclavicular joint subluxation and dislocation has been a source of controversy among orthopedic surgeons. At present, orthopedists are still divided into two equally committed and vociferous groups: those who report good results after surgical treatment using one of the numerous methods of fixation developed with or without biomechanical research, and those who report excellent results after closed (or non-) treatment and point to open management of these injuries as ". . . tantamount to shooting a dove with an elephant hunter's rifle . . . the antithesis of sound practice. . . ."[64]

CLASSIFICATION

The widely used tripartite classification of acromioclavicular dislocation was initially proposed by Tossy et al.[63] and later clarified by Allman.[2] Post[52] added three additional grades of injury. Table 40–5 summarizes this system of classification. Any of the rare, severe injuries of type IV–VI may be accompanied by fracture of the coracoid process, and few authors disagree with a need for surgical treatment of these injuries. However, Urist[64] advocates a trial of closed treatment for type IV injuries.

Table 40–5.

Classification of Acromioclavicular Dislocations

Type	Injury Pattern	Surgery
I	AC joint capsule partially disrupted	Not indicated
II	AC joint capsule and CC ligaments partially disrupted	Not indicated
III	AC joint capsule and CC ligaments completely disrupted	Optional (see text)
IV	Type III + avulsion of CC ligament from clavicle; penetration of clavicle through periosteal sleeve or major soft tissue injury	Indicated
V	Type III + posterior dislocation of clavicle behind acromion	Indicated
VI	Type III + infero-lateral dislocation of lateral end of clavicle	Indicated

Abbreviations: AC = acromioclavicular; CC = coracoclavicular

TREATMENT OF ACUTE ACROMIOCLAVICULAR DISLOCATIONS

Any discussion of management of acute injuries to the acromioclavicular joint must confront not only the question of which of the more than 30 methods of surgical treatment described[8] is best but also whether surgery should be considered at all for injury types I–III. Of the few statistically valid prospective series comparing closed treatment with surgical treatment of acromioclavicular dislocation, none shows superior results after surgical management. The majority of sur-geons are content to treat type I and II lesions with a sling and swathe and early motion based on symptoms. In some cases, type II injuries may best be treated with a Kenny Howard sling (Fig. 40–17).

When read closely, most studies have the same results, regardless of the authors' conclusions: longer recovery times and high local complication rates for surgically treated patients without any improvement in long-term function.[7,8,22,35,45,52,53,61,65] However, most authors hedge their conclusions, suggesting surgical treatment for patients whose work required frequent abduction to 90 degrees with forward flexion.

The Kenny Howard Sling: An Historical Note

During the late 1950s, the athletic trainer for the Auburn University football team, Kenny Howard, became dissatisfied with the treatment of what was then referred to as "knockdown shoulder,"[26] or acromioclavicular joint dislocation. The usual treatment was an adhesive tape bandage, which generally caused skin maceration after about 10 days' treatment, requiring therapy to be abandoned before healing was complete. In cooperation with Harvey's Brace Shop in Columbus, Georgia, Howard created a specialized sling, which, while not terribly comfortable to wear incessantly for three weeks, was a major improvement. The original sling was made with webbing straps and toothed clasps so that the patient's compliance could be monitored; more than one set of tooth marks at a clasp site indicated that the brace had been removed, which would compromise treatment. Dr. Fred Allman saw

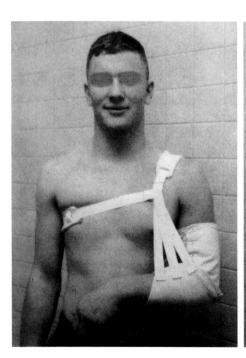
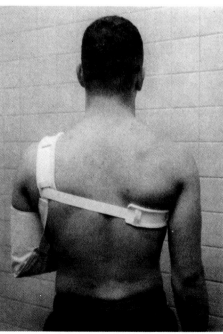

Figure 40–17

The Kenny Howard sling provides satisfactory closed treatment for the majority of acromioclavicular dislocations. (From Allman, F.L., Jr. J Bone Joint Surg 49(A):774–784, 1967.)

the brace at a sports medicine meeting and demonstrated its use in one of his articles.[2] The device has been used widely in the southeastern United States since the 1970s.

Surgical Techniques

Of the many types of surgical treatment described in the literature,[45] there are basically two general approaches: fixation of the acromioclavicular joint directly with transfixing wires, with or without cerclage or tension band wiring; and indirect purchase on the acromioclavicular joint with coracoclavicular fixation using screws, wire loops, woven Dacron loops, or other ligament substitutes. These procedures may be combined with debridement of the acromioclavicular joint and repair of the coracoclavicular ligaments, ligament transfer, or plication of the torn deltotrapezius mechanisms at the distal clavicle.[10,25,31,32,34,45]

Preferred Treatment

An orthopedic surgeon considering open management of *any* acromioclavicular injury of type I–III severity *must* justify operative management, as end-result studies simply do not support surgical intervention. We prefer to treat all of these injuries with a Kenny Howard sling or similar splint for three weeks, after which time range-of-motion exercises may be started, followed by resistive strengthening.

Type IV–VI injuries, which probably constitute less than 10% to 15% of the total number of acromioclavicular dislocations, should be managed surgically. We prefer coracoclavicular fixation, described in the following section.

Coracoclavicular Operative Technique

Place the patient in the "barber chair" (semisitting) position with a small roll under the affected scapula; prep and drape with the arm free in the operative field for necessary manipulation. An incision is made in the so-called Langer's line over the coracoid and clavicle (actually a medial "sabre cut" incision). The clavicular slip of the deltoid is dissected away and the clavipectoral fascia opened to gain access to the coracoid. By careful, deep undermining, the acromioclavicular joint is visualized and its contents debrided if the articular disk is damaged. If the acromioclavicular joint capsule appears repairable, stay sutures are inserted for later tying. The coracoclavicular ligament complex is inspected. It will frequently be "mop-ended" (attenuated) and difficult to suture. If so, repair of the ligaments is not attempted. If it is repairable, stay sutures of absorbable no. 1 material are placed for later tying. With an assistant holding the clavicle reduced using a bone-holding clamp, drill with a 3.2-mm bit from the clavicle through the coracoid and measure with a depth gauge. Tap with a 6.5-mm tap and insert a 6.5-mm AO type 16-mm thread (short-thread) cancellous bone screw with a washer. The short-thread screw is stronger than the 32-mm thread screw and thus less subject to breakage. Ensure that the screw has not malreduced the acromioclavicular joint and tie the previously placed sutures. With the acromioclavicular joint reduced, carefully inspect and repair the torn deltotrapezius insertion with absorbable suture. The wound is closed without a drain except in unusual circumstances.

A sling and swathe or Velpeau immobilizer is applied in the operating room. The patient may remove this to exercise the elbow and perform rotational exercises of the shoulder as soon as comfort allows. The sling can be discontinued within two weeks of surgery and full active range of motion regained within six weeks. The screw must be removed before any heavy labor or contact sports are started, or breakage of the screw may result. This is easily done under local anesthesia in an outpatient clinic setting.

The repair technique of Weaver and Dunn,[66] which combines distal clavicle resection with coracoclavicular ligament transfer, may also be used for acute injuries, but is discussed in the following section on nonacute problems.

TREATMENT OF NONACUTE INJURIES

For the patient with a chronic acromioclavicular joint dislocation or subluxation that remains painful after three to six months of closed treatment and rehabilitation, surgery is indicated to improve function and comfort. Only a minority of patients with untreated acromioclavicular joint injuries will actually choose to have surgical treatment.[47]

Most authors agree that resection of the lateral end of the clavicle will provide excellent relief for a painful acromioclavicular joint. This has been confirmed by long-term follow-up as well.[50] In neglected type II–III injuries, supplementary reconstruction of the coracoclavicular ligament complex should be based on the surgeon's perception of instability at the time of surgery; we feel that such reconstruction is needed only if instability of the distal clavicle is a contributor to the patient's pain or loss of function, and this is only rarely the case.

For sequelae of untreated type IV–VI injuries, a combination of distal clavicle resection and coracoclavicular ligament substitution is called for.

Preferred Treatment

The technique of Weaver and Dunn,[66] widely used in North America and simple to perform, is mechanically sound and fulfills its originators' criteria that "the ideal operative procedure should eliminate the possibility of migration of pins or failure of acromioclavicular reduction. Late degenerative changes should not be seen, and any further or secondary operative procedures should be unnecessary. In addition, the result should be cosmetically acceptable, and should allow the patient to have a fully functional shoulder in a short period of time." [66]

Operative Technique

The operation is accomplished through a longitudinal incision parallel to the inferior border of the clavicle and acromioclavicular joint. Because this is perpendicular to the so-called Langer's line, hypertrophy of the scar is to be expected. The deltoid and trapezius insertions on the clavicle are reflected, and through undermining and opening the clavipectoral fascia, the entire course of the coracoacromial ligament is visualized. The distal 1.5 to 2.0 cm of the clavicle is resected with an inferiorly facing osteotomy centered over the coracoid. The coracoacromial ligament is carefully dissected off of the undersurface of the acromion to preserve its maximum length. The clavicle is reduced into its desired position with a bone-holding clamp, and the approximate length of ligament to be transferred is measured. In exceptional circumstances, a small excess portion of coracoacromial ligament will need trimming, but in most cases, the full length is used. The medullary canal of the clavicle is debrided open with a curette, and two small holes are drilled in the overhanging superior cortex of the clavicle as far medially as will be accessible to the passage of sutures. A Bunnell stay suture of no. 1 nonabsorbable material is passed through the coracoacromial ligament and then upward through the drill holes in the clavicle while the bone is held reduced. Codman's circumduction and gravity exercises are started within one to two days after surgery, and full function should be restored at four to six weeks. Heavy labor and contact sports are possible at three to six months.

In some widely displaced dislocations, a supplemental coracoclavicular screw may be needed, with postoperative management as described in the previous section.

Fractures of the Distal Clavicle

In adults, fractures of the distal clavicle may be classified by the system of Neer,[45] which uses three types. Surgical treatment is occasionally indicated for only one of these types.

The distal clavicle is pinioned in place by the static

stabilization of the coracoclavicular ligament complex and the acromioclavicular joint capsule. Acting against these are the relatively weak dynamic downward forces of the pectoralis major and the stronger upward forces of the trapezius and sternocleidomastoid. Depending on the location of a fracture of the lateral end of the clavicle relative to these static and dynamic stabilizers, certain displacements and functional problems can be expected. Fracture types are based on these considerations.

Type I injuries, which occur lateral to the coracoclavicular ligament complex and are therefore quite stable, will heal with sling and swathe support. These fractures may be complicated by an undisplaced intraarticular component at the acromioclavicular joint, leading to some postfracture arthrosis and pain.

Type III injuries are intraarticular fractures of the distal clavicle at the acromioclavicular joint and are sometimes an occult source of posttraumatic arthritis and pain in injuries that might otherwise have been diagnosed as grade I acromioclavicular joint subluxations. Diagnosis may be made by anteroposterior tomography in patients with an unusual level of pain after an apparently trivial acromioclavicular joint injury. Acute treatment is supportive only.

Type II injuries are complex fracture-dislocations that leave the distal clavicle and the acromioclavicular joint intact but separate the clavicle from the underlying coracoclavicular ligament complex through an oblique fracture. Sometimes a small fragment of bone is left attached to the coracoclavicular ligaments, avulsed from the clavicle. The deformity is marked, and Neer[45] favors open treatment, with Kirschner wires transfixing the acromioclavicular joint into the displaced clavicle or suture loop fixation of the clavicle to the coracoid with no. 5 nonabsorbable material. Experience with these rare injuries is necessarily limited, but surgical treatment is probably unwarranted in most cases.

We have treated several of these injuries with the Kenny Howard sling, with excellent functional results. The deformity can be reduced somewhat, but a sizable lump will still be present, which in young women may be cosmetically distressing. The fact remains that these injuries, like other more routine clavicle fractures, heal readily, and splintage may be discontinued at three to four weeks. The result is generally a strong, painless shoulder with a cosmetic deformity.

REFERENCES

1. Ada, J.R.; Miller, M.E. Scapular fractures: Analysis of 113 cases. Clin Orthop 1991, in press.
2. Allman, F.L. Jr. Fractures and ligamentous injuries of the clavi-

cle and its articulations. J Bone Joint Surg 49(4):774–784, 1967.

3. Andersen, K.; Jensen, P.O.; Lauritzen, J. Treatment of clavicular fractures: Figure-of-eight bandage versus a simple sling. Acta Orthop Scand 58(1):71–74, 1987.

4. Aston, J.W.; Gregory, C.F. Dislocation of the shoulder with significant fracture of the glenoid. J Bone Joint Surg 55(7):1531–1533, 1973.

5. Aulicino, P.L.; Reinert, C.; Kornberg, M.; Williamson, S. Displaced intra-articular glenoid fractures treated by open reduction and internal fixation. J Trauma 26(12):1137–1141, 1986.

6. Barger, W.L.; Marcus, R.E.; Ittleman, F.P. Late thoracic outlet syndrome secondary to pseudarthrosis of the clavicle. J Trauma 24/9:857–859, 1984.

7. Bergfeld, J.A.; Amdrish, J.T.; Clancy, W.G. Evaluation of the acromioclavicular joint following first and second degree sprains. Am J Sports Med 6(4):153–159, 1978.

8. Bjerneld, H.; Hovelius, J.T.; Thorling, J. Acromioclavicular separations treated conservatively: A 5-year follow-up study. Acta Orthop Scand 54(5):743–745, 1983.

9. Booth, C.M.; Roper, M.A. Chronic dislocation of the sternoclavicular joint. Clin Orthop 140:17–20, 1979.

10. Bosworth, B.M. Acromioclavicular separation: A new method of repair. Surg Gynecol Obstet 73:866–871, 1941.

11. Brodsky, J.W.; Tullos, H.S.; Gartsman, G.M. Simplified posterior approach to the shoulder joint. J Bone Joint Surg 69(A):773–777, 1987.

12. Burrows, J.J. Tenodesis of the subclavius in the treatment of recurrent dislocation of the sterno-clavicular joint. J Bone Joint Surg 33-B:240–244, 1951.

13. Codman, E.A. The Shoulder. Boston, T. Todd and Co., 1934, pp. 32–64.

14. Dastgeer, G.M.; Mikolich, D.J. Fracture-dislocation of the manubristernal joint: An unusual complication of seizures. J Trauma 27(1):911–993, 1987.

15. Desault, P.J. A Treatise on Fractures, Luxations, and Other Affectations of the Bones. Translated by Charles Caldwell. Philadelphia, Fray and Kammerer, 1805, pp. 57–67.

16. Deutsch, A.L.; Resnick, D.; Mink, J.H. Computed tomography of the glenohumeral and sternoclavicular joints. Orthop Clin North Am 16:497–511, 1985.

17. Eskola, A. Sternoclavicular dislocation: A plea for open treatment. Acta Orthop Scand 57(3):227–228, 1986.

18. Eskola, A.; Vainionpaa, S.; Myllynen, P.; et al. Surgery for ununited clavicle fracture. Acta Orthop Scand 57:366–367, 1986.

19. Fischer, W.R. Fractures of the scapula requiring open reduction. J Bone Joint Surg 21:459–461, 1939.

20. Friedrich, B. Zur operativen therapie von frakturen der scapula. Chirurg 44:37–39, 1973.

21. Fromison, A.I. Fractures of the coracoid process of the scapula. J Bone Joint Surg 60-A:710–711, 1978.

22. Galpin, R.D.; Hawkins, R.J.; Grainger, R.W. A comparative analysis of acromioclavicular separations. Clin Orthop 193:150–155, 1985.

23. Gordes, W. Seltene Verletzungs folgen an der spina scapula. Arch Orthop Unfallchirurg 68:315–324, 1970.

24. Hardegger, F.H.; Simpson, L. The operative treatment of scapular fractures. J Bone Joint Surg 66-B:315–324, 1984.

25. Heitemeyer, U.; Hierholzer, G.; Schneppendahl, G.; Haines, J. The operative treatment of fresh ruptures of the acromioclavicular joint (Tossy III). Arch Orthop Trauma Surg 104:371–373, 1986.

26. Howard, K. Personal communication, 1989.

27. Ishizuki, M.; Yamura, I.; Isobe, Y.; et al. Avulsion fractures of the superior border of the scapula. J Bone Joint Surg 63-A:820–822, 1981.

28. Izadpanah, M. Osteosynthesis in scapular fractures. Arch Orthop Unfallchirurg 83:153–164, 1975.

29. Jupiter, J.B.; Leffert, R.D. Non-union of the clavicle: Associated complications and surgical management. J Bone Joint Surg 69-A:753–760, 1987.

30. Keferstein, R.; Frese, J. Intrathoracic dislocation of a metalpiece after the use of wires in bone surgery. Author's translation. Unfallchirurg 6:57–61, 1980.

31. Kennedy, J.C.; Cameron, H. Complete dislocation of the acromioclavicular joint. J Bone Joint Surg 36-B:202–208, 1954.

32. Kiefer, H.; Claes, L.; Burri, C.; Holzwarth, J. The stabilizing effect of various implants on the torn acromioclavicular joint. Arch Orthop Trauma Surg 106:42–46, 1986.

33. Kummel, B.M. Fractures of the glenoid causing chronic dislocation of the shoulder. Clin Orthop 69:189–191, 1970.

34. Lancaster, S.; Horowitz, M.; Alonso, J. Complete acromioclavicular separations: A comparison of operative methods. Clin Orthop 216:80–88, 1987.

35. Larsen, E.; Bjerg-Nielsen, A.; Christensen, P. Conservative or surgical treatment of acromioclavicular dislocation: A prospective, controlled, randomized study. J Bone Joint Surg 68-A:552–555, 1986.

36. Lasda, N.A.; Murray, D.G. Fracture separation of the coracoid process associated with acromioclavicular dislocation: Conservative treatment. A case report and review of the literature. Clin Orthop 134:222–224, 1978.

37. Lemire, L.; Rosman, M. Sternoclavicular epiphyseal separation with adjacent clavicular fractures. J Pediatr Orthop 4:118–120, 1984.

38. Levinsohn, E.M.; Bunnell, W.P.; Hansen, A.Y. Computed tomography in the diagnosis of dislocations of the sternoclavicular joint. Clin Orthop 140:12–14, 1979.

39. Manske, D.J.; Szabo, R. The operative treatment of mid-shaft clavicular non-unions. J Bone Joint Surg 67-A:1367–1371, 1985.

40. Matthews, R.E.; Cocke, T.B.; d'Ambrosia, B. A.; et al. Scapular fractures secondary to seizures in patients with osteodystrophy. J Bone Joint Surg 65-A:850–853, 1983.

41. Heyse-Moore, G.H.; Stoker, D.V. Avulsion fractures of the scapula. Skeletal Radiol 9:27–32, 1982.

42. Montgomery, S.P.; et al. Avulsion fractures of the coracoid epiphysis with acromioclavicular separation. J Bone Joint Surg 59-A:963–965, 1977.

43. Neer, C.S. Non-union of the clavicle. JAMA 172:1006–1011, 1960.

44. Neer, C.S. Injuries to the sternoclavicular joint. In: Rockwood, C.A., Jr.; Green, D.P., eds. Fractures in Adults. Philadelphia, J.B. Lippincott, 1984, pp. 910–950.

45. Neer, C.S. Injuries to the acromioclavicular joint. In: Rockwood, C.A., Jr.; Green, D.P., eds. Fractures in Adults. Philadelphia, J.B. Lippincott, 1984, p. 895.

46. Nevaiser, J.D. Injuries in and about the shoulder joint. A.A.O.S. Instr Course Lect 13:187–216, 1956.

47. Nevaiser, R.J. Injuries to the clavicle and acromioclavicular joint. Orthop Clin North Am 18:433–438, 1987.

48. Nordbeck, I.; Markula, H. Migration of Kirschner pin from clavicle into ascending aorta. Acta Chir Scand 151(3):177–179, 1985.

49. Oreck, S.L.; Burgess, A.; Levine, A. Traumatic lateral displacement of the scapula: A radiographic sign of neurovascular disruption. J Bone Joint Surg 66-A:758–763, 1984.

50. Petersson, C.J. Resection of the lateral end of the clavicle. A 3- to 30-year follow-up. Acta Orthop Scand 54(4):904–907, 1983.

51. Poigenfurst, J.; Reiler, T.; Fischer, W. Plating of fresh clavicular

fractures. Experience with 60 operations. Unfallchirurg 14(1):26–37, 1988.

52. Post, M. Current concepts in the diagnosis and management of acromioclavicular dislocations. Clin Orthop 200:234–247, 1985.

53. Powers, J.A.; Bach, P.J. Acromioclavicular separations: Closed or open treatment? Clin Orthop 104:213–223, 1974.

54. Protass, J.J.; Stampeli, E.V.; Osmaer, J.C.; et al. Coracoid process fracture diagnosis in acromioclavicular separation. Radiology 116:61–64, 1975.

55. Rowe, C.R.; Marble, H. Shoulder girdle injuries. In: Cave, E.F., ed. Fractures and Other Injuries. Chicago, Year Book Medical Publishers, 1958, pp. 263–264.

56. Rubenstein, J.D.; Ebraheim, N.A.; Kellam, J.F. Traumatic scapulothoracic dissociation. Radiology 157(2):297–298, 1985.

57. Sarrafian, S.K. Gross and functional anatomy of the shoulder. Clin Orthop 173:11–19, 1983.

58. Schuind, F.; Pay-Pay, E.; Andrianne, Y.; et al. External fixation of the clavicle for fracture or non-union in adults. J Bone Joint Surg 70-A:692–695, 1988.

59. Stanley, D.; Trowbridge, E.A.; Norris, S.H. The mechanism of clavicular fracture. J Bone Joint Surg 70-B:461–464, 1988.

60. Sturm, J.T.; Perry, J.F. Brachial plexus injuries from blunt trauma: A harbinger of vascular and thoracic injury. Ann Emerg Med 16(4):404–406, 1987.

61. Taft, T.N.; Wilson, F.C.; Oglesby, J.W. Dislocation of the acromioclavicular joint: An end-result study. J Bone Joint Surg 69-A:1045–1051, 1987.

62. Tarquinio, T.; Weinstein, M.E.; Virgilio, W. W. Bilateral scapular fractures from accidental electric. J Trauma 19:132–133, 1979.

63. Tossy, J.D.; Mead, N.C.; Sigmond, H.M. Acromioclavicular separations: Useful and practical classification for treatment. Clin Orthop 28:111–119, 1963.

64. Urist, M.R. The treatment of dislocations of the acromioclavicular joint: A survey of the past decade. Am J Surg 98:423–431, 1959.

65. Walsh, W.M.; Peterson, D.A.; Shelton, G.; Neumann, R.D. Shoulder strength following acromioclavicular injury. Am J Sports Med 13(3):153–158, 1985.

66. Weaver, J.K.; Dunn, H.K. Treatment of acromioclavicular injuries, especially complete acromioclavicular separation. J Bone Joint Surg 54-A:1187–1194, 1972.

67. White, R.R.; Anson, P.S.; Kristiansen, T.; Healy, W. Adult clavicle fractures: The relationship between mechanism of injury and healing. Orthop Trans 1988.

68. Wilkins, R.M.; Johnston, R.M. Un-united fractures of the clavicle. J Bone Joint Surg 65-A:773–778, 1983.

69. Wolf, A.W.; et al. Unusual fractures of the coracoid process. J Bone Joint Surg 58-A:423–424, 1976.

70. Wood, V.E. The results of total claviculectomy. Clin Orthop 207:186–190, 1986.

71. Zenni, E.; Krieg, J.; Rosen, M. Open reduction and internal fixation of clavicular fractures. J Bone Joint Surg 63-A:147–151, 1981.

72. Zettas, J.P.; et al. Fractures of the coracoid process base in acute acromioclavicular separation. Orthop Rev 11:77–79, 1976.

73. Zilberman, Z.; Rejovitsky, R. Fractures of the coracoid process of the scapula. Injury 13:203, 1981.

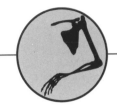

E.F. Shaw Wilgis, M.D.
Thomas M. Brushart, M.D.

41

Brachial Plexus and Shoulder Girdle Injuries

Basic Considerations

ANATOMY

This discussion of brachial plexus anatomy and relationships, except as specifically noted, is based on *Anatomy for Surgeons* by Hollinshead[15] and *Brachial Plexus Injuries* by Leffert.[23]

Neural Elements

The brachial plexus is usually formed from the ventral (anterior primary) rami of the fifth (C5) to eighth (C8) cervical nerves and the first thoracic (T1) nerve. Additional fibers from the fourth cervical nerve are received by 62% of plexi.[18] Contributions from the second thoracic nerve (T2) are infrequent but can be substantial when the first thoracic rib is rudimentary. Sympathetic fibers enter the brachial plexus largely through the C8 and T1 roots, although C7 can also contribute.[38] Brachial plexi receiving fibers from C4 are traditionally said to be "prefixed" and those receiving T2 contributions are termed "postfixed." Recent quantitative evaluations have shown, however, that a cephalad or caudad shift in brachial plexus formation can be defined most meaningfully by the relative cross-sectional areas of all contributing roots.[35]

In the most common form of the brachial plexus (Fig. 41–1), C5 and C6 roots join to form the upper trunk, C7 extends to become the middle trunk, and C8 and T1 are united to form the lower trunk. Three nerves arise at the root level: the phrenic nerve from C3 to C5, the dorsal scapular nerve from C5, and the long thoracic nerve from C5 to C7. The suprascapular nerve is the sole tributary at the trunk level. Each trunk then bifurcates into anterior and posterior divisions. This separation divides axons innervating the flexor muscles (anterior divisions) from those innervating the extensor muscles (posterior divisions). The lateral cord is formed from the anterior divisions of the upper and middle trunks and gives off the lateral pectoral and musculocutaneous nerves before terminating as a portion of the median nerve. The medial cord is the continuation of the anterior division of the lower trunk and contributes medial pectoral, medial brachial cutaneous, and medial antebrachial cutaneous nerves before joining the lateral cord in the formation of the median nerve. The posterior cord is the summation of all three posterior divisions and gives off subscapular and thoracodorsal nerves before terminating in the radial and axillary nerves.

There can be significant variations from this most common plexus configuration. The lateral cord was found to contribute to the ulnar nerve in 43% of dissections[18] and the musculocutaneous to the median nerve in 24%.[17] The medial pectoral and subscapular nerves can arise proximal to their normal location, the medial pectoral from the lower trunk and the subscapular from the posterior division of the upper trunk. No posterior cord was found in 20% of specimens,[18] with the radial and axillary nerves arising directly from the posterior divisions.

The internal anatomy of the brachial plexus elements is far more complex than their external form. Most are composed of multiple fascicles that intermingle to form an *intraneural* plexus. Attempts at tracing the path of fascicles through the brachial plexus are hampered by this intraneural plexus formation. A recent quantitative analysis of brachial plexus anatomy,[35] however, has yielded significant new informa-

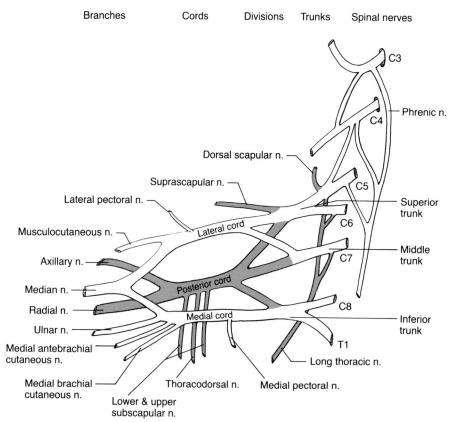

Branches   Cords   Divisions   Trunks   Spinal nerves

C3

Phrenic n.

C4

Dorsal scapular n.

Suprascapular n.

C5

Lateral pectoral n.

Superior
trunk

Lateral cord

C6

Musculocutaneous n.

Middle
trunk

C7

Axillary n.

Posterior cord

Median n.

Radial n.

C8

Ulnar n.

Medial cord

Inferior
trunk

Medial antebrachial
cutaneous n.

T1

Medial brachial
cutaneous n.

Long thoracic n.

Thoracodorsal n.   Medial pectoral n.

Lower & upper
subscapular n.

Figure 41–1

Schematic drawing of the brachial
plexus, including the formation of
the phrenic nerve. Deeper elements are shaded.

tion on its internal structure. An average of 65 to 70% of the cross-sectional area of brachial plexus elements was found to be neural tissue. The number of fascicles at a given location varied sixfold from plexus to plexus, with most specimens occupying the midrange. Several areas were consistently monofascicular (Fig. 41–2), whereas the posterior division of the lower trunk was usually bifascicular. Fascicles proceeded an average of 5 mm without branching or merging with other fascicles. Fascicular groups were more constant, however, averaging 15 mm without interaction with other fascicular groups and 25 mm without loss of localization within the brachial plexus element. Each terminal fascicular group retained its identity for an average of 2 cm proximal to its point of exit from the nerve. Fascicles supplying purely motor or cutaneous branches were less common than mixed fascicles but were found near branch points and spinal nerves. A schematic map of functional localization within the brachial plexus has been compiled from this collective experience (Fig. 41–3).

Relationships

The C5, C6, and C7 roots exit the intervertebral foramina and lie within grooves in the vertebral transverse

processes. Distal to this they emerge between the anterior and middle scalene muscles, although C5 and C6 might pierce the anterior scalene directly. The C8 root runs over the neck of the first rib directly posterior to the stellate ganglion and crosses the pleura between the posterior scalene and transversopleural muscles to join T1 on the superior surface of the first rib. The T1 root reaches this juncture by passing beneath the first rib neck and through the suprapleural membrane. The phrenic, long thoracic, and dorsal scapular nerves are formed at the root level (Fig. 41–1). The phrenic nerve receives C3, C4, and C5 contributions and crosses the anterior scalene laterally to medially to enter the chest between the subclavian artery and vein. The long thoracic nerve is formed from C5, C6, and C7 branches, which join on the anterolateral surface of the middle scalene and descend behind the brachial plexus to innervate the serratus anterior. The dorsal scapular nerve leaves the C5 root just distal to the intervertebral foramen, courses posteriorly and inferiorly on the middle scalene, and continues on or through the levator scapulae to innervate the rhomboid muscles.

The trunks of the brachial plexus lie within the posterior triangle of the neck (Fig. 41–4). C5 and C6 join to form the upper trunk at "Erb's point," 2 to 3 cm superior to the clavicle on the anterior surface of the middle

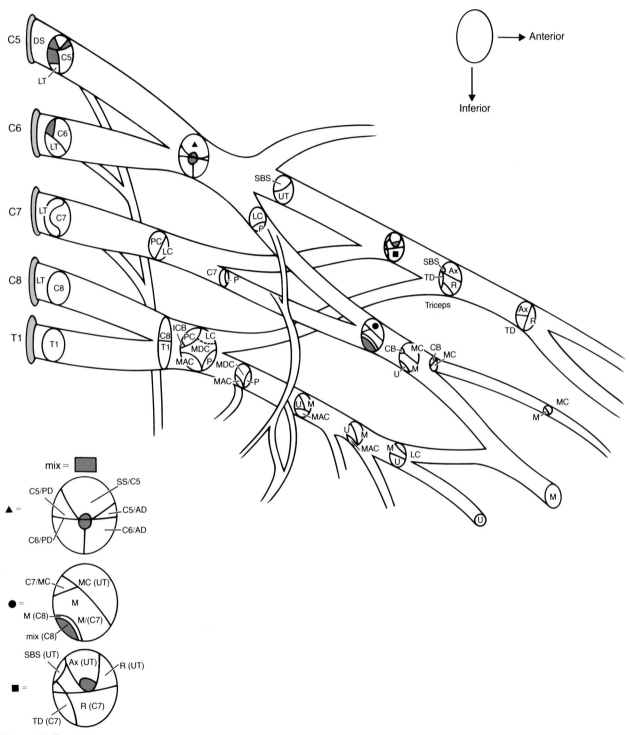

Figure 41–2

Schema of the brachial plexus showing monofascicular regions and "gray zones," areas in which fascicular localization cannot be determined. (Redrawn from Slingluff, C.L., et al. In: Terzis, J.K., ed. Microreconstruction of Nerve Injuries. W.B. Saunders, 1987, pp. 285–324.)

ZONES IN THE BRACHIAL PLEXUS

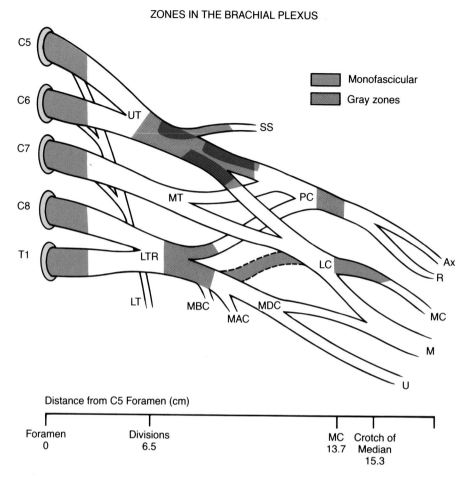

Figure 41–3

Schematic drawing of the localization of fascicular groups within plexus elements. This drawing is based on study of serial cross sections and represents the average of seven plexii. (Redrawn from Slingluff, C.L., et al. In Terzis, J.K., ed. Microreconstruction of Nerve Injuries. W.B. Saunders, 1987, pp. 285–324.)

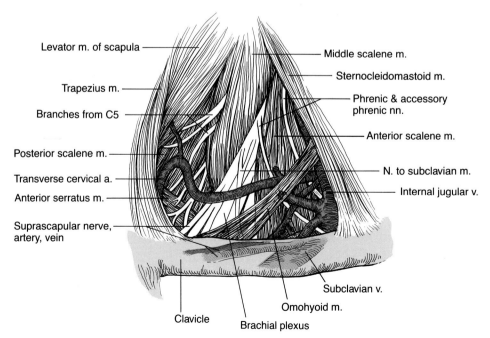

Figure 41–4

Right posterior cervical triangle, showing the landmarks encountered during initial exposure of the supraclavicular brachial plexus.

scalene. The upper and middle trunks are superior to the omohyoid muscle and the lower trunk is inferior to it. The transverse cervical artery crosses the superior portion of the upper and middle trunks, whereas the suprascapular artery crosses the inferior portion of the trunks just above the clavicle. The prevertebral layer of deep cervical fascia invests the nerve roots as they emerge from the scalenes and condenses over the trunks to form the axillary sheath at the level of the clavicle. The suprascapular nerve is the only surgically significant branch at the trunk level. It leaves the upper trunk just distal to Erb's point, coursing distally and posteriorly on the surface of the scalenus medius before passing deep to the trapezius near its origin from the clavicle. It traverses the scapular notch to innervate the supraspinatus and infraspinatus muscles.

The trunks of the brachial plexus split into anterior and posterior divisions beneath or just distal to the clavicle. These divisions, which do not normally give off branches, rearrange to form medial, lateral, and posterior cords that surround the axillary artery in the axilla (Fig. 41–5). The axilla is a pyramidal space with its apex superior. The pectoralis major and minor form the anterior wall, the subscapularis, teres major, and latissimus dorsi form the posterior wall, the rib cage and serratus anterior bound the axilla medially, and the coracobrachialis and biceps in the bicipital groove define the narrow lateral wall. Proximal formation of the lateral cord occurs lateral to the axillary artery within the axillary sheath. The highest branch is the lateral pectoral nerve, which passes anteriorly through the clavipectoral fascia to innervate the pectoralis major. As the lateral cord passes deep to the pectoralis minor, the

musculocutaneous nerve branches laterally to enter the coracobrachialis. Further distally, the lateral cord shifts anterior to the axillary artery, where it joins the medial cord to form the median nerve. The medial cord originates behind the axillary artery, where it gives off the medial pectoral nerve to the pectoralis major and minor. The medial brachial cutaneous and medial antebrachial cutaneous branches are generated as the medial cord shifts to a position medial to the artery.

Continuing distally, the ulnar nerve branches off, hugging the posteromedial side of the artery; the remaining, terminal portion of the lateral cord passes anterior to the artery to join in the formation of the median nerve. The posterior cord originates superior and lateral to the axillary artery. It rapidly assumes a posterior location, where it gives off the subscapular and thoracodorsal nerves. All are directly opposed to the subscapularis muscle, with the thoracodorsal nerve passing inferiorly to reach the latissimus dorsi. The posterior cord terminates in the axillary and radial nerves. The axillary nerve passes inferior to the subscapularis to enter the quadrangular space; the radial nerve continues posterior to the artery, crossing the tendons of the teres major and latissimus dorsi before passing deep between the long head of the triceps and the humerus.

Vascular Elements

The subclavian artery becomes the axillary artery as it crosses the superior surface of the first rib between the scalenus anticus and medius, inferior to the cords of the brachial plexus. The subclavian vein crosses the first rib

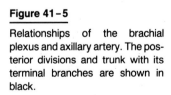

Figure 41–5

Relationships of the brachial plexus and axillary artery. The posterior divisions and trunk with its terminal branches are shown in black.

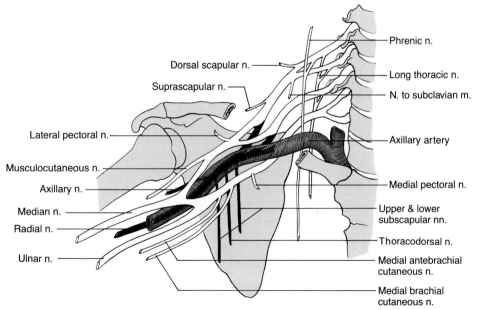

anterior to the scalenus anticus. The axillary artery can be divided into three parts, which lie superior, deep, and inferior to the pectoralis minor muscle. The first part has one branch, the supreme thoracic, the second part gives off thoracodorsal and lateral thoracic branches, and the third part gives rise to the subscapular and anterior and posterior humeral circumflex arteries. The first part of the axillary artery lies on the serratus anterior behind the clavipectoral fascia. Its neural relationships are as follows: posterior—medial cord, medial pectoral nerve; anterior—junction of the lateral and medial pectoral nerves; lateral—lateral and posterior cords of brachial plexus; medial—axillary vein. The second part, behind the pectoralis minor, lies on the subscapularis. The medial cord is medial or posteromedial, the lateral cord is lateral, and the posterior cord is posterior. The axillary vein is inferior and medial to the artery, with the medial cord sandwiched between the two. The third part of the axillary artery lies on the subscapularis and teres major muscles. Its neural relationships are as follows: posterior—axillary and radial nerves; anterior—medial cord contribution to the median nerve; lateral—median nerve, distally; medial—medial brachial cutaneous, medial antebrachial cutaneous, and ulnar nerves. The axillary vein is directly medial to these nerves.

Variations in the relationship between the brachial plexus and axillary artery were found in 8% of 480 specimens dissected by Miller.[27] In the most common variation the axillary artery was superior to the median nerve. In other cases the median nerve was divided by a branch of the artery, the artery originated from an abnormal segmental level and thus penetrated the plexus abnormally, the lateral cord was divided by an arterial branch, or nerves communicated around the axillary artery.

INCIDENCE

The incidence of brachial plexus lesions in the population has not been clearly defined. Narakas[30] has estimated, however, that 2% of those involved in motorcycle accidents suffer brachial plexus injury.[13] In his series of 114 patients with complete brachial plexus lesions, 76% resulted from motorcycle accidents, 6% from auto accidents, 4% each from bicycle and pedestrian accidents, and 11% from other causes. From his overall series[30] he generalized that approximately 70% of traumatic brachial plexus injuries are caused by traffic accidents, 70% involve the use of a motorcycle or bicycle, and 70% have associated injuries. Millesi's analysis of 247 patients with brachial plexus injuries[29] produced a similar breakdown, with 70% resulting from motorcycle accidents, 11% from auto accidents, 9% from pedestrian and bicycle accidents, and 9% from other causes.

CLASSIFICATION

Brachial plexus pathology can be classified according to the severity of damage to neural elements and to the location of that damage. The latter can be characterized further along two perpendicular axes; proximal-distal location with the plexus (e.g., root, trunk) and cervical root level of involvement.

Seddon[34] initially divided peripheral nerve injuries into three clinical categories based on their severity. *Neurapraxia,* the least severe, results in loss of function for days to a few weeks. The underlying pathology is presumed to be, at most, a segmental demyelination. This must involve larger fibers predominantly, because motor function is lost while sensory functions are often preserved. Axonal degeneration does not occur, and axonal conduction and EMG response are preserved distal to the lesion. A more prolonged deficit results from *axonotmesis,* in which both the myelin sheath and axon are interrupted, causing loss of conduction with wallerian degeneration and muscle atrophy. However, the endoneurial tube remains intact, regenerating axons are guided to appropriate end-organs, and regeneration is often quite satisfactory. The most severe lesion, *neurotmesis,* is produced when the nerve is completely severed or replaced by scar, so that spontaneous regeneration is not possible.

Sunderland[37] expanded this classification along more anatomic lines to include five degrees of injury. First- and second-degree lesions correspond to Seddon's neurapraxia and axonotmesis, with loss of conduction and axonal continuity, respectively. In third-degree injury, the entire nerve fiber is transected within an intact perineurium. Degeneration is similar to that seen in the second-degree injury, but regeneration can be hampered in degree by scar formation and in precision of reinnervation by interruption of the endoneurial tubes. Fourth-degree injury preserves only the epineurium, while fifth-degree injury results in anatomic separation of the nerve ends.

Millesi has further amplified this classification by localizing the fibrosis in grade 2 and 3 lesions.[29] Type A fibrosis thickens the external epineurium, potentially compressing the entire nerve. Type B fibrosis also compromises the internal epineurium, between fascicles, and type C fibrosis invades the endoneurium, within the fascicle itself. Types A and B can be present in a Sunderland grade 2 lesion and all types can be present in a grade 3 lesion. In current clinical practice the Sunderland classification is widely accepted as the standard for grading peripheral nerve pathology. Millesi's more recent additions, however, allow a more precise characterization of the lesion at the time of surgery and specifically guide surgical treatment based on the degree of fibrosis. Acceptance of this combined grading scale will depend on its subsequent correlation with clinical outcome.

The location of injury within the brachial plexus must be described on both the longitudinal (e.g., root, trunk) and vertical (e.g., C5, C6) axes. Current classification systems vary widely in anatomic precision, and no one system is applied uniformly. The simplest grading system on the longitudinal axis has been provided by Millesi,[28] who described four levels of injury. Level 1 injury, root avulsion, occurs proximal to the spinal ganglia, at the junction between peripheral and central nervous tissue. Sensory axons maintain contact with their cell bodies in the dorsal root ganglia and are preserved, whereas motor axons degenerate. Level 2 injuries interrupt the cervical roots. Both sensory and motor axons degenerate, but sensory axons in the central stump maintain contact with the CNS. A neuroma forms and gives rise to a positive Tinel's sign. Level 3 injury damages the trunks of the plexus, and level 4 injury damages the cords. The system used by Narakas[30] is slightly more specific as to location: (1) preganglionic (root avulsion); (2) root and proximal trunk; (3) retroclavicular; (4) distal cords; and (5) main extremity nerves. Cervical levels included in plexus injury (the vertical axis) can be grouped as follows: (1) C5, C6; (2) C5, C6, C7; (3) C7; (4) C8, T1; and (5) entire plexus. C5, C6 lesions are often described as Erb-Duchenne palsies and C8, T1 lesions as Klumpke palsies, although to be entirely accurate these terms should only be applied to the birth lesions originally described. Millesi[29] has also pointed out that peripheral lesions including the suprascapular, axillary, and musculocutaneous nerves as a group can mimic a C5, C6 lesion but have a better prognosis because of their more peripheral location.

The most complete anatomic classification of plexus lesions along both longitudinal and root axes has been provided by Kline and Judice,[20] who described 12 separate areas of partial plexus injury (e.g., C5, C6 to upper trunk, lateral cord, lateral cord to musculocutaneous, lateral cord to median). Use of this somewhat cumbersome system permits analysis of operative results by individual plexus elements, and thus provides the most specific information about surgical outcome.

MECHANISM OF INJURY

Traumatic injuries to the brachial plexus can be either closed or open. Closed injuries usually result from traction on the neural elements, although direct pressure by bones or bony fragments can also cause significant damage. The position of the arm and direction of force application determine the nature of the lesion. Motorcycle injury commonly results in forced distraction of the shoulder and head with the arm at the side, placing the greatest stress on the upper plexus roots. If the arm is abducted to 90° and forced posteriorly, traction will be applied equally at all root levels. Stress applied to the arm in full abduction results in progressively focal traction on the lower roots as they pass over the first rib. Any accompanying musculoskeletal disruption can allow the limb to lengthen, and further stretch the neural elements, which are anchored at both ends. Proximally, the epineurium of each nerve root is anchored firmly to the adjacent vertebral transverse process. Rupture of the epineurium, fracture of the transverse process, or rupture of the scalene muscles can directly expose the proximal neural elements to further traction. Fracture of the clavicle or humerus and dislocation of the humeral head all allow distraction of the arm itself, increasing traction on distal portions of the plexus. These injuries, and especially first rib fracture, can also be associated with direct trauma to the neural elements. In general, upper roots are more likely to be ruptured and lower roots to be avulsed, reflecting differences in the degree to which they are anchored to bony elements.[38] Narakas[30] has generalized that 70% of traumatic brachial plexus lesions are supraclavicular, 70% of supraclavicular lesions have at least one root avulsed, and 70% of these avulsions involve the lower roots.

Open plexus injuries are usually caused by sharp lacerations or gunshot wounds. Glass or knife stab wounds produce well-defined lesions with no traction component and little destruction of neural tissue adjacent to the wound; the acute neurologic deficit accurately reflects nerve transection. Blunter instruments such as fan blades, however, cause contusion in addition to transection, and the initial deficit can be greatly misleading. Heavy equipment and chain saws produce extensive open wounds, with massive damage to the plexus and adjacent structures. The lower trunk is partially shielded from stab wounds by the clavicle, so it is injured less frequently than the upper and middle trunks.[23] This is fortunate, given the juxtaposition of the lower trunk and axillary artery. Plexus stab wounds have also been found to involve predominantly the left side, presumably reflecting the hand dominance of an attacker.[6]

The severity of gunshot wounds varies with the caliber and nature of the wounding missile. Although complete plexus lesions are rare, injuries caused by a shotgun blast and high-caliber bullets can be extensive.[21] Most gunshot injuries result in incomplete damage to the neural elements; initial neurologic deficits reflect significant components of Sunderland grades 1 and 2 damage from concussive injury. In Brooks'[3] review of 170 gunshot wounds to the plexus during World War II, 54 patients required surgery; neural elements were found to be divided in only 16. Kline and Judice[20] operated on 46 of 77 patients with plexus gunshot wounds. In this group 17 elements could be sutured directly, whereas 38 required nerve grafting. Neurolysis alone was performed on 32 elements. The elements most frequently injured were the distal portions of the lateral and medial cords.

ASSOCIATED INJURIES

Brachial plexus trauma can be associated with severe, often life-threatening injury to other organ systems. Of 59 patients with blunt plexus trauma in a recent series,[36] 9 presented in shock. The subclavian artery was damaged in three patients, the axillary artery in two, and the internal carotid artery in one. Other associated injuries included rib fractures, hemopneumothorax, pulmonary contusion, head injury, and upper extremity fractures. Associated injuries were even more common in the 329 patients explored by Narakas for brachial plexus injury—23% had major vessel trauma and 80% had significant skeletal injuries.[30] A particularly severe consequence of blunt trauma to the shoulder girdle is scapulothoracic dissociation.[7] Fifteen patients with this injury were recently described; three of these died.[7] Eleven had vascular disruption and 12 suffered complete brachial plexus palsy. Associated injuries with open trauma to the plexus are more localized but can be equally serious. Eighteen stab wounds to the brachial plexus[6] resulted in eight severe vascular injuries and six instances of hemothorax or pneumothorax.

The most serious injuries directly related to brachial plexus trauma are those to the subclavian and axillary vessels. In the civilian population, 80 to 85% of subclavian-axillary injuries result from sharp wounds and the remainder from blunt trauma.[19,25] Of this entire group, 50 to 60% are accompanied by brachial plexus lesions. Fractures of the first rib and scapula are more common with subclavian artery injury, whereas fractures of the clavicle and humerus more often accompany injury to the axillary artery.[19] The latter can also be damaged, and even ruptured, by anterior shoulder dislocation, usually in older patients.[12] Most brachial plexus deficits accompanying vascular injury are the immediate result of direct trauma, but there are two potentially remediable situations in which the neural deficit is progressive. Seven of 40 patients treated by McCready and colleagues[25] for subclavian-axillary trauma had brachial plexus compromise secondary to compression by hematoma; this resolved in six of seven patients after decompression. Similarly, both axillary and subclavian artery trauma can lead to pseudoaneurysm formation and progressive neural deficit if not treated promptly.[9,40]

Injury to the brachial plexus is more commonly accompanied by skeletal injury in the absence of vascular disruption. Fractures of the cervical transverse processes are associated with severe supraclavicular lesions, fractures of the first rib with injuries to the lower trunk, and clavicular fractures with injuries to the cords. In contrast, brachial plexus palsies associated with more distal skeletal injuries are usually more benign. Gariepy and colleagues[10] described six patients with anterior shoulder dislocation and significant brachial plexus injuries, all of whom improved completely after reduction of the shoulder. They attributed the lesion to traction caused by the excursion of the humeral head but noted that direct pressure on the nerves could also be responsible. In analyzing 31 patients with infraclavicular plexus lesions, Leffert[23] found 17 shoulder dislocations, 12 of which were accompanied by fracture of the greater tuberosity, 11 by other humeral fractures, and 3 by scapular fractures. Recovery from these lesions was superior to that seen after supraclavicular lesions. Shoulder dislocation can also result in more focal injury to plexus elements or terminal branches. Although axillary nerve injury is commonly described, posterior cord and musculocutaneous nerve injury can also occur and should be sought out.

Rarely, brachial plexus injury can be accompanied by injury to the spinal cord or other peripheral nerves. Grundy and Silver[11] reported 11 patients with simultaneous brachial plexus and spinal cord damage. The injury was thought to involve forced separation of the head and neck from the shoulder in eight and upper limb abduction with traction on the lower trunk in two; a gunshot accounted for the remaining case. Rotation-flexion of the cervical spine has also been implicated in a case of simultaneous brachial plexus palsy–Brown-Sequard syndrome.[5] Brachial plexus palsy is particularly significant in the spinal cord injury patient, who already relies heavily on the upper limb function spared by the cord injury. Avulsion of cervical roots from the spinal cord can damage nearby fiber tracts leading to the lower extremities and, exceptionally, lead to subdural hematoma with acute spinal cord compression.[32] Individual peripheral nerves can also incur separate injury distal to a plexus lesion, as demonstrated by Narakas in 11 of his 329 operated cases.[30]

Diagnosis

HISTORY

Historical clues are often important in assessing brachial plexus injury. The severity of closed plexus injury is usually proportional to the violence of the trauma, with many severe cases involving high-speed motorcycle accidents. Unfortunately, these patients often cannot give a history because of their head injuries. The severity of gunshot wounds varies with the caliber and muzzle velocity of the projectile and that of stab wounds with the length and character of the knife. A history of profuse bleeding suggests major vascular injury. The time of onset of paralysis and sensory loss is also important; a previous deficit in the affected limb can confuse diagnosis, but progressive deterioration indicates a potentially remediable lesion such as compressive hematoma or pseudoaneurysm.

PHYSICAL EXAMINATION

Examination of the patient with acute brachial plexus injury begins with the identification of significant trauma to other areas and organ systems. When the patient has been stabilized, the skeletal and neurovascular status of the injured limb are determined. Skeletal stability is assessed first to guide radiographic examination and to prevent neurovascular injury during subsequent manipulations. The vascular supply to the limb is then evaluated. The absence or diminution of the radial pulse suggests vascular compromise. A strong pulse can persist in spite of axillary artery division, however, with flow redirected through collaterals around the scapula and shoulder. In patients with closed plexus trauma, a bruit or suprascapular hematoma also suggests major vascular injury. The latter is particularly worrisome, because it can be the first warning of life-threatening hemorrhage and can cause compression of the brachial plexus, with progressive neurologic deficit. With open injuries, significant vascular injury usually leads to profuse bleeding.

Horner's syndrome, or ptosis (drooped eyelid), meiosis (contracted pupil), and enophthalmos (sunken globe), is often the most obvious neurologic manifestation of brachial plexus injury. It results from interruption of the preganglionic sympathetic fibers to the eye as they exit the spinal cord through the C8 and/or T1 root(s). Narakas[30] correlated the presence or absence of Horner's syndrome with the findings at surgery in 114 cases of complete brachial plexus palsy. He found that C8 and/or T1 were avulsed in 75% of patients with Horner's syndrome but were still intact in 10%. Conversely, Horner's syndrome was absent in 25% of patients with clear C8, T1 pathology. Horner's syndrome is thus strongly suggestive but not absolutely diagnostic of C8 and/or T1 avulsion injury, and its absence does not guarantee the integrity of these roots. The sensory modalities of touch and pain are evaluated throughout the extremity, with the addition of two-point discrimination in the hand. Sensory dermatomes overlap, so

the most helpful information is obtained from the autonomous zone for each cervical root: C5, distal deltoid; C6, thenar eminence; C7, no autonomous zone; and C8, ulnar aspect of the elbow. Determination of sensory loss within the autonomous zones of major peripheral nerves can also be helpful, but correlation of sensory loss with injury to plexus elements is not usually of value.

Motor evaluation consists of manual examination of the muscles innervated by the C5 to T1 roots. The Medical Research Council[26] has published a pamphlet that demonstrates the proper technique of manual muscle testing. Table 41-1 shows the motor loss expected with various plexus lesions. Of particular importance is paralysis of the rhomboids and serratus anterior, which often correlates with proximal and usually irreparable damage to the C5 and C6 roots. The neurologic assessment should include examination of the lower and contralateral upper limbs to rule out long tract damage from root avulsion or Brown-Sequard syndrome (unilateral paralysis with contralateral loss of sensation).

Examination of the patient with chronic brachial plexus injury proceeds as described previously for acute injury. The passage of time, however, both unmasks diagnostic clues and introduces secondary pathology from denervation and disuse. The skeletal system is examined for bony defect secondary to fracture and for limitation of joint motion by contracture. Inferior subluxation of the shoulder, which increases traction on the neural elements, can result from shoulder girdle paralysis. Previous vascular injury can cause the trophic changes of vascular insufficiency, including nonhealing wounds, or the expanding mass of pseudoaneurysm. Neurologic examination reveals a Horner's syndrome if this was seen initially, although its early manifestations can become less prominent over time. Chronic denervation of the limb is manifested by cutaneous trophic changes and muscle atrophy; the distribution of atrophy should confirm the findings on motor examination. Similarly, reversal of atrophy and return of motor function are valuable clues to a Sunderland grade 1 or 2 (and potentially 3) injury, which might not require surgery. Perhaps the most significant delayed neurologic finding is a Tinel's sign or paresthesias elicited by tapping over a neural element. Tinel's sign signifies a potentially reconstructable lesion, because it requires regenerating sensory axons that have maintained contact with the spinal cord. Distal progression of Tinel's sign can occur as axons regenerate through a lesion in continuity, and the location of referred sensation is often a clue to the identity of the regenerating neural element. Tinel's sign can occur, however, even if the ventral (motor) root is avulsed,

Table 41–1.

Diagnostically Important Motor Findings in Lesions of the Brachial Plexus

	Level of Lesion			
	Supraganglionic Root Avulsion	*Spinal Nerve*	*Trunk*	*Cord*
Paralysis	All muscles served by injured root, including posterior cervical	C5: rhomboids, supraspinatus, infraspinatus, deltoid, biceps; C6: brachioradialis, supinator; C7: triceps, extensor digitorum communis, extensor carpi ulnaris; C8: flexor pollicis longus profundi; T1: intrinsic muscles	Upper: shoulder muscle, biceps; middle: triceps, wrist and digital extensors; lower: ulnar and most median innervated muscles	Posterior: deltoid, triceps, wrist and digital extensors, latissimus dorsi, teres major and minor, subscapularis; lateral: biceps, pronator teres, partial median forearm; medial: partial median forearm, intrinsics, complete ulnar forearm
Intact		Posterior cervical of involved root	Serratus anterior; rhomboids; pectoralis major	Supraspinatus; infraspinatus; pectoral muscles

and can be produced by a small number of axons with no significant reconstructive potential. Thus, it is *not* a guarantee of reconstructive potential.

RADIOLOGIC EVALUATION

Radiologic studies play a vital role in the diagnosis of brachial plexus lesions. Plain films of the chest, cervical spine, and arm should be obtained in all cases. Chest radiography can demonstrate first rib fracture, suggesting damage to the C8, T1 roots and the subclavian artery. Hematoma over the subclavian artery or widened superior mediastinum are further clues to arterial damage. Diaphragmatic paralysis, seen on inspiration-expiration films, results from avulsion of the C5 root, whereas hemothorax or pneumothorax can be found with open plexus injuries. Clavicular or scapular fractures should be identified and further views obtained, if necessary; lateral displacement of the scapula is especially worrisome, because it is often the harbinger of life-threatening scapulothoracic dissociation.[7] Cervical spine films are first examined for fracture or dislocation. The findings specifically related to brachial plexus injury are a transverse process fracture, usually accompanied by avulsion of the adjacent root, and lateral tilt from injury severe enough to separate vertebral bodies on the injured side. Proximal humeral and scapular fractures, often found with infraclavicular lesions, can also accompany multiple peripheral nerve injuries which, in concert, mimic a C5, C6 deficit.[30] Overall, Narakas has identified 16 patients with level 2 injuries, in 7 of whom the radiologic evaluation pinpointed an otherwise unsuspected lesion.[30]

Myelography is used to demonstrate root avulsions, which are usually seen as "traumatic meningoceles," or outpouchings of the meningeal sac, in which a root has been avulsed. Occasionally these pouches can be sealed over, producing a concave defect where the root sleeve would normally be seen. The relative distribution of traumatic meningoceles was studied by Yeoman in 60 patients with severe brachial plexus injury.[40] Single lesions were most common at the C7, C8, or T1 levels, double lesions at C8-T1, and triple lesions at C7-C8-T1. Unfortunately, root avulsion can occur in the presence of a normal myelogram[36] and intact roots can survive within a traumatic meningocele.[14] Frot[8] quantified these inaccuracies by correlating the myelographic appearance of 153 cervical roots with their condition at surgery. Of 63 myelographically normal roots, 5 were avulsed (8% false-negative) and 34 were injured distally. Of 90 myelographically abnormal roots, 4 were surgically normal, 16 were injured distally (total, 22% false-positive), and 70 were avulsed. Even though myelography yields both false-positive and false-negative results, it is still relied on by most brachial plexus surgeons to help diagnose root avulsion.

Of the newer radiologic techniques, computerized tomography (CT) scanning is extremely useful for the diagnosis of brachial plexus tumors but is only a supplement to myelography in the diagnosis of root avulsion.[1] Magnetic resonance imaging (MRI) provides excellent delineation of brachial plexus elements from the ventral rami to the peripheral nerves[2] and might prove to be an important component of the brachial plexus work-up when further experience has been gained with its use.

ELECTRODIAGNOSIS

Routine electrodiagnosis of brachial plexus lesions consists of the examination of muscle by electromyography (EMG) and the determination of peripheral sensory nerve conduction properties. EMG studies identify denervated muscle, confirming the distribution and severity of injury. Serial studies can demonstrate progressive reinnervation in Sunderland grade 2, and possibly grade 3, lesions. EMG evaluation of the deep posterior cervical muscles[4] is especially important. The traversus spinosus and interspinosus are segmentally innervated by the posterior branch of the anterior primary (motor) root, in close proximity to the vertebral foramen. They can thus remain innervated, even after proximal stretch injuries, but are denervated by root avulsion. Occasionally, however, overlapping innervation of these muscles can result in denervation at spinal levels at which there is a distal reparable lesion.[21] Paraspinal denervation is therefore a strong but not absolute indicator of root avulsion.

Examination of sensory nerve conduction also provides valuable information. Preganglionic root avulsion can occur without interrupting the continuity between the axon and parent cell body in the dorsal root ganglion. Peripheral sensory axons from this cervical level thus do not undergo wallerian degeneration; conduction is maintained, even in the total absence of peripheral sensation. Stimulating the digits and recording proximally from the median, radial, and ulnar nerves provides information about roots from C6 to T1; unfortunately, there are no good stimulating or recording sites for the C5 root. Furthermore, the absence of sensory conduction does not prove that damage is exclusively postganglionic, because preganglionic and postganglionic injury can be found within the same root.

Somatosensory evoked potentials have been used in the preoperative evaluation of brachial plexus injuries,[16,22] but this technique appears to share the fallibility of other electrodiagnostic studies and is more complex.[21] The current role of somatosensory studies thus appears to be limited to the intraoperative detection of root avulsion (see next section — Management: Operative Intervention).

Management

The management of the traumatized brachial plexus began with an initial wave of enthusiasm in the early 1900s, sparked by a few anecdotal reports, but with little in the way of results. During the world wars, particularly World War II, a very aggressive approach to nerve injuries and brachial plexus injuries was taken.

The initial reports gave a favorable outlook for recovery of function, and even in those days Sir Herbert Seddon[34] was advocating nerve grafting for brachial plexus repair. These cases, however, when followed for a sufficient length of time, showed gloomy results. Nulsen and Slade,[31] in 1956, reported on 117 patients with brachial plexus injuries sustained in World War II and concluded that the condition of patients with stretch injuries could not be improved. Further reports in the late 1950s and early 1960s indicated that surgical treatment was of little benefit for brachial plexus injuries. Thus, the surgical enthusiasm at the beginning of the century gave way to conservatism on the basis of six decades of generally unrewarding experiences. In 1963 Seddon, in the Watson-Jones address to the Royal College of Surgeons, reported that the results of repair of the brachial plexus were so disappointing that it should not be done, except in the upper trunk.

It was not until the advent of microsurgical techniques that a renewed interest was seen in the repair of the complex of structures known as the brachial plexus. More favorable reports emanated from Millesi,[28] Narakas,[30] and Samii,[33] among others. These reports from Europe were joined by those of Kline[20] in the United States, who reported satisfying results in adult patients suffering traction injuries and in patients with sharp injuries. When the results of all these reports were analyzed, there was agreement regarding patients with predominantly upper root involvement and, in particular, those with primarily infraclavicular injuries. It was found that patients with only C5 and C6 involvement possessed a well-functioning hand and that recovery of some shoulder stabilizers and elbow flexors, usually through nerve grafting or direct repair, was a worthy and frequently attainable goal, except when those roots were avulsed from the spinal cord. The reported results of repair of primarily infraclavicular lesions have been much more favorable than those of the more proximal supraclavicular lesion. Also, all the researchers agreed that patients with total brachial plexus palsy are destined to a nonfunctioning extremity.[20,28,30,33]

Today the wave of enthusiasm for microsurgical repair has become somewhat dampened, and most surgeons working in the field of brachial plexus injuries have become more realistic and present the patients with limited goals.

DETERMINATION OF TYPE OF TREATMENT

The treatment program proposed here deals with a goal-oriented approach that is not necessarily designed to restore full function to the extremity. For example, if an individual has good hand function and upper trunk involvement, a reasonable goal would be to restore elbow function through nerve reconstruction and shoulder stabilization by standard orthopedic technique. The promise of restoring some extrinsic function to the hand in the median nerve-innervated structures is a reasonable goal, but the chance for restoring intrinsic function or ulnar nerve extrinsic function to the paralyzed hand is unrealistic.

Open Injuries: Sharp

Most authors agree that the open, sharp laceration of the brachial plexus with or without vascular damage should undergo repair (Table 41-2). In patients with an expanding hematoma from a sharp laceration or vascular damage, immediate operative exploration of the vessels and vascular repair with decompression or repair of the nerve injury is mandatory. The operating surgeon must be familiar with the vascular and nerve repair; if not, a colleague who can perform any part that is not familiar to the treating physician should be on hand to assist.

The reports of stab wounds involving the brachial plexus show favorable results. Dunkerton and Boome[6] from South Africa operated on 64 patients with stab wounds involving the brachial plexus. The overall results of the operations were good; lesions of the C5 to C6 roots recovered better than those at the distal roots. Kline and Judice[20] reported recovery in 14 of 18 elements of the brachial plexus. They stressed that the reason for primary operation in the sharp laceration is

that the anatomy is relatively easy to identify, scar tissue secondary to other vascular procedures has not had time to develop, and end-to-end repair can be effective. It is also reasonable to expect that the exact lesion can be identified and repaired.

In an individual with nerve deficit in a vascular injury, decompression of the brachial plexus is mandatory in the supraclavicular (and particularly the infraclavicular) region, where the plexus is encased in a neural sheath with the structures. An axillary stab wound with injury to the axillary vein or artery and compression of the brachial plexus responds satisfactorily when operative decompression and appropriate repair are done early. If left beyond 12 hours, however, these patients will have unrecoverable nerve function and severe pain; moreover, they are not helped by neurolysis in the late stage.

Open Injuries: Blast

In patients with a gunshot wound or blast injury involving the supraclavicular and infraclavicular plexus, conservatism is the treatment of choice. In patients who have vascular damage or an expanding hematoma within the neural sheath, the decompression should be accomplished and the appropriate vascular repair done. Often a vascular graft must be used to reconstruct arterial and venous continuity in the gunshot wound. The area of intimal damage must be resected or eventual thrombosis can occur. The nerve should be inspected at operation and the exact damage assessed. Our recommendation, however, is *not* to resect nerve tissue on the basis of its appearance, because the vast majority of gunshot wounds of the brachial plexus show some degree of recovery in weeks.

In those patients *without* vascular damage and a gunshot wound, local wound care is the treatment of choice, with *no* attempt to explore or repair the neural damage. In Kline and Judice's[20] series, 46 of 77 patients with gunshot wounds were eventually operated on because there was some loss that persisted for two months or longer. Of these patients, there was approximately 50% recovery of useful function in the distribution of the repaired nerve.

Therefore, patients with open, sharp injury and nerve deficit, with or without vascular involvement, should undergo operative exploration and repair at the earliest convenience. It is incumbent on the treating surgeon to have the necessary resources available to deal with both the vascular and neural elements, if these lesions are identified. In patients with gunshot wounds, immediate operation is only recommended for repair of vascular injuries. Such patients should be closely followed postoperatively and the pattern of re-

---

Table 41–2.

Acute Brachial Plexus Injuries and Recommended Treatment

Condition	Recommended Treatment
Open injuries, sharp	
Vascular damage, nerve damage	Exploration and repair
Vascular damage, alone	Exploration and repair
Nerve damage, alone	Exploration and repair
Open injuries, blunt	
Vascular damage, alone	Explore and repair
Nerve damage, alone	Wound care, no exploration
Vascular and nerve damage, combined	Repair vessel, assess nerve
Closed injuries	
Scapulothoracic dissociation	Vascular control, consider amputation
Vascular damage, alone	Repair vessel
Nerve damage, alone	Observe
Vascular and nerve damage, combined	Repair vessel, assess nerve

covery observed for any signs of nerve deficit. After two months of observation, or when the patient's recovery has plateaued and no further advancement is noted, operative exploration and appropriate repair should be contemplated. In all the reported series the best results were with the upper trunk in the supraclavicular region and with the infraclavicular region. Generally, these involved median and radial nerve function, with very little recovery from the ulnar nerve.

Blunt Injury

Blunt injuries to the brachial plexus and vascular structures of the neck and shoulder girdle can be of varying severity. These can range from nerve injury alone, with a partial traction lesion of the brachial plexus that results in a mild, transient period of neural dysfunction, up to more complete types of nerve involvement, including traction and root avulsion. Because of the anatomic nature of the brachial plexus (described previously), a patient with avulsion of the lower roots often has a traction lesion of the upper roots and trunk. Conversely, those with an avulsion of the upper trunk, often have a traction lesion of the lower elements of the brachial plexus. This is a result of the mechanism of injury and of whether the shoulder is severely abducted or depressed.

Combination with a vascular injury complicates the entire situation, causes more difficulty in making the diagnosis in the early stage, and mandates surgical treatment. The most serious injury is a combination of rupture of the subclavian artery, brachial plexus avulsion of all roots, and scapulothoracic dissociation. This rare entity is caused by severe traction to the entire shoulder girdle. The lesion is characterized by massive soft tissue swelling, lateral displacement of the scapula, skeletal injury (acromioclavicular separation, fracture of the clavicle, or sternoclavicular disruption), and severe neurovascular injury. In a report by Ebraheim and associates,[7] 15 patients were described, 3 of whom had succumbed to the injury. Of the 12 patients who survived and were treated, all were left with a flail upper extremity. The scapulothoracic dissociation is accompanied by complete or partial tear of the deltoid, pectoralis minor, rhomboids, levator scapuli, trapezius, and latissimus dorsi muscles. The vascular disruption occurs most frequently at the level of the subclavian artery, but the axillary artery can be involved. The subclavian vein is usually torn and the neurologic deficit is usually the result of complete avulsion of the brachial plexus. The skin is always intact, but there is a complex spectrum of bony, ligamentous, and neurovascular injuries that constitute this lesion. The most important diagnostic sign is lateral displacement of the scapula,

which can be measured radiographically (Chapter 40). The major point of concern is that these are *unreconstructable* lesions, as well as life-threatening. We recommend that these patients be treated by vascular control and early amputation. We have treated two such patients and found that early amputation allows patients to accept their disability sooner and to proceed with their rehabilitation. If amputation is not done the hope might still remain that neural reconstruction can be accomplished, which leads to unrewarding pursuit of reconstructive techniques. Amputation should be done through a fracture of the humerus, if one exists, or at the above-elbow level. The subclavian or axillary artery should be tied off, as well as the vein.

The patient with vascular injury and complete or incomplete neural deficit without scapulothoracic dissociation should be evaluated with reconstruction in mind. In the acute phase the vascular injury must be repaired, usually by graft but occasionally by direct repair. At the time of vascular repair nerve damage should be assessed and, if possible, documentation of nerve root avulsion of one portion of the plexus should be obtained. This can be very helpful in planning later reconstruction. Traction injuries cannot be assessed by palpation or inspection but, if differentiation between traction and avulsion can be made at the time of the vascular exploration, it is most beneficial in planning the ultimate reconstructive procedure. Therefore, we recommend that an individual treating such a patient be able to repair both neural and vascular elements or to have someone available who can assess the damage and perform the appropriate repair.

The patient with a closed traction lesion of the brachial plexus, presenting with partial or complete neural deficit without vascular damage, should initially be evaluated and managed conservatively. Splinting the arm to decrease the weight of the force pulling on the arm in the depressed position is beneficial. The patient should be followed and studied for recovery patterns. It is important to carry out a complete evaluation and to chart the neural deficit so that the pattern of recovery or loss can be ascertained. All the diagnostic maneuvers discussed earlier should be used. After about three weeks, another thorough evaluation of the patient and deficit should be carried out. Patients with lesions in continuity without axon interruption begin to show recovery at this point. The patient should then be evaluated at three-week intervals for consideration of a possible surgical approach. In our opinion, the critical juncture occurs at three months. Those elements that do not show signs of recovery at three months should be evaluated with respect to surgical reconstruction. This is particularly relevant for a patient with an incomplete lesion in whom the deficit is manifested in a functional area, such as the patient with excellent hand function and no shoulder or elbow function. In such a case the goal would be restoration of elbow function to position the hand.

The patient with a complete nerve deficit should be evaluated at three months for the consideration of reconstruction of some of the functional areas, but with the realization that very little hand function will result. At this critical juncture all diagnostic measures should be employed to determine which roots are avulsed and which are torn apart and stretched. At the three-month interval, Kline and Judice[20] reported successful results of neurolysis of the incomplete lesions of the Sunderland II and III varieties, whereas others have questioned the usefulness of neurolysis on the basis that the nerve would eventually recover on its own.

OPERATIVE INTERVENTION

Surgical Options

Surgical options for the management of the traumatized brachial plexus include neurolysis, direct repair or graft, indirect nerve transfer, or a combination of nerve repair and nerve transfer.

Some early studies have reported transfer of a nerve graft with immediate vascularization, but the results are inconclusive at this time and do not indicate that this can produce improvement in function.[23]

The important aspect of management at this point is to establish a realistic goal and to devise the operation to attain this goal. If it is shoulder function, surgical treatment should be directed at repair of the suprascapular and axillary nerves, either by direct repair or by using an indirect nerve transfer, such as the intercostal nerves with or without prolongation with a graft. The intercostal nerves can be procured easily through the axilla and through the same surgical approach required to expose the brachial plexus.

In any operation on the brachial plexus, the entire plexus should be exposed. The supraclavicular region should be approached through a longitudinal incision along the course of the sternocleidomastoid. The incision should then curve laterally across the shoulder and down the arm. The clavicle can be mobilized and osteotomized, if necessary, to expose the divisions and axillary artery.

Faced with a patient who has one or more areas of nerve deficit for more than a year after injury, it is unlikely that primary reconstruction of the neural elements can restore that function because of the degradation of the motor neuron and motor end-plate and atrophy of the target muscle. An interesting development has occurred using microvascular techniques,

usually for restoration of elbow flexion. A new muscle can be taken as a direct microvascular transfer from the leg to replace the biceps and then it can be innervated by nerve transfer using the intercostal nerves. Preliminary reports are gratifying. The ideal case would be a patient with satisfactory hand function, no elbow function, and no muscles available for transfer to restore elbow function.

When approaching the patient with a traction lesion, intraoperative electrodiagnosis with nerve action potentials or spinal evoked responses is helpful. Surgeons faced with the need for this sophisticated technique should be familiar with the instrumentation or have a working relationship with an electromyographer who can be of assistance during the operative session. Although some surgeons do have experience in this field, most clinical surgeons must maintain this latter type of relationship.

The electrodiagnostic equipment used is of the standard type and is commercially available. A special probe for direct stimulation of the nerve can be modified from existing equipment or by using the probe from an existing nerve stimulator; the electromyographer can assist the surgeon with any modification necessary. There should be a minimum of background electrical activity in the operating room. Most modern operating rooms are well grounded, but it is best to try out the machine prior to the clinical situation. Sometimes one operating room in the corner of a surgical suite is more suitable for the electromyography than one in the center because of background electrical activity. The electromyographer can be scheduled to come into the operating room at the appointed time, and does not necessarily need to be available during the entire procedure. Because the equipment is fairly portable it can be stored on a cart and easily transported into the operating suite. In our experience, the electromyographer is usually needed for no longer than 30 minutes.

Kline and Judice[20] have popularized the use of intraoperative nerve action potential recordings across lesions in continuity. Those lesions with flat tracings would require resection, whereas those with evoked nerve action potentials would need only neurolysis. Kline and Judice[20] were able to do partial repairs because only a portion of the element is regenerating, and this is responsible for the recorded nerve action potential. Kline and associates[20,21] have recorded nerve action potentials for many years across all of their brachial plexus reconstructions and reported that this technique is a great aid in decision making. The involved area in the bracial plexus is exposed and the stimulating and recording electrodes are placed proximally. If the stimulating recording system is working correctly, a nerve action potential should be recorded from the proximal stump. Once the nerve action potential has been recorded proximally, the recording electrode is moved distally beyond the lesion to determine if the nerve action potential can be evoked throughout the area of injury. If a potential is recorded immediately distal to the neuroma in continuity, recording electrodes are moved further down the distal stump to determine how far the potential and presumably the regenerating fibers of adequate size have extended. If a nerve action potential cannot be recorded distal to the injury, voltage and amplification are gradually increased until it is difficult to visualize that portion of the tracing following the stimulus artifact. Attention must be paid to electrode contact and blood should be irrigated away from the region of the electrodes. It is generally best to elevate the nerve away from the surrounding soft tissue by means of the electrodes, but, if necessary, the nerve can be stimulated and recorded by isolating short segments on either side of the lesion and placing the electrodes on them.

VanBeek and co-workers[39] have described a technique in which cutaneous EEG electrodes are placed in the midfrontal region for reference, in the deltoid area for the ground, in the C4 posterior neck for recording the spinal cord evoked response, and at Erb's point for recording the peripheral nerve evoked response. The stimulating electrodes are positioned in the operative field and held mechanically. The wide separation of the intraoperative stimulator electrode and the cutaneously applied recording electrode permits differentiation from the stimulus artifact and the recording evoked response. The whole nerve, groups of fascicles, or fascicles can be stimulated and the recordings made using cutaneous recording electrodes placed at appropriate monitoring sites. In this technique, nerve dissection is minimized. Both a nerve's compound action potential from a near field by direct electrode application and response from a far field, taking advantage of volume conduction, can be measured with a computerized system. This technique is important in the supraclavicular region of the brachial plexus because stimulating the proximal nerve root and determining if a spinal cord evoked response can be obtained indicate whether live axons are present in the proximal stump. Stimulating across a lesion in continuity, such as a traction lesion at the trunk or cord level, is mandatory before resecting this particular nerve trunk or cord of the brachial plexus. If there is no recordable electrical response through the lesion after three months, that area can be resected with confidence and grafted. If, however, an electrical response is noted, neurolysis of the involved segment produces an anticipated good response. Thus, we believe that when approaching the brachial plexus for reconstruction, the intraoperative electrodiagnosis must be employed.

Postoperative Management

All these patients need psychological support throughout their care, especially in the perioperative period. During this time, their expectations are high and it is beneficial to provide some psychological support to accompany the surgical management.

The operated arm should be supported postoperatively which maintains any traction on the nerve juncture sites. With arm motion, the normal longitudinal excursion of the brachial plexus is approximately 1.5 cm. It is necessary to support the arm so that there is no traction at the suture site. The lungs should be evaluated, because an intraoperative injury to the pleura can cause a collapsed lung in the perioperative period. The patient should have adequate respiratory support. One complication that we have witnessed is an anesthetic injury to the contralateral uninjured arm during operation. This good arm should be protected and not be stretched; moreover, the ulnar nerve should be padded to help prevent the development of a stretched nerve in the uninjured arm.

Long-term postoperative care consists of evaluating the results of the nerve reconstruction.

Anticipated Results

The theme of this section has been for operating surgeons to limit their goals so that reasonable results can be anticipated and realized. This is important because such patients often imagine a normal, functioning extremity. If limited goals are entertained prior to surgical exploration, patients must be informed of these goals so that they will not be disappointed if their expectations are not met. Throughout the entire spectrum of reports on brachial plexus injury and surgical results, the upper plexus has been found to be more suitable to reconstruction than the lower plexus. In fact, there are *no* consistent results of the lower plexus showing recovery. The best possible results are obtained when an individual has excellent distal function in the hand and lacks only shoulder and elbow motion, because these can be effectively restored by one of the aforementiond measures.

Conclusions

In dealing with the patient with a traumatized brachial plexus in the supraclavicular, costoclavicular, and infraclavicular regions, a thorough knowledge of the anatomy and careful analysis of the problem can help the surgeon to make correct choices. Immediate repair of vascular injuries and sharp nerve injuries is gratifying. It is incumbent on the treating surgeon to diagnose an unreconstructable life-threatening injury such as scapulothoracic dissociation and to inform the patient. In such a case, we recommend ablation of the extremity. Above all, the overriding message is that the team of surgeons should be able to treat both the vascular and nerve injuries whenever exploration is entertained. It is useless to undertake vascular repair with no evaluation of the neural elements, and vice versa. Finally, if attempting to reconstruct a nonrecovering brachial plexus injury, it is important to establish functional goals so that the patient's and surgeon's expectations are the same. By so doing, the chances of realizing these expectations are maximized.

REFERENCES

1. Armington, W.R.; Harnsberger, H.R.; Osborn, A.G.; Seay, A.R. Radiographic evaluation of brachial plexopathy. Am J Neuroradiol 8:361–367, 1987.
2. Blair, D.N.; Rapoport, S.; Sostman, H.D.; Blair, O.C. Normal brachial plexus: MR imaging. Radiology 165:763–767, 1987.
3. Brooks, D.M. Open wounds of the brachial plexus. J Bone Joint Surg 31B:17–33, 1949.
4. Bufalini, C.; Pescatori, G. Posterior cervical electromyography in the diagnosis and prognosis of brachial plexus injuries. J Bone Joint Surg 51B:627–631, 1969.
5. Chechick, A.; Amit, Y.; Shaked, I.; et al. Brown-Sequard syndrome associated with brachial plexus injury in neck trauma. J Trauma 22:430–431, 1982.
6. Dunkerton, M.C.; Boome, R.S. Stab wounds involving the brachial plexus. J Bone Joint Surg 70B:566–570, 1988.
7. Ebraheim, N.A.; An, H.S.; Jackson, T.; et al. Scapulothoracic dissociation. J Bone Joint Surg 70B:428–432, 1988.
8. Frot, B. La myelographie cervicale opaque dans les paralysies traumatiques du plexus brachial. Rev Chir Orthop 63:67, 1977.
9. Gallen, J.; Wiss, D.A.; Cantelmo, N.; Mezoin, J.O. Traumatic pseudoaneurysm of the axillary artery: Report of three cases and literature review. J Trauma 24:350–354, 1984.
10. Gariepy, R.; Derome, A.; Laurin, C.A. Brachial plexus paralysis following shoulder dislocation. Can J Surg 5:418, 1962.
11. Grundy, D.J.; Silver J.R. Problems in the management of combined brachial plexus and spinal cord injuries. Int Rehabil Med 3:57–70, 1981.
12. Gugenheim, S.; Sanders, R.J. Axillary artery rupture caused by shoulder dislocation. Surgery 95:55–58, 1984.
13. Hentz, V.R.; Narakas, A. The results of microneurosurgical reconstruction in complete brachial plexus palsy. Orthop Clin North Am 19:107–114, 1988.
14. Heon, M. Myelogram: A questionable aid in diagnosis and prognosis of brachial plexus components in traction injuries. Conn Med 29:260–262, 1965.
15. Hollinshead, W.H. Anatomy for Surgeons. 3rd ed., Philadelphia, Harper & Row, 1982.
16. Jones, S.J. Diagnostic value of peripheral and spinal somatosensory evoked potentials in traction lesions of the brachial plexus. Clin Plast Surg 11:167–172, 1984.
17. Kaplan, E.B.; Spinner, M. Normal and anomalous innervation patterns in the upper extremity. In Omer, G.E.; Spinner, M., eds. Management of Peripheral Nerve Problems. Philadelphia, W.B. Saunders, 1980, p. 7599.
18. Kerr, A.T. The brachial plexus of nerves in man—the variations in its formation and its branches. Am J Anat 23:285–395, 1918.
19. Klein, S.R.; Bongard, F.S.; White, R.A. Neurovascular injuries of the thoracic outlet and axilla. Am J Surg 156:115–118, 1988.
20. Kline, D.G.; Judice, D.J. Operative management of selected brachial plexus lesions. J Neurosurg 58:631–649, 1983.
21. Kline, D.G.; Hackett, E.R.; Happel, L.H. Surgery for lesions of the brachial plexus. Arch Neurol 43:170–181, 1986.
22. Landi, A.; Copeland, S.A.; Wynn-Parry, C.B.; et al. The role of somatosensory evoked potentials and nerve conduction studies in the surgical management of brachial plexus injuries. J Bone Joint Surg 62B:9–22, 1980.
23. Leffert, R.D. Brachial Plexus Injuries. New York, Churchill Livingstone, 1985.
24. Liveson, J.A. Nerve lesions associated with shoulder dislocation; an electrodiagnostic study of 11 cases. J Neurol Neurosurg Psychiatry 47:742–744, 1984.
25. McCready, R.A.; Procter, C.D.; Hyde, G.L. Subclavian axillary vascular trauma. J Vasc Surg 3:24–31, 1986.
26. Medical Research Council: Aids to the Examination of the Peripheral Nervous System. London, Her Majesty's Stationery Office, 1976.
27. Miller, R.A. Observations on the arrangement of the axillary and brachial plexus. Am J Anat 64:143–163, 1939.
28. Millesi, H. Surgical management of brachial plexus injuries. J Hand Surg 2:367–379, 1977.
29. Millesi, H. Brachial plexus injuries. In Chapman, M., ed. Operative Orthopaedics. Philadelphia, J.B. Lippincott, 1988, pp. 1417–1426.
30. Narakas, A.O. The rreatment of brachial plexus injuries. Int Orthop 9:29–36, 1985.
31. Nulsen, F.E.; Slade, H.W. Peripheral nerve regeneration: VA medical myelograph. In Woodhall, B.; Beebe, G.W., eds. A follow-up study of 3,656 World War II injuries. Clin Orthop 133:71, 1975.
32. Russell, N.A.; Mangan, M.A. Acute spinal cord compression by subarachnoid and subdural hematoma occurring in association with brachial plexus avulsion. J Neurosurg 52:410–413, 1980.
33. Samii, M. Aspects of peripheral and cranial nerve surgery. In Krayenbuhl, H., ed. Advances in Technical Standards in Neurosurgery, Vol. 2. New York, Springer-Verlag, 1975, p. 53.
34. Seddon, H. Three types of nerve injury. Brain 66:237–288, 1943.
35. Slingluff, C.L.; Teriz, J.K.; Edgerton, M.T. The quantitative microanatomy of the brachial plexus in man: Reconstructive relevance. In Terzis, J.K., ed. Microreconstruction of Nerve Injuries. Philadelphia, W.B. Saunders, 1987, pp. 285–324.
36. Sturm, J.T.; Perry, J.F. Brachial plexus injuries from blunt trauma—a harbinger of vascular and thoracic injury. Ann Emerg Med 16:404–406, 1987.
37. Sunderland, S. A classification of peripheral nerve injuries producing loss of function. Brain 74:491–516, 1951.
38. Sunderland, S. Nerves and nerve injuries. 3rd ed. Edinburgh, Churchill Livingstone, 1978.
39. VanBeek, A.; Hubble, B.; Kinkead, L.; et al. Clinical use of nerve stimulation and reporting techniques. Plast Reconstr Surg 71:225, 1983.
40. Yeoman, P.M. Cervical myelography in traction injuries of the brachial plexus. J Bone Joint Surg 50B:253–260, 1968.
41. Zelenock, G.B.; Kazmers, A.; Graham, L.M.; et al. Nonpenetrating subclavian artery injuries. Arch Surg 120:685–692, 1985.

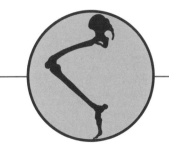

Section Editor
PETER G. TRAFTON, M.D., F.A.C.S.

IV

Lower Extremity

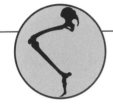

Paul Levin, M.D.

42

Hip Dislocations

*D*islocations of the hip encompass a spectrum of injuries with the potential for long-term disability and rapidly progressive joint degeneration. As the femoral head dislocates, the patient may also sustain a fracture to the femoral head, the femoral neck, the acetabulum, or a combination of any of these. The vascular supply may also be irreversibly damaged at the time of the injury. These associated injuries significantly diminish the prognosis for a normally functioning hip joint.

The first reports in the medical literature describing hip dislocations appeared in the second half of the nineteenth century prior to Wilhelm Roentgen's discovery of x-rays. These reports were based solely on clinical history and physical examination. Subsequent cadaveric studies defined the various anatomic injuries associated with hip dislocations.[1,6,7,137]

Funsten et al., in 1938, reported on a series of 20 hip dislocations and introduced the term "dashboard dislocation."[44] In this series, 13 dislocations were sustained by front seat occupants striking their knees against the dashboard. Subsequent to this report, Thompson and Epstein,[142] Stewart and Milford,[136] Brav,[12] Epstein,[36] and Stewart[134] have all reported on large series of hip dislocations. These reports have established the numerous complications and long-term disability associated with these injuries.

Presently, motor vehicle accidents still account for the majority of hip dislocations. The major series of hip dislocations report a range of 70% to nearly 100% of hip dislocations sustained in motor vehicle accidents.[12,13,36,73,110,114,135] Except for a few case reports, the vast majority of hip dislocations in motor vehicle crashes involve unrestrained vehicle occupants. Epstein reported two patients who dislocated their hips while wearing seat belts.[37] One patient apparently had not secured the seat belt properly, and the other was

ejected from the vehicle with seat and seat belt attached. Levin has reported two cases of hip dislocations in drivers restrained with both lap belt and shoulder harness.[84,85] One patient sustained an associated femoral head fracture and the other a comminuted posterior acetabular wall fracture. In each of these instances the accidents involved rapidly moving, compact model vehicles. Clearly, the regular use of appropriate passenger restraints would dramatically decrease the incidence of these major musculoskeletal injuries.

While these previously mentioned series as well as other reports[147,149] attest to the guarded prognosis of hip dislocations, it is hoped that recent technologic advancements will improve the outcome. Radiographic imaging techniques such as computerized tomography and magnetic resonance imaging allow the fracture surgeon to have a better understanding of the injury. New surgical approaches, improved instrumentation, and internal fixation devices permit more anatomically sound and stable fixation of this major weight-bearing joint.

This chapter will discuss the use of these newer technologies in evaluating and treating hip dislocations. The treatment of associated fractures of the femoral head and acetabulum will be reserved for those chapters addressing those injuries.

Pathology

RELEVANT ANATOMY

The hip joint and the glenohumeral joint are the two true ball-and-socket joints found in the human skeleton. The hip joint, unlike the glenohumeral joint, is an extraordinarily stable joint. This stability is related primarily to the bony and labral anatomy of the acetabulum and femoral head. The thick fibrous capsule with ligamentous condensations and the local muscular anatomy greatly supplement this stability.

Harty explains the inherent bony stability through the size and relationship of the femoral head and femoral neck to the acetabular socket, which has been deepened by an osteocartilaginous labrum.[57] The femoral head forms approximately two thirds of a sphere and is situated on a femoral neck approximately three quarters the diameter of the femoral head.

This relationship in size between the femoral head and femoral neck allows the femoral head to be deeply seated within its acetabular socket without compromising either stability or range of motion. The acetabulum is formed from the confluence of the ischium, ilium, and pubis at the triradiate cartilage. Biomechanical testing of newborn cadavers has found the joints to be extremely stable at birth, although some debate exists as to the actual stabilizing structures.[22,43] It is unclear whether the acetabulum deepens with development, but anatomic studies reveal that approximately

40% of the femoral head is covered by the bony acetabulum at any position of hip motion.[64] The articular surface of the acetabulum is horseshoe shaped, with articular cartilage covering the posterior, superior, and anterior portions of the acetabular cavity. The cartilaginous labrum is found attached to the perimeter of the portion of acetabulum covered by articular cartilage. In the midinferior portion of the acetabulum is the acetabular notch or cotyloid fossa. The transverse acetabular ligament traverses the most inferior portion of the acetabular notch extending from the most posteroinferior ridge of the labrum to the most anteroinferior edge of the labrum. The ligamentum teres originates from the acetabular notch.

The effect of the labrum is to deepen the acetabulum and increase the stability of the joint. The addition of the labrum ensures that at least 50% of the femoral head is covered by the osteocartilaginous labral-acetabular complex in any position of hip motion (Fig. 42–1). These motions include extension (from a prone position) of 20° to 30°, flexion of 120° to 135°, abduction

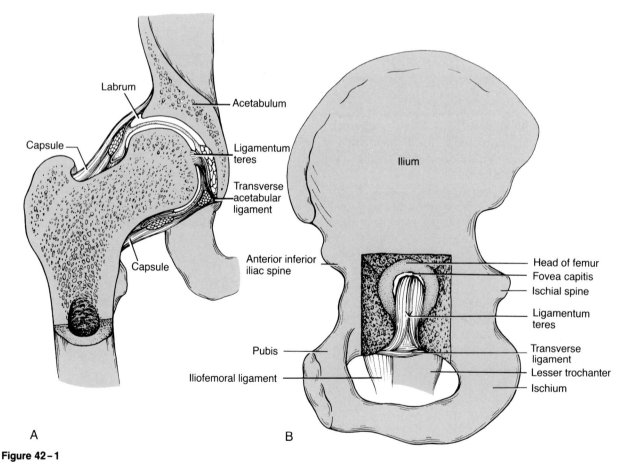

A

B

Figure 42–1

A and B, Schematic representation of the relationship of the femoral head, labrum, and acetabulum. The labrum extends beyond the equator of the femoral head, increasing excellent joint stability.

of 45° to 50°, adduction of 20° to 30°, and internal (medial) and external (lateral) rotation of 45° each. Definite individual variability is seen, and rotational measurements will differ if the rotation is tested in hip extension or hip flexion.[10,65,99,121]

The hip joint is surrounded by a capsule that extends posteriorly from the acetabular rim to the midfemoral neck and anteriorly from the acetabular rim to the intertrochanteric ridge. The primary capsular fibers run longitudinally and are supplemented by much stronger ligamentous condensations that run in a circular and spiral fashion. The iliofemoral ligament courses inferiorly from the iliac body and anteroinferior iliac spine in two distinct directions. One band continues directly inferiorly to insert on the intertrochanteric line just anterior to the lesser trochanter. The second band courses obliquely in a spiral fashion to insert on the intertrochanteric line overlying the greater trochanter. An additional anterior ligamentous condensation extends from the anterior border of the superior pubic ramus to the intertrochanteric line and is called the pubofemoral ligament. This ligament is believed to be a checkrein against pathologic extension of the hip. Posteriorly, the ischiofemoral ligament is a broad and less dense condensation extending in an oblique and horizontal fashion from the ischial border of the acetabulum to the superior base of the femoral neck and the region of the trochanteric fossa (Fig. 42–2).[64,96]

The femoral neck is normally anteverted in its relationship to the transcondylar axis of the femur. Hoagland and Low, in cadaveric studies, have demonstrated a significant variability in average anteversion and range of anteversion based on sex and genetic background.[62] Caucasian males were found to have an average of 7° of anteversion with a range of 2° of retroversion to 35° of anteversion. Caucasian females had an average anteversion of 10° with a range of 2° of retroversion to 25° of anteversion. Hong Kong Chinese males averaged 14° of anteversion with a range of −4° to 36°, and Hong Kong Chinese females averaged 16° of anteversion with a range of only 7° to 28°.

Upadhyay performed ultrasonographic measurements on a series of patients who had sustained a posterior hip dislocation. He found that this group of indi-

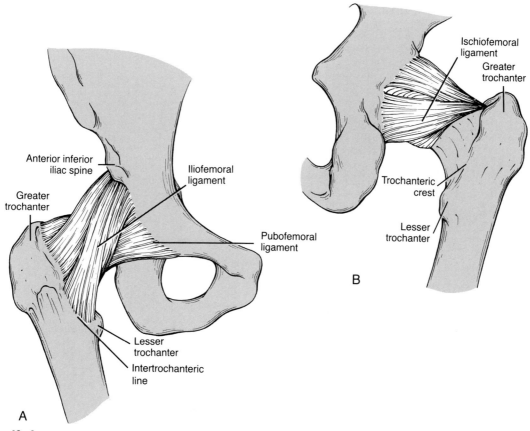

Figure 42–2

A and B, Ligamentous condensation about the hip capsule functions to supplement hip stability and to block pathologic motion.

viduals had significantly less anteversion on both the injured and uninjured sides when compared with a control group.[148] This may be a predisposing factor to hip dislocations and will be expanded on in the section on mechanisms and biomechanics.

The arterial supply of the femoral head has been widely studied, and a definite change in vascular patterns from infancy to adulthood has been identified. The main arterial supply of the adult femoral head originates from the medial and lateral femoral circumflex arteries, which are branches of either the femoral artery or deep femoral artery. The obturator artery and the inferior and superior gluteal arteries have also been demonstrated to contribute blood supply to the hip joint.[146]

An extracapsular vascular ring is formed at the base of the femoral neck. It is fed posteriorly by a branch at the medial circumflex artery and anteriorly by a branch of the lateral circumflex artery. Multiple ascending cervical branches arise from this arterial ring and pierce the hip joint at the level of the capsular insertion. From this point they ascend either along the femoral neck or laterally to supply the trochanter. Once these ascending cervical branches have entered the hip joint, they continue along the synovial reflections on the femoral neck and enter the bone just inferior to the articular cartilage of the femoral head (Fig. 42–3).[23,57,64]

Although this blood supply constitutes the major vascular supply in the human femoral head, Wertheimer and Lopes studied the variability of the vascular contribution of the artery of the ligamentum teres.[153] This vessel, when present, contributes blood supply to the epiphyseal region of the femoral head.

The sciatic nerve is formed from nerve roots from L4 to S3. As these nerve roots converge, there is an immediate division within the pelvis of the peroneal nerve and tibial nerve. These nerves exit the pelvis at the greater sciatic notch in a common sheath. A certain degree of variability exists in the relationship of the sciatic nerve with the piriformis muscle and short external rotators of the hip. Beaton and Anton demonstrated through anatomic dissections that in 85% of

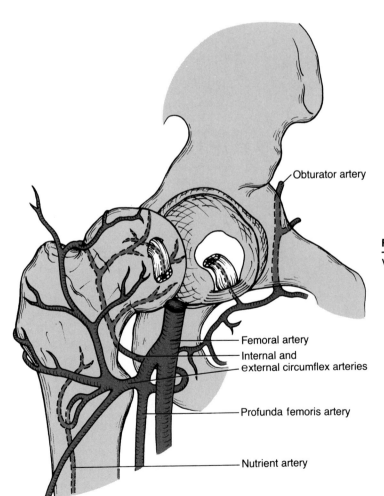

Obturator artery

Femoral artery
Internal and
external circumflex arteries

Profunda femoris artery

Nutrient artery

Figure 42–3

Vascular supply to femoral head.

individuals, the sciatic nerve exits the pelvis deep (anterior) to the muscle belly of the piriformis.[4] In 11% of individuals, the common peroneal nerve and tibial nerve are split by a portion of the piriformis muscle, with the peroneal nerve exiting through the substance of the muscle belly. In an additional 3% of individuals, the common peroneal nerve emerges superficial (posterior) to the piriformis, whereas the tibial nerve emerges deep (anterior) to the muscle belly. These anatomic variations are important considerations in extensile approaches to the posterior hip region (Fig. 42 – 4).

MECHANISMS OF INJURY

The anatomic configuration of the hip joint provides marked inherent stability. Consequently, hip dislocations are almost always due to high-energy trauma. Motor vehicle accidents account for the majority of hip dislocations; auto pedestrian accidents, falls from heights, industrial injuries, and sporting accidents are the other frequent mechanisms of injury.[37,43,136,140,142]

Regardless of the type of activity that results in the dislocation, the pathologic forces are transmitted to the hip joint from one of three common sources: (1) the anterior surface of the flexed knee striking an object; (2) the sole of the foot, with the ipsilateral knee extended; and (3) the greater trochanter. Less frequently, the dis-locating force may be applied to the posterior pelvis, with the ipsilateral foot or knee acting as the counter-force.[34,36,83,136]

The type of hip injury that an individual sustains depends on a number of factors, including the amount and direction of applied force, the quality of bone at both the proximal femur and acetabulum, and the position of the hip. Letournel has demonstrated through vector analysis the relationship of the position of the leg and pelvis to the injury sustained, thus explaining why an individual sustains an anterior dislocation, posterior dislocation, or fracture-dislocation of the hip.[82,83]

In the classic dislocation seen in unrestrained automobile drivers, the left hip tends to dislocate posteriorly, whereas the right hip will either develop a posterior fracture-dislocation or anterior dislocation. At the time of the rapid deceleration of the automobile, the right foot is positioned either on the brake pedal or on the accelerator pedal. The body pivots forward on this fixed foot, and the left knee strikes the dashboard in a knee 90°/hip 90° position. This tends to force the femoral head out posteriorly, usually without a fracture. With less flexion of the hip at the time of impact, the femoral head either strikes the posterior or posterosuperior aspect of the acetabulum, leading to a fracture-dislocation. Similarly, if the right foot is firmly pressed against the brake pedal at the moment of impact, the

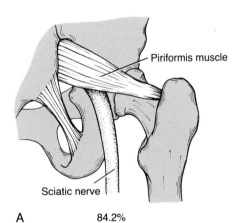

Piriformis muscle

Sciatic nerve

A   84.2%

Figure 42 – 4

Schematic representation of the most common relationships between the sciatic nerve and the piriformis muscle.

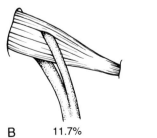

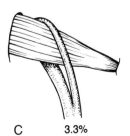

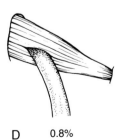

B   11.7%   C   3.3%   D   0.8%

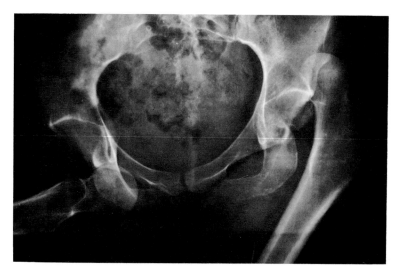

Figure 42–5

Bilateral hip dislocations sustained by an unrestrained intoxicated driver. The right hip was dislocated anteriorly and the left hip posteriorly (see text for explanation).

femoral head strikes the posterior or posterosuperior acetabulum. If an unsuspecting driver is involved in an accident, the right leg is often in a relaxed position on the gas pedal, with the hip externally rotated and abducted. In this position the inner aspect of the knee strikes the dashboard, resulting in accentuation of both abduction and external rotation. This extreme position results in anterior dislocation (Fig. 42–5).

In each of these previous examples, it is evident that the degree of hip rotation dramatically affects the position of the head within the acetabulum and therefore the ensuing injury complex. These mechanisms correlate with Upadhyay et al.'s sonographic analyses of hips in patients who had sustained posterior hip dislocations.[148] They demonstrated significantly less anteversion in patients who sustained posterior hip dislocations. In addition, those individuals with posterior fracture-dislocations had less anteversion than the control population but more than the pure dislocation group (Table 42–1). The retrospective data strongly suggest that the femoral head position, based on both an instantaneous position secondary to hip rotation

and the anatomic structure of the hip, dictates the type of injury.

Pringle was able to create anterior hip dislocations in cadavers through manipulation of the leg.[113] He demonstrated that extreme abduction with external rotation of the leg produces anterior dislocations. In a hip-flexed position, extreme abduction and external rotation lead to an anterior obturator dislocation. With the hip extended, these pathologic forces result in a superoanterior (pubic) dislocation. Epstein and Harvey have proposed that anterior dislocations are secondary to pathologic abduction of the hip.[38] It is their belief that in this position either the greater trochanter or the femoral neck impinges on the lateral ilium, which will then act as a lever to push the femoral head out of the acetabulum.

Femoral head fractures, impactions, and articular scorings are believed to occur as the femoral head exits the acetabulum. Actual shearing of the superior, anterosuperior, or posterosuperior femoral head can occur as the femoral head strikes the anterior or posterior acetabular lip.[21,27,39,111] Ligamentum teres avulsion

Table 42–1.		
Mean Femoral Anteversion as Measured by Ultrasonographic Techniques		
	Right Hip **Mean Anteversion (°)**	**Left Hip** **Mean Anteversion (°)**
Normal subjects	15.4	16.3
Type I dislocation, right hip	1.1	10.4
Type I dislocation, left hip	4.4	−3.2
Posterior fracture-dislocation, right hip	3.2	5.5
Posterior fracture-dislocation, left hip	5.0	6.1

Source: Adapted from Upadhyay, S.S.; et al. J Bone Joint Surg 67B:232–236, 1985.

fractures from the femoral head are frequently seen. These fragments can range in size from tiny cartilaginous avulsion fragments to major osteocartilaginous fragments of the femoral head (Fig. 42-6). Such loose fragments can become incarcerated between the femoral head and the acetabular articular surface following reduction of the dislocation. Failure to remove these fragments can lead to a rapidly destructive joint degeneration.

Femoral neck fractures associated with femoral head dislocations may result from two different mechanisms. Several case reports describing these associated injuries propose that the tremendous injury forces that initially dislocated the femoral head secondarily forced the femoral head against the pelvis. If, at that moment, the energy has not been fully dissipated, the continued application of pathologic forces to the leg while the femoral head is butting against the pelvis will fracture either the femoral neck or the femoral shaft.[41,74,95,112,126]

The second proposed mechanism of femoral neck fracture is "iatrogenic" and occurs at the time of manipulative reduction.[111,123,134] In most reported cases of iatrogenic neck fractures, there is an associated femoral head fracture. This may imply that the femoral neck absorbed a significant amount of energy and developed a nondisplaced or nonpropagated fracture that was not radiographically visible prior to the manipulation. Obviously, extreme care must be taken in reviewing the films prior to the reduction to ensure that a nondisplaced fracture is not present. In addition, reduction techniques must be gentle and well controlled; lever type manipulations must be avoided.

CONSEQUENCES OF INJURY

Normal articular cartilage is a highly resilient material that withstands both monotonic and cyclic loading.[116,120] Despite this resilience, Repo and Finley have demonstrated a threshold deformity that resulted in chondrocyte death.[120] They performed drop-tower testing on tibial plateau specimens harvested from renal transplant donors. Their results demonstrated that at cartilage strain of 20% to 30%, chondrocyte death occurred. The initial energy absorbed by the articular cartilage at the femoral head and acetabulum may in fact exceed this critical threshold for chondrocyte death and could be one possible explanation for the high incidence of traumatic arthritis reported following simple hip dislocations and the increasingly high rate of traumatic arthritis in the more extensive fracture-dislocations.[37,147,149]

Displacement or surgical excision of osteocartilaginous fragments also has significant biomechanical implications. Brown and Ferguson investigated the alteration in femoral head stress patterns in response to narrowing of the superior articular cartilage of the femoral head.[14] This loss of superior cartilage thickness created abnormally large transverse compressive stresses and increased stress concentration about the periphery of the femoral head. Brown and Ferguson proposed that this change in femoral head stress patterns secondary to loss of articular cartilage height was a predisposing factor to the development of osteoarthritis.

Bernard et al.[5] similarly studied the changes in femoral head stress patterns in relationship to varying thickness of the articular cartilage. They theorize that a built-in "incongruence" of the hip joint secondary to varying cartilage thickness is physiologically well tolerated and probably necessary for round joint mechanics. However, when cartilage thickness between the acetabulum and femoral head decreased to less than 1 mm total or 0.5 mm each (28% of normal), there was a dramatic increase in contact stresses.[5]

Although neither the study by Brown and Ferguson nor the one by Bernard et al. specifically addressed the question of loss of cartilage secondary to trauma, the situations seem to be analogous. Any significant loss of normal articular congruence or articular contact secondary to femoral head depressions or defects would also seem to predispose to similar changes in contact stresses and the development of early traumatic arthritis.

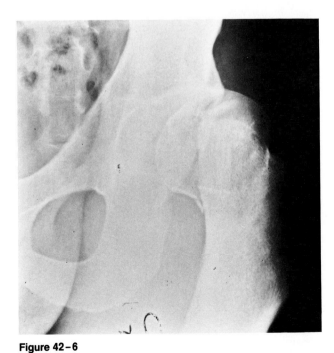

Figure 42-6

Large femoral head fracture associated with a posterior hip dislocation (comprehensive classification type V or Pipkin type II).

Studies on the ability of articular cartilage to heal defects and on the nature of the repair tissue also demonstrate the potential problems created by cartilaginous defects.[16,29,90,98,127,141] Suzuki produced surgical defects in rabbit patellae and subsequently studied the repair tissue.[141] The cartilage filling in the defects was found to be biochemically similar but with a slightly lower proteoglycan content. Mechanically it was found to be a "softer" substance than normal cartilage, which was attributed to the lower proteoglycan content. Abnormalities secondary to the loss of articular cartilage and alterations in contact stress seem likely to predispose to the development of traumatic arthritis.

Avascular necrosis (AVN) of the femoral head secondary to vascular embarrassment at the time of hip dislocation is the second most significant consequence. However, its incidence is controversial; some investigators suggest that previous radiologic diagnoses of avascular necrosis may in fact have been advanced traumatic arthritis.[36,124] Estimates of avascular necrosis vary in the literature from 1%–2% to 15%–17%.[93,97,107,114,136]

The specific anatomic lesion or lesions that are responsible for the development of avascular necrosis have never been identified. A strong correlation has been demonstrated by numerous authors between the incidence of avascular necrosis and the length of time the hip remains dislocated. The time threshold within which the hip should be reduced to prevent AVN is reported to be in the range of 6 to 24 hours.[36,60,68,110,135,144,150]

The association between avascular necrosis and dislocation time leads to a theory that three different mechanisms may cause AVN. The first mechanism is an immediate complete disruption of blood supply to the femoral head occurring at the time of a violent dislocation. The second mechanism is a slower process in which, because of the prolonged abnormal stretching of the arterial supply, the arteries develop vascular spasm or thrombosis. The third mechanism could be a venous phenomenon in which the tension on the vascular drainage leads to venous occlusion, back pressure, and ultimate arterial obstruction. These second two mechanisms can potentially be favorably affected through early reduction.

The possibility of early weight bearing following hip dislocation has been proposed as a cause of avascular necrosis.[26,34,77] This theory has been dispelled by numerous investigators, and no association has ever been demonstrated.[12,37,107,135]

Epstein et al. proposed that an anterior surgical approach to treat a posteriorly dislocated hip will place the patient at high risk for avascular necrosis.[36,39] Careful consideration of the vascular anatomy and T capsu-

lotomies with openings on the acetabular side of the joint should not compromise the vascular supply of the femoral head. Recent clinical experience of treatment of femoral head fractures through a variety of anterior surgical approaches (Smith-Petersen, Watson-Jones, transtrochanteric) have not demonstrated an increased incidence of avascular necrosis.[17,18,129,143]

The long-term significance of traumatic osteonecrosis is extremely variable. Glimcher and Kenzora have described significant pathologic and histologic differences among idiopathic and metabolic osteonecrosis and avascular osteonecrosis.[49–51] Unlike idiopathic varieties, not all hips affected with avascular osteonecrosis will progress to collapse and joint degeneration. At times, only a segment of the femoral head will be affected with avascular necrosis, and only this portion may undergo a segmental collapse (Fig. 42–7). This must be remembered prior to undertaking prophylactic or salvage procedures that may be appropriate to idiopathic varieties of osteonecrosis.

COMMONLY ASSOCIATED INJURIES

Hip dislocations are usually secondary to high-energy trauma and as a result are often associated with other

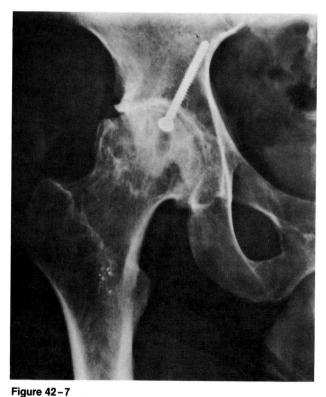

Figure 42–7

Segmental avascular necrosis of the femoral head following a posterior fracture-dislocation of the hip.

significant injuries. Concomitant neurologic injuries, musculoskeletal injuries, and intraabdominal and chest injuries have all been widely reported.[140]

Careful assessment of the patient is imperative to avoid missing associated injuries. It is important to establish the mechanism of injury so that all portions of the extremity that transmitted the energy are carefully examined. For example, if a patient suffered a posterior fracture-dislocation of the hip at the time his or her foot was jammed on the brake pedal, the foot must be carefully examined and radiographed for occult fractures or fracture-dislocations of Lisfranc's joint or the midtarsal joints.

A large variety of knee injuries are associated with hip dislocations. Gillespie reported on a series of 35 associated knee injuries; 25 were attributed to direct trauma to the knee region, and ten were associated with pathologic stresses applied to the knee ligaments.[48] Among the reported injuries were osteochondral fractures of the patella, tibia, and femur; posterior cruciate injuries; collateral ligament injuries; and traumatic patellofemoral chondrosis. A large percentage of these injuries were late diagnoses (two days to six months).

Sciatic nerve injuries are seen in association with hip dislocations in 8% to 19% of patients.[13,35,37,52,64,69,80,135,136] The mechanism of injury is presumed to be stretching of the nerve over the posteriorly dislocated, internally rotated femoral head.[39] Large posterior wall fragments can also stretch the nerve or even pierce or partially lacerate it. Intraoperatively, the nerve will often appear normal or have some mild associated hemorrhage. No cases of sciatic nerve injury have been reported secondary to anterior dislocations.

A complete disruption of the sciatic nerve is unusual. Most commonly, the peroneal portion is significantly involved, with little if any tibial nerve dysfunction. It is unknown why the peroneal nerve is injured and the tibial nerve is spared. Gregory has proposed that the unusual association of the peroneal portion of the nerve with the piriformis muscle places this portion of the nerve at risk.[52]

Nerve function must be carefully assessed prior to a manipulative reduction. Obviously, if the patient has sustained a head injury or is unconscious or uncooperative, neurologic examination will be incomplete. This should be noted on the patient's medical record.

It is imperative that a dislocated hip be reduced as soon as possible to relieve the stretching of the nerve. Surgical exploration is not indicated for associated neurologic injury. A possible exception to this rule is when initially normal neurologic function is lost following reduction.[26] In this situation the surgeon must ascertain whether the nerve has become incarcerated either in fracture fragments or in the hip joint. Some investigators recommend immediate surgical repair of displaced posterior wall fragments that are associated with sciatic nerve injuries. This is felt to relieve the stretching of the nerve by the fracture fragments.[114] Further discussion of the implications of sciatic nerve injury will be addressed later in the chapter.

Concomitant ipsilateral femur fractures have also been frequently reported.[32,42,59,131] Unfortunately, in many of these reported cases the diagnosis of hip dislocation was not made accurately. A femoral fracture masks the typical physical findings of a hip dislocation. Routine adherence to radiographic examination of the joint above and below the fracture should prevent missing this combination of injuries.

Classification of Hip Dislocations

EVOLUTION

Hip dislocations are subdivided into either anterior or posterior dislocations based on the location of the femoral head. A central dislocation is in fact a medial displacement of the femoral head secondary to a displaced acetabular fracture.[80,83,125,136] This poorly descriptive term, "central dislocation," is an outdated phrase and is no longer relevant in modern classification systems. Its ability to describe the injury complex is no better than calling a comminuted tibial pilon fracture a superior dislocation of the ankle.

Thompson and Epstein and, later, Stewart and Milford devised similar classification systems for posterior hip dislocations.[136,142] Both systems were based on the severity of the associated acetabular fracture as well as the presence of a femoral head fracture. A Thompson-Epstein type I dislocation is a pure dislocation with at most an insignificant posterior wall fragment. A type II dislocation is associated with a single large posterior wall fragment. A type III dislocation has a comminuted posterior wall fracture, and a type IV has an "acetabular floor" (more than posterior wall) fracture. Finally, a type V dislocation is complicated by a femoral head fracture (Fig. 42–8).

Stewart and Milford's system was based on the stability of the hip joint and the condition of the femoral head.[136] Type I dislocations have either no fracture or an insignificant acetabular rim fracture. A type II dislocation is associated with either a single or a comminuted posterior wall fracture, but the hip remains stable. Type III injuries are fracture-dislocations with gross instability of the hip joint secondary to loss of structural support, and a type IV dislocation is associated with a femoral head fracture.

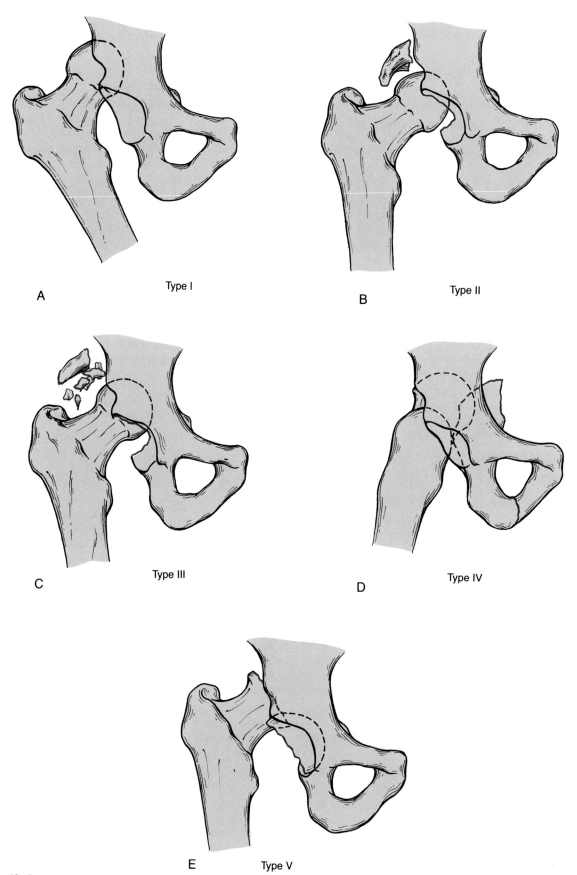

A   Type I

B   Type II

C   Type III

D   Type IV

E   Type V

Figure 42–8

Thompson-Epstein classification of posterior hip dislocations. (Redrawn from DeLee, J.C. Fractures and dislocations. In: Rockwood, C.A., Jr.; Green, D.P. Fractures, Vol. 2, 2nd ed. JB Lippincott, 1985.)

Pipkin classified posterior hip dislocations associated with femoral head fractures based on the location of the femoral head fracture.[111] A type I injury has a femoral head fracture inferior to the fovea centralis; a type II injury has a fracture line extending superior to the fovea centralis (and usually including the fovea); a type III injury is any femoral head fracture in association with a femoral neck fracture; and a type IV injury is any femoral head fracture associated with an acetabular fracture (Fig. 42–9).

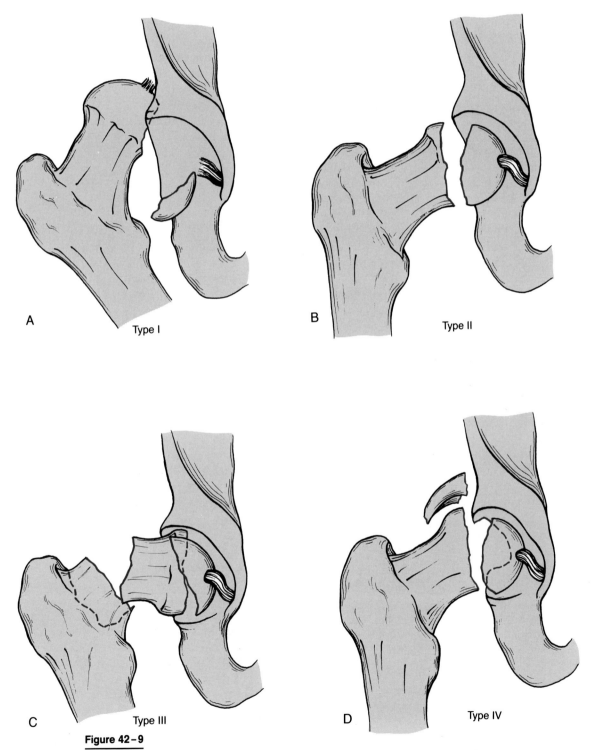

Figure 42–9

Pipkin classification system of posterior hip dislocations associated with femoral head fractures.

Each of these classification systems, at the time when they were devised, served the function of both setting a treatment protocol and predicting an outcome. Unfortunately, a recent study by Upadhyay et al. has reported that even in apparently simple dislocations the results are frequently poor.[149] It seems very likely that the discrepancies between type and outcome of hip dislocations are related to suboptimal initial evaluation. Recent advances in radiographic imaging offer the physician a better opportunity to accurately assess the initial injury and therefore to plan more appropriate treatment (see section on radiographic analysis).

POSTERIOR HIP DISLOCATIONS

These advances in imaging technology have necessitated the development of a new classification system (Table 42-2). The classification system incorporates the physical findings both before and after reduction, as well as the diagnostic information obtained through plain radiography, computed tomography (CT), and, possibly, magnetic resonance imaging (MRI). The definitive treatment can be derived primarily from the grading of the dislocation.

A type I posterior dislocation is either a pure dislocation or is associated with an insignificant posterior wall fracture. The postreduction CT scan demonstrates a concentric reduction, no widening of the joint, and no incarcerated fragments between articular surfaces. Occasionally a postreduction CT image will demonstrate a small bone fragment within the acetabular fossa secondary to a ligamentum teres avulsion. This fragment is of no clinical significance as long as it is not incarcerated between the articular surfaces of the femoral head and the acetabulum. The postreduction clinical exam in type I dislocations will demonstrate a hip that is stable at 90° of flexion when a posteriorly directed force is applied to the hip.

Type II posterior dislocations are pure dislocations without associated femoral head or acetabular fractures in which the femoral head is irreducible by closed manipulation. A hip will be presumed to be irreducible only if a closed reduction under general anesthesia with muscle paralysis fails to bring the femoral head back into the acetabulum. The eventual postreduction CT scan will demonstrate a normal relationship between the femoral head and the acetabulum. The joint spaces will be symmetric, without evidence of widening or incarcerated fragments.

A type III posterior dislocation is one in which the postreduction clinical exam reveals an unstable hip or one in which the postreduction imaging studies reveal a widened joint space or an incarcerated cartilaginous or osseous fragment. At times the instability will be the result of the failure to fully seat the femoral head secondary to an incarcerated fragment. On occasion the instability can be secondary to an extensive labral detachment or massive capsular and ligamentous disruption.

A type IV posterior dislocation is one that is associated with a significant acetabular fracture requiring reconstruction. Surgery in these patients is indicated to restore either joint stability or joint congruity. These fracture-dislocations of the hip are more appropriately classified according to their acetabular fracture pattern. The accepted indications for acetabular reconstruction as well as their classification will be discussed in chapter 32.

Type V posterior dislocations are associated with femoral head or femoral neck injuries. The femoral head injuries may be indentations, depressions, or cleavage fractures. These injuries will be classified further based on the femoral head fracture classification system (see chapter 43) (Fig. 42-10).

ANTERIOR HIP DISLOCATIONS

Anterior hip dislocations occur much less frequently than do posterior hip dislocations. Epstein has classified these injuries based on their anterior location (superior or inferior) as well as on the presence of associated acetabular fractures.[142] Recent long-term evaluations of these injuries have revealed a much less favorable prognosis than was previously believed.[27,38] A significant portion of the poor results may be related to associated femoral head injuries.

Previous classification systems have unnecessarily divided anterior dislocations into subgroups of superior and inferior types and then simply subdivided these into groups based on associated fractures. The

Table 42-2.

Comprehensive Classification of Posterior Hip Dislocations

Type I	No significant associated fractures; no clinical instability following concentric reduction.
Type II	Irreducible dislocation without significant femoral head or acetabular fractures (reduction must be attempted under general anesthesia).
Type III	Unstable hip following reduction or incarcerated fragments of cartilage, labrum, or bone.
Type IV	Associated acetabular fracture requiring reconstruction to restore hip stability or joint congruity.
Type V	Associated femoral head or femoral neck injury (fractures or impactions).

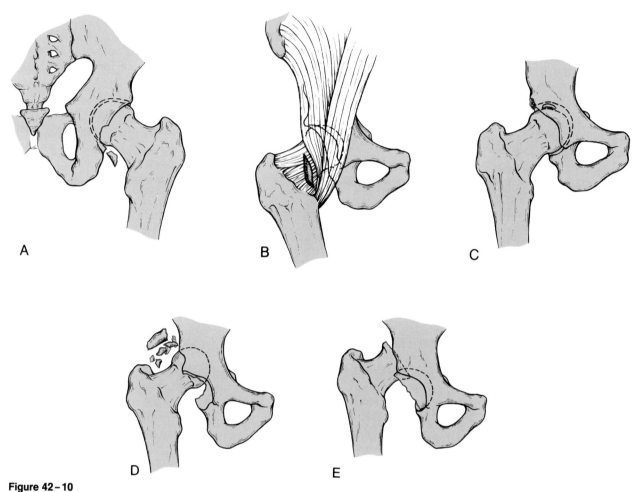

Figure 42-10

Comprehensive classification of posterior hip dislocations. *A* = type I; *B* = type II; *C* = type III; *D* = type IV; *E* = type V. See Table 42-2.

treatment plan is not altered by the subdivision of inferior or superior dislocation and has not, therefore, been incorporated into the current system. Again, the additional information obtained through postreduction imaging studies was not included in the previous classifications. The present system for classification of anterior dislocations is the same as that outlined for posterior dislocations but includes the suffix "anterior" following the subtype (e.g., type I anterior dislocation) (Fig. 42-11; Table 42-3).

Diagnosis

HISTORY

Patients presenting with dislocations and fracture-dislocations of the hip are in severe discomfort. They complain of inability to move their lower extremity and may also complain of numbness throughout the leg. These patients have usually been involved in high-

energy trauma such as motor vehicle accidents, industrial trauma, or falls from heights.

Individuals suffering multiple injuries often experience pain at numerous sites and as a result may not be able to localize specific injuries. Associated injuries to the chest, abdomen, spine, and extremities all compromise the ability of the patients to isolate and differentiate their symptoms. A high percentage of these patients will be obtunded or unconscious when they arrive in the emergency department and as a result will be unable to assist the physician in their initial evaluation.

PHYSICAL EXAMINATION

The classic appearance of an individual with a posterior hip dislocation is a patient in severe pain with the hip fixed in a position of flexion, internal rotation, and adduction (Fig. 42-12). Patients with an anterior dislocation hold their hip in marked external rotation with mild flexion and abduction (Fig. 42-13).

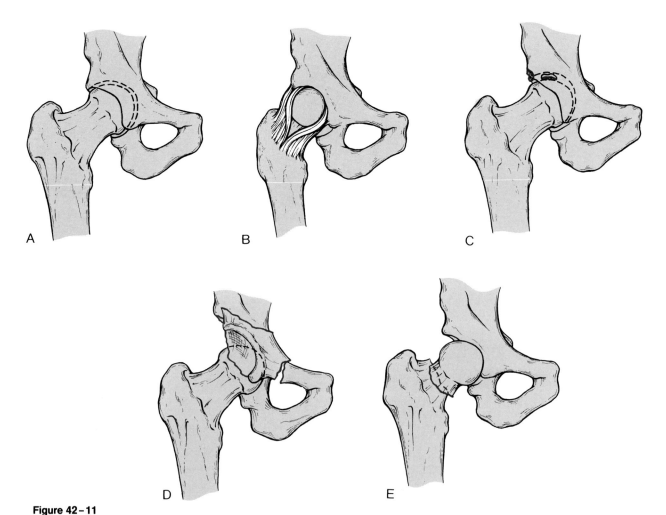

Figure 42-11

Comprehensive classification of anterior hip dislocations. *A* = type I; *B* = type II; *C* = type III; *D* = type IV; *E* = type V. See Tale 42-3.

Despite these classic descriptions, the appearance and alignment of the extremity can be dramatically altered by ipsilateral extremity injuries. The leg may be seen to lie in a near-neutral position in a posterior hip

Table 42-3.
Comprehensive Classification of Anterior Hip Dislocations

Type I	No significant associated fractures; no clinical instability following concentric reduction.
Type II	Irreducible dislocation without significant femoral head or acetabular fractures (reduction must be attempted under general anesthesia).
Type III	Unstable hip following reduction or incarcerated fragments of cartilage, labrum, or bone.
Type IV	Associated acetabular fracture requiring reconstruction to restore hip stability or joint congruity.
Type V	Associated femoral head or femoral neck injury (fractures or impactions).

dislocation associated with a displaced posterior wall or posterior column fracture. Shortening of the extremity will be present in these cases but may be difficult to demonstrate. Obviously ipsilateral femur or tibia fractures also affect the appearance of the extremity.

The initial physical examination must include an evaluation of the entire involved limb. Care must be taken to check for the presence of a partial or complete sciatic nerve injury. Sciatic nerve injuries are frequently seen, and an accurate diagnosis must be made prior to any closed or open manipulation of the hip.[13,37,69,80,135,136] Lumbosacral plexus injuries are associated with major pelvic trauma, and a careful neurologic examination in a cooperative patient may reveal their presence.[33]

Abrasions overlying the patella or proximal anterior tibia are often evidence of the site of application of the injury force.[32,42,52] These findings should alert the physician to the possibility of occult knee ligament injuries, patella fractures, or osteochondral fractures of the distal femur.[48] Pelvic fractures and spine injuries may also

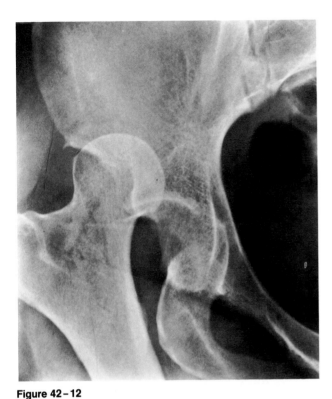

Figure 42-12

Type I posterior dislocation, with classic position of leg in adduction and internal rotation.

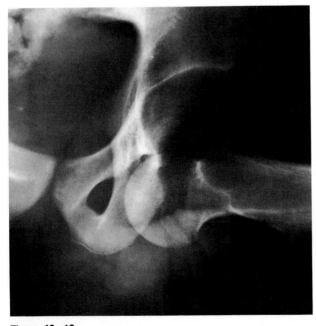

Figure 42-13

Anterior dislocation of the hip. Note that the leg is widely abducted and externally rotated.

be seen in association with hip dislocations, and these areas must be carefully assessed.

IMAGING STUDIES

The association of hip dislocations with high-energy trauma and multiple injuries should maintain the physician's high index of suspicion for such injuries. All trauma patients with an altered mental state, or local signs or symptoms, must have a screening anteroposterior (AP) radiograph of the pelvis. Patients with significant lower extremity injuries, spine fractures, or abdominal or chest injuries should undergo an anteroposterior pelvic radiograph. Alert and fully cooperative injured patients may not need pelvic radiographs if they are hemodynamically stable and no physical finding suggests an occult pelvic fracture or hip joint injury.

The review of the initial screening AP pelvic radiograph must be done carefully and systematically. The femoral heads should appear symmetric in size, and the joint spaces should be symmetric throughout the arc of the acetabulum as well as when comparing left to right. In the presence of a posterior hip dislocation, the femoral head will appear smaller on the AP radiograph. In an anterior dislocation, the femoral head will appear slightly larger than that in the normal hip. Shenton's line should be smooth and continuous. The relative appearance of the greater and lesser trochanters may indicate pathologic internal or external rotation of the hip. The adducted or abducted position of the femoral shaft should also be noted. Finally, careful evaluation of the femoral neck must rule out the presence of a femoral neck fracture prior to any manipulative reduction.

Following the diagnosis of a hip dislocation, additional imaging studies are necessary prior to any definitive surgical treatment. In general, these additional studies are obtained after a closed reduction has been achieved. The precise timing and techniques of reduction will be discussed in the section of this chapter concerning treatment.

Plain Film Analysis

Once the diagnosis of a hip dislocation is made, it is imperative that additional radiographs be obtained prior to any open surgical intervention. Usually these films are obtained following a successful closed reduction, but on occasion they are obtained prior to an open reduction of an irreducible femoral head.

Plain film analysis should include an AP radiograph centered on the affected hip and internal and external oblique views (Judet views) at 45° centered on the af-

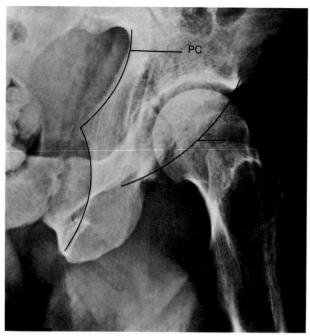

Figure 42–14

The iliac oblique radiograph brings the posterior column and anterior wall of the acetabulum into profile. PC = posterior column; AW = anterior wall.

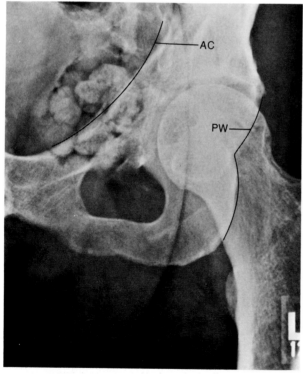

Figure 42–15

The obturator oblique radiograph brings the anterior column and posterior wall of the acetabulum into profile. AC = anterior column; PW = posterior wall.

fected hip. The AP radiograph should be carefully reviewed to ascertain the presence of incarcerated osteochondral fragments and asymmetry of the joint space. The iliac oblique (medial anterior oblique) view brings the beam perpendicular to the posterior column and is best for evaluation of the integrity of the posterior column and the anterior wall. The obturator oblique (lateral anterior oblique) view brings the anterior column into profile and is the best view for evaluating the integrity of the anterior column and posterior wall (Figs. 42–14 and 42–15).[56]

In addition, each one of these views will present a different profile of the femoral head. Femoral head depressions and fractures should be noted. Precise interpretation of these initial films is crucial in the event that open surgery will be required prior to obtaining CT analysis. Proper choice of surgical approach may depend on correct preoperative identification of associated acetabular or femoral head fractures.

Computerized Tomography

Computerized tomography should be routinely obtained following successful closed reduction of a dislocated hip. If a successful closed reduction is not possible and an open reduction is planned, a CT scan should be obtained if no undue delay is required. Emergency CT scanning has become readily available and more accessible and has demonstrated accuracy in the evaluation of the traumatized abdomen.[40,108] A specific request for multiple cuts through the hips and sacroiliac joints may be required.

The value of CT scanning is its ability to assess the femoral head, demonstrate the presence of small intra-articular fragments, and assess the congruence of the femoral head and acetabulum.[3,56,88,130,133,151,155] Baird placed 2-mm and 4-mm methylmethacrylate spacers in cadaver hip joints and then performed plain radiographs and CT scans on these specimens. The CT scans routinely revealed the 2-mm spacers, whereas the plain radiographs failed to demonstrate their presence. Figure 42–16 demonstrates an incarcerated osteochondral fragment not visualized on postreduction plain radiographs.

CT imaging better visualizes the size and displacement of acetabular wall fractures. Calkins et al. have devised a scale that correlates the percentage of displaced acetabular wall as measured on CT scan with hip stability.[19] Although some basic parameters can be developed from this study, a significant degree of variability exists, making precise correlations impossible (Figs. 42–17A,B and 42–18A,B). CT scanning has also proven to be invaluable in demonstrating major de-

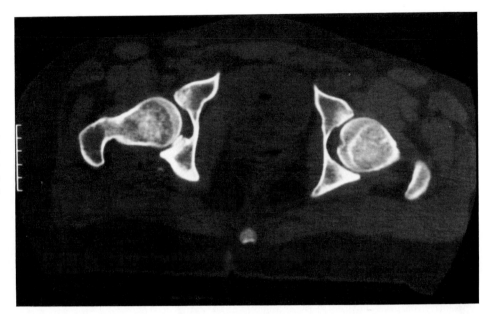

Figure 42–16

Following reduction of a posterior hip dislocation, CT scan demonstrates an incarcerated osteochondral fragment. This fragment requires removal (comprehensive classification, type III).

pressions of the acetabular articular surface (Fig. 42–19*A,B*).

The value of CT scanning in demonstrating femoral head injury has been reported by a number of investigators.[88,105,133,155] Occult impactions, indentations, and other fractures have all been visualized on CT scanning. The severity of displacement of fractures is accurately assessed by CT scanning.

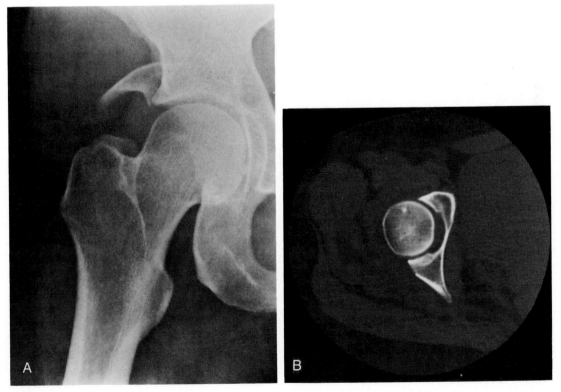

Figure 42–17

A displaced posterior wall fragment appears relatively large on a postreduction film *(A)*, but the CT scan *(B)* demonstrates that only a minimal portion of the posterior articular surface is involved.

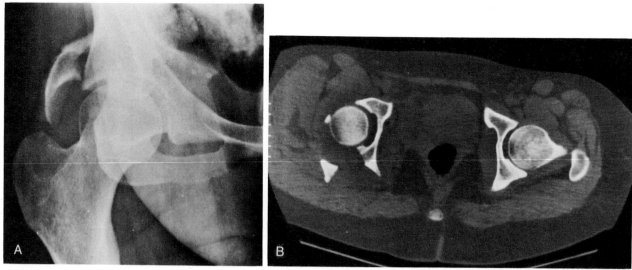

Figure 42–18

Displaced posterior wall fragment *(A)* is demonstrated on CT scan *(B)* to encompass a major portion of the posterior articular surface. Compare the contours of the normal and injured hips on the CT scan to gain an appreciation of the extent of the fracture.

Magnetic Resonance Imaging

The role of MRI in the posttraumatic imaging of the hip has yet to be established. Severe limitations in access to the patient during MRI make its use impossible in the acute evaluation of the multiply injured patient. Following stabilization of the patient, MRI may prove useful as an adjunct to CT scanning in the evaluation of the integrity of the labrum and vascularity of the femoral head. Stoller reports the diagnosis of a posterior

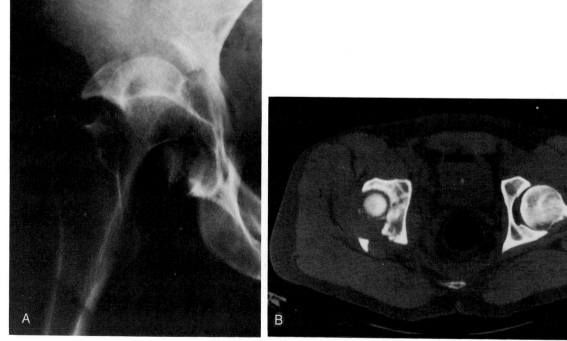

Figures 42–19

Injury film demonstrates a small displaced posterior wall fragment with some possible comminution. CT scan demonstrates extensive involvement of the posterior articular surface with major joint depression extending to the acetabular fossa.

labral disruption by high-resolution MRI with a surface coil.[138] The finding was subsequently verified by arthroscopic examination. This may prove helpful in the evaluation of unstable hips with no radiographic abnormalities (i.e., fractures, joint space widening).

Isotope Imaging

Isotope imaging with either technetium-labeled phosphate compounds or technetium 99m sulfur colloid is not indicated in the postinjury imaging of hip dislocations. Meyers et al. suggested using technetium 99m sulfur colloid to predict femoral head viability following hip dislocation.[96] However, current indications are that isotope imaging should not be used to determine treatment. The limited indications for these techniques will be discussed in chapter 43 on femoral head and neck fractures.

Management

The management of a patient with a hip dislocation is divided into an initial phase of achieving a reduction of the dislocation followed by a secondary phase of planning and performing definitive care. This division into phases is necessary because of the initial urgency of reducing the hip to prevent long-term complications. Numerous investigators have reported a strong correlation of avascular necrosis of the femoral head with the amount of time during which the hip remains dislocated.[12,68,136,142,144] Once the femoral head has been reduced, urgency is diminished. The appropriate diagnostic workup, including CT analysis of the hip, can then be completed. Surgical intervention, if necessary, can be undertaken when the patient has become hemodynamically stable, and safe for operative treatment.

INITIAL MANAGEMENT

Although it is generally agreed that dislocated hips should be reduced rapidly, some debate exists as to whether this should be by closed or open methods. Most investigators recommend an immediate attempt at a closed reduction.[12,68,69,78,79,83,114,135,144] Epstein[35] and DeLee[26] believe that closed reduction should be reserved for simple dislocations not associated with any fractures. They believe that all fracture-dislocations should be treated by immediate open surgery to remove loose fragments from the joint and to reconstruct fractures. Thompson and Epstein demonstrated dramatically improved long-term results when comparing open treatment with closed treatment.[37,142] Historically, it seems evident that the improved results with

the immediate open procedure were related to the ability to visually clear the acetabulum of all loose fragments, which at the time of Epstein's work could not be radiographically demonstrated. The introduction of CT scanning and its routine use in postreduction evaluation obviate this benefit of routine immediate open reduction.

Special Considerations in the Multiply Injured Patient

Hip dislocations are frequently encountered in patients with multiple injuries. The initial return of the femoral head to the acetabulum remains of utmost importance, whereas associated acetabular or femoral head fractures can be treated during the subacute phase of patient management.

Any patient requiring an immediate general anesthetic for surgical treatment of a head, abdominal, or thoracic injury can have a rapid closed reduction of the hip dislocation. A patient in the emergency department who has been intubated and immobilized for initial care of a closed head injury should also have a rapid closed reduction.

A hip that is stable following reduction can be placed in Buck's traction with a foam-cushioned boot; however, traction may not be necessary. An unstable hip secondary to an acetabular fracture should be placed in skeletal traction with care being taken to keep the leg slightly externally rotated and abducted when posterior instability is present and in neutral to mild internal rotation for anterior instability. The timing of surgery is discussed in chapter 32 on acetabular fractures. It is often helpful to treat those patients requiring traction in special rotating beds (e.g., Rotorest) while they await reconstructive acetabular surgery.

Algorithm for Initial Management

Prompt reduction of the femoral head is the goal of initial management. Regardless of the direction (anterior or posterior) of the dislocation, the reduction can be attempted with in-line traction with the patient lying supine. The preferred approach is to perform a closed reduction under general anesthesia if the anesthesiologist is readily available. An operating room does not necessarily need to be available, as reductions can be performed in a properly equipped emergency department with the benefit of general anesthesia.

If it is not feasible to immediately place the patient under general anesthesia, then an attempt at a closed reduction with intravenous sedation in the emergency department is performed using small doses of diazepam (2.5 to 5 mg) and larger doses of morphine (10 to

15 mg). A syringe of naloxone hydrochloride should be immediately available, along with an Ambu bag. The medications should be administered slowly over a few minutes' duration with the goal being a patient who is sleeping but relatively easily arousable. It is crucial that no attempt at reduction be performed until the patient is appropriately sedated. Intermittent attempts at reduction followed by incremental administration of medication are much less fruitful and usually fail to achieve an adequate level of sedation.

If closed reduction is unsuccessful using intravenous sedation, the patient must be brought to the operating room. In the operating room closed reduction should be attempted with the patient under general anesthesia and complete muscle paralysis. If closed reduction cannot be achieved in this setting, then an immediate open reduction must be performed.

It is incumbent on the orthopedic surgeon to stress the urgency of the situation to both the anesthesiologist and operating room personnel. It must be made clear that the prevention of long-term complications demands urgent treatment in the operating room. The urgency of treating a hip dislocation is greater than that of treating an open fracture.

The two most popular methods of achieving closed reduction are the supine method of Allis and the prone, gravity method of Stimson.[1,137] Both maneuvers are acceptable for all types of hip dislocations, with the exception of subspinous and pubic dislocations, which must be reduced with the Allis method.[26] The forceful rotational technique of Bigelow should be condemned, as it places the patient at an increased risk for an iatrogenic femoral neck fracture.[6]

The Allis method of reduction is essentially traction applied in line with the deformity. The patient is left supine, and the surgeon must be able to achieve a mechanical advantage by either standing on the stretcher or placing the patient on the floor. No attempt should be made to reduce the hip while the patient is lying on the stretcher and the surgeon standing on the floor. Initially the surgeon should apply in-line traction while the assistant applies countertraction by stabilizing the patient's pelvis. As in the reduction of any joint dislocation, a slow progressive increase in the traction force is much more effective than a rapid abrupt pull. While increasing the traction force, the surgeon should slowly increase the degree of flexion to approximately 60° to 70°. Gentle rotational motions of the hip as well as

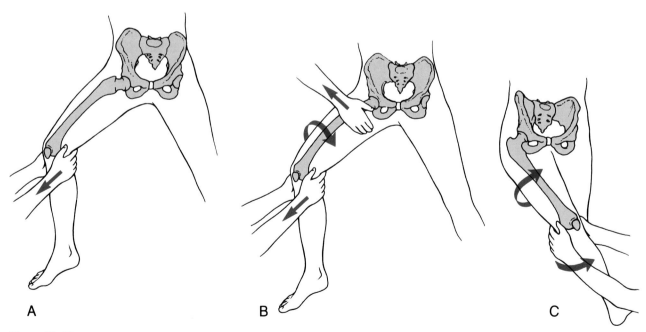

A   B   C

Figure 42-20

The Allis technique for reduction of a hip dislocation. The surgeon's position must provide a mechanical advantage for the application of traction. *A,* Internal and external rotation is gently alternated, perhaps with lateral traction by an assistant on the proximal thigh. *B,* In-line traction with hip flexes. *C,* Adduction is often a helpful adjunct to in-line traction. (Redrawn from DeLee, J.C. Fractures and dislocations. In: Rockwood, C.A., Jr.; Green, D.P. Fractures, Vol. 2, 2nd ed. JB Lippincott, 1985.)

slight adduction will often help the femoral head clear the lip of the acetabulum. Some authors recommend application of a lateral force to the proximal thigh to assist in the reduction. The successful closed reduction is usually clinically evident by an audible "clunk" as well as return of the leg to a neutral alignment. An awake patient will have an immediate improvement in symptoms (Fig. 42–20).

The Stimson gravity technique of reduction is preferred by some surgeons because of the ease of reduction (from the surgeon's perspective) and therefore the theoretic benefit of decreasing the risk of damage to the femoral head articular cartilage.[26,136,137] In this method the patient is placed prone on the stretcher with the affected leg hanging off the side of the stretcher. This brings the extremity into a position of hip flexion and knee flexion at 90° each. In this position the surgeon can easily apply an anteriorly directed force on the proximal calf. In actuality, the Allis and Stimson maneuvers are precisely the same, with the ultimate reduction force being applied to the hip in a flexed position. The apparent benefit lies in the surgeon's position (Fig. 42–21).

My preference is the technique of Allis. I feel more comfortable in administering intravenous sedation to a supine patient, as resuscitation is easier. Furthermore, because a large percentage of these patients have multiple injuries, placing them in the prone position may risk additional complications.

If the hip cannot be reduced by closed manipulation under general anesthesia, then an immediate open reduction must be performed. Prior to open reduction, Judet views of the hip should be obtained while the patient is in the operating room. These two oblique radiographs are crucial for surgical planning. In general, anterior acetabular fractures or femoral head injuries will require an anterior exposure of the hip joint regardless of the direction of the hip dislocation. Posterior acetabular fractures will require repair through a posterior hip exposure. The overall integrity of the acetabulum can be readily assessed with the Judet views.

It is also preferable to obtain a CT scan prior to undertaking an open surgical procedure. Unfortunately, this cannot always be obtained because of the unavailability of the CT scanner or the tactical problem of transporting an anesthetized patient to the CT suite. A CT scan provides valuable preoperative information regarding intraarticular fragments or a femoral head injury that was not appreciated on plain films.

MANAGEMENT AFTER REDUCTION

Postreduction management of hip dislocations is controversial. Recommendations have run the spectrum from short periods of simple bed rest to hip spica cast immobilization or various durations of skeletal traction.[2,13,142,152] Although some authors contend that early weight bearing predisposes the patient to avascular necrosis, most have found no such correlation.[12,26,34,37,107,135,144]

Algorithm for Postreduction Management

Management following successful closed reduction will depend on the postreduction physical examination and imaging studies. The location of the femoral head at its time of dislocation is not a factor in determining postreduction management. The grading of the injury, the

Figure 42–21

The Stimson gravity reduction technique. This method has limited application in patients with multiple injuries. (Redrawn from DeLee, J.C. Fractures and dislocations. In: Rockwood, C.A., Jr.; Green, D.P. Fractures, Vol. 2, 2nd ed. JB Lippincott, 1985.)

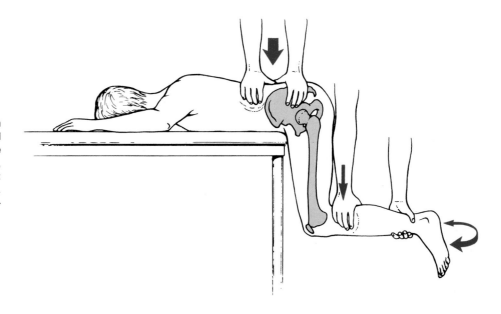

presence and location of femoral head or acetabular fractures, and the presence and direction of instability will determine the appropriate surgical approach. Obviously, a hip that demonstrates posterior instability without fracture following posterior dislocation will most probably require a posterior soft tissue repair. A hip that demonstrates anterior instability without fracture following an anterior dislocation may require an anterior exploration and repair.

Immediately following reduction, an anteroposterior and lateral radiograph of the involved hip as well as an anteroposterior radiograph of the pelvis should be obtained. Systematic analysis of the radiographs should be carried out to verify that the hip has been concentrically reduced (i.e., by looking for subtle widening of the hip joint). If there are significant acetabular fractures (fractures other than small avulsion fractures), Judet views should also be obtained (Fig. 42–22A,B).

Once radiographic verification of reduction has been obtained, an examination for hip stability is performed. This is performed while the patient is still sedated or under anesthesia, depending on the method used for the initial closed reduction. If there is an obvious large, displaced posterior or posterosuperior acetabular wall fracture, the stability examination is not performed. The examination is also deferred in the presence of displaced acetabular column fractures.

The capsule and supporting ligamentous condensations of the hip supply secondary stabilization, and a portion of these structures is presumed to be damaged at the time of dislocation. Despite this relative loss of stability, the combined bony and cartilaginous acetabulum should leave the hip relatively stable. Following verification of reduction, the hip is flexed to between 90° and 95° in neutral abduction/adduction and neutral rotation. A strong posteriorly directed force is then applied.[52] If any sensation of subluxation is detected, the patient will require additional diagnostic studies and possibly either surgical exploration or traction. If the patient is awake during this examination, he or she may be able to assist the surgeon in detecting instability. Larson retrospectively reviewed a series of hip dislocations and found that 17 hips treated in traction had obvious radiographic signs of instability or incongruity.[80] Each one of these patients developed traumatic arthritis. The most important principle to remember is that if there is any question of instability, surgical exploration and repair are warranted.

Following successful closed reduction and completion of the stability examination, the patient is placed in traction while awaiting a CT evaluation. If the hip has been demonstrated to be stable, simple traction with a Buck's traction boot or skin traction is sufficient. If the hip is unstable, it is preferable to use skeletal traction with a tibial pin. The angle of inclination of the

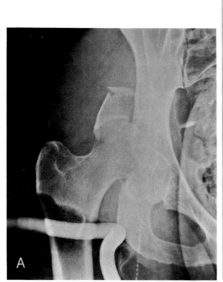
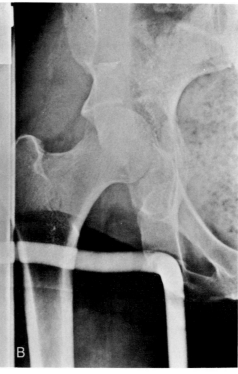

Figure 42–22

A, Careful assessment of postreduction films must be undertaken to avoid errors. Obturator oblique view shows posterior dislocation. B, AP radiograph was initially misinterpreted owing to the apparent congruence of the femoral head with the displaced acetabular fragment. Note abnormal appearance of Shenton's line.

traction pin should be planned to control rotation of the hip when the traction weight is applied. A hip with posterior instability should have the pin angled in a slightly posteromedial direction from an anterolateral starting point. This will externally rotate the leg when the traction weight is applied and therefore bring the femoral head into a more stable position. The reverse angle is planned for a hip with anterior instability. Alternatively, the traction pull can be split medially and laterally to obtain the appropriate rotation of the leg.

A CT scan should be expediently obtained within a day or two of admission. Three-millimeter sections through the entire acetabulum should be obtained and processed for both bone and soft tissue windows. The femoral head must be carefully analyzed for the presence of fractures or depressions. The acetabulum should be examined for depression fractures as well. Finally, the presence of incarcerated osteochondral fragments between the acetabular articular cartilage and femoral articular cartilage should be noted (see Fig. 42–16).

Magnetic resonance (MR) scanning plays a role in two circumstances, one of which is in the analysis of an unstable hip in which CT scanning has not demonstrated an intraarticular fragment and in which no acetabular wall fracture exists. Rashleigh-Belcher reported on a case of recurrent hip dislocation following an initial traumatic dislocation in which surgical exploration revealed a labral detachment.[117] MR scanning does visualize the acetabular labrum and therefore may demonstrate such a detachment.[8,97] Second, if both plain radiographs and CT images demonstrate unexplained joint widening, MR scanning may reveal the cause. Canale and Manugian,[20] Dameron,[25] and Paterson[106] have all reported cases in which the acetabular labrum either blocked reduction or became incarcerated in the joint. MR scanning is the ideal modality to analyze unexplained widening, as it is able to differentiate among a labral incarceration, a pure articular cartilage incarceration, and a simple hematoma. This investigation is indicated only in an unstable or widened hip with no other obvious etiology (i.e., fractures or intraarticular fragments).

Final grading of the injury can be performed following completion of the physical examination and imaging studies. The ultimate grade is based on the most severe injury. For example, an irreducible hip (type II) that is also noted to have a femoral head injury (type V) is graded as a type V fracture-dislocation of the hip.

The definitive management is based entirely on the type of dislocation. The direction of the dislocation (anterior or posterior) may or may not determine the actual surgical approach. The final decisions regarding surgical exploration and specific surgical approach must be determined by the pathology. The classification (type) of dislocation as well as the location of the fractures and the direction of the instability determines the optimal surgical approach. It is therefore unnecessary to separately discuss the treatment of anterior and posterior dislocations.

Posterior Approach to the Hip

The standard posterior approach to the hip joint is the Kocher-Langenbeck approach. My preference is to perform the procedure in the straight lateral decubitus position without use of the traction table. I have not found the fracture table necessary, but I do require two scrubbed surgical assistants. One assistant maintains the position of the leg and ensures that the hip remains extended and the knee remains flexed to avoid excess tension on the sciatic nerve. Letournel recommends prone positioning with a femoral traction pin.[82,83] After splitting the gluteus maximus muscle, the sciatic nerve must be identified. The nerve should be examined for contusion, hemorrhage, and partial or complete laceration. Care must be taken not to split the gluteus maximus too proximally, as this can lead to denervation secondary to injury of the inferior gluteal nerve. After identifying the sciatic nerve, the tendinous insertions of the piriformis muscle and obturator internus are identified and tagged with a heavy absorbable suture. If not torn, they are detached and retracted posteriorly. The piriformis muscle is usually posterior to the nerve and thus does not protect it when reflected. The obturator internus and other short external rotators lie anterior to the sciatic nerve and protect it when retracted. The need for further surgical dissection and capsulotomy is determined by the condition that is being treated. Care is taken not to injure the labrum when performing capsulotomies. Capsulotomy, if not already created by the injury, is always performed by removing the capsule adjacent to its acetabular insertion to prevent injury to the vascular supply to the femoral head at the base of the femoral neck. Depending on the procedure, the hip joint may require distraction by an assistant's traction, by a bone distractor (from iliac crest to proximal femur), or by traction with a fracture table. On occasion the hip may actually require dislocation for a successful surgical approach (Fig. 42–23).[72]

Following completion of the procedure, the wound is irrigated thoroughly with a power pulsatile lavage system. Intraoperative radiographs are obtained to verify concentric hip reduction without widening. The capsule is closed with heavy absorbable sutures, and the piriformis and obturator internus tendons are reattached. A suction drain is placed deep to the gluteus maximus. The gluteus maximus and tensor fasciae are

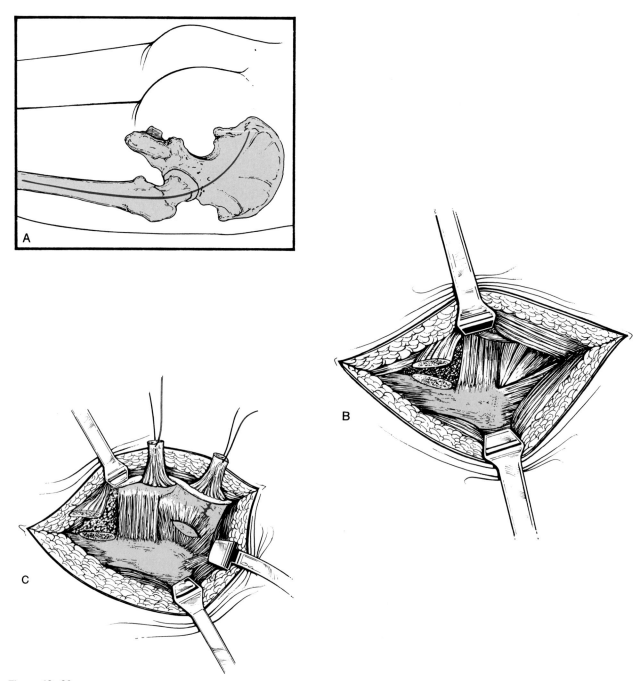

Figure 42–23

Kocher-Langenbeck posterior approach to the hip. The approach is used for removal of posteriorly incarcerated fragments, treatment of major posterior labral disruptions or instability, and repair of posterior acetabular fractures. *D*, External iliac view of posterior wall fracture of the right acetabulum following internal fixation through a Kocher-Langenbeck approach. *E*, Internal iliac view of the same hemipelvis showing the location of screw types.

closed with heavy absorbable interrupted sutures. A second suction drain is placed in the subcutaneous layer, and the skin is closed with mattress sutures to help close the dead space. The procedure is performed under antibiotic prophylaxis with cefazolin. One gram

is administered by intravenous bolus just prior to the skin incision. An additional gram is administered every 2 to 3 hours during surgery, and finally, 1 g is given every 8 hours for three postoperative doses. Suction drains remain in place until drainage has decreased to

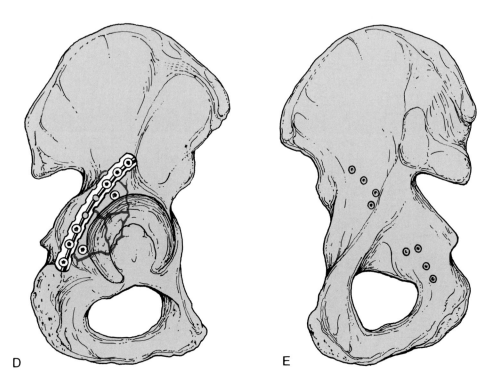

Figure 42-23 *Continued*

D   E

less than 30 ml during an 8-hour shift. The rehabilitative regimen will then vary depending on the surgical procedure performed. This will be discussed further in the specific sections detailing treatment of each type of injury.

Anterior Approach to the Hip

The surgical approach utilized to expose the hip joint anteriorly will be determined by the injury complex. Thorpe et al. recommend the Smith-Petersen approach for fixation of isolated femoral head fractures.[143] A Watson-Jones incision may be better if there is a combined fracture of both femoral head and neck (see chapter 43).

In my experience, the direct lateral approach of Hardinge and the anterolateral approach of Watson-Jones have both afforded excellent access to femoral head fractures following an anterior capsulotomy and anterior dislocation or subluxation of the hip.[66,70] When performed with the patient in the lateral decubitus position, an additional exposure of the posterior hip can be achieved through the same skin incision. The main advantage of the anterior approach of Smith-Petersen is that it allows more direct visualization of the anterior femoral head and, as a result, reduction and screw insertion may be somewhat easier. Extensive stripping of the abductors from the lateral ilium may increase the risk of heterotopic bone.

Direct Lateral and Anterolateral Approach to the Hip

The patient is placed in either the lateral decubitus position or the semilateral position with a sandbag under the affected side. If the surgeon feels that posterior exposure may be necessary, then the lateral position is mandatory. The affected leg is draped free.

A straight lateral incision is made extending from the iliac crest to 4 cm to 6 cm distal to the tip of the greater trochanter. The fascia lata is incised longitudinally, with care being taken to remain just posterior to the palpable muscle belly of the tensor fasciae muscle. If an anterolateral approach is used, the anterior third of the gluteus medius muscle is subperiosteally freed off the trochanter, and the gluteus minimus tendon is incised. If a direct lateral approach is used, the tendon of the gluteus medius is longitudinally split for 3 cm to 4 cm proximal to the tip of the trochanter. The fascia of the vastus lateralis is split longitudinally for approximately 4 cm distal to the vastus ridge, and the anterior vastus insertion is subperiosteally dissected off the base of the trochanter. The proximal and distal incisions are then connected (medius tendon to vastus lateralis), cutting sharply down to the greater trochanter. A large, curved osteotome is then used to remove an anterior sliver of bone, ensuring that the soft tissues of the anterior gluteus medius and anterior vastus lateralis remain as a continuous sleeve.

Regardless of the initial dissection plane, the remainder of the surgical dissection is the same. A Hoh-

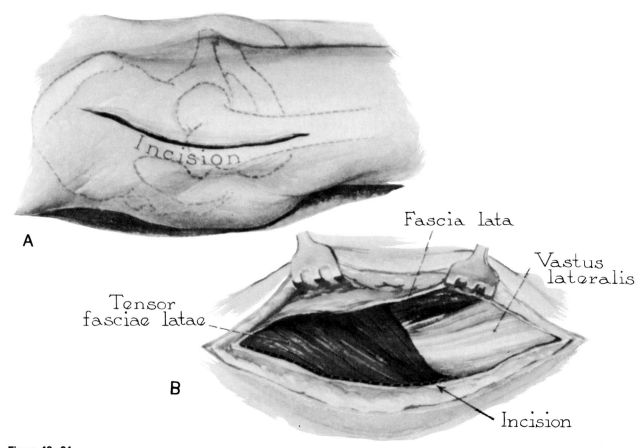

Figure 42–24

Exposure of the hip joint and the subtro chanteric region of the femur through a lateral hip and thigh incision. This approach can be used for treatment of femoral head fractures. (From Banks, S.W.; Laufman, H. An Atlas of Surgical Exposures of the Extremeties, 2nd ed. Philadelphia, W.B. Saunders, 1987.)

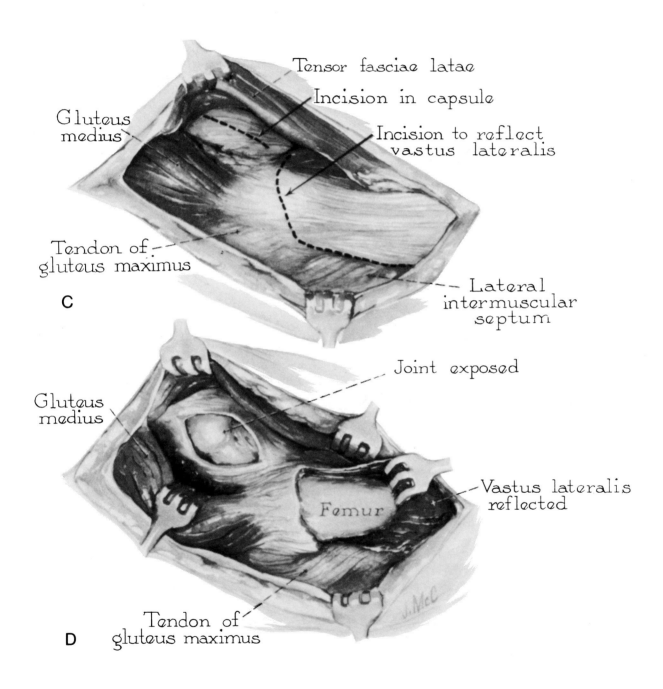

Tensor fasciae latae

Incision in capsule

Incision to reflect
vastus lateralis

Gluteus
medius

Tendon of
gluteus maximus

Lateral
intermuscular
septum

C

Joint exposed

Gluteus
medius

Vastus lateralis
reflected

Femur

Tendon of
gluteus maximus

D

mann retractor is placed anteromedially over the femoral neck superficial to the capsule, and a second retractor is placed in the trochanteric fossa lateral to the neck. If necessary, the capsule can be removed from its acetabular side, leaving a cuff of tissue for repair. The joint can be distracted with an AO/ASIF distractor or manually by an assistant with a bone hook. If necessary, the hip can be gently dislocated anteriorly following a wide capsulotomy (Fig. 42–24).

At the completion of the procedure, the wound is irrigated with a power pulse lavage. The capsule is closed with heavy absorbable sutures, and a deep suction drain is placed in the wound. The gluteus medius is reattached with interrupted sutures, and the bone sliver is reattached through drill holes with a heavy nonabsorbable suture. The fascia of the tensor is closed with heavy interrupted sutures, and the skin is closed with deep mattress sutures after placing a subcutaneous suction drain. Prophylactic cefazolin is used for three postoperative doses at 8-hour intervals, and drains are left in place until drainage has decreased to less than 30 ml during an 8-hour period. The rehabilitative regimen will vary depending on the procedure performed.

MANAGEMENT OF SPECIFIC TYPES OF HIP DISLOCATIONS

The treatment of each type of hip dislocation should be based on the type of dislocation and the location of the pathologic manifestations. As discussed previously the surgical approach chosen must not be determined by the direction of the dislocation. Epstein et al. have raised concerns over using an anterior approach following posterior dislocation, believing that complete vascular disruption will occur.[39] This belief is not supported by either a careful analysis of the vascular supply of the femoral head or by a review of the recent literature. Injury should not occur to the lateral femoral circumflex artery or its branches if the dissection avoids removal of the capsule from the femoral neck and trochanters. Clinical support of this approach can be found in the works of Butler[17] and Thorpe.[143] The following sections will address the treatment of each type of hip dislocation, regardless of the initial position of the dislocated femoral head.

Type I

Type I injuries are essentially pure dislocations with either no associated fractures or small acetabular rim fractures. The physical examination verifies inherent stability, and no surgical stabilization is indicated. These individuals are treated in gentle Buck's traction (5 lb) and begun on an active and passive range-of-motion protocol. Flexion beyond 90° and internal rotation beyond 10° are not permitted for six weeks. The traction is used until the majority of the hip irritability resolves. The patient is instructed in weight bearing–as-tolerated ambulation and is advised to use crutches for six to eight weeks, pending restoration of near normal hip muscle strength. Follow-up radiographs are obtained only if the patient's symptoms are not resolving in the expected chronology.

A small bone fragment noted to be in the acetabular fossa on CT scanning but not incarcerated between the articular surfaces of the femoral head and acetabulum is felt not to be significant. This is a nonarticular region of the hip joint, and a bone fragment in this location should not create any more symptoms than a fragment in the lateral gutter of the knee. If the patient later develops symptoms of a loose intraarticular fragment (e.g., catching, locking, pain, or the hip giving way), then consideration should be given to possible removal of the fragment. The section on the treatment of type III dislocations will discuss the appropriate surgical approach for removal.

Type II

The type II dislocation is one in which a successful closed reduction cannot be achieved. If the femoral head has been returned to the confines of the acetabulum but the joint space is widened, then the ultimate grading of the dislocation will be type III, IV, or V depending on the cause of the widening.

A hip that is irreducible purely for reasons of soft tissue interposition (e.g., capsular, tendinous, or muscular) will be demonstrated during open reduction of the dislocation. In this instance the grading will remain type II.

Proctor has reported a case in which the piriformis tendon became wrapped around the femoral neck, preventing reduction.[114] I have noted a similar finding while attempting to reduce a posterior dislocation associated with a transverse acetabular fracture. Epstein has described a case in which the iliopsoas tendon prevented reduction of an anterior dislocation.[37]

Bucholz and Wheeless have reported a series of six irreducible posterior hip fracture dislocations.[15] Surgical exploration of these six hips and cadaveric dissection and analysis revealed that a portion of the broad base of the iliofemoral ligament remained tethered between the displaced wall fragment and the posterosuperior ilium just proximal to the acetabulum. This tethering effect left the displaced posterior wall fragment caught between the femoral head and acetabulum, thus preventing reduction (Fig. 42–25).

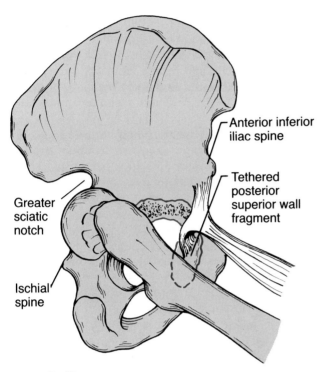

Figure 42-25

Tethering of the displaced posterior wall fragment by the iliofemoral ligament (Y ligament of Bigelow) is blocking the reduction of the hip dislocation.

No matter what the cause for the type II dislocation, immediate open surgical reduction must be performed. Preoperative radiographs (Judet views) should be obtained to determine the surgical approach. If logistically possible without excessive delay in treatment, it is also desirable to obtain a CT scan prior to the surgical procedure.

If there are no associated acetabular or femoral head fractures, the surgical approach should expose the hip joint on the side of the dislocation. In the event of an irreducible posterior dislocation, a standard Kocher-Langenbeck approach is performed. An irreducible anterior dislocation is exposed through a surgical approach that visualizes the anterior hip capsule (e.g., Watson-Jones or Hardinge).[55,66] It is advisable to avoid a straight anterior exposure such as the Smith-Petersen approach in order to avoid the possibility of damaging the taut and displaced femoral nerve, artery, and vein.

Prior to the actual reduction of the femoral head, the hip joint should be examined. Femoral head and acetabular depressions should be elevated and grafted if of appropriate size (see chapters 32 and 43). The joint should be profusely irrigated to remove all loose fragments and debris. The status of the articular cartilage of the femoral head and acetabulum should be noted. Gentle manipulation of the hip with appropriate trac-

tion on the leg may then be performed. A bone hook on the proximal femur will help the femoral head gain clearance over the acetabular margin. Manual pressure on the femoral head when guiding it into the acetabulum will obviate the need for aggressive traction and torsion to the leg.

Following successful open reduction, a stability examination is performed prior to wound closure. If the hip is stable at 90° of flexion with a strong posteriorly applied force, then the postoperative regimen is the same as for the type I dislocation. The patient is placed in gentle Buck's traction and instructed in the use of crutches for weight bearing–as-tolerated ambulation. Aggressive rehabilitation of hip musculature is begun, and crutches are used for six weeks.

If the postreduction examination reveals instability, additional surgical exploration is essential to uncover the cause. Extensive capsular tears or labral disruptions should be repaired. Intraoperative radiographs should be obtained to evaluate for a widened hip joint secondary to incarcerated fragments. These are the most common causes of failure to achieve stability.

If the irreducible hip dislocation is associated with a femoral head or acetabular fracture, the fracture pattern must be fully understood prior to performing open reduction of the femoral head. In this situation, the surgical approach used should be appropriate for the osteosynthesis of the associated fractures. A Kocher-Langenbeck approach is used for posterior wall, posterior column, and most transverse fractures. An ilioinguinal approach is used for anterior wall or anterior column fractures. Complex acetabular fractures may require extensile or combined surgical approaches. The reader is referred to chapter 32 for more detailed information on the treatment of acetabular fractures.

When faced with an extensive acetabular fracture and an irreducible hip, it is often most prudent to perform a limited surgical procedure to reduce the femoral head. Definitive fracture management can then be performed in three to ten days following hemodynamic stabilization of the patient and formulation of a precise surgical plan. This staged reconstruction is warranted for a number of reasons. First, major acetabular reconstruction with a prolonged anesthetic is not advisable early in the care of a critically injured patient. Second, immediate acetabular surgery carries greater blood loss and includes the potential for massive hemorrhage. Finally, reconstruction of difficult acetabular fractures requires careful preoperative analysis and planning as well as a rested surgeon for optimal results. The incision used for preliminary reduction should be planned not to compromise the subsequent definitive procedure. The reader is referred to chapter 32 for details.

Treatment of an irreducible dislocation associated

with a femoral head fracture requires precise localization of the femoral head injury. The femoral head injury is almost always located anteriorly, and therefore an anterior exposure of the hip joint will be necessary. In this situation it is advisable to approach the hip through either a direct lateral or an anterolateral approach. This will allow posterior hip exposure through the same skin incision, which may be necessary to release soft tissues that are incarcerating the femoral head. The reader is referred to chapter 43 for a more detailed discussion of the treatment of femoral head injury.

The final situation in which the femoral head will be irreducible by closed manipulation is in the instance of an ipsilateral displaced femoral neck fracture. In this situation an open manipulation of the femoral head into the acetabulum will be required, followed by internal fixation of the femoral neck fracture. This is usually best accomplished through a direct lateral approach to the hip, with the patient on a fracture table to allow for fluoroscopic control of femoral neck fracture fixation.

A patient noted to have a nondisplaced femoral neck fracture is best treated as if the hip is irreducible by closed means. Although it is possible to achieve a reduction by closed manipulation under general anesthesia, the risks of displacing the fracture and dramatically affecting the prognosis mandate fixation of the femoral neck fracture prior to reduction of the dislocation. In this situation the patient is placed on a fracture table, and a direct lateral approach to the hip is performed. It is preferable to place at least one screw across the fracture prior to manipulative reduction. Following the provisional fixation of the femoral neck fracture, a gentle reduction of the dislocation is performed by controlling the proximal femur with a bone-holding forceps. Additional parallel screws are then placed to complete the fixation of the femoral neck fracture. Further discussion of this injury is in chapter 43.

Type III

In type III dislocations, either the postreduction physical examination demonstrates an unacceptably unstable hip with no associated fractures or the postreduction imaging studies (CT or MRI) demonstrate an osteochondral or purely cartilaginous fragment or displaced labrum incarcerated between the articular surfaces of the femoral head and acetabulum.

In the circumstance of the unstable hip with no associated fractures and no incarcerated fragment preventing full seating of the femoral head, MRI is recommended. The surgeon will then be faced with several treatment options. If imaging studies reveal an extensive detachment of the acetabular labrum, then surgical

repair is considered.[117] Minor labral detachments, labral tears, or ligamentous and capsular disruptions are more suitably treated by bracing the hip with stops on the hip hinge that limit the hip to its stable arc of motion. If the hip remains unstable following six weeks of bracing, then surgical exploration and repair are indicated.

Intraarticular fragments prevent complete reduction of the femoral head and also act as an abrasive, damaging the articular surfaces. In either circumstance the fragment must be removed if it is too small to be surgically replaced. Surgical removal is best planned through a surgical approach that will bring the surgeon most directly to the fragment (Fig. 42–16).

When opening the hip, the capsulotomy must be performed on the acetabular side of the joint so as to preserve the blood supply to the femoral head. The hip joint can be distracted with the AO/ASIF distractor from iliac crest to proximal femur or with traction placed by an assistant. Be sure to remove all the fragments visualized on the CT scan. A number of fine instruments (e.g., a mosquito or tonsil forceps) are excellent aids for removing the fragments. On occasion, dislocation of the hip must be performed to allow for removal of the fragments. A forceful pulsatile lavage system may also help flush out fine debris. An intraoperative radiograph must be obtained to verify that the reduction is concentric and symmetric to the unaffected hip joint. A stability examination should be performed following reduction to determine the stable arc of hip motion. Fracture bracing can again be utilized, if necessary, for six weeks to maintain the hip in a stable arc of motion. The patient is instructed in use of crutches with a weight bearing–as-tolerated protocol and begun on aggressive rehabilitation of all hip muscle groups. Crutches may be discontinued at six weeks if good hip strength has been regained.

Arthroscopic surgery of the hip is presently in development stages but may ultimately prove to be valuable for removal of loose fragments. In this procedure a distracting force is required, again either through the use of a fracture table or the AO/ASIF femoral distractor. Fluoroscopic guidance is used for the safe placement of the arthroscope and instruments.[71,103,154] The postoperative regimen is the same as that following open arthrotomy.

Type IV

Type IV dislocations are associated with significant acetabular fractures that require reconstruction. Surgical stabilization may be warranted to restore the anterior or posterior wall to correct instability (Fig. 42–26). Displaced acetabular column fractures will require os-

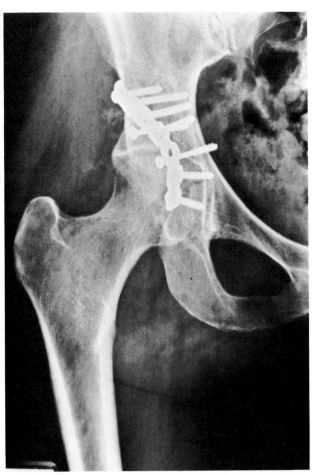

Figure 42–26

Comminuted posterosuperior acetabular fracture reconstructed with a lag screw in each main fracture fragment and buttressed with a 3.5-mm pelvic reconstruction plate. Injury films are seen in Figure 42–18.

teosynthesis to restore articular congruity. Letournel and Judet,[83] Mears,[94] and Matta[92] have demonstrated the gratifying results that can be achieved through successful acetabular osteosynthesis. The precise indications and surgical techniques for acetabular reconstruction are discussed in chapter 32.

Type V

Femoral head injuries associated with hip dislocations, as occur in type V dislocations, dramatically affect the long-term prognosis. Some investigators have recommended excision of femoral head fragments, but the results are generally poor.[39] Butler developed a prospective protocol for treatment of displaced femoral head fractures.[17] Fragments that were not anatomically reduced by closed reduction were treated by internal fixation. Nine of ten patients ultimately had excellent results (Fig. 42–27).

Mast has described a technique for elevation of femoral head depressions.[91] The depressed fragment is elevated, and cancellous bone packed deep to the subchondral bone. No internal fixation is required.

It is hoped that these more aggressive approaches to evaluation and treatment of femoral head injuries will improve the long-term prognosis. Details are discussed in chapter 43.

Assessment of Results

The functional outcome following hip dislocations ranges from an essentially normal hip both clinically and radiographically to a severely painful and degenerated joint. The applicability of numerous published series is compromised by both insufficient follow-up and small patient populations. Even those series that report all good and excellent results following type I dislocations have a high percentage of good rather than excellent results (i.e., abnormal hips) (Table 42–4).

Most series utilize the criteria established by Stewart and Milford to analyze results.[136] A determination of excellent is reserved for those hips with no symptoms, normal physical exam, and normal radiographs. A

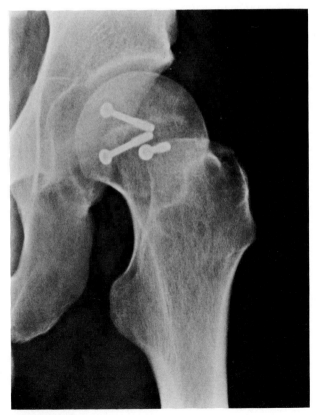

Figure 42–27

The femoral head fracture demonstrated in Figure 42–6, repaired through a direct lateral approach.

Table 42–4.

Long-Term Results and Average Follow-up Reported in Literature for Simple Posterior Hip Dislocations

Investigator	Total No. Cases	Results				Average Follow-Up (yrs)
		Excellent	Good	Fair	Poor	
Upadhyay et al., 1983[149]	74	43	13	8	10	14.65
Upadhyay et al., 1981[147]	53	33	7	4	9	12.5
Epstein, 1980[37]	134	17	70	20	27	6.5
Reigstad, 1980[118]	20	20	—	—	—	9.9
Kristensen and Stougaard, 1974[78]	11	7	4	—	—	4.5
Lamke, 1970[79]	34	—	24	8	2	6.8

Referenced articles used similar classification systems and based results on both clinical and radiographic findings.

good result is considered to be a hip with minimal stiffness after sitting, slight pain after a long day of work, no more than 25% loss of motion, and minimal arthritic changes. Fair results had mild to moderate pain, slight limp, 25% to 50% loss of motion, and moderate degenerative changes. A poor result had persistent pain and limp, marked limitation of motion, and severe joint degeneration.

Based on these guidelines, a review of the literature will highlight the difficulties encountered in treating simple type I (Thompson-Epstein type I) dislocations. Upadhyay et al. retrospectively reviewed 74 cases of simple posterior dislocations with an average 14½-year follow-up.[149] They found a 16% incidence of osteoarthritis and an 8% incidence of avascular necrosis. Manual laborers were at nearly twice the risk of developing traumatic arthritis when compared with sedentary workers. In general, most large retrospective series report a 70% to 80% good or excellent outcome in simple posterior dislocations.[37,79,91,107,135] Other series by Hunter,[69] Kristensen and Stougaard,[78] and Reigstad[118] also report good and excellent results in retrospective analyses of type I dislocations. However, in these studies the length of follow-up varied, and the total number of patients reviewed was only 66.

When posterior dislocations are associated with femoral head fractures or acetabular fractures, the associated fractures generally compromise the outcome. Epstein reported no excellent results in his extensive review of fracture-dislocations of the hip (type II–type V, Thompson-Epstein classification) (Table 42–5).[34,36,37,142]

Anterior dislocations of the hip have been noted to have a high incidence of associated femoral head injuries. DeLee et al. reported on a series of 15 anterior dislocations, 13 of which were noted to have femoral

head injuries.[27] The only patients with excellent results in these series were those without femoral head injuries. Ten of 15 patients developed traumatic arthritis. Among the five with radiographically normal hips were two without fractures, two with indentations less than 4 mm, and one with a 6-mm indentation. Epstein and Harvey[38] and, later, Epstein[37] reported on a series of anterior hip dislocations and noted only 70% good and excellent results. There were eight associated femoral head fractures in this series.

Complications

AVASCULAR NECROSIS

Avascular necrosis of the femoral head following hip dislocations has been reported to occur in 1%–2% to 15%–17% of injuries.[93,97,107,114,136] Numerous investigators have reported that the risk of avascular necrosis increases when the hip remains dislocated for a period of time. This threshold time has been reported to be from 6 to 24 hours.[36,60,68,101,110,135,144] More recent investigators suggest that the incidence of avascular necrosis is much less than previously reported and may in fact result from the initial injury and not from a prolonged dislocation. However, no well-controlled studies support this hypothesis, and thus prompt reduction is still considered vital. Avoiding this complication is paramount and may make the difference between a normal, functioning hip and a severely painful and degenerating hip.

TRAUMATIC ARTHRITIS

Traumatic arthritis is the most frequent long-term complication of hip dislocations. The symptoms can

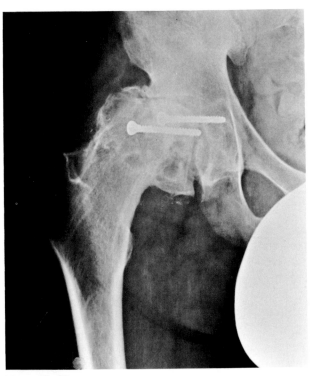

Figure 42-28

Traumatic arthritis following a posterior fracture-dislocation of the hip.

vary greatly. Those individuals most severely affected may ultimately be unable to remain gainfully employed; this often occurs at an early, productive age. Upadhyay reported a 14½-year follow-up of 74 cases of apparently uncomplicated hip dislocations with no associated fractures.[149] Surprisingly, 16% developed traumatic arthritis, and an additional 8% developed arthritis secondary to avascular necrosis. Manual laborers were nearly twice as likely as sedentary workers to develop traumatic arthritis.

The incidence of traumatic arthritis becomes dramatically higher when dislocations with associated acetabular fractures are reviewed (Fig. 42-28). Upadhyay and Moulton report incidences as high as 88% in those dislocations associated with severe acetabular fractures.[147] Epstein has also reported much higher rates of traumatic arthritis in this group of injuries (Table 42-5).[37]

Matta,[92] Mears,[94] and Letournel[82] have all reported series of acetabular fractures treated by open reduction and internal fixation. In each series good to excellent results were reported when reduction within 3 mm was obtained. These impressive results by separate investigators demonstrate that the improved diagnostic and surgical approaches outlined in this chapter as well as in

chapters 32 and 43 can lead to a dramatic improvement in long-term results.

RECURRENT DISLOCATION

Recurrent dislocation of the hip is exceedingly rare. The literature related to this subject is limited to simple case reports, with approximately half involving children and half involving adults.[24,47,54,58,63,76,86,87,100,115,117,121,132,139,145] The cases reported include only pure dislocations, without associated femoral head or acetabular fractures. Many of the initial injuries described in these reports are secondary to relatively minor low-energy injuries such as sporting injuries, simple falls, and falls off tricycles.[47,54,63,76,86,87,100,117,132,139]

Arthrograms and CT arthrograms have been successful diagnostic modalities in demonstrating capsular defects and large sacular expansions of the capsule.[54,76,87,122] CT arthrography has an additional benefit of demonstrating cartilaginous fragments not visualized on plain CT. MRI may augment these modalities because of its ability to detect cartilaginous fragments, fluid-filled regions, and soft tissue injuries.

Upadhyay et al. have demonstrated a correlation of decreased femoral anteversion in patients who have suffered posterior dislocations when compared with a control group.[148] They proposed that people are prone to posterior hip dislocation secondary to their relative retroversion. This anatomic variation could also be a predisposing factor in recurrent hip dislocations. Dall et al. reported the case of an adult with recurrent anterior hip dislocation.[24] Operative exploration revealed "moderate" anteversion that was treated by a derotation osteotomy. This report suggests that osseous anatomic variations could predispose to acute and recurrent dislocations.

Surgical exploration usually reveals a capsular defect with a large synovial sac. The capsular defects and synovial evaginations were found at different muscular intervals between the short rotators of the hip. The femoral head was always visualized through this sac and could usually be dislocated into it. Rashleigh-Belcher reported a "Bankart type" lesion in a patient with recurrent dislocation. The intraoperative findings noted a posterosuperior labral detachment.[117] Nelson has reported a similar labral detachment.[100]

Various surgical reconstructive procedures have been described to treat recurrent dislocations. Most authors describe imbrication procedures at the site of capsular tear and redundancy. The piriformis tendon has been reattached in the area of the defect to support the repair. Lutter[87] and Rashleigh-Belcher[117] have described the use of a bone block to buttress the area with the capsular or labral deficiency.

Table 42–5.

Long-Term Results Reported in the Literature for Posterior Hip Dislocations Associated With Acetabular Fractures or Femoral Head Fractures

Investigator	Total No. Cases	Results				Average Follow-Up (yrs)
		Excellent	Good	Fair	Poor	
Upadhyay et al., 1981[147]	28	5	4	4	15	12.5
Epstein, 1980[37]						
Closed reduction						
Dislocation with acetabular fracture	102	0	13	33	56	6.5
Dislocation with femoral head fracture	14	0	0	6	8	
Epstein, 1980						
Closed followed by open reduction						
Dislocation with acetabular fracture	78	0	34	15	29	6.5
Dislocation with femoral head fracture	15	0	5	3	7	6.5
Primary open reduction						
Dislocation with acetabular fracture	66	0	42	12	12	6.5
Dislocation with femoral head fracture	17	0	8	2	7	6.5
Reigstad, 1980[118] Mixed treatment						
Dislocation with acetabular fracture	22	16	—	6	0	9.9
Dislocation with femoral head fracture	5	2	—	3	0	9.9
Kristensen and Stougaard, 1974[78]						
Closed reduction, skeletal traction						
Dislocation with acetabular fracture	29	8	15	4	2	4.5
Dislocation with femoral head fracture	5	1	1	1	2	4.5

The dislocations associated with acetabular fractures have been grouped together, regardless of the fracture pattern, in an effort to compare the reported results in various series.

Although the operative findings in these numerous case reports are surprisingly similar, the surgeon should search for predisposing osseous abnormalities. This recommendation is supported by Upadhyay's sonographic studies as well as by the fact that the majority of individuals reported had relatively minor accidents leading to the first episode of dislocation.[148] In addition, all patients suffering hip dislocations are presumed to suffer capsular tears at the time of the initial dislocation. Possibly, patients with less-than-average anteversion place abnormal stresses on the healing capsule, resulting in capsular redundancy and laxity.

Preoperative evaluation should include MRI to evaluate for intraarticular chondral fragments, labral detachments, and capsular outpockets filled with synovial fluid. Femoral anteversion should be measured by one of the described radiographic techniques.[61,109,119] CT scanning may demonstrate deficiency of the anterior or posterior acetabular wall. The acetabular stress patterns as described by Bombelli must be carefully examined; abnormalities may be representative of acetabular dysplasia.[9] If no obvious osseous abnormality is uncovered, then repair of a labral detachment capsular plication or placement of a posterior bone block may be performed, as described in various case reports. Each report claims no recurrence of a dislocation, but follow-up time is not sufficient, and the series are not large enough to recommend a specific procedure.[87,100,117]

MISSED AND DELAYED DIAGNOSES

Failure to obtain adequate routine radiographs of the pelvis in the multiply injured patient may delay diagnosis of hip dislocation. This delays treatment and places the patient at increased risk for developing avascular necrosis, sciatic nerve injury, joint stiffness, and traumatic arthritis.[36,37,135,136]

Nixon has described the treatment of three patients following delayed diagnosis of 4 to 13 weeks. These three patients were treated with open reduction, and all achieved excellent clinical results.[102]

Gupta and Shravat described the treatment of seven hip dislocations in which the diagnosis was delayed for 26 to 75 days.[53] This group of patients was treated with skeletal traction until length was achieved, and then the legs were brought into abduction. One hip associated with extensive pelvic fracture failed to reduce by this method. Oni et al.[104] and Sarkar[128] described a similar technique using three weeks of traction followed by open reduction if closed reduction is not accomplished.

Garrett et al. report far less encouraging results in a group of 39 dislocations that had not been treated for a period ranging from three days to nine years after injury.[46] Eleven of 18 patients who had successful closed or open reduction developed avascular necrosis within one year. Six hips that were left dislocated all had poor results. The best results occurred in the group of patients who underwent primary reconstructive procedures.[46] Malkin and Tauber reported two cases that were treated with primary total hip arthroplasty using the femoral head to reconstruct the deficient posterior acetabulum.[89]

Despite the guarded prognosis resulting from a delay in treatment of hip dislocations, an aggressive attempt should be made to salvage the hip in a young patient. Use of skeletal traction has been successful in a number of patients and seems to be a prudent approach. Arthrodesis or total joint arthroplasty, if necessary, can be performed at a future time.

Obviously, optimal treatment for the delayed diagnosis of hip dislocation is to prevent it by maintaining a high level of suspicion to avoid missing the diagnosis. All unconscious and multiply injured patients must have an AP pelvic radiograph. Any radiographic uncertainty or abnormality should be immediately followed up with a CT scan.

SCIATIC NERVE INJURY

Sciatic nerve injuries occur in 8% to 19% of hip dislocations. As previously mentioned, this is usually caused by stretching of the nerve from a posteriorly dislocated femoral head or from a displaced fracture fragment.

The prognosis for nerve recovery is extremely variable and unpredictable. Epstein has reported a 43% incidence of recovery, whereas Gregory reports a 40% full recovery and 30% partial recovery.[37,52]

Patients with significant neurologic injury must have meticulous nursing care to prevent skin breakdown in the areas with sensory compromise. The patient should be placed in a well-padded neutral ankle splint to prevent the rapid onset of a fixed equinus deformity. Electromyographic (EMG) and nerve conduction studies are indicated at three to four weeks for baseline information and prognostic guidance. In addition, the precise level of the neurologic injury, including possible lumbosacral plexus injury, can be determined.

Because of the variability of nerve recovery, no definitive surgical procedure addressing the disability should be considered for at least one year. Patients tolerate a lightweight ankle/foot orthosis (AFO) well with only slight disability. Follow-up EMGs can be obtained at three months to evaluate for electrical evidence of repair. If no clinical or electrical improvement is seen by one year, then a posterior tibial transfer may be considered.[11] Often patients would rather continue with the AFO rather than undergo an additional surgical procedure that requires immobilization and extensive rehabilitation. Such transfers are less successful if there is significant weakness of the tibialis posterior muscle from injury to the tibial portion of the sciatic nerve, which may not be demonstrated by a casual examination.

SURGICAL COMPLICATIONS

Infection

Postoperative infection rates are relatively low in the operative treatment of simple dislocations or minor posterior wall fractures. More extensive fractures requiring large surgical exposures and prolonged operative time have an increased incidence of infection. Average rates of infection are 3% to 5% for the Kocher-Langenbeck and anterolateral approaches and 5% to 10% for the extended iliofemoral or ilioinguinal approaches. Prophylactic antibiotics are routinely used for 24 hours. Suction drains are left in place, often for three to five days, until drainage has dropped to a minimal amount.

If an infection develops, immediate surgical irrigation and drainage is carried out. A superficial hematoma can be drained without opening the deeper layers. The wounds are packed open. If no implants or bones are exposed, the dressings are changed daily, and a delayed wound closure is performed in five to seven days. In the event of exposed bone or implants, dressing changes are performed in the operating room every two to three days and delayed closure is performed at five to seven days. Bacteria-specific antibiotics are used for 10 to 14 days, or longer if necessary.

Sciatic Nerve Injury

Sciatic nerve injury in extensive posterior approaches to the hip is reported to occur in approximately 11% of cases.[83] This is usually temporary neurapraxia, and the treatment should be the same as outlined for immediate sciatic nerve injuries. Intraoperative measures should be undertaken to limit the occurrence. The knee should remain flexed throughout the procedure, and whenever possible, the hip should be extended. When using a Hohmann retractor behind the posterior column, care must be taken to maintain the retractor parallel to the nerve. As the retractor rotates, its edge will press against the nerve and may injure it.

Late Sciatic Nerve Palsy

A number of cases of delayed sciatic neurapraxia have been reported. This is thought to be secondary to a hematoma, to scar formation, or to heterotopic ossification.[28,75,83] I have revised an attempted open reduction and internal fixation of a posterior fracture-dislocation of the hip at two weeks and found the sciatic nerve encased in scar. Decompression of the nerve resulted in immediate return of nerve function postoperatively.

The physician must carefully watch for development of sciatic neurapraxia. Any significant neurologic deficit should be treated with an immediate nerve exploration and decompression. The few cases reported with delayed exploration had no significant return of nerve function.

Heterotopic Ossification

Heterotopic ossification is primarily associated with acetabular fractures and not with simple dislocations. The exception to this rule is the patient with a head injury.[45] The most effective prophylactic measures are low-dose radiation and indomethacin. The present recommendation for indomethacin prophylaxis is 25 mg t.i.d. for six weeks (see chapter 32).

Thromboembolism

No effective method for preventing thromboembolic disease has been convincingly established for trauma patients. Low-dose warfarin is the method of choice following total joint arthroplasty. If possible, patients with hip dislocations should be up in a chair on the first postreduction day if the hip is stable or on the first postoperative day if the hip was unstable. Physical therapy is instituted to work on ankle pump exercises and quadriceps-setting exercises. Patients are all placed in compressive stockings and in sequential compressive boots while in bed. In the event of a pulmonary embolism, the patients are appropriately treated with anticoagulants, first with heparin and then warfarin, unless the risk of bleeding is excessive. Vena caval filters may on occasion have to be considered in the immediate preoperative period or to control continued showering of emboli.

Conclusion

The treatment of dislocations of the hip presents a significant clinical challenge to the physician. Reports to date in the literature have indicated a rather high incidence of long-term disability. The routine use of radiographic imaging modalities followed by appropriate management of hip joint widening, instability, and articular incongruity may improve long-term results. Confirmation of this approach will require further studies.

REFERENCES

1. Allis, O.H. An Inquiry Into the Difficulties Encountered in the Reduction of Dislocations of the Hip. Philadelphia, Dornan Printer, 1986.
2. Armstrong, J.R. Traumatic dislocation of the hip joint. Review of one hundred and one disorders. J Bone Joint Surg 30B:430–445, 1948.
3. Baird, R.A.; Schobert, W.E.; Pais, M.J.; et al. Radiographic identification of loose bodies in the traumatized hip joint. Radiology 145:661–665, 1982.
4. Beaton, L.E.; Anson, B.J. The relation of the sciatic nerve and of its subdivisions to the piriformis muscle. Anat Rec 70(1):1–5, 1937.
5. Bernard, R.F.; Christel, R.S.; Meearier, A.; et al. Role of articular incongruence and cartilage thickness in hip joint stresses distribution: A biphasic and two dimensional photoelastic study. Acta Orthop Belgia 48(2):335–344, 1982.
6. Bigelow, H.J. Luxations of the hip joint. Boston Med Surg J 5:1–3, 1870.
7. Birkett, J. Description of a dislocation of the head of the femur complicated with its fractures. Trans Med Chir Soc 52:133, 1869.
8. Bisese, J.H. MRI: A Teaching File Approach. New York, McGraw-Hill, 1988, pp. 203–305.
9. Bombelli, R. Osteoarthritis of the Hip. New York, Springer-Verlag, 1983, pp. 13–31.
10. Bosce, A.R. The range of active abduction and lateral rotation of the hip joint of men. J Bone Joint Surg 14:325–331, 1932.
11. Brand, P.W. The insensitive foot (including leprosy). In: Jahss, M.H., ed. Disorders of the Foot. Philadelphia, W.B. Saunders, 1982, pp. 1281–1282.
12. Brav, E.A. Traumatic dislocation of the hip. Army experience and results over a twelve year period. J Bone Joint Surg 44A:1115–1134, 1962.
13. Bromberg, E.; Weiss, A.B. Posterior fracture-dislocation of the hip. South Med J 70:8–11, 1977.
14. Brown, T.D.; Ferguson, A.B. The effect of hip contact aberrations on stress patterns within the human femoral head. Ann Biomed Eng 8:75–92, 1980.
15. Bucholz, R.W.; Wheeless, G. Irreducible posterior fracture-dislocations of the hip. The role of the iliofemoral ligament and the rectus femoris muscle. Clin Orthop 167:118–122, 1982.

16. Buckwalter, J.A. Articular cartilage. AAOS Instr Course Lect 1983 32:349–370.

17. Butler, J.E. Pipkin type II fractures of the femoral head. J Bone Joint Surg 63A:1292–1296, 1981.

18. Butler, J.E. Personal communication, Houston, Texas, 1986.

19. Calkins, M.S.; Zych, G.; Latta, L.; et al. Computed tomography evaluation of stability: Posterior fracture dislocation of the hip. Clin Orthop 227:152–163, 1988.

20. Canale, S.T.; Manugian, A.H. Irreducible traumatic dislocations of the hip. J Bone Joint Surg 61A:7–14, 1979.

21. Chakraborti, S.; Miller, I.M. Dislocation of the hip associated with fracture of the femoral head. Injury 7:134–142, 1975.

22. Crelin, E.S. An experimental study of hip stability in human newborn cadavers. Yale Biol Med 49:109–121, 1976.

23. Crock, H.V. An atlas of the arterial supply of the head and neck of the femur in man. Clin Orthop 152:17–27, 1980.

24. Dall, D.; MacNab, I.; Gross, A. Recurrent anterior dislocations of the hip. J Bone Joint Surg 52A:574–576, 1970.

25. Dameron, T.B. Bucket-handle tear of acetabular labrum accompanying posterior dislocation of the hip. J Bone Joint Surg 41A:131, 134, 1959.

26. DeLee, J.C. Dislocations and fracture-dislocations of the hip. In: Rockwood, C.A.; Green, D.P., eds. Fractures and Dislocations, ed. 2. Philadelphia, J.B. Lippincott, 1984, pp. 1287–1327.

27. DeLee, J.C.; Evans, J.A.; Thomas, J. Anterior dislocation of the hip and associated femoral head fractures. J Bone Joint Surg 62A:960–964, 1980.

28. Derian, P.S.; Bibighaus, A.J. Sciatic nerve entrapment by ectopic bone after posterior fracture-dislocation of the hip. South Med J 67:209–210, 1974.

29. Donohue, J.M.; Buss, D.; Oegema, T.R.; Thompson, R.C. The effects of indirect blunt trauma on adult canine articular cartilage. J Bone Joint Surg 65A:948–957, 1983.

30. Dowd, G.S.E.; Johnson, R. Successful conservative treatment of a fracture-dislocation of the femoral head. A case report. J Bone Joint Surg 61A:1244–1246, 1979.

31. Dussault, R.G.; Beauregard, G.; Fauteaux, P.; et al. Femoral head defect following anterior hip dislocation. Radiology 135:627–629, 1980.

32. Ehtisham, S.M.A. Traumatic dislocation of the hip joint with fracture of shaft of femur on the same side. J Trauma 16:196–205, 1976.

33. Eisenberg, K.S.; Scheft, D.J.; Murray, W.R. Posterior dislocation of the hip producing lumbosacral nerve root avulsion. A case report. J Bone Joint Surg 54A:1083–1086, 1972.

34. Epstein, H.C. Traumatic dislocations of the hip. Clin Orthop 92:116–142, 1973.

35. Epstein, H.C. Traumatic anterior and simple posterior dislocations of the hip in adults and children. AAOS Instr Course Lect 22:115–145, 1973.

36. Epstein, H.C. Posterior fracture-dislocations of the hip: Long-term follow-up. J Bone Joint Surg 56A:1103–1127, 1974.

37. Epstein, H.C. Traumatic Dislocation of the Hip. Baltimore, Williams and Wilkins, 1980.

38. Epstein, H.C.; Harvey, J.P. Traumatic anterior dislocations of the hip. Management and results. An analysis of fifty-five cases. J Bone Joint Surg 54A:1561–1562, 1972.

39. Epstein, H.C.; Wiss, D.A.; Coze, L. Posterior fracture-dislocation of the hip with fractures of the femoral head. Clin Orthop 201:9–17, 1985.

40. Fabian, T.C.; Mangiante, E.C.; White, T.J.; et al. A prospective study of 91 patients undergoing both computed tomography and peritoneal lavage following blunt abdominal trauma. J Trauma 26:602–608, 1986.

41. Fernandes, A. Traumatic posterior dislocation of hip joint with a fracture of the head and neck of the femur on the same side: A case report. Injury 12:487–490, 1981.

42. Fina, C.P.; Kelly, P.J. Dislocations of the hip with fractures of the proximal femur. J Trauma 10:77–87, 1970.

43. Frankel, V.H.; Pugh, J.W. Biomechanics of the hip. In: Tronzo, R.G., ed. Surgery of the Hip Joint. Philadelphia, Lea and Febiger, 1973, pp. 115–131.

44. Funsten, R.V.; Kinser, P.; Frankel, C.J. Dashboard dislocation of the hip: A report of twenty cases of traumatic dislocations. J Bone Joint Surg 20:124–132, 1938.

45. Garland, D.E.; Miller, G. Fractures and dislocations about the hip in head injured adults. Clin Orthop 186:154–158, 1984.

46. Garrett, J.C.; Epstein, H.C.; Harris, W.H.; et al. Treatment of unreduced traumatic posterior dislocations of the hip. J Bone Joint Surg 61A:2–6, 1979.

47. Gaul, R.W. Recurrent traumatic dislocation of the hip in children. Clin Orthop 90:107–109, 1977.

48. Gillespie, W.J. The incidence and pattern of knee injury associated with dislocation of the hip. J Bone Joint Surg 57B:376–378, 1975.

49. Glimcher, M.J.; Kenzora, J.E. The biology of osteonecrosis of the human femoral head and its clinical implications: Chap. I tissue biology. Clin Orthop 138:284–309, 1979.

50. Glimcher, M.J.; Kenzora, J.E. The pathologic changes in the femoral head as an organ and in the hip joint. 139:283–312, 1979.

51. Glimcher, M.J.; Kenzora, J.E. Chap. III. Discussion of the etiology and genesis of the pathologic sequelae: Comments and treatment. 140:273–312, 1979.

52. Gregory, C.F. Early complications of dislocation and fracture-dislocations of the hip joint. AAOS Instr Course Lect 22:105–114, 1973.

53. Gupta, R.C.; Shravat, B.P. Reduction of neglected traumatic dislocation of the hip by heavy traction. J Bone Joint Surg 59A:249–251, 1977.

54. Guyer, B.; Lainsohn, E.M. Recurrent anterior dislocation of the hip: Case report with arthrographic findings. Skeletal Radiol 10:262–264, 1983.

55. Hardinge, K. The direct lateral approach to the hip. J Bone Joint Surg 64B:17–19, 1982.

56. Harley, J.C.; Mack, L.A.; Winquist, R.A. CT of acetabular fractures: Comparison with conventional radiography. AJR 138:413–417, 1982.

57. Harty, M. The anatomy of the hip joint. In: Tronzo, R.G., ed. Surgery of the Hip Joint, ed 2. New York, Springer-Verlag, 1984, pp. 45–74.

58. Heikkinen, E.S.; Sulamaa, R. Recurrent dislocation of the hip: Report of two children. Acta Orthop Scand 42:58–62, 1971.

59. Helal, B.; Skevis, X. Unrecognized dislocation of the hip in fractures of the femoral shaft. J Bone Joint Surg 49B:293–300, 1967.

60. Herndon, J.H.; Aufranc, O.E. Avascular necrosis of the femoral head in the adult. A review of its incidence in a variety of conditions. Clin Orthop 86:43–62, 1977.

61. Herrlin, K.; Ekelund, L. Radiographic measurements of the femoral neck anteversion. Comparison of two simplified procedures. Acta Orthop Scand 54:141–147, 1983.

62. Hoaglund, F.T.; Low, W.D. Anatomy of the femoral neck and head with comparative data from caucasians and Hong Kong Chinese. Clin Orthop 152:10–16, 1980.

63. Hollingdale, J.P.; Aichroth, P.M. Recurrent post-traumatic dislocation of the hip in children. J R Soc Med 74:545–546, 1981.

64. Hollingshead, W.H. Anatomy for Surgeons, Vol. 3, ed. 3. Philadelphia, Harper and Row, 1982, pp. 563–732.

65. Hoppenfeld, S. Physical Examination of the Extremities. New York, Appleton-Century-Crofts, 1976, pp. 155–159.

66. Hoppenfeld, S.; deBoer, P. Surgical Exposures in Orthopaedics. Philadelphia, J.B. Lippincott, 1984, pp. 301–356.

67. Hougaard, K.; Lindequist, S.; Nielsen, L.B. Computerized tomography after posterior dislocation of the hip. J Bone Joint Surg 69B:556–557, 1987.

68. Hougaard, K.; Thomsen, P.B. Traumatic posterior dislocation of the hip—prognostic factors influencing the incidence of avascular necrosis of the femoral head. Arch Orthop Trauma Surg 106:32–35, 1986.

69. Hunter, G.A. Posterior dislocation and fracture-dislocations of the hip. A review of fifty-seven patients. J Bone Joint Surg 51B:38–44, 1969.

70. Johnson, K.D.; Cadambi, A.; Seibert, B. Incidence of adult respiratory distress syndrome in patients with multiple musculoskeletal injuries. Effect of early operative stabilization of fractures. J Trauma 25:375–383, 1985.

71. Johnson, L.L. Arthroscopic Surgery: Principles and Practice. St. Louis, C.V. Mosby, 1986, pp. 1491–1516.

72. Judet, R.; Judet, J.; LeTournel, E. Fractures of the acetabulum: Classification and surgical approaches for open reduction. J Bone Joint Surg 46A:1615–1646, 1964.

73. Kelly, R.P.; Yarbrough, S.H. Posterior fracture-dislocation of the femoral head with retained medial head fragment. J Trauma 11:97–108, 1971.

74. Klasen, H.J.; Binndndijk, B. Fracture of the neck of the femur associated with posterior dislocation of the hip. J Bone Joint Surg 66B:45–48, 1984.

75. Kleiman, S.G.; Stevens, J.; Kolb, L.; Pankovich, A. Late sciatic nerve palsy following posterior fracture-dislocation of the hip. J Bone Joint Surg 53A:781–782, 1971.

76. Klein, A.; Sumner, T.E.; Volberg, F.M.; Orbon, R.J. Combined CT-arthrography in recurrent traumatic hip dislocation. AJR 138:963–964, 1982.

77. Kleinberg, S. Aseptic necrosis of the femoral head following traumatic dislocation. Arch Surg 39:637–646, 1939.

78. Kristensen, O.; Stougaard, J. Traumatic dislocation of the hip: results of conservative treatment. Acta Orthop Scand 45:206–212, 1974.

79. Lamke, L. Traumatic dislocations of the hip; Follow-up on cases from Stockholm area. Acta Orthop Scand 41:188–198, 1970.

80. Larson, C.B. Fracture-dislocations of the hip. Clin Orthop 92:147–154, 1973.

81. Lawson, T.L.; Middleton, W.D. The hip. In: Middleton, W.D.; Lawson, T.L., eds. Anatomy and MRI of the Joints. A Multiplanar Atlas. New York, Raven Press, 1989, pp. 153–204.

82. Letournel, E. Fractures of the Acetabulum and Pelvis. Fourth Course and Workshop. Paris, 1986.

83. Letournel, E.; Judet, R. Fractures of the Acetabulum. New York, Springer-Verlag, 1981.

84. Levin, P. Femoral head fracture associated with a posterior hip dislocation in a restrained passenger. Case report. 1990 (in preparation).

85. Levin, P. Posterior fracture dislocation of hip in a restrained passenger. Case report. 1990 (in preparation).

86. Liebenberg, F.; Dommisse, G.F. Recurrent post-traumatic dislocation of the hip. J Bone Joint Surg 51B:632–637, 1969.

87. Lutter, L.D. Post-traumatic hip redislocation. J Bone Joint Surg 55A:391–399, 1977.

88. Mack, L.A.; Harvey, J.D.; Winquist, R.A. CT of acetabular fractures: Analysis of fracture patterns. AJR 138:407–412, 1982.

89. Malkin, C.; Tauber, C. Total hip arthroplasty and acetabular bone grafting for unreduced fracture-dislocation of the hip. Clin Orthop 201:57–59, 1985.

90. Mankin, H.J. The response of articular cartilage to mechanical injury. J Bone Joint Surg 64A:460–466, 1982.

91. Mast, J. Fractures of the Acetabulum and Pelvis. Fourth Course and Workshop. Paris, 1986.

92. Matta, J.M. Fractures of the Acetabulum and Pelvis. Fourth Course and Workshop. Paris, 1986.

93. Mears, D.C. Personal communication, 1986.

94. Mears, D.C. Fractures of the Acetabulum and Pelvis. Fourth Course and Workshop. Paris, 1986.

95. Meller, Y.; Tennenbaum, Y.; Torok, G. Subcapital fracture of neck of femur with complete posterior dislocation of the hip. J Trauma 22:327–329, 1982.

96. Meyers, M.H. Anatomy of the hip. In: Fractures of the Hip. Chicago, Year Book Medical, 1985, pp. 12–22.

97. Meyers, M.H.; Telfer, N.; Moore, T.M. Determination of the vascularity of the femoral head with technetium 99 mm-sulfur colloid: Diagnostic and prognostic significance. J Bone Joint Surg 59A:658–664, 1977.

98. Mitchell, N.; Shepard, N. Healing of articular cartilage in intra-articular fractures in rabbits. J Bone Joint Surg 62A(4):628–634, 1980.

99. Mundale, M.O.; Hislop, H.J.; Rabidean, R.J.; Kottke, F.J. Evaluation of extension at hip. Arch Phys Med 37:75–80, 1956.

100. Nelson, C.L. Traumatic recurrent dislocation of the hip: Report of a case. J Bone Joint Surg 52A:128–130, 1970.

101. Nicoll, E.A. Proceedings and reports of councils and associations: Traumatic dislocation of the hip joint. J Bone Joint Surg 34B:503–505, 1952.

102. Nixon, J.R. Late open reduction of traumatic dislocation of the hip: Report of three cases. J Bone Joint Surg 58B:41–43, 1976.

103. Nordt, W.; Giangarra, C.E.; Levy, I.M.J.; Habermann, E.T. Arthroscopic retrieval of entrapped debris following dislocation of a total hip arthroplasty. Arthroscopy 3(3):196–198, 1987.

104. Oni, O.O.A.; Orhewee, F.A.; Keswani, H. The treatment of old unreduced traumatic dislocations of the hip. Injury 15:219–223, 1984.

105. Ordway, C.B.; Xeller, C.F. Transverse computerized axial tomography of patients with posterior dislocation of the hip. J Trauma 24:76–79, 1989.

106. Paterson, I. The torn acetabular labrum. A block to reduction of a dislocated hip. J Bone Joint Surg 39B:306–309, 1957.

107. Paus, B. Traumatic dislocation of the hip. Late results in 76 cases. Acta Orthop Scand 21:99–112, 1951.

108. Peitzman, A.B.; Makaroon, M.S.; Slasky, B.S.; Ritter, P. Prospective study of computed tomography in initial management of blunt abdominal trauma. J Trauma 26:585–592, 1986.

109. Peterson, H.A.; Krassen, R.A.; McLeod, R.A.; Hoffman, A.D. The use of computerized tomography in dislocation of the hip and femoral neck anteversion in children. J Bone Joint Surg 63B:198–208, 1981.

110. Pietratesa, C.A.; Hoffman, J.R. Traumatic dislocation of the hip. JAMA 249:3342–3346, 1983.

111. Pipkin, G. Treatment of grade IV fracture-dislocation of the hip. J Bone Joint Surg 39A:1027–1042, 1957.

112. Polesky, R.E.; Polesky, F.A. Intrapelvic dislocation of the femoral head following anterior dislocation of the hip. J Bone Joint Surg 54A:1097–1098, 1972.

113. Pringle, J.H. Traumatic dislocation of the hip joint. An experimental study on the cadaver. Glasgow Med J 21:25–40, 1943.

114. Proctor, H. Dislocations of the hip joint (excluding central dislocations) and their complications. Injury 5:1–12, 1973.

115. Provenzano, M.P.; Holmes, P.F.; Tullos, H.S. Atraumatic recurrent dislocation of the hip: A case report. J Bone Joint Surg 69A:938–940, 1987.

116. Radin, E.L.; Ehrlich, M.G.; Chernack, R.; et al. Effect of repetitive impulsive loading on the knee joints of rabbits. Clin Orthop 131:288–293, 1978.

117. Rashleigh-Belcher, H.J.C.; Cannon, S.R. Recurrent dislocation of the hip with a "Bankart-type" lesion. J Bone Joint Surg 68B:398–399, 1986.

118. Reigstad, A. Traumatic dislocation of the hip. J Trauma 20:603–606, 1980.

119. Reikeras, O.; Bjerkreim, I.; Kolbenstuedt, A. Anteversion of the acetabulum in patients with idiopathic increased anteversion of the femoral neck. Acta Orthop Scand 53:847–852, 1982.

120. Repo, R.V.; Finley, J.B. Survival of articular cartilage after controlled impact. J Bone Joint Surg 59A(8):1068–1076, 1977.

121. Roberts, W. The locking mechanism at the hip joint. Anat Rec 147:321–324, 1963.

122. Roberts, J.M.; Taylor, J.; Burke, S. Recurrent dislocation of the hip in congenital indifference to pain. J Bone Joint Surg 62A:829–831, 1980.

123. Roeder, L.F.; DeLee, J.C. Femoral head fractures associated with posterior hip dislocations. Clin Orthop 147:121–130, 1980.

124. Rosenthal, R.E.; Coker, W.L. Posterior fracture-dislocation of the hip. J Trauma 19:572–581, 1979.

125. Rowe, C.R.; Lowell, J.D. Prognosis of fractures of the acetabulum. J Bone Joint Surg 43A:30–59, 1961.

126. Sadler, A.H.; Distefano, M. Anterior dislocation of the hip with ipsilateral basicervical fracture. J Bone Joint Surg 67A:326–329, 1985.

127. Salter, R.B.; Simmonds, D.F.; Malcolm, B.W.; et al. The biologic effects of continuous passive motion on the healing of full-thickness defects in articular cartilage. An experimental investigation in the rabbit. J Bone Joint Surg 62A:1232–1251, 1980.

128. Sarkar, S.D. Delayed open reduction of traumatic dislocation of the hip: A case report and historical review. Clin Orthop 186:38–41, 1989.

129. Sarmiento, A.; Laird, C.A. Posterior fracture-dislocation of the femoral head. Clin Orthop 92:143–146, 1973.

130. Sauser, D.B.; Billimoria, P.E.; Rouse, G.A.; Mudge, K. CT evaluation of hip trauma. AJR 135:269–274, 1980.

131. Schoenecker, P.L.; Manske, P.R.; Sertl, G.O. Traumatic hip dislocation with ipsilateral femoral shaft fractures. Clin Orthop 130:233–238, 1978.

132. Scudese, V.A. Traumatic anterior hip redislocation. A case report. Clin Orthop 88:60–63, 1972.

133. Stein, H. Computerized tomography for ascertaining osteocartilaginous intra-articular (slice) fractures of the femoral head. Isr J Med Sci 19:180–184, 1983.

134. Stewart, M.J. Management of fractures of the head of the femur complicated by dislocation of the hip. Orthop Clin North Am 5:793–798, 1974.

135. Stewart, M.J.; McCarroll, H.R.; Mulhollan, J.S. Fracture-dislocation of the hip. Acta Orthop Scand 46:507–525, 1975.

136. Stewart, M.J.; Milford, L.W. Fracture-dislocation of the hip. J Bone Joint Surg 36A:315–342, 1954.

137. Stimson, L.A. A Treatise on Fractures. Philadelphia, H.C. Leas Son, 1883.

138. Stoller, D.W. Personal communication. Los Angeles, 1989.

139. Sullivan, C.R.; Bickel, W.H.; Lipscomb, P.R. Recurrent dislocation of the hip. J Bone Joint Surg 37A:1266–1270, 1955.

140. Suraci, A.J. Distribution and severity of injuries associated with hip dislocations secondary to motor vehicle accidents. J Trauma 26:458–460, 1986.

141. Suzuki, Y. Studies on repair tissue of injured articular cartilage; Biochemical and biomechanical properties. Nippon Seiheigeka Gakkai Zasshi 57:741–752, 1983.

142. Thompson, V.P.; Epstein, H.C. Traumatic dislocation of the hip. J Bone Joint Surg 33A:746–778, 1951.

143. Thorpe, M.; Swiontkowski, M.F.; Seiler, J.; Hansen, S.T. Operative management of femoral head fractures. Orthop Trans 13:51, 1989.

144. Toni, A.; Gulino, G.; Baldini, N.; Gulino, F. Clinical and Radiographic long term results of acetabular fractures associated with dislocations of the hip. Ital J Orthop Traumatol 11:443–454, 1985.

145. Townsend, R.G.; Edwards, G.E.; Bazant, F.J. Post-traumatic recurrent dislocation of the hip without fracture. J Bone Joint Surg 51B:194, 1969.

146. Trueta, J.; Harrison, M.H.M. The normal vascular anatomy of the femoral head in adult man. J Bone Joint Surg 35B:442–461, 1953.

147. Upadhyay, S.S.; Moulton, A. The long-term results of traumatic posterior dislocation of the hip. J Bone Joint Surg 63B:548–551, 1981.

148. Upadhyay, S.S.; Moulton, A.; Burwell, R.G. Biological factors predisposing to traumatic posterior dislocation of the hip. J Bone Joint Surg 67B:232–236, 1985.

149. Upadhyay, S.S.; Moulton, A.; Srikrishnamurthy, K. An analysis of the late effects of traumatic posterior dislocation of the hip without fractures. J Bone Joint Surg 65B:150–157, 1983.

150. Urist, M.R. Fracture-dislocation of the hip joint: The nature of the traumatic lesion, treatment, late complications, and end results. J Bone Joint Surg 30A:699–727, 1948.

151. Walker, R.H.; Burton, D.S. Computerized tomography in assessment of acetabular fractures. J Trauma 22:227–234, 1982.

152. Watson-Jones, R. Fractures and Joint Injuries, Ed. 5. New York, Churchill Livingstone, 1976, pp. 885–926.

153. Wertheimer, L.G.; Lopes, S.D.F. Arterial supply of the femoral head. A combined angiographic and histological study. J Bone Joint Surg 53A:545–555, 1971.

154. Witwity, T.; Uhlmann, R.D.; Fisher, J. Arthroscopic management of chondromatosis of the hip: A case report. Arthroscopy 4(1):55–56, 1988.

155. Yandown, D.R.; Austin, C.W. Femoral defect after anterior dislocation. J Comput Assist Tomogr 7(6):1112–1113, 1983.

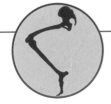

Marc F. Swiontkowski, M.D.

43

Intracapsular Hip Fractures

Femoral Head Fractures

PATHOLOGY

Relevant Anatomy

Because femoral head fractures nearly exclusively occur as a result of hip dislocations or fracture-dislocations, the anatomy, particularly the vascular anatomy, of the proximal femur plays a critical role in determining outcome. The end results of fracture healing, fragment resorption, or femoral head necrosis are determined by the traumatic effect of the hip dislocation on the vascular anatomy and are influenced to some degree by management of the injury. Similarly, the effects of the traumatic dislocation on the femoral and acetabular articular cartilage may result in arthrosis, which may be functionally limiting. This, too, can be affected to some degree by management of the injury. Finally, damage to the hip capsule and hip musculature may lead to periarticular fibrosis and heterotopic ossification, which can produce functional limitations.

The femoral head is supplied by three terminal arterial sources: the artery of the ligamentum teres; a terminal branch of the lateral femoral circumflex artery; and the terminal branch of the medial femoral circumflex artery, the lateral epiphyseal artery (Fig. 43–1).[38] The last is the critical blood supply to the majority of the weight-bearing superior portions of the femoral head. In the majority of cases where hip dislocation is associated with a femoral head fracture, the direction of the dislocation is posterior.[3] The medial femoral circumflex artery is stretched, and the lateral epiphyseal artery may be occluded because of pressure from the edge of the disrupted posterior hip capsule. Intracapsular hematoma does not result because of loss of capsular integrity. The anteroinferior femoral head fragment generally remains within the acetabulum attached to the ligamentum teres. The intact blood supply to this fragment, the artery of the ligamentum teres from the obturator artery, allows fracture healing to occur. The plane of the fracture, especially in posterior hip dislocation, most likely disrupts the osseous branches of the terminal branches of the lateral femoral circumflex artery. The tension or occlusive pressure on the lateral epiphyseal artery makes prompt reduction of the femoral head within the acetabulum critical. As noted in chapter 42 on hip dislocation, avascular necrosis of the femoral head increases in incidence with the number of hours that the hip remains dislocated.[13,14] These concepts also apply when the dislocation is associated with a femoral head fracture.

Articular Cartilage

Articular cartilage covers the proximal femoral epiphysis, which involves roughly the weight-bearing hemisphere.[5,21] The cartilage reaches a maximum thickness of 4 mm in the superiormost region and tapers as it approaches the equator of the hemisphere. It thins in the region of the insertion of the ligamentum teres. At the periphery of the cartilage, the retinacular vessels penetrate the bone.

Approximately 70% of the entire femoral head articular surface is involved in load transfer.[21] Damage to this surface such as that produced by a femoral head fracture decreases the total surface of the femoral head available for load transfer. Accompanying increases in peak compressive forces may lead to breakdown of the articular cartilage matrix, loss of the articular seal, and development of posttraumatic osteoarthritis. Femoral head indentation fractures, which are associated with acetabular fractures and anterior hip dislocations, pro-

1369

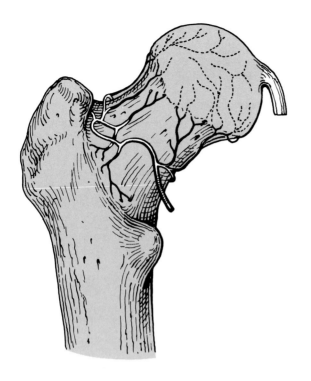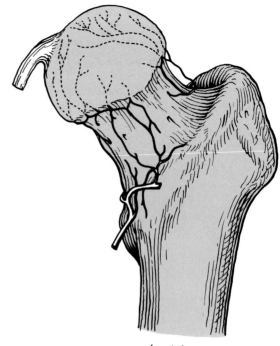

J. Klausmeyer

Figure 43-1

Arterial blood supply to the adult proximal femur. The lateral epiphyseal artery supplies the majority of the weight-bearing surface of the femoral head in 90% of adults. Note the lack of significant arterial supply along the anterior capsule.

duce focal crush of cartilage matrix as well as loss of total contact area with the same result.[11,30]

Osseous Anatomy

The adult human femoral head ranges in diameter from approximately 40 mm to 60 mm and is not a perfect sphere. Out-of-round estimates are in the 1- to 1.5-mm range. [5] This subtle asphericity is reflected on the acetabular side. Previously this was thought to be an important factor in prosthetic design.[5] Accurate reduction of femoral head fragments that involve the articular cartilage is necessary to maximize the contact between the femoral head and acetabulum and minimize the peak stresses across the articular cartilage.

The maintenance of an optimal femoral head-acetabular contact requires the entire femoral head. The loss of a significant piece of the femoral head will allow radial-lateral, noncongruent motion. How large the anteroinferior fragment has to be to allow the loss of this "shim" effect is not known. Short-term clinical results from resection of small fragments have been satisfactory in some series and poor in others.[3,25,37]

Incidence

Femoral head fractures occur in association with hip dislocations. Of the 238 published cases identified by

Brumback et al., only 24 (10%) were associated with anterior hip dislocations.[3] In a series of reported anterior hip dislocations, 15 of 22 (68%) had associated femoral head fractures.[11] Because anterior dislocations occur infrequently, additional data on the association of femoral head fractures is inadequate.[11,15,30]

Eighty-five to ninety percent of hip dislocations are posterior. In the largest series of posterior hip dislocations, the incidence of associated femoral head fractures was 7%[14,16] In much of the published literature on femoral head fractures, no attempt is made to identify the type of hip dislocations that produce femoral head fractures.

Most of the 265 cases of femoral head fractures published are of the shear or cleavage type.[3,14] Recently the phenomenon of indentation or crush fractures has been recognized.[3] The results in this group of patients seem to be worse than those in the cleavage group. These have been reported to be commonly associated with anterior hip dislocation but are now being recognized frequently in association with acetabular fractures.

Mechanism

The vast majority of the 265 reported cases of femoral head fractures are secondary to motor vehicle crashes.

The mechanism in the majority of cases associated with posterior hip dislocation is similar to that thought to produce femoral neck, shaft, or combination fractures.[17,18] The thigh is axially loaded on impact through the dashboard, and if the femoral shaft does not fracture, a hip injury will result if sufficient force is present. If the thigh is abducted, a femoral neck fracture may result; if neutral or adducted, a posterior hip dislocation with or without a concomitant femoral head or acetabular posterior wall fracture may result. Femoral head fractures may be the result of avulsion by the ligamentum teres or of cleavage over the posterior acetabular edge. Especially in anterior dislocations, impacted femoral head fractures may occur because of a direct blow from the acetabular margin.

Consequences of Injury

Degenerative Joint Disease

Hip dislocations occur as a result of high-velocity injury. Significant force is required to disrupt the posterior hip capsule, and more may be required to add a shearing injury producing a femoral head fracture as the head is impaled on the posterior acetabular rim. Crushed, indented, or fragmented articular cartilage results in loss of function of this critical material. If the injury is associated with poor reduction, loss of bone stock, or excision, the mechanical environment for the remaining articular cartilage will be negatively affected, adding further impetus to the breakdown of cartilage matrix. If significant posterior wall bone loss is also seen, posterior hip instability will add to the deterioration of hip function.[10,19] The loss of the medial "shim" effect will, in the same way, produce a poor environment for survival of the remaining intact femoral head cartilage. The end result of the trauma and subsequent poor conditions for articular cartilage will be degenerative arthritis of the hip.[32,37,39] As the majority of these injuries occur in young adults, subsequent reconstruction becomes problematic. Total hip replacement has not been successful in the long term for this patient population.[6] Hip arthrodesis, although effective at limiting pain and optimizing function, is not an attractive option for the majority of patients.

Avascular Necrosis

Avascular necrosis is frequently seen in association with posterior hip dislocation. It accompanies 13% of posterior hip dislocations and is seen in 18% of posterior hip dislocations associated with femoral head fractures.[14,16] The higher incidence may be the result of the greater amount of force required to produce the accompanying fracture, which produces more soft tissue disruption. Additionally, delay in closed reduction may occur because of the fracture surfaces or interposed frag-

ments. Optimum management of the hip dislocation is required to minimize the risk of this complication, as avascular necrosis in the young adult is a devastating problem without good options for treatment.

Limited Motion

Poor functional results frequently occur following dislocation of the hip complicated by femoral head fracture. In addition to joint arthrosis and avascular necrosis of the femoral head, femoral head fracture is often associated with heterotopic ossification.[37] This results from disruption of the joint capsule and contusion, tearing, and avulsion of the abductor musculature. Heterotopic ossification can also be associated with a surgical exposure.

Associated Injuries

The association of femoral head fracture with hip dislocations is strong. It is difficult to conceive how a shearing fracture of the femoral head could be produced without dislocation.[7] Indentation fractures do frequently accompany acetabular fractures and result from "central dislocation" with impaction of the head of the femur on acetabular fragments. Management of the hip dislocation can have an impact on the incidence of sciatic nerve palsy, as delayed reduction of the hip dislocation results in increasing incidence and severity of sciatic neuropraxia.

The axial loading mechanism described previously explains the not-infrequent association of knee ligament injury, patella fracture, and femoral shaft fracture. The knee and femur must be carefully examined in patients with femoral head fractures, as the force is usually transmitted through these structures. Radiographic examination is mandatory for the ipsilateral limb.

Because these injuries are a result of high-energy trauma, injury to other body systems is frequent. An early report on these fractures revealed a 47% mortality rate overall.[8] Critical evaluation of the whole patient by the trauma team must be performed as outlined in chapter 5.

Classification

The first recognition of femoral head fracture as a unique entity was published in 1869 by Birkett.[1] Thompson and Epstein's classification of posterior hip dislocations, published in 1951,[36] included the following classification of femoral head fractures as a separate entity:

Type I: With or without minor fracture of the acetabulum.

Type II: With a large single fracture of the posterior acetabular rim.
Type III: With comminuted fractures of the acetabular rim (with or without a major fragment).
Type IV: With fracture of the acetabular rim and floor.
Type V: With fracture of the femoral head.

This classification did not include anterior hip dislocation, nor did it include fractures of both the acetabulum and femoral head.

Stewart and Milford's classification, published in 1954,[33] did include the distinction between anterior and posterior hip dislocations. The associated fractures were classified as follows:

Grade I: No acetabular fracture or only a minor chip.
Grade II: Posterior rim fracture, but stable after reduction.
Grade III: Posterior rim fracture with hip instability after reduction.
Grade IV: Dislocation accompanied by fracture of the femoral head or neck.

Again the system was limited by the inability to include fractures of the acetabulum with femoral head fractures. Additionally, the classification of the acetabulum component was lacking in detail. Because of the fact that more conditions are clearly included, the Thompson-Epstein classification was used in most publications of the 1950s and 1960s.

Pipkin's landmark article on femoral head fractures included his classification system (Fig. 43–2).[25] This article remains the most significant contribution on the subject more than 30 years after its publication. The Pipkin classification is as follows:

Type I: (Hip) dislocation with fracture of the femoral head caudad to the fovea capitis femoris.
Type II: (Hip) dislocation with fracture of the femoral head cephalad to the fovea capitis femoris.
Type III: Type 1 or type 2 injury associated with fracture of the femoral neck.
Type IV: Type 1 or type 2 injury associated with fracture of the acetabular rim.

The major deficiencies of this classification are the lack of differentiation of anterior hip dislocation and insufficient expansion of the acetabular fracture categorization. The latter is a minor point, and the need for the former was not apparent to Pipkin, as the cases, collected from his Kansas City associates, on which this classification was based were probably all associated with posterior hip dislocation.

As the association of femoral head fractures with anterior hip dislocations has become more apparent in recent years, Brumback et al. have published the most complete classification[3]:

Type 1: Posterior hip dislocation with femoral head fracture involving the inferomedial, non–weight-bearing portion of the femoral head.
Type 1A: With minimum or no fracture of the acetabular rim and stable hip joint after reduction.
Type 1B: With significant acetabular fracture and hip joint instability.
Type 2: Posterior hip dislocation with femoral head fracture involving the superomedial, weight-bearing portion of the femoral head.
Type 2A: With minimum or no fracture of the acetabular rim and stable hip joint after reduction.
Type 2B: With significant acetabular fracture and hip joint instability.
Type 3: Dislocation of the hip (unspecified direction) with associated femoral neck fracture.
Type 3A: Without fracture of the femoral head.
Type 3B: With fracture of the femoral head.
Type 4: Anterior dislocation of the hip with fracture of the femoral head.
Type 4A: Indentation type; depression of the superolateral weight-bearing surface of the femoral head.
Type 4B: Transchondral type; osteocartilaginous shear fracture of the weight-bearing surface of the femoral head.
Type 5: Central fracture-dislocation of the hip with fracture of the femoral head.

Although most authors have used Pipkin's classification since its publication, Brumback et al.'s classification is more complete and includes fractures of the femoral head reorganized with associated fractures. Although somewhat cumbersome, its precision warrants the use of this system in future publications.

DIAGNOSIS

History

The vast majority of patients with femoral head fracture occur as a result of high-velocity motor vehicle accidents. Although the mechanism of posterior dislocation is thought to be axial loading of a flexed and adducted hip and that of anterior dislocation to be abduction, flexion, and external rotation, most patients are unable to give these detailed descriptions. Especially where multiple trauma is involved, the type and direction of the force are difficult to ascertain and are not germane to the problems at hand.

Physical Exam

The associated hip dislocation, if it remains unreduced, will determine the findings of the examination on admission. The posterior dislocation will leave the limb

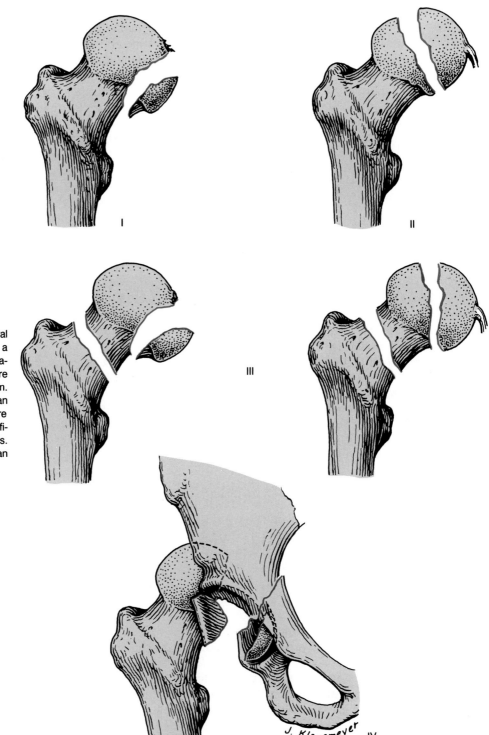

Figure 43–2

Pipkin's classification of femoral head fractures. Pipkin's type I is a fracture fragment below the ligamentum teres; type II is a fracture fragment above the ligamentum. Type III is either of these with an associated femoral neck fracture —a combination with a significantly poorer patient prognosis. Type IV is either of these with an associated acetabular fracture.

shortened, slightly flexed, adducted, and internally rotated. The anterior obturator type of dislocation will result in the injured limb being flexed, abducted, and externally rotated. The position of the limb should be noted, and then a rapid assessment of the circulatory status, including pulses, capillary refill, and skin temperature, should be performed. This must be followed with a thorough assessment of sciatic and femoral nerve function. The ability or lack thereof to dorsiflex and plantar flex the ankle, invert and evert the foot, and flex and extend the knee should be evaluated by palpating muscle bellies as the indicated motion is attempted. This should be followed by a careful sensory examination using light touch and pin prick modalities. No reduction of the hip joint should be attempted until this examination is complete.

Radiographic Imaging

An anteroposterior (AP) pelvic radiograph is a routine part of the evaluation of the multiply injured patient (See chapter 5). In any case of suspected hip dislocation, proximal femur fracture, or pelvis fracture, this critical radiograph must be obtained. The findings of this radiograph will determine which other radiographic studies are needed. In the case of posterior hip dislocation, the radiograph must be scrutinized with regard to femoral head fragments remaining in the acetabular fossa. The femoral head defect is not obvious unless the angle of the beam catches the plane of the femoral head fracture in profile. The femoral neck should be carefully scrutinized before the decision is made to reduce the hip to avoid displacement of an undisplaced femoral neck component of a Pipkin Type III fracture. If the radiograph clearly demonstrates a hip dislocation with or without a concomitant femoral head fracture, the surgeon should proceed with a closed reduction maneuver. If there is an associated disruption of the anterior or posterior pelvic ring, the prereduction evaluation should also include pelvic inlet and outlet views. Similarly, if an associated acetabular fracture is suspected either on the contralateral side or as in a Pipkin type IV fracture, the prereduction radiographic evaluation should include the 45° oblique views described by Judet and Letournel.

After obtaining the best possible plain radiographs, usually an attempt is made at a closed reduction. This may be done in the emergency department with analgesia and sedation or in the operating room with a general anesthetic and complete muscle relaxation. Although the latter is probably less traumatic, it may not be an available option without excessive (45 to 60 minutes) delay. Thus it is often appropriate to attempt a gentle closed reduction in the emergency department.

If this is unsuccessful, and if further studies do not delay a general anesthetic, a computed tomography (CT) scan through the acetabulum and femoral head at 1- to 3-mm cut intervals should be rapidly obtained. If an open reduction becomes necessary, this will alert the surgeon to search for loose bodies and interposed soft tissue[9] or perform open reduction and internal fixation of an associated femoral head or acetabulum fracture.[13,14,16] This will also serve as a valuable piece of information for the surgeon as to choice of surgical approach.

If the closed reduction is successful in either setting, it must be confirmed by a follow-up AP pelvic radiograph. The follow-up studies should also include a pelvic CT with 1.5-mm cuts through the acetabulum to search for loose bodies, check for acetabular integrity, and evaluate the reduction status of associated femoral head fractures.

Other Studies

In certain settings, electromyography, contrast venography, cystography and urethrography, bone scans, and magnetic resonance imaging may be useful aids as part of the pre- or postreduction evaluation. Hip dislocations, especially those that remain out for long periods of time, may have associated sciatic nerve palsies. Electromyography can play an important role in determining the specific areas of the nerve that are involved and the degree of involvement. This information is helpful in relating the prognosis for recovery to the patient, especially if the electromyograms are repeated serially. The initial study should not be obtained until three weeks after injury to allow accurate diagnosis. Compression ultrasound is a convenient and reliable test for deep venous thrombosis in the thigh and popliteal fossa, whereas contrast venography remains the confirmatory "gold standard."[74a] Urethrography and cystography are seldom indicated in pure hip dislocation with associated femoral head fracture but may be indicated where there is an associated anterior pelvic ring fracture with significant displacement (see chapter 40). Technetium bone scanning can offer some predictive information as to the chances of later avascular necrosis.[164] If femoral head uptake is significantly lower than that of the contralateral normal hip as measured by quantitative scintimetry, the risk of later avascular necrosis may be as high as 80% to 90% but is dependent on multiple factors. Finally, magnetic resonance imaging (MRI) may offer some prognostic information in regard to the risk of femoral head avascular necrosis. The exact clinical implications of an abnormal femoral head MRI signal are yet to be clearly defined.

MANAGEMENT

Two significant problems are evident in attempting to analyze the published series of femoral head fractures; inadequate follow-up both in percentage of series and length, and lack of a uniform classification. Since Pipkin's important article of 1957, the majority of authors have attempted to use his classification, and it will therefore be utilized here. Brumback's classification is more expansive and complete but has not been applied to a series of published patients. This classification should be utilized in future publications.

Of the 265 published cases of hip dislocation with associated femoral head fracture, 170 are classifiable by the Pipkin scheme.[1,3,4,7,12,18–20,22,23,27,29,33,35] Femoral head fractures associated with anterior hip dislocation are not included, as they do not fall into the Pipkin categories. There are 37 (22%) type I fractures, 72 (42%) type II, 25 (15%) type III, and 36 (21%) type IV femoral head fractures in the published literature. Multiple treatment regimens were employed for each classification and will be discussed independently. Although Pipkin categorized results as excellent, good, serviceable, and poor, the criteria were not clearly defined. Other authors used similar softly defined classifications of results, which makes comparison of series difficult. The evaluation of these series is made more complex by the fact that multiple treating surgeons were involved in all series. Limitation of follow-up is a more serious qualifying factor. Because of these problems, conclusions regarding treatment remain uncertain.

Of the 26 Pipkin I femoral head fractures reported with adequate follow-up, 18 were treated with closed reduction and traction. Of these, 13 had excellent/good results, two fair, one poor, and two were lost to follow-up. The length of traction varied but generally was from four to six weeks. Eight patients were treated with fragment excision because of a noncongruent reduction, fragmentation, or other intraarticular fragments. Two had excellent/good results, three fair, two poor, and one was lost to follow-up. No patient in any published series has been treated with open reduction and internal fixation.

Of the 36 Pipkin II cases published with follow-up, 13 were treated with closed reduction and traction. Of these, eight had excellent/good results, three fair, and two poor. Six were treated with closed reduction and excision of the fragment. Four had excellent/good results, two fair, and none poor. Seventeen were treated with open reduction and internal fixation; ten had excellent/good results, three fair, and four poor. The large size of the fragment would seem to lend itself to internal fixation.[4,37] Surgical sectioning of the ligamentum teres facilitates reduction and has not resulted in an increase

in poor results.[3,37] Loss of the uniform contact of the femoral head with the acetabulum (the "shim effect") that occurs with fragment excision adds motivation to attempt open reduction and internal fixation, especially when the reduction of the fragment on CT scan reveals a nonanatomic reduction.

The segmental femoral head fracture classified as Pipkin III has been reported in 17 patients with adequate follow-up. Three received primary arthroplasty because of the anticipated high risk of complications. Three underwent closed reduction and traction, all with poor results, and one underwent closed reduction and excision with a poor result. Of the ten who underwent open reduction and internal fixation, five had excellent/good results, two fair, and three poor. In this situation, long-term (minimum 3 to 5 years) follow-up is necessary because of the anticipated complication of avascular necrosis, and this was not available in a significant number of these cases. Of interest is the fact that 5 of 17 cases were situations where the femoral neck fracture was produced by the closed reduction. Although these may have been simply displacement of nondisplaced neck fractures, the consequences of displacement are significant, and the prereduction radiographs should be reviewed carefully to search for a femoral neck fracture. If the closed reduction attempt requires significant force, the surgeon should proceed with open reduction to maneuver interposed soft tissue out of the way.[9,14,16]

Pipkin's type IV category introduces the variable of the acetabular fracture. The management of the femoral head fracture must be included in the overall decision making for the management of the acetabular fracture. Of the 28 type IV femoral neck fractures with associated acetabulum fractures and adequate follow-up, 12 were treated with closed reduction and traction, with six excellent/good results, one fair, three poor, and two lost to follow-up. Eight were treated with closed reduction and excision with no good results, three fair, three poor, and two lost to follow-up. Eight were treated with open reduction and internal fixation, with two excellent/good results, one fair, four poor, and two with no follow-up. The difficulty in evaluating these results is that details regarding the classification of the acetabular fracture are lacking and are of extreme importance in the final outcome. This fracture type similarly suffers from unclear reporting of the final results in relationship to the treatment used.

Recently, Thorpe et al. have reported 37 cases of femoral head fractures.[37] Seventeen were Pipkin type I, nine were type II, eight were type IV, and three were unclassifiable fractures. All but five patients were treated with open reduction and internal fixation, and one patient with a bilateral type IV fracture died. In evaluating anterior versus posterior approaches for internal fixation of Type I and Type II fractures, the authors concluded that the anterior approach offered better visualization and opportunity to internally fix the femoral head fragment while offering no increase in risk of femoral head avascular necrosis (two cases of avascular necrosis occurred with posterior approaches, 0 of 12 with anterior approaches). The incidence of functionally significant heterotopic ossification in Pipkin I and II fractures treated with the anterior approach was 2 of 12 versus 0 of 12 posteriorly. The two cases treated with closed reduction and traction had excellent results in this series.

Anterior dislocation of the hip associated with superior indentation or shear fracture is a more recently reported phenomenon and is not included in Pipkin's classification. It is becoming an increasingly recognized phenomenon with acetabular fractures as well. The association of superior femoral head fracture with anterior hip dislocation was initially reported by Funsten et al.[18] and more recently delineated by DeLee et al.[11] The indentation of the superior weight-bearing femoral head occurs as it levers off the anterior wall of the acetabulum or possibly as it impacts against the superior margin of the obturator ring. Similarly, shear fractures occur as the superior femoral head impacts the anterior acetabular rim and is cleaved off. Of the ten published cases of impaction type femoral head fractures associated with anterior hip dislocation, seven had evidence of significant posttraumatic arthritis at follow-up. Of the four cleavage or shear fractures, all had significant joint space narrowing at follow-up. It is fortunate that anterior hip dislocations with their associated femoral head fractures are rare, as such patients have a high risk of developing posttraumatic arthritis.

Algorithm

After adequate physical examination, review of the AP pelvic radiograph for location of the femoral head fracture, and evaluation of the femoral neck and acetabulum, an emergent gentle closed reduction is recommended as outlined in chapter 42. If closed reduction is unsuccessful, an open reduction is indicated. A preoperative CT scan (if it can be obtained without delay of more than 45 to 60 minutes) is helpful to evaluate the acetabulum and femoral neck and to check for the size of the femoral head fragment and for loose bodies. If the closed reduction is successful, a postreduction CT scan is indicated. This is then reviewed for reduction of the fragment, status of the femoral neck and acetabulum, and loose bodies. The treatment recommendations are then based on the classification, reduction of the fracture, and general considerations.

For isolated Pipkin type I fractures with an excellent (less than 1-mm step-off) reduction, closed treatment is recommended. Four weeks of light traction (Buck's skin traction or skeletal traction) followed by touchdown weight bearing on crutches for four weeks has produced good results in the majority of patients.[3] If the reduction is not adequate, open reduction and internal fixation with small cancellous[37] or Herbert[24] screws using an anterior approach is recommended. In the case of polytrauma, this may also be indicated, even when reduction is good, to allow mobilization of the younger patient. The same recommendations apply to type II fractures, but because of the involvement of the superior femoral head, only an anatomic reduction on repeated radiographic evaluations should be accepted for conservative care.

For cleavage femoral head fractures associated with a femoral neck fracture (Pipkin type III), the prognosis is poor (Fig. 43–3). The prognosis for the injury in regard to posttraumatic avascular necrosis of the femoral head is related to the degree of displacement of the femoral neck fracture. For this reason, care must be taken with the closed reduction to prevent displacement of a recognized or unrecognized femoral neck fracture. In the younger, more active patient, an emergent open reduction and internal fixation of the type I or II femoral head fracture using an anterior Watson-Jones approach is recommended, followed by screw fixation of the femoral neck fracture. The decision to proceed in this manner should be weighted toward treating those who are active, physiologically young, and have minimally displaced or nondisplaced femoral neck fractures. In those patients who do not fulfill these criteria a bipolar endoprosthesis should be inserted.

Pipkin type IV fractures must be treated in tandem with their associated acetabular fractures. The acetabular fracture should dictate the surgical approach, and the femoral head fracture, even if it is nondisplaced, should be internally fixed to allow early motion of the hip joint. Management of the associated acetabulum fracture is covered in chapter 32.

Femoral head fractures associated with anterior hip dislocations are very difficult to manage. Elevation of the indentation fragment has recently been advocated by Mears,[24a] but the long-term results are not known. The prognosis is poor because of the risk of posttraumatic arthritis, and the patient should be so informed. Cleavage fractures, if they are large and noncommunited, may be internally fixed. This should be done with an anterior approach if the CT scan indicates the major portion of the fragment is anterior and with a posterior approach if the fragment involves the posterior weight-bearing femoral head. No results with this treatment have been published.

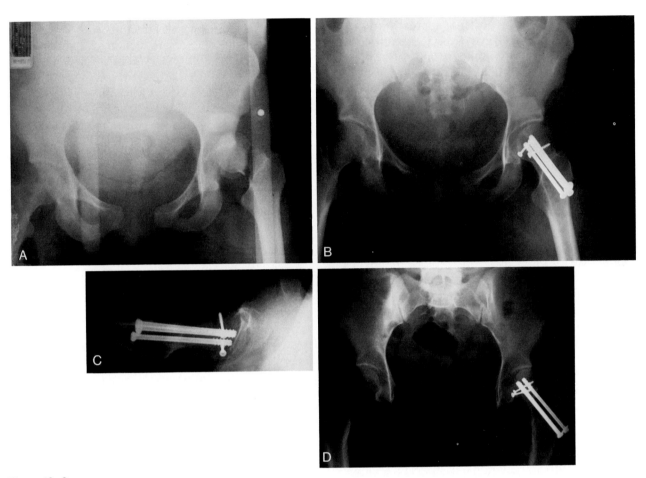

Figure 43-3

Combined fractures of the femoral head and neck. *A,* This 22-year-old female, 20 weeks pregnant, was involved in a motor vehicle accident and sustained a Pipkin type III fracture-dislocation of the femoral neck and femoral head. *B,C,* After being cleared for an anesthetic by the obstetrics department, the patient was taken for an emergent open reduction and internal fixation, which was done using an anterior approach. The femoral head major fragment was trapped within the subgluteal fascial space and was devoid of all soft tissue attachments. The anteroinferior femoral head fragment was reduced and fixed to the major head fragment, which was then stabilized to the neck with multiple cannulated screws. An anatomic reduction was achieved. *D,* At 1½ years follow-up the patient had some groin pain and had developed changes consistent with osteonecrosis of the proximal femur, a complication that was not unexpected. To date she has not undergone hip arthroplasty, which is the expected outcome.

Polytrauma Patient: Special Considerations

An unreduced hip dislocation, because of the consequences of posttraumatic femoral head necrosis, which increases with the duration of the dislocations, represents a musculoskeletal emergency. An AP pelvic radiograph is part of the initial evaluation of the multiply injured patient and will reveal the hip dislocation with the femoral head fracture. If the patient is going to the operating room for head, abdominal, or chest procedures, closed reduction of the hip dislocation can be expedited by the orthopedist's presence during induction of anesthesia. As soon as muscle relaxation has been achieved and the airway secured, closed reduction of the hip is performed as described in chapter 42. If this is unsuccessful, an open reduction should be performed as soon as other lifesaving procedures are completed. If the closed reduction is successful, the same algorithm of postreduction CT followed by open reduction and internal fixation of a poorly reduced fracture, debridement of loose bodies, or open reduction and internal fixation of the femoral neck or acetabulum is carried out. In the case of the associated unrecognized femoral neck fracture or loose bodies, the open procedure should follow as soon as the patient can tolerate a second anesthetic. This is to avoid damage to the articular surfaces in the case of small loose fragments of bone or cartilage and to improve the risk of avascular necrosis of the femoral head in the case of the femoral neck fracture. Skeletal traction should be added in the interim when loose fragments are identified to minimize the articular cartilage damage.

In the case of well-reduced femoral head fractures of the Pipkin I or II classification, it may be advisable to perform an open reduction and internal fixation of the femoral head fragment to allow the patient to be mobilized. Traction, in general, should be avoided in the case of serious thoracic trauma or pulmonary dysfunction. The ability to mobilize the multiply injured patient has a proven positive benefit of reducing the incidence of pulmonary failure and sepsis.[31]

Treatment

Closed Reduction

An urgent closed reduction of the hip is indicated in *all* hip dislocations regardless of whether there is an asso-

ciated femoral head fracture.[13] The techniques for closed reduction are outlined in chapter 42. Delay must be avoided to optimize the risk of posttraumatic avascular necrosis of the femoral head. If a femoral neck fracture is identified, it is probably better to forego any attempt at closed reduction and to proceed with open surgery, with an urgent preoperative CT scan if possible. Such an approach may decrease the risk of displacement of the femoral neck fracture with further injury to the vascular supply of the femoral head.

Open Reduction Alone

The indication for open reduction of the dislocated hip is failure of closed reduction. A preoperative CT scan, whenever possible, helps alert the surgeon to intraartic-

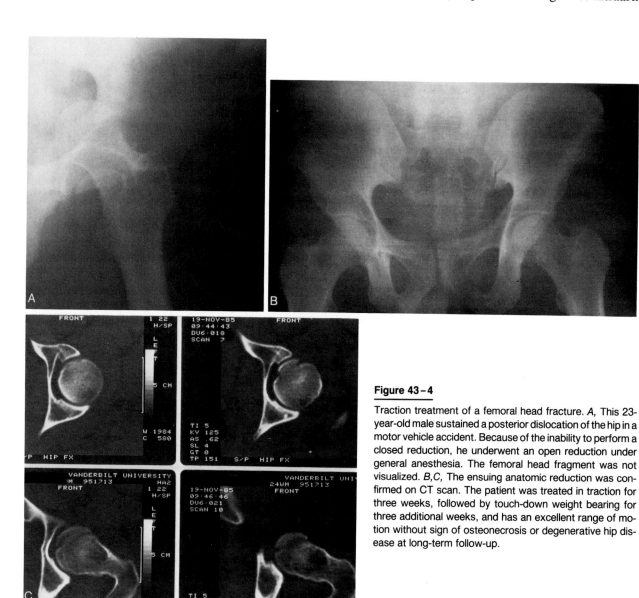

Figure 43-4

Traction treatment of a femoral head fracture. *A,* This 23-year-old male sustained a posterior dislocation of the hip in a motor vehicle accident. Because of the inability to perform a closed reduction, he underwent an open reduction under general anesthesia. The femoral head fragment was not visualized. *B,C,* The ensuing anatomic reduction was confirmed on CT scan. The patient was treated in traction for three weeks, followed by touch-down weight bearing for three additional weeks, and has an excellent range of motion without sign of osteonecrosis or degenerative hip disease at long-term follow-up.

ular fragments, acetabular or femoral neck fractures, and the size of the femoral head fragment. A delay of more than 45 to 50 minutes to allow the CT scan to be completed should be avoided. In general, posterior dislocations should be reduced using a posterior approach. The external rotators and button-holed capsule are the usual structures blocking reduction. Intraarticular fragments can be removed with this approach and posterior wall acetabular fractures can be operatively reduced under direct vision. Internal fixation of the femoral neck and head, as well as the reduction of these fractures, is difficult with this approach.[37] The patient should be placed in the lateral decubitus position to allow access to the anterior pelvis should a simultaneous approach be necessary to reduce and internally fix the femoral head fragment. A femoral distractor applied from the iliac crest to the proximal femoral shaft helps gain distraction of the hip joint to improve visualization of the reduction. If the surgeon chooses to leave the femoral head fragment unfixed, the patient should be treated in skin or light skeletal traction for four to six weeks (Fig. 43–4).

Fragment Excision

In combination with closed reduction or open reduction, the indications for fragment excision are severe comminution and interposition of a small femoral head fragment between the femoral head and acetabulum. This can be done through the same surgical approach used for the open reduction. If done after reviewing the post–closed-reduction CT scan, the approach is dictated by the location of the fragments. Anterior and inferior fragments should be approached using the Smith-Petersen interval. In the case of inter-

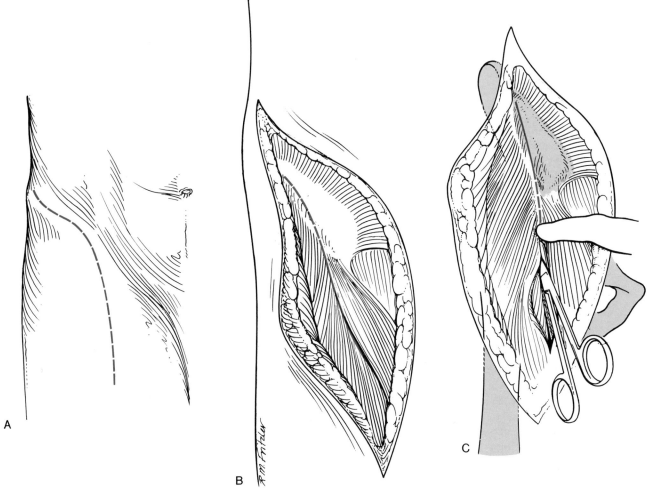

Figure 43–5

Anterior (Smith-Petersen) approach for open reduction and internal fixation of a femoral head fracture. *A*, Skin incision. The leg is draped free for manipulation. *B*, Exposure of deep fascia and release of abductors from the iliac crest. *C*, Development of interval between the sartorius and the tensor fascia lata, which is usually palpable with a finger.

Illustration continued on following page

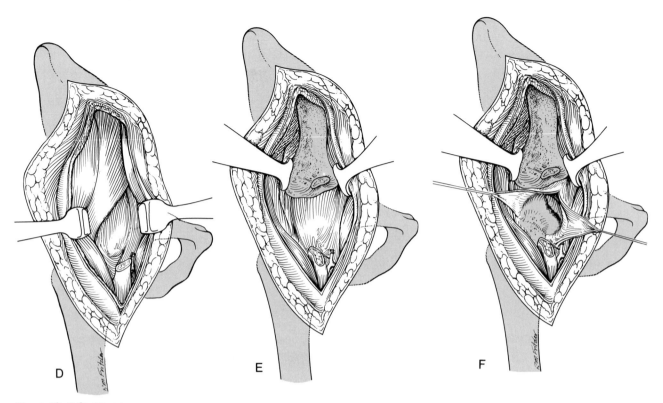

Figure 43–5 *Continued*

D, Identification, division, and ligation of ascending branches of lateral femoral circumflex vessels; release and suture tag of direct and reflected heads of the rectus femoris to define hip capsule. *E,* Elevation and reflection of the tensor fascia lata, gluteus medius, and gluteus minimus from the anterolateral ilium to improve access to the hip capsule. This lateral stripping of musculature should be minimized to limit the extent of heterotopic ossification. *F,* Arthrotomy by releasing the hip capsule from its acetabular marginal attachment and incising longitudinally along the anterior femoral neck reveals the femoral head fracture. Sutures placed at the edges of the capsulotomy are useful for retraction to enhance exposure. By flexing and maximally externally rotating the limb, the reduction can be assessed and adjusted. This exposure permits fixation with small lag screws recessed below the articular surface.

posed fragments, excision is urgent, and the procedure must be done quickly to avoid further damage to the articular surfaces. General or spinal anesthesia is utilized for fragment excision regardless of the approach used.

Open Reduction and Internal Fixation

Open reduction and internal fixation are indicated for all fractures with residual displacement of 1 mm or more, those associated with femoral neck or acetabular fractures, and those large femoral head fragments that are associated with a need for an open reduction of the associated hip dislocation. For most Pipkin I and II fractures, this should be done using an anterior Smith-Petersen approach. (Fig. 43–5).[37] The surgery is performed with the patient in the "semilateral" position with a large pad underneath the affected hip. These procedures can be performed within several days after the closed reduction and postreduction CT scan. In the

case of a posterior approach, the fragments off the anterior femoral head are difficult to visualize, harder to reduce, and can be nearly impossible to fix internally. This approach was recommended by Epstein because of fear of damage to the blood supply to the femoral head from the anterior capsule.[16] The blood supply to the femoral head from this source is negligible, and because of these operative difficulties, the anterior approach is favored.[37,38] The patient may be treated in a continuous passive motion machine postoperatively,[28] along with eight weeks of touch-down weight bearing and avoidance of extreme hip flexion ($>70°$) for four to six weeks. The anterior approach may be accompanied by heterotopic ossification of functional significance.[37] This can be avoided by minimizing the stripping of the tensor fascia lata and abductor musculature. Indocin 25 mg orally t.i.d. for six weeks or low-dose irradiation may also have a favorable influence, but diphosphonates are probably of limited therapeutic value (Fig. 43–6).[2,26,35]

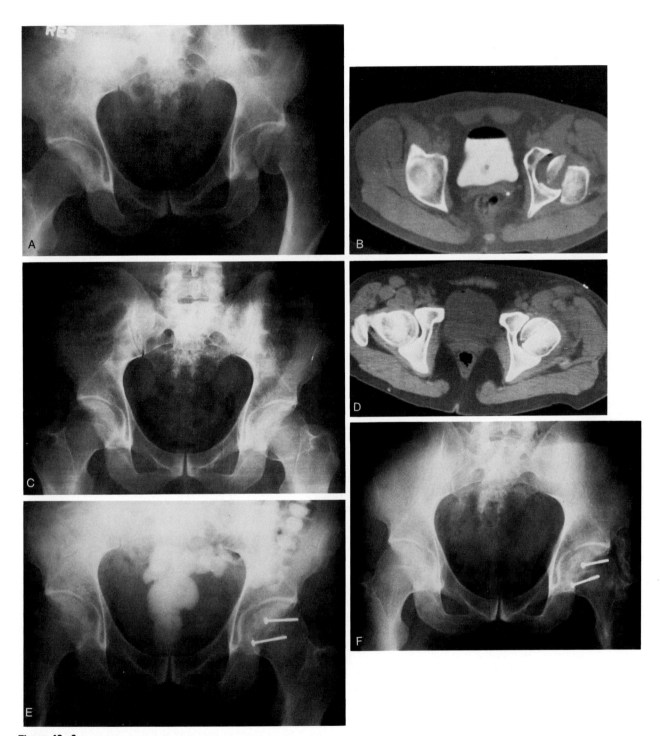

Figure 43–6

Internal fixation of a femoral head fracture using an anterior approach. *A,B,* This 44-year-old male was involved in a high-speed motor vehicle accident in which he sustained an open mandible fracture, multiple rib fractures, pneumothorax, and this posterior hip dislocation with a Pipkin type II femoral head fracture. On admission he was taken emergently to the CT scanner for an intraabdominal scan prior to reduction of the hip. *C,D,* Closed reduction was successful. *E,* Because of his pulmonary injuries, which required ventilation, it was felt that open reduction and internal fixation were indicated to mobilize the patient. Therefore he underwent open reduction and internal fixation using an anterior Smith-Petersen approach on the day of admission. *F,* The patient was mobilized postoperatively, was extubated on the fourth postoperative day, and remained at touch-down weight bearing for 12 weeks. At three years follow-up, flexion was limited to 80° because of heterotopic ossification. The patient has no pain and does not desire to have the heterotopic ossification resected.

Prosthetic Replacement

Prosthetic replacement is indicated in a Pipkin III fracture where the patient is physiologically elderly or the femoral neck fracture is markedly displaced in patients over 50 or 60 years of age.[3,23] Primary femoral head replacement is otherwise contraindicated and should only be performed following a trial of conservative care when the end result of internal fixation is joint incongruity or degenerative arthritis. When the treatment chosen results in the latter, total hip replacement is indicated. Details regarding the procedure of endoprosthetic replacement are discussed in the section on femoral neck fractures (Fig 43–7).

Open Reduction and Internal Fixation of Associated Acetabular Fractures

Open reduction and internal fixation of the acetabular fracture in a Pipkin type IV fracture are indicated when the fracture is displaced or the hip reduction is unstable. The femoral head fragment should also be internally fixed to gain the benefits of early, relatively unrestricted joint motion. Whereas the main component of the acetabular fracture will dictate the surgical approach, the femoral head fracture may require a separate anterior approach to accomplish the reduction and fixation. The details of the operative management of the acetabular fracture are in chapter 32.

Early Mobilization

Disregard of femoral head fracture reduction and mobilization of the patient should only be performed when the patient is extremely debilitated and unable to undergo surgery. In the elderly patient this may be a reasonable approach with the concept that if posttraumatic arthritis develops, the patient can undergo secondary replacement after optimization of his or her general medical condition. Hip flexion precautions should be followed for 6 to 8 weeks.

Follow-up Care and Rehabilitation

In the situation where closed reduction and traction treatment is selected, the four to six weeks of skin or light skeletal traction should be followed by an additional four to six weeks of crutch ambulation with touch-down weight bearing. In general, hip flexion of more than 70° should be avoided for the same period of time. At three months, supervised active and passive range-of-motion exercises as well as abduction strengthening can be initiated.

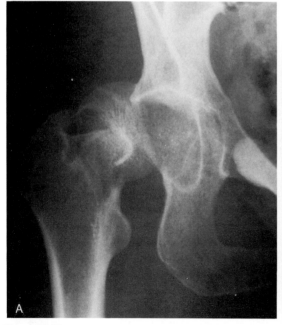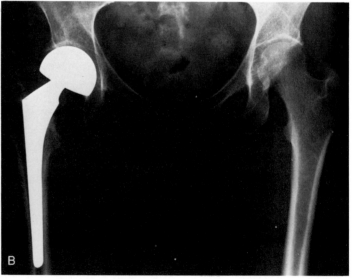

Figure 43–7

Prosthetic replacement for femoral head and neck fracture. *A,* This 55-year-old female was involved in a rollover motor vehicle accident, sustaining a fracture of the femoral neck with an inferior femoral head fragment and a dislocation of the major femoral headpiece. This is not, strictly speaking, a Pipkin type III lesion because of the dislocation of the femoral head. *B,* Because of the age of the patient, an uncemented bipolar prosthesis was selected as the treatment of choice. The patient had done reasonably well at three years follow-up; she has an occasional aching groin, but treatment has not been revised to a total hip replacement.

For open reduction and internal fixation of femoral head fractures, the patient should be immediately mobilized and treated with six to eight weeks of touch-down weight-bearing using crutch ambulation, followed by motion exercises and strengthening as previously noted. Continuous passive motion can be utilized in the early postoperative period.[28]

In the case of fragment excision, the patient should be asked to limit hip flexion to 60° to 70° for 8 to 12 weeks and should be treated with crutch ambulation during this period of time, followed by strengthening and motion exercises.

When femoral head fractures are internally fixed in connection with femoral neck or acetabular fractures, early range-of-motion exercises are indicated. The patient should also be treated with touch-down weight bearing with crutches for 8 to 12 weeks.

Postoperative care in patients who have undergone prosthetic replacement is covered in the section of femoral neck fractures.

Assessment of Results

A standardized system for evaluating end results is necessary to facilitate communications regarding treatment and results. This is especially true for femoral head fractures, as very few surgeons treat more than four or five such fractures in a career. The following system developed by Brumback et al.[3] is the most comprehensive system utilized in the literature yet is not overly complex.

Excellent: Normal hip motion, no pain, no significant radiographic changes.
Good: 75% of normal hip motion, no pain, minimum degenerative changes of the hip joint on radiographic evaluation.
Fair/Poor: Painful hip with moderate or severe restriction of hip motion, moderate or severe radiographic joint incongruity, or degenerative joint disease.

Because of the necessary linkage with hip dislocation, optimum follow-up should be a minimum of three to five years to definitively rule out posttraumatic osteonecrosis of the femoral head.

COMPLICATIONS

Chronic Instability

Chronic instability is most likely to occur in the setting of fragment excision, especially where this is accompanied by an unreduced or excised acetabular posterior wall fragment. This is best avoided by internal fixation of femoral head and acetabular fragments when they are of adequate size. When instability is recognized early, a posterior wall bone graft with tricortical iliac crest bone graft can be attempted. Chronic subluxation may result in degenerative arthritis with joint space narrowing, which requires hip arthroplasty or arthrodesis.

Wound Infection

Wound infection can result from any operative procedure and in general should occur in no more than 1% of patients in whom open reduction of femoral head fragments is performed. Postoperative hip infections are usually occult, so a high index of suspicion is requried. Joint aspiration is necessary for early diagnosis. The treatment for a deep wound infection is prompt and thorough surgical debridement of necrotic tissue and systemic administration of appropriate antibiotics. (see chapter 18 for more details).

Heterotopic Ossification

Heterotopic ossification may follow either the anterior or posterior approach utilized for reduction and internal fixation of femoral head fractures. In Pipkin type IV fractures in which extended surgical exposures are required to reduce and internally fix the acetabular fracture, the incidence of heterotopic ossification may be significant and is approach related (see chapter 32). For Pipkin type I and II fractures, the incidence of functionally significant heterotopic ossification is higher with anterior approaches.[37] Resection of the heterotopic mass at 18 to 24 months post injury, when alkaline phosphatase levels are declining toward normal and bone scan activity is decreasing, will generally yield an improvement in hip motion. While diphosphonates play no role in the prophylaxis against this complication, indomethacin 25 mg orally t.i.d. or low-dose radiation prophylaxis may be helpful.[2,26,35] The latter should probably be avoided until some long-term follow-up data regarding its use in young patients are available.

Sciatic Nerve Palsy

Sciatic nerve palsy is usually related to a delayed reduction of a posterior hip dislocation and is best avoided by prompt reduction. When it occurs, the dysesthesias in the early recovery period are aided by treatment with Carbamazepine or amitriptyline. Carbamazepine must be gradually increased to dosages in the range of 200 mg orally t.i.d. These patients must be followed with monthly or bimonthly liver function tests and complete blood cell (CBC) analysis because of potential marrow and liver toxicity. Serial electromyograms can yield prognostic information regarding return of function. Ankle dorsiflexion is generally the last function to return, and therefore a posterior split or plastic ankle-foot orthosis must be utilized. A dense sciatic nerve palsy that follows a hip fracture-dislocation generally carries a poor prognosis.

Avascular Necrosis

The incidence of avascular necrosis increases with the length of time the hip remains unreduced. It is also slightly more frequent when hip dislocation is associated with femoral head fracture, probably indicative of the greater degree of trauma required to fracture the femoral head. Treatment is difficult. If the area of subchondral resorption and subsequent fracture is limited, flexion osteotomy may play a role in avoiding hip arthroplasty or arthrodesis in younger patients.

Degenerative Arthritis

Degenerative arthritis occurs in the vast majority of cases associated with anterior hip dislocation. Similarly, it occurs in about half of the Pipkin type II, most of the Pipkin type III, and about half of the type IV injuries reported. The treatment for this complication is weight control, walking aids, and antiinflammatory medications. In physiologically older patients, the treatment for severe symptoms is total hip replacement. In younger patients with manual labor professions, hip arthrodesis should be considered. In general, total hip arthroplasty should be delayed as long as possible.

Femoral Neck Fractures

PATHOLOGY

Relevant Anatomy

Osseous Anatomy

The upper femoral ephiphysis generally is closed by age 16 years, thus establishing the adult proximal femoral anatomy.[76, 184] The neck shaft angle in adults does not seem to vary significantly between the sexes and is approximately $130\pm7°$.[143] The femoral neck is normally anteverted with respect to the femoral shaft and has been measured at $10.4\pm6.7°$ in normal specimens, again with no differences between the sexes.[141,142] Proximal femoral anteversion does not change after skeletal maturity. The femoral head diameter varies according to the size of the individual and ranges from 40 to 60 mm. Hoaglund and Low have measured the

articular cartilage covering the femoral head and found that it averages 4 mm at the superior portion and tapers to 3 mm at the periphery.[94] A substantial synovial membrane covers the entire anterior femoral neck, but only the most proximal half posteriorly.[187] The femoral neck has a wide variability in length and shape. There is a large posterior overhang of the greater trochanter, which locates the femoral neck in the anterior half of the proximal femur when viewed from the lateral orientation, a fact that must be recognized for the accurate placement of internal fixation devices. The calcar femorale is a condensed, vertically oriented plate of bone within the proximal femur. It originates in the posteromedial portion of the femoral shaft, radiates superiorly toward the greater trochanter, and fuses with the cortex of the posterior femoral neck.[90] This structure has been frequently misunderstood and mislabeled in the hip arthroplasty literature. As pointed out by Harty and later Griffin, it plays a central role in the development of upper femoral fracture patterns.[84,90]

Bone Density

It is generally agreed that bone density within the upper femur declines with age.[2] Certainly chronic disease, surgical or biologic menopause and medications (i.e., steroids, barbiturates, calcium- or magnesium-binding agents, seizure control medications, and hormonal therapy) have an adverse effect on bone metabolism and may affect the mechanical properties of the proximal femur. Freeman et al. identified trabecular fatigue fractures within the femoral head and at the head-neck junction in cadavers and within specimens removed at surgery (arthroplasty) for femoral neck fracture.[73] Only one necropsy specimen (from a 20-year-old patient) did not have any recognizable trabecular fatigue fractures in the upper femur, whereas all ten of the surgically removed specimens had them. The highest concentration of fatigue fractures (56%) was at the head-neck junction. The threshold density value below which fatigue fractures were associated was 0.5 gm/ml. Femoral neck fractures have been similarly associated with declining bone density by Singh et al., but more than just simple aging trends seem to be responsible for this phenomenon.[155]

Vascular Anatomy and Physiology

Trueta and Harrison expanded on the work of Howe et al. utilizing injection techniques to study the vascular anatomy of the proximal femur.[104,185] The lateral epiphyseal artery, which is the terminal branch of the medial femoral circumflex artery of the profunda femoris circulation, supplies the majority of the femoral head (see Fig. 43–1). In 15 of Trueta and Harrison's high-quality injection studies (barium suspensions examined in 15-micron sections studied with light microscopy), the lateral epiphyseal artery supplied $\frac{3}{4}$ of the femoral head in seven cases, $\frac{2}{3}$ in another seven, and slightly more than half in one case. The inferior metaphyseal artery is the terminal branch of the ascending portion of the lateral femoral circumflex artery, which pierces the midportion of the anterior hip capsule. This vessel supplies the more distal metaphyseal bone anteriorly and inferiorly in $\frac{2}{3}$ of the cases studied. The third major blood supply of the femoral head is the medial epiphyseal artery of the ligamentum teres from the obturator arterial system. This vessel generally connects with the lateral epiphyseal artery system. This anastomotic system formed by the two minor vessels may play a role in revascularization of the femoral head following femoral neck fracture. There seems to be no evidence in multiple other injection studies to support the concept that the metaphyseal vessels extending proximally from the nutrient artery system play a role in supply of nutrition to the proximal femoral neck or femoral head. The distribution of the minor arterioles from the lateral epiphyseal artery system is preferentially toward the subchondral bone of the femoral head articular surface. Multiple authors have noted that the important vessels supplying the majority of the femoral head (the lateral epiphyseal system) are contained within the retinacular reflection at the superior femoral neck (the retinacular arteries of Weitbrecht).[26,35,38,47,48,89,111,150,186]

Effect of Femoral Neck Fracture on Vascular Supply

A femoral neck fracture produces a devastating effect on the blood supply to the femoral head.[5,6,164,177] Displacement is generally related to the severity of the damage to the major blood supply, which is the lateral epiphyseal artery system.[32] In Sevitt's series of 25 patients who died following femoral neck fracture, only four femoral heads had a normal vascular pattern when studied with standard injection techniques.[149] Several authors have noted that after a femoral neck fracture compromises the retinacular vessels, the ligamentum teres system provides a source of blood supply for revascularization of the femoral head by creeping substitution. Focal mechanical failure of the femoral head during this process accounts for the development of segmental collapse in avascular necrosis.

Catto examined 188 femoral heads removed at necropsy or at surgery for femoral neck fracture and compared them with 50 control femoral heads.[32] The study was primarily a histologic analysis and confirmed that the control specimens had no evidence of marrow cellular changes or osteocyte death. In all 109 femoral heads removed more than 16 days after femoral neck fracture, some damage to the vascular supply as revealed by histologic changes was found. The cellular changes are detectable from 48 hours on, but it is generally agreed that osteocyte loss proceeds slowly after ischemia and that the cellular changes are irreversible after 12 hours. That cellular death proceeds slowly was confirmed by the fact that osteocyte "dropout" was not complete in uncrushed trabeculae proximal to the femoral neck fracture until the third week following fracture. Using dynamic blood flow studies, it has been recently documented for adult miniature swine that a femoral neck fracture, displaced 5 to 7 mm with an osteotome and then reduced anatomically, produces a 60% decrease in femoral head blood flow.[177]

Although the adverse effect of femoral neck fracture on femoral head blood flow has been documented with certainty, there are some elements of the situation that remain under the surgeon's control. Optimum reduction of the femoral neck fracture has been shown in numerous studies to be associated with a lower incidence of femoral head avascular necrosis.[12,61,77,78,160] This may be a result of the fact that all of the vessels of the lateral epiphyseal artery system may not be torn and that reduction may "unkink" the vessel or, when performed beyond the acute phase, may allow for rapid recanalization of the vessel. Claffey has shown that a complete, displaced femoral neck fracture can occur without disruption of this critical vascular supply.[38] Similarly, stabilization of the fracture with internal fixation allows revascularization to proceed under an optimum mechanical environment. Although further vascular damage to the femoral head is unlikely with standard techniques of fixation, Brodetti has demonstrated that the posterior and superior femoral head quadrant should be avoided.[26]

Marked displacement of a femoral neck fracture will disrupt the posterior hip capsule.[58] In cases where the displacement is not greater than half the diameter of the neck, the hip capsule may remain intact. Intracapsular hematoma may produce a pressure elevation significant enough to occlude the venous drainage system within the capsule or actually limit arteriolar flow in the retinacular reflection of the superior femoral neck. Several authors have shown by utilizing different techniques for measuring femoral head blood flow that increased intracapsular pressure has an adverse effect on femoral head blood flow and may produce cellular death.[176,177] Increased intracapsular pressures have been documented by numerous authors in clinical studies and in patients with femoral neck fracture.[46,98,107,126,162,194] Reduction of femoral head blood flow in association with elevated intracapsular pressure has been confirmed clinically using technetium bone scanning by Stromqvist et al.[171] Most authors have confirmed that extension and internal rotation of the hip elevate the intracapsular pressure to a significant degree by limiting the capsular volume. This position should be avoided in the preoperative phase of treatment, and the position of flexion and external rotation should be encouraged. Because pressures that exceed the local arteriolar pressures have been frequently documented by multiple authors, anterior capsulotomy may play a positive role in minimizing femoral head ischemia.[178,179] This surgical maneuver, along with rapid and accurate reduction, remains within the surgeon's control, and to the extent that they may limit the risk of necrosis of the femoral head following acute ischemia resulting from femoral neck fracture, these maneuvers are encouraged.

Incidence

Femoral neck fracture is primarily a disease of individuals older than 50 years.[12,195] Published reports in the early 1980s have indicated that femoral neck fracture in patients younger than age 50 makes up 2% to 3% of the total population.[195] It is the impression of many individuals working in United States trauma centers that the incidence of femoral neck fractures in younger, active adults involved in vehicular trauma is increasing. Some have pointed to the increased incidence of femoral neck fracture associated with femoral shaft fracture as evidence. It has also been suggested that smaller automobiles with lower dashboards increase the risk of forces being applied to the distal femur in a way that causes fractures of the femoral neck.

Femoral neck fractures occur more frequently in females. Zetterberg et al. found the female-to-male ratio for femoral neck fracture over the 43-year period from 1940–1983 to be 3.4:1.[195] The incidence of femoral neck fracture has been seen to be greater than is explainable by aging trends in the population in multiple studies.[49,70,195] The aging trend of the population does explain some of the increase, as the mean age for patients sustaining femoral neck fracture has increased from 71.7 to 74.3 years for males and from 72.6 to 79 years for females from 1965 to 1981.[101] The annual incidence of femoral neck fracture for 1000 persons in 1981 was 7.4 for females and 3.6 for males. The increase in annual incidence has been higher in urban (6%) than in rural (3%) populations[67,125] and has been confirmed in Great Britain.[49] Most of the literature published on femoral neck fracture is based on population studies done in Scandinavia. Since osteoporosis is associated with fair skin and northern, female smokers, these studies may not be strictly applicable to North American populations. Although Melton et al. did not identify an increasing incidence of femoral neck frac-

tures in the United States population, the incidence of the fracture in the late 1970s, 9.2 per 1000 person-years, is not dissimilar.[127]

Mechanism of Injury

The less common femoral neck fracture associated with vehicular trauma or falls from significant heights is thought to be caused by axial loading of the thigh (by the dashboard in an automobile) with the hip positioned in abduction.[179] This "high-energy" loading will fracture a femoral neck of normal density. If the hip were adducted, the most likely injury would be a hip dislocation, with or without an associated posterior acetabular wall or femoral head fracture.

The most common (in excess of 90%) type of trauma associated with femoral neck fractures is a fall from a standing position.[37] This "low-energy" type of injury will generally not produce a fracture in a femoral neck of normal density. The issue has been raised as to whether the fracture precedes the fall or the fall causes the fracture. Sloan and Holloway identified 13 of 54 patients (24%) who complained of increasing groin pain prior to their leg "giving way."[156] Freeman et al. found numerous fatigue fractures in control specimens, with the highest concentration in the subcapital region.[73] Although fatigue fractures of the femoral neck do occur and fairly frequently displace, most authors feel that the trauma of the fall does play a role in creating the fracture in the majority of cases. Because the number of fatigue fractures of trabeculae in the femoral neck do increase with decreasing bone density, fractures occurring before falling or without falling occur most often in the setting of severe osteoporosis.

Neuromuscular conditions exclusive of Parkinson's disease[44,166] are more frequently associated with intertrochanteric than femoral neck fractures.[37,59] Rashiq and Logan recently investigated the role of drugs as a cause of femoral neck fracture in 102 patients and 204 age-matched controls.[140] One hypothesis that has been advanced is that hypnotic or sedating drugs impair postural control and result in falls. Although the association between femoral neck fracture and sedative use has not been consistent, emerging evidence strongly suggests that it plays a role.[140a]

Bone Density

Singh et al. developed a classification scheme for severity of osteoporosis that focused on the changes in the trabecular patterns as seen on radiographs of the intact proximal femur (Fig. 43–8).[155] The radiographic changes were compared with graded iliac crest biopsies and correlation identified. A Singh grade IV or lower

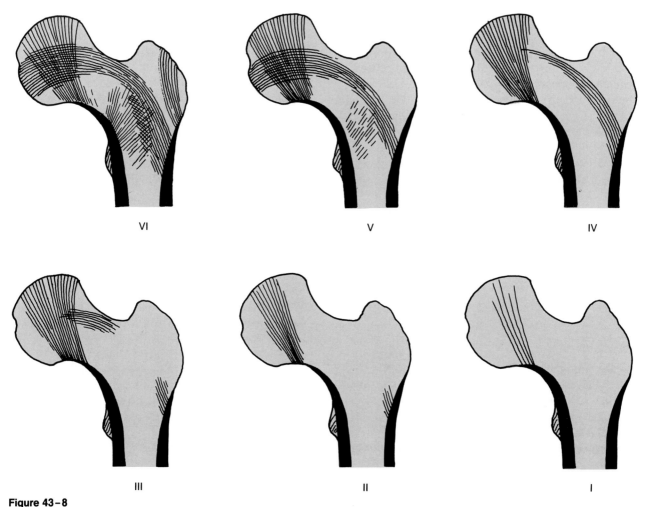

Figure 43-8

The Singh index of proximal femoral osteopenia. Progression is from normal grade VI with well-defined primary and secondary tension and compression trabeculae to severely osteopenic grade I with only a few residual primary compression trabeculae. Although extremely useful in determining suitability for reduction and internal fixation, the scheme has limited application as a research tool because of interobserver variability and difficulty in interpreting many radiographs.

represents some degree of osteoporosis. Although associations have been identified between osteoporosis as defined by this method and fracture displacement,[51,102] strong correlations between osteoporosis and incidence of femoral neck fracture are lacking.[68] Similarly, Wilton et al. sought to identify osteomalacia as an association with femoral neck fracture by doing iliac crest biopsies on nearly 1000 patients with femoral neck fracture and found an incidence of 2%.[193] In an aged-matched population of acutely ill patients, the incidence was 3.7%. The lack of a strong association was also found by Hoikka et al. and Lund et al.[96,124]

Aitken studied bone density utilizing metacarpal morphometry in a population of 195 women who had sustained a hip fracture in a minor fall, comparing them with a control population who had similar bone mass measurements.[2] Only 16% were not osteoporotic

by this method. Femoral neck fractures were more common than trochanteric injuries in the patients who were not osteoporotic. Aitken felt that osteoporosis was not a significant cause of hip fracture, even though it might influence the fracture type. Firooznia et al. looked at spinal bone mineral content using computed tomography in a series of 74 women with vertebral fractures, 83 with hip fractures, and 28 with both.[68] Only 4% of patients had spinal bone mineral content below that of their age-matched peers. Although osteoporosis plays a significant role in the severity of fracture displacement and the ability to obtain stable internal fixation, it seems safe to conclude that, by itself, it does not play a major role in causing femoral neck fracture. Although level of physical activity prior to fracture has been proven to have a role (i.e., greater activity = lower incidence) and may well be related to bone density and quality of trabecular organization, falls are the initial factor in the production of femoral neck fracture.[10,156]

Consequences of Injury

Nonunion

The problem of nonunion is rare following a nondisplaced or impacted fracture. The incidence of nonunion following displaced fracture is in the range of 50% to 60% with traction or cast treatment[42,43,190,191] and 15% to 33% following internal fixation.[12,21,77] Several studies have shown that nonunion is a rare problem in patients with normal bone density and in whom stable fixation is achieved.[95,179,196] In the vast majority of cases, a femoral neck nonunion will be associated with moderate to severe groin or proximal thigh pain and related limp and Trendelenburg gait. Because of these symptoms, most will require a reconstructive procedure.

Avascular Necrosis

The ischemic event of the femoral neck fracture that leads to revascularization and subsequent trabecular thinning and collapse has been called posttraumatic osteonecrosis, aseptic necrosis of the femoral head, late segmental collapse, and avascular necrosis.[3,13,20,80] It is associated with an impacted or nondisplaced fracture in about 10% to 15% of patients and in 30% to 35% of displaced fractures.[12] Fracture displacement with damage to the arteriolar supply, as well as intracapsular tamponade, plays a causative role. Some reports indicate that patients with normal bone density are at greater risk for this complication.[22] This implies that a greater amount of force is involved with the cause of the fracture, and the displacement and soft tissue injury are therefore greater.[93] Certainly the incidence of avascular necrosis has been reported to be higher in younger adults with high-energy injuries.[52,138,179,186] Older individuals with lower functional demands will have symptoms of groin and proximal thigh pain severe enough to warrant a reconstructive procedure in 35% to 50% of cases.[12] Most agree that the higher the functional demands, the more likely it is that the patient will require a secondary procedure. Patients younger than 50 years who develop this complication nearly all require a reconstructive procedure.[138]

Pain

Pain following a femoral neck fracture is minimized by stable internal fixation. Groin or buttock pain that develops in the recovery period is generally associated with impending nonunion (with loss of stability) or avascular necrosis. However, with modern fixation techniques the incidence of nonunion is well below 10%, and thus the latter is more likely.[95,196] The pain is probably caused by revascularization of the femoral head with resorption of dead trabeculae and associated microfractures in the subchondral region, which leads to segmental collapse.[16] An acute increase in pain not related to a traumatic event is frequently associated with the final collapse of the segment. Pain can be rarely associated with postsurgical sepsis or injury to the sciatic nerve. In the late stages, pain can be related to the development of posttraumatic degenerative arthritis, which is most frequently related to avascular necrosis and resultant loss of femoral head sphericity.[21,81,145]

Limited Motion

Limited motion is commonly associated with pain, as the position of maximal hip extension is avoided. This position decreases capsular volume and raises intraarticular pressure while placing maximal stress across the femoral neck. This symptom therefore is generally associated with nonunion or avascular necrosis. In the remote phase, true loss of motion caused by capsular fibrosis and osteophyte formation is a result of posttraumatic degenerative hip arthritis.

Impaired Mobility

After hip fractures, half or more of patients fail to regain their preoperative level of mobility.[108a,129a] In some patients this may result from complications of the fracture; in others, from deterioration of their overall mental or physical condition. In many cases, the impaired mobility that results from a femoral neck fracture will result in the loss of independent living for an older patient. Holmberg and colleagues reviewed 3053 consecutive femoral neck fracture patients from Stockholm. A relatively large percentage (79%) were living in their own homes, 16% were in chronic care hospitals, and 5% were in homes for the elderly. Mortality was lowest in those patients admitted from home: 9% at four months, 16% at one year, and 22% at two years, compared with 16%, 22%, and 30% respectively for the entire series, illustrating the greater impact of the injury on institutionalized patients.

By four months, 69% of those living at home when injured had returned there, 20% were in chronic care hospitals, and 2% in acute care institutions. Most of those patients initially discharged to convalescent facilities returned home after two months. Concomitant illness, rather than the hip fracture itself, was the reason for long-term institutionalization.[99a] It may be assumed that differences among societies and medical care systems will influence the course and site of rehabilitation after femoral neck fracture. No convincing data have been published demonstrating the superiority of any given form of treatment for femoral neck fracture with regard to outcome measured by ability to walk, or by rate of institutionalization.

Medical Complications

Medical complications associated with femoral neck fractures increase in incidence with the age of the patient at injury. Potential complications include urinary tract infection; wound infection; ileus, occasionally with risk of cecal rupture; mental status changes; stroke; myocardial infarction; pneumonia; deep venous thrombosis; pulmonary embolus; and death. When patients present after fracture, a full medical evaluation must be performed and treatment instituted to deal with dehydration, electrolyte imbalance, and pulmonary dysfunction. The risk of medical complications is favorably influenced by early surgery and mobilization.[151] However, Kenzora et al.'s demonstration of a higher rate of mortality in patients operated on during the first day after injury emphasizes the need for adequate medical evaluation and preoperative treatment of correctable medical conditions.[116]

The vast majority of investigators have identified a favorable influence on the rate of deep venous thrombosis with prophylaxis.[31,85,86,87,137] Dextran, warfarin, subcutaneous heparin therapy, phenindione, aspirin, dihydroergotamine, and intermittent compression boots have all been reported to decrease the incidence of deep venous thrombosis. Limb elevation and early patient mobilization also favorably influence the rate of thrombosis.[88,116] Some form of prophylaxis against deep venous thrombosis and pulmonary embolism should be instituted in the preoperative or early postoperative period.

Nutritional supplements have been shown to play an important role in aiding recovery and minimizing wound healing complications.[14,14a,165,186a] Medical consultation should be sought preoperatively and again with any sign of postoperative complication to minimize the effect of these problems.

Mortality

An increased mortality rate over that of the general population following femoral neck fracture has been confirmed in numerous studies. In the large series of Barnes et al., the mortality rate in the first month after surgery was 13.3% in men and 7.4% in women.[12] The mortality rate increased significantly when the surgery was delayed beyond 72 hours. Similarly, in a large Norwegian series published by Dahl, the figures were 17.1% for males and 9.8% for females in the first month following fracture.[50] The mortality rate when compared with an age-matched population was 15 times greater in the first month, seven times greater in the second month, and thereafter followed the population trends. Kenzora et al. found a mortality rate at one year of 13% in the femoral neck fracture population compared with 9% for the age-matched controls.[116] Holmberg et al. confirmed the clinical suspicion that patients who sustain their femoral neck fractures in institutions have a higher mortality (three times) than those who are injured at home.[97] Those patients who sustain a second femoral neck fracture have a higher mortality rate than those with a single fracture. This was confirmed by Boston, who found a three-month mortality of 30% after the second fracture compared with 13% for a single such injury.[22] Several studies have suggested that the mortality rate is higher following prosthetic replacement than after internal fixation.[146,105,106] Additionally, Chan and Hoskinson found a higher mortality rate after a posterior approach for prosthetic replacement (20.6%) than after an anterior approach (6.5%).[34] Because many of the deaths following these fractures are attributable to thromboemboli and nutritional and pulmonary dysfunction, efforts toward prophylaxis against deep venous thrombosis, supplemental nutrition, and early mobilization of the patient are warranted.

Commonly Associated Injuries

In the "high-energy" femoral neck fracture population, associated injuries are common. Most series reporting on patients younger than 50 with nonpathologic femoral neck fractures report an incidence of head, chest, abdominal, or extremity fractures or dislocations in the range of 50% to 60%.[8,52,138,179,182] Closed head injury, cervical or thoracic spine fractures, pneumothorax or hemopneumothorax, and splenic or bowel injury occur commonly in association with a high-energy femoral neck fracture. Because of the axial loading mechanism, the most frequent musculoskeletal injury associations are ipsilateral tibial or femoral fractures, patellar fracture or knee ligament injury, and ipsilateral pelvic fracture or acetabular fracture or hip dislocation.[74]

In the more common "low-energy" femoral neck fractures, which are related to falls from a standing position, associated injuries are less common. Head injury, including subdural or epidural hematoma, may occasionally occur. Ipsilateral injury to the upper extremity (commonly the distal radius or proximal humerus), which occurs in an attempt to break the fall, occurs in 1% to 2% of cases. Far more common is the situation in which a medical problem such as cerebrovascular accident or myocardial infarction is responsible for the fall.

Evolution of Classification

When Senn, in 1889, became the first to advocate immediate reduction and internal fixation, a need was created for a classification system with which to compare and report results.[148] Speed advocated the formation of groups to study this fracture, noting that "in comparison to practically all other (fractures) this fracture remains unsolved."[163] Pauwels' classification system, reported in 1928, classified femoral neck fractures in reference to the inclination of the fracture relative to the horizontal axis of the hip joint.[135] His type I was a horizontal fracture which, because of the forces of impaction, had the lowest risk of nonunion. Whereas his type II has an intermediate inclination, the type III fracture is a more vertical fracture that produces a high risk of nonunion. Because the more horizontal fractures tended to be impacted fractures and the more vertically oriented fractures were generally associated with higher energy and displacement, the classification system was somewhat prognostic.

Garden's classification was an attempt to classify fractures according to their prognosis and incidence of complications.[12] His grade I is an incomplete fracture impacted in a valgus position; II is a nondisplaced fracture; III is a fracture displaced in a varus position; and IV is a completely displaced fracture in which the bony trabeculae within the head have realigned themselves with the trabecular system within the acetabulum (Fig. 43–9). It is probable that many, if not most, grade I injuries are actually complete fractures impacted in a valgus position. Nondisplaced, nonimpacted fractures are only occasionally seen. Because of their high risk of displacement, these grade II fractures deserve to remain a separate category. The difference between a Garden grade III and a Garden grade IV in displaced fractures is frequently difficult to delineate on radiographic review. Furthermore, the large clinical series of Barnes et al. failed to demonstrate a significant difference in terms of the risk of nonunion and avascular necrosis between these two groups.[12] In terms of the results and incidence of complication when utilizing the Garden classification in this large series, the I and II grades (nondisplaced) and the III and IV grades (dis-

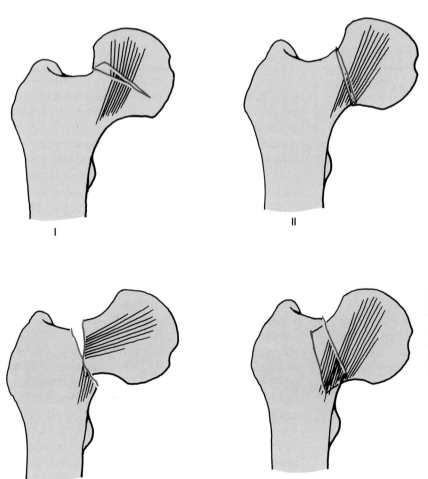

I

II

III

IV

Figure 43–9

The Garden classification for femoral neck fractures. Grade I is an incomplete, impacted fracture in valgus malalignment (generally stable); grade II is a nondisplaced fracture; Grade III is an incompletely displaced fracture in varus malalignment; grade IV is a completely displaced fracture with no engagement of the two fragments. The compression trabeculae in the femoral head line up with the trabeculae in the acetabular side. Displacement is generally more evident on the lateral view in grade IV. For prognostic purposes, these groupings can be lumped into nondisplaced/impacted (grades I and II) and displaced (grades III and IV), as the risks of nonunion and aseptic necrosis are similar within these grouped stages.

placed) fell together with little confirmation of a need to distinguish between them.

Femoral neck fractures with associated femoral shaft, femoral head, or acetabular fractures need to be classified separately. In the case of ipsilateral femoral shaft–femoral neck fracture, the risk of avascular necrosis is 5%, far lower than without the associated shaft fracture.[172] Casey and Chapman have offered the hypothesis that much of the energy producing the fractures is dissipated through the femoral shaft, which frequently makes the femoral neck injury a lower energy, minimally displaced fracture.[30] Femoral neck fractures associated with femoral head fractures carry a very poor overall prognosis in terms of high risk of avascular necrosis and joint degeneration and therefore are included with the classification of femoral head fractures (see preceding section). Finally, the outcome of a femoral neck fracture associated with an acetabular fracture is as dependent on the pattern of the acetabular fracture (perhaps more so) as it is on the outcome of the femoral neck injury and should therefore be classified with the acetabular injury (see chapter 32).

Current Classification

Nondisplaced

Nondisplaced fractures include both the truly nondisplaced fracture that occurs after a traumatic event and the impacted valgus femoral neck fracture. The lack of displacement places this fracture type into a much better prognostic situation in terms of nonunion or avascular necrosis.[9] Biologically, this results from the fact that the main arterial supply to the femoral head is seldom (if ever) disrupted with these fracture patterns. Similarly, because of the lower amount of energy involved in producing the fracture and the resultant lack of displacement, intracapsular tamponade may play a more central role in producing avascular necrosis when it occurs.[171]

Displaced

Displaced fractures include all femoral neck fractures with any detectable displacement. In the strictest sense this would indicate any alignment offset between the distal intertrochanteric fragment and the proximal femoral head fragment. There are important prognostic factors that accompany this designation, as with the fracture offset the major arterial supply to the femoral head may be disrupted, which has implications in regard to both avascular necrosis and nonunion. Additionally, when fracture management is delayed, synovial fluid may bathe the fracture surfaces and negatively influence the rate of union. The higher risk of both complication categories plays a major role in determining fracture treatment, especially in the older, more sedentary patient.

Fatigue

Fatigue fractures result from repetitive loading in pathologic (rheumatoid arthritis, osteoporosis) and nonpathologic (military recruits) bone.[7,19,62,91,108,183] Devas subclassified stress or fatigue fractures into two subgroups, transverse (tension) and compression, based on prognostic factors.[55] It is important to recognize that fatigue fractures occur more often in patients with osteoporosis than in those with normal bone density.[101,113]

Transverse (Tension) Fractures. Transverse fractures start as a crack at the superior neck, apparent on the internally rotated AP pelvic radiograph, and become complete over days to weeks. If left untreated, there is a significant risk of displacement in patients in this fracture subgroup.[11,45,134] These fractures are distinct from the nondisplaced type in that they are not associated with a single traumatic event.[57]

Compression. Compression fractures are seen radiographically as a haze of internal callus at the inferior neck. There is essentially no risk of displacement without additional trauma, so most authors agree these should be treated with crutch ambulation.[55]

Pathologic

The treatment of pathologic fractures, including those of the femoral neck, is covered in chapter 17.

Young Adults

The treatment of fractures of the femoral neck in patients with open physes in the proximal femur is beyond the scope of this text. In adolescents and younger adults (younger than 50), femoral neck fractures do occur in patients with normal bone density because of high-velocity trauma. The same classification applies as noted previously, but the prognosis is worse in these younger patients.[138] Especially in the case of displaced femoral neck fractures in these individuals, extreme trauma has produced displacement of the fracture fragments. This explains the increased incidence of avascular necrosis and nonunion in series of young patients. Smith documented loads of 900 to 2000 pounds to produce femoral neck fractures in cadavers.[157] Based on the supposition that the articulated hips in his study were probably from older individuals, one can extrapolate even higher forces to produce femoral neck fractures in young adults.

Special Cases

There are conditions of abnormal bone metabolism that can make the diagnosis and treatment recommendations quite different. For these reasons, the standard classification can be applied but with modifications as noted in the following two sections.

Rheumatoid Arthritis. Because of the severe hip synovitis that can occur with this disease, bone density is generally poor and chronic hip symptoms can mask acute femoral neck fractures.[170] Williams et al. reported that four of five patients with rheumatoid arthritis and a femoral neck fracture did not have a fall in their medical history.[192] This implies that fatigue fractures through severely osteoporotic bone are a common occurrence in this setting. Femoral neck fracture can also be occasionally seen in an osteoarthritic hip.[189] Treatment in both situations, because of the underlying articular disease, should generally be total hip arthroplasty.[40,53,153,154,180]

Renal Failure. Patients on chronic renal dialysis have metabolic bone disease and develop femoral neck fatigue fractures as outlined previously. Treatment, when the fractures are displaced, is generally total hip arthroplasty. Internal fixation of displaced fractures in the setting of severe osteoporosis will be mechanically suboptimal.[175] Biological factors may interfere with healing as well.

Basilar Neck Fracture

The low femoral neck/high intertrochanteric hip fracture represents an area of transition. Although generally true, it cannot be universally assured that these fractures are extracapsular and carry a better prognosis. A severely displaced low femoral neck fracture can still result in the disruption of the lateral epiphyseal artery complex. Based on laboratory studies, Claffey determined this degree of displacement to be half the diameter of the femoral head superiorly (distal fragment relative to femoral head).[38] Because the fracture is not frequently viewed radiographically at the extreme of displacement that occurs at the time of the injury, this is a distinct possibility in the case of the basilar neck fracture. Although most surgeons may favor an internal fixation construct that would be selected for an intertrochanteric hip fracture,[39,133] the fracture should be viewed biologically as a femoral neck fracture (with its attendant risk of avascular necrosis of the femoral head) and treated as such with urgent fixation and capsulotomy.

DIAGNOSIS

Clinical Suspicion

In the most common setting of low-velocity femoral neck fractures resulting from falls, clinical suspicion is based on the history, complaint, and physical exam. In the case of a high-velocity femoral neck fracture, suspicion is often based on the history alone, as the complaint and physical exam may be unavailable because of central nervous system injury or may be masked by other musculoskeletal injury. When high-quality plain radiographs in two planes fail to demonstrate the fracture, a high index of suspicion mandates further evaluation. In the low-energy case, tomography or CT scanning can be employed to evaluate critically the femoral neck region. If still inconclusive, the patient should be treated with bed rest and evaluated with a technetium bone scan at 48 to 72 hours following injury.[64] If the scan is negative, the patient can be safely treated symptomatically.

In the case of the high-energy injury, clinical suspicion should be high when there is an associated patellar fracture or knee ligament (especially posterior cruciate) injury; midshaft femoral shaft fracture; or an ipsilateral calcaneus, distal tibia, or tibial or femoral shaft fracture resulting from vehicular trauma or a jump or fall from a significant height.[172] If high-quality films do not reveal the fracture and the associated injuries require urgent care, the physician should proceed. Whenever there are procedures done with the femur (i.e., intramedullary nailing), the femoral neck should be quickly reevaluated with the image intensifier. When treatment of other injuries is not pressing, the surgeon can proceed with tomography, CT, or bone scanning as outlined previously.

History

In the case of the young patient involved in a high-velocity event, information about the event is helpful in directing the clinical and radiographic evaluation. The physical and radiographic exams, however, are usually more valuable than the history for directing the evaluation and treatment. An accurate history is more important in the more common situation, the low-energy femoral neck fracture that usually occurs in older individuals. For these elderly, occasionally demented patients, it is essential to obtain a reliable description of the activity level prior to injury. Did the patient ambulate independently? Was he or she able to assist with transfers from bed to chair and so forth? This information can help the physician in making the choice between internal fixation of the fracture and prosthetic replacement. Prognosis is influenced by the patient's preinjury functional level, preexisting medical problems, and, especially, mental status.

Additionally in the older patient, it is critical to seek information about the potential for the fracture to be associated with significant osteoporosis. Information concerning medications, medical conditions, and activity level is helpful in this regard. Finally, investigating whether there was pain in the groin or proximal thigh prior to the fracture may suggest the presence of some type of pathologic fracture.

Physical Examination

The evaluation of the patient involved in high-energy trauma is covered in chapter 5. In the case of the femoral neck fracture associated with a minor fall, the examination can be conducted in a more methodical manner. The presence of a femoral neck fracture may be apparent from the attitude of the affected leg, with obvious shortening, external rotation, and reluctance to move the limb. Alternatively, usually with an undisplaced fracture, the injury may be occult, suggested only by the patient's complaints of groin, thigh, or (rarely) lateral hip pain. Tenderness in the hip region produced by percussion on the sole of the foot with the fist or pain at extremes of hip motion, particularly rotation, may be the only local physical findings to suggest such an occult hip fracture.

After evaluating vital signs and mental status, the head and neck exam should focus on areas of tenderness, evidence of contusions or abrasions, and decreased cervical range of motion. If any of these are present, a hard cervical collar should be applied until the cervical spine can be cleared radiographically. The chest should be palpated for signs of rib fracture and auscultated to rule out pneumothorax. A screening exam of the upper and lower extremities should follow with palpation and with the patient, if alert, putting the joints through a range of motion. The examination should then focus on the affected lower extremity. The trochanteric region should be evaluated for contusions and for traumatic or nontraumatic skin conditions that might influence surgical management. The knee should be examined for tenderness, effusion, and instability. If this is not possible because of thigh pain, the knee exam must be repeated prior to the surgical procedure after initiation of anesthesia. The thigh and leg should be palpated and the foot and ankle examined for signs of trauma. The circulatory status of both limbs should be assessed as a baseline for follow-up evaluations and the status of the pulses carefully recorded. Finally, a complete sensory and motor examination of the limb should be performed and the findings of the physical examination detailed in the medical record.

When the patient's complaints and history suggest a femoral neck fracture, but physical findings are lacking, the patient should be evaluated with a technetium bone scan as outlined earlier.

Radiographic Imaging

Plain Films

For patients involved in high-energy injuries, an AP radiograph of the pelvis is routinely obtained as a part of the early trauma series of radiographs. The area of the femoral neck should always be carefully scrutinized. When possible, the legs should be taped in internal rotation prior to obtaining this film. Physical or radiographic findings of ipsilateral trauma in the leg and a history of injury from a dashboard type of mechanism or fall from a significant height should alert the consulting orthopaedist to obtain the routine anteroposterior (AP) pelvic radiograph.

In the low-energy setting, an AP pelvic radiograph, with the legs gently internally rotated, should be obtained and observed for the potential of a femoral neck fracture. If a hip fracture is suspected from history and physical findings, but is not evident on this initial radiograph, it is important to obtain an AP radiograph of the symptomatic hip with the femur sufficiently internally rotated to show a maximal profile of the anteverted femoral neck region, as this will be the projection most likely to demonstrate an occult fracture.

An estimate of osteoporosis should be made using the Singh index, as it has some predictive value regarding the degree of osteoporosis and the potential for obtaining stable internal fixation.[155] If a fracture is evident or suspected on clinical grounds, a cross-table lateral radiograph of the affected limb is also required. This radiograph is made with the affected limb remaining on the stretcher while the good limb is flexed up to obtain the proper angle. The lateral view should be scrutinized for posterior femoral neck comminution, as this, too, affects the prognosis for obtaining stable internal fixation.

Tomography

Tomography is helpful in identifying a nondisplaced femoral neck fracture when it is not radiographically apparent but is suspected on clinical grounds (e.g., history, complaint, or pain on rotation of the hip). Tomography also can provide critical information with regard to typing fatigue fractures for treatment purposes. Generally, AP tomography of the proximal femur is obtained with the feet taped together to internally rotate the involved hip. This positions the axis of the femoral neck perpendicular to the tomographic beam and improves the quality of the study. Occult and pathologic fractures of the upper femur can be detected with this technique.

Radionuclide Studies

Radionuclide uptake has been studied for more than 50 years with the concept of using this technique to detect avascular necrosis at an early stage. Radioactive calcium, phosphorus, and iodine were injected and Geiger counter systems utilized to obtain data that could be assessed in terms of femoral head blood flow.[23,25,100] These miniature injection systems, although they showed some early promise, were not consistently reliable and involved high radiation burdens for the patient.

The two techniques that remain in use for assessment of femoral neck fractures are sulfur colloid scans and technetium 99m diphosphonate scans.[129,168] The former is a compound that demonstrates bone marrow viability and has been used with good success as a predictor of avascular necrosis. Unfortunately a large series of patients has not been followed after use of this technique. It has been considered to be accurate, and the data obtained have been utilized for decision making for performing prosthetic replacement.[129] It has the drawbacks of a significantly higher radiation burden, less detailed images, and a longer delay after injection before the images are obtained.

Technetium 99m diphosphonate scanning is the method of choice for both diagnosing an undisplaced femoral neck fracture when radiographs are negative and obtaining predictive data in regard to the risk of nonunion and avascular necrosis.[15,82,83,123] Stromqvist[164] and Stromqvist et al.[168] have published results from 468 patients who underwent serial bone scans after femoral neck fractures. They determined that visual evaluation of pictorial images (scintigrams) is neither reproducible nor reliable. Quantitative scans (scintimetry) allow side-to-side comparison based on carefully defined regions of interest (ROI). Preoperative bone scans were not helpful as predictors of avascular necrosis or nonunion, as internal fixation procedures could be followed by either deterioration of perfusion with avascular necrosis or recovery of an apparently unperfused femoral head. They also reported that screw-type implants have a much more favorable influence on femoral head circulation than do triflanged nails that are hammered into the bone.[169] Data on femoral head uptake is expressed as a ratio relative to the intact side. The best prediction of result after internal fixation of a femoral neck fracture is provided by scintimetry performed between two and three weeks after injury and fixation. If the ratio of the injured to the uninjured ROI is less than 0.9, patients had an 84% chance of developing nonunion, avascular necrosis, or both. For patients with an abnormal contralateral hip, the uptake ratio of femoral head to ipsilateral femoral

shaft can be measured. If this ratio is at least 1.4, uneventful healing is likely. By four weeks after injury, those who go on to develop nonunion or avascular necrosis have equal or higher femoral head uptake, which lasts up to 24 months after injury. These data integrate well with the hypothesis that revascularization follows an avascular episode and produces trabecular resorption and weakening, which allows mechanical failure in the subchondral plate and femoral head collapse.[80]

Scintigraphic images produced by nuclear medicine scanning cameras can be helpful for diagnosing occult problems of the proximal femur. When plain radiographs are normal, osteoblastic activity in the region of the femoral neck, demonstrated by a technetium phosphate scan, may indicate the presence of a nondisplaced or fatigue femoral neck fracture.[64] In this setting, visual inspection of scintigrams, rather than scintimetric data, is most helpful, as it is in searching for additional occult metastases of a primary lesion when planning treatment of a pathologic fracture. Thus scintigraphic bone scans can be valuable for localizing and identifying lesions, but unlike scintimetric data, they have not proved helpful in the effort to preoperatively establish the prognosis for uneventful healing of a given femoral neck fracture (Fig. 43–10).

Other Studies

CT Scanning

Computerized tomography can function in the same way as plain tomography in demonstrating a nondisplaced femoral neck fracture. This may be most useful in the high-energy fracture patient who is undergoing an examination for abdominal, pelvic, or spine trauma. This technique is also of use in differentiating pathologic (nonosteoporotic) femoral neck fractures from nonpathologic fractures. Although good studies are available that confirm that the stability of the postfixation construct is most dependent on bone density, there are as yet no clinical data using CT-measured density to determine the potential for stability of internal fixation of femoral neck fractures.[175]

Dual-Photon Absorptiometry

Dual-photon absorptiometry has been shown to provide an accurate determination of spinal osteoporosis. However, some published reports indicate that spinal bone density is not directly related to femoral neck bone density.[68] The technique is being adapted to more accurately determine femoral neck bone density, and data regarding the bone density necessary to achieve a stable internal fixation may be forthcoming.

Magnetic Resonance Imaging

Magnetic resonance imaging has been shown to be a sensitive indicator of avascular change within the femoral head in nontraumatic forms of avascular necrosis. Severe distortion of the images is produced by proximal femoral internal fixation devices. Pure titanium or nearly pure titanium fixation devices must be utilized to study femoral head signals following internal fixation. This technique will most certainly allow a greater understanding of the pathologic processes of posttraumatic avascular necrosis, but whether it will have any predictive value or aid in decision making remains to be seen.

Compression Ultrasound

High-resolution, real-time ultrasonography has recently attracted interest as a simple, repeatable, noninvasive means for diagnosis of deep venous thrombosis. A variety of criteria have been proposed for the ultrasonographic diagnosis of venous thrombosis. Froehlich et al., in a prospective study of 40 hip fracture patients, used a single test: noncompressibility of the vein lumen.[74a] This was applied from the calf veins to the common femoral artery and validated with venography. Five patients (12.5%) had major thrombi; all were

asymptomatic. Compression ultrasound had an accuracy of 97%, a sensitivity of 100%, and a specificity of 97%. It is well tolerated and is significantly less expensive than venography.

Nutritional Assessment

Malnutrition is more common than expected in elderly patients with hip fractures, even in those with adequate resources.[14,14a,78a,164] Improved outcome after hip fracture has been demonstrated when dietary supplements are provided. Screening studies that may be used to evaluate nutritional status are absolute lymphocyte count, serum albumin, transferrin, and skin fold thickness.[14,14a,157a]

Essential Studies

The diagnostic algorithms for multiply injured patients are presented in chapter 5. To prevent missing a femoral neck fracture (which occurs most frequently in midshaft femoral neck fractures), the femoral neck must be carefully scrutinized as outlined previously. Spine and extremity radiographs are obtained based on the initial assessment, which includes the history of the injury and the physical exam. A preoperative electrocardiogram

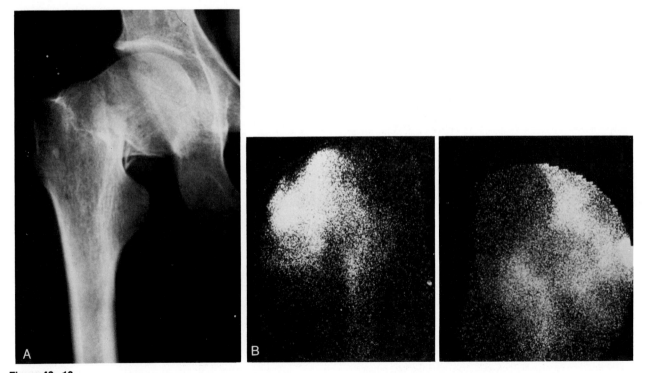

Figure 43–10

Scintigraphy after femoral neck fracture. *A,* A 23-year-old male fell off a bunk bed, sustaining this displaced Garden grade III femoral neck fracture. *B,* The patient underwent a preoperative bone scan at 8 hours after injury with the right side showing lower femoral head uptake than the left.

Illustration continued on following page

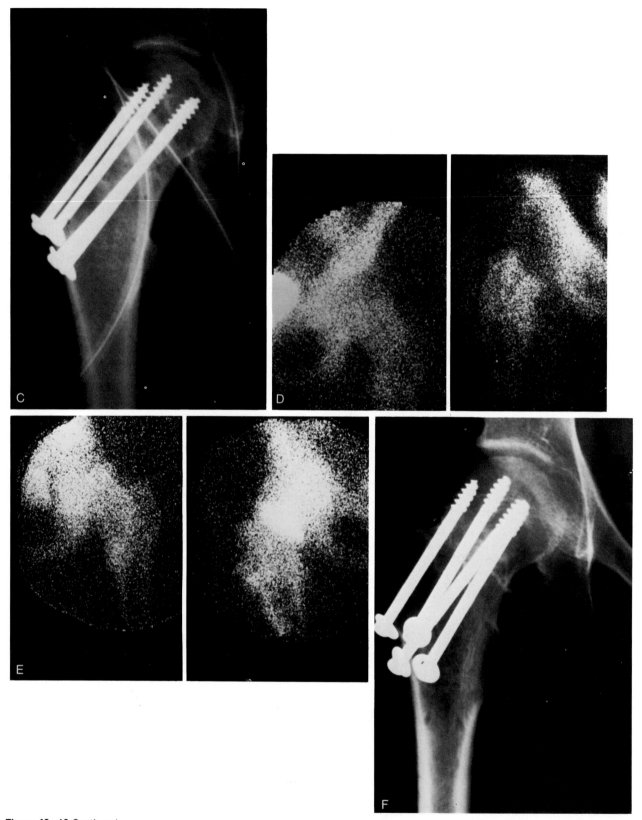

Figure 43–10 *Continued*

C, He underwent emergent open reduction using the Watson-Jones approach, with evacuation of intracapsulary hematoma and screw fixation with four cancellous screws. *D,* A bone scan obtained the day after surgery shows an even lower amount of femoral head uptake than previously when compared with the normal side. *E,* At three weeks, a bone scan shows a high degree of uptake, greater than on the intact side. *F,* An 18-month follow-up scan shows the fracture to be united with no evidence of osteonecrosis. This was confirmed at ten years.

(EKG); chest radiograph; screening CBC count, and serum electrolyte, creatinine, serum albumin, and urine analyses should be obtained in all patients older than 40 years. See discussion of evaluation of patient in chapter 44.

Differential Diagnosis

The differential diagnosis for a femoral neck fracture in a high-energy trauma patient must include a pelvic fracture, acetabular fracture, hip dislocation intratrochanteric or subtrochanteric femur fracture, and a contusion or muscle avulsion without fracture. The differential diagnosis of the patient with a low-energy femoral neck fracture should include intertrochanteric or subtrochanteric femur fracture, pelvic fracture, acetabular fracture, and hip contusion/traumatic trochanteric bursitis. The potential for pathologic lesions, nondisplaced fractures, fatigue fracture of the proximal femur or pelvis, and hip arthritis must be considered based on both the history and the physical exam.

MANAGEMENT

Evolution of Treatment

Nonunion and avascular necrosis of the femoral head have long been recognized to be the major problems associated with femoral neck fractures. Senn, in 1901, stated, "We are not only justified but warranted in assessing that the only cause for nonunion in the case of an intracapsular fracture is to be found in our inability to maintain coaption and immobilization of the fragments during the time required for boney union to take place."[163] He had previously advocated immediate reduction and internal fixation of these fractures in 1889 and had published animal data to support the concept that these fractures would heal with internal fixation.[148] Whitman, in 1902 and 1933, and Cotton, in 1927 and 1934, advocated closed reduction and impaction followed by placement into a spica cast in internal rotation as the method of choice for the management of femoral neck fractures.[42,43,190,191] Leadbetter further detailed the method of closed reduction and stated that "plaster fixation cannot be expected to yield good results consistently and logically in more than 65 or 75 percent of these (femoral neck fracture) cases."[121] Phemister outlined the pathophysiology of "creeping substitution" as it pertains to avascular necrosis of the femoral head following femoral neck fracture.[136]

The first widely accepted method for internal fixation was reported by Smith-Petersen et al. in 1931.[159] Use of this device was reported on in many publications until the mid 1970s. The most highly documented series was that of Fielding et al., published in 1962, which revealed a nonunion rate of 18% and an avascular necrosis rate of 29% in a series of 284 displaced and nondisplaced femoral neck fractures.[66] Moore published a report on the first multiple pin implant (adjustable nails) in 1937.[130] He thought the advantage of this type of implant was that no special tools were necessary for insertion. A 96% rate of union was reported. Multiple pin implants of several designs followed shortly thereafter. Moore then developed the prosthetic replacement for the femoral head and published on its use in 33 cases in 1952.[131] The Thompson prosthesis was developed shortly thereafter, and the current debate of whether to fix the femoral neck fracture or replace the femoral head began.[181] Sliding devices such as the Pugh nail (1955)[139] and the Richards screw (1964)[39] were developed for controlled impaction of the femoral neck fracture. More multiple pin and screw designs were added to the already numerous devices in the late 1960s and 1970s. The debate rages on regarding the replacement of the femoral head versus internal fixation and the indications for both.[24] When internal fixation is deemed warranted, most surgeons now utilize some type of multiple pins or screws, including a compression hip screw with an added screw or pin to prevent rotation of the femoral head.

Judet developed a method for placing a viable bone graft across the posterior aspect of the femoral neck fracture and into the femoral head to decrease the incidence of avascular necrosis and nonunion.[112] This quadratus femoris muscle pedicle graft was popularized by Meyers, who reported an 8% incidence of posttraumatic avascular necrosis and an 11% incidence of nonunion.[128a] Recent reports have not confirmed these results (Fig. 43–11).[110a]

Current Algorithm

Initial Treatment

During initial evaluation and care of the patient with a femoral neck fracture, it is important to splint the injured limb to protect it from additional damage as well as to minimize the patient's discomfort. Moderate flexion and external rotation increase the volume of the hip capsule and may thus decrease intracapsular pressure, with potential improvement of femoral head perfusion. A pillow under the knee, perhaps with gentle (five pounds) Buck's traction using a corrugated foam traction boot, will provide this. It is important that the leg be elevated enough from the mattress to protect the heel from pressure and the resulting skin breakdown.

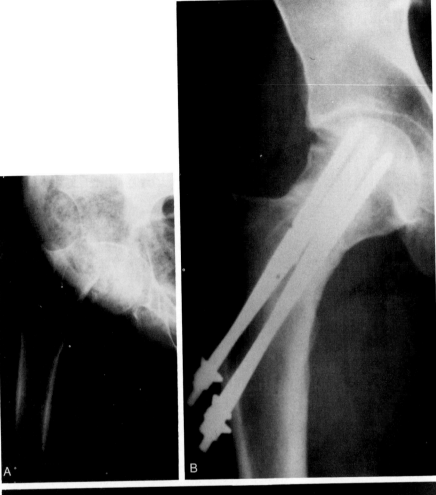

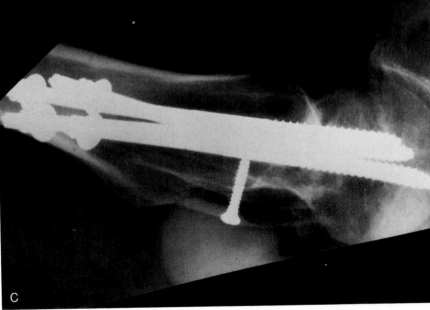

Figure 43–11

Quadratus femoris muscle pedicle graft for femoral neck fracture. *A*, A 63-year-old male was treated for a Garden grade III femoral neck fracture with a Judet quadratus femoris muscle pedicle graft. The patient was treated on a fracture table in the prone position using multiple modified Hagie pins. The quadratus femoris graft was placed posteriorly and fixed with a single screw. *B,C,* The result at 2½ years. The patient is ambulatory with a cane and is not complaining of hip symptoms.

Undisplaced Femoral Neck Fractures

As defined previously, undisplaced femoral neck fractures include both valgus-impacted (Garden grade I) and complete (Garden grade II) femoral neck fractures, because of the similar prognosis of both fracture types. Their treatment is the same. *Internal fixation is indicated for all undisplaced femoral neck fractures.* It has been clearly shown that mobilization of the patient results in a lower mortality rate.[151] Internal fixation allows mobilization of the patient without loss of fracture reduction in most cases (osteoporotic femoral heads are infrequently an exception). With conservative treatment (recumbant position for seven weeks), the displacement rate or disimpaction rate has been shown to be 10% to 27% by Bentley,[17] Hilleboe et al.,[91] and Jensen and Hogh.[109] Bentley reported that the avascular necrosis rates following nondisplaced femoral neck fracture were 14% for conservative treatment and 18% for internal fixation.[17] If displacement occurs, the rates more than double, and prosthetic replacement may become the treatment of choice for an older patient. Therefore internal fixation with a multiple pin or screw implant of the surgeon's choice seems justified. Because insertion of a nail type device might displace the fracture, nails should *not* be used. Several laboratory and clinical publications support the concept of performing a capsulotomy to release excessive pressure from fracture bleeding into the hip joint capsule.[98,107]

Displaced Femoral Neck Fracture

As previously discussed, the treatment of displaced femoral neck fractures is aimed at restoring hip function. Rapid mobilization of the patient is thought to reduce the risks of medical complications and improve the ultimate functional outcome. Additionally, it decreases the costly length of stay in an acute care hospital. Failure of fracture fixation, nonunion, and avascular necrosis with symptomatic late segmental collapse have long been recognized as serious complications that compromise the results of treatment for femoral neck fractures. Striving to provide mobilization while avoiding these and other complications, the treatment scheme has evolved from closed reduction and casting, to internal fixation, to prosthetic replacement and presently to a selective use of both prosthetic replacement and internal fixation. The currently offered algorithm for displaced femoral neck fractures employs internal fixation, after closed or open reduction, for the majority of cases. Prosthetic replacement is reserved for those chronologically older patients in whom internal fixation is unlikely to succeed—those with marked osteopenia, fracture comminution, or both. In general, such patients are physiologically elderly, with low functional

demands. Their ambulation is at best restricted to their domicile, they may be unable to assist with their own care, and their life expectancy is often limited. They are thus less at risk of developing late complications that might require revision of an arthroplasty. Although different types of prosthetic replacement for the proximal femur have relative advantages and disadvantages, none can provide as durable and functional a hip as that regained by satisfactory bone healing. Furthermore, failure after internal fixation of a femoral neck fracture can be satisfactorily salvaged by total hip arthroplasty, which has a low rate of complications.[85b] Failed hemiarthroplasties require a similar procedure, though a more difficult one with possibly poorer results.[63]

Indications. Surgical treatment is warranted for all but the most medically fragile and bed-bound patients with displaced femoral neck fractures. The basic choice of treatment is between internal fixation and arthroplasty. This controversy will be discussed further in the following section. It is recommended that several factors be considered when choosing a treatment for patients with displaced femoral neck fractures.

Age alone is a poor predictor of activity level, bone quality, and life expectancy, all of which should also be considered when deciding between reduction/fixation and replacement arthroplasty. If they succeed, reduction (either closed or open) and internal fixation provide the best and most durable result after displaced femoral neck fracture. Failure of reduction and fixation results from early loss of fixation, from nonunion, and from symptomatic segmental collapse resulting from avascular necrosis. Although not always predictable, fixation problems are most common in patients with osteopenic bone and comminution. Prosthetic replacement of the proximal femur avoids the problems of nonunion and avascular necrosis but may have a higher perioperative morbidity than internal fixation.[105] Additionally, it poses late problems of loosening and acetabular erosion, either of which may need revision surgery. Results after revision of failed hemiarthroplasties are not as good as those following primary total hip arthroplasty, and the procedure may be quite difficult.[63] Therefore the initial treatment for a displaced femoral neck fracture should seek to minimize the likelihood of needing to revise a failed arthroplasty in the future. In general this is best accomplished by restricting hemiarthroplasties to low-demand users with limited life spans. Variations in arthroplasty implants and technique may increase their durability and ease of revision, though the data to support this assertion are not yet conclusive.

Factors that suggest the advisability of prosthetic replacement include pathologic bone, severe chronic illness (especially rheumatoid arthritis[192] and chronic renal failure), and a very limited life span. Advanced chronologic age alone is a questionable indication for hemiarthroplasty. Average life expectancy for 75-year-olds is more than 10 years.[4a] Therefore many would extend the indications for internal fixation into the early and mid 70s for active individuals with good bone density and without chronic illness. Inactive, osteoporotic elderly patients with a limited life span are candidates for simple unipolar hemiarthroplasties. Those with displaced femoral neck fractures who can ambulate functionally outside their homes (community ambulators), and whose likelihood of success with internal fixation is low should receive modern bipolar hemiarthroplasties, with the awareness that revision may be required in the future because of loosening of the femoral component or acetabular degenerative changes, including protrusio. These problems are greater in younger and more active patients. It is currently felt that the bipolar hemiarthroplasty may survive longer in more active patients and that its Morse taper modular design might make revision easier without removal of a securely fixed femoral component.[85a] Primary total hip arthroplasty may be an alternative for such individuals.[40,53,153,154,180]

Controversy. The debate regarding prosthetic replacement versus internal fixation for femoral neck fractures in older patients is widespread.[152,161] Hunter reviewed the subject in detail.[106] The literature on prosthetic replacement reveals the rate of clinically poor results to be 28%; dislocations, 0.3% to 11%; infection, 2% to 42%; and six-month mortality, 14% to 39%, all of which are significantly higher than corresponding rates for internal fixation. (Tables 43–1 and 43–2).[106] However, Sikorski and Barrington found that anterior approach hemiarthroplasty had a lower six-month mortality than did internal fixation.[152] Holmberg et al. found complication rates to be lower after prosthetic replacement (15%) than after internal fixation (37%).[99] In a retrospective nonrandomized study, Johnson and Crothers found the incidence of unsatisfactory results to be lower after prosthetic replacement. Rodriguez et al. reviewed multiple factors and concentrated on morbidity and mortality. They found internal fixation to be the most innocuous method of treatment.[146] Other reports of hemiarthroplasty suggest that perioperative complications might be less frequent than reported in earlier series (see Tables 43–1 and 43–2).[19a,61a,152,161]

Insistence on an adequate reduction and proper use of multiple screw or pin fixation has decreased the rate of fixation failure and nonunion to 10% or less in most recent series. Although avascular necrosis occurs in 10% to 30% of united, initially displaced femoral neck fractures, it may not become symptomatic enough to

require treatment, especially in low-demand users. If it does occur, salvage with total hip arthroplasty is safe and successful.[85a]

When the costs and potential complications of modern hip prostheses are considered, it appears wise to limit the use of bicentric and total hip arthroplasties to those patients who are most likely to benefit from them. In fact, many patients will not survive long enough after their hip fractures to justify procedures with higher risks and higher costs. White et al. reported

Table 43–1.

Reported Incidence of Dislocation of the Prosthesis After Primary Prosthetic Arthroplasty

Investigator	Percent
Hinchey and Day (1964)[92]	0.3
Glass (1965)[79b]	5
Hunter (1969)[105]	3
Lunt (1971)[124a]	10
Wrighton and Woodyard (1971)[194a]	3
Raine (1973)[139a]	8
Hunter (1974)[105a]	7
Chan and Hoskinson (1975)[34]	8
D'Arcy and Devas (1976)[51a]	2
Hunter (1980)[106]	11
Long and Knight (1980)[122]	2.6
Franklin and Gallannaugh (1983)[72]	0
Staeheli et al. (1988)[166]	2

Table 43–2.

Reported Incidence of Infection After Prosthetic Arthroplasty

Investigator	Percent
Garcia et al. (1961)[75a]	6
Hinchey and Day (1964)[92]	2
Glass (1965)[79b]	10
Niemann and Mankin (1968)[132a]	42
Hunter (1969)[105]	8
Lunt (1971)[124a]	19
Riska (1971)[143a]	5
Wrighton and Woodyard (1971)[194a]	9
Chan and Hoskinson (1973)[34]	2
Raine (1973)[139a]	6
Arnold et al. (1974)[4d]	16
Fielding et al. (1974)[65a]	8
Hunter (1974)[105a]	8
Kavlie and Sundal (1974)[114a]	3
Salvati et al. (1974)[146a]	17
Long and Knight (1980)[122]	0.5
Franklin and Gallannaugh (1983)[72]	0
Staeheli et al. (1988)[166]	0

that increased mortality is seen during the first year after hip fracture.[189a] This effect is greater for those with more severe preoperative medical problems. For 75-year-old patients, they found an approximately 6.5-fold increase in mortality during the first year after hip fracture. Applying this figure to the U.S. population with mortality rates identified in 1986,[4b] it can be calculated that only 10% of patients with hip fractures at age 75 will still be alive ten years later. A therapeutic strategy that advocates routine bipolar or total hip arthroplasty for 75-year-olds with femoral neck fractures will result in many patients receiving operations that they do not need to obtain comfortable function for the rest of their lives. Bauer and his group from the University of Lund, Sweden, have demonstrated the efficacy and safety of a therapeutic strategy that relies on initial internal fixation of all femoral neck fractures.[15] From their department, Stromqvist et al. recently reported 215 displaced femoral neck fractures treated with internal fixation.[168a] At two-year follow-up, 63 (29%) had died. Of the survivors, 53 had fracture healing complications: redisplacement or nonunion in 39 (18% of original group) and avascular necrosis with segmental collapse in 14 (6.5% of original group). These complications led to reoperations in 36 (17%) of the original group: 28 total hip arthroplasties and four hardware removals in the redisplacement/nonunion category; three total hip arthroplasties and one osteotomy in those with segmental collapse. The authors point out that if they had chosen routine arthroplasty for their displaced femoral neck fractures, the procedure would have been done unnecessarily for the 83% of patients who did not require revision operations. The end result in these patients was uneventful healing, death from other problems, or complications with tolerable symptoms. It is tempting to speculate that the 17% incidence of reoperations, mostly caused by loss of fixation and nonunion, could have been further decreased if those markedly osteopenic individuals with the greatest risk of such fixation problems had been treated instead with primary hemiarthroplasty. Note, however, that this is a small proportion of the whole group, whose average age was 78 years.

Orthopedists who take the middle ground seem to agree that the patient is best off with a healed femoral neck fracture, his or her own femoral head, and no avascular necrosis. When factors such as limited life span, chronic disease, and poor bone quality intervene, most North American surgeons would recommend prosthetic replacement.

Timing of Surgery. Numerous laboratory and clinical studies indicate that reduction of a displaced femoral neck fracture improves femoral head blood flow. This is probably because of "unkinking" the lateral epiphyseal artery complex in patients in whom these remain intact. Claffey showed that there can be superior displacement of the femoral head of up to one half the femoral neck diameter without disruption of these vessels.[38] These data all indicate the need for urgent, if not emergent, reduction of the femoral neck fracture. In one series of patients younger than 50 years with displaced femoral neck fractures, the rate of nonunion was 0% and avascular necrosis 20% when the femoral neck fractures were reduced and internally fixed with compression within eight hours.[179]

Intracapsular tamponade has similarly been found to have a negative influence of femoral head blood flow in numerous laboratory and clinical studies.[98] Although some authors disagree, the current recommendation is to extend the standard lateral approach into the Watson-Jones interval between the tensor fascia lata and gluteus medius and perform an anterior capsulotomy under direct vision (see Fig. 43–13). Although there may be only 5% to 10% of fractures in which the hip capsule is not disrupted by the original fracture displacement and sufficient intracapsular pressure has accumulated to impede the femoral head venous drainage or arteriolar supply, these can be effectively treated by this simple maneuver. This adds 5–10 minutes to the dissection and exposes the patient to no further risk. Furthermore, an anatomic reduction can then be achieved under direct vision.

Many older patients with femoral neck fractures have significant medical problems. Correcting these preoperatively may greatly reduce the risks of complications. Therefore extreme care should be taken to optimize the patient's condition for surgery. The time that this requires is well spent. Medical consultation should be obtained and the patient's fluid status evaluated. The cardiac and pulmonary status should be optimized and any indicated drug or respiratory therapy instituted as soon as possible. Nutritional factors should also be assessed so that they can be addressed early in the postoperative period. Bastow et al. has emphasized that mortality after hip fractures is increased in thin and very thin patients and that nutritional supplements can reduce both length of hospitalization and mortality.[14,14a] As soon as the patient is optimally prepared, surgery should be carried out. If internal fixation has been chosen, early surgery may be especially beneficial, since, as noted previously, there is evidence that early reduction of a displaced femoral neck fracture can improve the circulation of the femoral head.[179] This benefit may be of greatest value in minimizing the risk of symptomatic avascular necrosis in young patients with femoral neck fractures. However, the large series of Barnes et al. did not demonstrate a time-related difference in the complication rate (avascular necrosis, nonunion) among fractures fixed within the first 72 hours.[12]

If arthroplasty has been selected as the treatment of choice, early surgery after optimal patient evaluation and preparation is also beneficial because of the medical deterioration that is likely to occur as a result of immobility and pain in a bed-bound patient.

Treatment for Displaced Femoral Neck Fractures by Patient's Status

Young patients with normal bone and high-energy injuries: urgent closed or open reduction and internal fixation with multiple pins or screws, and with simultaneous capsulotomy.

Older patients with high functional demands and good bone density: rapid medical evaluation followed promptly by closed or open reduction and internal fixation with multiple pins or screws and with simultaneous capsulotomy.

Older patients with normal or intermediate longevity, poor bone density, chronic illness, and lower functional demands: bipolar hemiarthroplasty or possibly total hip arthroplasty.

Elderly, low-demand users with poor bone density: unipolar hemiarthroplasty.

Bed-bound, nonambulatory patients: trial of nonoperative treatment with consideration of early surgery (internal fixation, unipolar hemiarthroplasty, or excisional arthroplasty) if sufficient comfort for routine nursing care is not regained within a few days.

Fatigue Fractures

Devas classified fatigue fractures into compression and transverse fractures.[55] The latter appear as a crack at the superior femoral neck and are at significant risk (10% to 15%) for displacement, with resultant increased risk of avascular necrosis. A compression fracture starts at the inferior neck and gradually over many weeks appears as a haze of internal callus. These are much more common in the osteoporotic elderly woman and are less likely to displace.[101]

Treatment of Fatigue Fractures of the Femoral Neck by Type of Fracture

Transverse type: urgent internal fixation with multiple pins.

Compression type: mobilization with limited weight bearing using crutches or walker.

Pathologic Femoral Neck Fractures

The reader is referred to chapter 17 for details of diagnosis and treatment of pathologic fracture of the femoral neck. If surgery is indicated, some form of arthroplasty is necessary.

Polytrauma Patient

Associated Injuries

Nearly all femoral neck fractures in young patients with normal bone are secondary to high-velocity trauma. Fifty percent to seventy percent of patients younger than 50 years with a nonfatigue, displaced femoral neck fracture will have other organ system injuries.[138,179] The young patient with a displaced femoral neck fracture should be assumed to have other injuries until definitely proven otherwise.

Timing of Femoral Neck Fracture Management

Because of the significant risk of avascular necrosis with segmental collapse and the limited therapeutic alternatives for managing it, reduction and fixation of displaced femoral neck fractures are matters of great urgency for young individuals. Therefore, in the orthopedic management of the multiply injured patient, femoral neck fracture treatment should only be superceded by the debridement (not stabilization) of contaminated open fracture wounds and reduction of cervical spine subluxations or dislocations. A displaced femoral neck fracture in a young patient represents a true orthopedic emergency.

Associated Injury Protocols

Femoral Shaft Fractures. Ipsilateral femoral neck fractures occur with approximately 2.5% of femoral shaft fractures. Generally femoral neck fracture displacement is minimal, but it can be severe. Most often the hip injury is associated with a fracture within the middle third of the femoral shaft (greater than 80% of the reported cases).[172] The femoral neck fracture was missed on initial evaluation in 34% of published cases.[172] Initial radiographs of a patient with a femoral shaft fracture must include high-quality AP and lateral views of the femoral neck.

The femoral neck fracture must take precedence over the femoral shaft fracture because of the poor results of treatment of posttraumatic avascular necrosis in young patients. Optimal surgical management must be carried out to minimize the risk of avascular necrosis. The femoral neck should be treated as outlined previously with emergent reduction, capsulotomy, and internal fixation with three multiple pins or screws. In no case should an antegrade femoral nail be inserted adjacent to the femoral neck fracture without initially stabilizing the femoral neck, because of the high risk of displacing it. After the femoral neck is fixed, the femoral shaft may be fixed with plate and screws, flexible retrograde intramedullary nails, or a retrograde Küntscher or interlocking nail (Fig. 43–12).[30,172,174] If the femoral neck can be stabilized with screws or pins anterior to the standard intramedullary starting portal,

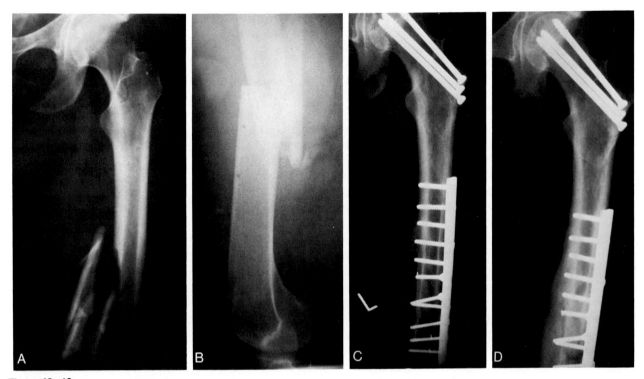

Figure 43-12

Associated femoral neck and shaft fractures. *A,B,* A 24-year-old female sustained this highly comminuted femoral shaft fracture with an ipsilateral vertical femoral neck fracture. *C,* She had an intraarticular distal femur fracture on the opposite side and a splenic rupture. Following her laparotomy, she underwent a Watson-Jones open reduction internal fixation of the femoral neck with cannulated screws, followed by plating of the femoral shaft. *D,* A radiograph at eight months shows complete healing of the femoral shaft fracture and femoral neck fracture. At 2½ years, the patient had not developed posttraumatic osteonecrosis. To diminish the risk of osteonecrosis, the femoral neck fracture should receive priority regardless of the treatment selected for the femoral shaft fracture in this injury combination.

then an antegrade standard or interlocking nail can be safely introduced. Recently developed cephalomedullary nails with proximal locking screws directed into the femoral head have also been advocated for fixation of ipsilateral neck and shaft fractures of the femur.[40a,79a,90a] There is a risk of displacing the neck fracture during insertion of such a nail, and location of the entry portal is critical. Initial reduction and provisional wire or pin fixation of the neck fracture should precede preparation of the femur for insertion of the cephalomedullary device.

Femoral Neck and Head Fractures. The reader is referred to the previous section on femoral head fractures for management of this injury combination. First priority is urgent reduction of the hip dislocation. Femoral head fracture fixation should be considered seriously in such a multiply injured patient. The shaft fracture should also be fixed but not in a manner that compromises treatment of the hip injury. In older patients, prosthetic replacement may be advisable for more severe femoral head fractures (Pipkin grades 2 and 3).

Femoral Neck-Acetabular Fractures. The treatment principles for the femoral neck fracture remain the

same. The femoral neck fracture should be treated urgently with operative stabilization; the acetabular fracture can be managed at a later time if indications for open reduction are present. Operative management of both fractures by an experienced surgeon is usually important for optimal results. See chapter 32 for details regarding the management of the acetabular portion of this fracture combination.

Individual Treatment Modalities

Nonoperative Management. The indications for nonoperative treatment are limited primarily to the compression type of fatigue fracture. The risk of displacement with its attendant higher risk of avascular necrosis is great enough that nonoperative treatment should not be considered for impacted acute or transverse fatigue femoral neck fractures. Nonoperative treatment for fatigue fractures consists of limiting activity to a pain-free level, often with crutches and partial weight bearing initially. Risky activities should also be avoided. Once symptoms have resolved and sufficient time (6 to 12 weeks) has elapsed for mechanically secure healing, progressive resumption of normal activity is begun.

Occasionally nonoperative treatment may be indicated for debilitated, usually demented, nonambulatory bed-ridden patients, possibly including those who, with significant assistance, may be able to transfer to a chair.[193a] Although it is relatively easy to forgo operation for such patients if they have severe cardiopulmonary illness and a very limited life span, some do not appear to be on the verge of demise. For these individuals, it is hard to justify surgical treatment in view of the limited benefits it offers and its high risks. A good test for the adequacy of nonoperative treatment in such patients is the achievement of comfort sufficient to tolerate routine nursing care. A few days with analgesia and careful logrolling will often suffice and may permit the patient to remain in a chronic care setting. In other circumstances, the patient may be transferred to a hospital emergency room, where the treating surgeon is faced with deciding between admitting the patient or sending him or her back to the chronic care facility. Good communication and collaboration between the surgeon and the patient's caretakers are essential. If the patient appears quite uncomfortable, it may be best to hospitalize the patient for a few days, often using a special low-pressure bed so that frequent turning is not necessary to avoid skin breakdown. With small doses of narcotics initially, the patient will usually become comfortable enough to tolerate routine nursing and may then return to his or her prior situation. Occasionally this is not well tolerated, and consideration should be given to unipolar hemiarthroplasty, excisional arthroplasty, or possibly closed reduction and multiple pin fixation. A drawback of internal fixation in such patients, especially if flexion contractures restrict them to a lateral decubitus position, is the risk of skin breakdown over prominent hardware, but it may offer the least invasive form of treatment.

In Situ Fixation

INDICATIONS. Indications include nondisplaced femoral neck fractures, fatigue fractures, and impacted femoral neck fractures.

TIMING OF SURGERY. Stabilization should be done as soon as the patient can be medically cleared. Because there is some evidence that intracapsular hematoma can be involved in the pathophysiology of avascular necrosis following this fracture, the need for internal fixation combined with a decompressive anterior capsulotomy is urgent.

PREOPERATIVE PLANNING AND PREPARATION. The radiographs of the fracture must be carefully evaluated in both planes to be sure there is no reduction indicated. A multiple screw (cannulated or noncannulated) or pin implant must be available in several lengths. The equipment must be available for screw or pin insertion (e.g., guides, depth measuring systems, etc.). A C-arm image intensifier fluoroscope is required. Perioperative

systemic antistaphylococcal antibiotics should be administered to reduce the frequency of postoperative infection.

ANESTHESIA AND POSITIONING. The patient should be positioned supine on the fracture table with the well leg in the lithotomy position or abducted in gentle traction. Radiographic control in the AP and lateral planes must be confirmed before starting the procedure. If this is not absolutely clear on the fluoroscope monitor, permanent films should be made using the appropriate attachment on the C arm. These actual radiographs, rather than digital copies of the fluoroscopic image, provide the best detail and often aid in interpreting the CRT image. Either spinal or general anesthesia is equally appropriate.[18,41]

SURGICAL TECHNIQUE. Percutaneous fixation can be achieved through small stab incisions, but this is not recommended, especially in younger patients in whom an anterior capsulotomy is indicated.[103,117] A straight lateral incision is made from the top of the trochanter to a point 1 cm distal to the lesser trochanter. The fascia lata is incised longitudinally and the vastus lateralis either split or lifted anteriorly. The capsular attachments at the trochanteric ridge/vastus tubercle can be exposed with anterior retraction and the capsule incised in line with the neck of the femur and released proximally and distally from the intertrochanteric ridge to produce a T-shaped capsulotomy. This will allow release of hematoma and palpation of the fracture if indicated. Extending this lateral incision into a femoral Watson-Jones approach through the interval between tensor fascia lata and gluteus medius will aid visualization of the fracture (Fig. 43–13).

A guide pin is placed centrally in the neck under fluoroscopic control in two planes. A multiholed guide can then be placed over the guide pin and used to predrill and insert three parallel screws (Fig. 43–14). There is insignificant mechanical advantage to adding more implants.[175] Sliding hip screws and telescoping nails are not recommended for femoral neck fractures.[27] Implant position must be verified with permanent AP and lateral radiographs, readily made with the C-arm fluoroscope as well as by careful fluoroscopy in different positions of hip rotation.

INTRAOPERATIVE COMPLICATIONS

Displacement of the Fracture. This can be avoided by gentle handling of the patient in positioning. If the fracture displaces, it is suggested that reduction and internal fixation be performed in active patients with good bone stock. If displacement is recognized before the procedure is initiated and the patient is not a candidate for internal fixation, he or she should be moved to a regular operating table and prepared for insertion of a prosthesis instead.

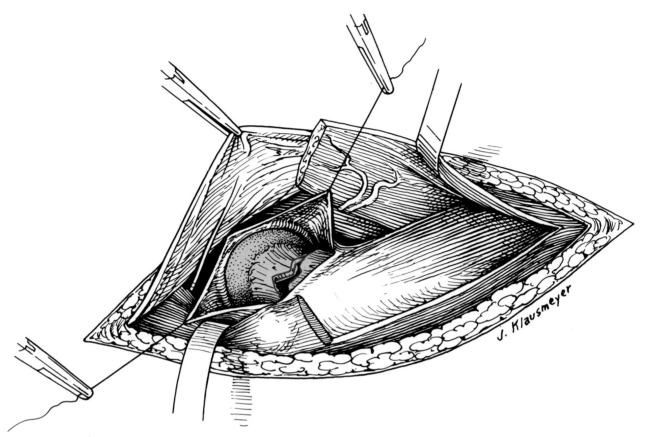

Figure 43-13

The Watson-Jones anterolateral exposure to the hip for open reduction of femoral neck fractures. The interval between the tensor fascia lata and the abductors is bluntly developed, and the vastus lateralis is elevated off the intertrochanteric ridge. The capsule is divided anteriorly along the axis of the neck of the femur and transversely released from its insertion into the proximal femur. With sutures as retracting aids, the fracture can be visualized. A bone hook can be used to disimpact the fracture by applying a laterally directed force, and a blunt instrument can be inserted to improve the reduction (i.e., lift the proximal fragment anteriorly). The insertion area for internal fixation devices on the lateral aspect of the proximal femur is easily exposed.

Intraarticular Pin Placement. Placement of pins or screws into the hip joint may easily go unrecognized, as a two-dimensional monitoring technique is used for a three-dimensional problem.[188] Thus the tips of intraarticular pins can appear to be inside the shadow of the femoral head. This fact should remind the surgeon to beware of subchondral pin positioning, especially in the periphery of the femoral head. Visualizing the joint in different rotational positions helps identify intraarticular pins. If recognized, replacement rather than partial withdrawal is best to avoid repenetration of the joint should the femoral neck shorten by impaction during fracture healing.

AFTERCARE. The patient should be out of bed in a chair two to three times daily beginning on the first postoperative day. Physical therapy should begin on the second or third postoperative day and the patient instructed in touch-down weight bearing with a walker (for most elderly patients) or crutches (for younger pa-

tients). This should be continued for 8 to 12 weeks following injury. Many older patients are unable to comply with restricted weight bearing, and this restriction appears to be of limited additional benefit, especially after internal fixation of undisplaced fractures. Most patients can be mobilized safely, with weight bearing as tolerated, using external support for the first four to six weeks after fixation. Long-term follow-up is advisable because of the risk of avascular necrosis, which may not be manifest for two or even three years.

HARDWARE REMOVAL. Hardware removal is generally not indicated for elderly patients. If, after one year has elapsed, the patient is unable to lie on the injured side because of pain over prominent hardware, the implants may be removed if fracture healing has been clinically and radiographically confirmed.

Reduction of Displaced Fractures

CLOSED REDUCTION. Closed reduction of displaced femoral neck fractures has been described by numer-

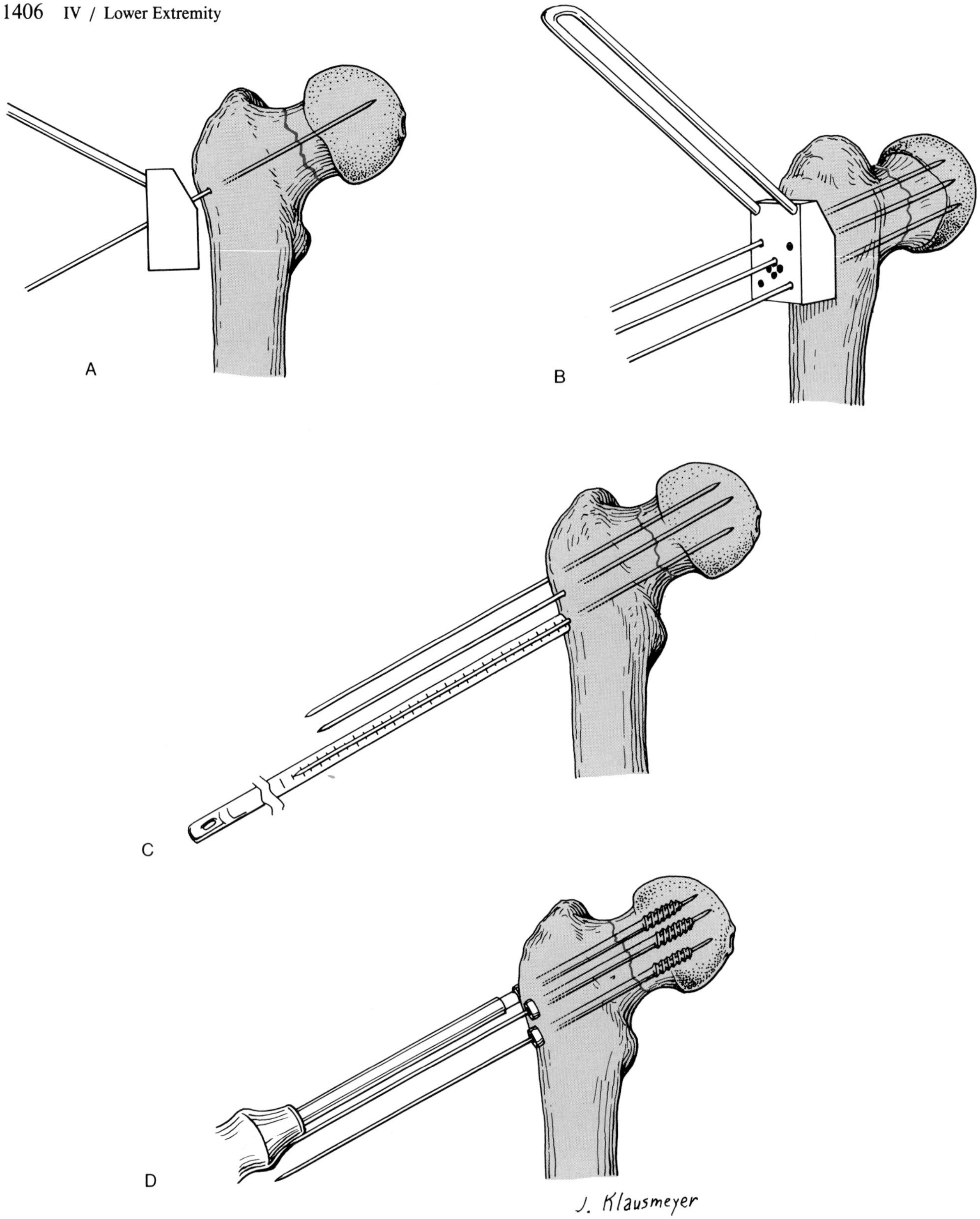

Figure 43–14

Internal fixation of a femoral neck fracture with a cannulated screw system. *A*, After satisfactory reduction is confirmed, the lateral aspect of the proximal femur is exposed and a control guide wire inserted. The guide is placed over the initial guide wire, and using the multiple holes available, adjustments are made to allow placement of all screws within the femoral neck. *B*, Remaining guide wires are inserted through the guide; drilling at high revolutions per minute (rpms) with a light hand will allow optimal control of the wires. *C*, Once three satisfactory parallel guide wires have been inserted using fluoroscopic control, then the length of the wires is determined. A cannulated drill may be used and should be inserted to 10 mm less than the total length of the wire to prevent the wire from being removed. *D*, A cannulated tap can be used in dense cancellous bone, and screws of appropriate length are inserted over guide wires to the preselected depth.

ous authors, including Speed, Smith-Petersen, Cotton, Leadbetter, and Deyerle, with minor differences in technique.[42,43,56,121,158,163] A good technique is to flex the externally rotated hip to 45° in slight abduction, extend it while gently increasing traction, and then internally rotate to 30° to 45° in full extension. Alternatively, traction can be applied with the hip in extension, slight abduction, and external rotation. After length is appropriately restored, the leg is internally rotated until the neck axis is properly aligned with the femoral head. If the neck is too anterior, external rotation "unlocks" the reduction, and internal rotation is repeated with posteriorly directed pressure applied manually to the front of the upper thigh (Fig. 43 – 15).

A number of criteria have been advanced for a satisfactory reduction. Although restoration of normal anatomy is desirable, posterior comminution and osteoporosis can make such a reduction less stable than a slightly valgus, overreduced alignment (i.e., what Brunner and Weber called a "hat-hook" reduction).[27a]

Excessive valgus can increase the risk of avascular necrosis; AP and lateral radiographs should be inspected carefully. On the AP view, ensure that length has been restored and that an anatomic or slight valgus alignment exists. Garden has emphasized the crucial nature of the reduction on the lateral view. This should demonstrate neither anterior (the usual) nor posterior displacement of the femoral neck relative to the head. Especially important is correction of angulation seen on the lateral radiograph. Garden demonstrated that absence of angulation produced the best results and that angulation of more than 20° produced a high incidence of failures (Fig. 43 – 16).[78]

If the reduction maneuver, which should rely primarily on extension and internal rotation, is not producing satisfactory alignment, then rather than repeating closed manipulations with greater force (which could potentially damage the femoral head blood supply), the surgeon should proceed to an open reduction.[115]

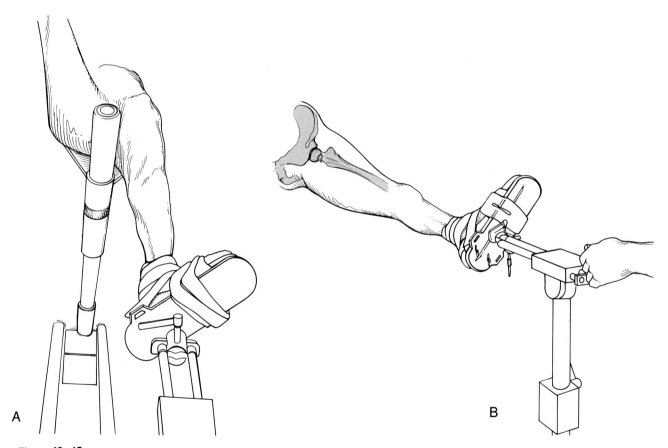

A   B

Figure 43–15

Closed reduction of a femoral neck fracture. *A,* The patient is positioned supine on a fracture table with the uninjured leg in a lithotomy position to allow the C-arm image intensifier access to the injured hip in AP and lateral projections. The injured leg is attached to the footpiece securely, but with adequate padding. It is slightly abducted and flexed and externally rotated with minimal traction initially. *B,* Traction is increased to correct length and varus deformity at the fracture site, as revealed by the AP fluoroscopic view.

Illustration continued on following page

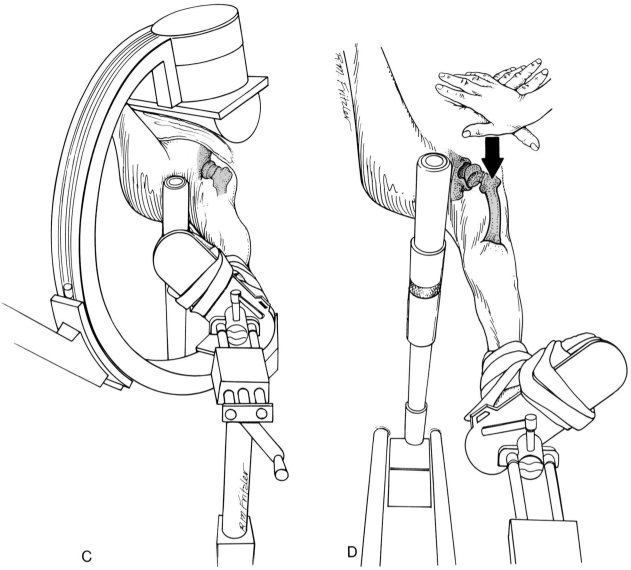

C

D

Figure 43–15 *Continued*

C, The leg is internally rotated and adducted to a neutral position to correct apex anterior angulation and to oppose the fracture surfaces. *D,* If the distal fragment is too anterior, then the leg is externally rotated again, and pressure is applied firmly to the proximal thigh while the leg is rotated internally.

OPEN REDUCTION. The Watson-Jones incision, recommended for open reduction of a femoral neck fracture, was illustrated earlier in Figure 43–13. The full technique is shown here (Fig. 43–17). The initial lateral incision is extended proximally in the interval between the tensor fascia and the gluteus medius muscles. This interval is split bluntly down to the anterior hip capsule while the vastus lateralis origin is elevated off the intertrochanteric ridge. The hip capsule is split onto the femoral neck anteriorly and then dissected off the intertrochanteric ridge 1 cm inferiorly and 1 cm superiorly. By inserting a small pointed (Hohmann) retractor

intracapsularly onto the anterior acetabulum rim, the fracture can be easily visualized. For reduction, a bone hook is placed onto the greater trochanter and the hip brought into external rotation by adjusting the fracture table. With lateral traction using the bone hook, the fracture is disimpacted. The femoral neck (distal fragment) is usually found anterior to the femoral head (proximal fragment). This is corrected with leverage from a blunt curved instrument placed between the fracture surfaces as the lateral traction is released, and the limb is returned into maximum internal rotation. The reduction is provisionally held by a 2.0-mm

Figure 43–16

Fluoroscopic images during closed reduction of a displaced femoral neck fracture. *A,* With the hip slightly abducted, slightly flexed, externally rotated, and initially in minimal traction. Initial AP fluoroscopic view shows varus malalignment and shortening. *B,* Traction is applied with intermittent fluoroscopic views taken until length is restored and anatomic or slight valgus alignment is achieved. *C,D,* Internal rotation and adduction oppose fracture surfaces and correct apex anterior angulation on lateral view. *E,* The final AP view should show anatomic or slight valgus reduction. The angle between the axes of the head and shaft should be 150° to 155° or, using Garden's landmarks, the angle between the femoral shaft and the axis of the trabecular stream in the femoral head (which is not always visible, especially on the fluoroscopic image) should be 160° to 180°. *F,* Final lateral fluoroscopic view. The subchondral bone of femoral head should be visible on both views to permit placing screws at proper depth. Internal rotation should correct apex anterior angulation. There should be no angulation between the head and shaft.

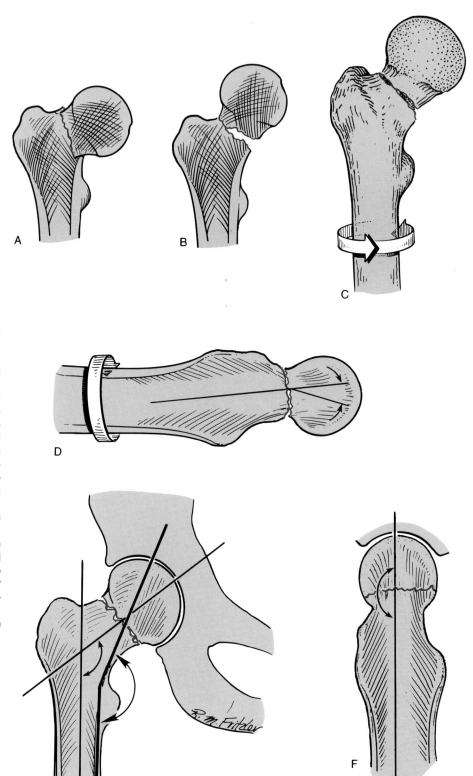

Illustration continued on following page

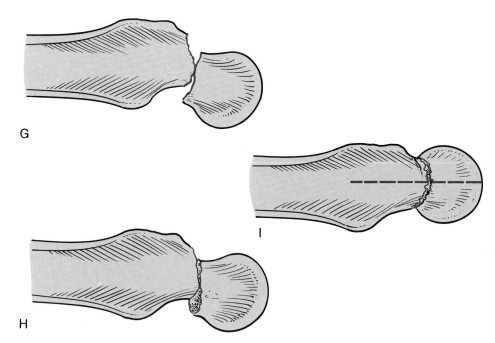

Figure 43-16 *Continued*

G, Adjustment may be required to eliminate angulation between the neck and shaft. *H,* Anterior displacement of the distal neck relative to the head is not uncommon and also requires correction to maximize contact of the fracture surfaces. Both anterior and posterior neck profiles should appear concave on the lateral radiograph. To correct anterior displacement, first externally rotate the distal femur, and then apply posteriorly directed pressure to the subtrochanteric region of the thigh. Then reapproximate the fracture surfaces by restoring internal rotation. *I,* Finally, recheck the AP image to ensure that the reduction has remained satisfactory during correction of displacement using the lateral view.

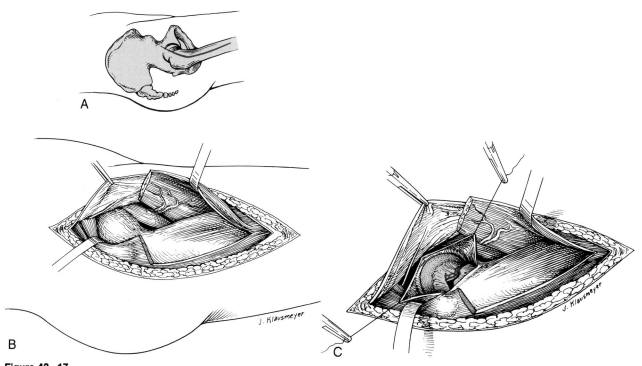

Figure 43-17

Open reduction of a femoral neck fracture. *A,* Watson-Jones skin incision. *B,* Blunt dissection to develop the interval between the tensor fascia lata muscle and the abductors. The vastus lateralis is dissected from the intertrochanteric ridge. *C,* The capsule is divided in line with the femoral neck and transected off its insertion at the base of the femoral neck. Sutures function as retractors.

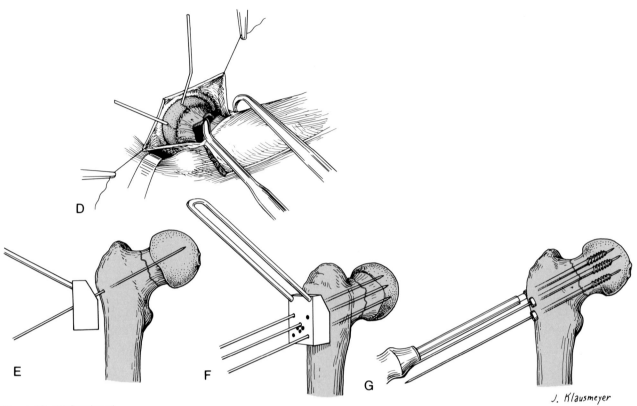

J. Klausmeyer

Figure 43-17 Continued

D, A curved retractor can be inserted into the joint to lift the proximal femoral head fragment as the fracture is disimpacted using lateral traction applied with a bone hook in the greater trochanter. E, A guide wire for a cannulated screw is inserted up the femoral neck across the fracture line under fluoroscopic control to stabilize the fracture. F, Additional wires are inserted in a parallel fashion using the drill guide, as in Figure 43-14. G, The screws are inserted one at a time; tapping may be necessary in dense bone. The fluoroscope is used to confirm that each screw is within the femoral head. This is done by checking AP and lateral views with the hip at both extremes of rotation.

Kirschner wire placed centrally in the neck in both planes (see Fig. 43-17). The reduction should then be confirmed visually, by palpation and radiograph, in both planes.

Fixation of Femoral Neck Fractures. More than 100 different internal fixation devices have been utilized for stabilizing femoral neck fractures. Triflanged nails, either with or without femoral shaft side plates, should not be used to internally fix femoral neck fractures. Distraction produced when utilizing these devices has been shown to have an adverse effect on femoral head blood flow.[167,169] The device chosen should have a mechanism for producing compression across the fracture site.

In general, large hip compression screws such as those recommended for intertrochanteric hip fractures should not be used. They sacrifice large amounts of central bone in the femoral neck, which can make reconstruction of an eventual nonunion very difficult. Furthermore, Brodetti has shown that these large implants, if placed suboptimally in the posterior and supe-

rior femoral head, can damage the blood supply to the femoral head.[26] However, Ort and Lamont have reported results with compression screws that are equal to those of other techniques.[133] If these are selected, a second pin or screw should be inserted superiorly to the centrally placed guide wire for the large compression screw to control rotation of the femoral head fragment during insertion of the screw. Because the hip compression screw by itself controls rotation poorly when compared with multiple screw or pin implants, this superior screw should remain as part of the definitive fixation.

Recommended Fixation Technique. The recommended implant for internal fixation of a femoral neck fracture is a multiple pin implant (e.g., Knowles, Gouffon) or some type of cannulated or noncannulated cancellous screw (e.g., Ace, AO/ASIF, Asnis, Richards). Screw cannulation allows for guide wire use, thereby allowing more sophisticated guide systems with which to ensure parallel placement of the implants. In general, the amount of compression generated across the fracture is proportional to the thread area of the screw (length of thread × maximum width of thread − core diameter at thread). The critical element in fracture stability is the density of the bone. There does not seem to be an increased mechanical advantage to using more than three implants.[175] The general technique for inserting multiple screws is depicted earlier in Fig. 43–14. The drill guide device is placed over the centrally positioned guide wire. Three parallel drills or guide wires are then inserted and the length measured for screw insertion. If appropriate for the selected implant system, a cannulated drill is then placed over each pin and drilling carried out to a depth of 8 to 10 mm short of the tip of the pin to keep the guide wire from coming out. In very dense bone, a tap should be utilized into the femoral head, but generally it is only necessary to tap the lateral cortex. The screws are then inserted and retightened after any traction that has been placed on the limb has been released. The guide wire should be removed after a screw has passed across the fracture to prevent advancing the guide wire into the hip joint. Reinsertion of such a guide wire permits easy exchange of the screw if its length is inappropriate. Care should be exercised to avoid stripping the screw threads through osteopenic cancellous bone and also to avoid penetration into the joint space. When the bone is very dense, impaction of the fracture can be performed after the traction is released by applying mallet blows to a broad bone tamp placed on the lateral surface of the proximal femur adjacent to the screws. Following such impaction, the screws should be retightened in hopes of maintaining interfragmentary compression. Fracture reduction and implant location are confirmed with multiple-plane fluoroscopy and with permanent radiographs. After removal of the central guide wire and all screw guide wires, the wound is closed in layers over a drain, leaving the hip capsule open.

With the exception of fracture reduction, the essential considerations of internal fixation procedures for displaced femoral neck fractures are similar to those for internal fixation of undisplaced fractures as discussed previously. Urgent reduction and decompressive capsulotomy may be valuable for reducing the risks of avascular necrosis and are thus especially important in the younger patient. Proper general preoperative assessment and patient preparation are also essential, particularly for older patients. Preoperative planning must include the possible need for prosthetic arthroplasty. In general, this decision should be made preoperatively, because of the logistic problems posed by the different operating table, position, and surgical instruments and implants. Failure to gain a satisfactory reduction with closed manipulation should indicate open reduction rather than arthroplasty. The details of implant insertion have been discussed previously. Peri-operative antibiotics are probably of greater value in implant insertion because of the longer procedure with the possibility of extensive exposure.

Postoperative management is also similar to that of undisplaced injuries, but the potential for increased fracture instability raises additional concerns about weight-bearing after fixation of displaced femoral neck fractures. A limited weight-bearing regimen, if the patient is able to cooperate, is preferable until fracture healing has progressed significantly (8 to 12 weeks). If the patient is unable to comply with limited weight-bearing ambulation, the surgeon must decide among restricting the patient to bed and chair activity, to ambulation only under supervision, or to acceptance of a greater or lesser amount of weight bearing. Various reports have indicated that weight bearing can be permitted for most patients after satisfactory reduction and fixation of femoral neck fractures.[4c,33] Furthermore, the forces applied to the hip during bed rest are essentially the same as those with protected ambulation (Fig. 43–18).[94a]

Displaced fractures, especially in the elderly, may heal more slowly than undisplaced fractures. This must be appreciated if premature removal of symptomatic hardware is to be avoided.

Hemiarthroplasty

INDICATIONS AND IMPLANT CHOICE. As noted previously, prosthetic replacement is selected for management of a femoral neck fracture when the patient has preexisting hip joint pathology, a medical condition that precludes fracture healing, low functional demands, poor bone stock, and is physiologically older. Note that this consideration is based on an estimate of the patient's physiologic, not chronologic, age.

Although prostheses eliminate concerns about fixation failure, nonunion, and avascular necrosis, they also introduce problems related to prosthetic loosening, acetabular erosion, dislocation, infection, and the potential perioperative consequences of a more extensive surgical procedure. These difficulties were recognized soon after introduction of the first generation of well-accepted endoprostheses by Moore, Thompson, and others. The most frequent problems were loosening and protrusion with late pain, primarily in younger and more active patients who provided significant challenges to the durability of hip prostheses. Continuing efforts have led to improvements in prosthetic design and technique.

Beginning in 1974, prostheses with internal ball-and-socket bearings were developed.[54,60,72,119,120–147] These consisted of a femoral component with a smaller head onto which fitted a plastic socket with a rounded external metal shell available in several graduated sizes to fit the acetabulum. The anticipated advantages of

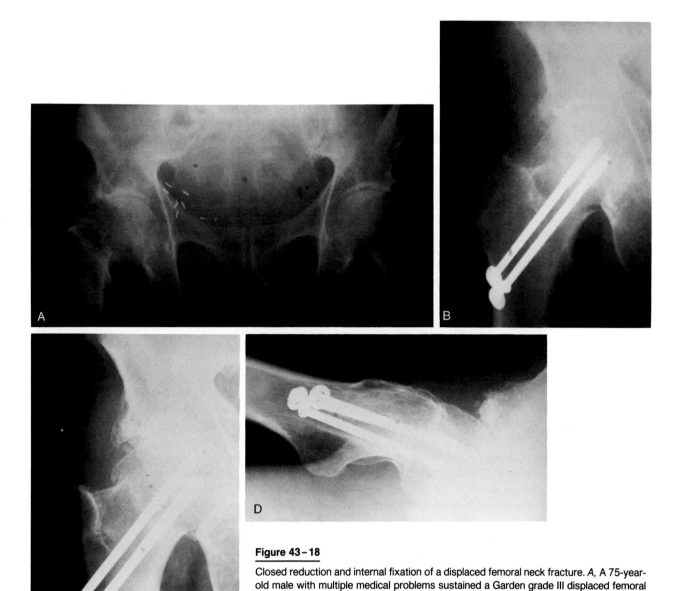

Figure 43–18

Closed reduction and internal fixation of a displaced femoral neck fracture. *A,* A 75-year-old male with multiple medical problems sustained a Garden grade III displaced femoral neck fracture in a low-energy fall. *B,* He was treated with closed reduction and cannulated screw fixation with a good reduction in the AP and lateral plane. At four days postoperatively the screws had settled, as the fracture site had undergone physiologic compression. *C,D,* A successful clinical result was achieved because of an anatomic reduction in the AP and lateral planes.

such so-called bipolar or bicentric devices were reduced frictional wear between the prosthesis and the acetabular articular cartilage, as well as possibly improved cushioning of weight-bearing forces by the plastic insert between metal stem and cup. It has also been claimed that the two articulating surfaces provide more resistance to postoperative dislocation than do other types of prostheses.

Subsequently, the bipolar implants were improved by the development of locking head components to increase stability and prevent dislocation of the prosthetic head from the femur. Additionally, modification of the head component so that its axis of rotation around the femoral implant was medial to the center of the external acetabular cup also provided better stability. This avoids an abduction moment, which tends to make the cup impinge on the medial side of the femoral neck, and tends instead to position the cup concentrically about the femoral implant's head.

Hemiarthroplasty design has also benefited from improvements associated with the evolution of total hip replacement. Changes have focused on improving the stability of the prosthesis in the proximal femur. Three different modes of stem fixation have emerged: press fit, polymethylmethacrylate (PMMA) cement, and bony ingrowth. The Austin-Moore original endoprosthesis design incorporated a window in the stem in hopes that bone would fill it and provide an anchor to the proximal femur. It was advocated that this window be filled with bone graft (from the femoral head) when the prosthesis was inserted. The first generation of femoral endoprostheses relied on interference fit between the stem and the medullary canal, which was enlarged by removal of cancellous bone to accommodate the chosen stem. Some osteoporotic individuals have such large medullary diameters, however, that a snug press fit cannot be achieved. With the adoption of PMMA bone cement for fixation of total hip prostheses, it soon became common to fix nonfenestrated endoprostheses in place with cement. This technique is of obvious value in maintaining satisfactory alignment of a prosthesis that does not fill the medullary canal. It has been claimed to increase patient comfort and improve early results. However, in active patients with unipolar prostheses, it is associated with progressive acetabular wear, painful arthropathy, and protrusio, all of which often require revision surgery.[136a]

Recent femoral stem designs offer an evolving collection of prostheses that may be considered for treatment of displaced femoral neck fractures in suitable individuals. Larger, anatomically shaped stems better match the medullary cavity and may improve on results achieved with early press fit prostheses; in addition, these are better suited to cement fixation.

The third approach to implant fixation, in addition to press fit and PMMA cement, is fabrication of endoprosthetic femoral stems with one of a variety of microporous surfaces. Bony ingrowth into the pores of such implants can provide secure fixation of a prosthesis without the use of PMMA cement. However, this method necessitates meticulous bone tailoring to obtain intimate bone contact and a tight interference fit (with increased risk of femoral shaft fracture). Bony ingrowth requires avoidance of micromotion of the implant within the femur. Therefore careful abstention from weight bearing is initially required. These prostheses have an increased incidence of thigh pain and are costly when compared with less elaborate implants. Their long-term performance remains uncertain, although for many orthopedic surgeons, they have gained a role in the management of youthful patients and in revision surgery. Given the known durability of cemented prostheses and their acknowledged success rate, it is hard to justify using a bony ingrowth prosthesis for a femoral neck fracture, except in the most unusual circumstances.

It is not known whether there are sufficient benefits for elderly, low-demand ambulators to justify the use of modern, modular press fit femoral stems, which often are costly and require more complex femoral canal preparation when compared with first-generation endoprostheses. Furthermore, there is no proof that they are more successful than cemented implants in the slightly younger, moderate-demand ambulators who are the usual recipients of bipolar hemiarthroplasties for displaced femoral neck fractures.

There is presently an ever-changing array of modern hip prostheses developed and produced by a number of different manufacturers. The following design features have become well accepted:

1. A specific system of instruments provided to prepare the femoral canal to the size and shape of the prosthesis.

2. Modular components with morse-taper junctions that permit custom adjustment of prosthetic neck length and head size, thus reducing the inventory required to obtain optimal fit and also providing the possibility for later revision of a stable femoral component to a total hip arthroplasty, should acetabular problems occur after a hemiarthroplasty. Both unipolar and bipolar prosthetic femoral head components are available for many modern hemiarthroplasty systems.

3. Use of high-performance alloys with great strength and fatigue life.

In addition to improvements in prosthetic design, newer cementing techniques probably offer more durable fixation than that first achieved with PMMA, which initially was manually packed into the proximal femur in a doughy consistency. Modern techniques of cement application include (1) preliminary canal shaping to a uniformly larger size than the stem, (2) thorough cleansing to remove blood and fat, (3) use of a distal plug to contain the cement, (4) injection and pressurization of semiliquid cement to fill bony interstices and increase fixation, (5) use of PMMA or other spacers to maintain a uniform thickness of the cement mantle, and (6) improved mixing techniques to avoid air bubbles and lack of homogeneity.

In summary, there are at present two major categories of hemiarthroplasty to be considered for femoral neck fractures: first-generation implants like the Austin-Moore and current-generation implants with femoral stems designed for cement fixation (or possibly press fit insertion). Although many authors have reported superior results with bipolar designs when compared with unipolar historical prostheses, this has not been proven conclusively.[19a,61a,72,120,161] Even with the improved stem design and newer cementing techniques, radiolucent lines around the cement mantle have been reported in up to 80% of cases. Long-term follow-up information is lacking. The majority of dislocations of bipolar prostheses, although less frequent than with unipolar designs, have to be treated with open reduction because of the inner and outer components.[60] Revision to total hip arthroplasty has not been as easy as anticipated.[63]

Despite these uncertainties, the recommendation at this time is for cemented bipolar prosthetic replacement for displaced femoral neck fractures in the elderly but moderately active patient. For younger patients who develop symptomatic avascular necrosis, many surgeons would consider modern uncemented stem designs in anticipation of better long-term function. For the debilitated elderly patient with limited activity and life expectancy, an older unipolar design should be used. The physician should be aware of the higher reported difficulty with revision of these older stem designs.[63]

Finally, it must be noted that some authors are now recommending total hip replacement for selected active older patients with displaced femoral neck fractures and preexisting hip disorders, such as significant osteoarthritis, rheumatoid arthritis, and Paget's disease.[40,53,153,154,188] In such patients, hemiarthroplasty is less likely to provide a satisfactory result. Long-term outcome and more detailed indications for total hip replacement as primary treatment for femoral neck fractures remain topics for further study.

SURGICAL APPROACH. Hemiarthroplasty for femoral neck fracture can be done through any of a variety of posterior or anterior surgical approaches. In anterior approaches, including the so-called direct lateral, an anterior capsulotomy is performed, and the proximal femur is delivered through it by externally rotating the thigh, which may be done with the hip extended or flexed. In posterior approaches, flexion and internal rotation are used to expose the proximal femur through a posterior capsulotomy. The surgeon's prior experience appears to be the most common reason for choosing one approach over the other. However, there have been reports of lower rates of serious complications following anterior approaches for prosthetic replacement.[34] This may be because such approaches spare the posterior capsule so that postoperatively the hip is more stable in the flexed, sitting position, thus diminishing the chances of dislocation. It is also claimed that the anterior incision's greater distance for the perineum reduces the frequency of wound contamination and infection.

The posterolateral modified Gibson approach, for which the patient is placed the lateral decubitus position, is illustrated in Fig. 43–19. The important elements of this approach include (1) a lateral skin incision, the proximal portion of which may be directed somewhat posteriorly; (2) longitudinal, lateral division of the fascia lata, beginning distally and extending proximally posterior to the tensor fascia lata, with (3) deepening of the proximal part of the wound by splitting the muscle fibers of gluteus maximus; (4) going posterior to gluteus medius, dividing the tendons of the short external rotators; (5) performing a T-shaped posterior hip capsulotomy; and (6) delivering the distal fragment through the capsulotomy by flexing and internally rotating the thigh. After completion of the procedure, the posterior capsulotomy is repaired with stout sutures. This may not be a significant preventive measure against posterior dislocation because of the tenuous reattachment of the capsule to the femur.

As mentioned previously, anterior approaches leave the capsule intact posteriorly. Examples are that of Smith-Petersen, through the interval between sartorius and tensor fascia lata (Fig. 43–20); that of Watson-Jones, between tensor and gluteus medius (see Fig. 43–13); and also the "direct lateral" of Hardinge, which proximally passes between the anterior and posterior halves of the gluteus medius (Fig. 43–21). In each of these, an anterior capsulotomy provides access to the hip for removal of the femoral head and insertion of the prosthesis. Each can be done with the patient supine. Burwell and Scott modified Watson-Jones's technique by placing the patient on the side, angling the proximal part of the skin incision posteriorly to improve access to the proximal femur through the wound, and delivering it through the anterior capsulotomy by externally rotating the flexed hip and knee, with good muscle relaxation. The direct lateral approach is also well suited to the lateral decubitus position, in which an anteriorly placed sterile envelope receives the leg when the knee is flexed to a right angle and the extended hip is externally rotated. Familiarity with the chosen approach greatly facilitates positioning, placement of retractors, and minor variations in extent and location of dissection, all of which aid in gaining an atraumatic exposure.

PROCEDURE

Indications and Contraindications. As discussed earlier, hemiarthroplasty is recommended for those ambulatory (generally elderly) individuals who, because of osteopenia and/or pre-existing hip disease, are not able to do well with internal fixation. Please see previous sections.

Timing of Surgery. In the case of prosthetic replacement, surgery should be performed within 48 hours of admission whenever possible. This amount of time should allow for medical clearance and optimization of hydration, cardiorespiratory status, and electrolyte and hematologic balance.

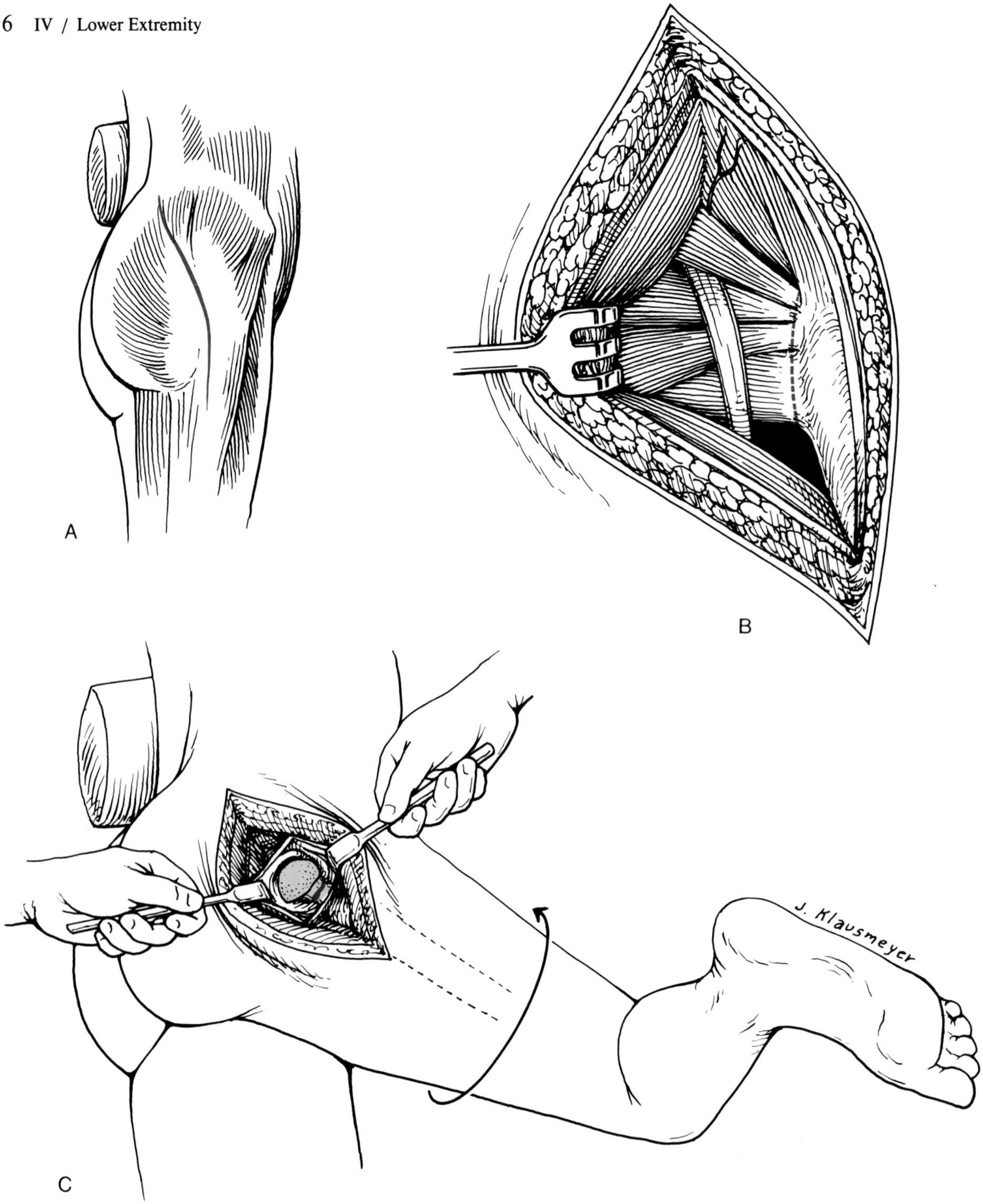

Figure 43–19

Posterolateral (Kocher-Gibson) approach to the hip. The frequently chosen posterolateral approach to the hip has been modified by so many authors that eponyms poorly denote the exact procedure. *A,* The lateral decubitus position is used. Typical skin and fascial incisions are made over the proximal femur for 15 cm to the tip of the greater trochanter and then angled slightly posteriorly toward the posterosuperior iliac spine for another 10 cm. The fascial incision is made first through the fascia lata directly over the proximal femoral shaft. The thinnest part of the superficial muscular cover is palpated between the index finger (inserted proximally through the fasciotomy) and the thumb (placed outside the fascia). This locates a spot anterior to the bulk of the gluteus maximus and posterior to the tensor fascia lata. The overlying fascia is incised, and the muscle fibers are spread bluntly, watching for crossing vessels that may need to be divided and coagulated. *B,* The gluteal bursa is reflected posteriorly or excised to reveal the trochanteric attachments of the short external rotators. The sciatic nerve is illustrated here but is not usually exposed at surgery. Note that the piriformis is usually superficial to the nerve, so that only the more distal muscles protect it when it is reflected posteriorly. *C,* The hip capsule is exposed by reflecting the short external rotators; for hemiarthroplasty it is usually incised in a manner suitable for subsequent closure. The proximal femur is delivered through the capsulotomy by flexing, adducting, and internally rotating the hip. Closure involves capsular repair, reattachment of the short rotators, and suture of the fascia and skin. Suction drains are employed.

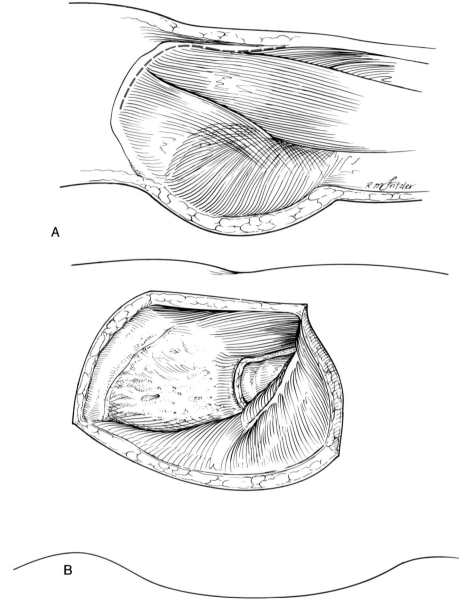

Figure 43-20

Anterior (Smith-Petersen) approach to the hip. This approach employs the interval between the sartorius and the tensor fascia lata. *A,* That patient is supine. This skin incision overlies that in the fascia, following the iliac crest from its highest point to the anteriosuperior spine and then directly distally approximately 15 cm. *B,* The abductors are released and reflected as shown from the lateral surface of the ilium, but only as much as necessary to minimize the risk of heterotopic bone formation. The anterior edge of the tensor fascia lata is followed distally. Branches of the lateral femoral circumflex artery crossing the interval between this and the sartorius must be identified and controlled. The capsule is incised longitudinally and released along its acetabular margin, sparing the labrum, to permit retraction and visualization of the hip joint. Closure involves repair of the capsulotomy, reattachment of the abductors to the iliac crest, and closure of the anterior fascia. Suction drains are used.

Preoperative Planning. High-quality radiographs made with a magnification marker should be available for every patient undergoing prosthetic replacement. Templates for the chosen stem system should be matched to the radiograph to guide in selecting stem, neck, and outer bearing size. Preoperative selection of implant type and size is essential for current-generation systems with femoral stems designed to fit within close tolerances. With first-generation implants, radiographic templates are usually not available, and there is only one stem size. It is still valuable to determine preoperatively whether there will be problems with the femoral anatomy or fracture level, either of which might require a different choice of implant.

Whenever possible, cell saver systems should be arranged for intraoperatively. If unavailable, the patient should be typed and crossmatched for two units of blood. A perioperative antibiotic should be chosen and made available for administration when anesthesia is induced.

Anesthesia and Positioning. The patient is positioned laterally with the pelvis perpendicular to the floor and held there with an inflatable bean bag, kidney rests, or hip positioner. Alternatively, with anterior approaches, the surgeon may choose a supine position with the affected buttock just over the edge of the table to allow the soft tissues to hang posteriorly. The hind quarter and leg are draped free. Spinal or general anesthesia are equally efficacious.

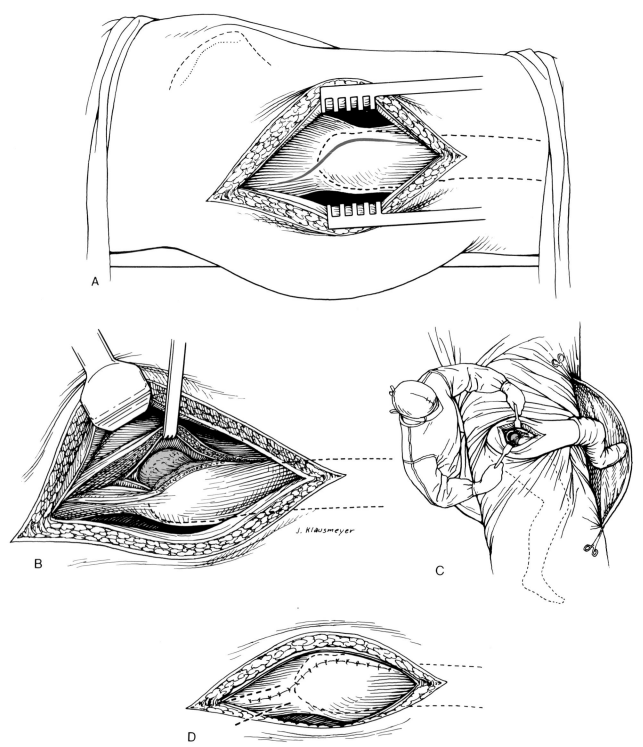

Figure 43–21

Direct lateral (Hardinge) approach to the hip. This approach gains access to the anterior hip capsule through a longitudinal incision along the anterior edge of the greater trochanter that releases the anterior bulk of the gluteus medius in continuity with the vastus lateralis fascia. *A,* A straight lateral skin incision is deepened through the fascia lata and extended proximally, splitting the anterior fibers of the gluteus maximus. The incision in the gluteus medius, through tendon anterior and just proximal to the greater trochanter, is shown. Its proximal extent is limited by the superior gluteal neurovascular structures. *B,* The incision is deepened, and with retraction an anterior capsulotomy is performed. *C,* The proximal femur is delivered by externally rotating the flexed, adducted hip. *D,* The abductor repair is effected by closure of the tenotomy, including direct reattachment to the trochanter if soft tissues are tenuous. Stout nonabsorbable sutures are used.

Surgical Technique

FIRST-GENERATION ENDOPROSTHESIS. Insertion of a first-generation Austin-Moore endoprosthesis is depicted in Figure 43–22. In this example, a posterolateral incision is illustrated. After splitting the fascia lata and gluteus maximus, the external rotators are tagged and divided. A T-shaped incision is made in the hip capsule, in line with the femoral neck and across its base and is retracted with sutures. The labrum must be preserved. The femoral head is removed intact if possible using a cork screw, and its outside diameter is measured as a guide in choosing the proper size prosthesis. The femoral neck is delivered with a bone hook, cleared of soft tissue, and inspected. Sufficient neck length (at least 0.5 in) is required for an Austin-Moore prosthesis. If the fracture is lower, another implant (e.g., Thompson) may provide a better fit. Using the prosthesis as a guide, tailor the neck appropriately with rongeurs or a power saw to fit the flange of the prosthesis and to support it with an appropriate degree of anteversion.

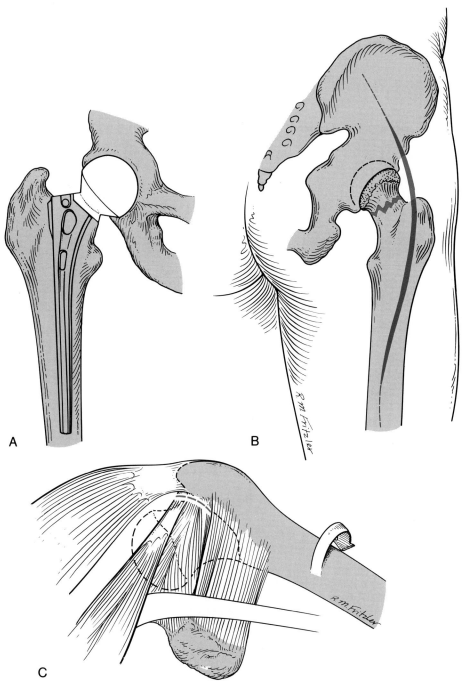

Figure 43–22

Insertion of an Austin-Moore prosthesis using a posterolateral approach. *A,* The prosthesis in place. *B,* Skin incision for the posterolateral approach. Patient is in the lateral decubitus position with the affected side up and the leg draped free. This procedure can also be done with other suitable hip incisions, depending on the surgeon's preference (see text). The fascia lata is divided in line with the skin, and the incision is extended proximally through the gluteus maximus, the fibers of which must be spread bluntly. The inferior gluteal neurovascular bundle defines the proximal extent of the split. *C,* The gluteal bursa is reflected or excised, and the short external rotators are released from the greater trochanter and reflected posteriorly, protecting the sciatic nerve, which usualy lies ventral to the piriformis and dorsal to the more distal rotators. This is aided by internal rotation of the thigh, being cautious not to injure the osteopenic limb.

Illustration continued on following page

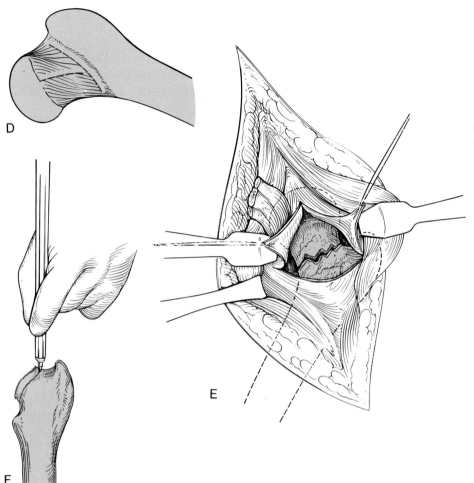

Figure 43–22 *Continued*

D,E, The posterior hip capsule, thus exposed, is incised in a manner suitable for later repair. This reveals the fractured femoral neck. *F,* The femoral neck is thus delivered into the wound by internal rotation of the thigh with the knee flexed. It is marked and osteotomized (most easily with a power saw) about 1.0 to 1.5 cm proximal to the lesser trochanter's flare, on a line suitable for the flange of the prosthesis, positioned with its stem down the femoral canal. The plane of the osteotomy should be inclined anteriorly, or anteverted, so that the flange of the prosthesis receives bony support in this position.

After any necessary neck osteotomy, access to the acetabulum is easier, and it can be inspected for degenerative changes; the ligamentum teres, if especially large, can be resected, and a trial or definitive prosthesis can be checked for fit. The head size should be neither too loose nor too tight. Its fit in the acetabulum, rather than suction produced by the labrum, should be assessed.

Next, use the box chisel to start the medullary preparation by excising adequate bone extending from the medial neck (calcar) into the substance of the greater trochanter. An awl or straight curette inserted in line with the femoral shaft will aid in entering the diaphyseal medullary canal. The appropriate broach or rasp is used to enlarge the canal. Its rotational alignment will determine the ultimate anteversion of the prosthesis. This should be directed approximately 10° to 15° anteriorly relative to a line perpendicular to the tibia if the knee is flexed to a right angle. Using the rasp, and curettes and other tools as needed, remove enough medullary bone to allow the prosthesis to be inserted with a snug but not overly tight press fit. Do not force the prosthesis into the femur, which can be fractured by

such a maneuver. Once the flange of the prosthesis seats on the calcar, the implant position, including version, and stability are checked and the prosthetic femoral head carefully and gently inserted into the acetabulum. Forcing the head in or out of the acetabulum, and especially using the femur as a lever, may fracture the proximal femoral shaft; little force is needed to produce such a fracture in an osteopenic elderly patient. If a fenestrated prosthesis such as the Austin-Moore is used, the holes in the stem may be filled with bone to aid in maintaining fixation. Stability and range of motion are documented. Confirm that full extension is possible, flexion is at least 90°, and there is no tendency to dislocate in functional positions of rotation and adduction. Length should be adequate to maintain tension on the soft tissues that cross the hip. Preexisting contractures may benefit from release of iliopsoas or adductor tendons. The capsule is repaired, the external rotators reattached, and the wound closed in layers over suction drains (Figs. 43–22 and 43–23).

CURRENT-GENERATION BIPOLAR ENDOPROSTHESIS. Insertion of a modern bipolar prosthesis is shown in

Figure 43–22 *Continued*

G, After shortening the neck, there is more room for removal of the femoral head fragment from the acetabulum using a "corkscrew." It may be necessary to transect the ligamentum teres. The head diameter must then be measured in order to choose the size of the prosthesis. *H,* Holding the femur internally rotated, with a retractor under the base of the neck, the medullary canal of the proximal femoral shaft is entered with an awl or straight curette. Next a box chisel and Austin-Moore rasp are used to prepare the medullary canal. The flexed leg can be used to guide rotational alignment of these instruments so that version remains appropriate (10° to 15° anteverted). The prosthetic stem is placed centrally in the medullary canal. Gentleness is required to avoid damaging the proximal femur, especially if osteoporosis is profound. *I,* Centralize the entry site by ensuring that the rasp works adequately against the medial border of the greater trochanter. *J,* If desired, the fenestrations of the prosthetic stem are filled with morcellized cancellous graft prepared from the patient's femoral head, and the prosthesis is securely impacted into the proximal femur. Its rotational stability as well as its alignment must be assessed. Problems with either may require further tailoring of the proximal femur or use of bone cement or another prosthesis. The prosthetic head is gently guided into the acetabulum while the capsule is retracted and after all debris has been irrigated and removed with suction. Range of motion and stability are assessed, and if satisfactory, the capsule is closed, the short rotators are reattached to the base of the trochanter if desired, and the deep fascia, subcutaneous tissue, and skin are closed, with suction drains left posteriorly in the region of the hip capsule.

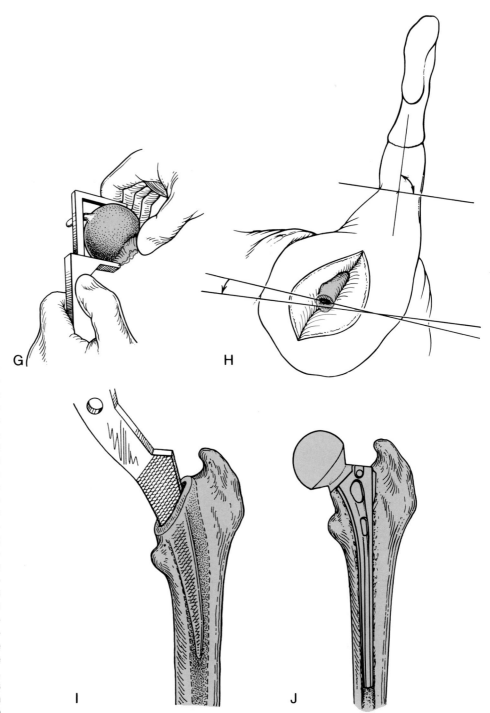

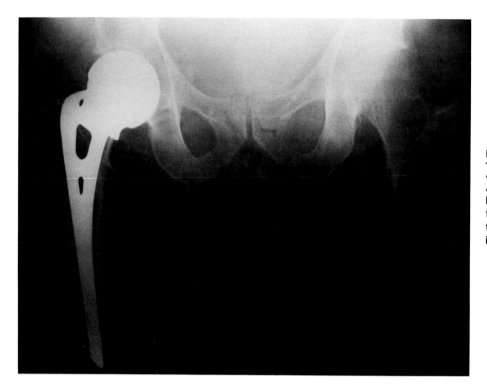

Figure 43-23

Anteroposterior radiograph of an Austin-Moore unipolar femoral head and neck prosthesis inserted for a displaced femoral neck fracture in an elderly patient with limited ambulation outside the home.

Figure 43-24. Because implants and instrumentation systems are evolving rapidly, reference must be made to the appropriate product literature, and the surgeon should have hands-on familiarity with the chosen system prior to using it clinically. A direct lateral approach is illustrated with the patient in the lateral position (see also Fig. 42-24, chapter 42). After anterior capsulotomy, the femoral head is removed with a corkscrew extractor, and its diameter is measured. An osteotomy of the femoral neck is performed with the aid of the appropriate guide. A box chisel and tapered Charnley awl are used to begin preparation of the femoral canal. Depending on the system used and the size of the proximal femur, reaming of the medullary canal may be required. A rasp or broach of size chosen according to preoperative radiographs and templates is used to complete canal preparation. Care is taken to avoid fracturing the proximal femur during insertion of the rasp with a mallet. For a press fit application, the rasp should be essentially the same size as the implant stem and should fit snugly with the femur. Its alignment and rotational stability must be confirmed. In some systems the rasp handle is removable, and the rasp doubles as a trial prosthesis, with proximal attachments of varying lengths and diameters. Such a rasp may also be provided with an attachment for final planing of the femoral neck osteotomy to gain optimal contact with the flange of the prosthesis. In any event, an effort should be made to ensure appropriate contact between the calcar and the flange of the prosthesis.

Once the bone is prepared, the trial rasp combination or a separate trial prosthesis is used to check neck length and stem alignment as well as fit into the acetabulum. Range of motion, stability, and length are assessed. If the fit is satisfactory, the definitive prosthesis is inserted directly into the femur, if press fit, or with cement, if this option is selected. There are as yet no convincing data regarding the relative indications of press fit versus cemented endoprostheses for femoral neck fractures, except that if a stable press fit cannot be achieved, then the use of cement is advisable. The prosthetic stem is inserted after or before the chosen head-neck component is driven onto its morse taper. The appropriate diameter bipolar head component is applied over this, and the hip is reduced after lavaging the acetabulum to remove any debris. Alternatively, the bipolar component may be placed into the acetabulum and the prosthetic head reduced into it. This may be easier if exposure is limited. If required, the bipolar component is locked onto the modular stem.

CEMENT INSERTION. A solid rather than fenestrated stem should be used with cement. Some prostheses are now being provided with acrylic obturators that effectively convert a windowed stem to a solid one. Modern cement application techniques have been developed in an effort to decrease the risks of mechanical loosening of the cement-bone interface. The manufacturer's recommendations should be reviewed and followed for a given cement and cement insertion system. General principles include (1) preparation of the canal to a uni-

Text continued on page 1427

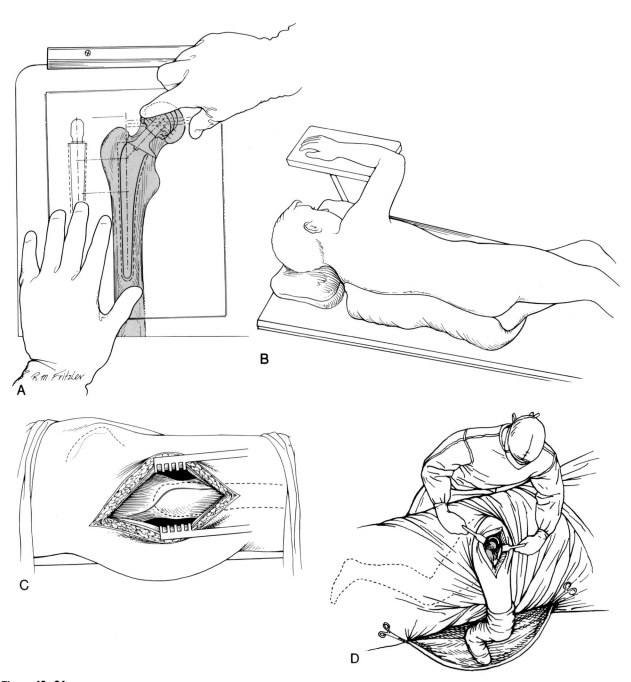

Figure 43–24

Insertion of a modular bipolar prosthesis using a direct lateral approach with cement fixation. *A,* Preoperative planning using radiographs and outline drawings of proposed implants allows provisional choice of prosthesis, stem size and neck length, as well as the appropriate site and orientation of the femoral neck osteotomy. Availability of necessary implants and instruments is thus confirmed before surgery. *B,* The patient is placed in the lateral decubitus position. The affected limb is prepared and draped free. *C,* The skin incision is made as shown. Details of the incision are shown in Figure 43–21. *D,* Anterior dislocation in external rotation permits ready access to the proximal femur, the rotational orientation of which is demonstrated by the flexed knee, with the leg perpendicular to the frontal plane.

Illustration continued on following page

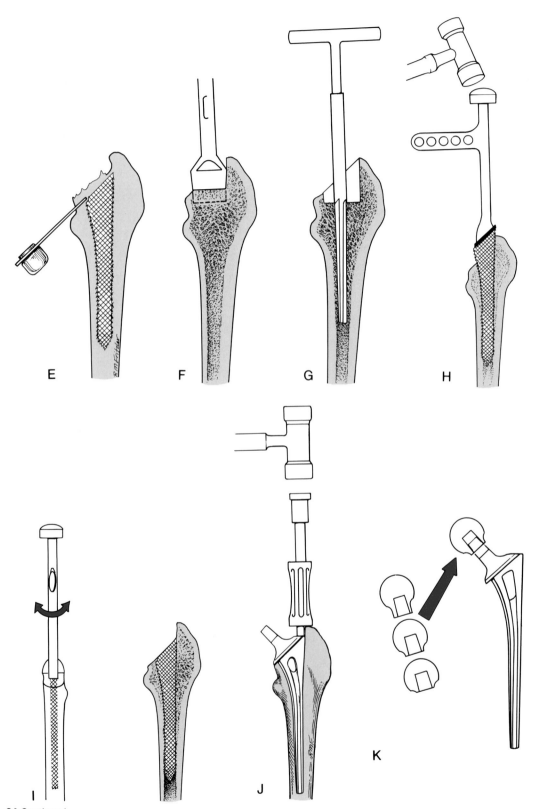

E   F   G   H

I   J   K

Figure 43-24 *Continued*

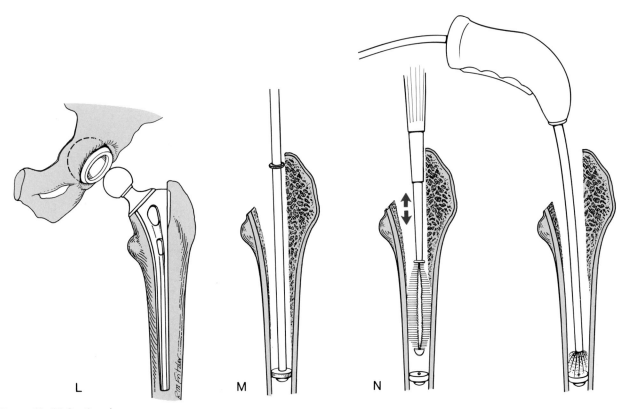

L   M   N

Figure 43–24 *Continued*

E, The rasp or trial prosthesis is used to orient the femoral neck osteotomy at the level determined by preoperative planning. The plane of the osteotomy should be anteverted 10° to 15° from the plane of the knee axis. The femoral head is removed and its diameter measured to estimate an appropriate size for the bipolar prosthetic head. A trial bipolar head is selected and attached to its handle. It should fit the acetabulum closely, turning freely but not permitting ''sloppy'' sideways mobility. *F,G,* The femoral canal is opened with a box chisel centered over the axis of the femoral shaft. This requires encroaching on the medial wall of the greater trochanter. Additionally, anteversion should be appropriately adjusted. The canal is defined and deepened with a straight awl. *H,* The handle is attached to a rasp of appropriate size for the prosthesis chosen preoperatively. The rasp is inserted into the medullary canal, maintaining 10° to 15° anteversion and proceeding slowly and cautiously so as not to fracture the proximal femur. If the rasp is too large, a smaller one should be selected. If it is too loose, a larger size and a correspondingly larger prosthesis will be needed to obtain a secure fit. Advancing and withdrawing the rasp intermittently aids removal of bone debris. *I,* Confirm that the rasp fits snugly enough to provide rotational control and that the femoral neck is trimmed to the level of the top of the rasp. Some rasps have provision for a femoral neck planing attachment to facilitate final preparation of the neck osteotomy. A precise fit of the flange of the prosthesis against the top of the femur may enhance its stability. *J,K,* Next an appropriate trial prosthesis is inserted. At this point the surgeon makes a final choice between cement and press fit fixation. A snug fit must be maintained if cement is not to be used. Use of cement usually requires a rasp one size larger than the prosthesis. Neck length is provisionally chosen by mounting a trial head of appropriate height. *L,* A provisional reduction is performed by first placing the trial bipolar head in the acetabulum and then reducing the trial prosthetic head into the bipolar trial. Next the surgeon assesses range of motion, stability, and leg length, making adjustments in the prosthesis or its orientation if needed. There should be a nearly normal range of motion and no tendency to dislocate, especially in flexion, adduction, and external rotation. Length is assessed by soft tissue tension, by the ability to ''shuck'' the prosthesis distally from the acetabulum with manual traction on the limb, and by the relative positions of the tip of the trochanter and the top of the femoral head. At the conclusion of this step, the surgeon chooses the definitive prosthesis. *M,* Assuming that cement fixation is chosen, an appropriately sized cement restrictor is inserted into the femoral canal 1 cm distal to where the tip of the prosthetic stem will rest. *N,* The canal is prepared with a brush and pulsatile lavage spray to remove fat and blood.

Illustration continued on following page

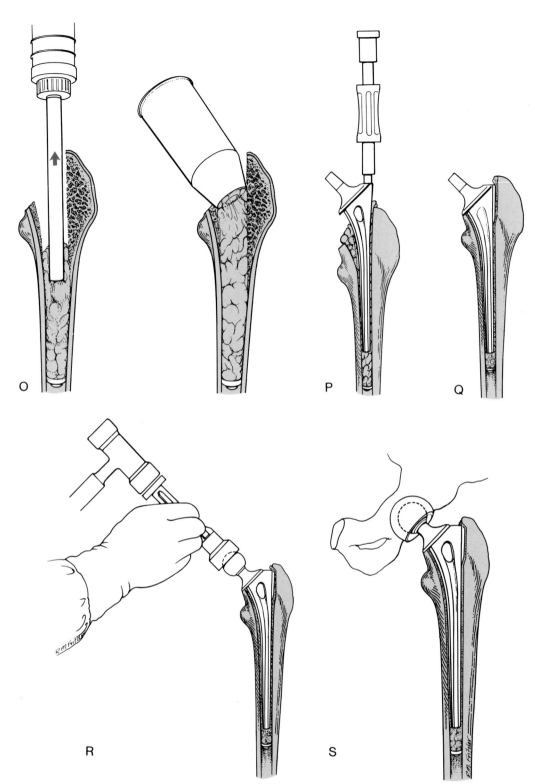

O   P   Q

R   S

Figure 43–24 *Continued*

O, Viscous liquid cement is inserted into the femoral canal, starting at the distal end, with a long-tipped cement delivery syringe. Once the canal is full of cement, a pressurizing nozzle may be used to gain further penetration of the cement into the bony interstices to improve fixation and stability of the cement envelope relative to the femur. *P,Q,* Next the prosthesis is inserted into the proximal femur, ensuring that its rotational alignment provides the desired 10° to 15° of anteversion and that it is driven into the prepared channel so that its collar rests squarely on the osteotomized proximal femur. It is held in place until the cement hardens. A nonfenestrated, or plugged, stem is used with cement. All excess cement is removed from the acetabulum and adjacent wound. *R,* Based on the selected trial components, the appropriate prosthetic modular head is placed onto the Morse taper fitting of the stem and impacted lightly but firmly with the appropriate instrument. *S,* The trial bipolar component can be rechecked, or the definite one placed, unlocked, into the acetabulum, and the femoral head reduced into it. The bipolar assembly is locked, if required, and the surgeon once again confirms leg length, stability, and range of motion. It is important to check for excess cement, interposed soft tissues, and prominent osteophytes that might affect mobility and stability. Once satisfactory joint alignment and mechanics are confirmed, the wound is closed over a suction drain, reattaching the anterior abductors to the proximal femur as shown in Figure 43–21.

formly larger size than the prosthetic stem to accommodate the cement mantle; (2) insertion of a prefabricated plastic, bone, or PMMA plug several centimeters distal to the intended location of the stem tip; (3) cleansing and drying the medullary canal using a pulsating lavage system, a bone brush, and dry sponges; (4) preparation of the cement in ways that avoid bubbles and other discontinuities; and (5) pressurized application of semiliquid, viscous cement, filling the canal with a syringe from the bottom up so that the cement mantle interdigitates with the porous structure of residual cancellous bone and completely fills the canal. Compared with earlier techniques using doughy cement, a larger volume of PMMA is often required, and insertion of the prosthesis is more difficult, requiring final impaction with a mallet and inserter. During insertion of the prosthesis, it is important that there be free and adequate access to the proximal femur so that appropriate alignment can be achieved and evaluated before the cement has hardened. Cement extruded around the prosthesis is removed with a curette. A small sponge in the acetabulum helps to collect the extra cement. After the cement has set, all excess PMMA, both free fragments and overhanging pieces that might fracture later, must be removed to avoid potential loose bodies that might cause acetabular erosion. The head-neck assembly is then placed on the morse taper and the outer bearing snapped on. The hip is reduced after irrigating and recovering any fragments. Motion and stability are confirmed. If these are satisfactory, the wound is closed over suction drains. Secure repair of the capsulotomy helps decrease the risk of early dislocation. Reattachment of the gluteus medius tendon, released from the femur anteriorly in the direct lateral approach, should be secure enough to permit immediate mobilization of the patient (Fig. 43–25).

Intraoperative Complications

Femoral Shaft Fracture. Femoral shaft fracture is avoided by obtaining a well-lateralized starting point for the femoral broach; by correctly estimating the size of the stem; and by being cautious with broaching, component insertion, and relocation-dislocation maneuvers. If a shaft fracture occurs, it should be treated by cerclage wire fixation if it is the usual longitudinal pattern. If it occurs prior to cementing, a longer stem should be considered in addition to cerclage wiring.

Incorrect Sizing of the Outer Bearing. Incorrect sizing may lead to acetabular erosion and is preventable by careful preoperative and intraoperative measurement. Most authorities agree it is better for long-term hip function for the bearing to be 1 mm larger rather than 1 mm smaller than measured size.

Poor Implant Position. Errors in insertion can result

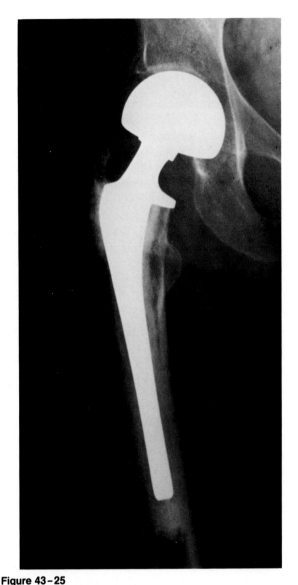

Figure 43–25

Anteroposterior radiograph of a bicentric femoral head and neck prosthesis inserted for a displaced femoral neck fracture in an active, independently ambulatory, elderly individual with osteopenic bone stock.

in a malaligned femoral prosthesis. Often this is because of inappropriate version (malrotation about the long axis of the femur). Most prostheses are designed to be anteverted 10° to 20° relative to the coronal plane of the femur. Insertion in a varus position that is too proximal or too distal and, occasionally, penetration of the femoral cortex may also occur. Attention to prosthetic alignment during preparation of the femur, trial insertion, and definitive prosthesis insertion should identify such problems. When any question exists, intraoperative radiographs can be quite helpful. Inappropriate prosthetic alignment usually requires removal and reinsertion of the device, often with cement if it was not initially used.

AFTERCARE. Intraoperative assessment of stability helps in selecting any restrictions that may be advisable to prevent dislocation. After a posterior approach, flexion of greater than 70°, particularly with adduction, should be avoided for six weeks. Low chairs and toilets, as well as crossing the legs, must be avoided. The patient may sit in an elevated chair. An abduction pillow, Buck's traction, a knee immobilizer that blocks hip flexion by preventing knee flexion, and pillow suspension all have been advocated for postoperative management. If stability is adequate, no external support is required. It is essential to protect the patient's heel from pressure on the bed by supporting the weight of the leg with a pillow under the calf. After an anterior approach, hip stability in flexion is of less concern, and mobilization may be facilitated. Such a patient should, however, be cautioned against abducting and externally rotating the extended hip during the first few weeks.

Progressive weight bearing as tolerated is encouraged with the help of the physical therapy team beginning on the second postoperative day. Prophylactic anticoagulation with warfarin is probably indicated for the period of time the patient is inactive (7 to 21 days) with prothrombin time maintained at 1.5 times the control values. Alternatives are intermittent compression boots or elastic stockings.

Total Hip Arthroplasty. As previously noted, because of acetabular erosion, some surgeons are currently recommending total hip arthroplasty for acute femoral neck fractures. There is a higher dislocation rate in such cases than when the arthroplasty is done for some form of arthritis, because the native hip, prior to the fracture, had a normal range of motion.[53,153,154] Certainly, when the femoral neck fracture occurs in the setting of prior hip disease, rheumatoid arthritis, osteoarthritis, or Paget's disease, total hip arthroplasty is indicated. For the vast majority of patients receiving a total hip replacement for a femoral neck fracture, it is best to use a cemented stem technique because of the greater long-term experience with this method. Many surgeons recommend an uncemented acetabular component because of its greater stability. For details regarding surgical technique for total arthroplasty, the reader is referred to standard texts.[21a,27b,131a,166]

Follow-up Care and Rehabilitation. The comments in this section will, when necessary, differentiate between patients who have had internal fixation of femoral neck fractures and those who have undergone bipolar replacement for such injuries.

Immobilization. Neither the patient nor the injured extremity should be immobilized after a femoral neck fracture. Surgery is performed to allow mobilization of the patient. Any positioning aids or other devices used in bed should promote patient mobilization with comfort and safety. After either internal fixation or arthroplasty, a patient should be out of bed and in a chair on the first postoperative day. Hip flexion beyond 70° is to be avoided initially after prosthetic replacement using a posterior approach.

Mobilization. As noted previously, the patient should be mobilized with assistance from the nursing staff on the first postoperative day. A totally assisted transfer or mechanical lift may be required for debilitated or uncooperative patients. Patients treated with internal fixation should pivot off the nonoperated limb, as should patients treated with prosthetic replacement; however, it is not as critical in the latter group. Full weight bearing can be tolerated as rapidly as the patient can progress in the setting of prosthetic replacement. Touch-down weight bearing may be wiser for 8 to 12 weeks after internal fixation of a displaced femoral neck fracture. This can be liberalized to six to eight weeks or less for impacted or nondisplaced fractures.[1] Some surgeons have reported results that suggest that little if anything is lost by allowing weight bearing as tolerated for most patients after either displaced or undisplaced injuries.[4b,33] Unless fixation is especially tenuous, it may be best to avoid placing restrictions that cannot be followed on elderly, uncooperative patients. Younger individuals, with more to lose from loss of fixation and usually with much more ability to cooperate, are the most obvious candidates for ambulation with limited weight bearing until fracture healing is confirmed.

Physical Therapy. The role of physical therapy during the acute phase following surgery for a femoral neck fracture is to assist with gait training, to provide reminders of flexion restriction in the case of prosthetic replacement, and to identify the need for and instruct in the use of aids for ambulation and activities of daily living. As the fracture heals, the therapist should progress with muscle strengthening and gait training regimens. Similarly, abductor/adductor strengthening and gait training rehabilitation are indicated beginning at three months following prosthetic replacement.

Duration and Extent of Disability. It must be remembered that loss of function is very common after hip fracture. Miller showed that only 51% of patients in his region returned to the ambulatory status they possessed prior to injury.[129a] Jette and colleagues prospectively studied a group of 75 hip fracture patients, 71% of whom survived a year after fracture.[108a] Only 33% of survivors returned to their preinjury function in five basic activities of daily living (ADL): indoor walking, bed-to-chair transfers, donning shoes and socks, and getting on and off a toilet. Only 21% returned to their prior level of instrumental ADL: climbing stairs, outdoor walking, getting in and out of the bathtub, preparing meals, washing dishes, and doing light housework. As expected, these disabilities resulted in significant disturbance of social role function, which was recovered by only 26% of survivors.

Recovery is not clearly related to the type of fracture or to fracture treatment. Rather, it depends on the age of the patient, his or her mental status, preexisting medical problems, and number of close social contacts.[48a,129a] Barring complications, the healthy patient in the age range of 50 to 60 years will generally return to near full function by six to eight months after a displaced fracture and in half that time after undisplaced injuries. Initial recovery may be more rapid in displaced fractures treated with prosthetic replacement, depending on limp caused by abductor weakness.

Assistance/Living Arrangements. In the case of the older patient group suffering femoral neck fracture, the advent of the diagnosis-related grouping (DRG) payment program for Medicare has resulted in less in-hospital therapy, earlier discharge, and much lower rates of return to function.[69,144] Assistance of hospital social services must be requested on the day of admission for essentially all patients with femoral neck fractures. Specifically, this involves development of a discharge plan in terms of where and when the patient will be discharged, type of assistance needed, equipment needed, and a schedule for follow-up appointments. Early involvement of family and friends, regardless of the type of surgery done for the femoral neck fracture, will optimize outcome.

Assessment of Results. The functional ratings that are of importance include hip motion, presence of pain or limp, walking, sitting, and stair climbing functions. The radiographic ratings are different for internal fixation (neck shaft angle, fracture healing, avascular necrosis) than for prosthetic replacement (stem loosening, acetabular wear). The hip rating scale developed by Harris is suggested for functional rating (Table 43–3).

Expected results. Impacted or nondisplaced femoral neck fractures will heal uneventfully in the majority of cases. Avascular necrosis occurs in 5% to 15% of these fractures and nonunion in 2% to 5%. For displaced femoral neck fractures, the result are dependent on multiple factors.

For example, prosthetic replacement for femoral neck fractures has a wide range of reported complications. These can be seen in Tables 43–1 and 43–2.

COMPLICATIONS

Identification and Treatment

Avascular Necrosis

The majority of patients who eventually develop avascular necrosis of the femoral head have groin, buttock, or proximal thigh pain. This may not be functionally significant.[12] It is generally true that the higher the functional demands on the hip, the more significant are the symptoms. This is manifested by the fact that the majority of patients younger than 50 years who develop posttraumatic femoral head osteonecrosis are symptomatic enough to require a reconstructive procedure.[138] Only one third of older patients in Barnes et al.'s extensive series had symptoms severe enough to warrant a second surgical procedure.[12]

The risk of avascular necrosis generally corresponds to the degree of displacement of the femoral neck fracture on the presenting radiographs.[61] Patients with normal bone stock have a higher risk of avascular necrosis. Although some estimation of the risk of this complication can be made based on the radiographs, more detailed information can be obtained from technetium bone scans. Stromqvist has been able to document the risk of developing avascular necrosis or nonunion based on quantitative bone scans obtained one to two weeks after injury. A femoral head uptake ratio of 90% of the intact side or less was found to carry an 84% risk of avascular necrosis or nonunion.[164]

Tomograms or computed tomography can show, with higher resolution, the bony appearance of stippled areas of bone sclerosis, trabecular resorption, microfracture, and subchondral collapse at an earlier stage than can plain radiographs. Magnetic resonance imaging may offer the potential for very early diagnosis of the condition. Because ferrous metals distort the magnetic resonance images, titanium or nonmetallic implants must be developed to obtain good postfixation images. Signal changes in the femoral head are produced by marrow and osteocyte ischemia. Prospective data on the use of these scans for predictive purposes have not yet been reported.

Once the diagnosis is established, the problem of posttraumatic avascular necrosis is extremely difficult to treat. Core decompression as a means for treating nontraumatic avascular necrosis has provided mixed results.[28,65] Natural history data on nontreated avascular necrosis is insufficient. Most authors doubt any favorable influence of core decompression on posttraumatic avascular necrosis, but adequate data are unavailable. In older patients, where radiographic findings may not correlate with function, observation is

Table 43–3.

Harris Hip Rating Scale

Index	Rating
I. PAIN (44 Possible)	
A. None or ignores it	44
B. Slight or occasional; no compromise in activities	40
C. Mild pain, no effect on average activities; rarely, moderate pain with unusual activity, may take aspirin	30
D. Moderate pain, tolerable but makes concessions to pain; some limitation of ordinary activity or work; may require occasional pain medicine stronger than aspirin	20
E. Marked pain, serious limitation of activities	10
F. Totally disabled, crippled, pain in bed, bedridden	0
II. FUNCTION (47 Possible)	
A. Gait (33 Possible)	
1. Limp	
a. None	11
b. Slight	8
c. Moderate	5
d. Severe	0
2. Support	
a. None	11
b. Cane for long walks	7
c. Cane most of the time	5
d. One crutch	3
e. Two canes	2
f. Two crutches	0
g. Not able to walk (specify reason)	0
B. Activities (14 Possible)	
1. Stairs	
a. Normally without using a railing	4
b. Normally using a railing	2
c. In any manner	1
d. Unable to do stairs	0
2. Shoes and Socks	
a. With ease	4
b. With difficulty	2
c. Unable	0
3. Sitting	
a. Comfortable in ordinary chair one hour	5
b. Comfortable in a high chair for one half hour	3
c. Unable to sit comfortably in any chair	0
4. Enter public transportation	1

III. ABSENCE-OF-DEFORMITY; POINTS (4) ARE GIVEN IF THE PATIENT DEMONSTRATES THE FOLLOWING:
  A. Less than 30° fixed flexion contracture
  B. Less than 10° fixed adduction
  C. Less than 10° fixed internal rotation in extension
  D. Limb length discrepancy less than 3.2 cm

IV. RANGE OF MOTION; INDEX VALUES ARE DETERMINED BY MULTIPLYING THE DEGREES OF MOTION POSSIBLE IN EACH ARC BY THE APPROPRIATE INDEX
  A. Flexion:
    $0° - 45° \times 1.0$
    $45° - 90° \times 0.6$
    $90° - 110° \times 0.3$
  B. Abduction
    $0° - 15° \times 0.8$
    $15° - 20° \times 0.3$
    $>20° \times 0$
  C. External rotation in extension
    $0° - 15° \times 0.4$
    $>15° \times 0$
  D. Internal rotation in extension
    Any amount $\times 0$
  E. Adduction
    $0° - 15° \times 0.2$

To determine the overall rating for range of motion, multiply the sum of the index values $\times 0.05$.

Record Trendelenburg test as positive, level, or neutral.

Source: Data from Harris, W.H. J Bone Joint Surg 51A:737–755, 1969.

probably indicated with arthroplasty as a backup. In younger patients, no good option is available. If the area of collapse is found to involve less than 50% of the femoral head based on tomograms, CT, or plane radiographs in various degrees of flexion and abduction, a flexion osteotomy may provide acceptable improvement in function.[75] Hip arthrodesis is an option in the younger patient with high functional demands but is made more difficult by the presence of avascular bone. Many authors have advocated bipolar endoprosthetic replacement for this complication, but long-term functional results are lacking. Because of the difficulty with acetabular wear, total hip arthroplasty may be the procedure of choice even in patients younger than 50 years. In the past, this procedure has produced a high incidence of early failures in younger patients, but data are unavailable for newer, uncemented techniques. All things considered, with the lack of reliable reconstructive options, the best method of dealing with this problem is prevention.

Fixation Failure

Fixation failure is suspected based on the clinical exam in the early postoperative period. The patient with unstable fixation will generally have symptoms of groin or buttock pain.[173] The suspicion is confirmed on plain radiographic studies or tomograms that confirm displacement or angulation of the fracture, usually inferiorly and posteriorly; radiolucency around the implants; or backing out of the implants. The last finding can, however, occur with settling of the fracture as healing progresses and is encouraged by parallel insertion of multiple implants. Some degree of fracture settling is often associated with otherwise uneventful healing.

Because loss of fixation is probably related to failure of osteoporotic bone around the implants, it may perhaps best be seen as a problem of patient selection. In the future, bone density studies may aid in assigning patients to internal fixation or prosthetic replacement treatments. Technical problems, such as malreduction or the use of implants that are too short, have threads that cross the fracture line, or are widely divergent and prevent fracture settling, play a role in fixation failures. Similarly, implants that do not provide adequate stability of the fragments may play a role. This is best avoided by selecting a pin or screw that provides adequate fracture stabilization (Fig. 43–26).

Posttraumatic arthritis can also result from fixation problems. Implant penetration into the joint can occur with femoral neck fixation.[36,173] This problem has been most clearly defined in reference to pin fixation of slipped capital femoral epiphysis but has also been reported in reference to femoral neck fracture fixation.[188]

The risk increases as the number of implants increases; thus no more than three implants should be used. The screw tips must be carefully observed radiographically at surgery. The safe-zone concept of Walters and Simon, with the central axis being the area where screws can be the closest to the joint, applies to femoral neck fixation as well.[188] If screws are intraoperatively recognized to penetrate the femoral head, they should be exchanged for a shorter screw inserted through a new tract. If the old tract is used and fracture settling begins to develop, the screw, rather than backing out of the lateral cortex, may repenetrate the hip joint.[56] Screw penetration recognized in the early postoperative period should be managed in the same way. If it is recognized late, after posttraumatic degenerative arthritis has developed, then the surgeon may elect to remove the implant and treat the arthritis conservatively. Total hip arthroplasty or arthrodesis are the other main surgical options.

With loss of reduction caused by fixation failure, the choice of procedure is again related to patient age, functional demand, medical condition, and bone density. When these factors are favorable in the active individual with good bone quality, the surgeon should elect to re-reduce and internally fix (Fig 43–27). When the failure occurs in association with nonunion, valgus osteotomy may be indicated.[125] When these factors involve an older patient with poor bone density and lower functional demands, bipolar or total hip arthroplasty becomes the procedure of choice.

Nonunion

The diagnosis of nonunion is initially suspected on a clinical basis. The symptoms of groin or buttock pain, pain on hip extension, or pain with weight bearing all suggest the potential for this complication. In comparison with avascular necrosis, these symptoms occur earlier and are more severe. Radiographs suggest a lucent zone, and tomography will confirm the lack of healing. If bone scanning is performed, increased uptake will be seen in the area of nonunion.

As with fixation failure, the decision as to how to proceed is based on consideration of the patient's age, function, medical history, and bone density. In the younger patient, if adequate bone remains in the femoral head, a refixation with cancellous or muscle pedicle grafting is indicated.[112,128,132] Many have advocated valgus osteotomy to improve the mechanical loading of the nonunion, with good results (Fig. 43–28).[125a] If the physiologic neck-shaft axis remains intact, however, refixation with bone grafting without osteotomy has similarly produced good radiographic and clinical results. Where a short limb is involved, the valgus osteotomy is the procedure of choice.

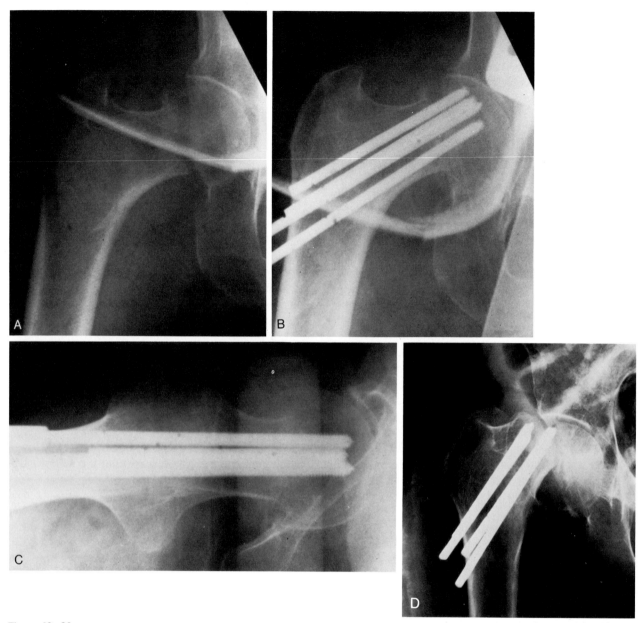

Figure 43–26

Loss of fixation of a femoral neck fracture. *A,* This 78-eight-year-old female sustained a displaced Garden grade IV femoral neck fracture in a low-energy fall. *B,C,* She underwent Neufeld pinning with four pins. A good reduction was apparent on the lateral view, but the AP view revealed a varus malreduction. *D,* By ten days postoperatively she was complaining of pain while ambulating with a walker, and the femoral head had fallen off the femoral neck. This illustrates the importance of a good reduction in the AP view, something that is especially critical in osteoporotic individuals.

In the case of the older, osteoporotic patient or in the situation where instability has produced loss of bone in the femoral head, hip arthroplasty is the procedure of choice. Good to excellent functional results in this setting have been reported.[85b,125a] Again, prevention is the best method of treatment. Conservative treatment of undisplaced fractures should be avoided. Internal fixation with multiple implants of adequate thread or with a sliding hip screw with a second cancellous screw for rotation control should provide stability for fracture union in at least 90% of displaced fractures with adequate bone stock. Internal fixation is relatively contraindicated in osteopenic patients.

Figure 43–27

Loss of fixation of a femoral neck fracture. *A,* This 44-year-old male fell off a roof, sustaining this displaced Garden grade II femoral neck fracture with an associated intraarticular distal radius fracture. *B,C,* He was treated with an anterior capsulotomy using a Watson-Jones approach, with the findings of a hematoma under pressure. He was fixed with three cancellous screws. *D,* The patient began immediate full weight bearing against advice and was doing lumbar hyperextension exercises at three weeks when he felt a snap in his groin. *E,* Salvage with a compression hip screw. The patient developed posttraumatic osteonecrosis with collapse at nine months. He is symptomatic but has not undergone revision surgery. This emphasizes the importance of a careful postoperative plan and touch-down weight bearing until fracture union occurs.

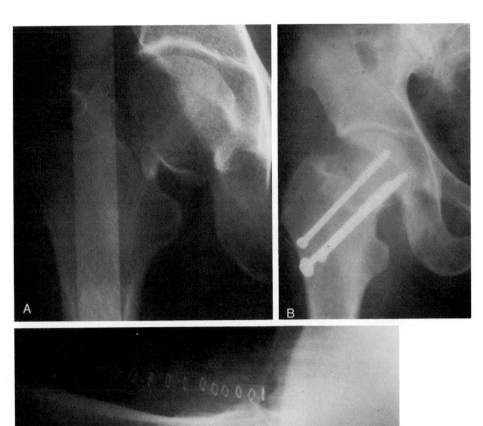

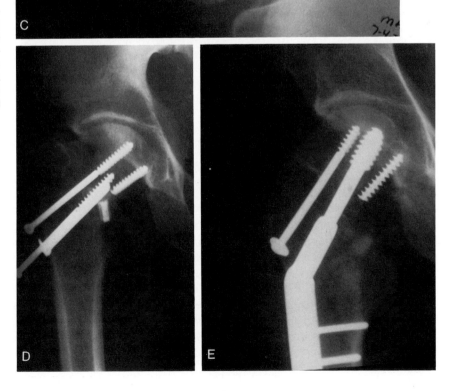

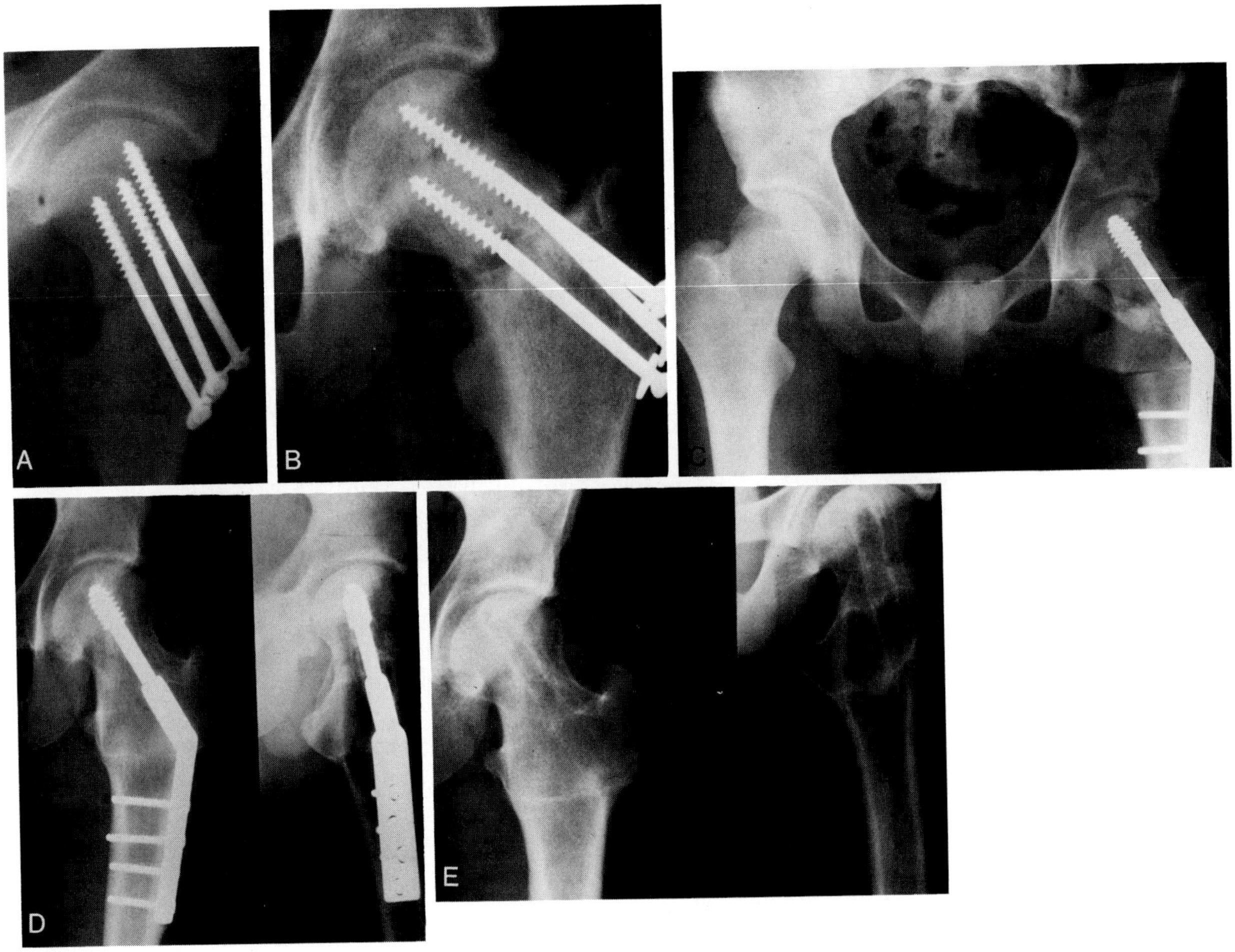

Figure 43-28

Nonunion of a femoral neck fracture. *A,* This 26-year-old male underwent an open reduction and internal fixation of a displaced femoral neck fracture, with a poor reduction resulting. *B,* This reduction showed excessive valgus malalignment, and with touch-down weight bearing and active motion of the hip, followed by progressive weight bearing beginning at 12 weeks, the patient developed a varus deformity with nonunion at six months. *C,* This was salvaged by a valgus intertrochanteric/subtrochanteric osteotomy and hip screw fixation. *D,* Union of the osteotomy and the femoral neck fracture occurred. *E,* At 22 months follow-up the patient has no evidence of osteonecrosis.

Failed Arthroplasty

Failure of primary prosthetic replacement for femoral neck fractures has been reported to be caused by infection, acetabular wear (protrusio), stem loosening, and dislocation.[54,118]

Infection following prosthetic replacement has been reported in 0% to 10% or more of cases (Table 43–2).[106] Superficial infection is best managed by antibiotic treatment and local debridement and appropriate wound care. Early deep infection (i.e., in the first one to two weeks) in a relatively healthy patient may be managed with deep debridement, closure over suction drains, and prolonged intravenous antibiotic treatment. If this regimen fails or the patient becomes septic, the prosthesis and all cement must be removed, followed by debridement, closure of the wound over

drains, and prolonged antibiotic treatment. In the younger, healthy patient, reimplantation of a prosthesis utilizing antibiotic-impregnated cement may be considered at a later date. This is most frequently chosen in the setting of a gram-positive infection. An excellent review of the management of infected hip prostheses has been published by Canner et al.[29]

Failure of older unipolar prosthetic designs (Austin-Moore, Thompson) as a result of acetabular wear was a major impetus in developing bipolar designs. This radiographic complication has been reported to be as common as 20%.[4] Symptomatic acetabular erosion occurs in approximately 6% to 8% of patients with Thompson or Austin-Moore prostheses, although it has been reported to be as high as 37%.[54] Although theoretically biopolar designs, because of their inner bearing motion, decrease acetabular wear, this has not been documented in a large series with long-term follow-up; the functional results for both unipolar and bipolar designs are similar.[122] Short-term improvement on acetabular wear in 161 cases was reported by Devas and Hinves.[54] The feeling that this complication is unaltered by bipolar endoprosthetic design has led many surgeons to recommend total hip arthroplasty for displaced femoral neck fractures in selected patients.

When acetabular erosion occurs and is symptomatic, conversion to a total hip arthroplasty is indicated. If there is no concomitant stem loosening and the prosthesis is bipolar, then the femoral component can be retained and an acetabular component placed. There is some debate over the issue of using cemented versus noncemented acetabular components in this setting. There is good evidence to indicate that revision of a unipolar Thompson or Austin-Moore prosthesis to a total hip arthroplasty is difficult and has a high incidence of both later loosening of the new femoral component and shaft fracture on insertion. This has led some authors to condemn the use of these components in patients with a life expectancy in excess of one to two years.

Failure of prosthetic replacement can also occur with stem loosening. This generally is present on radiographic examination prior to the development of clinical symptoms. Sinking or subsidence of the prosthesis, radiolucent lines around the cement mantle, and scalloping around the cement or prosthesis are radiographic signs of loosening of the prostheses. In Long and Knight's study, some radiolucency around the cement was present in 81% of the 156 Bateman prostheses with a minimum of one year follow-up.[122] In the series reported by Lausten et al., these lines exceeded 2 mm in 15% of 77 cases.[120] When this radiographic picture is present and the patient presents with a complaint of thigh or buttock pain, revision is generally indicated. In general, revision should be to a total hip prosthesis. In the occasion that component loosening is identified by a proximal femur fracture, revision should be to a long-stem femoral component. The reader is referred to Kavanaugh and Fitzgerald's review of revision arthroplasty.[114]

Subtrochanteric Fracture Below Screws

Subtrochanteric fracture below screws is readily apparent based on the history and presentation of the patient with the subtrochanteric femur fracture. Usually it is the result of a minor fall or twisting with unprotected, full weight bearing after femoral neck fracture fixation. The diagnosis is confirmed by plain radiographs. Factors thought to play a role in this phenomenon are unfilled drill holes (from attempted screw or pin placement) in the subtrochanteric region and pins inserted from too distal a location. Very low angle implants that start in the region of the proximal femur where the cortical bone is thick (distal to the point opposite the middle of the lesser trochanter) pass through bone that is in an area of high stress during weight bearing. If the pins have not been predrilled, radial cracks may develop during insertion. Small cracks, unfilled holes, or the implants themselves concentrate the stresses in this region and may lead to propagation of a subtrochanteric fracture. The factors mentioned are generally visible on radiographs or at inspection of the fracture site during reoperation.

When this complication occurs in the early postoperative phase (which it generally does), treatment consists of reoperation. Conservative treatment of minimally displaced or nondisplaced fractures will generally result in fracture displacement, and operative stabilization is therefore recommended. The implant selected must allow continued stabilization of the femoral neck fracture while extending fixation to the subtrochanteric fracture. This is best accomplished by leaving one or two of the screws or pins in place and fixing the subtrochanteric fracture by inserting a compression hip screw with a side plate long enough to obtain four good screws distal to the fracture or an equivalently angled blade plate. Lag screws should be added to stabilize the subtrochanteric femur fracture wherever possible. Primary autogenous bone grafting of the subtrochanteric injury, especially where there is any gapping of the medial cortex, is mandatory. In general, changing to an intramedullary device is to be avoided unless the main portion of the neck fixation can be left during insertion of the device. The triflanged nail (Zickel) and one-piece nail plate (Jewett) should not generally be used because of the distraction force applied to the femoral neck during their insertion. Although large series of patients treated for this complication have not been published, successful healing of the subtrochanteric fracture usually occurs when the preceding principles are followed.

Pressure Sores

Pressure sores occur too frequently in patients with femoral neck fractures. Occasionally they are the result of a debilitated patient lying unassisted on the floor for a prolonged period after a fall. More often they develop in the hospital before, during, or after surgery for hip fracture and thus should be preventable. Jensen and Junker reported a 30% incidence of pressure sores after hip fracture.[109a] They are most common in elderly women, appear within a week of surgery, increase hospital stay, and are associated with higher mortality. Pressure sores occur most frequently on the sacrum or posterior heel, especially of the injured limb. Most can be prevented by turning the patient at least every two hours and by supporting the legs with pillows placed longitudinally under the calf so that the heel does not contact the mattress. Rarely, a special bed with a flotation or air cushion mattress may be required. Close monitoring for the persisting erythema of a low-grade pressure sore, with prompt, complete relief of pressure on affected areas, can significantly decrease the severity and cost of these troublesome problems.[186a]

REFERENCES

Femoral Head Fractures

1. Birkett, J. Traumatic dislocation of the head of the femur complicated with its fracture. Med Chir Trans 52:133, 1869.
2. Bosse, M.J.; Poka, A.; Reinert, C.M.; et al. Heterotopic ossification as a complication of acetabular fracture. J Bone Joint Surg 70A:1231–1237, 1988.
3. Brumback, R.J.; Kenzora, J.E.; Levitt, L.E.; et al. Proceedings of the Hip Society, 1986, St. Louis, C.V. Mosby, 1987, pp. 181–206.
4. Butler, J.E. Pipkin type II fractures of the femoral head. J Bone Joint Surg 63A(8):1292, 1981.
5. Cathcart, R.F. The shape of the femoral head and preliminary results of clinical use of a non-spherical hip prosthesis. J Bone Joint Surg 53A:397, 1971.
6. Chandler, H.P.; Reineck, F.T.; Wixson, R.L.; McCarthy, J.C. Total hip replacement in patients younger than thirty years old; a five year follow up study. J Bone Joint Surg 63A:1426–1434, 1981.
7. Chakraborti, S.; Miller, I.M. Dislocation of the hip associated with fracture of the femoral head. Injury 7(2):134, 1975.
8. Christopher, F. Fractures of the head of the femur. Arch Surg 12:1049, 1926
9. Connolly, J.F. Acetabular labrum entrapment associated with a femoral head fracture-dislocation. J Bone Joint Surg 56A(8):1735, 1974
10. Coventry, M.B. The treatment of fracture-dislocation of the hip by total hip arthroplasty. J Bone Joint Surg 56A(6):1128, 1974
11. DeLee, J.C.; Evans, J.A.; Thomas, J. Anterior dislocation of the hip and associated femoral head fractures. J Bone Joint Surg 62A(6):960, 1980
12. Dowd, G.S.E.; Johnson, R. Successful conservative treatment of a fracture dislocation of the femoral head: A case report. J Bone Joint Surg 61A(8):1244, 1979
13. Epstein, H.C. Posterior fracture-dislocation of the femoral head: A case report. J Bone Joint Surg 43A(8):1079, 1961.
14. Epstein, H.C. Posterior fracture-dislocation of the hip: long term follow-up. J Bone Joint Surg 56A(6):1103, 1974.
15. Epstein, H.C.; Harvey, J.P. Jr. Traumatic anterior dislocation of the hip. (Abstract) J Bone Joint Surg 56A(1):1103, 1974.
16. Epstein, H.C.; Wiss, D.A.; Cozen, L. Posterior fracture dislocation of the hip with fractures of the femoral head. Clin Orthop 201:9, 1985.
17. Fina, C.P.; Kelly, P.J. Dislocations of the hip with fractures of the proximal femur. J Trauma 10(1):77, 1970.
18. Funsten, R.V.; Kinser, P.; Frankel, C.H. Dashboard dislocation of the hip: A report of twenty cases of traumatic dislocation. J Bone Joint Surg 20(1):124, 1938.
19. Garrett, J.C.; Epstein, H.C.; Harris, W.H.; et al. Treatment of unreduced traumatic posterior dislocations of the hip. J Bone Joint Surg 61(A)91:2, 1979.
20. Gordon, E.J.; Freiberg, J.A. Posterior dislocation of the hip with fracture of the head of the femur. J Bone Joint Surg 31A(4):869, 1949.
21. Greenwald, A.S.; Haynes, D.W. Weight bearing areas in the human hip joint. J Bone Joint Surg 54B:157–163, 1972
22. Johnstone, G. Posterior dislocation of the hip with fracture of the femoral head. East Afr Med J 42(8):429, 1965.
23. Kelly, P.J.; Lipscomb, P.R. Primary vitallium-mold arthroplasty for posterior dislocation of the hip with fracture of the femoral head. J Bone Joint Surg 40A(3):675, 1958.
24. Lange, R.H.; Engber, W.D.; Clancy, W.G. Expanding application for the Herbert scaphoid screw. Orthopaedics 9:1393–1397, 1986.
24a. Mears, D.C. Personal communication.
25. Pipkin, G. Treatment of grade IV fracture-dislocation of the hip: A review. J Bone Joint Surg 39A(5):1027, 1957.
26. Ritter, M.A.; Gioe, T.J. The effect of indomethacin on para-articular ectopic ossification following total hip arthroplasty. Clin Orthop 167:113–117, 1982.
27. Roeder, L.F. Jr.; DeLee, J.C. Femoral head fractures associated with posterior hip dislocations. Clin Orthop 147:121, 1980.
28. Salter, R.B.; Simmonds, D.F.; Malcolm, B.W.; et al. The biologic effect of continuous passive motion on the healing of full thickness defects in articular cartilage. J Bone Joint Surg 62A:1232, 1980
29. Sarmiento, A.; Laird, C.A. Posterior fracture-dislocation of the femoral head. Clin Orthop 92:143, 1973.
30. Scham, S.M.; Fry, L.R. Traumatic anterior dislocation of the hip with fracture of the femoral head: A case report. Clin Orthop 62:133, 1969.
31. Seibel, R.; LaDuca, J.; Hassett, J.M.; et al. Blunt multiple trauma (ISS 36), femur traction, and the pulmonary failure-septic state. Ann Surg 202:283–295, 1985.
32. Stewart, M.J. Management of the fractures of the head of the femur complicated by dislocation of the hip. Orthop Clin North Am 5(4):793, 1974.
33. Stewart, M.J.; Milford, L.W. Fracture-dislocation of the hip: An end-result study. J Bone Joint Surg 36A(92):315, 1954.
34. Stromqvist, B. Femoral head vitality after intracapsular hip fracture; 490 cases studied by intravital tetracycline labeling and TC-MDP radionuclide imaging. ACTA Orthop Scand 54(suppl 200):5–71, 1983.
35. Thomas, B.J.; Amstutz, H.C. Results of the administration of diphosphonate for the prevention of heterotopic ossification after total hip arthroplasty. J Bone Joint Surg 67A:400–403, 1984.
36. Thompson, V.P.; Epstein, H.C. Traumatic dislocation of the hip: A survey of 204 cases covering a period of 21 years. J Bone Joint Surg 33A(3):746, 1951.
37. Thorpe, M.; Swiontkowski, M.F.; Seiler, J.G.; Hansen, S.T. Operative management of femoral head fractures. Orthop Trans 13:51, 1989.
38. Trueta, J.; Harrison, M.H.M. The normal vascular anatomy of the femoral head in adult man. J Bone Joint Surg 35B:442–461, 1953.
39. Upadhyay, S.S.; Moulton, A. The long-term results of traumatic posterior dislocation of the hip. J Bone Joint Surg 63B(4):548, 1981.

Femoral Neck Fractures

1. Abrami, G.; Stevens J. Early weight bearing after internal fixation of transcervical fracture of the femur; preliminary report of a clinical trial. J Bone Joint Surg 46B:204–205, 1965.
2. Aitken, J.M. Relevance of osteoporosis in women with fracture of the femoral neck. Br Med J 288:597–601, 1984.

3. Alberts, K.A.; Dahlborn, M.; Glas, J.E.; et al. Radionuclide scintigraphy of femoral head specimens removed at arthroplasty for failed femoral neck fractures. Clin Orthop 205:222–229, 1986.

4. Anderson, L.D.; Hamsa, W.R.; Waring, T.L. Femoral-head prosthesis; a review of three hundred and fifty-six operations and their results. J Bone Joint Surg 46A:1049–1065, 1964.

4a. Andersson, G. Hip assessment: a comparison of nine different methods. J Bone Joint Surg 54B:621, 1972.

4b. Anonymous: Life expectancy remains at record level. Statist Bull 70:26–30, 1989.

4c. Arnold, W.D. The effect of early weight-bearing on the stability of femoral neck fractures treated with Knowles pins. J Bone Joint Surg 66A:847–852, 1984.

4d. Arnold, W.D.; Lynden, J.P.; Minkoff, J. Treatment of intracapsular fractures of the femoral neck. J Bone Joint Surg 56A:254, 1974.

5. Arnoldi, C.C.; Lemperg, R.K. Fracture of the femoral neck. II. Relative importance of primary vascular damage and surgical procedure for the development of necrosis of the femoral head. Clin Orthop 129:217–222, 1977.

6. Arnoldi, C.C.; Linderholm, H. Fracture of the femoral neck, I. Vascular disturbances in different types of fractures, assessed by measurements of intraosseous pressure. Clin Orthop 84:116–127, 1972.

7. Aro, H.; Dahlstrom, S. Conservative management of distraction-type stress fractures of the femoral neck. J Bone Joint Surg 68B:65–67, 1986.

8. Askin, S.R.; Bryan, R.S. Femoral neck fractures in young adults. Clin Orthop 114:259–264, 1976.

9. Asser Hansen, B.; Solgaard, S. Impacted fractures of the femoral neck treated by early mobilization and weight-bearing. Acta Orthop Scand 49:180–185, 1978.

10. Astrom, J.; Ahnqvist, S.; Beertema, J.; Jonsson, B. Physical activity in women sustaining fracture of the neck of the femur. J Bone Joint Surg 69B:381–383, 1987.

11. Bargren, J.H.; Tilson, D.H.; Bridgeford, O.E. Prevention of displaced fatigue fractures of the femur. J Bone Joint Surg 53A:1115–1117, 1971.

12. Barnes, J.T.; Brown, J.T.; Garden, R.S.; Nicoll, E.A. Subcapital fractures of the femur; a prospective review. J Bone Joint Surg 58B:2–24, 1976.

13. Barnes, R. The diagnosis of ischaemia of the capital fragment in femoral neck fractures. J Bone Joint Surg 44B:760–761, 1962.

14. Bastow, M.D.; Rawlings, J.; Allison, S.P. Benefits of supplemental tube feeding after fractured neck of femur: A randomized controlled trial. Br Med J 287:1589–1592, 1983.

14a. Bastow, M.D.; Rawlings, J.; Allison, S.P. Undernutrition, hypothermia, and injury in elderly women with fractured femur: An injury response to altered metabolism? Lancet 1:143–146, 1983.

15. Bauer, G.; Weber, D.A.; Ceder, L.; et al. Dynamics of technetium-99m methylenediphosphonate imaging of the femoral head after femoral neck fracture. Clin Orthop 152:85–92, 1982.

16. Bayliss, A.P.; Davidson, J.K. Traumatic osteonecrosis of the femoral head following intracapsular fracture: Incidence and earliest radiological features. Clin Radiol 28:407–414, 1977.

17. Bentley, G. Impacted fractures of the neck of the femur. J Bone Joint Surg 50B:551–561, 1968.

18. Bigler, D.; Adelhoj, B.; Petring, O.U.; et al. Mental function and morbidity after acute hip surgery during spinal and general anesthesia. Anesthesia 40:672–676, 1985.

19. Blickenstaff, L.D.; Morris, J.M. Fatigue fracture of the femoral neck. J Bone Joint Surg 48A:1031–1047, 1966.

19a. Bochner, R.M.; Pellici, P.M.; Lyden, J.P. Bipolar hemiarthroplasty for fracture of the femoral neck. J Bone Joint Surg 70A:1001–1010, 1988.

20. Bohr, H.; Larsen, E.H. On necrosis of the femoral head after fracture of the neck of the femur—a microradiographic and histologic study. J Bone Joint Surg 47B:330–338, 1965.

21. Bonfiglio, M.; Voke, E.M. Aseptic necrosis of the femoral head and non-union of the femoral neck; effect of treatment of drilling and bone-grafting (Phemister technique). J Bone Joint Surg 50A:48–66, 1968.

21a. Booth, R.E.; Balderston, R.A.; Rothman, R.H. Total Hip Arthroplasty. Philadelphia, W.B. Saunders, 1987.

22. Boston, D.A. Bilateral fractures of the femoral neck. Injury 14:207–210, 1982.

23. Boyd, H.B.; Calandruccio, R.A. Further observations on the use of radioactive phosphorous (P32) to determine the viability of the head of the femur; correlation of clinical and experimental data in 130 patients with fractures of the femoral neck. J Bone Joint Surg 45A:445–460, 1963.

24. Boyd, H.B.; Salvatore, J.E. Acute fracture of the femoral neck: Internal fixation or prosthesis? J Bone Joint Surg 46A:1066–1068, 1964.

25. Boyd, H.B.; Zilversmit, D.B.; Calandruccio, R.A. The use of radio-active phosphorous (P32) to determine the viability of the head of the femur. J Bone Joint Surg 37A:260–269, 1960.

26. Brodetti, A. The blood supply of the femoral neck and head in relation to the damaging effects of nails and screws. J Bone Joint Surg 42B:794–801, 1960.

27. Brown, T.I.S.; Court-Brown, C. Failure of sliding nail-plate fixation in subcapital fractures of the femoral neck. J Bone Joint Surg 61B:342–346, 1979.

27a. Brunner, C.F.; Weber, B.G. Special Techniques in Internal Fixation. Berlin, Springer-Verlag, 1982, p. 34.

27b. Calandruccio, R.A. Arthroplasty of the hip. In: Crenshaw,A.H., ed. Campbell's Operative Orthopaedics, Ed. 7. St. Louis, C.V. Mosby, 1987.

28. Camp, J.F.; Colwell, C.E. Core decompression of the femoral head for osteonecrosis. J Bone Joint Surg 68A:1313–1319, 1986.

29. Canner, G.C.; Steinberg, M.E.; Heppenstall, R.B.; Balderston, R. The infected hip after total hip arthroplasty, J Bone Joint Surg 66A:1393–1399, 1984.

30. Casey, M.J.; Chapman, M.W. Ipsilateral concomitant fractures of the hip and femoral shaft, J Bone Joint Surg 61A:503–509, 1979.

31. Castle, M.E.; Orinion, E.A. Prophylactic anticoagulation in fractures. J Bone Joint Surg 52A:521–528, 1970.

32. Catto, M. A histological study of avascular necrosis of the femoral head after transcervical fracture. J Bone Joint Surg 47B:749–776, 1965.

33. Ceder, L.; Stromqvist, B.; Hansson, L.I. Effects of strategy changes in the treatment of femoral neck fractures during a 17-year period. Clin Orthop 218:53–57, 1987.

34. Chan, R.N.W.; Hoskinson, J. Thompson prosthesis for fractures of the neck of the femur; a comparison of surgical approaches. J Bone Joint Surg 57B:437–443, 1975.

35. Chandler, S.B.; Kreuscher, P.H. A study of the blood supply of the ligamentum teres and its relation to the circulation of the head of the femur. J Bone Joint Surg 14:834–846, 1932.

36. Chapman, M.W.; Stehr, J.H.; Eberle, C.F.; et al. Treatment of intracapsular hip fractures by the Deyerle method; a comparative review of 119 cases. J Bone Joint Surg 57A:735–744, 1975.

37. Christodoulou, N.A.; Dretakis, E.K. Significance of muscular disturbances in the localization of fractures of the proximal femur. Clin Orthop 187:215–217, 1984.

38. Claffey, T.J. Avascular necrosis of the femoral head; an anatomical study. J Bone Joint Surg 42B:802–809, 1960.

39. Clawson, D.K. Intracapsular fractures of the femur treated by the sliding screw plate fixation method. J Trauma 4:753–756, 1964.

40. Coates, R.L.; Armour, P. Treatment of subcapital femoral fractures by primary total hip replacement. Injury 11:132–135, 1979.

40a. Cole, J.D.; Browner, B.D.; Cotler, H.B.; et al. Initial experience with a second-generation locking nail. Orthop Trans 14:269, 1990.

41. Coleman, S.A.; Boyce, W.J.; Cosh, P.H.; McKenzie, P.J. Outcome after general anesthesia for repair of fractured neck of femur—a randomized trial of spontaneous v. controlled ventilation. Br J Anaesth 60:43–47, 1988.

42. Cotton, F.J. Artificial impaction in hip fractures. Surg Gynecol Obstet 45:307–319, 1927.

43. Cotton, F.J. Intracapsular hip fracture. J Bone Joint Surg 16:105–109, 1934.

44. Coughlin, L.; Templeton, J. Hip fractures in patients with Parkinson's disease. Clin Orthop 148:192–195, 1980.

45. Crawford, H.B. Conservative treatment of impacted fractures of the femoral neck; a report of fifty cases. J Bone Joint Surg 42A:471–479, 1960.

46. Crawfurd, E.J.P.; Emery, R.J.H.; Hansell, D.M.; et al. Capsular distension and intracapsular pressure in subcapital fractures of the femur. J Bone Joint Surg 70B:195–198, 1988.

47. Crock, H.V. A revision of the anatomy of the arteries supplying the upper end of the human femur. J Anat 99:77–88, 1965.

48. Crock, H.V. An atlas of the arterial supply of the head and neck of the femur in man. Clin Orthop 152:17–27, 1980.

48a. Cummings, S.R.; Phillips, S.L.; Wheat, M.E.; et al. Recovery of function after hip fracture. The role of social supports. J Am Geriatr Soc 36:801–806, 1988.

49. Currie, A.L.; Reid, D.M.; Brown, N.; Nuki, G. An epidemiological study of fracture of the neck of the femur. Health Bull 44:143–148, 1986.

50. Dahl, E. Mortality and life expectancy after hip fractures. Acta Orthop Scand 51:163–170, 1980.

51. Dalen, N.; Jacobsson, B. Rarefied femoral neck trabecular patterns, fracture displacement, and femoral head vitality in femoral neck fractures. Clin Orthop 205:97–98, 1986.

51a. Arcy, L.; Devas, M. Treatment of fractures of the femoral neck by replacement with the Thompson prosthesis. J Bone Joint Surg 58B:279, 1976.

52. Dedrick, D.K.; Mackenzie, J.R.; Burney, R.E. Complications of femoral neck fractures in young adults. J Trauma 26:932–937, 1986.

53. Delamarter, R.; Moreland, J.R. Treatment of acute femoral neck fractures with total hip arthroplasty. Clin Orthop 218:68–74, 1987.

54. Devas, M.; Hinves, B. Prevention of acetabular erosion after hemiarthroplasty for fractured neck of femur. J Bone Joint Surg 65B:548–551, 1983.

55. Devas, M.B. Stress fractures of the femoral neck. J Bone Joint Surg 47B:728–738, 1965.

56. Deyerle, W.M. Impacted fixation over resilient multiple pins. Clin Orthop 152:102–122, 1980.

57. Dorne, H.L.; Lander, P.H. Spontaneous stress fractures of the femoral neck. Am J Radiol 144:343–347, 1984.

58. Drake, J.K.; Meyers, M.H. Intracapsular pressure and hemarthrosis following femoral neck fracture. Clin Orthop 182:172–176, 1984.

59. Dretakis, E.K.; Christodoulou, N.A. Significance of endogenic factors in the location of fractures of the proximal femur. Acta Orthop Scand 54:198–203, 1983.

60. Drinker, H.; Murray, W.R. The universal proximal femoral endoprosthesis; a short term comparison with conventional hemiarthroplasty. J Bone Joint Surg 61A:1167–1174, 1979.

61. Edholm, P.; Lindblom, K.; Maurseth, K. Angulations in the fractures of the femoral neck with and without subsequent necrosis of the head. Acta Radiol Scand 6:329–336, 1967.

61a. Eiskjaer, S.; Gelineck, J.; Soballe, K. Fractures of the femoral neck treated with cemented bipolar hemiarthroplasty. Orthopedics 12:1545–1550, 1989.

62. Ernst, J. Stress fractures of the neck of the femur. J Trauma 4:71–83, 1964.

63. Ewald, F.C.; Christie, M.J.; Thomas, W.H.; et al. Total hip arthroplasty for failed hemiarthroplasty. Presented at the AAOS 52nd Annual Meeting, Las Vegas, January 28, 1985.

64. Fairclough, J.; Colhoun, E.; Johnston, D.; Williams, L.A. Bone scanning for suspected hip fractures—a prospective study in elderly patients. J Bone Joint Surg 69B:251–253, 1987.

65. Ficat, R.P. Idiopathic bone necrosis of the femoral head. Early diagnosis and treatment. J Bone Joint Surg 67B:3–9, 1985.

65a. Fielding, J.W.; Wilson, S.A.; Ratzaw, S. A continuing end-result study of displaced intracapsular fractures of the neck of the femur treated with the Pugh nail. J Bone Joint Surg 56A:1464, 1974.

66. Fielding, J.W.; Wilson, H.J.; Zickel, R.E. A continuing end-result study of intracapsular fracture of the neck of the femur. J Bone Joint Surg 44A:965–974, 1962.

67. Finsen, V.; Benum, P. Changing incidence of hip fractures in rural and urban areas of central Norway. Clin Orthop 218:104–110, 1987.

68. Firooznia, H.; Rafii, M.; Golimbu, C.; et al. Trabecular mineral content of the spine in women with hip fracture: CT measurement. Radiology 159:737–740, 1986.

69. Fitzgerald, J.F.; Fagan, L.F.; Tierny, W.M.; Dittus, R.S. Changing patterns of hip fracture care before and after implementation of the prospective payment system. JAMA 258:218–221, 1987.

70. Frandsen, P.A.; Kruse, T. Hip fractures in the county of Funen, Denmark; implications of demographic aging and changes in incidence rates. Acta Orthop Scand 54:681–686, 1983.

71. Frangakis, E.K. Intracapsular fractures of the neck of the femur-factors influencing non-union and ischaemic necrosis. J Bone Joint Surg 48B:17–30, 1966.

72. Franklin, A.; Gallannaugh, S.C. The bi-articular hip prosthesis for fractures of the femoral neck—a preliminary report. Injury 15:159–162, 1983.

73. Freeman, M.A.R.; Todd, R.C.; Pirie, C.J. The role of fatigue in the pathogenesis of senile femoral neck fractures. J Bone Joint Surg 56B:698–702, 1974.

74. Friedman, R.J.; Wyman, E.T. Ipsilateral hip and femoral shaft fractures. Clin Orthop 208:188–194, 1986.

74a. Froehlich, J.A.; Dorfman, G.S.; Cronan, J.J.; et al. Compression ultrasonography for detection of deep venous thrombosis in patients who have a fracture of the hip. J Bone Joint Surg 71A:249–256, 1989.

75. Ganz, R.; Büchler, U. Overview of attempts to revitalize the dead head in aseptic necrosis of the femoral head—osteotomy and revascularization. In: Proceedings of the Eleventh Hip Society. St. Louis, C.V. Mosby, 1983, pp. 296–305.

75a. Garcia, A.; Meer, E.S.; Ambrose, G.B. Displaced intracapsular fractures of the neck of the femur. J Trauma 1:128, 1961.

76. Garden, R.S. The structure and function of the proximal end of the femur. J Bone Joint Surg 43B:576–589, 1961.

77. Garden, R.S. Stability and union in subcapital fractures of the femur. J Bone Joint Surg 46B:630–647, 1964.

78. Garden, R.S. Malreduction and avascular necrosis in subcapital fractures of the femur. J Bone Joint Surg 53B:183–197, 1971.

78a. Gegerle, P.; Bengoa, J.M.; Delmi, M.; et al. Enquete alimentaire apres fracture du col du femur: Effet d'un supplement dietetique sur les apports nutritionels. Schweiz Rundsch Med Prax 75:933–935, 1986.

79. Gilberty, R.P. Hemiarthroplasty of the hip using a low-friction bipolar endoprosthesis. Clin Orthop 175:86–92, 1983.

79a. Giordani, M.; Sarmiento, A.; Wiss, D.A.; et al. Complex fractures of the hip treated with a second-generation locking nail. Orthop Trans 14:269, 1990.

79b. Glass, K.E. Moore arthroplasty operations. J Bone Joint Surg 47B:598, 1965.

80. Glimcher, M.J.; Kenzora, J.E. The biology of osteonecrosis of the human femoral head and its clinical implications; III. Discussion of the etiology and genesis of the pathological sequelae; comments on treatment. Clin Orthop 140:273–312, 1979.

81. Greenwald, A.S.; Haynes, D.W. Weight-bearing areas in the human hip joint. J Bone Joint Surg 54B:157–163, 1972.

82. Greiff, J.; Lanng, S.; Hoilund-Carlsen, P.F.; et al. Early detection by 99m tc-sn-pyrophosphate scintigraphy of femoral head necrosis following medial femoral neck fractures. Acta Orthop Scand 51:119–125, 1980.

83. Grieff, J. Determination of the vitality of the femoral head with 99m tc-sn-pyrophosphate scintigraphy. Acta Orthop Scand 51:109–117, 1980.

84. Griffin, J.B. The calcar femorale redefined. Clin Orthop 164:211–214, 1982.

85. Gruber, U.F. Prevention of fatal pulmonary embolism in patients with fractures of the neck of the femur. Surg Gynecol Obstet 161:37–42, 1985.

85a. Gustke, K. The treatment of intracapsular hip fractures. Techn Orthop 4:19–29, 1989.

85b. Hagglund, G.; Nordstrom, B.; Lidgren, L. Total hip replacement after nailing failure in femoral neck fractures. Arch Orthop Trauma Surg 103:125–127, 1984.

86. Hamilton, H.W.; Crawford, J.S.; Gardiner, J.H.; Wiley, A.M. Venous thrombosis in patients with fracture of the upper end of the femur; a phlebographic study of the effect of prophylactic anticoagulation. J Bone Joint Surg 52B:268–289, 1970.

86a. Harris, W.H. Traumatic arthritis of the hip after dislocation and acetabular fractures: treatment by mold arthroplasty. J Bone Joint Surg 51A:737–755, 1969.

87. Harris, W.H.; Athanasoulis, C.A.; Waltman, A.C.; Salzman, E.W. High and low-dose aspirin prophylaxis against venous thromboembolic disease in total hip replacement. J Bone Joint Surg 64A:63–66, 1982.

88. Hartman, J.T.; Altner, P.C.; Freeark, R.J. The effect of limb elevation in preventing venous thrombosis; a venographic study. J Bone Joint Surg 52A:1618–1622, 1970.

89. Harty, M. Blood supply of the femoral head. Br Med J 7:1236–1237, 1953.

90. Harty, M. The calcar femorale and the femoral neck. J Bone Joint Surg 39A:625–630, 1957.

90a. Henry, S.L.; Seligson, D. Ipsilateral femoral neck–shaft fractures: a comparison of therapeutic devices. Orthop Trans 14:269, 1990.

91. Hilleboe, J.W.; Staple, T.W.; Lansche, E.W.; Reynolds, F.C. The nonoperative treatment of impacted fractures of the femoral neck. South Med J 63:1103–1109, 1970.

92. Hinchey, J.J.; Day, P.L. Primary prosthetic replacement in fresh femoral-neck fractures. J Bone Joint Surg 46A:223–240, 1964.

93. Hirsch, C.; Frankel, V.H. Analysis of forces producing fractures of the proximal end of the femur. J Bone Joint Surg 42B:633–640, 1960.

94. Hoaglund, F.T.; Low, W.D. Anatomy of the femoral neck and head, with comparative data from Caucasians and Hong Kong Chinese. Clin Orthop 152:10–16, 1980.

94a. Hodge, W.A.; Carlson, K.L.; Fijan, R.S.; et al. Contact pressures from an instrumented hip endoprosthesis. J Bone Joint Surg 71A:1378–1386, 1989.

95. Hogh, J.; Jensen, J.; Lauritzen, J. Dislocated femoral neck fractures; a follow-up study of 98 cases treated by multiple AO (ASIF) cancellous bone screws. Acta Orthop Scand 53:245–249, 1982.

96. Hoikka, V; Alhava, E.M.; Savolainen, K.; Parviainen, M. Osteomalacia in fractures of the proximal femur. Acta Orthop Scand 53:255–260, 1982.

97. Holmberg, S.; Conradi, P.; Kalen, R.; Thorngren, K.G. Mortality after cervical hip fracture; 3002 patients followed for 6 years. Acta Orthop Scand 57:8–11, 1986.

98. Holmberg, S.; Dalen, N. Intracapsular pressure and caput circulation in nondisplaced femoral neck fractures. Clin Orthop 219:124–126, 1987.

99. Holmberg, S.; Kalen, R.; Thorngren, K-G. Treatment and outcome of femoral neck fractures—an analysis of 2418 patients admitted from their own homes. Clin Orthop 218:42–52, 1987.

99a. Holmberg, S.; Thorngren, K-G. Rehabilitation after femoral neck fracture. Acta Orthop Scand 56:305–308, 1985.

100. Holmquist, B,; Alffram, P.A. Prediction of avascular necrosis following cervical fracture of the femur based on clearance of radioactive iodine from the head of the femur. Acta Orthop Scand 36:62–69, 1965.

101. Horiuchi, T.; Igarashi, M.; Karube, S.; et al. Spontaneous fractures of the hip in the elderly. Orthopedics 11:1277–1280, 1988.

102. Horsman, A.H.; Nordin, B.E.; Simpson, M.; Speed, R. Cortical and trabecular bone status in elderly women with femoral neck fracture. Clin Orthop 166:143–151. 1982.

103. Howard, C.B.; Mackie, I.G.; Fairclough, J. Femoral neck surgery using a local anesthetic technique. Anesthesia 38:993–994, 1983.

104. Howe, W.W.; Lacey, T.; Scwartz, R.P. A study of the gross anatomy of the arteries supplying the proximal portion of the femur and acetabulum. J Bone Joint Surg 32A:856–866, 1950.

105. Hunter, G.A. A comparison of the use of internal fixation and prosthetic replacement for fresh fractures of the neck of the femur. Br J Surg 56:229–232, 1969.

105a. Hunter, G.A. A further comparison of the use of internal fixation and prosthetic replacement for fresh fractures of the femur. Br J Surg 61:382, 1974.

106. Hunter, G.A. Should we abandon primary prosthetic replacement for fresh displaced fractures of the neck of the femur? Clin Orthop 152:158–161, 1980.

107. Jacobsson, B.; Dalen, N.; Jonsson, B.; Ackerholm, P. Intraarticular pressure during operation of cervical hip fractures. Acta Orthop Scand 59:16–18, 1988.

108. Jeffery, C.C. Spontaneous fractures of the femoral neck. J Bone Joint Surg 44B:543–549, 1962.

108a. Jette, A.M.; Harris, B.A.; Cleary, P.D.; Campion, E.W. Functional recovery after hip fracture. Arch Phys Med Rehabil 68:735–740, 1987.

109. Jensen, J.; Hogh, J. Fractures of the femoral neck; a follow-up

study after non-operative treatment of Garden's stage 1 and 2 fractures. Injury 14:339–342, 1982.

109a. Jensen, T.T.; Junker, Y. Pressure sores common after hip operations. Acta Orthop Scand 58:209–211, 1987.

110. Johnson, J.T.H.; Crothers, O. Nailing versus prosthesis for femoral neck fractures; a critical review of long-term results in two hundred and thirty-nine consecutive private patients. J Bone Joint Surg 57A:686–692, 1975.

110a. Johnson, K.D.; Brock, G. A review of reduction and internal fixation of adult femoral neck fractures in a county hospital. J Orthop Trauma 2:83–96, 1989.

111. Judet, J.; Judet, R.; Langrange, J.; Dunoyer, J. A study of the arterial vascularization of the femoral neck in the adult. J Bone Joint Surg 37A:663–680, 1955.

112. Judet, R. Traitment des fractures du col du femur par greffe pediculee. Acta Orthop Scand 23:421–427, 1952.

113. Kaltsas, D-K. Stress fractures of the femoral neck in young adults; a report of seven cases. J Bone Joint Surg 63B:33–37, 1981.

114. Kavanaugh, B.F.; Fitzgerald, R.H. Multiple revisions for failed total hip arthroplasty not associated with infection. J Bone Joint Surg 69A:1144–1149, 1987.

114a. Kaulie, H.; Sundal, B. Primary arthroplasty in femoral neck fractures. Acta Orthop Scand 45:579, 1974.

115. Keller, C.S.; Laros, G.S. Indications for open reduction of femoral neck fractures. Clin Orthop 152:131–137, 1980.

116. Kenzora, J.E.; McCarthy, R.E.; Lowell, J.D.; Sledge, C.B. Hip fracture mortality—relation to age, treatment, preoperative illness, time of surgery, and complications. Clin Orthop 186:45–56, 1984.

117. Kofoed, H.; Alberts, A. Femoral neck fractures; 165 cases treated by multiple percutaneous pinning. Acta Orthop Scand 51:127–136, 1980.

118. Kofoed, H.; Kofod, J. Moore prosthesis in the treatment of fresh femoral neck fractures—a critical review with special attention to secondary acetabular degeneration. Injury 14:531–540, 1981.

119. Langan, P. The Gilberty bipolar prosthesis; a clinical and radiographical review. Clin Orthop 141:169–175, 1979.

120. Lausten, G.S.; Vedel, P.; Nielsen, P.M. Fractures of the femoral neck treated with a bipolar endoprosthesis. Clin Orthop 218:63–67, 1987.

121. Leadbettter, G.W. Closed reduction of fractures of the neck of the femur. J Bone Joint Surg 20:108–113, 1938.

122. Long, J.W.; Knight, W. Bateman UPF prosthesis in fractures of the femoral neck. Clin Orthop 152:198–201, 1980.

123. Lucie, R.S.; Fuller, S.; Burdick, D.C.; Johnston, R.M. Early prediction of avascular necrosis of the femoral head following femoral neck fractures. Clin Orthop 161:207–214, 1981.

124. Lund, B.; Sorensen, O.H.; Melsen, F.; Mosekilde, L. Vitamin D metabolism and osteomalacia in patients with fractures of the proximal femur. Acta Orthop Scand 53:251–254, 1982.

124a. Lunt, H.R. The use of prosthetic replacement of the head of the femur as primary treatment for subcapital fractures. Injury 3:107, 1971.

125. Mannius, S.; Mellstrom, D; Oden, A.; et al. Incidence of hip fracture in Western Sweden 1974–1982—comparison of rural and urban populations. Acta Orthop Scand 58:38–42, 1987.

125a. Marti, R.K.; Schüller, H.M.; Raaymakers, E.L. Intertrochanteric osteotomy for non-union of the femoral neck. J Bone Joint Surg 71B:782–787, 1989.

126. Melberg, P.E.; Korner, L.; Lansinger, O. Hip joint pressure after femoral neck fracture. Acta Orthop Scand 57:501–504, 1986.

127. Melton, J.L.; Ilstrup, D.M.; Riggs, B.L.; Beckenbaugh, R.D. Fifty-year trend in hip fracture incidence. Clin Orthop 162:144–149, 1982.

128. Meyers, M.H.; Harvey, J.P. Jr.; Moore, T.M. Delayed treatment of subcapital and transcervical fractures of the neck of the femur with internal fixation and a muscle-pedicle bone graft. Orthop Clin North Am 5:743–756, 1974.

128a. Meyers, M.H.; Harvey, J.P. Jr.; Moore, T.M. Treatment of displaced subcapital and transcervical fractures of the femoral neck by muscle-pedicle bone grafts and internal fixation. J Bone Joint Surg 55A:257, 1973.

129. Meyers, M.H.; Telfer, N.; Moore, T.M. Determination of the vascularity of the femoral head with technetium 99m-sulfur-colloid; diagnostic and prognostic significance. J Bone Joint Surg 59A:658–664, 1977.

129a. Miller, C.W. Survival and ambulation following hip fracture. J Bone Joint Surg 60A:930–934, 1978.

130. Moore, A.T. Fracture of the hip joint; treatment by extra-articular fixation with adjustable nails. Surg Gynecol Obstet 64:420–436, 1937.

131. Moore, A.T. Metal hip joint: A new self-locking vitallium prosthesis. South Med J 45:1015–1018, 1952.

131a. Moreland, J.R. Primary total hip arthroplasty. In: Chapman, M.W., ed. Operative Orthopaedics. Philadelphia, J.B. Lippincott, 1988.

132. Morwessel, R.; Evarts, C.M. The use of quadratus femoris muscle pedicle bone graft for the treatment of displaced femoral neck fractures. Orthopedics 8:972–976, 1985.

132a. Niemann, K.M.W.; Mankin, H. Fractures about the hip in an institutionalized patient population. II. Survival and ability to walk again. J Bone Joint Surg 50A:1327–1340, 1968.

133. Ort, P.J.; Lamont, J. Treatment of femoral neck fractures with a sliding hip screw and two Knowles pins. Clin Orthop 190:158–162, 1984.

134. Pankovich, A.M. Primary internal fixation of femoral neck fractures. Arch Surg 110:20–26, 1975.

135. Pauwels, F. Biomechanics of the Normal and Diseased Hip. New York, Springer-Verlag, 1976, p. 83.

136. Phemister, D.B. Fractures of neck of femur, dislocations of hip, and obscure vascular disturbances producing aseptic necrosis of head of femur. Surg Gynecol Obstet 59:415–440, 1934.

136a. Phillips, T.W. Thompson hemiarthroplasty and acetabular erosion. J Bone Joint Surg 71A:913–917, 1989.

137. Pini, M.; Spadini, E.; Carluccio, L.; et al. Dextran/aspirin versus heparin/dihydroergotamine in preventing thrombosis after hip fractures. J Bone Joint Surg 67B:305–309, 1985.

138. Protzman, R.F.; Burkhalter, W.E. Femoral-neck fractures in young adults. J Bone Joint Surg 58A:689–695, 1976.

139. Pugh, W.L. A self-adjusting nail-plate for fractures about the hip joint. J Bone Joint Surg 37A:1085–1093, 1955.

139a. Raine, G.E. A comparison of internal fixation and prosthetic replacement for recent displaced subcapital fractures of the neck of the femur. Injury 5:25, 1973.

140. Rashiq, S.; Logan, R.F.A. Role of drugs in fractures of the femoral neck. Br Med J 292:861–863, 1986.

140a. Ray, W.A.; Griffin, M.R.; Downey, W. Benzodiazepines of long and short elimination half-life and the risk of hip fracture. JAMA 262:3303–3307, 1989.

141. Reikeras, O.; Hoiseth, A. Femoral neck angles in osteoarthritis of the hip. Acta Orthop Scand 53:781–784, 1982.

142. Reikeras, O.; Bjerkreim, I.; Kolbenstvedt, A. Anteversion of the acetabulum and femoral neck in normals and in patients with osteoarthritis of the hip. Acta Orthop Scand 54:18–23, 1983.

143. Reikeras, O.; Hoiseth, A.; Reigstad, A.; Fonstein, E. Femoral neck angles; a specimen study with special regard to bilateral differences. Acta Orthop Scand 53:775–779, 1982.

143a. Riska, E.B. Prosthetic replacement in the treatment of subcapital fractures of the femur. Acta Orthop Scand 42:281, 1971.

144. Robbins, J.A.; Donaldson, L.J. Analyzing stages of care in hospital stay for fractured neck of femur. Lancet 239:1028–1029, 1984.

145. Roberts, S.; Weightman, B.; Urban, J.; Chappell, D. Mechanical and biochemical properties of human articular cartilage from the femoral head after subcapital fracture. J Bone Joint Surg 68B:418–422, 1986.

146. Rodriguez, J.; Herrara, A.; Canales, V.; Serrano, S. Epidemiologic factors, morbidity and mortality after femoral neck fractures in the elderly—a comparative study: Internal fixation vs. hemiarthroplasty. Acta Orthop Belgica 53:472–479, 1987.

146a. Salvati, E.A.; Artz, T.; Aglietti, P.; Asnis, S.E. Endoprostheses in the treatment of femoral neck fractures. Orthop Clin North Am 5:757, 1977.

147. Scales, J.T. Prosthetic replacement of the femoral head for femoral neck fractures; which design? J Bone Joint Surg 65B:530–531, 1983.

148. Senn, N. The treatment of fractures of the neck of the femur by immediate reduction and permanent fixation. JAMA 13:150, 1889.

149. Sevitt, S. Avascular necrosis and revascularization of the femoral head after intracapsular fractures; a combined arteriographic and histological necropsy study. J Bone Joint Surg 46B:270–296, 1964.

150. Sevitt, S.; Thompson, R.G. The distribution and anastomoses of arteries supplying the head and neck of the femur. J Bone Joint Surg 47B:560–573, 1965.

151. Sherk, H.H.; Snape, W.J.; Loprette, F.L. Internal fixation versus nontreatment of hip fractures in senile patients. Clin Orthop 141:196–198, 1979,

152. Sikorski, J.M.; Barrington, R. Internal fixation versus hemiarthroplasty for the displaced subcapital fracture of the femur; a prospective randomized study. J Bone Joint Surg 63B:357–361, 1981.

153. Sim, F.H.; Sigmond, E.R. Acute fractures of the femoral neck, managed by total hip replacement. Orthopedics 9:35–38, 1986.

154. Sim, F.H.; Stauffer, R.N. Management of hip fractures by total hip arthroplasty. Clin Orthop 152:191–197, 1980.

155. Singh, M.; Nagrath, A.R.; Maini, P.S. Changes in trabecular pattern of the upper end of the femur as an index of osteoporosis. J Bone Joint Surg 52A:457–467, 1970.

156. Sloan, J.; Holloway, G. Fractured neck of the femur: The cause of the fall? Injury 113:230–232, 1982.

157. Smith, L.D. Hip fractures; the role of muscle contraction or intrinsic forces in the causation of fractures of the femoral neck. J Bone Joint Surg 35A:367–383, 1953.

157a. Smith, T.K. Prevention of complications in orthopedic surgery secondary to nutritional depletion. Clin Orthop 222:91–97, 1987.

158. Smith-Petersen, M.N. Treatment of fractures of the neck of the femur by internal fixation. Surg Gynecol Obstet 64:287–295, 1937.

159. Smith-Petersen, M.N.; Cave, E.F.; Vangorder, G.W. Intracapsular fractures of the neck of the femur—treatment by internal fixation. Arch Surg 23:715–759, 1931.

160. Smyth, E.H.J.; Shah, V.M. The significance of good reduction and fixation in displaced subcapital fractures of the femur. Injury 5:197–209, 1974.

161. Soreide, O.; Molster, A.; Raugstad, S. Internal fixation versus primary prosthetic replacement in acute femoral neck fractures: A prospective, randomized clinical study, Br J Surg 66:56–60, 1979.

162. Soto-Hall, R.; Johnson, L.H.; Johnson, R.A. Variations in the intra-articular pressure of the hip joint in injury and disease: A probable factor in avascular necrosis. J Bone Joint Surg 46A:509–516, 1964.

163. Speed, D. The unsolved fracture. Surg Gynecol Obstet 60:341–351, 1935.

164. Stableforth, P.G. Supplement feeds and nitrogen and calorie balance following femoral neck fracture. Br J Surg 73:651–655, 1986.

165. Staeheli, J.W.; Frassica, F.J.; Sim, F.H. Prosthetic replacement of the femoral head for fracture of the femoral neck in patients who have Parkinson's disease. J Bone Joint Surg 70A:565–568, 1988.

166. Stillwell, W.T. The Art of Total Hip Arthroplasty. Orlando, FL, Grune and Stratton, 1987.

166a. Stromqvist, B. Femoral head vitality after intracapsular hip fracture; 490 cases studied by intravital tetracycline labeling and tc-mdp radionuclide imaging. Acta Orthop Scand 54(suppl 200):5–71, 1983.

167. Stromqvist, B.; Hansson, L.I. Avascular necrosis associated with nailing of femoral neck fracture—two cases examined pre and postoperatively by tetracycline and radionuclide tracer techniques. Acta Orthop Scand 54:687–694, 1983.

168. Stromqvist, B.; Hansson, L.I.; Ljung, P.; et al. Pre-operative and postoperative scintimetry after femoral neck fracture. J Bone Joint Surg 66B:49–54, 1984.

168a. Stromqvist, B.; Hansson, L.I.; Nilsson, L.T.; Thorngren, K.G. Hook-pin fixation in femoral neck fractures. A two-year follow-up study of 300 cases. Clin Orthop 218:58–62, 1987.

169. Stromqvist, B.; Hansson, L.T.; Palmer, J.; et al. Scintimetric evaluation of nailed femoral neck fractures with special reference to type of osteosynthesis. Acta Orthop Scand 54:340–347, 1983.

170. Stromqvist, B.; Kelly, I.; Lidgren, L. Treatment of hip fractures in rheumatoid arthritis. Clin Orthop 28:75–78, 1988.

171. Stromqvist, B.; Nilsson, L.T.; Egund, N.; et al. Intracapsular pressures in undisplaced fractures of the femoral neck. J Bone Joint Surg 70B:192–194, 1988.

172. Swiontkowski, M.F. Ipsilateral femoral shaft and hip fractures. Orthop Clin North Am 18:73–84, 1987.

173. Swiontkowski, M.F.; Hansen, S.T. The Deyerle device for fixation of femoral neck fractures; a review of one hundred twenty-five consecutive cases. Clin Orthop 206:248–252, 1986.

174. Swiontkowski, M.F.; Hansen, S.T.; Kellam, J. Ipsilateral fractures of the femoral neck and shaft; a treatment protocol. J Bone Joint Surg 66A:260–268, 1984.

175. Swiontkowski, M.F.; Harrington, R.N.; Keller, T.S.; Van Patten, P.K. Torsion and bending analysis of internal fixation techniques for femoral neck fractures: The role of implant design and bone density. J Orthop Res 5:433–444, 1987.

176. Swiontkowski, M.F.; Tepic, S.; Perren, S.M.; et al. Laser Doppler flowmetry for bone blood flow measurement: Correlation with microsphere estimates and evaluation of the effect of intracapsular pressure on femoral head blood flow. J Orthop Res 4:362–371, 1986.

177. Swiontkowski, M.F.; Tepic, S.; Rahn, B.A.; Perren, S.M. The effect of femoral neck fracture on femoral head blood flow. Orthop Trans 11:344–345, 1987.

178. Swiontkowski, M.F.; Winquist, R.A. Displaced hip fractures in children and adolescents. J Trauma 26:384–388, 1986.

179. Swiontkowski, M.F.; Winquist, R.A.; Hansen, S.T. Fractures of the femoral neck in patients between the ages of twelve and forty-nine years. J Bone Joint Surg 66A:837–846, 1984.

180. Taine, W.H.; Armour, P.C. Primary total hip replacement for displaced subcapital fractures of the femur. J Bone Joint Surg 67B:214–217, 1985.

181. Thompson, F.R. Two and a half years' experience with a vitallium intramedullary hip prosthesis. J Bone Joint Surg 36A:489–502, 1954.

182. Tooke, S.M.; Favero, K.J. Femoral neck fractures in skeletally mature patients, fifty years old or less. J Bone Joint Surg 67A:1255–1260, 1985.

183. Tountas, A.A.; Wadell, J.P. Stress fractures of the femoral neck; a report of seven cases. Clin Orthop 210:160–165, 1986.

184. Trueta, J. The normal vascular anatomy of the human femoral head during growth. J Bone Joint Surg 39B:358–393, 1957.

185. Trueta, J.; Harrison, M.H.M. The normal vascular anatomy of the femoral head in adult man. J Bone Joint Surg 35B:442–461, 1953.

186. Tucker, F.R. Arterial supply to the femoral head and its clinical importance. J Bone Joint Surg 31B:82–93, 1949.

186a. Versluysen, M. Pressure sores in elderly patients. The epidemiology related to hip operations. J Bone Joint Surg 67B:10–13, 1985.

187. Walmsley, M.B. A note on the retinacula of Weitbrecht. J Anat 51:61–64, 1917.

188. Walters, R.; Simon, S. Joint destruction: A sequel of unrecognized pin penetration in patients with slipped capital femoral epiphysis. In: 1980 Proceedings of the Hip Society. St. Louis, C.V. Mosby, 1980.

189. Weintraub, S.; Papo, J.; Ashkenazi, R.; et al. Osteoarthritis of the hip and fractures of the proximal end of the femur. Acta Orthop Scand 53:261–264, 1982.

189a. White, B.L.; Fisher, W.D.; Laurin, C.A. Rate of mortality for elderly patients after fracture of the hip in the 1980s. J Bone Joint Surg 69A:1335–1340, 1987.

190. Whitman, R. A new method of treatment for fracture of the neck of the femur, together with remarks on coxa vara. Ann Surg 36:746–761, 1902.

191. Whitman, R. The abduction method; considered as the exponent of a treatment for all forms of fracture at the hip in accord with surgical principles. Am J Surg 21:335–344, 1933.

192. Williams, P.L.; Amin, N.K.; Young, A. Unsuspected fractures of the femoral neck in patients with chronic hip pain due to rheumatoid arthritis. Br Med J 292:1125–1126, 1986.

193. Wilton, T.J.; Hosking, D.J.; Pawley, E.; et al. Osteomalacia and femoral neck fractures in the elderly patient. J Bone Joint Surg 69B:388–390, 1987.

193a. Winter, W.G. Nonoperative treatment of proximal femoral fractures in the demented nonambulatory patient. Clin Orthop 218:97–103, 1987.

194. Wingstrand, H.; Stromqvist, B.; Egund, N.; et al. Hemarthrosis in undisplaced cervical fractures; tamponade may cause reversible femoral head ischemia. Acta Orthop Scand 57:305–308, 1986.

194a. Wrighton, L.D.; Woodyard, J.E. Prosthetic replacement for subcapital fractures of the femur: a comparative study. Injury 2:287, 1971.

195. Zetterberg, C.; Elmerson, S.; Andersson, G.B.J. Epidemiology of hip fractures in Goteborg, Sweden, 1940–1983. Clin Orthop 191:43–52, 1984.

196. Zetterberg, C.H.; Irstram, L.; Andersson, G.B. Femoral neck fractures in young adults. Acta Orthop Scand 53:427–435, 1982.

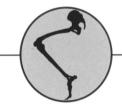

Roger N. Levy, M.D.
James D. Capozzi, M.D.
Michael A. Mont, M.D.

44

Intertrochanteric Hip Fractures

The intertrochanteric area of the hip is defined as that region adjacent to the distal femoral neck proximally and the distal edge of the lesser trochanter distally. This chapter reviews fractures in this area, including the relatively proximal basicervical fracture and the intertrochanteric fracture with distal subtrochanteric extension. (Fig. 44–1).

In an intertrochanteric hip fracture, not only is bone continuity disrupted, but there is also a disturbance of a delicate homeostasis involving physical health, mental vigor, emotional well-being, and balance with the environment. The treatment of hip fractures must address all these issues.

The specific surgical treatment of intertrochanteric fractures requires stable fixation of the fracture with an appropriate device. The stability of the fracture-implant assembly depends on five factors: the quality of the bone, the fracture pattern, the reduction achieved, the design of the implant selected, and the position of the implant in the bone. Each of these will be reviewed in detail in this chapter. The surgeon can influence only the last three but must diagnose the first two factors and plan treatment accordingly.

Incidence

The incidence of intertrochanteric fractures appears to be increasing. Particularly the more unstable, comminuted fracture types are increasing, paralleling increased longevity in the world's population. Postural and gait disturbances of old age cause these individuals to fall more frequently. Their diminished bone mass predisposes to the multiple fragment patterns characteristic of the unstable intertrochanteric fracture (Fig. 44–2).

Data can be derived from studies performed in the United States, England, and the Scandinavian nations.[44,47,56,102,105–107,115,167,173] Areas of agreement include the increasing incidence of intertrochanteric fracture, especially the more unstable types. These occur at a rate of 16.6 per 100 person-years in women with a bone density of 0.6 g/cm³ or less and rarely occur with a bone density of 1.0 g/cm³ or more. This relationship of osteopenia to age is not related to sex or, as popularly supposed, to the menopause. Most fractures occur with moderate trauma at home, but hospitalized patients had 11 times the frequency of fracture of age-matched controls living at home.[63,64,116,127]

Relevant Anatomy

The hip is a ball-and-socket joint comprising the acetabulum and the head of the femur. Linking the femoral head to the shaft of the femur is the femoral neck. The angle that the femoral neck subtends with the long axis of the femur is the angle of inclination. In the adult population, this angle is usually between 125° and 135°. Noble et al.'s recent anthropometric studies have shown a gradual decrease in the neck-shaft angle with age; the average angle is just under 125° (Fig. 44–3).[123]

In addition to its angle in the frontal plane relative to the vertical axis, the femoral neck is slightly anteverted or forward facing in relation to the position of the femo-

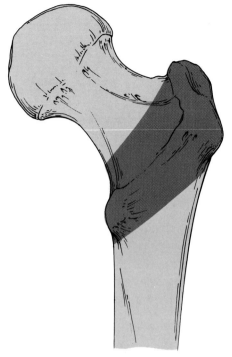

Figure 44–1

Intertrochanteric fracture zone. The major portion of an intertrochanteric fracture lies within this region. Extension into the proximal intracapsular region is rare. However, comminution frequently involves the area just distal to the trochanters, especially medially, with no sharp distinction between intertrochanteric and subtrochanteric fractures.

ral condyles in the horizontal or transverse plane. In adults, femoral anteversion averages about 15°, decreased from approximately 30° during infancy.

Supporting the femoral head and neck is an internal scaffolding system of trabecular bone. This internal trabecular system was originally described by Ward in 1838.[174] Fanning out under the superior dome of the femoral head and concentrating at the medial femoral neck are the primary compressive trabeculae. Arching from the area of the fovea to the lateral femoral cortex just distal to the greater trochanter is the primary tensile group. Secondary compressive and tensile trabecular groups, as well as a greater trochanteric group, are oriented along stress lines in the lateral femoral neck, with a relative paucity of trabecular scaffolding in the central area known as Ward's Triangle.[54]

It is the presence or absence of these primary and secondary trabecular groups that Singh et al. and Obrant have used as an index of osteopenia.[125,152] In addition to fracture stability and surgical technique, the degree of osteopenia affects the ultimate success or failure of fracture fixation. Singh et al. graded femoral neck cancellous bone quality from I to VI. Grade VI is normal bone with all five trabecular groups present, and grade I is severe osteopenia with evident loss of a portion of the primary compressive group (Fig. 44–4).

Laros and Moore have determined that a Singh index of grade III or less is associated with increased complications of fracture fixation.[99] Anteroposterior hip radiographs demonstrating a break in the continuity of the principal tensile trabeculae (Singh grade III)

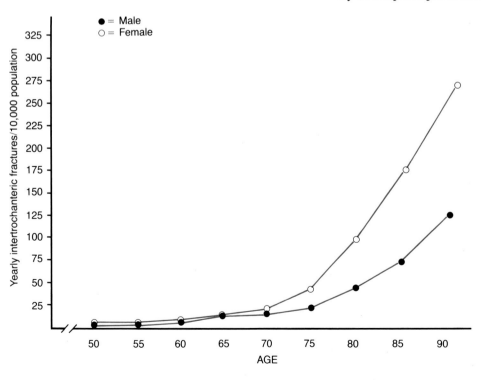

Figure 44–2

Frequency of intertrochanteric fractures increases with age, especially for women. The increase is due almost entirely to low-energy injuries in osteopenic patients.

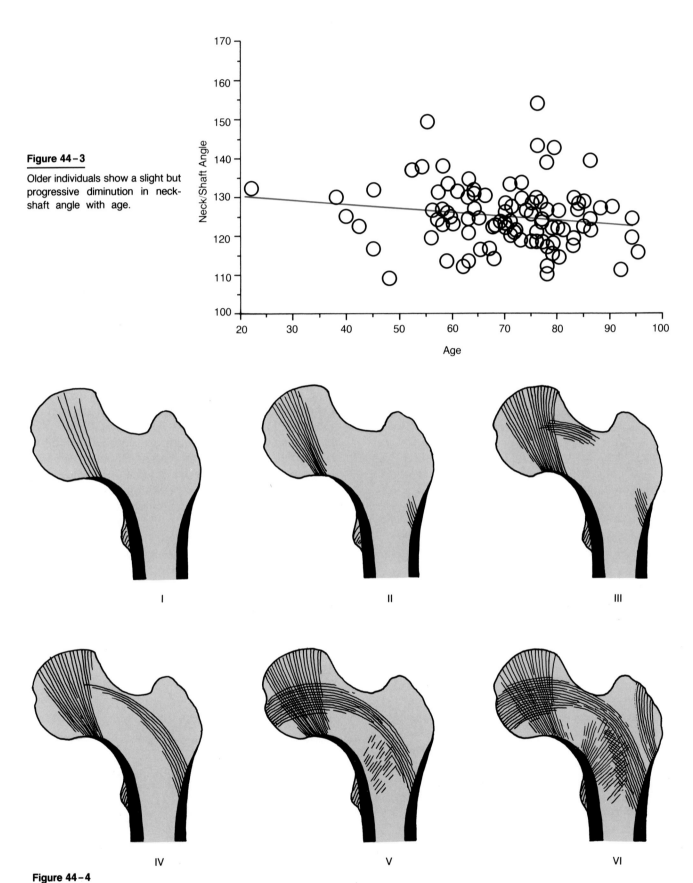

Figure 44–3

Older individuals show a slight but progressive diminution in neck-shaft angle with age.

I

II

III

IV

V

VI

Figure 44–4

Singh classification of osteopenia of proximal femur. Grades I through III represent clinically significant osteopenia. Grade I: only primary compression trabeculae are present, and they are reduced in volume. Grade II: primary tension trabeculae are absent. Grade III: interruption of primary tension trabeculae in the greater trochanteric region. Grade IV: loss of secondary compression and tension trabeculae. Grade V: loss of trabecular bone in Ward's triangle. Grade VI: all secondary and primary trabecular groups are present including the region of Ward's triangle.

indicate significant osteopenia that will affect fracture stability. In fact, Laros and Moore found the complication rate of osteopenic patients with stable hip fractures to be equal to that of patients with unstable fracture patterns in normal bone. Unfortunately, the reproducibility and reliability of Singh's classification is limited, and it is often hard to classify a given clinical radiograph. Needless to say, the highest complication rates are found in patients with osteopenic bone and unstable fracture patterns.[2,40] Zain-Elabdien et al. noted a continuous decrease in bone quantity with age and a direct relationship between bone quality and the severity of intertrochanteric fracture patterns.[180] They suggest that with the increasing age of the population and the longer survival of the aged, more unstable, comminuted intertrochanteric fractures will be seen.

In addition to the reduction of proximal femoral strength associated with reduced bone mass, bone microstructure may also play a role.[117,135] Ferris et al. examined undecalcified bone specimens from proximal femoral fracture sites under polarized light microscopy.[45] They found changes in the nature of the bone at the fracture site when compared with control specimens. Larger hydroxyapatite crystals and altered molecular orientation of the bone matrix proteoglycans were noted in the fracture group.[35,96,97,104,168]

Mechanism of Injury

Although a small percentage of intertrochanteric hip fractures occur with high-energy injuries such as motor vehicle and motorcycle accidents, the vast majority of these fractures are associated with a simple fall. The patient usually describes a fall with direct trauma to the hip or may report a twisting activity immediately followed by a fall. In addition to the direct forces acting on the hip to produce the intertrochanteric fracture pattern, indirect muscle forces also contribute.[88] The iliopsoas muscle pulls on its insertion at the lesser trochanter, and the abductors and short rotator muscles act through their attachments on the greater trochanter. The magnitude of force applied, the direction of force, and the degree of osteoporosis all contribute to the variations in fracture pattern that may be encountered.[30]

Anatomic and Functional Consequences of Intertrochanteric Fractures

For ambulatory patients, intertrochanteric fractures are severely disabling injuries. They are painful and render the patient unable to walk or even to transfer from bed to chair. Thus disabled, the bed-bound patient is at risk of complications such as pneumonia, pressure sores, venous thrombosis and its sequellae, gastrointestinal disturbances, urinary infections, and dementia. Although relatively normal anatomy may be preserved in occasional undisplaced intertrochanteric fractures, more commonly a varus deformity occurs along with shortening and external rotation of the leg below the fracture. Untreated fractures usually heal in this position, if the patient survives the two to three months required for healing. A patient who is sufficiently fit and agile may then resume walking, with a limp, with or without external support, and usually without much pain.

Whether a patient will be able to resume ambulation after an intertrochanteric fracture is significantly related to a number of factors other than fracture healing. The importance of mental and emotional status, previous functional level, social situation, and nutrition, as well as chronologic age, has been well documented.[18,26,119]

Need for assistance is common and may be temporary or permanent. Outpatient rehabilitation in the home environment may be optimally successful for some patients,[133a] but limited family and home resources may preclude such a program. In various studies, 25% to 75% of patients have been discharged directly home from hospital, but whether at home, in a rehabilitation unit, or a chronic care facility, the patient who has sustained an intertrochanteric fracture exhibits a greater reliance on social welfare systems. Intertrochanteric fractures affect a more biologically aged group of patients than do femoral neck fractures. In poorer health and having an increased dependence on assistance with self-care and other activities of daily living, these patients place a large and increasing demand on our health care system.

Commonly Associated Injuries

Most elderly patients with low-energy intertrochanteric femur fractures do not have other injuries. However, their fracture is rarely an isolated event because of the frequency of preexisting and acute medical problems, compounded by the systemic effects of the injury. When the injury is the result of a high-energy mechanism, the possibility of one or more potentially occult associated injuries is the same as for any trauma patient. Occasionally, the intertrochanteric fracture itself can be occult. Barquet and others have reported that 15% of such injuries associated with ipsilateral femoral shaft fractures were missed during initial assessment of the patient.[6,7,49]

Hemodynamic challenges may be posed by bleeding into the fracture site or by dehydration. The trochanteric area of the femur is well-perfused cancellous bone. Its disruption may result in the loss of two to three units of blood into the fracture hematoma. Dehydration and secondary fluid shifts as a result of immobility and pressure are not uncommon in solitary elderly individuals who sustain a hip fracture and lie helpless for many hours before being discovered. The resulting hemoconcentration may overwhelm the limited reserves of a geriatric patient.

Associated fractures do occur in 7% to 15% of older patients with intertrochanteric fractures. Commonly affected bones include those most susceptible to osteopenia: the distal radius, proximal humerus, ribs, pubis, and spine. These injuries may be missed if not carefully sought after during initial evaluation in the emergency department.

Fifty percent of geriatric patients with hip fractures suffer from cardiopulmonary problems, senility and other neurologic problems, deafness, blindness, or a combination of any of these, all of which may be directly associated with the injury. These deserve a full medical evaluation. McClure and Goldsborough found contralateral intracerebral lesions in 20% of patients with hip fractures.[114] They hypothesized that these brain lesions produce a neurologic deficit that causes a fall resulting in a contralateral hip fracture.

Classification of Intertrochanteric Fractures

Considerable attention will be devoted in this chapter to radiographic classification based on anatomic fracture patterns. We can introduce here the observation that the fracture pattern, as a result of its inherent stability or instability, has a direct predictive effect on the surgeon's ability to achieve a stable fracture reduction. Secondary displacement of the fracture fragments after fixation is also related to the type of reduction achieved (i.e., the location and extent of persistent fracture gaps larger than 4 mm). Comminution increases the likelihood of such gaps.

A classification system must be practical, clinically relevant, and well enough accepted to provide a common language.[12,13] As part of the preparation for this chapter, we queried 25 American orthopedic surgeons with a documented interest in the treatment of hip fractures. Of those who replied, almost all agreed that a critical determinant in the care of patients with intertrochanteric fractures was a classification of the fracture as stable or unstable.

Two factors are important in determining stability of intertrochanteric fractures. These are (1) the likelihood of achieving accurate reduction of fracture fragments prior to fixation and (2) the likelihood of loss of reduction after fixation. However, it must be kept in mind that other critical factors come into play. Although the relative accuracy of the Singh index in evaluating mechanical bone strength and structural properties of the hip bone has been questioned, it remains a useful guide for planning treatment. Interruption of the primary (superolateral) tension trabeculae on an anteroposterior radiograph of the proximal femur signifies osteopenia of Singh grade III or worse. This degree of osteopenia is clinically relevant and significantly increases intertrochanteric fracture instability.[99] The type and technique of fixation are also important. Frank fixation failures, manifested by implant breakage, protrusion into the hip, or loss of purchase on the femoral shaft, are much less frequent with modern sliding hip fixation devices. Instability is usually manifested by controlled and inconsequential collapse of the fracture site with maintenance of overall alignment and only slight shortening. Nonetheless, fractures that are, by pattern, unstable are more at risk of failure and demand the surgeon's awareness.

Evans offered a classification system based on the presence or absence of displacement and the number of fragments (Fig. 44–5).[42,43] Evans also included the reverse oblique fracture as a special category. Although the significance of the reverse oblique fracture pattern is often overlooked, it does require our attention. This precarious pattern often has disastrous results following fixation. This appears to be particularly true if the reverse oblique fracture is combined with significant osteopenia. Reverse oblique intertrochanteric fractures are intrinsically unstable with sliding hip screws or nails (Fig. 44–6).

Jensen reviewed 234 patients treated by contemporary methods and applied five different classification systems retrospectively.[77-79] He utilized the fracture reduction initially achieved and the possibility of later loss of reduction as measures to evaluate the validity and reliability of various classifications.

The modified Evans system, based on associated fractures of the lesser trochanter, the greater trochanter, or both trochanters and utilizing a five-part system, proved to be significantly the most informative in Jensen's review (Fig. 44–7).

Type I and II fractures could be anatomically reduced (no fracture gap greater than 4 mm in either plane) in 94% of patients and were followed by loss of position of 9% of patients. These were stable fractures; the remaining types III, IV, and V were unstable. Type III (greater trochanter detached) fractures could be anatomically reduced in 33% of all patients, and 55% of

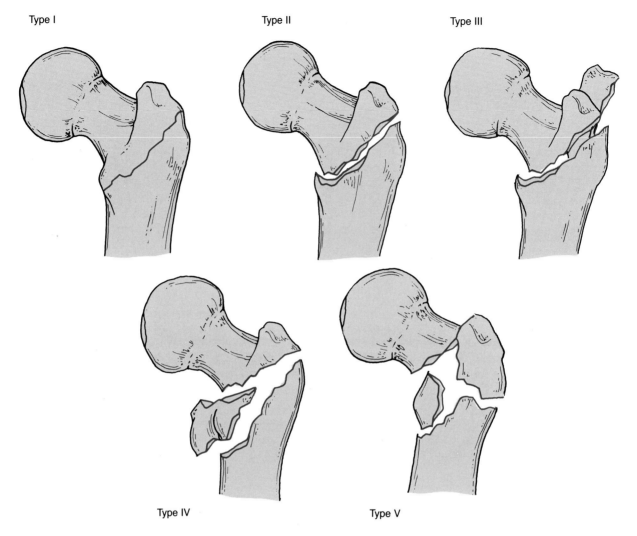

Type I   Type II   Type III

Type IV   Type V

Figure 44-5

Evans classification of intertrochanteric fractures. The primary fracture line runs between the lesser and greater trochanters. Increasing comminution, involving the greater and/or lesser trochanteric region, increases instability and thus the fracture grade. A *small* lesser trochanteric fragment is conventionally ignored. Type I: undisplaced two-part fracture. Type II: displaced two-part fracture. Type III: displaced three-part fracture with posterolateral comminution. Type IV: displaced three-part fracture with large posteromedial comminuted fragment. Type V: displaced four-part fracture, with comminution involving both trochanters.

all type II fractures lost some position after fixation. The problem was largely a result of the inability to reduce the fracture anatomically in the lateral plane (Fig. 44-8). Type IV (lesser trochanter detached) fractures could be anatomically reduced in only 21% of all patients, with displacement occurring in 61%. The problem primarily resulted from an inability to completely close the medial diastasis (Fig. 44-9). Type V fractures (greater and lesser trochanter detached) could be reduced in only 8% of patients and tended to displace later in 78% of these very comminuted fractures. These four-part comminuted fractures are even more difficult to reduce anatomically and often have persistent fracture gaps in both planes.

In all categories of fracture classifications, secondary

displacement may lead to increased impaction of fragments as an internal fixation device telescopes and may also be associated with technical failure (Fig. 44-10).

Jensen also assessed four other classification systems. The next most predictive system was one that only divided fractures into nondisplaced or displaced fractures. However, such a system lacks the sensitivity to add enough information to aid either the patient or surgeon. The Tronzo classification, the Ender classification, and assessment of instability by use of medial comminution alone do not add any additional information to that gained from observing displaced versus nondisplaced fractures.[39,66]

The predictive ability of the modified Evans system justifies its use for classifying intertrochanteric frac-

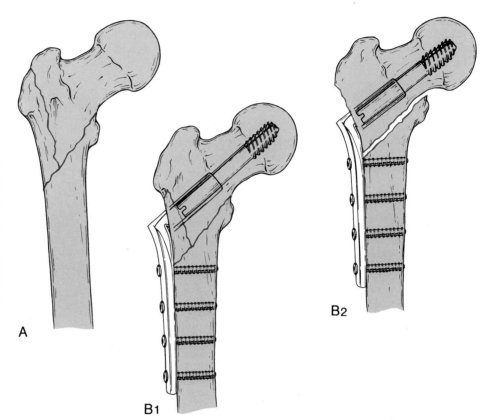

Figure 44–6

A, Reverse oblique intertrochanteric fracture. Lateral comminution is common. *B*, Telescoping of the sliding hip screw does not promote interfragmentary compression because of the orientation of the fracture plane. Stability requires secure impaction of the fracture, with either osteotomy of the distal piece to provide mechanical engagement or an implant that resists progressive medial displacement of the shaft.

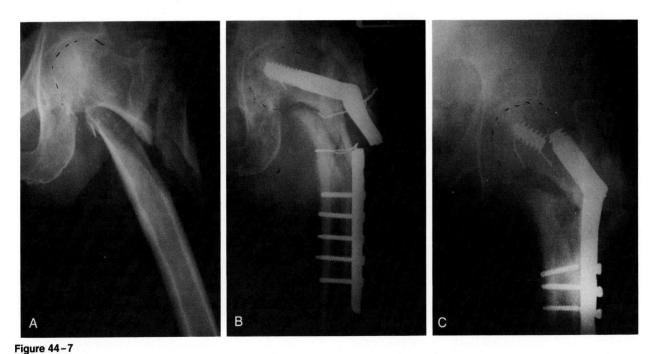

Figure 44–7

A, Reverse oblique intertrochanteric fracture in an elderly woman. *B*, Medial displalcement, nonunion, and fixation failure after complete telescoping of sliding hip screw. *C*, Several months after revision with a similar sliding hip screw, medial displacement and nonunion persist, and fixation has failed again.

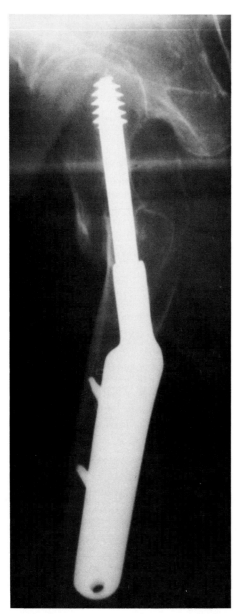

Figure 44-8

Evans-Jensen type III (greater trochanteric comminution) intertrochanteric fracture with typical unsatisfactory reduction demonstrated by a lateral radiograph.

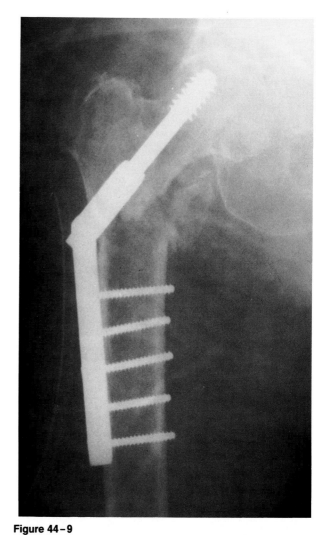

Figure 44-9

Evans-Jensen type IV intertrochanteric fracture (greater and lesser, four-part trochanteric comminution) with inadequate reduction (and malpositioned lag screw in superolateral femoral head).

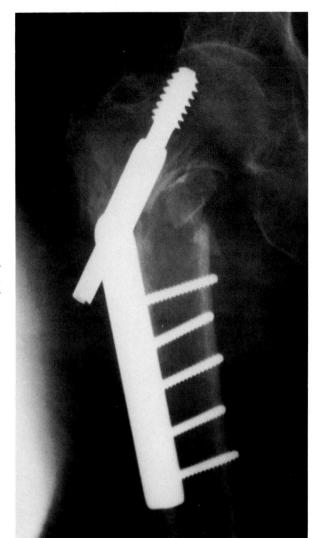

Figure 44–10

Technical failure of sliding screw fixation for unstable intertrochanteric fracture, with absent medial buttress, varus collapse, loss of lag screw purchase in the femoral head, and likely nonunion.

I

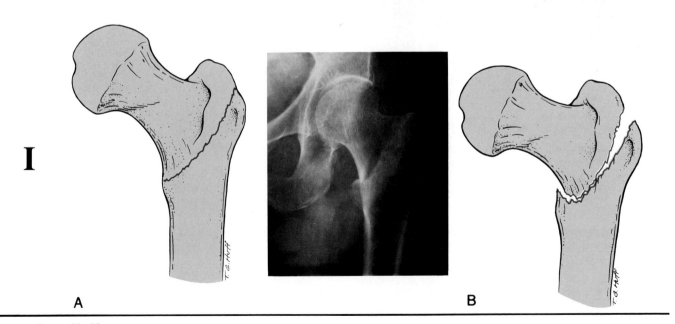

A   B

Figure 44–11

Simplified Evans-Jensen classification of intertrochanteric fractures. Type I (two-part) fractures may be undisplaced or in varus.

Illustration and legend continued on page 1452

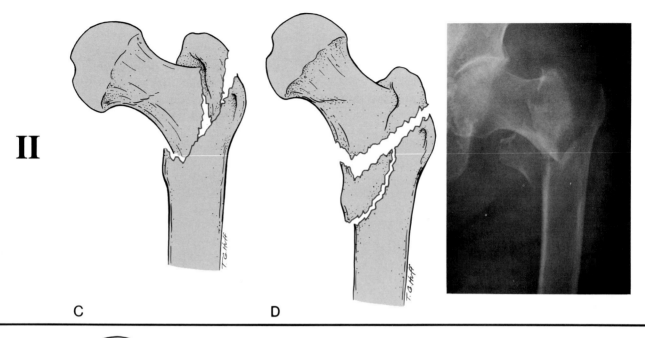

II

C   D

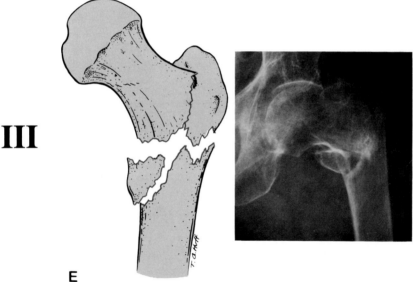

III

E

Figure 44–11 *Continued*

Type II (three-part) fractures may have comminution of either lesser or greater trochanteric regions. Type III (four-part) fractures have comminution of both trochanteric regions. Reduction problems and instability increase with fracture type.

tures. Review of Jensen's data reveals that this system essentially predicts the quality of reduction. Therefore one may also infer that the quality of reduction determines likelihood of secondary displacement. It is the reduced fragment position, rather than the fracture type itself, that is most predictive of secondary displacement.

As suggested by Jensen, the five types may be simplified to three based on likelihood of anatomic reduction:

type I nondisplaced and type I displaced (Evans types I and II) can usually be reduced anatomically in both planes (94%) and are therefore stable (Fig. 44–11A,B). Type II greater and type II lesser trochanter fractures (Evans types III and IV) can usually be reduced in only one plane and are therefore unstable (Fig. 44–11C,D). Type III fractures (Evans type V) are difficult to reduce in any plane and are therefore very unstable (Fig. 44–11E).

Diagnosis

HISTORY

The vast majority of patients with intertrochanteric hip fracture are elderly. Women outnumber men by a ratio of 2:1, and most patients report a fall at home involving only moderate trauma. A history regarding dizziness or a temporary loss of consciousness should be sought. Inability to bear weight on the affected extremity is present from the instant of injury. Preexisting pain may indicate a pathologic lesion or symptomatic arthritis. In addition, the patient should be queried for pain in other extremities or the axial skeleton, as fractures of the humeral head, distal radius, ipsilateral femoral shaft, knee, or ankle can occur concurrently with hip fractures.

Perhaps the most important part of the patient's history is the documentation of preexisting medical problems. These must be carefully determined and enumerated. Collaboration with the patient's primary physician and others, if appropriate, may be crucial for obtaining a complete history, including allergies and drug sensitivities, medications and dosage, and results of previous laboratory studies. The number of significant preexisting medical conditions is one of the most important factors relating to patient mortality following hip fracture surgery.

PHYSICAL EXAMINATION

The examination for the diagnosis of intertrochanteric hip fracture follows the classic components of physical examination. On inspection of the involved lower extremity, a relative shortening and external rotation will be noted, if the fracture is displaced. Depending on the period of time from injury, local ecchymosis from the fracture hematoma can be observed. This is usually found at the posterolateral aspect of the trochanteric area. Local skin conditions, as well as pressure point areas such as the sacrum, buttocks, and heels, should be inspected for evidence of breakdown. These areas can cause significant postoperative morbidity, dramatically increasing the patient's hospital course and length of stay.

On palpation, local tenderness should be noted over the trochanteric area but not over the femoral shaft or the pubis. Crepitus of mobile fracture fragments may be present to palpation on motion of the hip, which will be resisted because of obvious pain.

Percussion auscultation of the hip for the detection of fracture is a valuable test that is not widely appreciated. This method of evaluating fractures was first reported by Dr. Robert K. Lippmann of the Mount Sinai Hospital in New York and was taught as a standard part of examination for more than 25 years by Dr. Robert S. Siffert of the same institution. The examining physician should place the stethoscope over the prominence of the pubis and listen to the comparative transmission of sound as the examining percussion finger taps sharply over each patella. If a discontinuity of bone exists on one side, an obvious difference of tone and pitch will be apparent.[151]

RADIOGRAPHIC IMAGING

Standard anteroposterior (AP) and lateral radiographs remain the benchmark of intertrochanteric hip fracture imaging. In most cases, these films confirm the diagnosis of trochanteric hip fractures and also demonstrate the fracture pattern. The anteroposterior view is used to evaluate the fracture obliquity and location, the presence or absence of a medial buttress, and the quality of the patient's bone stock. To exclude a fracture and to evaluate the trabecular pattern of the proximal femur (on the uninjured side), this film should be taken with the leg internally rotated to obtain a true AP profile of the involved femur. The lateral view is most useful in determining the status of the posterior fracture fragments.

On occasion, intertrochanteric fractures may not be apparent on initial radiographs. If the patient's history and physical examination are consistent with a hip fracture but radiographs fail to confirm the diagnosis, then nuclear imaging is helpful in confirming the diagnosis.[68] In patients older than 65 years, approximately 80% of technetium bone scans are positive one day after fracture; 95% are positive in patients younger than 65 years. By three days after fracture, close to 100% of the scans are said to be positive. However, we have seen negative results in a significant number of bone scans in elderly patients even at five days following fracture, but if a fracture is present, these scans all become positive between the fifth and tenth day after injury. In patients in whom a hip fracture is strongly suspected despite initial negative radiographs, a technetium bone scan is obtained at 48 to 72 hours following injury. If the initial bone scan is negative and pain persists, the bone scan is repeated seven to ten days later.

Except for evaluating impending pathologic hip fractures, computed tomography (CT) scanning and magnetic resonance imaging (MRI) appear to have little value in routine intertrochanteric hip fractures. MRI may prove to be helpful in the nondisplaced, insufficiency hip fracture, but at present no studies have confirmed its usefulness. Likewise, CT scans may be used to delineate complex fracture patterns or the location of fracture fragments. It must be remembered, however, that the definitive diagnosis of intertrochanteric fractures is made at surgery. In evaluating the fracture pattern, there can be no substitute for intraoperative palpation of the fracture site, the femoral neck, the anterior and posterior buttresses, and the subtrochanteric region. A well-placed finger at surgery will provide more information regarding fracture anatomy than any imaging technique.

EVALUATION OF MEDICAL PROBLEMS

The initial evaluation of medical problems involves a thorough history and physical examination of the patient for associated injuries, illness, and prior medical conditions. A thorough workup also includes laboratory evaluation, with complete blood count (CBC) with differential, platelets, and full serum chemistries (SMA-6, SMA-12). Frontal and lateral chest radiographs should be obtained. A urinalysis (UA) should be obtained with culture and sensitivity if the patient is symptomatic. In patients with a history of pulmonary disorders or current respiratory symptoms, baseline arterial blood gases should be drawn prior to surgery. Table 44–1 provides a guide to the laboratory evaluation of the patient with a hip fracture. Any abnormal values should be identified, evaluated, and treated, if necessary, preoperatively. It should be noted that the guidelines suggested are not all-inclusive and must be individualized for each patient, doctor, and institution.

EVALUATION OF PREINJURY FUNCTION

It is important to determine the patient's level of function prior to hip fracture. Under the best circumstances, this level is the most the patient can expect to achieve on recovery, but there will more likely be some loss of preinjury-level functioning. The patient's social function prior to injury has great significance. Miller documented that the patient's preinjury social function (i.e., socioenvironmental level) not only determined the level achievable after surgery, but also had great impact on mortality rate after hip fracture surgery.[119] Recovery is also related to the number of close social contacts a patient has before hip fracture.[26] Patients who have a greater number of social supports tend to have a more complete recovery of their prefracture level of function. Additional indicators such as arm strength, mental status, ability to pull oneself to a sitting position, and serum albumin levels have all been shown to correlate with functional recovery following hip fractures.

Campion showed that preinjury functional impair-

Table 44–1.

Preoperative Tests for Patients with Hip Fractures

Complete Blood Cell Count
- Anemia (primary and secondary)
- Infection (white cell count)
- Malignancy (myelodysplasia, myeloma)
- Thrombocytopenia

Prothrombin Time; Partial Thromboplastin Time
- Bleeding disorders, including anticoagulant medications

Urinalysis
- Urinary tract infection (cells, bacteria)
- Other abnormalities (check pH, protein, hematuria, etc)
- follow-up with culture and sensitivities if necessary

Serum Chemistries (SMA-12, SMA-6, etc.)
- Hypo/hypernatremia, rule out dehydration
- Potassium; may need to be repeated and then rechecked
- Blood urea nitrogen and creatinine for dehydration, renal failure
- Glucose; rule out diabetes
- Calcium; rule out parathyroid disease, etc.
- Alkaline phosphatase; rule out Paget's disease,
Osteomalacia, metastatic disease, liver problems, etc.
- Liver function tests; rule out hepatitis, cirrhosis
- Creatinine phosphokinase; rule out myocardial infarction; may need to fractionate into myocardial and skeletal muscle fractions
- Drug levels, as indicated.

Chest Radiograph
- Pneumonia
- Congestive heart failure
- Tumor; may choose to evaluate postoperatively to work up at later time

Electrocardiogram
- Ischemia
- Arrhythmias
- Electrolyte effects
- Drug effects (i.e., digitalis)

ments in elderly patients with trochanteric hip fractures are common.[18] Before their hip fractures, his patients had problems with community ambulation (49%), using a bath tub (40%), walking outdoors (26%), and stair climbing (18%). These preinjury functional impairments were reliable predictors of hospital stay. As previously emphasized, preexisting medical conditions are prime determinants of postfracture mortality.

EVALUATION FOR PATHOLOGIC FRACTURE

In evaluation for pathologic fracture, the history is of great importance. A prior history of malignancy, especially breast, lung, prostate, or bone marrow, raises the index of suspicion. However, the first presentation of a tumor may be a pathologic fracture. Conversely, not every fracture in a patient with cancer is a result of metastatic spread.

Pathologic fractures usually occur with only trivial trauma. Prior to fracture, pain at rest as well as with weight bearing may have been present at the hip. Every patient presenting with a hip fracture should be questioned about such symptoms.

Radiographic examination may demonstrate striking findings that make diagnosis obvious or may only reveal localized bone lysis or, occasionally, sclerosis.

In the presence of a so-called impending fracture, we have used the following 12-point scale to determine the need for prophylactic fixation:

Location = 3, hip; 2, lower extremity; 1, upper extremity.
Lesion = 3, lytic; 2, mixed lytic/blastic; 1, blastic.
Size = 3, $\frac{2}{3}$ shaft; 2, $>\frac{1}{3}$; 1, $<\frac{1}{3}$.
Pain = 3, narcotics required; 2, nonnarcotic analgesics required; 1, no pain-relieving drugs required.

Patients with a score of nine or more are highly likely to experience fracture and should have the benefit of prophylactic treatment. Prophylactic fixation usually provides a better prognosis than treatment after fracture.

Fracture treatment usually consists of debulking the tumor tissue, followed by internal fixation with a sliding hip screw assembly augmented with bone cement. If the lesion has extended into the femoral neck and head, hip replacement may be indicated. If the femoral diaphysis is involved, a long stem component is required. A bipolar prosthesis will suffice, unless acetabular involvement is present. Proximal femoral replacement components are best avoided except by highly experienced tumor or reconstructive surgeons. This procedure is palliative, not curative, and there is an unacceptably high incidence of dislocation with the use of segmental replacements.

The goal of surgery for pathologic fractures is to permit immediate weight bearing and improve the quality of remaining life. Postoperative radiotherapy should be utilized to prevent tumor recurrence in the entire operative field. The presence of metal and cement does not interfere with the radiation effect, and radiation does not mechanically weaken the implant-cement system.

Management of Intertrochanteric Fractures

Intertrochanteric hip fractures are serious injuries. Extensive blood loss frequently occurs in older, more debilitated patients who often have other medical problems. These fractures may initiate a patient's demise, both medically and psychologically. Therefore the goal of treatment should be early mobilization of the patient, with a prompt return of that patient to his or her prefracture level of functioning. This goal is rarely, if ever, achieved through nonoperative methods. Closed treatment of intertrochanteric hip fractures has been associated with high mortality rates. Horowitz reported a 35% mortality rate, though Murray and Parrish reported only a 10% rate within the first year in patients treated nonoperatively.[70,122]

Hornby et al.'s prospective trial of skeletal traction vs. sliding hip screw fixation demonstrated low complications with both treatments. Mortality at six months, pain, leg swelling, and nonhealed pressure sores occurred at similar rates following both procedures. The demonstrated advantages of surgical fixation were its shorter hospitalization, its better restoration of normal anatomy, and its better preservation of the ability to live independently when compared with traction.[69b]

Closed treatment methods should be the rare exception in treating intertrochanteric fractures. Indications for closed treatment methods include patients in whom the risks of surgical intervention outweigh the benefits of early fixation, the nonambulatory patient with minimal pain from the fracture, or the end-stage terminally ill patient who can be nursed satisfactorily without fracture fixation. In general, such patients are not maintained in traction unless the goal is healing with nearly anatomic alignment. Instead, these patients are mobilized in bed or in a bed and chair as soon as this can be done without excessive discomfort.

Closed fracture treatment thus falls into one of two categories: stabilization of the fracture in an attempt to achieve near anatomic union or early mobilization with no attempt at preserving normal anatomy. The first approach has been attempted by a variety of methods, but skeletal traction with x-ray monitoring has withstood the test of time. In the second method of treatment, the patient is mobilized from bed to chair. Most such patients will never walk. Initial pain is controlled as needed with analgesics. Transfers and ambulation begin as soon as the patient's fracture and medical conditions permit. For any given patient, the potential medical complications of nonoperative treatment and the loss of independence it may entail, combined with the potential for significant malunion, must be weighed against the risks of surgery.

Open treatment of an intertrochanteric fracture is the treatment of choice for most patients. Historically, straight nails, screw bolts, fixed nail plates, intramedullary devices, and osteotomies have all been advocated to reduce and maintain these fractures. In the early 1970s, sliding nail and screw devices were introduced. Their purpose was to maintain alignment of the fracture while still permitting it to impact into a stable configuration. These devices are strong enough to control bending and rotation in almost all situations and have sufficient fatigue life to last until the intertrochanteric fracture is healed. Fracture fixation depends on the durability of a composite made from the fixation device and bone. With modern sliding hip screws, the patient's bone, rather than the metallic implant, is the "weak link" in the system. Its well-documented clinical success has made sliding screw fixation the preferred implant for almost all intertrochanteric fractures.

NONOPERATIVE TREATMENT

Most reports have shown an increased mortality in patients treated without operative stabilization. Early operation ensures optimum rehabilitation and purportedly decreases the risk of pulmonary complications, urinary tract infections, deep venous thromboses, and decubiti. However, as mentioned, there are certain relative indications for nonoperative treatment of intertrochanteric fractures. These indications include the nonambulatory demented patient with little evidence of pain, a patient with an old fracture, a terminally ill patient, or a patient with unstable medical problems.[150,178] Lyons and Nevins believe that if the patient is nonambulatory or has little chance to walk again, then a nonsurgical treatment regimen in the nursing home is safer, more humane, and less expensive than hospitalization with surgical treatment.[108] Many regimens for nonoperative treatment have been advocated, including early mobilization, Buck's traction, spica cast immobilization, and skeletal traction through the distal femur or proximal tibia.

In patients who are nonoperative treatment candidates with a potential for ambulation, we commonly utilize skeletal traction through a proximal tibial Steinmann pin. Approximately 15% of body weight is used to maintain traction on the hip. The leg is placed in balanced suspension with minimal abduction. The traction maintains alignment and prevents varus angulation or shortening with external rotation. Serial roentgenograms are obtained to check position. Traction is maintained for 8 to 12 weeks, at which time

mobilization to partial weight bearing is allowed until full union occurs. Special low-pressure or air suspension beds may be used to prevent skin breakdown and decubitus ulcer formation. An aggressive physical therapy program for the bed-bound patient can aid in maximizing recovery. Once the intertrochanteric fracture has consolidated, this can include assisted hip and knee motion.

SPECIAL CONSIDERATIONS FOR POLYTRAUMA PATIENTS

Young adults with hip fractures are often the victims of high-energy trauma resulting from motor vehicle collisions and falls of more than 15 feet.[17] It has already been mentioned that hip fractures may be missed in the multiply injured patient. Polytrauma patients should generally have immediate stabilization of all long-bone fractures. Several studies have stressed the advantage of early fixation of all fractures, as it lessens morbidity and mortality. This allows early mobilization and decreases the risk of pulmonary complications, thromboembolic phenomena, and decubitus ulcers and the necessity for imported nutrition. Fat embolism syndrome has been found to be almost nonexistent in patients with multiple trauma who were operatively stabilized within 12 hours of injury.

When the hip has been fractured along with other long bones in the same or contralateral lower extremity, priority should be given to fixation of the hip fracture. Once the hip is stabilized, early nursing care is far easier and usually requires a lower dosage of narcotic analgesics.

Ipsilateral femoral shaft and intertrochanteric hip fractures occur less frequently than do concomitant shaft and femoral neck fractures.[163] Wellin et al., in a recent review of associated hip and femoral shaft fractures, found that rigid fixation of both fractures allows early mobilization, facilitates nursing care, and permits rapid rehabilitation.[175] The choice of fixation for ipsilateral hip and shaft fractures depends on the fracture patterns, as well as on patient considerations and the surgeon's expertise.

If the hip and shaft fractures are within close proximity of each other, a sliding hip screw with a long side plate may suffice. This is by far the simplest and most effective means of stabilizing closely related fractures. As the distance between the intertrochanteric fracture and shaft fracture increases, fixation techniques become more complicated and success rates more variable. Multiple stacked pins (Ender pins) usually require supplementary cerclage wiring. These pins usually improve fracture alignment but offer insufficient stability for unprotected early mobility. Locked intramedullary nails may be difficult to pass with intertrochanteric fractures. Reconstruction nails, with screws anchored in the femoral head and neck, may have a role but are not usually recommended in patients with greater trochanteric comminution. A separate compression plate, although biomechanically not ideal, may provide the best solution for fixation of a femoral shaft fracture significantly distal to an intertrochanteric fracture.

Fractures involving the supracondylar region can frequently be treated as two separate fractures. The intertrochanteric hip fracture is fixed with a sliding hip screw. The distal fracture can then be treated with a blade plate, screws, Ender pins, or Zickle supracondylar nails. Distal intramedullary pins can often be inserted past the proximal side plate with little difficulty.

OPEN TREATMENT

The goal of surgical treatment of an intertrochanteric hip fracture is to obtain a stable reduction of the fracture fragments and internally fix them with a well-placed, mechanically strong implant. Ideally, the result of surgical intervention should be secure enough to permit early or immediate protected weight bearing. This immediate protected return to ambulation is critical to the functional recovery of the aged and very aged patients who form a large proportion of this fracture population. Additionally, early weight bearing may stimulate bone healing and helps retard the progression of disuse osteoporosis.

Because of the frequency of intertrochanteric fractures, the health care needs of our society will be best served by treatment methods that are simple, reproducible, and characterized by minimal technical complications. It would indeed be desirable if these objectives could be routinely achieved. Unfortunately, some of the most challenging problems of fracture fixation occur in this population of often sick, frail individuals. Consequently, despite the most diligent preoperative planning and attention to surgical detail, an undesirable outcome, including failure of fixation or death of the patient, can occur.

Kaufer et al. were among the first to point out that the strength of the composite of fracture fragments plus fixation implants depends on five factors: bone quality, fracture pattern, fracture reduction, implant design, and implant placement.[87]

Bone quality and fracture pattern are predetermined for a given patient. The surgeon can influence the reduction of the fracture and the choice and placement of the implants. However, even the best conceived and executed internal fixation may be insufficient to compensate for highly comminuted, osteopenic bone. In some patients, bone stock may be augmented with methylmethacrylate bone cement to improve fixation. In others, prosthetic replacement of the proximal femur may need to be considered.[52,153]

Fracture Reduction

The following sections review specific methods for operative treatment of intertrochanteric fractures, focusing on fracture reduction, implant design and selection, and implant insertion. Modern techniques for managing intertrochanteric fractures offer a high percentage of successful results.

Fracture reduction remains in some dispute but is of paramount importance to the successful treatment of intertrochanteric hip fractures.[73,75] No internal fixation device, regardless of how clever the design, will improve the result of a poorly reduced fracture. It is true that the reasonably reliable sliding characteristics of most present-generation tube-plate-screw designs allow for progressive impaction of fracture surfaces.[34] This encourages closure of gaps between fragments that remained at surgery or developed secondary to bone resorption at the fracture site, as the hip and fracture are progressively mechanically loaded in the postoperation period. This is not to be confused with converting a poor reduction into a good one. The choices available to the surgeon are either to attempt to reduce the fragments in an anatomic position or to select a nonanatomic position with which to achieve a goal of improved fracture stability.

Stable Fractures

Anatomic reduction of the fracture fragments can usually be achieved, or may even be present, with an obvious stable position in type I undisplaced and type I displaced stable intertrochanteric fractures.[15,36] Care should be exercised, however, to avoid overreducing these stable fractures into unstable positions (see next section). These fracture patterns, with little if any comminution, permit relatively easy fixation of the fracture fragments in a manner that reproduces the original prefracture anatomy. In fact, type I fractures are inherently stable enough that they respond well to a variety of well-executed fixation techniques. Kyle et al., Levy and co-workers, and Steinberg and co-workers all obtained similar superior results in stable fracture patterns with different surgical techniques.[95,103,158] MacEachern and Heyse-Moore did note that postoperative impaction occurred in approximately one fourth of these injuries.[109] However, the small amount of displacement that may occur after adequate fixation of stable intertrochanteric fractures is rarely of any consequence to the patient.[69]

Unstable Fractures

A more difficult treatment choice exists in dealing with the unstable intertrochanteric fractures: type II (greater trochanteric), type II (lesser trochanteric), and type III. A considerable amount of clinical and some laboratory data exist to aid in decision making, but some conflicting conclusions are evident. One alternative that can be selected is so-called "anatomic" reduction of the unstable fracture, recognizing that the posteromedial lesser trochanter fragment and the lateral greater trochanter fragment may not actually be anatomically reduced. The likelihood of gaps greater than 4 mm between fragments is the basis for classification into stable (I), unstable (II), and very unstable (III) fracture patterns. The anatomic alternative assumes that the addition of the rigid internal fixation device will sufficiently augment the relative stability of the fracture reduction and that the sliding mechanism of the lag screw in the tube plate will allow for a progressive controlled impaction of the irregular fracture surfaces as muscle forces and body weight mechanically load the hip joint in the postoperative period. Clinical support for this method exists in various reports, such as those of Clawson,[23] Kyle,[93] Heyse-Moore et al.,[66] and Rao et al.[134] Laboratory support from the work of Chang and co-workers found that anatomic reduction of a four-part fracture model prepared from cadaver bone consistently provided higher compression forces across the medial calcar bone area and lower tensile stresses on the sliding hip screw compared with reduction by medial displacement osteotomy.[20] These mechanical advantages were present even if the posteromedial lesser trochanter fragment was not anatomically reduced. Its fixation in a relatively appropriate position, however, did contribute to the stability of the montage. In applying Chang's laboratory data to clinical situations, it is important to remember that comminuted intertrochanteric fractures can seldom be reduced so that every fragment is anatomically repositioned. In the 162 unstable fractures treated by "anatomic reduction" and compression screw fixation reported by Rao and co-workers, only 2% retained the anatomic reduction.[134] Ninety percent were reported to have moved to a medial displacement position and 8% to a lateral displacement position. The clinical success rate was still high. Anatomic reduction requires further definition, especially in stable fracture patterns in older patients. Most surgeons are accustomed to regarding 135° as the most common angle for neck-shaft angle at the hip. In a pivotal anthropometric study, Noble and associates found that the femoral neck-shaft angle gradually decreased with increasing age. In 325 hips, the average neck-shaft angle was just under 125°.[123] Several alternatives to the so-called anatomic reduction are also worthy of mention and will next be considered. A number have been proposed as means of reducing rates of hardware failure and loss of fixation. These were much more common with earlier trochanteric fracture fixation devices, particularly various side plate attachments for Smith-Petersen nails and one-piece nail-plate appliances such as Jewett's, even in its reinforced design.[57] Knowledge of these techniques may help the surgeon solve a particular fracture problem, but it should be remembered that their development preceded that of the sliding hip screw. In general, results using this implant and an anatomic reduction are at least as good as those achieved with other approaches to reduction and fixation.

High-Angle Fixation. High-angle fixation may be performed with an anatomic reduction, but screw placement is made easier if the neck and femoral shaft are repositioned in a valgus reduction.[140,141] To achieve a position of postoperative stability, the use of a high-angle tube plate assembly (i.e., 150°) has been advocated. The increased tube-plate angle encourages sliding of the hip screw in the tube and thereby allows postoperative impaction of fracture surfaces. The higher angle also decreases bending stress on the tube plate assembly.

Medial Displacement Osteotomy. Medial displacement osteotomy has been advocated to convert the pathologic anatomy of the unstable fracture into a stable but nonanatomic position.[1,14,101,124,139,145] Dimon and Hughston reported improved results with Jewett nail fixation of unstable intertrochanteric fractures by displacing the distal shaft fragment medially and inserting the medial spike of the major proximal fragment into the medullary canal of the distal fragment.[31,32] This technique is illustrated below. If the fragments are firmly impacted proximal into distal, then a stable position can be obtained from a previously unstable fracture pattern. To the extent that the proximal fragment is impacted into the distal, femoral shortening will occur. This can be at least partially counteracted by a valgus positioning of the proximal fragment. However, such a valgus alignment at the hip may adversely affect the function and appearance of the knee. In spite of its reduction in the rate of fixation failure after Jewett nailing,[84] medial displacement osteotomy has found limited acceptance in the current treatment of intertrochanteric fractures because of its technical difficulties, poorer functional results, and greater alteration of normal anatomy when compared with sliding hip screw fixation. Roberts et al.[139] found higher rates of shortening and external rotation deformity, as well as impaired gait. Other clinical reviews confirm that medial displacement osteotomy is of no

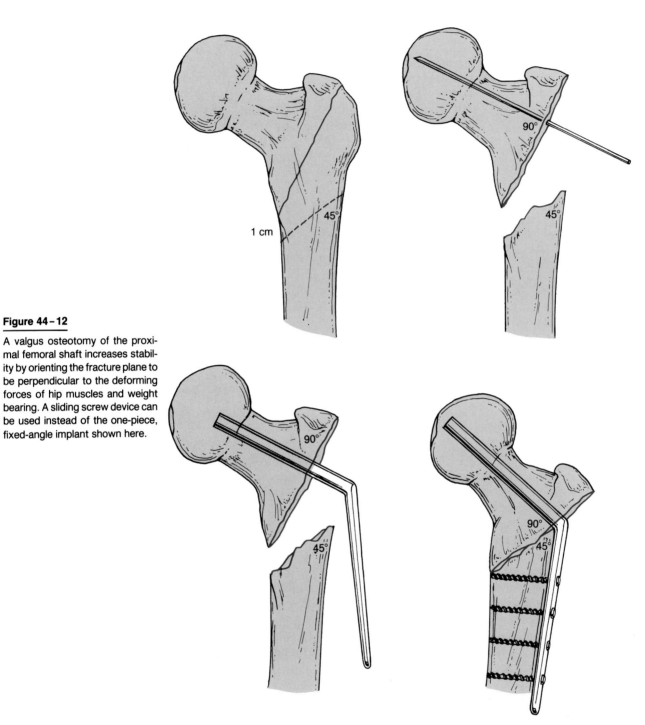

Figure 44–12

A valgus osteotomy of the proximal femoral shaft increases stability by orienting the fracture plane to be perpendicular to the deforming forces of hip muscles and weight bearing. A sliding screw device can be used instead of the one-piece, fixed-angle implant shown here.

value unless a stable reduction is actually achieved in the process.

Valgus Osteotomy. Sarmiento recommended removing a wedge of bone, with the base lateral and apex medial, so that the plane of the fracture is made more transverse to improve stability. He initially reported good results, but these have rarely been reproduced elsewhere.[142] Possible problems include excessive valgus of the proximal fragment causing a subjective perception of instability at the hip, excessive shortening, and external rotation deformity of the limb (Fig. 44–12).[71]

Implant Choice and Placement

A variety of contemporary hip fracture fixation devices are available for selection by the surgeon (Fig. 44–13).[113] These can be divided into four categories: (1)

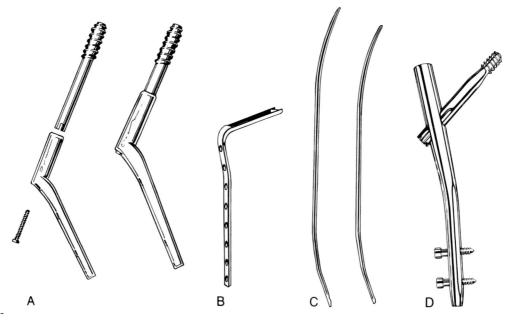

Figure 44–13

Examples of implants currently used for treatment of intertrochanteric fractures. *A*, Sliding hip screw, with separate screw for compression. *B*, Fixed-angle blade plate; the 95° angle shown might be used for a reverse-oblique intertrochanteric fracture. A 95° condylar compression screw could be used instead and may be easier to insert. *C*, Condylocephalic nails, represented by those of Ender. *D*, Cephalomedullary implants similar to the gamma nail, which has recently been introduced.

tube-plate-screw (or nail) designs, (2) fixed nail or blade plate designs, (3) condylocephalic sliding ("telescoping," "compression") plate and screw (or nail) devices, and (4) cephalomedullary implants such as the Zickle nail or the newer gamma nail, with distal interlocking screws. Prosthetic replacement, an alternative to fracture fixation, is ordinarily restricted to treatment of severely comminuted fractures in elderly or osteopenic patients.[41,62,165]

Tube plate designs provide a much stronger margin of safety for withstanding the bending stresses encountered after surgery than do previous one- or two-part nail plate designs. Thus fatigue fracture of the tube plate is a rarity. By decreasing the bending moment, a high-angle device is also more secure. For example, the Arbeitsgemeinschaft für Osteosynthesefragen/Association for the Study of Internal Fixation (AO/ASIF) dynamic hip screw was found to have a safety factor 3.6 times that of an angled blade plate for the 150° angle and 1.5 times for the 135° angle. No matter which implant is chosen, external walking support is advisable during the postoperative period to provide the greatest possible margin of safety against fatigue failure.

Postoperative impaction may be necessary to maintain contact of fracture surfaces. Thus the sliding characteristics of the lag screw within the side plate must be considered. Higher angles enhance sliding of the screw

in the tube. Conversely, with angles less than 135°, sliding and fracture impaction deteriorate significantly. Sliding of the screw within its tube is also impeded by inadequate engagement of the screw shaft in the tube. Insufficient overlap allows the screw to toggle within the barrel and jam, or gall, against it so that sliding friction is markedly increased. This effect is less with higher tube plate angles but should always be considered when choosing and evaluating the lengths of lag screw and side plate barrel during insertion of a sliding hip fixation device.[95]

Many of the newer designs utilize new stainless steel formulations that offer increased yield strength, greater corrosion resistance, and improved fatigue life over the same design fabricated in 316L stainless steel. New designs made of titanium may also offer advantages related to greater fatigue life and corrosion resistance and perhaps to lower modulus. Mizrahi studied biomechanical parameters of gait in patients treated with a variety of compression screw devices and found no significant difference among them.[119a]

Ample clinical experience has shown that fatigue failure of the tube-plate portion of a sliding hip implant is quite rare. With a significant delay to union or significant repetitive loading, failure of the fixation composite is, of course, inevitable. This most often occurs with loss of screw fixation, either in the head-neck fragment, as discussed later, or by loss of purchase of the screws affixing the side plate to the shaft of the femur. A fairly unusual mode of failure is fracture of the hip lag screw shaft.

Occasionally, failure of hip screw-implants occurs because of spontaneous postoperative disassembly of the device, with the lag screw shaft disengaging from the side plate barrel. This only occurs when the compressing screw was not used or was removed after use to avoid excessive lateral prominence of the implant, which may be painful or rarely may produce a pressure sore. When the compressing screw is omitted, there is no mechanical block to disassembly other than tissue tension across the fracture site. To prevent implant disassembly with associated loss of fracture reduction, it is important to ensure that there is ample engagement of the screw shaft within the barrel of the implant and to leave the compressing screw in place in especially unstable situations or when neuromuscular problems might contribute to disassembly.

The most common fixation problem currently encountered is "cutout" of the device from the head fragment. Instability at the fracture site is necessary for this to occur. It is most commonly associated with poor positioning of the lag screw in the femur head, as well as with unstable reduction. Implant design features that can reduce the incidence of failure include an adequate sliding mechanism and the avoidance of excessively sharp knifelike edges on the hip screw threads. Several of the newer designs have used more rounded edges. Other methods to present a broader surface area in the femoral head include replacing the screw threads with an expansion bolt (ALTA hip fixation device, Howmedica, Inc.). Haig has incorporated the broad paddlelike surfaces of a tri-finned nail, instead of a screw, combined with a low-angle tube plate.[55] Haig reported that 237 hip fractures followed to healing after this method of fixation were without a single instance of nail cutout. Thus this represents a standard for other methods to be measured against.

Another method for increasing implant surface area and thus preventing cutout is the incorporation of polymethylmethacrylate (PMMA) bone cement as part of the fracture fixation montage. PMMA is typically confined to the proximal fragment but can be used in the distal portion as well. Both expansion bolt and the device developed by Haig have special ports to allow cement injection after the implant is placed into the femoral head. The use of bone cement in osteopenic, comminuted intertrochanteric fractures has been reported on positively by Harrington and by Bartucci et al., among others.[8,59]

Condylocephalic Fixation

Intramedullary devices possess a theoretical advantage in that by being closer to the neutral mechanical axis of the femur, they are subject to lower mechanical stresses than are laterally applied plates and screws.[4,21,25,28,80-82,130,131,136,138,165] Ender flexible pins rarely break, but complications relating to retrograde migration of the pins have been reported by Levy et al., Kuderna et al., and others.[19,91,103] Because the pins do not telescope, any postoperative impaction and shortening must be associated with either proximal penetration or distal backing out, which leads to problems with soft tissue impingement and knee pain. This explains why the best results with this method are obtained in stable intertrochanteric fractures, where little postsurgical impaction occurs. In addition, there is only a random relationship between the endosteal diameter of the femur proximal to the lesser trochanter (a limiting factor to the number of pins to be passed proximal) and the endosteal diameter of the diaphyseal isthmus; as a result, additional short pins may be required to better fill the diaphysis and thus stabilize the pins crossing the metaphysis. Jacobs et al. studied unstable hip fractures in cadaver femurs and noted that multiple Ender pins were modestly stronger than a single Harris condylocephalic nail for those fractures.[73] They noted compression hip screws to be three times stronger than the Harris nail, two and one-half times stronger then Ender pins, and five times more rigid than either of them. The Harris nail has proven less successful clinically than sliding hip screws. Some authors have reported excellent results with condylocephalic nails in all classes of fracture, and it may be that extensive experience with this technique does improve results.[24]

Prosthetic replacement has been advocated as a reasonable alternative to internal fixation of severely comminuted, markedly osteopenic, intertrochanteric fracture.[132,157] Green et al. report good results with cemented bipolar hip replacements, and similar results were reported by Stern and Angerman utilizing a Leinbach type prosthesis.[53,159] However, reattachment of the greater trochanter may pose a problem. In selecting a prosthetic component for this purpose, attention must be paid to assuring ample stem length for long-term component stability. The stem tip must extend beyond the most distal point of apparent stress concentration by an amount of least two to three times the diameter of the canal. If a much larger posteromedial fragment is deficient, an intermediate or long-stem component may be required.

Implant Placement

There is considerable agreement as to the optimal location of the proximal tip of an internal fixation device. Most surgeons agree that it should be in the firm cancellous bone of the subchondral portion of the head, which is usually within 10 mm of the articular cartilage. In patients with ample bone stock, this point may range to as much as 20 mm from the articular margin. Leaving the proximal tip of a device in the relatively empty area of Ward's triangle provides limited fixation in the proximal fragment and invites disaster. Placing the tip closer than 4 mm to the subchondral bone may lead to penetration of the head if the compression screw does not telescope at the same rate as fragment impaction occurs or if the intramedullary pins do not extrude from the distal medial femoral entry port.

A compression screw or nail should be placed in the central axis of the head and neck. Slight deviation posteriorly or inferiorly may be acceptable, but the central position offers the best fixation. Superior and anterior quadrant placement is much less desirable. An inherent problem is that fixation in the proximal fragment is intramedullary, and the lag screw gains purchase only in cancellous bone with cortical support. Multiple Ender pins should fan out in the femoral head to improve purchase.

Techniques for Operative Treatment

This section describes in detail the operative techniques recommended for treatment of intertrochanteric fractures. These include (1) sliding hip screw fixation with anatomic reduction, (2) medial displacement osteotomy, (3) use of bone cement to augment internal fixation, (4) condylocephalic (Ender) nail fixation, and (5) proximal femoral replacement. Their advantages and disadvantages and relative indications have been discussed previously and must be considered when choosing and performing each of the surgical procedures.

PREOPERATIVE PLANNING AND PREPARATION

The importance of preoperative planning and preparation prior to the commencement of surgery cannot be emphasized enough. These steps seem elementary but are often omitted, frequently to the detriment of the patient. They include (1) medical and anesthesia evaluations, (2) assessment of local soft tissue and concomitant skeletal injuries, (3) adequate preoperative radiographs, (4) determination of the availability of sufficient blood for transfusion, (5) determination of the availability of the desired implant, as well as alternative implants, and (6) assessment of the capacity for intraoperative imaging. Although the insertion of hip fixation screws is possible with portable x-ray machines, a C-arm image intensifier offers faster surgery and better

results. The achievable radiographic control is far superior with the image intensifier. The C arm allows for an accurate assessment of fracture reduction, guide pin position, and screw placement.

PATIENT POSITIONING

A fracture table is strongly recommended to aid with the fracture reduction, as well as for optimal fluoroscopic visualization. The appropriate anesthetic can be administered on the fracture table or in the bed in which the patient is transported to the operating room. The patient should be transferred from the bed to the table with as much assistance as possible and carefully placed in a supine position. The physician should ascertain the normal position of slight external rotation that characterizes the uninjured hip.

Secure attachment of the contralateral lower extremity to the table's foot piece is required if strong traction must be applied with a fracture table; otherwise the pelvis rotates. The normal leg must be positioned to avoid interference with the cross-table lateral fluoroscopic view, which is important for proper reduction and implant placement. This can be achieved with wide abduction of the unaffected leg or, less satisfactorily, with hyperextension of the normal hip and acceptance of an oblique approximation of a lateral view (Fig. 44–14). Many elderly patients have limited hip abduction, and this option is not available. Fortunately, most low-energy intertrochanteric fractures require little intraoperative traction, unless surgery is delayed and significant shortening has occurred. (This is a good argument for skeletal traction in such cases.) When traction

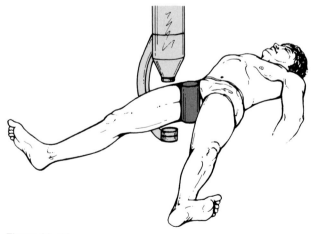

Figure 44–14

The patient is positioned on the fracture table with the uninjured leg widely abducted to allow clearance of the C-arm when it is positioned for a lateral radiograph. The image intensifier is shown in position for condylocephalic nailing. Flexion, abduction, and internal rotation of the uninjured limb can improve access for the fluoroscope.

is not required, the unaffected leg can almost always be flexed at the hip and knee to permit a highly satisfactory cross-table lateral radiograph. If strong traction should be needed with the patient in this position, the AO distractor can be applied across the fracture without requiring traction on the normal leg.

Both feet must be well padded. The foot of the affected side is securely attached to the traction foot piece, or traction is applied through a skeletal traction pin, if the pin remains securely in place. The unaffected limb is positioned and secured as chosen according to the preceding considerations. The perineal post and the sacral area should also be well padded. The patient's perineum, with genitals displaced in males, should rest against the padded perineal post. Many fracture tables provide improved access to the fractured hip by allowing a portion of the table under the involved hip to be shifted down or laterally toward the other side. This allows the buttock to sag and prevents a bulging of compressed tissue in the posterior aspect of the wound.

FRACTURE REDUCTION

Undisplaced fractures require no reduction maneuver. The patient is positioned on the fracture table with the unaffected leg flexed or abducted, and the injured limb supported in extension and slight abduction (5 to 10°), with minimal traction. Slight internal rotation to place the femoral neck horizontal will aid the procedure, as long as it does not result in fracture displacement. After positioning the patient and before scrubbing, the surgeon should supervise positioning the C-arm fluoroscope and ensure that adequate AP and lateral radiographs demonstrate an acceptable reduction. Whether C-arm image intensifier or two portable x-ray machines are used, it is essential to see clearly the outline of the femoral head and neck in both AP and lateral planes before proceeding.

Stable displaced fractures generally reduce well with firm traction (sufficient to prevent attempted passive knee flexion). No more than 10° of abduction should be utilized. The hip can be externally rotated to match the resting position of the uninjured limb or slightly internally rotated to a neutral position (patella points vertically). Posterior displacement of the distal fragment or apex posterior angulation may require correction with a crutch placed between limb and floor under the drapes. Alternatively, these deformities may be corrected manually after exposure of the fracture.

Unstable fractures may often be acceptably reduced with the preceding traction technique. Alternatively, valgus overcorrection and internal rotation may be attempted. Valgus overcorrection is performed by applying longitudinal traction to both limbs, greater on the

injured side, followed by release of traction on the uninjured leg. This allows the pelvis to rotate, increasing abduction of the injured hip. Significant internal rotation is defined as that required to internally rotate the femur so that the knee faces medially. To accomplish this, the foot must be rotated even more internally, because of laxity of ankle and knee ligaments.

If an adequate closed reduction cannot be achieved, it will be necessary to improve fracture alignment and fragment apposition once the wound is open. The need for appropriate instruments and assistance can be anticipated based on the radiographically observed results of closed manipulation.

Lateral Approach to the Proximal Femur

After appropriate skin preparation, the wound is surgically draped. The use of special transparent sterile plastic drapes suspended vertically from fracture table attachments or other suitable frames is a convenience.

A straight incision paralleling the shaft of the femur should begin proximally over the prominence of the greater trochanter and proceed distally for approximately 15 cm. The length should be adequate to allow insertion of the side plate to be used or for manipulation of comminuted fragments if required. The incision should continue through the subcutaneous tissue and the longitudinal thick fibers of the fascia lata. The tensor fascia femoris muscle, which may be incised in the proximal end of the wound, may be the site of a brisk bleeding vessel to be cauterized or tied at this point. The tensor muscle can be avoided by beginning the fascia lata incision distally and sufficiently posteriorly. The tensor is then palpated within the fascia between thumb and index finger, and the fascial incision is extended proximally posterior to the palpable muscle.

Beneath the fascia lata, a variably sized hematoma is usually present. Evacuate this with a slightly moistened laparotomy pad spread over a finger. By this method the posterior junction of the fascia lata and the vastus lateralis muscle will be visualized. Pull the vastus anteriorly with a retractor and select a line to incise its intrinsic fascia, splitting between the obvious fascial fibers, the white horizontal fascial fibers of the muscle itself. This is done with gentle scalpel strokes about 1 to 2 cm anterior to the linea aspera junction with the fascia lata. This incision goes through a thin part of the vastus muscle, avoiding the perforating vessels passing through the linea aspera attachments, and leaves adequate tissue to hold a suture at time of closure. Split the underlying muscle with two clamps inserted tip to tip down to the femur, and then spread apart longitudinally. Finish the deep dissection with an elevator, and then gently place lever retractors (e.g. the Hohmann, Bennett, or cobra retractors) over the anterior femur. If additional exposure is required, as in some comminuted fractures, release the nonmuscular vastus tendon aponeurotic origin from the vastus ridge on the greater trochanter by a transverse incision extending anteriorly from the proximal end of the incision in the vastus.

The surgeon who is gentle with exposure and retraction for fracture fixation is repaid with reduced complications of wound and fracture healing. Although adequate visualization is necessary for assessment, reduction, and fixation of the patient's fracture, nonessential trauma to soft tissue should be avoided. This includes crushing and tearing of soft tissues with overly vigorous blunt dissection, prolonged forceful retraction with self-retaining or manual retractors held long in position, as well as detachment of nourishing soft tissues from bone and indiscriminate use of the electrocautery.

Indirect reduction techniques using the fracture table or a bone distractor, supplemented with fluoroscopic control and guided by proper preoperative planning, will help to minimize the unavoidable trauma of fracture fixation procedures.

FRACTURE ASSESSMENT

Next, confirm the preoperative diagnostic assessment with visual and digital examination of the fracture site. The intertrochanteric line can be easily assessed by running a fingertip along the intertrochanteric line from greater to lesser trochanter. Is this main fragment aligned? Palpate medially for the lesser trochanter. Is it intact, displaced, or displaced with a major posteromedial fragment? Palpate posteriorly behind the greater trochanter. Is there a large displaced posterolateral fragment? Inspect the proximal shaft area for vertical extensions of the primary fracture.

If a stable reduction is present, proceed to guide pin insertion. If a suitable reduction is not present, the fracture can sometimes be improved by manipulation of the limb by an unscrubbed assistant. Consider the value of rotating the limb externally if a large posterior gap is present. Increased traction may possibly be required. Alternatively, if the fracture sags posteriorly, reduction can be improved by placing a broad elevator, a Bennett retractor, or a hip skid under the trochanter and lifting the fracture. Provisional fixation with one or more small Steinmann pines (e.g., extra guide pins) placed so as not to interfere with insertion of the fixation device will often aid reduction and fixation of difficult intertrochanteric fractures. If an acceptable open reduction cannot be achieved, then consideration must be given to medial displacement osteotomy, which will be addressed in a later section.

GUIDE PIN INSERTION

For a 135°-angle device, select an entry point about 2.0 cm below the vastus ridge. Three landmarks assist in locating this point: (1) it is directly opposite the lesser trochanter, (2) it is at the same level as the most proximal posterior osseous insertion of the gluteus maximus tendon, and (3) it is generally about two fingerbreadths below the vastus ridge. Add about 0.1 mm per degree for higher angle devices. Another rule-of-thumb is to move 20 mm distally if a 150° implant is to be used.

Make a drill hole in the lateral cortex from 4.8 to 6.5 mm ($\frac{3}{16}$ to $\frac{1}{4}$ in.) in diameter. First penetrate the cortex at 90°, and then redirect the drill to 45°. This entry hole should lie midway between anterior and posterior on the "equator" or midlateral line of the femoral shaft.

To assist in guide pin placement, first place a free guide pin along the anterior surface of the femoral neck paralleling the intended angle of the implant, and impact it gently with a mallet in the AP plane. It will offer a good visual guide to the anteversion of the proximal fragment (Fig. 44–15A,B).

Utilize the pin guide assembly for the specific implant to be used. Set the angle for the desired plate angle (i.e., 130°, 135°, 140°, 145°, 150°). Do not use a 130° implant unless required by a patient's abnormal varus anatomy. Politely request a moment of quiet, and gently hammer the guide pin into place until a change in resonance and in resistance signifies entry into firm subchondral bone. Check the pin position on both AP and lateral radiographs.

The guide pin is advanced under fluoroscopic control until it makes contact with the subchondral bone of the femoral head and its final position is once more confirmed as satisfactory. A truly central position on both AP and lateral views is optimal. Modest posterior and inferior positioning is acceptable. If the pin position is suitable, proceed to the next step. If the position is unsuitable, analyze what improvement is needed, and revise the pin position accordingly. Make certain that the real problem is not an unreduced fracture. Replacement of the hip lag screw after unsatisfactory positioning seriously compromises its purchase. One of the major advantages of the fluoroscopically guided hip screw system is that the position of the implant may be confirmed with the guide pin before any irreversible bone damage has occurred. Thus precise guide pin placement must be assured at this point before going any further with the procedure.

Radiographic imaging should allow great precision and avoidance of penetration, if the guide wire is placed in the middle of the femoral head and the central ray of the fluoroscope is perpendicular to the guide wire and femoral neck axis on both AP and Lateral views. Inser-

Figure 44–15

A, A guide pin is inserted by hand through the anterior hip capsule and is advanced along and in line with the femoral neck until it encounters the head of the femur. This serves as a radiographic marker for positioning the definitive guide wire on the AP view. *B*, Demonstration of the version of the femoral neck in this way is also a visual aid to orientation on the lateral view.

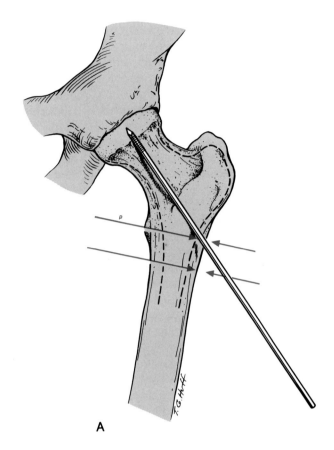

A

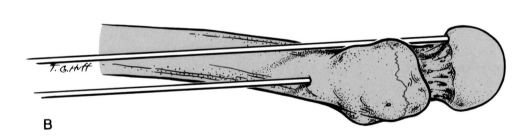

B

tion of the guide pin into the subchondral bone minimizes its risk of displacement during placement of the femoral head lag screw. It is important, however, not to penetrate the hip joint if liquid bone cement is to be used in the femoral head and to avoid fracturing a guide pin that is, for any reason, inserted across the hip joint.

An alternative to hammer insertion is advisable if the system's guide pin is thin and insufficiently rigid. Some systems use a guide pin that has a very sharp, self-tapping tip with a short, threaded segment at the end to be inserted. These are inserted with a power drill and may often be placed directly through an older patient's lateral femoral cortex without predrilling. Removal of such threaded-tip guide pins usually requires counterclockwise application of the drill. The guide pin can be inserted freehand, without use of an angle guide, but

such a guide often improves the ability to match the pin-shaft angle precisely to that of the chosen implant. This improves implant fit and avoids altering the alignment of a minimally displaced fracture.

Most contemporary systems provide for a direct reading of the intraosseous length of the guide pin with a special ruler. Another simple method is to place an identical pin alongside the protruding portion of the guide pin. Measure the amount of identical pin extending beyond the guide pin used. This is the length of pin in the bone.

LAG SCREW SELECTION

The length of the hip lag screw is estimated from the depth of the guide pin by subtraction of (1) the distance that the tip of the pin extends beyond the desired screw position and (2) the surgeon's estimate of the amount of excessive telescoping of the screw in the side plate that will produce lateral prominence of the screw shaft. Generally the hip screw should be inserted so it is 5 to 10 mm from the subchondral bone. If the bone is very firm and the fracture very stable, a distance of up to 20 mm from the subchondral bone may be acceptable, but it is important not to leave the screw tip within the sparse cancellous bone of Ward's triangle. Approaching closer than 5 mm to the subchondral bone probably leaves too little margin for error.

To obtain the lag screw length, measure the depth of the guide pin within the bone by subtraction using an identical pin positioned outside the cortex or by using an appropriate ruler. It is important to be familiar with the system being used, as some rulers have built-in correction factors. If the tip of the guide pin is positioned just inside the subchondral bone as previously advocated, subtract 5 to 10 mm to determine the desired screw tip position. From this figure, calculate the required screw length by subtracting any apparent fracture gap that will be closed by fixation and an estimate of any further telescoping that will occur postoperatively. However, ensure that an adequate amount of screw shaft remains within the barrel to facilitate sliding of the screw and postoperative fracture impaction. Rarely, if ever, should the end of the screw be more than 1 cm from the outside of the plate barrel. It is important to recognize that the screw length is an estimate that should be confirmed intraoperatively, the tip position with the image intensifier and the lateral end by direct inspection after the side plate is positioned and all traction has been released. Some sliding hip screw systems have optional shorter barrels or shorter screw threads to permit more telescoping before the screw threads abut against the barrel, converting the sliding device into a fixed one with increased risk of fatigue failure or joint penetration. Such an option ought to be considered at this time, but with the realization that a shorter barrel may decrease the ease with which the screw slides because of jamming of the shaft within the barrel, and a shorter screw thread length may possibly reduce its purchase in the femoral head.

Preparation of the Channel for the Lag Screw

Preparation of the channel for the lag screw should not be undertaken until the surgeon is completely satisfied with the position of the guide pin in the head-neck fragment. It may also be wise, if the reduction is satisfactory, to reconfirm by fluoroscopy the angle the guide wire makes with the lateral femoral cortex, as fixation with a device of a different angle will change the rela-

tionship of proximal to distal fragments. After this has been confirmed, the angle of the side plate may be chosen. The length of the side plate should be sufficient to ensure that a minimum of four screws are placed in intact bone distal to the fracture site.

Most contemporary hip screw systems use a so-called "triple reamer," which drills a hole in the femoral head for the lag screw, increases its diameter laterally for the barrel of the side plate, and chamfers the lateral femoral cortex to accommodate the barrel-plate junction. The triple reamer is adjusted by setting the length of the central drill so that is penetrates as deep as desired for final screw placement. This depth has previously been calculated in the first step of determining lag screw length. In very osteopenic patients, one may drill a few millimeters less than the desired depth and insert the screw into undrilled cancellous bone for improved purchase. It is important to realize that the triple reamer must accomplish three not necessarily related tasks and that its length adjustment is an estimate. Use

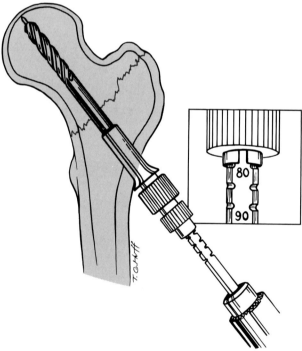

Figure 44-16

The compression screw triple reamer is adjusted appropriately, based on guide wire depth and fracture. See text. It is then advanced over the previously placed guide wire, under fluoroscopic and visual control, (1) to create a channel of appropriate (but not excessive) length for the lag screw; (2) to prepare a shorter, wider channel for the tube of the side plate; and (3) to bevel, or chamfer, the inferior edge of the hole in the lateral femoral cortex to improve apposition of the side plate to the bone. Intermittent fluoroscopy confirms the depth of the central reamer and provides reassurance that the guide wire has not become incarcerated in the drill, so that it is advanced as well.

fluoroscopy to ensure that the drill tip penetrates just to the chosen depth. Direct inspection laterally is required to ensure that the second and third stages of the reamer satisfactorily prepare the lateral femur. In very soft bone, it is possible to overream the lateral femoral cortex while concentrating on drilling far enough into the femoral head. Adjustment of the triple reamer may be required during this procedure (Fig. 44–16).

In physiologically younger patients with dense cancellous bone, it may be necessary to cut threads into the bone by tapping it prior to insertion of the lag screw. Most sliding hip screw sets provide a tap for this purpose. Like the triple reamer and the lag screw itself, the tap is inserted over the guide pin, which must remain in place until the lag screw is inserted far enough to follow the prepared channel without difficulty.

Tapping lag screw threads is unnecessary in osteopenic cancellous bone, as it decreases pull-out strength. If a threaded-tip guide pin is used and is inserted to the subchondral bone, it rarely displaces during the insertion of the lag screw. Should this occur, the pin must be carefully and concentrically reinserted. This can be done by nesting suitable instruments from the insertion set or by placing the shaft of the lag screw backward through the side plate and using this to guide the pin back into its track.

INSERTION OF LAG SCREW AND TUBE-PLATE

The surgeon should be familiar with the selected implant and its instrumentation in order to facilitate proper insertion of the device. A "trial run" with the system on a plastic bone model in a motor skills laboratory or an instructional course is an appropriate way to gain familiarity with a new hip fixation system.

Whereas some sliding screw devices permit free rotation of the screw shaft within the side plate barrel, others block this rotation with a noncircular cross section or occasionally an optional mechanical "key." If a locked (e.g., Synthes, "DHS") or lockable (e.g., Richards, "AMBI") device is chosen, the screw must be inserted so that its rotational alignment centers the side plate over the femoral shaft. This is usually accomplished by turning the T-handled wrench for the lag screw until its handle is parallel with the shaft of the femur when viewed from the side. This need for gaining rotational alignment of the lag screw appears to be the only "disadvantage" related to blocking rotation of the hip screw shaft within the barrel. It is possible that such systems provide better rotational control of the proximal fragment, even though the fragment may rotate around the screw itself. Nonlocked systems have been

shown to provide poor rotational control of fractures with subtrochanteric extension.

With the guide pin's position confirmed by fluoroscopy, the lag screw is inserted with care (Fig. 44–17). A palpating finger over the femoral neck ensures that the proximal fragment is not torqued excessively. If extreme resistance is met, tapping may be required. Fluoroscopy verifies proper insertion and ensures that the guide pin is not bent or advanced ahead of the screw. Once screw position is satisfactory, the guide pin is removed, but it should be replaced if the screw must be changed for any reason. The depth of the screw relative to the lateral cortex is confirmed, and the barrel is slid over the screw so that the plate is approximated to the lateral cortex of the femoral shaft.

Once the assembly is properly positioned, check to ensure that the screw shaft engages the barrel sufficiently. If a locking key is to be used, it should be placed now, prior to fixing the plate to the shaft. A perfectly apposed plate may be attached to the femoral shaft with cortical bone screws. Alignment may be improved by clamping the plate to the femoral shaft before attaching it with screws. At this point, all traction can usually be released and the distal femur slid proximally to gain optimal impaction of the fracture (Fig. 44–18A,B).

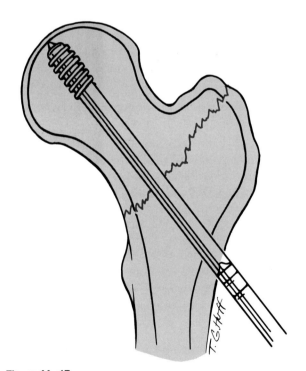

Figure 44–17

The lag screw is inserted to a depth of 5 to 10 mm from the subchondral bone and centrally in the femoral head on both AP and lateral radiographs. Proper guide wire placement is essential to this step. This must be confirmed first on both views. In dense bone, threads for the lag screw should preliminarily be tapped.

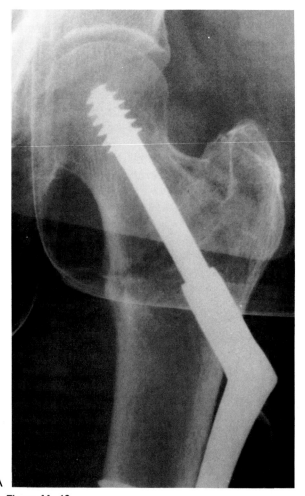

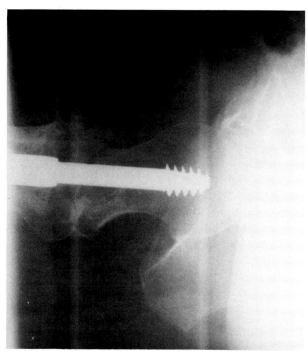

Figure 44–18

A, Anteroposterior and *B,* lateral radiographs of a satisfactorily inserted sliding hip screw in a two-part (type I) intertrochanteric fracture.

The implant acts as an aid to reduction, controlling alignment during this impaction process, which may occur in two ways. The first is by telescoping of the lag screw within the side plate barrel, which can be encouraged by using the separate compression screw that is inserted through the end of the barrel into the shaft of the lag screw (Fig. 44–19). Excessive tightening of this screw may pull the lag screw out of an osteopenic femoral head. The second type of fracture impaction is by relative proximal displacement of the femoral shaft along the plate. These two modes of impaction of the fracture site represent the completion of reduction maneuvers and should, if at all possible, gain stable impaction of the proximal against the distal fragment. If this cannot be achieved without excessive shortening, it must be recognized that the plate is acting in a buttress mode and is at high risk of failure unless fracture healing is rapid and adequate postoperative protection is provided. Such a situation should, if possible, be iden-

tified by preoperative planning so that treatment can be modified, as indicated, with bone grafting, a nontelescoping implant, a nonanatomic reduction, cement, or a prosthesis. Fixation of comminuted proximal femur fractures with subtrochanteric involvement is described in the next chapter.

The wound should be debrided of devitalized tissue and thoroughly irrigated. Closed suction drains are placed for 24 to 48 hours. The muscular, fascial, subcutaneous, and skin layers are separately closed. An elastic bandage spica dressing may protect the wound from a disoriented patient's exploring fingers, but we have not been very impressed with the value of this. Elastic stockings should be applied to the lower extremities and heel protection provided by placing pillows under the calves so that the heels do not touch the bed.

Extensively comminuted subtrochanteric extensions of intertrochanteric fractures can be great problems. It is our feeling that if the fracture is basically an

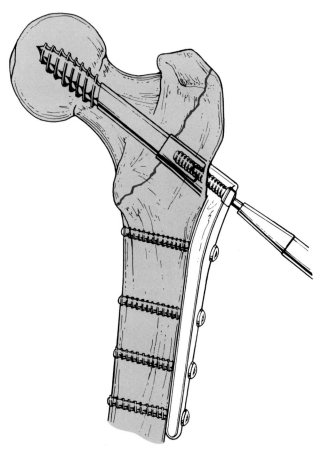

Figure 44-19

The separate compressing screw pulls the lag screw into the barrel of the sliding hip screw's side plate. Note that adequate length of the lag screw is present to minimize jamming of the lag screw within its tube. There is also sufficient length of the shaft between the lag screw threads and the end of the barrel. If with telescoping the threads come to rest on the barrel, the device will become the equivalent of a fixed-length implant, preventing further impaction, with adverse consequences for fixation and fracture healing. See text. Overtightening the compressing screw may impair fixation in osteopenic bone. Although it may project laterally after telescoping, it also provides a margin of safety against disassembly of the implant during the early stages of fracture healing.

intertrochanteric fracture, it should be treated as such. A major subtrochanteric fracture fragment extension, usually posteromedially, can first be anatomically reduced and held with interfragmentary screws. In such a circumstance, the physician should attempt to place the interfragmentary screws so that they will not prevent the nail plate assembly from touching the lateral cortex. Typically, the interfragmentary screws will enter from a more anterior or anterolateral position. More extensive exposure may be required. A longer side plate is typically necessary to bypass the stress riser effect of the distal fracture extension. The physician should inspect the extent of soft tissue stripping re-

quired to expose and reduce the fragments, the size of the subtrochanteric fracture extension, and the bone quality present. Primary medial bone grafting can be of considerable value in such cases. Subtrochanteric fractures with intertrochanteric extension are discussed in the next chapter.

MEDIAL DISPLACEMENT OSTEOTOMY

When a stable anatomic reduction of an intertrochanteric fracture cannot be obtained by closed or open methods, a medial displacement osteotomy may be indicated. Some four-fragment fractures with prominent palpable posteromedial defects are amenable to this approach. There should not be a major vertical subtrochanteric extension. The method of Dimon and Hughston is occasionally used for difficult fractures in elderly, osteopenic patients.[32] The surgeon should decide promptly if the osteotomy is to be used and should be quite certain to achieve a stable impaction after performing the osteotomy. Dimon currently believes displacement osteotomy should be used only for very unstable fractures and stresses the need to perform it properly.[69a] Merely displacing the femoral shaft medially without gaining a stable impacted realignment of the medial cortex is not a properly performed medial displacement osteotomy (Fig. 44-20).

If the lateral cortex extends proximally, start a transverse cut 1.5 cm distal to the vastus ridge with drill holes and complete it with a straight osteotome. Alternatively, an oscillating saw can be used. Hold the distal fragment with a clamp after subperiosteally clearing its proximal end of the soft tissue. Push the distal fragment medially. Remove any bony spikes that impede reduction with a rongeur, and reduce the proximal medial spike into the shaft of the distal fragment securely against the medial endosteal surface. Undo the reduction to facilitate guide wire placement. Pass a guide wire into the open bony surface of the proximal fragment in a slight varus position. Check the guide pin position and length by imaging in two planes. A short lag screw will almost always be required. Prepare the lag screw channel in standard fashion.

Prior to reducing the fragments, make a semicircular notch in the midlateral point of the lateral proximal cortex of the distal fragment. This will permit the tube plate device to rest snugly in place when the fracture is reduced. Insert the short lag screw into the proximal fragment along with a 135° tube plate. The proximal fragment will be abducted as the fracture is reduced, and high angles are seldom required. Repeat, securing the distal fragment to the plate by abduction. Hold the plate in position against the femoral shaft with an appropriate clamp such as a Verbrugge or Lohmann but

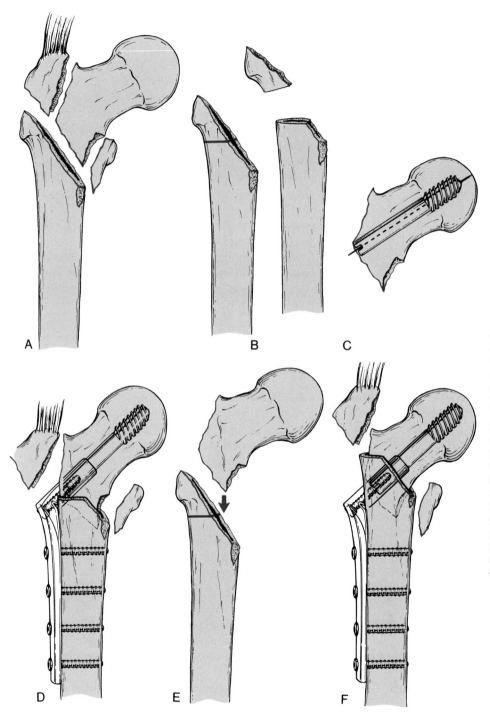

A

B

C

D

E

F

Figure 44–20

Medial displacement osteotomy for unstable intertrochanteric fracture. *A,* Four-part unstable (type III) intertrochanteric fracture. *B,* The proximal spike of the shaft fragment is osteotomized, and its lateral cortex is notched to accept the barrel of the side plate. *C,* A lag screw is inserted into the center of the femoral head over a guide wire, with fluoroscopic control. *D,* The femoral shaft is displaced medially, *impacted against the proximal fragment,* and fixed in valgus with the sliding hip screw. The compressing screw is used to maintain apposition. Fracture stability is provided by good bone contact. Without this, excessive telescoping of the implant might occur, resulting in the screw threads contacting the barrel of the side plate, with potential for penetration of the screw into the hip. A short barrel may better allow telescoping of the hip screw. *E,* Alternatively, medial displacement and impaction are performed *before* the fixation is applied. *F,* The fixation device is inserted through the intact lateral cortex distal to the osteotomy site.

without completely tightening it. An unscrubbed assistant releases the traction and forcibly impacts the fragments into each other under the surgeon's observation and control. A very stable impaction should result. The plate can be fixed to the femur in the usual manner, and additional compression can be added if it will increase stability.

BONE CEMENT AUGMENTATION

Polymethylmethacrylate bone cement (PMMA) can be used as an adjunct to internal fixation to increase fracture stability. The following four methods are available:

1. Individual screw purchase can be improved by injecting liquid cement into the hole of a loose screw, as suggested by Schatzker and Haeri, which is then replaced and tightened after the cement has hardened.[144]

2. Bertucci et al. have reported on Laros's technique of excavating osteopenic cancellous bone from the head and neck fragment and then injecting liquid PMMA, under fluoroscopic control, followed by replacement of the previously prepared sliding hip screw.[8,98]

3. Doughy PMMA can be used to recreate a noncompressible medial buttress, as described by Harrington.[59]

4. Some hip fixation implants (ALTA, Haig) permit injection of liquid PMMA through special ports in the lag screw. Results of this technique are not yet available.

INTRAMEDULLARY FIXATION

Intramedullary devices for the fixation of hip fractures gained popularity in the early 1970s.[27] Dissatisfied with the complications of malunion, nonunion, joint penetration, and implant breakage encountered with the fixed-angle nail plate, surgeons looked for alternative solutions. The theoretic advantages of intramedullary devices were shortened operation time; decreased infection rates, as the operative site is far removed from the fracture site; and a lowered bending moment across the proximal fragment. It was hoped that the intramedullary placement of these nails, which more closely approximates the lines of force in the hip, would lead to stable bone healing.

The most commonly used intramedullary devices are the multiple curved pins described by Ender and the single, more rigid, condylocephalic nail, originally introduced by Küntscher and later modified by Harris.[37–39,60,61] Both single and multiple devices are inserted through a portal in the medial femoral condyle and driven up toward the femoral head. The increased

flexibility and "stacking" potential of the Ender pins allow for easier insertion than the single nail device, as well as more stable fixations. Multiple pin fixation can be augmented by inserting some of the pins from a lateral distal femoral portal.

Overall, however, the results of intertrochanteric hip fractures fixed with intermedullary nails have been disappointing. In Sherk and Foster's review of condylocephalic rods, 51% of the patients lost rigid fixation when compared with those undergoing compression screw fixation.[149] In addition, none of the proposed advantages of condylocephalic rods were noted. Harris[60] ultimately suggested that condylocephalic nailing should be reserve for debilitated patients with stable intertrochanteric fractures.

Ender's method of multiple pin fixation has also met with mixed success (see Fig. 44–13). Levy et al. reported a series of 200 hip fractures fixed with Ender pins.[103] There was a 50% incidence of distal pin migration. Seventy-six percent of patients experienced knee pain, and 36% developed significant external malrotation. In addition, there was a failure of fixation in all of the basicervical type fractures. Knee pain, loss of knee motion, external malrotation, and pin migration seem to be prevalent in the vast majority of reported series. The reoperation rate in three separate series varied from 12% to 31%. Marsh, in his series of 80 patients, found an 80% malposition rate resulting in severe disability.[112] He questioned the continued use of Ender pins. Kuokkanen, after reviewing his complications, categorized intramedullary fixation as a semiconservative method that should be reserved for elderly people with systemic illnesses or poor general health precluding other surgery.[92a]

Several series, however, do report success with Ender pins. Waddell, reviewing 723 patients treated with Ender pins, found a less than 1% reoperation rate.[171] He stated that many of the reported fixation failures can be overcome by proper technique. Harper and Walsh reported good results when an anatomic reduction was made and four more pins were used.[58] The choice of intramedullary nail fixation is probably best described in the concluding remarks of Zukur et al., who stated that the ultimate choice of fixation should be based on the surgeon's experience and tailored to the patient's needs.[182]

Ender Pin Surgical Technique

The patient is placed in a supine position on the fracture table. The feet are fastened and the legs placed in sufficient abduction to allow enough room for the surgeon and for C-arm positioning (see Fig. 44–14). A valgus reduction facilitates nail insertion, especially when the patient has a narrow medullary canal, which tends to remove the proximal curve from the implants. A 7-cm longitudinal skin incision is made just anterior to the medial femoral condyle. The fascia is incised, and the vastus medialis is retracted anteriorly. Care is taken to avoid entering the knee joint. The medial femoral cortex just proximal to the condyle is exposed. This area is almost always crossed by the superior medial geniculate artery.

A $\frac{1}{4}$-in drill hole is made through the medial femoral cortex 1 to 2 cm proximal to the medial condyle. The hole should be at the midportion of the femoral shaft in the coronal plane and is enlarged using the curved awl. To avoid splitting the femoral shaft with the awl, a bone clamp can be placed around the femoral shaft just proximal to the hole.

An Ender nail of appropriate length is placed over the draped thigh. The distal end of the nail should extend 1 cm beyond the pilot hole, and the proximal tip should be at the level of the hip joint, as confirmed by fluoroscopy. Additional bending of the nail may be necessary to facilitate accurate nail placement. Use a nail 1 cm longer than the original estimate if the curvature of the pin must be increased. Bending should follow a gradual sloping curve; avoid sharp bends, and use the bending instruments.

The first nail is inserted into the hole and driven proximally. The nail will deflect off the lateral femoral cortex and pass medially into the femoral head. We routinely avoid final seating of the nails until several nails are in place. This prevents the first nail from being carried across the hip joint or disappearing into the medullary canal as subsequent nails are passed. We have also attached a towel clip through the proximal nail eyelet to prevent the nail from dropping into the canal.

The ends of the Ender nails should fan out into the femoral head and neck fragment on AP and lateral views. Usually four pins are sufficient to fill the medullary canal and adequately control fracture alignment. In patients with small medullary canals, two or three pins may be sufficient; when the medullary canal is wide, as in osteoporotic patients, five or more pins may be needed.

Reverse Oblique Intertrochanteric Fractures

Reverse oblique intertrochanteric fractures are not reliably fixed with sliding hip screws because telescoping of the implant promotes fracture separation rather than impaction. Several approaches reduce the risk of

failure: (1) Axial impaction of the shaft against the major proximal fragment *may* provide stability because of this. This is probably least safe, and may be improved upon by (2) an osteotomy of the proximal shaft to augment fracture contact and allow the hooking of the proximal fragment against the shaft; (3) the fracture can be reduced anatomically and buttressed with a 95° blade plate or condylar compression screw device; the proximal extent of these implants resists fracture displacement but may be mechanically stressed by unprotected weight bearing; (4) a cephalomedullary implant such as a Zickle or a gamma nail can be used to prevent displacement (Fig. 44–21).

GAMMA (CEPHALOMEDULLARY) NAIL

The recently developed gamma locking nail for proximal femur fractures consists of a short, proximal intramedullary nail for the femoral shaft, about the length of a conventional sliding hip screw side plate, with holes for two distal locking screws and a larger proximal hole through which is inserted a stout sliding femoral head lag screw. This screw is placed over a guide wire, the position of which is determined by a guide attached to the intramedullary nail. Obtaining proper nail depth and rotational alignment are thus key surgical steps. After insertion of the lag screw, the same guide assembly is used for placing the distal locking screws. The implant appears biomechanically sound, but only preliminary clinical experience is yet available.[54a,109a] A learning curve can be expected, especially for surgeons not well versed in use of other locked intramedullary nails.

Subtrochanteric Fractures

Intertrochanteric fractures often extend into the subtrochanteric region of the proximal femur.[148] Although subtrochanteric fractures per se will be covered in the following chapter, we mention this fracture pattern here for the sake of completeness. Subtrochanteric fractures are traditionally treated with the intramedullary Zickle nail. We have had good success, however, in treating intertrochanteric-subtrochanteric fracture patterns using the sliding screw with long side plate attachments. Previous sliding screw devices were not recommended for fractures extending into the subtrochanteric region, but newer side plate devices with improved designs and components made of high-strength alloys seem to provide the additional strength needed to control these fracture patterns. Results from reported series of subtrochanteric fractures treated with these newer fixation devices are pending.[67,134,165a]

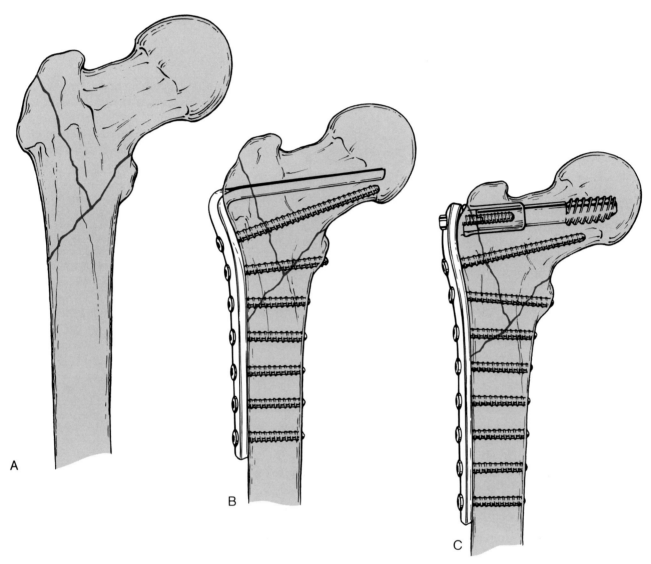

Figure 44-21

A, Reverse oblique intertrochanteric fracture, illustrating typical lateral comminution. *B*, Anatomic reduction and fixation with 95° blade plate. *C*, Anatomic reduction and fixation with 95° condylar compression screw.

Endoprosthesis

Prosthetic replacement may be considered as a treatment option for the highly comminuted intertrochanteric fracture in the elderly patient (Fig. 44-22). Early mobilization and weight bearing are usually achieved, thereby minimizing the risks of pneumonia and thromboembolic complications. Infection and dislocation of the prosthesis are potential complications. However, recent series do not seem to demonstrate unacceptable rates of these complications. Binns reported one dislocation in his series of 100 patients treated with Thompson hemiarthroplasty and no increased infection rate when compared with other fixation devices.[10] Green et al. reported 20 comminuted intertrochanteric fractures treated with cemented bipolar prostheses.[53] Full unrestricted weight bearing occurred at an average of five days after surgery. By using the greater trochanter as a landmark, correct limb length was easily achieved. Using Leinbach prosthetic replacements, Stern and Angerman also found early unrestricted weight bearing and markedly shortened hospital stay.[159] In their series retrospectively comparing prosthetic replacement to Ender nails and blade plate fixation of unstable peritrochanteric fractures, Claes et al. found superior results with endoprostheses.[22] Patients with prosthetic re-

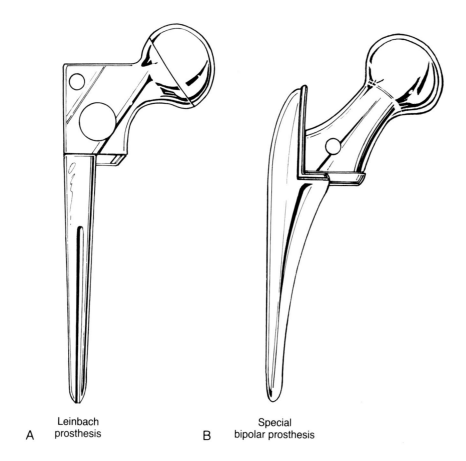

A   Leinbach
      prosthesis

B   Special
      bipolar prosthesis

Figure 44–22

Proximal femoral endoprostheses designed for intertrochanteric fracture patterns. Note the "calcar replacement" modification of these components. *A*, Leinbach-type prosthesis. *B*, Modified bipolar prosthesis. Attention must be paid to fixation of the greater trochanter, to minimize the risk of painful nonunion.

placements had fewer mechanical complications and the best walking ability. Technique is important, especially with regard to trochanteric reattachment. For details see references 53 and 159.

Aftercare

Antibiotics, begun with the induction of anesthesia, are continued for at most 24 to 48 hours after surgery, unless a documented infection is being treated.

We encourage all patients to be out of bed to a chair the day after surgery. Deep breathing exercises and the use of an incentive spirometer are recommended. Venous thrombosis prophylaxis should be in progress at this time, but the best form of prophylaxis is not yet clear. This is further discussed in chapter 18.

If fracture fixation is stable and comorbidities permit, protected weight bearing with crutches or a walker is begun on the second or third postoperative day. It is not recommended that patients be kept non–weight bearing on the affected side. Older patients are frequently unable to comply with non–weight bearing and may be frustrated in their physical therapy efforts. In addition, forces produced across the hip joint to maintain the limb in a non–weight-bearing state are

higher than those produced in protected weight-bearing situations. By 8 to 12 weeks, most patients are bearing full weight. However, many hip fracture patients continue to use a cane for at least several months following their surgery.

NUTRITIONAL SUPPORT

Even in wealthy societies, unrecognized malnutrition is frequent among the elderly and increases morbidity after hip fractures.[156] Nutritional screening is important to identify patients at risk. This may be done by history, physical exam, and laboratory tests, including cluding total lymphocyte count ($N > 1500$), serum albumin level ($N > 3.4$), and transferrin ($N > 199$). Evaluation by a dietitian should be routine, and a good case can be made for dietary supplementation for any patient who presents evidence of impaired nutrition preoperatively.

Rehabilitation and Discharge Planning

Ideally, hip fracture patients progress satisfactorily with inpatient therapy and leave the hospital within approximately two weeks.[133] However, in dealing with an older patient population, often with medical comorbidities, this goal may be difficult to achieve. Vigorous but supportive physical therapy is encouraged. It is strongly recommended that the social services department become actively involved with hip fracture patients promptly on hospitalization. Patients with slower progress following hip fracture surgery may be excellent candidates for short-term placement in rehabilitation facilities. These centers can act as an intermediary step between hospitalization and the patient's return home. If a rehabilitation center is not needed or is unavailable, physical therapy should be provided in the home. Jarnlo et al. found that the majority of patients receiving at-home physical therapy regained their preoperative level of function within four months.[76] The cost of therapy at home was found to be one tenth the cost of a nursing home facility. Pryor et al. have similarly demonstrated effective outpatient rehabilitation after hip fractures and emphasize the value of an organized, team management approach for such patients.[133,133a] In view of the present medicoeconomic climate, early involvement of social service and home care personnel has become an essential aspect of treating hip fracture patients. An organized geriatric hip fracture program has much to offer these patients.

Assessment of Results

Intertrochanteric fractures are commonly reported on retrospectively. The parameters most obvious to the surgeon are the status of the fracture, the course of healing after internal fixation, and the patient's walking ability. Other studies have focused on the patient's ultimate level of function, which may be assessed in various ways. These may range from the fundamental question of whether the hip fracture patient returned home, or when they returned home, to the patient's ability to perform various activities of daily living.[9] Health care economists study effects on patient survival and function for the purpose of eliminating or reducing expenses for services to the patient whose efficacy can not be documented.

It has become clear that standard methods of reporting surgical results may not accurately reflect the full picture of intertrochanteric fractures, including the effects on the patient's family, the local community, and the larger society that supports and maintains the delivery of care generally.

Health outcome has been defined as the description of what actually happened to the patient as compared with the surgical results alone. Health outcome studies include a scaling system to evaluate death, physical and psychological pain, physical and psychological disability, and financial cost.

Several scaling systems of this type have been attempted in the area of arthritis with the objective of better evaluating the true effect of a medical or surgical intervention. Examples include the Harris, HSS, and Mayo Clinic hip rating scores which all measure pain, walking ability, function, and disability. The difference between a chronic disease (arthritis) and an acute problem (an intertrochanteric hip fracture) must be appreciated. The hip fracture patient does not arrive with a well-documented evaluation of preinjury function expressed as a numeric score. History-taking may yield a somewhat unrealistic picture from the patient of preinjury function, which can vary significantly, ranging from patients in long-term placement in nursing homes to those living and functioning successfully in the community.

Unresolved questions include: Should fracture treatment outcome be compared to preinjury function only, or should the injury itself be factored into any postinjury evaluation? Should all studies be of a prospective randomized nature, applying the same end-criteria to all groups? And should one uniform rating system be applied for all studies?

Expected Results

Expected results relate to the functional status ultimately achieved by the patient both personally and in the social environment, and not just to the fate of the fracture itself.[50,51,72]

It must be recognized that comments made about expected results are generalizations about populations of patients with intertrochanteric hip fractures. These comments are based on our own personal experience and data derived from a broad base available in the orthopedic literature. We have not included every study reported, and each study we have utilized is not entirely comparable to others. For these reasons, although this section can serve as a guide, it may not be predictive of outcome for each individual, unique patient with a trochanteric hip fracture.

It has been observed that intertrochanteric hip fractures occur in a more biologically aged group of patients than do femoral neck fractures; this group of patients has poorer health and a higher mortality rate and puts greater demand on the health care system.

Mortality rates reported for patients with hip fractures range from 7% to 27% within three months of injury.[29,176] Mortality risk after hip fracture is increased compared with that of the age-matched control population for a period of from at least four months to as long as one year in various reports. In our own experience, hip fracture mortality is approximately 10% at one year. In a well-documented study, Kenzora et al. noted a 15% mortality after intertrochanteric hip fractures, compared with 9% for the age-matched population group. In addition, mortality rates will vary with the source of hip fracture patient referral. Miller noted a 20% mortality rate to be related more to preinjury functional status than to age.[119] Kenzora noted mortality to be related to the number of preoperative significant medical problems presented, as well as to postoperative significant medical complications.[90] It is likely that preinjury medical problems and functional status are interrelated (Table 44–2).

Return of preinjury function is subject to many interpretations, varying from a list of tasks to the ability to live alone. In an evaluation of the contribution of intensive rehabilitation efforts, Jette et al. observed that only 33% of patients recovered preinjury function.[83] This contrasts with a 69% good or excellent hip function noted by Miller, and an optimistic report of Jarnio et al. that "most" patients regained preinjury function by four months.[76,119] The individual elderly patient is unlikely to regain full preinjury function. Close to one half of patients will experience some transient mental confusion, and the incidence of in-hospital pulmonary, urinary tract, and cardiac problems will range from one fourth to one third of the patient group. Only 40% will walk as well as they did prior to injury. As many as two thirds to three fourths of patients will ultimately return to their own home, but the majority will not do so directly. Of those who do return home, at least 50% will be more dependent than before.

As the patient's mortality and functional outcome are related to preexisting factors, so too is the fate of the fracture itself related to a variety of factors. The factors influencing postoperative stability of the fracture fragment–internal fixation device complex have been emphasized throughout this chapter.[100] These factors are bone quality, fracture type, the reduction achieved, the implant selected, and the position of the implant.

The marked influence of fracture classification type has been emphasized. When inherent fracture instability is combined with radiographic osteoporosis (Singh grade III or less) the problems of loss of position and implant migration or penetration are compounded.

It is our opinion that fixed-angle nail plate devices (i.e., Jewett nail, McLaughlin nail and plate) are currently of historical interest and have been replaced by telescoping (sliding or compressing) implants. No change in mortality or morbidity has clearly accompanied this technical development, but the incidence of nail penetration, nail cutout, and implant breakage has been greatly diminished. Although fracture complications are less frequent with sliding hip fixation implants, they still occur and may significantly increase morbidity or cost of care.[1] The most obvious way to minimize fracture complications is avoidance of technical errors in reduction and fixation. Further studies may better define the roles of cement augmentation, prosthetic replacement, and intramedullary fixation. Perhaps such approaches will provide fewer complications and more cost-effective care for certain subcategories of patients with intertrochanteric fractures.

Stable fractures, type I undisplaced and type I displaced (Evans I and II), tend to heal with minimal collapse and deformity. Affected patients return rapidly to weight-bearing status. The surgeon should expect minimal settling of a stable fracture and uneventful healing with early weight bearing. The addition of

---

Table 44–2.

Prehospitalization Functional Status*

	No.	Performed Unassisted (%)	Performed with Equipment (%)	Performed with Help (%)	Unable to Perform (%)
Walking indoors	77	70	23	5	1
Transfers	77	82	13	4	1
Climbing stairs	75	63	19	1	17
Walking outdoors	77	51	23	9	17
Shopping	61	43	11	8	38
Community mobility	56	41	11	4	45
Dressing	77	88	—	6	5
Toileting	77	79	14	4	3
Tub use	70	59	1	7	33
Meal preparation	63	78	—	—	22

*Percentages do not always add to 100% because of rounding error.
Data from Campion, E.W., et al. Hip fracture: A prospective study of hospital course, complications, and cost. J Gen Intern Med 2(2):78, 1987.

bone cement to the head-neck fragment of a stable trochanteric fracture in osteopenic bone will not improve the result.

Treatment of unstable type II medial and type II lateral (Evans type III) and very unstable type III (Evans type IV) fractures is more difficult. Significant fracture fragment movement and impaction will likely occur. Despite this, nonunion has been only infrequently reported after compression screw fixation, as will be discussed in the section on nonunion.

In earlier years, failures of fixation averaged approximately 10%, ranging from a low of 5.6% to a high of 18.5%. However, these are largely unrefined figures, without separate analysis of different fracture types. Rao et al. noted a 4% failure rate in 124 unstable fractures.[134] Kyle et al. noted a 9.6% loss of fixation in unstable fractures.[94] The "gold standard" reported to date is a 0% cutout incidence with the Haig sliding nail–tube plate device in 257 fractures, 50% of which were classified as unstable or very unstable (see complication section).

Bartucci et al. noted that the addition of bone cement to the head-neck fragment significantly reduced the incidence of fixation failure in osteoporotic unstable fractures. Failure occurred in only 1 of 29 in which PMMA was added and in a surprisingly high 10 of 17 in which it was not.[8] The remarkably high failure rate of the control patients makes this study difficult to interpret.

The use of Ender pins for unstable fractures yields unacceptable complication rates for most surgeons.[86] Levy et al. reported a 76% incidence of knee pain related to distal pin migration in unstable fractures and 36% external malrotation.[103] Strathy and Johnson noted a 41% incidence of knee pain.[160] A high complication rate with this method has been reported in many studies around the world. In direct contrast are the excellent results reported by Waddell, who noted that 644 of 773 patients lived beyond six months, and of these, only one required revision surgery.[170] In very stable fractures, the average surgeon can expect results roughly comparable to those of other methods, providing sufficient experience can be gained to ensure precise and accurate surgical technique and at least four pins are inserted.

Prosthetic replacement for very unstable intertrochanteric fractures can yield good results. In separate reports, Green et al., Stern and Angerman, and Claes et al. noted good results and low complication rates with prosthetic replacements.[22,53,159] Much of this was attributed to patients resuming walking early, at an average of 5.5 days, according to Green et al. Claes et al. retrospectively compared this method to the use of Ender pins and a blade plate device and found that the

prosthesis patients walked better and had fewer complications.[22] It is clear that prosthetic replacement can be useful for the elderly patient with a very unstable intertrochanteric fracture. However, a prospective randomized study is needed comparing contemporary methods of fracture stabilization to contemporary prosthetic devices for patients with a high risk of failure of fixation. This study must consider the cost, loss of function, and complications of each method.

Complications

NONUNION

Nonunion of intertrochanteric fractures is reported to occur in 1% to 2% of patients regardless of the initial treatment.[3,89] Nonunions are uncommon, as these fractures occur in cancellous bone with an abundant blood supply. Union generally occurs 12 to 20 weeks postfracture by radiographic and clinical criteria. However, nonunion rates may approach 10% after complex fixation of comminuted fractures.

In most series, nonunion occurred only in those patients with severely comminuted fractures with bone loss. Marianni and Rand found that 19 of their 20 nonunions occurred in unstable fractures with loss of medial calcar continuity.[111] Most reported nonunions follow unsuccessful attempts at operative stabilization of fractures, with subsequent collapse into the varus position. This collapse leads to increased tensile stresses on the implant with subsequent implant failure or perforation through the femoral head or neck.

A diagnosis of nonunion is made in the patient with persistent pain in the hip with radiographs revealing a change in the neck-shaft angle with a radiolucent defect at the fracture site. Often the diagnosis is not obvious. It may require demonstration of fracture fragment mobility by fluoroscopy, perhaps with anesthesia, or by surgical exploration. Progressive loss of alignment strongly suggests nonunion, although healing may occur after an initial change in alignment, particularly if fragment contact is thus improved. Fixation failure is often associated with nonunion either as a cause or an effect. As with any nonunion, the possibility of an occult infection must be considered.

The treatment of nonunions generally consists of a second operative procedure combining stable bony apposition (preferably in a valgus position) and fixation with bone grafting. A hemiarthroplasty or total hip arthroplasty can be performed, but these usually require the use of a custom femoral component to compensate for bone loss. Selected patients with painless nonunion may not require reoperation.

FIXATION FAILURE

In general, any patient complaining of persistent pain, gait disturbance, or loss of fracture alignment (shortening or rotational deformity) should be evaluated for problems with fracture fixation. This should include a full clinical examination and radiographs in multiple projections to assess fracture alignment, implant loosening or failure, fracture healing, and possible acetabular penetration.[5,74,110] The entire sequence of radiographs, not only the current ones, should be studied. Tomograms may help assess fracture healing. If fixation failure is noted, it is important to determine the status of fracture healing in order to plan further therapy. If union has not occurred, skeletal traction may correct the deformity and can be continued until healing is secure.

Alternatives are to accept deformity and treat the patient symptomatically until union occurs, to revise the reduction and fixation, or to attempt salvage with a prosthesis.

MALUNION

Various factors may be responsible for varus displacement or rotational deformity. Varus displacement occurs frequently in unstable fractures with inadequate reduction. Moller et al. have related this to osteoporosis with the nail cutting out weak bone.[120] Others, such as Kyle and associates, have shown that poor placement of the screw or inadequate depth of screw insertion is primarily responsible.[94] Varus displacement is associated with failure of nail fixation, implant bending, breaking of the screw, or screw cutout of the head. These complications are usually diagnosed early (within two months of operation), with the patient complaining of pain, weakness of the hip, and a shortened extremity. Treatment must be individualized as outlined previously for nonunions, but correction of the malalignment requires an operation.

ACETABULAR PENETRATION

The use of a compression screw has decreased the frequency of screw penetration through the femoral head, which was common with earlier noncollapsing devices.[85] Telescoping of the device allows it to adapt to impaction at the fracture site rather than preventing it. However, upward penetration of the sliding screw through the osteoporotic bone of the superior aspect of the head may still occur, especially after the device has telescoped to its limit. Such penetration was noted in 5.4% of unstable fractures by Kyle and associates.[95]

Occasionally the telescoping action of the sliding screw fails, resulting in slight penetration of the femoral head but without clinical symptoms. Penetration of the nail may not lead to arthritis. It is generally recommended that slightly protruding implants with otherwise satisfactory alignment and fixation be left in place until union is obtained. Removal is in fact rarely necessary for elderly, inactive patients.

THROMBOEMBOLIC PHENOMENA

Venous thromboembolic disease is probably the most common complication of hip fractures in the geriatric patient.[146] The incidence of venography-proven deep vein thrombosis (DVT) after hip fracture varies between 40% and 90% if no prophylaxis is used. The incidence of fatal pulmonary embolism may be greater than 2% even with prophylactic measures. Froehlich and others have recently shown that compression ultrasound is a reliable, noninvasive screening test that is readily applied to the hip fracture patient. Studies with this technique indicate that 45% of patients who developed DVT after hip fractures already had formed a clot in veins near the fracture before an initial preoperative ultrasound study. The most appropriate treatment for such previously unrecognized patients is not yet clear.

The diagnosis of DVT may be difficult. Fatal pulmonary embolism (PE) may occur without previous clinical signs of DVT. Clinical assessment includes checks of calf and thighs daily for pain, swelling, tenderness, and increased temperature.

Venography remains the time-honored gold standard for diagnosing deep venous thrombosis. Newer methods utilizing radioactive-labeled platelets, fibrinogen, ultrasound, and impedance plethysmography have been reported. Only ultrasonography is readily applicable in the clinical situation. For detection of a pulmonary embolism, a chest radiograph and arterial blood gas test followed by a ventilation-perfusion scan and, occasionally, pulmonary angiography are utilized when clinical status warrants evaluation.

Prophylactic methods proposed for DVT and PE include the use of aspirin, warfarin, low-dose heparin, dextran, and other chemical agents, as well as external pneumatic compression, elastic stockings, early mobilization, and occasional uses of a vena caval filter.[16,48,126,129,154] A full discussion of these regimens and their efficacy is not possible here. The reader is referred to chapter 18 in this text, as well as to other publications in this intensively studied field. Prevention of thromboembolism with a prophylactic regimen is less expensive and more medically effective than the alternative of withholding prophylaxis and treating only recognized disease.

INFECTION

The incidence of postoperative wound infections varies from 0.15% to 15%. Lower figures have been obtained in most recent studies that used perioperative prophylactic antibiotics.[65,164] Burnett demonstrated in a double-blind prospective study the value of prophylactic antibiotics in reducing wound infections.[16a] The value of perioperative antibiotics in operations for hip fracture is now generally, but not universally, accepted.[66a,123a] Less clear is the optimal duration of prophylaxis. A single day's treatment may be sufficient.[122a] Because most infecting organisms are *Staphylococcus aureus* and other gram-positive cocci, a first-generation cephalosporin is commonly utilized, with an initial preoperative dose followed by doses for 24 to 48 hours postoperatively.

Infections can be divided into superficial and deep. Superficial wound infections are characterized by wound swelling, erythema, and discharge with or without persistent fever. These infections should be treated with appropriate antibiotics, open drainage with debridement as needed, and secondary closure. The most important goal is to prevent deep infection.

Deep infections may arise before or after fracture healing, even several years after initial surgery. They have a high morbidity and mortality. It may be hard to diagnose late deep infection. Symptoms include fever, pain in the hip, decreased range of motion, and an increased sedimentation rate. These infections also require debridement and antibiotics. If the fracture is not yet healed and fixation is stable, the implant should not be removed.[94,120] If there is hip joint involvement, most authors recommend removal of the internal fixation device and debridement to produce an excisional arthroplasty.

Wound hematomas or seromas may cause persisting hip wound drainage during the first several days after fixation of an intertrochanteric fracture. With reduced activity and sterile dressings, such drainage often resolves without development of an infection. However, if it persists, this may be the first sign of a deep infection, or a superinfection may occur. Patients should be watched closely for such wound drainage. If it is copious, increasing, or does not resolve within seven to ten days, reoperation is advisable. This involves a return to the operating room and formal wound exploration, often best done in the lateral decubitus position with the leg draped free. Deep cultures and Gram-stained slides of the exudate are obtained. Appropriate antibiotics are then begun intraoperatively, and after thorough debridement and irrigation, the wound is closed over suction drains. Closure may need to be delayed if an obvious infection is present. Antibiotics are soon discontinued if the final intraoperative culture results are negative. However, if bacterial organisms are recovered, the adjunctive antibiotic treatment may need modification according to sensitivity tests and should be continued for several weeks, perhaps with outpatient intravenous therapy or with conversion to an oral agent, if appropriate.

PRESSURE SORES

Skin ulcers are a common problem encountered in the hip fracture patient. Agarwal et al. reported an incidence of 20%. Common sites include the sacrum, heels, and buttocks, with most patients having more than one sore. The mortality rate among patients with pressure sores is reported to be 27% by Versluysen.[169a] Thus careful attention to prevention and treatment of this problem is necessary.

A total team approach to this complication is imperative. Pressure caused by the weight of the involved part will create tissue necrosis, if it is maintained for more than two hours or is repeated too frequently. Pressure sores are prevented by avoiding such pressure. Their early stage is indicated by localized erythema that persists for more than a few minutes after removing pressure on the area. The usual pressure points must be protected from contact with firm mattresses by increasing the surface area that supports the limbs of a patient at risk and by bridging high-pressure areas. This is especially important when skin sensation or protective mobility are impaired. Frequent turning of the patient is a time-honored protective measure but is difficult and painful for a patient with a hip fracture. Special beds, flotation mattresses, early fracture fixation, and constant vigilance by physicians, nurses, and therapists are all helpful ways to decrease the incidence and severity of pressure sores after hip fractures.

REFERENCES

1. Agarwal, N.; Reyes, J.D.; Westerman, D.A.; Cayter, C.G. Factors influencing DRG 201 chip fractures reimbursement. Trauma 26(1):426, 1986.
2. Aitken, J.M. Relevance of osteoporosis in women with fracture of the femoral neck. Br Med J 288(6417):597, 1984.
3. Altner, P.C. Reasons for failure in treatment of intertrochanteric fractures. Orthop Rev 11(8):117, 1982.
4. Arpin, H.; Kilfoyle, R.M. Treatment of trochanteric fractures with Ender rods. J Trauma 20:32, 1980.
5. Baker, D.M. Fractures of the femoral neck after healed intertrochanteric fractures: A complication of too short a nail plate fixation. J Trauma 15:73, 1975.
6. Barquet, A.; Fernandez, A.; Leon, H. Simultaneous ipsilateral trochanteric and femoral shaft fracture. Acta Orthop Scand 56(1):36, 1985.
7. Barquet, A.; Mussio, A. Fracture-dislocation of the femoral head with associated ipsilateral trochanteric and shaft fracture of the femur. Arch Orthop Trauma Surg 102:61, 1983.

8. Bartucci, E.J.; Gonzalez, M.H.; Cooperman, D.R.; et al. The effect of adjunctive methylmethacrylate on failures of fixation and function in patients with intertrochanteric fractures and osteoporosis. J Bone Joint Surg 67A:1094, 1985.

9. Beringer, T.R.; McSherry, D.M.; Taggart, H.M. A microcomputer base audit of fracture of the proximal femur in the elderly. Age Ageing 13(6):344, 1984.

10. Binns, M. Thompson hemiarthroplasty through a trochanteric osteotomy approach. Injury 16(9):595, 1985.

11. Bong, S.C.; Lau, H.K.; Leong, J.C.; et al. The treatment of unstable intertrochanteric fractures of the hip: a prospective trial of 150 cases. Injury 13:139, 1981.

12. Boyd, H.B.; Anderson, L.D. Management of unstable trochanteric fractures. Surg Gynecol Obstet 112:663, 1961.

13. Boyd, H.B.; Griffin, L.L. Classification and treatment of trochanteric fractures. Arch Surg 112:663, 1961.

14. Bray, T.J.; Esser, M.; Mulkerson, L. Osteotomy of the trochanter in open reduction and internal fixation of acetabular fractures. J Bone Joint Surg 69A(5):711, 1987.

15. Brink, P.R.; Bolhuis, R.J.; Runne, W.C.; Devries, A.C. Low nail-plate fixation and early weight-bearing ambulation for stable trochanteric fractures. J Trauma 27(5):491, 1987.

16. Brooks, R.L.; Winslow, M.C.; Kenmore, P.I. The week old hop fracture: Indication for prophylactic use of a vena cava filter? Orthopedics 10(9):1287, 1987.

16a. Burnett, J.W.; Gustilo, R.B.; Williams, D.N.; et al. Prophylactic antibiotics in hip fractures. J Bone Joint Surg 62A:457, 1980.

17. Callahan, D.J.; Burton, S.R. Bilateral hip and femur fractures. J Trauma 26(6):571, 1986.

18. Campion, E.W.; Jette, A.M.; Cleary, P.D.; Harris, B.A. Hip fracture: A prospective study of hospital course, complications, and cost. J Gen Internal Med 2(2):78, 1987.

19. Chan, K.M.; Tse, P.Y. Late subcapital fracture of the neck of the femur — a rare complication of the Ender nailing. J Trauma 26(2):196, 1986.

20. Chang, W.S.; Zuckerman, J.D.; Kummer, F.J.; Frankel, V.H. Biomechanical evaluation of anatomic reduction versus medial displacement osteotomy in unstable intertrochanteric fractures. Clin Orthop 225:141, 1987.

21. Chapman, M.W.; Bowman, W.E.; Songradi, J.J.; et al. The use of Ender's pins in extracapsular fractures of the hip. J Bone Joint Surg 63A:14, 1981.

22. Claes, H.; Broos, P.; Stappaerts, K. Petrochanteric fractures in elderly patients: Treatment with Ender's nails, blade-plate or endoprosthesis? Injury 16(4):261, 1985.

23. Clawson, D.K. Introcapsular fractures of the femur treated by the sliding screw plate fixation method. J Trauma 4:753, 1964.

24. Cobelli, N.J.; Sadler, A.H. Ender rod vs. compression hip screw fixation of hip fractures. Clin Orthop 201:123, 1985.

25. Collado, F.; Vila, J.; Beltran, J.E. Condylo-cephalic nail fixation for trochanteric fractures of the femur. J Bone Joint Surg 55A:578, 1969.

26. Cummings, S.R.; Phillips, S.L.; Wheat, M.E.; et al. Recovery of function of the hip fracture. The role of clinical social supports. J Am Geriatric Soc 36:801, 1988.

27. Cuthbert, H.; Howat, T.W. The use of Küntscher Y nail in the treatment of intertrochanteric and subtrochanteric fractures of the femur. Injury 8:135, 1976.

28. Dalen, N.; Jacobsson, B.; Eriksson, P.A. A comparison of nail-plate fixation and Ender's nailing in pertrochanteric fractures. J Trauma 28(3):405, 1988.

29. Davidson, T.I.; Bodey, W.N. Factors influencing survival following fractures of the upper end of the femur. Injury 17:12, 1986.

30. Dias, J.J.; Robbins, J.A.; Steigold, R.F.; Donaldson, L.J. Subcapital vs. intertrochanteric fracture of the neck of the femur: Are there two distinct populations? J R Coll Surg Edinb (5)303,1987.

31. Dimon, J.H. III. The unstable intertrochanteric fracture. Clin Orthop 92:100, 1973.

32. Dimon, J.H. III; Hughston, J.C. Unstable intertrochanteric fractures of the hip. J Bone Joint Surg 49A:440, 1967.

33. Doherty, J.H.; Lyden, J.P. Intertrochanteric fractures of the hip treated with hip compression screw. Clin Orthop 141:184, 1979.

34. Doppelt, S.H. The sliding compression screw today's best answer for stabilization of intertrochanteric hip fractures. Orthop Clin North Am II:507, 1980.

35. Dretakis, E.K.; Christodoulou, N.A. Significance of endogenic factors in the lication of fractures of the proximal femur. Acta Orthop Scand 54(2):198, 1983.

36. Ecker, M.L.; Joyce, J.J.; Johl, E.J. The treatment of trochanteric hip fractures with a compression screw. J Bone Joint Surg 57A:23, 1975.

37. Ender, H.G. Fixation trochanterer frakturen mit elastichen kondylennageln. Chir Praxis 18:81, 1974.

38. Ibid.

39. Ender, H.G. Treatment of pertrochanteric and subtrochanteric hip fractures with Ender pins. In: The Hip. St. Louis, C.V. Mosby, 1978.

40. Eriksson, S.A.; Widhe, T.L. Bone mass in women with hip fracture. Acta Orthop Scand 59(1):19, 1988.

41. Esser, M.P.; Kassab, J.Y.; Jones, D.H. Trochanteric fractures of the femur. A randomised prospective trial comparing the Jewett nail-plate with the dynamic hip screw. J Bone Joint Surg 68B:557, 1986.

42. Evans, E.M. The treatment of trochanteric fractures of the femur. J Bone Joint Surg 31B:190, 1949.

43. Evans, E.M. Trochanteric fractures. J Bone Joint Surg 33B:192, 1951.

44. Falch, J.A.; Ilebekk, A.; Slungaard, U.Y. Epidemiology of hip fractures in Norway. Acta Orthop Scand 56:12, 1985.

45. Ferris, B.B.; Dodds, R.A.; Klenerman, L.; Bitensky, L. Major components of bone in subcapital and trochanteric fractures. J Bone Joint Surg 69B:234, 1987.

46. Fitzgerald, J.F.; Fagan, L.F.; Tienney, W.M.; et al. Changing patterns of hip fracture care before and after implementation of the prospective payment system. JAMA 258:218, 1987.

47. Finsen, V.; Benum, P. The second hip fracture. An epidemiological study. Acta Orthop Scand 57(5):431, 1986.

48. Fredin, H.; Lindblad, B.; Jaroszewski, H.; Bergqvist, D. Prevention of thrombosis after hip fracture surgery. Acta Chir Scand 151:681, 1985.

49. Friedman, R.J.; Wyman, E.T. Ipsilateral hip and femoral shaft fractures. Clin Orthop 208:188, 1986.

50. Furstenberg, A. Expectations about outcome following hip fracture among older people. Social Work Health Care 11(4):33, 1986.

51. Ganz, R.; Thomas, R.J.; Hammele, C.D. Trochanteric fractures of femur: Treatment and results. Clin Orthop 138:30, 1979.

52. Gotfried, Y.; Frish, E.; Mendes, D.G.; Roffman, M.; et al. Intertrochanteric hip fractures in high risk geriatric patients treated by external fixation. Orthopaedics 8(6):769, 1985.

53. Green, S.; Moore, T.; Proano, F. Bipolar prosthetic replacement for the management of unstable intertrochanteric hip fractures in the elderly. Clin Orthop 224:169, 1987.

54. Griffin, J.B. The calcar femorale redefined. Clin Orthop 164:211, 1982.

54a. Grosse, A.; Taglong, G. A new device for treatment of trochanteric fractures—the intramedullary gamma locking nail. Presented at the Annual Meeting of AAOS, New Orleans, February 10, 1990.

55. Haig, A.C.: Haig, S.V.: Results of intertrochanteric fracture fixation with the Haig torque-free nail. Orthop Trans vol. 12, No. 3, Fall 1988.

56. Hammer, A.J. Intertrochanteric fractures in elderly white South Africans. S. Afr Med J 74:124, 1988.

57. Harding, A.F.; Cook, S.D.; Thomas, K.A.; et al. A clinical and metallurgical analysis of retrieved Jewett and Richards hip plate devices. Clin Orthop 195:261, 1985.

58. Harper, M.C.; Walsh, T. Ender nailing for peritrochanteric fractures of the femur. An analysis of indications, factors related to mechanical failure, and postoperative results. J Bone Joint Surg 67A:79, 1985.

59. Harrington, K.D.; Johnston, J.O.; Turner, R.H.; Green, D.L. The use of methylmethacrylate as an adjunct in the internal fixation of malignant neoplastic fractures. J Bone Joint Surg 54A:1665, 1972.

60. Harris, L.J. Condylocephalic nailing of intertrochanteric and subtrochanteric fractures of the femur, part 1. Closed intramedullary nailing of intertrochanteric and subtrochanteric fractures of the femur. Instr Course Lect 29:29, 1980.

61. Harris, L.J. Closed retrograde intramedullary nailing of peritrochanteric fractures of the femur with a new nail. J Bone Joint Surg 62A:1185, 1980.

62. Hayward, S.J.; Lowe, L.W.; Tzevelekos, S. Intertrochanteric fractures: A comparison between fixation with a two-piece nail plate and Ender's nails. Int Orthop 7(3):153, 1983.

63. Hedlund, R.; Lindgren, U. Trauma type, age, and gender as determinants of hip fracture. J Orthop Res 5(2):242, 1987.

64. Hedlund, R.; Lindgren, U.; Ahlbom, A. Age- and sex-specific incidence of femoral neck and trochanteric fractures. An analysis based on 20,538 fractures in Stockholm County, Sweden, 1972–1981. Clin Orthop 222:132, 1987.

65. Hedstrom, S.A.; Lidgren, L.; Serneo, I.; et al. Cefuroxime prophylaxis in trochanteric hip fracture operations. Acta Orthop Scand 58(4):361, 1987.

66. Heyse-Moore, G.H.; MacEachern, A.G.; Evans, D.D. Treatment of intertrochanteric fractures of the femur. A comparison of the Richards screw-plate with the Jewett nail-plate. J Bone Joint Surg 65B:262, 1983.

66a. Hjortrup A.; Sorensen C.; Mejdahl S.; et al. Antibiotic prophylaxis in surgery for hip fractures. Acta Orthop Scand 61:152–153, 1990.

67. Hogh, J.; Lund, B.; Lucht, U.; et al. Trochanteric and subtrochanteric fractures—Enders vs. McLaughlin osteosynthesis. Acta Orthop Scand 52:639, 1981.

68. Holmberg, S.; Thorngren, K.G. Preoperative 99mTc-MDP scintimery of femoral neck fractures. Acta Orthop Scand 52:639, 1981.

69. Holt, E.P. Jr. Rigid fixation by use of the Holt nail. Orthop Clin North Am 5:601, 1974.

69a. Hopkins, C.T.; Nugent, J.T.; Dimon, J.H., III. Medial displacement for unstable intertrochanteric fractures twenty years later. Clin Orthop 245:169, 1989.

69b. Hornby, R.; Grimley-Evans, J.; Vardon, V. Operative or conservative treatment for trochanteric fractures of the femur. A randomized epidemiological trial in elderly patients. J Bone Joint Surg 71B:619, 1989.

70. Horowitz, B.G. Retrospective analysis of hip fractures. Surg Gynecol Obstet 123:565, 1966.

71. Hubbard, M.J.; Burke, F.D.; Houghton, G.R.; et al. A prospective controlled trial of valgus osteotomy for unstable intertrochanteric fractures. Injury 11:228, 1980.

72. Hughes, S.L.; et al. Hospital volumes and patient outcomes. Hip fractures. Med Care 26:1057, 1988.

73. Jacobs, R.R.; McClain, O.; Armstrong, H.J. Internal fixation of intertrochanteric hip fractures: A clinical and biomechanical study. Clin Orthop 26:1057, 1988.

74. Jakobsen, B.W. Breakage of a sliding hip screw. A case report. Acta Orthop Scand 58(3):292, 1987.

75. James, E.T.; Hunter, G.A. The treatment of intertrochanteric fractures—a review article. Injury 14(5):421, 1983.

76. Jarnlo, G.B.; Ceder, L.; Throngren, K.G. Early rehabilitation at home of elderly patients with hip fractures and consumption of resources in primary care. Scand J Primary Health Care 2(3):105, 1984.

77. Jensen, J.S. Trochanteric fractures. Acta Orthop Scand [suppl] 188:1, 1981.

78. Jensen, J.S. Classification of trochanteric fractures. Acta Orthop Scand 51:949, 1980a.

79. Jensen, J.S. Mechanical strength of sliding-screw hip implants. Acta Orthop Scand 51:625, 1980b.

80. Jensen, J.S.; Sonne-Holm, S. Critical analysis of Ender nailing in the treatment of trochanteric fractures. Acta Orthop Scand 51:817, 1980.

81. Jensen, J.S.; Sonne-Holm, S.; Tondevold, E. Unstable trochanteric fractures: A comparative of four methods of internal fixation. Acta Orthop Scand 51:949, 1980.

82. Jensen, J.S.; Tondevold, E.; Sonne-Holm, S. Stable trochanteric fractures: A comparative analysis of four methods of internal fixation. Acta Orthop Scand 51:811, 1980.

83. Jette, A.M.; Harris, B.A.; Cleary, P.D.; Campion, E.W. Functional recovery after hip fracture. Arch Phys Med Rehab 68(10):735, 1987.

84. Jewett, E.L. One piece angle nail for trochanteric fractures. J Bone Joint Surg 23:803, 1941.

85. Joseph, K.N. Acetabular penetration of sliding screw. A case of trochanteric hip fracture. Acta Orthop Scand 57(3):245, 1986.

86. Juhn, A.; Krimerman, J.; Mendes, D.G.; et al. Intertrochanteric fracture. CHS vs. Enders. Arch Orthop Trauma Surg 107:136, 1988.

87. Kaufer, H.; Matthews, L.S.; Sontegard, D. Stable fixation of intertrochanteric fractures: A biomechanical evaluation. J Bone Joint Surg 56A:899, 1974.

88. Kaufer, H. Mechanics of treatment of hip injuries. Clin Orthop 146:53, 1980.

89. Kelbel, J.M.; Connolly, J.F. Avascular necrosis following a "routine" intertrochanteric fracture of the femur. Nebr Med J 69(5):156, 1984.

90. Kenzora, J.E.; McCarthy, R.E.; Lowell, J.D.; Sledge, C.B. Hip fracture mortality. Relation to age, treatment, preoperative illness, time of surgery, and complication. Clin Orthop 186:45, 1986.

91. Kuderna, H.; Bohler, N.; Collan, D.J. Treatment of intertrochanteric and subtrochanteric fractures by the Ender method. J Bone Joint Surg 58A:604, 1976.

92. Kuntscher, G. A new method of treatment of pertrochanteric fractures. Proc R Soc Med 63:1120, 1970.

92a. Kuokkanen, H.; Korkala, O.; Lautamus, L. Ender nailing of trochanteric fracture. A review of 73 cases. Arch Orthop Trauma Surg 105:46, 1986.

93. Kyle, R.F. Fixation of intertrochanteric hip fractures with sliding device. Instr Course Lect 32:303, 1983.

94. Kyle, R.F.; Gustilo, R.B.; Premer, R.F. Analysis of six hundred and twenty-two interchanteric hip fractures. J Bone Joint Surg 61A:216, 1979.

95. Kyle, R.F.; Wright, T.M.; Burnstein, A.H. Biomechanical analysis of the sliding characteristics of compression screws. J Bone Joint Surg 62A:1308, 1980.

96. Laros, G.S. Intertrochanteric fractures. (Editorial) Clin Orthop 138:3, 1979.

97. Laros, G.S. The role of osteoporosis in intertrochanteric fractures. Orthop Clin North Am 11:25, 1980.

98. Laros, G.S. Intertrochanteric fractures. In: Evarts, C.M., ed. Surgery of the musculoskeletal system, 2nd ed., Vol. 3. New York, Churchill-Livingstone, 1990, p. 2613.

99. Laros, G.S.; Moore, J.F. Complications of fixation in intertrochanteric fractures. Clin Orthop 101:110, 1974.

100. Larson, S.; Elloy, M.; Hansson, L.I. Stability of osteosynthesis intertrochanteric fracture: Comparison of three fixation devices in cadavers. Acta Orthop Scand 59(4):386–370, 1988.

101. Lau, H.K.; Lee, P.C.; Tang, S.C.; et al. Treatment of comminuted intertrochanter femoral fractures with Dimon Hughston displacement fixation and acrylic cement—a preliminary report of sixteen cases. Injury 15(2):129, 1983.

102. Lawton, J.O.; Baker, M.R.; Dickson, R.A. Femoral neck fractures—two populations. Lancet 2(8341):70, 1983.

103. Levy, R.N.; Siegel, M.; Sedlin, E.D.; Siffert, R.S. Complications of Ender-pin fixation in basicervical, intertrochanteric, and subtrochanteric fractures of the hip. J Bone Joint Surg 65A:66, 1983.

104. Lips, P.; Taconis, W.K.; van-Ginkel, F.C.; Netelenbos, J.C. Radiologic morphometry in patients with femoral neck fractures and elderly control subjects. Comparison with histomorphometric parameters. Clin Orthop 183:64, 1984.

105. Lizaur-Utrilla, A.; Puchades-Orts, A.; Sanchez-del-Campo, F. Epidemiology of trochanteric fractures of the femur in Alicante, Spain, 1974–1982. Clin Orthop 218:24, 1987.

106. Luthje, P. Incidence of hip fracture in Finland. A forecast for 1990. Acta Orthop Scand 56(3):223, 1985.

107. Luthje, P. Fractures of the proximal femur in Finland in 1980. Ann Chir Gynecol 72(5):282, 1983.

108. Lyons, J.W.; Nevins, M.C. Non-treatment of hip fractures in senile patients. JAMA 238:1175, 1977.

109. MacEachern, A.G.; Heyse-Moore, G.H. Stable intertrochanteric fractures. A misnomer? J Bone Joint Surg 65B:582, 1983.

109a. Mohamed, W.; Kellam, J.; Harrington, I.; et al. Biomechanical comparison of the gamma nail and sliding hip screw. Presented at the 6th Annual Meeting of the Orthopaedic Trauma Association, Toronto, November 9, 1990.

110. Manoli, A. II. Malassembly of the sliding screw-plate device. J Trauma 26(10):916, 1986.

111. Mariani, E.M.; Rand, J.A. Nonunion of intertrochanteric fractures of the femur following open reduction and internal fixation. Results of second attempts to gain union. Clin Orthop 218:81, 1987.

112. Marsh, C.H. Use of Ender's nails in unstable intertrochanteric femoral fractures. J R Soc Med 76(7):550, 1983.

113. Massie, W.K. Extracapsular fractures of the hip treated by impaction using a sliding nail-plate fixation. Clin Orthop 92:16, 1973.

114. McClure, J.; Goldsborough, S. Fractured neck of femur and contralateral intracerebral lesions. J Clin Pathol 39(8):920, 1986.

115. Melton, L.J.; Ilstrup, D.M.; Riggs, B.L.; Beckenbaugh, R.D. Fifty-year trend in hip fracture incidence. Clin Orthop 162:144, 1982.

116. Ibid.

117. Melton, L.J. III; Wahner, H.W.; Richelson, L.S.; et al. Osteoporosis and the risk of hip fracture. Am J Epidemiol 124(2):254, 1986.

118. Miller, B.N.; Lucht, U.; Grymer, F.; Bartholdy, N.J. Instability of trochanteric hip fractures following internal fixation. A radiographic comparison of the Richards sliding screw-plate and the McLaughlin nail-plate. Acta Orthop Scand 55(5):517, 1984.

119. Miller, C.W. Survival and ambulation following hip fracture. J Bone Joint Surg 60A:930, 1978.

119a. Mizrahi, J.; Kantarovski, A.; Najenson T.; et al. In vivo biomechanical evaluation of nail-plate fixation of femoral neck fractures of rehabilitated patients. Scand J Rehab Med [Suppl] 12:112, 1985.

120. Moller, B.N.; Lucht, U.; Grymer, F.; Bartholdy, N.J. Early rehabilitation following osteosynthesis with the sliding hip screw for trochanteric fractures. Scand J Rehab Med 17:39, 1985.

121. Muhr, G.; Tscherne, H.; Thomas R. Comminuted trochanteric femoral fractures in geriatric patients: The results of 231 cases with internal fixation and acrylic cement. Clin Orthop 138:41, 1979.

122. Murray, J.A.; Parrish, F.F. Surgical management of secondary neoplastic fractures of the hip. Orthop Clin North Am 5:88, 1974.

122a. Nelson, C.L.: Green, T.G.; Porter, R.A.; et al. One day versus seven days of preventive antibiotic therapy in orthopaedic surgery. Clin Orthop 176:258–263, 1983.

123. Noble, P.C.; Alexander, J.W.; Lindahl, L.J.; et al. The anatomic basis of femoral component design. Clin Orthop 235:148, 1988.

123a. Norden, C.W. Prevention of bone and joint infections. Am J Med. 78:229, 1985.

124. Nunn, D. Sliding hip screws and medial displacement osteotomy. J R Soc Med 81(3):140, 1988.

125. Obrant, K.J. Trabecular bone changes in the greater trochanter after fracture of the femoral neck. Acta Orthop Scand 55(1):78, 1984.

126. Oster, G.; Tuden, R.L.; Colditz, G.A. A cost-effectiveness analysis of prophylaxic against deep-vein thrombosis in major orthopedic surgery. JAMA 257(2):203, 1987.

127. Owen, R.A.; Melton, L.J. III; Gallagher, J.C.; Riggs, B.L. The national cost of acute care of hip fractures associated with osteoporosis. Clin Orthop 150:172, 1980.

128. Paachsburg-Nielson, B.; Jelnes, R.; Rasmussen, L.B.; Ebling, A. Trochanteric fractures treated by the McLaughlin nail and plate. Injury 16(5):333, 1985.

129. Paiement, G.D.; Wessinger, S.J.; Harris, W.H. Survey of prophylaxis against thromboembolism in adults undergoing hip surgery. Clin Orthop 223:188, 1987.

130. Pankovich, A.M.; Tarabishy, I.E. Ender nailing of intertrochanteric and subtrochanteric fractures of the femur. J Bone Joint Surg 62A:635, 1980.

131. Passoff, T.L.; Schein, A.J. Ender's flexible intramedullary pins for the treatment of pertrochanteric hip fractures: Preliminary report of the first 100 cases. J Trauma 20:876, 1980.

132. Pho, R.W.H.; Nather, A.; Tong, G.O.; Korku, C.T. Endoprosthetic replacement of unstable, comminuted intertrochanteric

fracture of the femur in the elderly, osteoporotic patient. J Trauma 21(9):792, 1981.

133. Pryor, G.A.; Myles, J.W.; Williams, D.R.R.; Anand, J.K. Team management of the elderly patient with hip fracture. Lancet 20:401, 1988.

133a. Pryor, G.A.; Williams, D.R.R. Rehabilitation after hip fractures. Home and hospital management compared. J Bone Joint Surg 71B:471, 1989.

134. Rao, J.P.; Banzon, M.T.; Weiss, A.B.; Raychack, J. Treatment of unstable intertrochanteric fractures with anatomic reduction and compression hip screw fixation. Clin Orthop 175:65, 1983.

135. Rapin, C.H.; Lagier, R.; Boivin, G.; et al. Is a certain degree of osteomalacia involved in femoral neck fractures of the elderly? Histological approach to the problem and practical applications. Z Gerontol 16(6):277, 1983.

136. Raugstad, T.S.; Molster, A.; Haukeland, W.; et al. Treatment of pertrochanteric and subtrochanteric fractures of the femur by the Ender method. Clin Orthop 138:231, 1979.

137. Rennie, W.; Mitchell, N. Compression fixation of peritrochanteric fractures and early weight-bearing. Clin Orthop 121:157, 1976.

138. Richmond, W.W.; Kazes, J.A.; MacAusland, W.R. An evaluation of three current techniques of internal fixation for intertrochanteric and subtrochanteric fractures of the hip. Orthopaedics 4:895, 1981.

139. Roberts, A.; Rooney, T.; Loone, J.; et al. A comparison of the functional results of anatomic and medial displacement valgus nailing of intertrochanteric fractures of the femur. J Trauma 12:341, 1972.

140. Sarmiento, A. Intertrochanteric fractures of the femur: 150-degree-angle nail-plate fixation and early rehabilitation: A preliminary report of 100 cases. J Bone Joint Surg 45A:706. 1093.

141. Sarmiento, A. Avoidance of complication of internal fixation of intertrochanteric fractures: Experience with 250 consecutive cases. Clin Orthop 53:47, 1967.

142. Sarmiento, A. Valgus osteotomy technique for unstable intertrochanteric fractures. In: The Hip. St. Louis, The C.V. Mosby, 1975.

143. Sartoris, D.J.; Kerr, R.; Goergen, T.; Resnick, D. Sliding-screw fixation of proximal femoral fractures: radiographic assessment. Skeletal Radiol 14(2):104, 1985.

144. Schatzker, J.; Haeri, G.B. Meta as an adjunct in internal fixation of pathologic fractures. Can J Surg 22:179, 1979.

145. Scher, M.A. Intertrochanteric osteotomies for degenerative hip conditions. Case reports. S Afr Med J 69(2):125, 1986.

146. Schlag, G.; Gaudernak, T.; Pelinka, H.; et al. Thromboembolic prophylaxis in hip fracture. Acta Orthop Scand 57:340, 1986.

147. Schultz, R.J.; Whitfield, G.F.; Lamura, J.J.; et al. The role of physiologic monitoring in patients with fractures of the hip. J Trauma 25(4):309, 1985.

148. Seinsheimer, F. III. Subtrochanteric fractures of the femur. J Bone Joint Surg 60A:300, 1978.

149. Sherk, H.H.; Foster, M.D. Hip fractures: Condylocephalic rod versus compression screw. Clin Orthop 192:255, 1985.

150. Sherk, H.H.; Snape, W.J.; Loprete, F.L. Internal fixation versus nontreatment of hip fractures in senile patient. Clin Orthop 141:196, 1979.

151. Siffert, R.S.; Lattuga, S.; Figueirdo, M.; et al. Noninvasive Acoustic Assessment of Fracture Healing. Int. Soc. for Fracture Repair, 2nd Conf., Mayo Clinic, Sept. 6–8, 1990.

152. Singh, M.; Nagrath, A.R.; Maini, P.S. Changes in the trabecular pattern of upper end of the femur as an index of osteoporosis. J Bone Joint Surg 52A:457, 1970.

153. Skinner, P.W.; Powles, D. Compression screw fixation for displaced subcapital fracture of the femur. Success or failure? J Bone Joint Surg 68B:78, 1986.

154. Snook, G.A.; Crisman, O.D.; Wilson, T.C. Thromboembolism after surgical treatment of hip fractures. Clin Orthop 155:21, 1981.

155. Sontesgard, D.A.; Kaufer, H.; Matthews, L.S. A biomechanical evaluation of implants, reduction, and prosthesis in the treatment of intertrochanteric hip fractures. Orthop Clin North Am 5:551, 1974.

156. Stableforth, P.G. Supplement feeds and nitrogen and calorie balance following femoral neck fracture. Br J Surg 73(8):651, 1986.

157. Staeheli, J.W.: Frassica, F.J.: Fitzgerald, R.H.; et al. Comparison study of primary endoprosthetic replacement vs. CLAS for unstable intertrochanteric fractures. Orthop Trans 10:481, 1986.

158. Steinberg, G.G.; Desai, S.S.; Kornwitz, N.A.; Sullivan, T.J. The intertrochanteric hip fracture. A retrospective analysis. Orthopaedics 11(2):265, 1988.

159. Stern, M.D.; Angerman, A. Comminuted intertrochanteric fractures treated with a Leinbach prosthesis. Clin Orthop 218:75, 1987.

160. Strathy, G.M.; Johnson, E.W. Jr. Ender's pinning for fractures about the hip. Mayo Clin Proc 59(6):411, 1984.

161. Street, D.M. Condylocephalic nailing of intertrochanteric fractures. Part II. Condylocephalic nailing of intertrochanteric and subtrochanteric fractures of the femur. Instr Course Lect 29:29, 1980.

162. Stromqvist, B. Hip fracture in rheumatoid arthritis. Acta Orthop Scand 55(6):624, 1984.

163. Swiontkowski, M.F. Ipsilateral femoral shaft and hip fractures. Ortho Clin North Am 18(1):73, 1987.

164. Tengve, B.; Kjellander, J. Antibiotic prophylaxis in operations on trochanteric femoral fractures. J Bone Joint Surg 60A:97, 1978.

165. Trafton, P.G.; Day, L.J.; Cohen, H.A.; et al. A comparative study of compression hip screw and condylocephalic nail for intertrochanteric fractures of the femur. Orthop Trans 8:391, 1984.

165a. Trafton, P.G. Subtrochanteric-intertrochanteric femoral fractures. Orthop Clin North Am 18:59–71, 1987.

166. Tronzo, R.B. Hip nails for all occasions. Orthop Clin North Am 5:479, 1974.

167. Uden, G.; Nilsson, B. Hip fracture frequent in hospital. Acta Orthop Scand 57(5):428.

168. Urovitz, E.P.M.; Fornasier, V.L.; Risen, M.I.; MacNab, I. Etiological factors in the pathogenesis of femoral trabecular fatigue fractures. Clin Orthop 127:275, 1977.

169. Valentin, N.; Lomholt, B.; Jensen, J.S.; et al. Spinal or general anesthesia for surgery of the fractured hip? A prospective study of mortality in 578 patients. Br J Anaesth 58(3):284, 1986.

169a. Versluyjen, M. Pressure sores in elderly patients. The epidemiology related to hip operations. J Bone Joint Surg 67B:10, 1985.

170. Waddell, J.P.; Czitrom, A.; Simmons, E.H. Ender nailing in fractures of the proximal femur. J Trauma 27(8):911, 1987.

171. Waddell, J.P. Ender nailing in intertrochanteric fractures of the femur. Instr Course Lect 33:218, 1984.

172. Waddell, J.P. Remote nailing of intertrochanteric and subtrochanteric fractures of the femur. Instr Course Lect 32:303, 1983.

173. Walloe, A.; Andersson, S.; Herrlin, K.; Lidgren, L. Incidence and stability of trochanteric femoral fractures. Acta Orthop Scand 54(4):622, 1983.

174. Ward, F.O. Human Anatomy. London, Renshaw, 1838.

175. Wellin, D.E.; Galloni, L; Gelb, R.I. Ipsilateral intertrochanteric and diaphyseal femoral fractures. Four patients treated by one technique. Clin Orthop 183:71, 1984.

176. White, B.L.; Fisher, W.D.; Laurin, C.A.; et al. Rate of mortality for elderly patients after hip fractures in 1980's. J Bone Joint Surg 69A:1335, 1987.

177. Whitman, R. A new treatment for fractures of the femoral neck. Med Rec 65:441, 1904.

178. Winter, W.G. Nonoperative treatment of proximal femoral fractures in the demented, nonambulatory patient. Clin Orthop 218:97, 1987.

179. Zain-Elabdien, B.S.; Olerud, S.; Karlstrom, G. Ender nailing of pertrochanteric fractures. Complications related to technical failures and bone quality. Acta Orthop Scand 56(2):138, 1985.

180. Zain-Elabdien, B.S.; Olerud, S.; Karlstrom, G. The influence of age on the morphology of trochanteric fractures. Arch Orthop Trauma Surg 103(3):156, 1984.

181. Zetterberg, C.; Elmersson, S.; Andersson, G.B. Reoperations of hip fractures. Acta Orthop Scand 56(1):8, 1985.

181a. Zuckerman, J.D., ed. Comprehensive Care of Orthopaedic Injuries in the Elderly. Baltimore, Urban & Schwarzenberg, 1990.

182. Zukor, D.J.; Miller, B.J.; Hadjipavolou, A.J.; Lander, P. Hip pinning, past and present: Richard's compression-screw fixation versus Ender's nailing. Can J Surg 28(5):391, 1985.

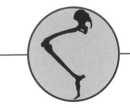

Thomas A. Russell, M.D.
J. Charles Taylor, M.D.

45

Subtrochanteric Fractures of the Femur

Subtrochanteric fractures of the femur have always been difficult to treat.[9,16,25] During this century a better understanding of the biomechanics of the fracture and the development of better implants have led to radical changes in treatment modalities. Emphasis on preservation of the blood supply to the fracture fragments and autogenous bone grafting have improved biologic results, while improved engineering and manufacturing capabilities have yielded implants of greater strength and longer fatigue life. With a thorough understanding of the variants of the subtrochanteric fractures and the available treatment options, the optimal treatment can be selected for each patient.

Pathology

ANATOMY AND BIOMECHANICS

The plane of the femoral head and neck is anteverted 15° to 20° to the plane of the femoral shaft in most adults. This plane of the femoral neck and head is also anteriorly positioned 1 cm to 1.5 cm compared with the center axis of the femoral shaft. The normal neck-shaft axis is 127° to 130°. If the center line of the femoral shaft is continued through the intertrochanteric region, it emerges from the femur in the region of the piriformis fossa. On an anteroposterior radiographic projection, this line appears to transect the femur at the medial wall of the greater trochanter, but on the lateral projection, the line crosses the piriformis fossa. The lesser trochanter is a posteromedial prominence at the termination of the intertrochanteric ridge and serves as the prominent insertion point of the iliacus and psoas

tendons. Its prominence in the anteroposterior radiographic projection helps assess the anteversion of the proximal fragment in fractures with an intact lesser trochanter. This portion of the medial femoral cortex involving the lesser trochanter and an area just anterior to it are important in obtaining stable fixation with proximal locking screws in interlocking nailing techniques. The inclusion of the region of the lesser trochanter in the fracture generally precludes the use of standard interlocking femoral nails and necessitates the use of specialized cephalomedullary nails (nails with proximal locking screws that can be inserted up into the femoral head). The femoral shaft is bowed primarily anteriorly but also slightly laterally. The plane of the bow is situated approximately 15° lateral to the pure anteroposterior plane. When nailing an impending pathologic fracture of the femoral shaft, the intramedullary nail tends to align itself along this plane in a slightly lateral rather than a purely anteroposterior plane.

In the subtrochanteric and shaft regions, the femur is covered circumferentially by well-vascularized muscle groups (Fig. 45–1). The primary direct surgical exposure of the subtrochanteric shaft region involves either splitting the vastus lateralis muscle or reflecting it anteriorly from the lateral intermuscular septum. Profuse bleeding from the perforating branches of the profundus femoris artery can complicate this exposure (Fig. 45–2). The attachments of the hip muscles (iliacus and psoas, gluteus medius and minimus, gluteus maximus and adductors) all contribute to the powerful forces that act on the individual fragments in the subtrochanteric fracture.

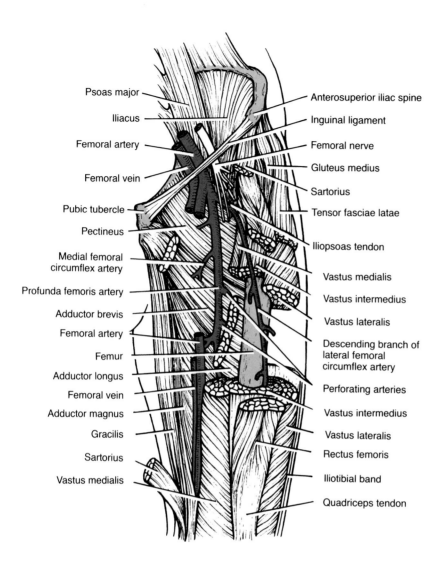

Psoas major

Iliacus

Femoral artery

Femoral vein

Pubic tubercle

Pectineus

Medial femoral
circumflex artery

Profunda femoris artery

Adductor brevis

Femoral artery

Femur

Adductor longus

Femoral vein

Adductor magnus

Gracilis

Sartorius

Vastus medialis

Anterosuperior iliac spine

Inguinal ligament

Femoral nerve

Gluteus medius

Sartorius

Tensor fasciae latae

Iliopsoas tendon

Vastus medialis

Vastus intermedius

Vastus lateralis

Descending branch of
lateral femoral
circumflex artery

Perforating arteries

Vastus intermedius

Vastus lateralis

Rectus femoris

Iliotibial band

Quadriceps tendon

Figure 45–1

Anterior anatomy of the hip and
subtrochanteric area.

The major neurologic structures in this region are the sciatic nerve posteriorly and the femoral nerve anteriorly; they are rarely involved in closed injuries in the subtrochanteric region (Fig. 45–3). For more anatomic detail of this area, the reader is referred to chapters 43 and 44. It should be noted that the transition between the cancellous bone of the intertrochanteric region to the thick cortical bone in the diaphysis makes the subtrochanteric area the most attenuated area of cortical bone with the narrowest cortical wall thickness.[27]

Koch,[43] in the early twentieth century, was one of the first to analyze mechanical stresses on the femur during weight bearing. He showed that up to 1200 pounds/in^2 of force could be generated in a 200-pound male. Compression stresses exceeded 1200 pounds/in^2 in the medial subtrochanteric area one to three inches distal to the level of the lesser trochanter. The lateral tensile stresses were approximately 20% less. His analysis did not take into account the additional stresses of muscle

forces.[57] Frankel and Burstein[25] demonstrated significant forces on the hip and proximal femur with activities such as flexing and extending the hip in bed, indicating continuous stresses on the implant system even with the patient at bed rest. Fielding et al.,[23] in an analysis of the biomechanics of subtrochanteric fractures, called attention to the necessity of a medial cortical buttress to minimize the implant stresses. They noted that nonunion would inevitably result in fatigue failure of some component of the fixation system and that nonunion is the cause of implant failure. Higher forces are generated on an implant applied eccentrically from the line of reaction forces (e.g., a plate and screw device) than on a centromedullary device.[56] Froimson's[26] description of the forces generated by the muscles aids in understanding the displacement of the fracture and also indicates mechanisms for reduction of the fracture fragments (Fig. 45–4). The proximal fragment of the greater trochanteric attachment is abducted by the gluteus medius and minimus muscles. The iliopsoas flexes

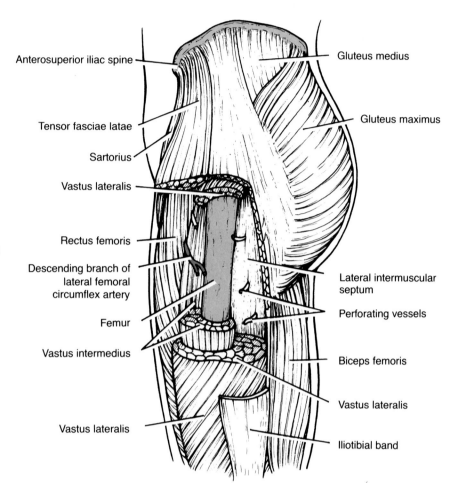

Anterosuperior iliac spine

Tensor fasciae latae

Sartorius

Vastus lateralis

Gluteus medius

Gluteus maximus

Figure 45–2

Lateral anatomy of the hip and subtrochanteric area.

Rectus femoris

Descending branch of lateral femoral circumflex artery

Femur

Vastus intermedius

Vastus lateralis

Lateral intermuscular septum

Perforating vessels

Biceps femoris

Vastus lateralis

Iliotibial band

and externally rotates the proximal fragment if the lesser trochanter is attached. The adductors and hamstrings cause shortening and adduction of the distal fragment, resulting in relative varus of the hip. All three forces must be neutralized for successful immobilization of the fracture. In 1969, Toridis[74] noted the torsional effects of stresses in the subtrochanteric region, an important development in relation to current concepts of static interlocking techniques to reduce the rotational shear forces that may lead to implant failure from cyclic loading. Tencer et al.[72] in 1984 presented a detailed evaluation of implant devices used for subtrochanteric fractures at that time (Fig. 45–5). Their studies included evaluation of Ender pins, the Klemm-Schellmann nail, the Zickle nail, the Grosse-Kempf interlocking nail, the Brooker-Wills nail, and a hip compression screw and blade plate device. They evaluated bending stresses, torsional stresses, and load to axial failure in cadavers with simulated subtrochanteric femoral fractures, evaluating transverse osteotomy and segmental defect models. Interestingly, they reported their results in relation to the femoral bending stiffness of the cadaver femur. They found that inter-

locking nails and Zickle nails approached 75% to 80% of the relative general bending stiffness and Ender pins less than 50% of bending stiffness in the transverse osteotomies. In the fracture with segmental defect, the compression hip screw, which permitted free rotation of the screw shaft inside the side plate barrel, resulted in a marked diminution of stiffness as a result of rotation of the femoral head. With torsional testing, all of the slotted, open-section nails and Ender nails restored less than 5% of the normal femoral torsional stiffness. The plate and screw devices restored approximately 40% of femoral torsional stiffness. When tested in a single load to failure, the Grosse-Kempf and Klemm-Schellmann devices failed at loads of 350% to 400% of body weight. Plate and screw devices failed at approximately 200% of body weight and the Ender system, blade plate, and Brooker-Wills failed at less than 150% body weight. To reduce implant failure and maximize torsional stability, we developed, in 1984, a closed-section, cloverleaf, interlocking centromedullary nail and subsequently a closed-section, interlocking, cephalomedullary nail, the reconstruction nail. The design goals of these implants was to improve fatigue performance and de-

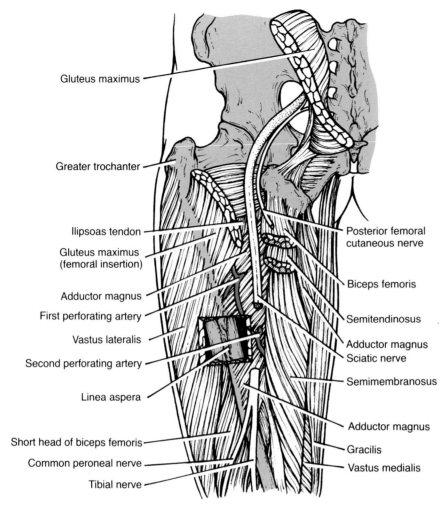

Gluteus maximus

Greater trochanter

Ilipsoas tendon

Gluteus maximus
(femoral insertion)

Adductor magnus

First perforating artery

Vastus lateralis

Second perforating artery

Linea aspera

Short head of biceps femoris

Common peroneal nerve

Tibial nerve

Posterior femoral
cutaneous nerve

Biceps femoris

Semitendinosus

Adductor magnus
Sciatic nerve

Semimembranosus

Adductor magnus

Gracilis

Vastus medialis

Figure 45–3

Posterior anatomy of the hip and
subtrochanteric area.

crease shear at the fracture site by eliminating the longitudinal slot and by varying the wall thickness of the implant to approximate more closely the stiffness of the intact femur. In a subsequent study by Tencer et al.[71] in which the Russell-Taylor femoral nail was tested in the same manner as previous implants, the 15-mm Russell-Taylor femoral nail approximated the intact femur at 106% bending stiffness. Because of the closed-section design, 58% of the intact torsional stiffness of the cadaver femurs was restored. This is a tenfold increase over the torsional stiffness of open-section interlocking nails. When tested for axial load to failure, the Russell-Taylor closed-section femoral nail was the strongest implant tested, failing at 450% of body weight. The Russell-Taylor reconstruction nail was tested in a similar fashion using a 13-mm diameter nail. Because of its greater wall thickness it restored approximately 96% of the bending stiffness of the cadaver femurs, torsional stiffness was the same as for the closed-section, standard Russell-Taylor nail (58% of the intact femur), and axial load to failure was 500% of body weight.

Recently developed compression screws and side plates have sufficient strength and fatigue life that manufacturers are approving their use for subtrochanteric fractures, but only those hip compression screws and side plates indicated for subtrochanteric fractures should be used, as all are not the same with respect to bending strength and fatigue life.

INCIDENCE

Subtrochanteric fractures have been variously defined, but most authors limit the term to fractures occurring between the lesser trochanter and the isthmus of the diaphysis of the femoral shaft. Subtrochanteric fractures account for approximately 10% to 34% of all hip fractures. Boyd and Griffin[8] classified 26.7% as subtrochanteric in their review of 300 hip fractures. Retrospective reviews have noted a bimodal age distribution for these fractures.[6,54,76,77] In their study of subtrochanteric fractures Velasco and Comfort[76] found 63% of subtrochanteric fractures occurred in patients from 51 to more than 70 years old and 24% in patients between 17 and 50 years old. Waddell[77] found a 33% incidence

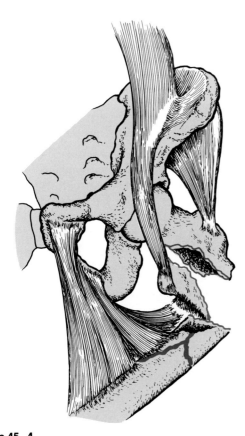

Figure 45–4

Pathologic anatomy: additional deforming forces on subtrochanteric fracture. (Modified from Froimson, A.I.: Surg Gynecol Obstet 131:465, 1970, by permission of SURGERY, GYNECOLOGY, & OBSTETRICS.)

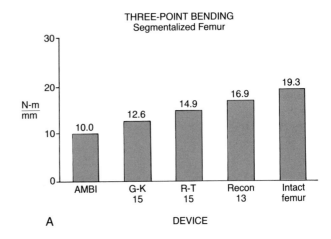

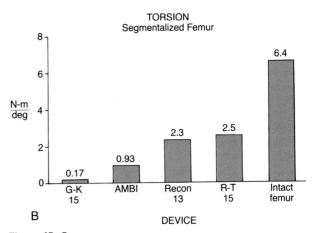

Figure 45–5

A, Three-point bend testing of devices indicated for the use in subtrochanteric fractures in relation to the stiffness of an intact cadaver femur as studied by Tencer et al. *B,* Results of testing of various implants denoting poor resistance to torsional stresses in open section to medullary devices. (Modified from Tencer, A.F., et al. Orthop Biomed Lab Report #002. Memphis, Richards Medical Co., 1985.)

of subtrochanteric fractures in patients 20 to 49 years old and a 7% incidence in patients between 50 and 100 years old in their review of proximal femoral fractures. The mechanism of injury is also different in these different age groups. In younger patients the fracture is more commonly caused by high-energy trauma such as motor vehicle accidents, vehicular-pedestrian accidents, falls from significant heights, or penetrating injuries. In the older age group, fractures occur with low-energy trauma, as in a simple fall. Bergman et al.,[6] in a review of subtrochanteric fractures at a Level I trauma center, noted an average age of 40.6 years in the high-energy trauma group and 76.2 years in the low-energy trauma group. A review of our patients at the Presley Trauma Center (also a Level I trauma center) in Memphis, Tennessee, from 1984 to 1985 revealed that 17% to 44% of proximal third femoral fractures were subtrochanteric, depending on the classification system used. It is anticipated that the increased population of the United States from the "baby boomers" will result in a significant increase in the number of low-energy subtrochanteric fractures over the next two decades.

A third group of patients not considered in detail in this chapter are those with subtrochanteric fractures occurring as a result of pathologic states of the bone (tumors, metastatic bone disease, primary neoplastic processes, or metabolic bone disease). The reader is referred to chapter 17 for more information on the specifics of treatment of these particular injuries.

MECHANISMS OF INJURY

Fractures from low-energy trauma usually involve minimal comminution, and spiral fractures are relatively common. Frequently these fractures occur in more osteopenic bone with widened medullary canals and thinner cortices. Subtrochanteric fractures from high-energy trauma are often associated with comminution over large areas of the proximal femur, indicating significant damage to the soft tissues, even in closed injuries, and frequent compromise of the vascularity of the fracture fragments. Gunshot wounds are a frequent source of high-energy trauma in the subtrochanteric region. In our series, over the past six years approximately 10% of high-energy subtrochanteric fractures were caused by gunshot or shotgun. Excluding penetrating trauma, the majority of subtrochanteric fractures are caused either by direct lateral forces to the proximal thigh (as in side impacts from motor vehicle accidents or from falls from a height) or by axial loading failure in the subtrochanteric region. Low-energy trauma usually results in transverse, short, oblique or spiral fractures. As with femoral shaft fractures, hemorrhage into the soft tissues may be significant. The physician should be attentive to the possible complications of hemorrhage and also compartment syndromes.

ANATOMIC AND FUNCTIONAL CONSEQUENCES OF INJURY

A subtrochanteric fracture results in shortening of the affected extremity and varus positioning of the femoral head and neck, effectively creating a functionally weakened abductor muscle group. If not corrected, the shortening and varus deformity will cause a significant limp and an abductor lurch because of the shortened working length of the abductor muscles. Thus the goals of subtrochanteric fracture management are restoration of normal length and rotation as well as correction of the femoral head and neck angulation to restore adequate tension to the abductor muscles.

COMMONLY ASSOCIATED INJURIES

Significant associated injuries are unusual in patients with low-energy trauma. Contusions and abrasions are most common, but cranial or vertebral injury must be considered. Older patients are frequently on medications that affect their mentation and coordination and may impair their ability to call attention to significant trauma in the cranial or vertebral area. When subtrochanteric fracture is caused by high-energy trauma, total system examination is required, as with all polytrauma patients. Bergman et al.[6] noted that 16 of 31 patients had other injuries to the long bones, pelvis, spine, or viscus. Waddell's[77] retrospective review of eight different hospitals over a six-year period found associated injuries of the cranium, thorax, and abdomen that required surgical treatment in 27 of 130 patients. Twenty of these 27 patients had more than one injury. We have noted a high incidence of ipsilateral patellar and tibial fractures associated wth subtrochan-

teric fractures. These are particularly serious, as they may compromise knee flexion and ankle motion and, coupled with the possible loss of hip flexion, may severely limit the patient's functional ability.

CLASSIFICATION

Boyd and Griffin[8] originally called attention to the subtrochanteric fracture as a variant of peritrochanteric fractures and noted a higher incidence of unsatisfactory results following operative treatment. They also first proposed open reduction and two-plane fixation of complex subtrochanteric injuries.

Classification schemes are useful if they alert the surgeon to potential complications or if they recommend specific treatment options. A review of classification schemes gives insight into the evolution of treatment options for subtrochanteric fractures. Fielding and Magliato[24] devised a three-part classification in 1966 with type I fractures at the level of the lesser trochanter, type II fractures within one inch below the lesser trochanter, and type III fractures within one to two inches of the lesser trochanter. This classification did not take into account extension over a large area or comminution. The Arbeitsgemeinschaft für Osteosysthesefragen/Association for the Study of Internal Fixation (AO/ASIF) group, in the *Manual of Internal Fixation*[51] in 1969, also recommended a three-part classification: simple transverse and oblique fractures, fractures with three major fragments and one fragment being either a medial or lateral butterfly, and fractures with marked comminution. This classification also did not consider trochanteric extension. Zickle,[83] in 1976, reported a six-part classification system that added long spiral fractures and trochanteric extension. He used his classification to help determine whether adjunctive fixation with his interlocking device would be necessary. Seinsheimer,[62] in 1978, presented a rather complex, though concise, classification involving eight subgroups: type I, nondisplaced fractures; type II, fractures with three parts consisting of transverse, oblique, noncomminuted fractures; type III, oblique fractures with medial or lateral butterfly comminution; type IV, fractures with bicortical comminution; and type V, fractures involving bicortical comminution with extension into the trochanteric mass. The significance of Seinsheimer's classification is that it predicted a higher rate of implant failure in those fractures with loss of medial cortical stability. Waddell,[77] in 1979, presented yet another classification with three major subgroups: transverse or short oblique fractures, long oblique fractures, and comminuted fractures with possible extension into the trochanteric mass. Johnson,[37] in 1988, suggested the concept of regionalization based on involvement of the greater trochanteric area, lesser trochanteric area, or area below the lesser trochanter and recomended intramedullary fixation of fractures involving the lesser trochanteric area and below and hip screw fixation of fractures with any evidence of greater trochanteric extension.

The following classification is based on the type of internal fixation that allows the best biomechanical construct with the least vascular damage to the fracture. This classification is based on current techniques of closed intramedullary nailing and interlocking principles and emphasizes the biologic imperatives of preserving vascularity to the fracture fragments and, when appropriate, augmenting fracture repair with bone grafting, as recommended initially by Stewart.[67] Because we believe all fractures with shaft extension, including subtrochanteric fractures, are best treated with a static interlocking nail, comminution of the shaft does not have a direct role in this classification system. The important variables are continuity of the lesser trochanter and extension of the fracture into the greater trochanter and posteriorly involving the piriformis fossa. This region is critical, because it actually dictates whether closed intramedullary techniques requiring an intact starting portal are possible. Extension into the greater trochanter not involving the piriformis fossa

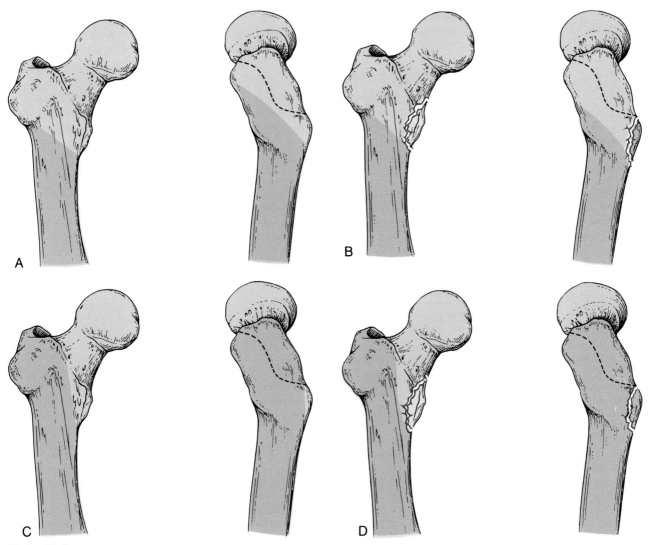

Figure 45–6

Russell-Taylor classification of subtrochanteric fractures. *A,* Type IA: fracture extension with any degree of comminution from below the level of the lesser trochanter to the isthmus with no extension into the piriformis fossa. *B,* Type IB: fracture extension involving the lesser trochanter to the isthmus with no extension into the piriformis fossa. *C,* Type IIA: fracture extension into the piriformis fossa. Stable medial construct. *D,* Type IIB: fracture extension into the piriformis fossa in the lesser trochanteric area with no stability of the medial femoral cortex. (Modified from Tencer, A.F., et al. Orthop Biomed Lab Report #002. Memphis, Richards Medical Co., 1985.)

does not affect the use of closed interlocking nailing. This classification divides subtrochanteric fractures into two major groups, each of which has two subgroups. Group I fractures do not extend into the piriformis fossa, so intramedullary nailing techniques are possible. In type IA fractures, comminution and fracture lines extend from below the lesser trochanter to the femoral isthmus; any degree of comminution may be involved in this area, including bicortical comminution (Fig. 45–6A). Type IB fractures have fracture lines and comminution involving the area of the lesser trochanter to the isthmus (Fig. 45–6B). Because the lesser trochanter is not intact and is out of continuity with the proximal fragment, conventional diagonal interlocking screw techniques are not effective, and a cephalomedullary interlocking nail technique is required. In both types IA and IB, however, closed intramedullary nailing techniques have the biologic advantage of minimizing vascular compromise of the fracture fragments. Group II fractures extend proximally into the greater trochanter and involve the piriformis fossa, as detected on the lateral radiograph of the hip; such involvement of the greater trochanter complicates closed nailing techniques. Type IIA fractures extend from the lesser trochanter to the isthmus with extension into the piriformis fossa, but significant comminution or major fracture of the lesser trochanter is not present (Fig. 45–6C). In a type IIB fracture there is extension into the greater trochanteric area with significant comminution of the medial femoral cortex and loss of continuity of the lesser trochanter (Fig. 45–6D).

Diagnosis

HISTORY

The patient's history is most significant in determining whether the fracture occurred from high-energy or low-energy trauma. Patients who report minimal trauma or no trauma associated with their subtrochanteric fracture should be extensively evaluated to rule out preexisting pathologic bone disease. The common complaint of all patients with subtrochanteric fractures is the inability to bear weight on the affected extremity. Most patients require transport to the hospital by ambulance because of pain with any attempted movement of the extremity.

PHYSICAL EXAMINATION

The patient is usually apprehensive and in pain from the injury. Examination most often reveals a shortened extremity and swelling of the thigh. Internal or external rotation of the foot results from loss of continuity at the fracture site. Patients are unable to flex the hip actively or move it through a range of motion. Neurologic or vascular deficits are unusual with these fractures unless they are the result of a penetrating injury. On palpation, prominence of the proximal fragment as a result of flexion, abduction, and external rotation of the hip is common.

RADIOGRAPHIC IMAGING

Radiographic evaluation consists of full length views of the femur from the hip to the knee in both the anteroposterior and lateral views. Scrutiny of the pelvis and knee on radiograph is essential because of the frequency of associated injuries. We obtain a cross-table lateral radiograph of the affected hip to detect any trochanteric extension that may exit either anteriorly or posteriorly into the piriformis fossa. Because of treatment ramifications, attention to the inner and outer diameter of the medullary canal, the curvature of the femoral shaft, the neck-shaft angle of the unaffected side, and any preexisting deformities or implants of the femur should be noted. Further radiographic views are usually unnecessary except to rule out associated injuries. In patients with neurologic deficits, further evaluation is indicated to rule out intraspinal or lumbosacral plexus injury, as sciatic nerve injury is rare in subtrochanteric fractures. In severely comminuted fractures, we use an intraoperative scanogram ruler on the normal side to measure length, then use the traction table or the femoral distractor to obtain proper length of the affected extremity. In penetrating trauma, arteriograms may be required to diagnose vascular injury.

DIFFERENTIAL DIAGNOSIS

Differential diagnosis of subtrochanteric fractures essentially requires only discrimination between purely traumatic lesions and underlying pathologic lesions. When the patient gives a history of preinjury pain or limp or of metastatic disease, the surgeon should always be prepared to perform a biopsy of the proximal femur during surgical repair.

Management

As with any complex fracture, subtrochanteric femoral fractures require the surgeon to assess his or her own abilities when choosing operative or nonoperative treatment. The most pertinent question is by which method can sufficient stabilization of the fracture be obtained without vascular compromise of the fracture

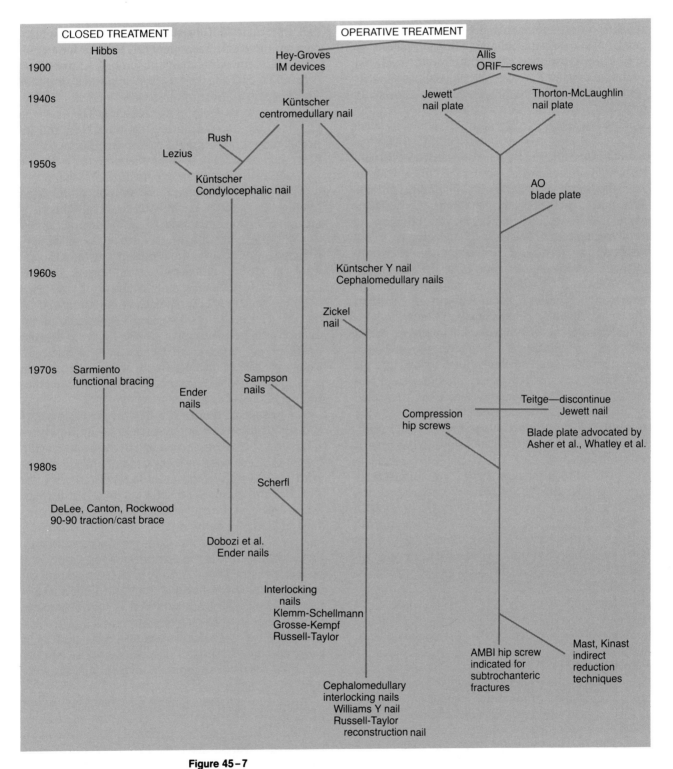

Figure 45–7

Evolution of treatment of subtrochanteric fracture since the 1900s.

fragments. Because of the high level of mechanical stress about the proximal third of the femur, longevity of the implant has been a major concern. Nonoperative modalities such as traction and bracing have been advocated to avoid complications of implant failure, especially in young active patients, and several variations of internal fixation have been developed and popularized for treatment of this difficult fracture (Fig. 45–7).

EVOLUTION OF TREATMENT

In 1891, Allis[1] analyzed the deforming forces on subtrochanteric fractures and, noting the difficulty in obtaining satisfactory reducton with longitudinal traction alone, advised surgical treatment. Hibbs,[34] in 1902, attempted to improve traction results by bringing the distal fragment to the deviated proximal fragment. Recent comparative series have shown rather dismal results with conventional traction treatment. In a retrospective review of traction treatment of nondisplaced fractures and fractures in patients unsuited for surgical treatment, Waddell[77] noted that although nondisplaced fractures did well with traction treatment, only 4 of 11 patients with displaced fractures obtained satisfactory results with Thomas splint traction. Of four patients treated with 90-90 skeletal traction, three had satisfactory results. Velasco and Comfort[76] reported that of 22 adult subtrochanteric fractures treated with traction, half had unsatisfactory results, with significant shortening, varus or valgus deformity, or persistent peroneal palsy.

In the late 1960s and early 1970s, femoral cast bracing was popularized by Sarmiento,[59] but most reports indicated frequent poor results with this method in proximal femoral fractures.[50] However, Sarmiento stated that cast bracing was not indicated for fractures of the proximal third of the femur. DeLee et al.[19] reported 15 subtrochanteric fractures treated with 90-90 traction followed by fracture bracing with a hinged-knee, single-hip spica cast. All fractures united, and there were no refractures. They recommended this treatment protocol for patients with inoperable or open fractures.

Boyd and Griffin[8] identified subtrochanteric fractures as having the highest incidence of loss of reduction and migration of the distal fragment medially as well as frequent coxa vara deformity after healing (Fig. 45–8A). They reported good preliminary results with the use of the Jewett nail.[36] From the 1940s to the 1960s, the Jewett nail was probably the most frequently used device for fixation of subtrochanteric femoral fractures. Concerns about fatigue failure led Jewett to design, specifically for subtrochanteric fractures, a special nail consisting of two plates welded together for

anterior and lateral fixation; however, this nail did not gain widespread acceptance. Reports documented failure rates of approximately 20% to 30% with the Jewett nail, and in 1976 Teitge,[69] in a study of 155 subtrochanteric fractures, recommended that the Jewett nail not be used for subtrochanteric femoral fractures.

In 1978, Hanson and Tullos[31] reported an 87.5% union rate in 42 fractures treated with a nail-plate device and prolonged non–weight bearing. The AO blade plate became popular during the late 1970s, and reported success rates with the device varied from 65% to 85%, with most authors recommending the AO plate for transverse subtrochanteric fractures.[80] Asher et al.[5] recommended its primary use in noncomminuted fractures and stressed the importance of interfragmentary compression, anatomic reduction, and placement of the blade under tension. In 1989, Kinast et al.[42] reported union in all fractures treated with the AO plate when (1) extensive preoperative planning was done, (2) the AO blade plate and femoral distractor were used without dissection of the medial comminution, and (3) prophylactic antibiotics were used. When anatomic reduction required dissection of the fracture, delayed union or nonunion occurred in 16.6% of fractures. They also stressed the importance of obtaining a stable construct with interfragmentary compression and tensioning of the AO plate.

The popularization of the compression hip screw and sliding hip screw in the early 1970s improved results because of the impaction and dynamization at the fracture site provided by these implants. Waddell[77] reported a 10% failure or nonunion rate in 21 fractures with the hip compression screw, noting that it functioned as an intramedullary nail in the femoral neck. Wile et al.[81] and Berman et al.[7] reported no implant failures in 25 and 38 subtrochanteric fractures, respectively, with the use of the compression hip screw. Berman et al.[7] added bone grafting in all fractures and lag screw fixation when possible. Ruff and Lubbers[55] obtained union in 95% of their series of subtrochanteric fractures, most of which were comminuted. They recommended valgus reduction, medial displacement of the shaft, and insertion of only the lag screw into the proximal fragment to promote impaction of the fracture.

Intramedullary nails can be designated as *centromedullary*, *condylocephalic*, or *cephalomedullary*. *Centromedullary* nails are contained within the medullary canal and are usually inserted from the piriformis fossa; if of interlocking design, the screws are inserted into the metaphyseal-diaphyseal area proximally and distally. *Condylocephalic* nails (e.g., Ender nails) are inserted into the femoral condyle and extend into the femoral head and neck. *Cephalomedullary* nails are

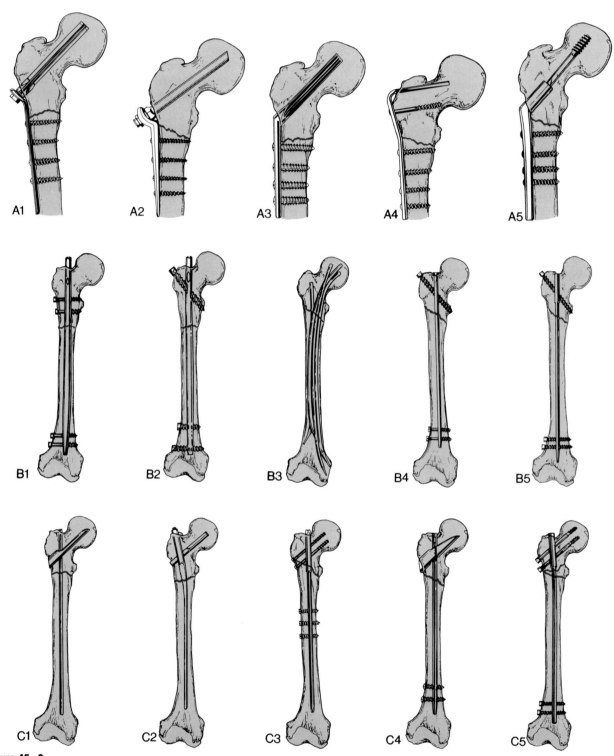

Figure 45–8

A, Evolution of plate design. (1) Thornton device. (2) McLaughlin nail plate. (3) Jewett nail plate. (4) AO blade plate. (5) Richards hip compression screw. *B,* Centromedullary and condylocephalic devices. (1) Küntscher interlocking screws and detensor. (2) Klemm-Schellmann device with diagonal proximal locking screw. (3) Ender condylocephalic devices. (4) Grosse-Kempf interlocking device. (5) Russell-Taylor closed section interlocking femoral nail. *C,* Cephalomedullary implants with proximal fragment stabilization by internal fixation into the femoral head and neck. (1) Küntscher Y nail, (2) Zickle device, (3) Huckstep nail, (4) Williams Y nail, (5) Russell-Taylor reconstruction interlocking nail. (Redrawn from Calandruccio, R.A., Chairman, AAOS Committee on the History of Orthopaedic Surgery. Internal fixation devices for fractures of the proximal femur. Exhibit at the 55th Annual Meeting, Atlanta, February 4–9, 1988.)

interlocking centromedullary nails with screw devices that can be inserted cephalad into the femoral head and neck, such as the Zickle nail and the Russell-Taylor reconstruction nail.

Anecdotal reports of intramedullary nailing techniques were present as early as 1918 when Hey-Groves[33] reported centromedullary nailing of a subtrochanteric fracture resulting from a gunshot wound. Küntscher[44] first reported intramedullary nailing of subtrochanteric fractures in 1939. Aronoff et al.[4] reported good results with centromedullary nails, particularly for reoperation of nonunions of subtrochanteric fractures. Interest in these techniques was revived in the late 1960s and early 1970s, particularly for the Zickle and Ender nails. The Zickle device, introduced in 1967,[84] consisted of a strong, solid, rectangular rod with a cross bolt engaging the femoral head. Küntscher had designed a Y nail with similar biomechanical principles but not with the strength of Zickle's device. In 1976, Zickle[83] reported nine years' experience with his cephalomedullary interlocking nail and reported union in 75 of 76 fractures, 26 of which required accessory fixation for either obliquity or comminution. During the late 1970s and early 1980s, the Zickle device became the treatment of choice for pathologic subtrochanteric fractures.[70] In 1987, Bergman et al.[6] classified 154 subtrochanteric fractures treated with the Zickle device as high-energy trauma, pathologic fractures, low-energy trauma, or previous failures of internal fixation. Union was obtained in approximately 90% in each group. They recommended the Zickle device for low-energy trauma but preferred other forms of fixation for high-energy trauma because of frequent comminution; they suggested the use of interlocking nail techniques that control shortening and rotation.

Proponents of the Ender technique suggested that this resulted in lower morbidity and less blood loss when compared with the open technique. Some reports, however, suggested high incidences of knee pain, rotational deformity, and instability.[46] Those familiar with the Ender technique obtained good results if certain criteria were met.[22,53] Common factors in most reports of successful use of the Ender technique included low-energy fractures, minimal comminution, and elderly patients. The larger medullary canals in these patients allow entry into the canal with four or five Ender pins from both medial and lateral portals.

Other intramedullary nailing techniques reported include that of Heiple et al.,[32] who modified the Sampson nail by expanding it proximally in an attempt to control rotation. Scherfel[61] reported good results in 16 fractures treated with a special nail with fins in the proximal portion to control rotation.

The biomechanical advantages of centromedullary,

condylocephalic, and cephalomedullary implants were well recognized, as were their shortcomings in controlling rotation and shortening. In three large series[10,28,66] of subtrochanteric fractures presented at the 1987 American Academy of Orthopaedic Surgeons (AAOS) meeting, the addition of interlocking capability to intramedullary nails achieved the highest union rates ever reported in high-energy trauma. These nails were limited, however, by the requirements of an intact entry portal in the greater trochanter in relation to the piriformis fossa and an intact lesser trochanter for proximal fixation (Fig. 45–8B).

The Russell-Taylor reconstruction interlocking nail combines the advantages of cephalomedullary implants with distal interlocking to prevent rotation and shortening. As with earlier implants, preoperative planning includes evaluation for fracture extension into the greater trochanter and particularly into the piriformis fossa, which is the entry portal for this device. Because of two-screw fixation in the femoral head, however, rotation is well maintained, and the lesser trochanter does not have to be intact (Fig. 45–8C).

CURRENT ALGORITHM

The choice of treatment for subtrochanteric fractures depends on several factors (Fig. 45–9). Balanced (90-90) traction, possibly followed with a hinged-knee hip spica cast brace, as advocated by DeLee et al.,[19] remains a viable option, although it does not provide for early mobilization of the multiply injured patient. Furthermore, in elderly patients, nonoperative treatment of subtrochanteric fractures should generally be limited to situations in which the patient's medical situation makes the risks of surgery excessive or in which bone quality is so poor that there is no hope of secure fixation.

Fixation for subtrochanteric fractures is determined according to fracture configuration. Type IA fractures, with intact trochanters, are most effectively managed with closed insertion of a conventional interlocked centromedullary IM nail (Fig. 45–10). In type IB subtrochanteric fractures, with extension into the lesser trochanter, the cephalomedullary reconstruction interlocking nail is indicated (Fig. 45–11).

For type IIA and IIB fractures, with comminution of the greater trochanter including the piriformis fossa, modern hip compression screws offer reliable fixation. A hip compression screw with a locking barrel should be used to limit rotation of the femoral head (Fig. 45–12). If the hip compression screw is to function as a dynamically interlocked device, then placement of the screws through the plate and into the proximal frag-

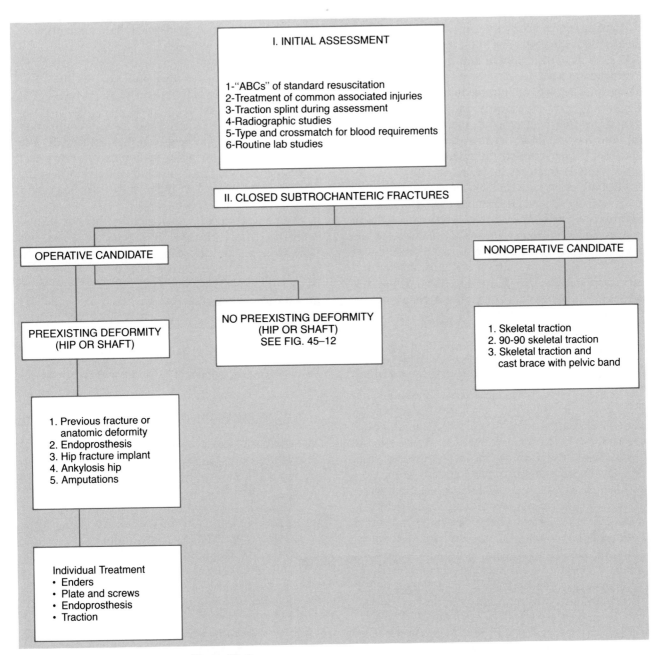

Figure 45–9

Algorithm for the treatment of closed subtrochanteric fractures.

ment must be avoided, as they could maintain distraction of the fracture.

Other alternatives may be considered, although they appear to offer less predictable results. Kinast et al.[42] achieved a 100% success rate using a blade-plate with the indirect reduction technique. Sanders et al.[58] were less successful when this technique was used with a 95° condylar screw device. The Zickle nail has been advocated for type II fractures, with adjunctive fixation of the comminuted greater trochanteric region.[6,83] Ceph-

alomedullary nailing is more difficult when comminution involves the nail insertion site. Experience with cerclage wiring techniques may be helpful for gaining secure fixation of the trochanteric fragments.

Ender nailing should be reserved for those patients in whom other treatment options are not feasible, such as those with severe soft tissue trauma about the proximal buttock and hip that prohibits a direct approach to the proximal femur. Plate and screw fixation of subtrochanteric fractures probably is indicated only for frac-

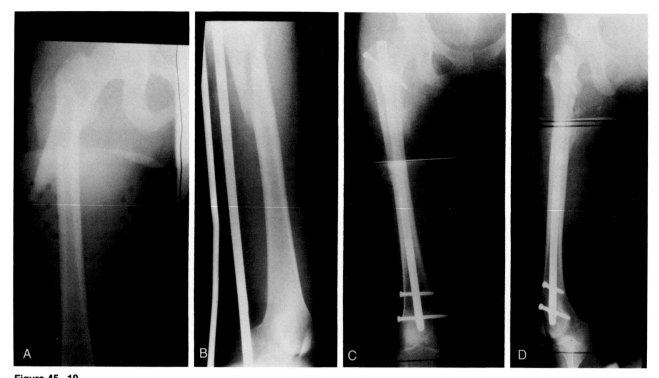

Figure 45–10

Eighty-year-old female with a type IA subtrochanteric fracture from motor vehicle accident. *A* and *B*, Anteroposterior preoperative radiographs; lesser trochanter is intact and in continuity with the proximal fragment. *C* and *D*, Anteroposterior radiographs five months after fracture showing healing.

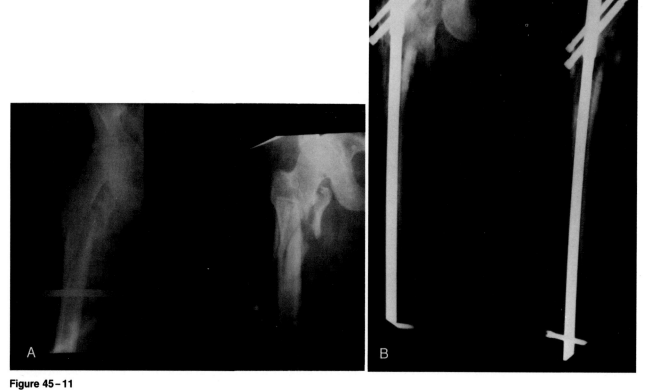

Figure 45–11

Russell-Taylor type 1B fracture in 39-year-old male, sustained while parachuting. *A*, Preoperative radiographs. *B*, Postoperative radiographs after immediate fixation with Russell-Taylor reconstruction nail in static locking mode.

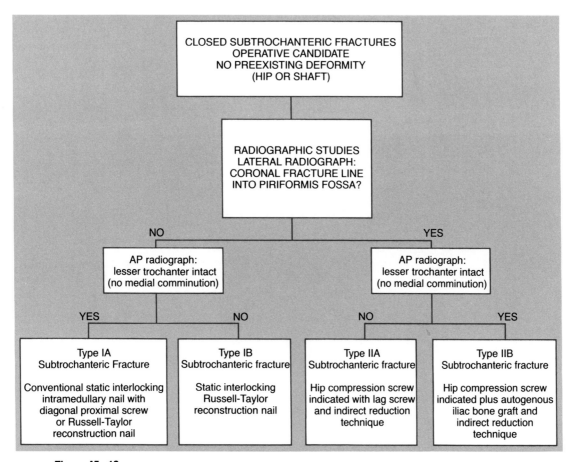

Figure 45-12

Algorithm for operative treatment of closed subtrochanteric fractures using Russell-Taylor classification.

tures associated with preexisting deformities of the proximal femur or previous implants (as in hip arthrodesis or arthroplasty). External fixation is reserved for open fractures with severe contamination or for intermediate treatment of complications from previous failed internal fixation. Pathologic fractures of the subtrochanteric area (see chapter 17) are best treated with cephalomedullary implants, such as the Zickle or reconstruction nail, that allow prophylactic stabilization of the entire femur from the knee to the femoral head.

INDICATIONS FOR BONE GRAFTING

The use of autogenous bone grafting in subtrochanteric fractures has been suggested by numerous authors since the 1960s, especially for revision of failed internal fixation. Stewart,[67] in a discussion of the presentation of Watson et al.[79] in 1964, advocated acute autogenous iliac bone grafting of traumatic subtrochanteric fractures in young patients. Autogenous bone grafting is indicated during open reduction of fractures with sig-

nificant comminution of the medial wall. Closed technique obviates the need for bone grafting, possibly because the fracture fragments are not devascularized as much as with open reduction.

OPEN SUBTROCHANTERIC FRACTURES

Open subtrochanteric fractures are rare and are almost always associated either with penetrating trauma or with high-energy trauma from motor vehicle accidents or falls from heights. The same principles that apply to all open fractures apply as well to subtrochanteric fractures: immediate surgical debridement and, after conversion to a clean contaminated wound, stabilization to help resist infection (Fig. 45-13). The goal is to use the minimum fixation necessary to adequately stabilize the subtrochanteric fracture. In the past, this has presented problems, because most methods for stabilization of subtrochanteric fractures involve further tissue dissection and contamination of tissue planes, prompting DeLee et al.[19] to recommend 90-90 traction and cast bracing for open subtrochanteric fractures. John-

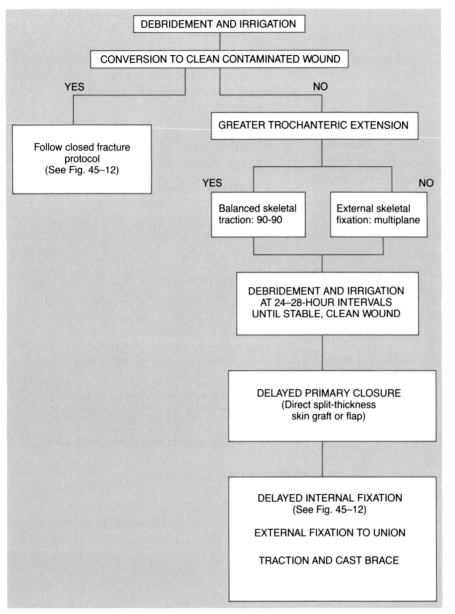

Figure 45-13

Algorithm for treatment of open subtrochanteric fractures.

son[37] recommended intramedullary fixation of subtrochanteric fractures after adequate debridement and conversion to a clean contaminated wound, either acutely or 10 to 21 days later, after delayed primary closure.

We prefer immediate internal fixation of open subtrochanteric fractures of types I though IIIA (Gustilo classification) after adequate debridement and with combined cephalosporin and aminoglycoside antibiotic coverage. We believe that all wounds should be left open, except for extensions, with repeat debridement at 24 to 48 hours and as often as necessary until either

delayed primary closure or plastic surgical wound coverage is obtained. We use external fixation for type IIIB or IIIC subtrochanteric fractures when the proximal fragment is large enough to insert pins in a delta configuration or when the fracture is accompanied by vascular injury requiring repair and the wound cannot be converted to a clean contaminated wound with the initial debridement and irrigation. With the advent of newer implants and techniques, we are exploring the option of nonreamed interlocking nail techniques for the treatment of open subtrochanteric fractures and believe that this will be a significant improvement over the standard operative management of these fractures as it allows a stable mechanical construct without the increased devascularization caused by reaming.

SPECIAL CONSIDERATIONS FOR POLYTRAUMA PATIENTS

There is now sufficient documentation in both retrospective and prospective studies to justify immediate (within the first 24 hours) stabilization of long-bone injuries in polytrauma patients.[20,47] The subtrochanteric fracture is certainly an injury requiring immediate stabilization to obtain the benefits of early mobilization and to avoid traction syndrome in the polytrauma patient. Maximum effort should be made to obtain stabilization, either internally or externally, in this group of patients because of their susceptibility to pulmonary failure and septic states.[13] When other injuries involve the ipsilateral extremity, we first attempt to stabilize the injury that will keep the patient in bed. If the patient's condition deteriorates (intraoperatively) and surgery cannot be continued, closed methods are used until the patient is stable enough for surgery.

DESCRIPTION OF INDIVIDUAL PROCEDURES

Traction

The technique of DeLee et al.[19] is recommended for treatment of subtrochanteric fractures with traction. Skeletal traction is applied with a femoral pin, if possible, to avoid traction through the knee; however, tibial traction has been used successfully. The hip is suspended in a 90-90 fashion, and the leg and foot are placed in a well-padded short-leg cast with the foot in a plantigrade position. This may be done with local or general anesthesia. For the average adult, initial traction is 30 to 40 pounds (13.6 to 18.2 kg). Appropriate adjustments are made under radiographic control until satisfactory reduction is obtained in both anteroposterior and lateral views: less than 5° of varus or valgus angulation and at least 25% apposition of the fracture fragments on both views. Shortening of more than 1 cm is avoided. After approximately three to four weeks, as the patient's symptoms subside, the leg is gradually lowered into a less flexed position, with abduction as necessary to prevent varus angulation. When clinical union has been obtained, as indicated by restoration of clinical continuity (rotation of the distal thigh yielding rotation of the greater trochanter) and early callus formation on radiographs, the patient may be placed in a cast brace with a pelvic band and a good quadrilateral

mold. We usually incorporate the traction pin in the cast. The patient is then taught transfers out of bed and touch-down weight-bearing ambulation is allowed with a built-up shoe on the contralateral leg. Radiographs should be made weekly and if signs of lost reduction occur, manipulation and recasting or traction should be performed as necessary.

Sliding Hip Screw

For open reduction and internal fixation of fractures with type IIA and IIB patterns, biomechanical and clinical studies indicate the use of a hip compression screw system that is approved for use in subtrochanteric fractures of the femur.[35,45,49,78] The newer hip screws and side plates have improved fatigue characteristics over the first generation devices. For example, we have had good results with the AMBI Hip Screw System (Richards) over the past several years and have no documented fatigue failures of this device. Fixation failures usually result from cutout of the screw from the femoral head rather than from fracture of the plate as with the first generation implants.[3,38,39] The general technique of insertion of the compression screw is described in chapter 44; only specific references to subtrochanteric fractures are included here. As noted previously, hip compression screws are preferred for open reduction and internal fixation of type IIA or IIB fractures for which interlocking nail techniques are complicated because of involvement of the piriformis fossa (Fig. 45–14). Contraindications to open reduction and internal fixation, other than general medical contraindications, are related to potential problems in obtaining stability. If the patient has osteoporosis to such a degree that internal fixation will not hold, the fracture should be considered pathologic. Adjunctive use of methylmethacrylate may permit secure fixation of such injuries. Surgery should be performed within 24 hours of injury if possible; if not, the patient is placed in skeletal traction. If this is not done, the hydraulic forces generated from the bleeding of the subtrochanteric fracture into the surrounding muscle groups may make intraoperative restoration of length quite difficult and may result in stretch injury to the neurologic structures or compartment syndrome.

Hip screw fixation of subtrochanteric fractures is difficult, and frequently 2 to 6 hours of surgery and several units of blood replacement are required. Detailed preoperative planning is mandatory, including measurement of the head and neck angle for selection of the hip screw device and correct length side plate. Lag screw fixation of major fragments should be carefully

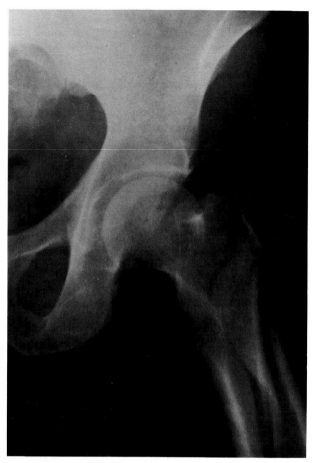

Figure 45-14

Russell-Taylor type IIA subtrochanteric fracture with fracture extension into the piriformis fossa; medial cortex stable after reduction.

planned to avoid placing the screws in areas that will compromise plate application.

The patient, usually under general anesthesia, is placed supine on a fracture table. The iliac crest is draped in the operative field to allow procurement of autogenous iliac bone graft if necessary. It is important to avoid internal rotation when securing the foot in the fracture table. We use the image intensifier to determine the correct position of the femoral head and match the rotation of the lower extremity to this; however, during reduction of the proximal femur, adjustments of the fracture table may be required before definitive fixation. A straight lateral incision is made over the hip. Rather than a muscle-splitting approach, we prefer to incise the fascia of the vastus lateralis and reflect the muscle from the intermuscular septum, trying to identify and individually ligate each perforating vessel. These vessels should not be cauterized, because they frequently retract, resume bleeding, and may be difficult to control. The relationship of the linea aspera should be noted as a further check of correct rotational

alignment of the fracture reduction. We prefer the AO femoral distractor and the technique of indirect reduction advocated by Kinast et al.[42] for open reduction and internal fixation of subtrochanteric fractures (Fig. 45-15). Avoiding dissection medially helps to preserve the vascularity of the fracture fragments. The femoral distractor is usually positioned anterior to the incision with Schanz screws proximally in the greater trochanteric area and distally in the shaft. Gradual distraction can then be carried out.

After provisional reduction is obtained and held with Kirschner wires, the hip compression screw is inserted in the standard manner. It is important to attach the plate to the distal fragment with at least four screws engaging a minimum of eight cortices. Lag screws may be used through the plate, but it is preferable to avoid fixing the plate to the proximal fragment, as this will prevent the compression screw from telescoping and thus interfere with impaction of the fracture (Fig. 45-16). We believe it is imperative to use a hip compression screw device that prevents rotation of the lag screw in the barrel. If medial dissection is necessary, autogenous iliac bone grafting should be performed. Most problems of implant fixation can be prevented by obtaining good quality radiographic control during internal fixation of the fracture. After debridement of any devitalized tissue, the wounds should be closed in layers over drainage tubes in the standard fashion (Figs. 45-17 and 45-18).

Follow-up Care and Rehabilitation

The patient is allowed to sit in a chair the day after surgery, and ambulation with touch-down weight bearing is begun when quadriceps control is regained. In the elderly patient, a walker may be preferable to crutches. We do not routinely remove hip compression scews in elderly patients. In young patients involved in competitive sports or employed in heavy manual labor, we offer implant removal two years after surgery if solid union is confirmed radiographically. The patient is cautioned to use crutches with weight bearing to tolerance for six weeks after removal of the implant and to avoid all contact sports for three months. This may be overly cautious, but with this protocol we have not experienced refracture of the subtrochanteric region.

Condylocephalic Nail

In our experience, indications for condylocephalic nailing of subtrochanteric fractures are few. We prefer it in patients who have traumatized skin over the proximal hip area that makes the incisions for either hip compression screws or closed nailing procedures undesirable. The technique may be useful in the elderly

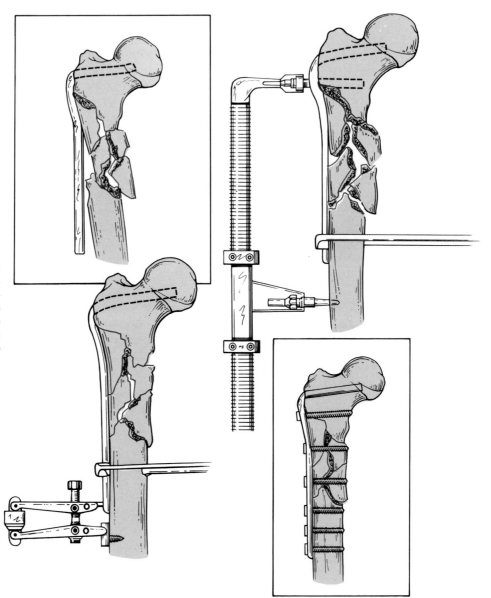

Figure 45-15

Indirect reduction technique using the AO femoral distractor described by Kinast et al.[42] allows satisfactory reduction of the fracture without devascularization of the major fragments. (Redrawn from Kinast, C., et al. Clin Orthop 238:122, 1989.)

patient with a large femoral canal that allows introduction of at least four or five Ender pins. As a rule, we believe the Ender technique for subtrochanteric fractures is contraindicated if more stable fixation techniques can be used. As with other techniques, condylocephalic nailing should be done within the first 24 hours, if possible, or as soon as the patient can be stabilized medically. For details of the procedure, the reader is referred to chapter 44. Following the recommendations of Dobozi et al.,[21] both medial and lateral entry portals should be used, along with a fracture table with image control with the patient supine. It is important to use a Lowman clamp about the femur just proximal to both entry portals to avoid fracture extension, which may cause a supracondylar fracture. Transverse or short oblique fractures with minimal comminution are the most suitable for this type of fixation; if adjunctive fixation is required, we prefer a more conventional form of stabilization—an interlocking nail or hip compression screw. Postoperative care may range from several weeks of traction to mobilization as described for hip compression screws. A frequent difficulty is obtaining full knee motion postoperatively, especially if pins are inserted too anteriorly or are allowed to protrude into the supracondylar region. Loss of fixation also is common.

Interlocked Intramedullary Nail

Femoral interlocking nail systems allow centromedullary fixation of most femoral fractures, including those

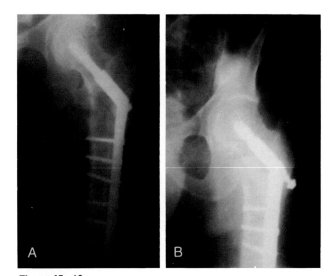

Figure 45-16

Russell-Taylor type IIA fracture. A, Postoperative stabilization with compression hip screw. B, Impaction of fracture fragments without loss of correct neck-shaft angle.

with severe or segmental comminution between the distal fifth of the femur and a point just distal to the lesser trochanter. Grosse et al.[29] established guidelines for intramedullary nailing of femoral fractures: stable fractures of the isthmus (transverse, short oblique, spiral, or mildly comminuted fractures of the lateral cortex) are treated with an unlocked nail; fractures proximal to the isthmus, with proximal locking; and more distal fractures, with one or two distal locking screws. Although excellent results have been reported when following these guidelines, most large series include some patients with postoperative shortening because of unrecognized nondisplaced cracks in the cortex or overestimation of fracture stability. In our experience and that of others, union can be achieved in almost all fractures with static interlocking and rotation, and length can be better controlled. Dynamization (removal of the distal screws) is seldom required for fracture healing.[11]

Preoperative Planning

Preoperative radiographs of the uninjured femur are used to estimate proper nail diameter, the expected amount of reaming, and the final nail length. Proper length of the extremity should be obtained with traction before closed antegrade intramedullary nailing, except in acute cases. Nail length should permit the proximal end to lie flush with the greater trochanter and the distal end to lie between the proximal pole of the patella and the distal femoral physeal scar. Subtrochanteric fractures should be stabilized immediately if the patient's general condition is stable. Most patients receive a perioperative cephalosporin antibiotic for 24 hours unless contraindicated by drug allergy. For open fractures, tobramycin is also given, usually for three days, pending the results of operative cultures.

Surgical Procedure (Russell-Taylor Femoral Intramedullary Nail System)

General anesthesia is most commonly used, but spinal or epidural anesthesia may be used if desired. Anesthesia is usually administered with the patient on the traction bed or stretcher, and then several assistants move the patient to the fracture table. The fracture table should permit easy access to the patient and complete exposure of the femur on both anteroposterior and lateral radiographic projections. Buttock supports can be used to gently internally rotate most patients with subtrochanteric fractures and give a more usual anteroposterior view rather than the frequent externally rotated

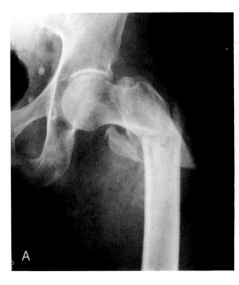

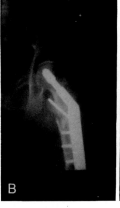

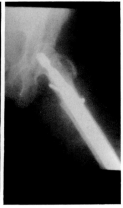

Figure 45-17

Russell-Taylor type IIB subtrochanteric fracture in 50-year-old female. A, Compression hip screw fixation two days after injury. B, Anteroposterior and lateral postoperative radiographs.

Figure 45–18

Russell-Taylor type IIB subtrochanteric fracture. *A*, Anteroposterior radiograph shows comminution of the medial femoral cortex and extension into the piriformis fossa. *B*, After treatment with hip compression screw (note reduction of extension into piriformis fossa on lateral view).

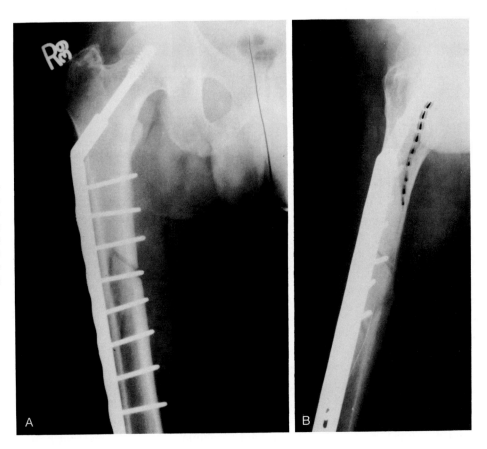

view (Fig. 45–19). If the standard centromedullary interlocking nail is used for a fracture distal to the lesser trochanter, either anteroposterior or lateral position is possible, but we strongly recommend the supine position because it is easier for the anesthesiologist, is more familiar to radiographic technicians, and allows for rapid preparation of patients with bilateral injuries. We recommend only the supine position for insertion of the reconstruction cephalomedullary nail.

With the patient in the supine position, adduct the affected extremity, bend the trunk laterally toward the opposite side, flex the affected hip approximately 10° to 15°, and apply traction through a skeletal pin or the foot (Fig. 45–20). Estimate correct rotational alignment with respect to the normal anteversion of the hip as determined with image intensification. With a normal anteversion of 15° to 20°, the plane of motion of the knee is in the sagittal plane (Fig. 45–21*A*). The second ray of the foot will usually be pointed vertically. When the patient is initially placed on the fracture table, the proximal fracture fragment may be externally rotated as much as 45° to 50° (Fig. 45–21*B*) and the plane of the femoral neck will not match that of the femoral condyles, requiring the foot to be turned out to match this external rotation (Fig. 45–21*C*). The buttock support can be used to internally rotate the proxi-

mal fragment somewhat, or a "cheater pin" or small guide wire drilled into the proximal fragment can be used. Another method of estimating rotation or anteversion of the proximal fragment is to place a small guide wire along the anterior femoral neck (Fig. 45–22*A,B*). A final check is made by placing the skin tension lines in their most relaxed position. The normal hip should be in neutral to very slight flexion. The entire femur from knee to hip should be examined on both anteroposterior and lateral image intensifier projections. The projected axis of the shaft is 1 to 1.5 cm posterior to the center of the femoral neck. The entry site for the guide wire must be placed in line with the shaft axis Fig. 45–23).

Scrub and prepare the affected extremity from several centimeters below the tibial tubercle to the peroneal post and from the midline to the fracture table as far proximally as the lower ribs. Drape the operative field from the level of the umbilicus proximally to the tibial tubercle distally and from approximately the midsagittal posterior and anterior lines of the extremity. A vertical isolation drape may be used, or the image intensifier may be covered with a sterile drape.

Make an oblique skin incision extending from the tip of the greater trochanter proximally and slightly posteriorly in line with the femur for 6 to 8 cm (Fig. 45–

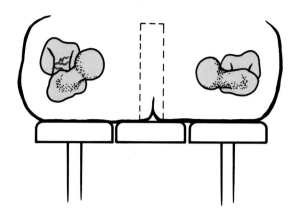

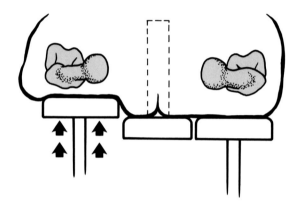

Figure 45–19

Buttock support used to internally rotate proximal fragment. (Courtesy of Campbell Clinic, Memphis, Tennessee.)

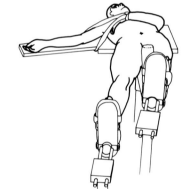

Figure 45–20

Patient in supine position with trunk and lower extremities adducted and affected hip flexed approximately 15°. (Courtesy of Smith and Nephew, Richards Co.)

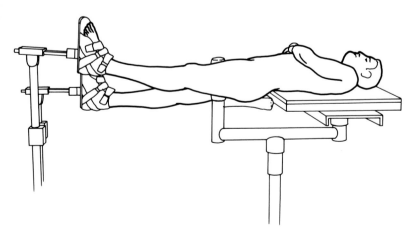

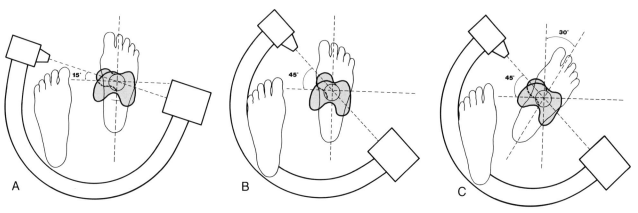

Figure 45–21

A, Normal radiographic anatomy with foot and knee aligned in midsagittal plane and femoral head and neck anteverted 15°. *B*, Typical radiographic anatomy of subtrochanteric fracture; proximal fragment is externally rotated an additional 30°. *C*, With additional external rotation of proximal fragment, foot and knee must be externally rotated to match. (Courtesy of Campbell Clinic, Memphis, Tennessee.)

24*A*). Incise the fascia of the gluteus maximus in line with the skin incision. Divide the gluteus maximus in line with its fibers, identify the subfascial plane, palpate the trochanteric region, and identify the piriformis fossa. Insert a 3.2-mm threaded guide pin into the piriformis fossa, taking care to place the pin in the midline of the femur in both anteroposterior and lateral projections (Fig. 45–24*B*). Enlarge the entry portal with a rigid cannulated reamer or introduce an awl into the piriformis fossa. Remove the small-tip threaded guide pin and reamer and, with the guide wire holder, insert the ball-tip reamer guide wire to the level of the fracture (Fig. 45–24*C*). Confirm containment of this guide wire in the femur on both anteroposterior and lateral views. If indicated, ream the proximal femur to a diameter of 12 mm, reaming in 0.5-mm increments with flexible cannulated reamers, using the skin protector. With the internal fracture alignment device or a

small intramedullary nail, reduce the proximal fragment to the distal fragment. A crutch or other supporting device under the distal fragment may be helpful. Advance the guide wire into the center of the distal fragment until the tip reaches the physeal scar (Fig. 45–24*D*). Remove the internal fracture alignment device and verify containment of the guide wire within the femur by image intensification. Determine proper nail length by using either a second guide wire or the nail length gauge. For the former method, with the distal end of the guide wire at the physeal scar, bring a second guide wire into the entry portal and measure the length of the second guide wire extending proximally beyond the first to determine proper nail length. Using the nail length gauge, position the gauge anterior to the femur with its distal end between the proximal pole of the patella and the distal femoral physeal scar. Move the C arm of the image intensifier to the proximal end

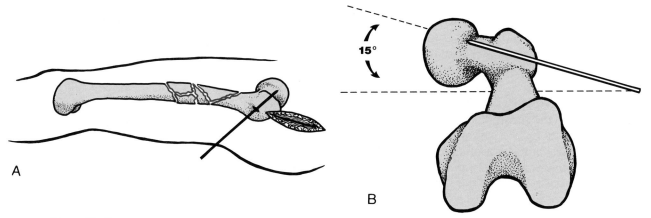

Figure 45–22

A, and *B*, Use of guide pin to determine anteversion of femoral neck. (Courtesy of Campbell Clinic, Memphis, Tennessee.)

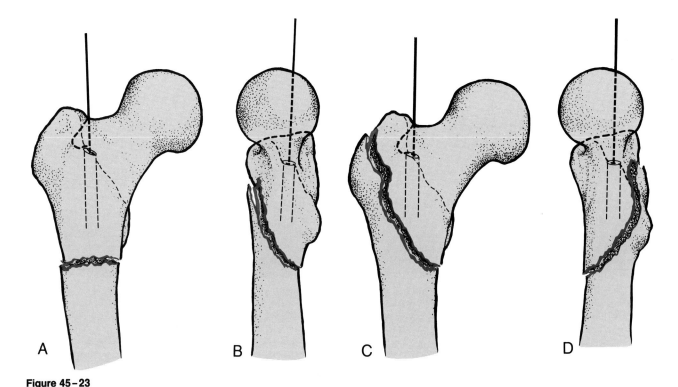

Figure 45–23

Guide wire centered on anteroposterior and lateral views of Russell-Taylor type IA (*A* and *B*) and type IIA (*C* and *D*) subtrochanteric fractures. (Courtesy of Campbell Clinic, Memphis, Tennessee.)

of the femur and read the correct nail length directly from the stamped measurements on the nail length gauge. Ream the remaining portion of the isthmus over the 3.2-mm guide wire in 0.5-mm increments until the desired diameter is reached (Fig. 45–24*E*). Verify final reamed diameter with the reamer template. Overreaming by at least 1 mm is essential with this intramedullary nail. With excessive anterior bowing, 1.5 mm of overreaming may be required. *Never* use a nail with a diameter larger than that of the last reamer. Because Russell-Taylor femoral nails are 0.3 mm larger than their stated size, slight overreaming is necessary. It is not necessary to exchange the reamer guide wire for the larger 4-mm driving wire, but a medullary alignment tube or exchange tube is provided if desired.

Hold the proximal nail guide with its cylindrical handle pointed away from the patient and position the locking nail horizontally so that the anterior curvature matches that of the femur. Attach the key on the guide with the keyway on the nail and securely screw the attachment bolt through the guide into the nail. Then attach the sliding hammer or supine position driver to the hexagonal bolt of the guide. Using the handle to control rotation, insert the nail. Never hit directly on the proximal drill guide; use the insertion instruments only. Confirm reduction and passage of the nail across the fracture site with biplane fluoroscopy during nail

insertion to avoid comminution. Retighten the handle of the proximal drill guide assembly as needed before final seating of the nail. The nail should advance with each hammer blow, or it must be withdrawn and additional reaming must be done. With proper orientation of the nail and femur, the handle will be 10° to 20° below horizontal. Withdraw the guide wire after the nail has entered the distal fragment by several centimeters. Drive the nail so that the proximal drill guide is flush with the tip of the greater trochanter (Fig. 45–24*F*). Remove the sliding hammer.

Proximal and distal interlocking with the 6.4-mm locking screws requires the 3.2-mm tip-threaded guide; 4.8-mm twist drill; red, blue, and green drill sleeves; and 3/16-inch femoral hexdriver. To insert the proximal locking screw, ensure that the hexagonal bolt is tightened, and place the 8-mm green and 4.8-mm blue drill sleeves into the proximal drill guide. Insert the 4.8-mm drill guide and drill through both cortices (Fig. 45–24*G*). Make a depth measurement using the 4.8-mm drill calibration and record the length against the top of the green drill sleeve (Fig. 45–24*H*). Drill sleeves must be against the cortex for accurate reading. Insert the selected 6.4-mm self-tapping locking screw through the green drill sleeve (Fig. 45–24*I*).

The Russell-Taylor distal targeting device permits control of four separate axes along the anteroposterior,

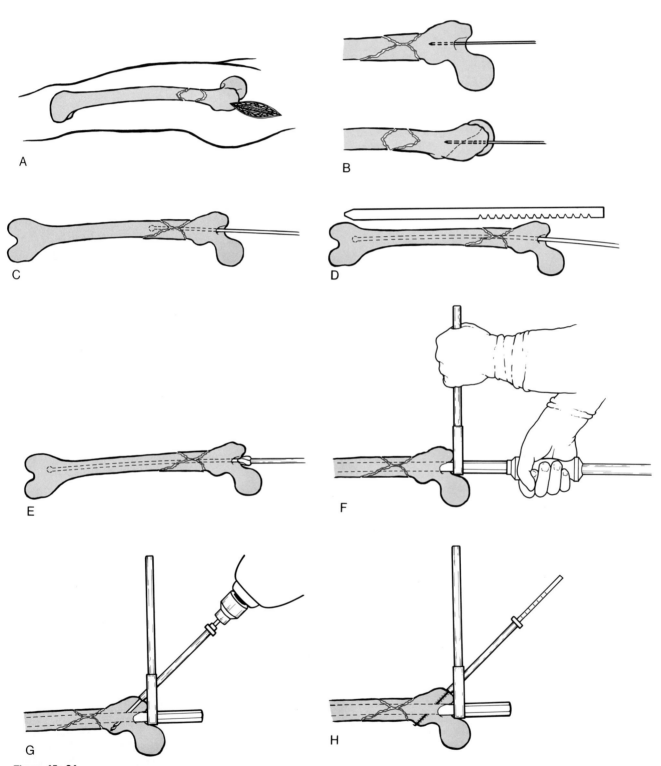

Figure 45-24

Technique for standard Russell-Taylor femoral nail. *A*, Skin incision. *B*, Insertion of guide wire. *C*, Reamer guide wire advanced to level of fracture. *D*, Guide wire advanced to physeal scar and determination of length using radiographic ruler. *E*, Remaining isthmus reamed. *F*, Insertion of nail. *G*, Predrilling for proximal screw. *H*, Determination of length of proximal screw.

Illustration continued on following page

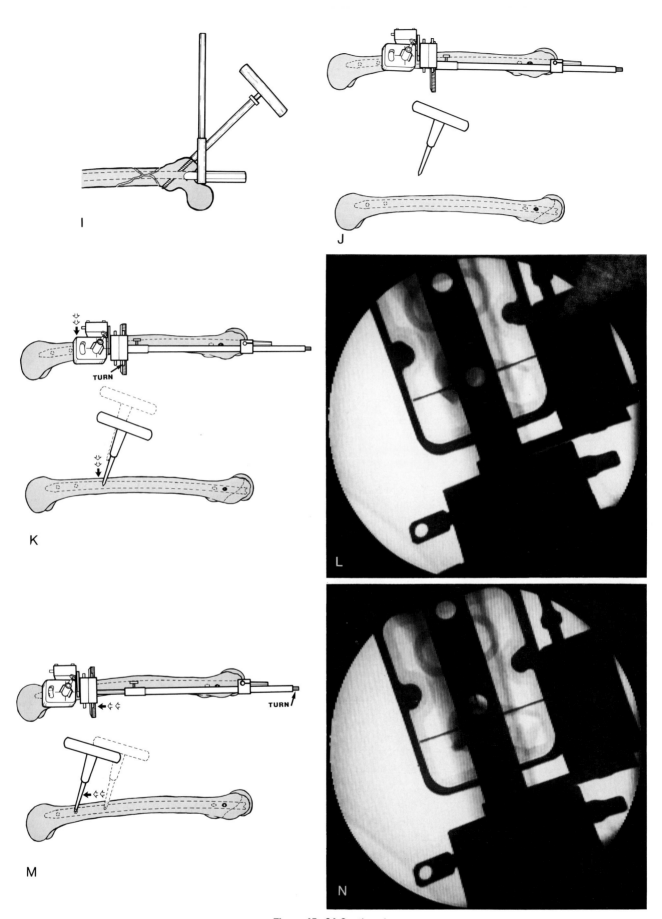

I

J

K

L

M

N

Figure 45–24 *Continued*

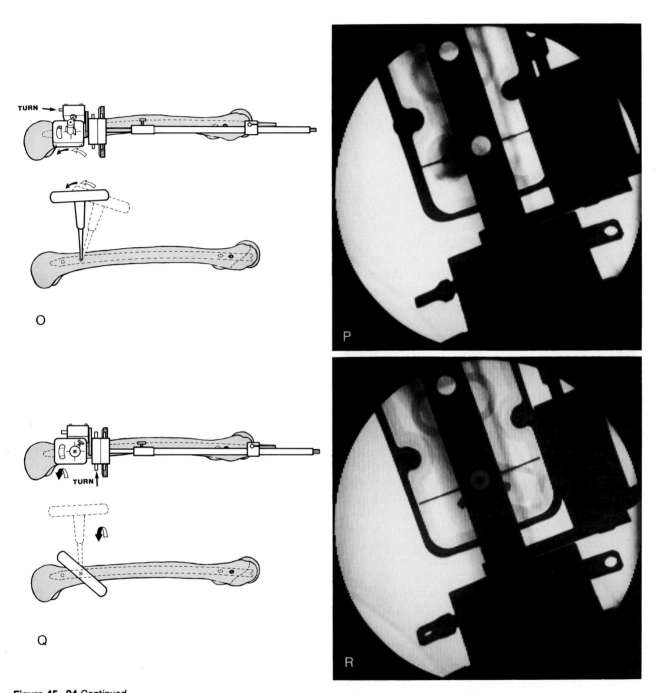

Figure 45–24 *Continued*

I, Insertion of proximal locking screw. *J*, Assembly of distal targeting device and schematic for freehand distal targeting with awl. *K*, Targeting device centered on intramedullary nail; awl aligned with center within hole. *N*, Radiographic appearance of targeting device with both cross hairs aligned on hole. *O*, Targeting device brought into transverse plane of proximal distal hole; awl and targeting device centered on hole in transverse plane. *P*, Radiographic appearance of both cross hairs aligned on hole and targeting bead centered on transverse cross hair. *Q*, Distal targeting device and awl aligned with hole and coincidental with hole in nail. *R*, Radiographic appearance of distal targeting device completely aligned with distal hole in nail.

Illustration and legend continued on following page

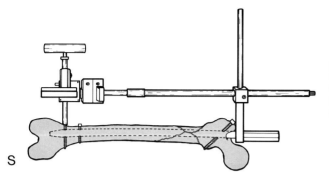

S

Figure 45-24 *Continued*

S, Seating of last distal screw for static interlocking in fracture with segmental comminution. (Courtesy of Smith and Nephew Richards Co.)

cephalic/caudal, transverse, and coronal planes and is recommended for use with these nails, although the freehand awl technique can be used (Fig. 45-24*J*).

To use the distal targeting device, first confirm with the image intensifier that the distal holes in the nail appear as perfect circles and are centered on the screen before attaching the device. Allow the maximum distance between the lateral thigh and the image intensifier. The C arm of the image intensifier should be positioned far enough from the thigh to allow drill sleeve insertion through the device. Attach the adaptor block to the handle of the proximal drill guide so the proper etched identification of "left" or "right" is facing the ceiling (or laterally if using the supine position). For additional stability, introduce a half pin unicortically into the distal femur, attach the swivel clamp, and tighten. Insert the shaft of the distal targeting device through the adaptor block until the shaft calibration (read from the proximal side of the block) equals the nail length. Lock the shaft in place by tightening the hexagonal screw with the hexdriver. Position the adaptor block/distal targeting device assembly so that the target platform is far enough from the skin to permit a 10° to 15° tilt, but close enough so that the six-inch drill sleeve will touch the lateral cortex. Lock the assembly by tightening the hexagonal screw with the hexdriver.

Using the adjustment instrument, rotate gear #1 to move the distal targeting device along the anteroposterior axis until the cross hair bisects the more proximal hole (Fig. 45-24*K, L*). To adjust along the cephalic/caudal axis, rotate adjustment knob #2 on the shaft of the distal targeting device until the perpendicular cross hair bisects the same hole (Fig. 45-24*M, N*). Insert the target bead and gently tighten the thumb screw. Rotate gear #4 until the bead is visible. Rotate gear #3 to move the bead in the coronal plane and center it over the cross hair (Fig. 45-24*O, P*), then rotate gear #4 to move the bead in the transverse plane and perfectly center it within the hole of the nail (Fig. 45-24*Q, R*). The axis of the distal targeting device should now be the same as that of the screw hole.

Remove the target bead and introduce the percutaneous knife through the plastic locating block; make a cruciate percutaneous incision to the lateral cortex. Insert the short green drill sleeve to the skin. Make a final image intensifier view at this time; a nearly perfect circle should still be seen; if not, repeat distal targeting. Insert the blue and red drill sleeves to the skin and drill with the tip-threaded guide pin to the lateral cortex. Confirm with the image intensifier that the guide pin is centered within the nail hole. Push the blue and red drill sleeves to the bone, then remove the guide pin and red drill sleeve. Use the 4.8-mm drill in the blue sleeve to drill through the lateral cortex, nail hole, and medial cortex. Make a depth measurement using the 4.8-mm drill calibrations and read the length against the top of the blue drill sleeve. Remove the drill and blue drill sleeve and insert the selected self-tapping screw through the green drill sleeve with the T-handle hexdriver (Fig. 45-24*S*). To place a second screw into the distal hole, repeat the targeting procedure. Remove the drill sleeves and disassemble the distal targeting device.

Instead of the distal targeting device, a free-hand technique may be used with a sharply pointed awl.

Reconstruction Nail (Russell-Taylor System)

The technique for insertion of the reconstruction (cephalomedullary) nail differs from that for the standard nail only at the proximal end. The proximal 8-cm section of the reconstruction nail is 15 mm in diameter; shaft diameters are 12, 13, and 14 mm. The femoral shaft must be reamed 1 mm larger than the diameter of the intended nail and the proximal 8 cm must be reamed to a diameter of 15 mm. The standard Russell-Taylor femoral nail may be used for either the right or left femur, but because of its additional 8° of anteversion, separate reconstruction nails are required for right and left femurs. An additional 1-cm offset on the proximal drill guide allows some adjustability for the proximal screws, allowing the 8-mm bolt to be placed low in the femoral neck and head to provide room for the second 6.4-mm screw. If only one screw is used for proximal interlocking, the larger 8-mm lag screw should always be used; a stronger mechanical construct is obtained with both screws.

With the patient supine, incise the skin from the tip of the trochanter proximally and slightly posteriorly for 6 to 8 cm (Fig. 45–25A). Insert the guide wire from a cannulated hip screw reamer set, centering it in the piriformis fossa on both anteroposterior and lateral projections (Fig. 45–25B). Ream over this with a cannulated 8-mm reamer (Fig. 45–25C). Keep in mind the anterior offset of the center of the head and neck as compared with the shaft (Fig. 45–25D). With the reconstruction nail, it is imperative to verify that the guide wire and reamer are centered on the true lateral projection of the proximal femur (Fig. 45–25E). Advance the guide wire to the level of the fracture (Fig. 45–25F) and ream the proximal fragment to approximately 11 mm. Using the internal fracture alignment device, reduce the fracture and advance the guide to the level of the physeal scar (Fig. 45–25G). Use a second guide wire or the nail length gauge to determine proper nail length. Ream any remaining isthmus to 1 mm larger than the selected nail shaft size (Fig. 45–25H). Ream the proximal 8 cm of the femur to 15 mm. Drive the nail over the reamer guide (Fig. 45–25I) (with the closed section nail, it is not necessary to exchange the reamer guide wire for the 4-mm driving wire). Rotational alignment of the nail must match that of the proximal fragment so that the cephalic screws are properly positioned in the femoral head. Final seating of the nail can be adjusted proximally and distally by approximately 1 cm to allow the 8-mm screw to lie on the calcar of the femoral neck (Fig. 45–25J). Using the image intensifier, bring the proximal driving and drill jig into alignment with the proximal end of the femur on the true lateral projection (Fig. 45–25 K,L).

Using the percutaneous knife, incise the skin and fascia through the inferior hole in the proximal drill guide and insert the stacked drill sleeves with all four sheaths (9.5-mm silver, 8.0-mm green, 4.8-mm blue, and 3.2-mm red) through this hole. Push the drill sleeve to the bone and insert the 3.2-mm tip-threaded guide pin through the red drill sleeve and advance it into the femoral head just superior to the calcar to a level approximately 5 mm from the subchondral bone (Fig. 45–25M). Confirm the position of the guide pin within the femoral head on anteroposterior, oblique, and lateral views (Fig. 45–25N, O). Even if only a single 8-mm screw is to be used, insert a second 3.2-mm tip-threaded guide pin in the superior hole to prevent movement of the proximal fragment when the lower screw is inserted. Incise the skin and fascia through the superior hole of the proximal drill guide and insert the stacked drill sleeves (8.0-mm green, 4.8-mm blue, and 3.2-mm red) through the superior hole. Push the drill sleeves to bone and insert the 3.2-mm tip-threaded guide pin through the drill sleeve and advance the guide pin to the femoral head (Fig. 45–25P). Confirm that the second guide pin is contained within the femoral head on anteroposterior, oblique, and lateral views (Fig. 45–25Q, R). Remove the inferior guide pin and red drill sleeve, leaving a pilot hole in which to center the 4.8-mm twist drill. Insert the 4.8-mm twist drill through the blue drill sleeve into the femoral head within 5 mm of subchondral bone; verify that the drill sleeves are against the bone (Fig. 45–25S). Measure screw length using the drill calibrations, reading the depth against the top of the blue drill sleeve. Remove the 4.8-mm twist drill and the blue drill sleeve. Using the large cortical reamer, ream the lateral cortex through the green drill sleeve until the blunt nose is within 5 mm of the subchondral bone (Fig. 45–25T). If the bone is especially dense, using the 6.5-mm cortical reamer first, followed by the 8.0-mm cortical reamer, may be helpful. Because of the sharp cutting flutes, the cortical reamer should always be pushed rather than advanced with power when it is within the nail. Remove the cortical reamer. In very dense bone, tapping may be required; use the large tap through the silver drill sleeve (Fig. 45–25U). Insert the selected 8.0-mm lag screw into the femoral head through the silver drill sleeve (Fig. 45–25V) and remove the silver drill sleeve. If not already in place, insert the red, blue, and green drill sleeves through the superior hole of the proximal drill guide. Advance the 3.2-mm tip-threaded guide pin to within the 5 mm of the subchondral bone. Remove the 3.2-mm tip-threaded guide pin and red drill sleeve. Insert the 4.8-mm twist drill through the blue drill sleeve into the femoral head within 5 mm of subchondral bone. Verify that the drill sleeves are against bone. Measure screw length using drill calibrations and read the depth against the top of the blue drill sleeve. Remove the 4.8-mm twist drill and the blue drill sleeve.

Using the small cortical reamer, ream the lateral cortex through the green drill sleeve until the blunt nose is within 5 mm of subchondral bone and then remove the small cortical reamer. In very dense bone, tapping may be required using the small tap through the green drill sleeve. Insert the selected 6.4-mm lag screw into the femoral head (Fig. 45–25W). Confirm containment of both screws within the femoral head on anteroposterior and lateral views. Proximal locking is now complete. Notice that the screws for proximal locking of the reconstruction nail have only a 2-cm threaded portion with smooth shanks to allow impaction if needed. Now perform distal interlocking with the distal targeting device or freehand technique as described for the Russell-Taylor standard femoral nail (Fig. 45–25X).

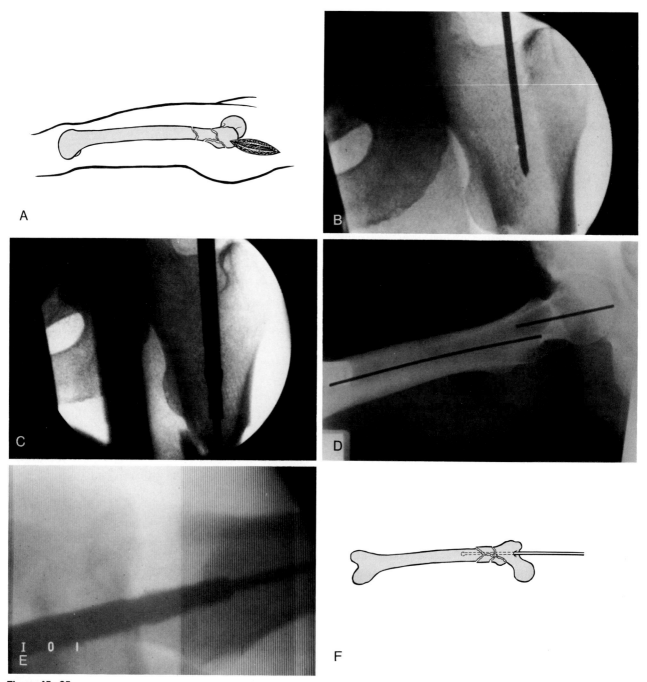

Figure 45 – 25

Technique for Russell-Taylor reconstruction nail. *A*, Skin incision. *B*, Guide pin centered on anteroposterior view. *C*, 8-mm cannulated reamer used to enlarge starting portal. *D*, Center lines of femoral neck and head and femoral shaft; note offset of approximately 1 cm. *E*, 8-mm reamer over guide wire in lateral projection. *F*, Reamer guide wire advanced to fracture.

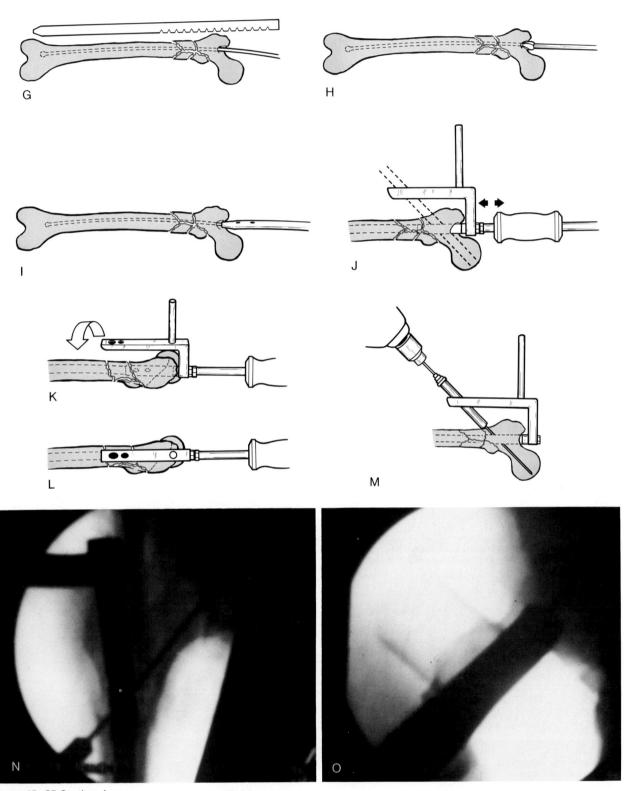

Figure 45–25 *Continued*

G, Reamer guide wire advanced to physeal scar. *H*, Remaining isthmus reamed. *I*, Nail is driven over reamer guide. *J*, Final seating of nail; note 1.5-cm adjustability with proximal seating to allow large 8-mm screw to lie on calcar. *K*, Proximal screw insertion jig brought to lie in true lateral plane of proximal femur. *L*, Proximal jig aligned with true lateral plane of proximal femur. *M*, Guide wire for 8-mm screw inserted. *N*, Anteroposterior view of first guide wire. *O*, Lateral view of first guide wire; note guide wire safely within femoral head and neck.

Illustration continued on following page

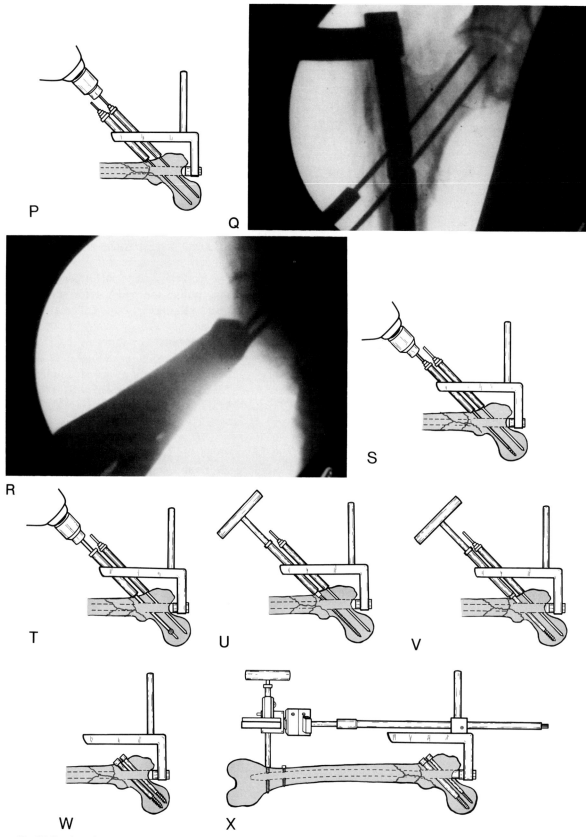

Figure 45–25 *Continued*

P, Second guide wire placed into femoral head. *Q*, Anteroposterior view of both guide wires in place. *R*, Lateral view of both guide wires in place; note safe placement within femoral head and neck. *S*, Predrilling with 4.8-mm drill for insertion of 8-mm screw. *T*, Lateral cortical reaming for 8-mm screw. *U*, Tapping for 8-mm screw. *V*, Insertion of 8-mm screw. *W*, Final seating of both proximal screws. *X*, Static locked reconstruction nail for comminuted subtrochanter fracture with final seating of second distal locking screw.

1516

Follow-up Care and Rehabilitation

Postoperative care depends on the stability achieved at surgery, determined by the strength of the implant and the quality of the bone (in particular the quality of the medial femoral cortex). As has been previously shown, forces of muscle contraction are essentially equal to those encountered with touch-down weight bearing, so we recommend ambulation with crutches or a walker with touch-down weight bearing up to 50 pounds. Monthly radiographic examinations should be performed to evaluate fracture healing. As fracture union progresses, the amount of weight bearing can be increased based on the patient's symptoms, so that by three months after surgery most patients are fully weight bearing. We recommend the routine use of prophylactic antibiotics and give one dose (usually a cephalosporin) before surgery and continue intravenous antibiotics for 24 to 48 hours. We do not routinely use anticoagulation in patients with subtrochanteric fractures due to high-energy trauma, but we do use mechanical procedures such as elastic stockings and early mobilization. In elderly patients, we prefer low-dose heparin, as it is easily reversible if bleeding studies indicate prolonged clotting times. Suction drains are usually removed at 48 hours. Isometric exercises and straight-leg raising exercises are begun on the first postoperative day.

When the patient has achieved sufficient quadriceps control, ambulation is begun. After the incisions have healed (three to four weeks postoperatively), progressive resistance exercises are begun with light weights and continued until the affected extremity is within 80% of the normal strength of the opposite extremity. Most patients with subtrochanteric fractures will be disabled for a minimum of four to six months before they can be evaluated for return to previous occupations. Other injuries and medical problems, however, may prolong the period of disability. Patients who are elderly or patients with multiple injuries may benefit from an intermediate stay at a rehabilitation center until they are sufficiently independent at home or can obtain assistance at home. If the patient is not fully weight bearing and walking without assistive devices by six months after fracture, tomograms should be obtained to assess the possibility of nonunion. If evidence of nonunion is present, then autogenous iliac bone grafting, perhaps with renailing using a larger implant, should be considered within 9 to 12 months. We have not used immobilization postoperatively for subtrochanteric fractures.

ASSESSMENT OF RESULTS

Successful treatment of a subtrochanteric fracture restores the patient to preinjury ambulatory status. This requires union and restoration of the normal neck shaft angle and correct length and rotation of the limb. Even with the best of treatment, some loss of motion about the hip can be expected. Most patients recover a functional range of motion, although some may have prolonged difficulty with squatting. Frequently, high-energy trauma injuries result in some type of liability or disability compensation. The most widely used source for evaluation of permanent impairment from these injuries is the American Medical Association's *Guide to the Evaluation of Permanent Physical Impairment*.[2] This guide focuses primarily on range of motion but also considers residual weakness and limb length inequality. Sanders et al.[58] have recommended a modification of The Hospital for Special Surgery Hip Grading Score, which, unlike the AMA guide, takes into account pain and walking capability and relates preinjury to postinjury status. It also considers the ability to perform such tasks as putting on shoes and socks and negotiating stairs and incorporates radiographic criteria for success. We believe this rating scale has much to offer in comparative studies and have begun to use it at our institution (Fig. 45–26).

Because of difficulties with Zickle nails in controlling length and rotation as well as with refracture after removal, Ovadia and Chess,[52] Shifflett and Bray,[66] Garbarino et al.,[28] and other authors[12,14,15,48,60,64,75] recommend interlocking intramedullary nail fixation as the treatment of choice for subtrochanteric fractures in which the lesser trochanter is intact. Brien et al.[10] reported a single nonunion in 66 subtrochanteric fractures, 75% of which were caused by high-energy trauma. In our treatment of nearly 200 subtrochanteric fractures, 100% have united without nail failure. Fifty complex subtrochanteric fractures with comminution of the lesser trochanteric region have been treated with the reconstruction nail. Twenty-eight percent of these fractures were open, usually because of motor vehicle accidents or gunshot wounds (Fig. 45–27). At three-year follow-up, all fractures have united. One patient required reoperation to correct external rotation deformity. Browner[11] also reported excellent results with the reconstruction nail in the treatment of 16 subtrochanteric fractures and nonunions. At follow-up ranging from six months to two years, there was 100% union, and all patients had excellent hip and knee motion.

Complications

General complications noted after subtrochanteric fractures in previous studies include pneumonia, urinary tract infections, decubiti, and cardiovascular complications, particularly in elderly patients. The causes of failure of fracture treatment can be grouped

TRAUMATIC HIP RATING SCALE

No. of points	Criteria	No. of points	Criteria
I. PAIN		**IV. MOTION-MUSCLE POWER**	
0	Constant; unbearable; uses strong medication frequently	0	Ankylosis with deformity
2	Constant but bearable; uses strong medication occasionally	2	Ankylosis with good functional position
4	Little or none at rest; with activities; uses salicylates frequently	4	Muscle power poor to fair; arc of flexion <60°; restricted lateral and rotary movement
6	When starting, then better, or after a certain activity; uses salicylates accasionally	6	Muscle power fair to good; arc of flexion as much as 90°; restricted lateral/rotary motion
8	Occasional and slight	8	Muscle power good or normal; arc of flexion >90°; fair lateral and rotary movement
10	None	10	Muscle power normal; motion normal or almost normal
II. WALKING			
(GAIT) 0	Bedridden	**V. DAILY ACTIVITIES**	
2	Uses a wheelchair; transfer activities with walker	A. Shoes 0	Unable
	Uses no support, housebound	& socks 3	With difficulty
(Markedly restricted) 4	Uses one support, less than one block	5	With ease
	Uses bilateral support, short distances	B. Stairs 0	Unable
(Moderately restricted) 6	Uses no support, less than one block	2	One at a time
	Uses one support, up to five blocks	4	With railing
	Uses bilateral support, unrestricted	5	Normal
(Mildly restricted) 8	Uses no support, limp		
	Uses one support, no limp	**VI. RADIOGRAPHIC EVALUATION**	
(Unretricted) 10	Uses no support, no appreciable limp	0	Nonunion/plate failure/arthritis
III. FUNCTION		2	Delayed union
A. Retired 0	Completely dependent and confined	4	Varus >10°, shortening >2.5 cm
Preinjury 2	Partially dependent	6	Varus >5° but <10°, shortening >1 cm but <2.5 cm
4	Independent; can do limited housework, limited shopping	8	Varus <5°, shortening <1 cm
6	Can do most housework; shops freely; can do desk-type work	10	Anatomic reduction
8	Very little restriction; can work on feet		
10	Normal activities	**TOTAL SCORE**	**RESULT**
B. Employed 0	Unemployed/retired secondary to injury	55–60	Excellent
Preinjury 2	Part-time/light duty	45–54	Good
4	Changed jobs secondary to injury	35–44	Poor
6	Altered job description somewhat	<35	Failure
8	Returned to work with some disability		
10	Returned to full work		

Figure 45–26

Traumatic hip rating score proposed by Sanders et al.[58] (Courtesy of R. Sanders, M.D.)

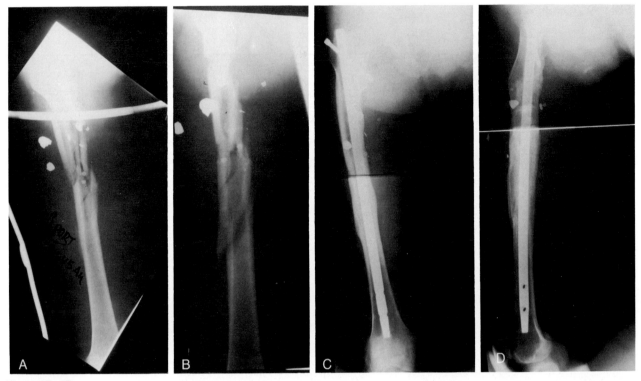

Figure 45-27

59-year-old male with open Russell-Taylor type IB fracture with marked comminution from gunshot wound to right femur. *A* and *B*, Anteroposterior and lateral preoperative radiographs. *C* and *D*, Anteroposterior and lateral radiographs after delayed fixation with Russell-Taylor standard femoral nail in static mode show fracture union.

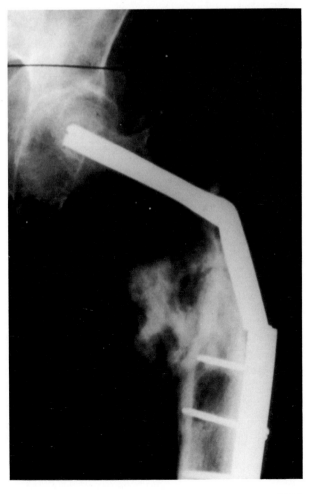

Figure 45-28

Nonunion with subsequent failure of Jewett nail that required revision surgery.

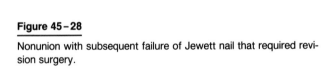

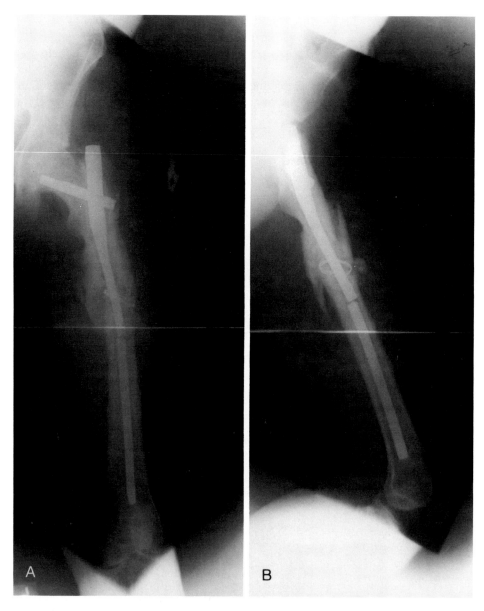

Figure 45–29

Two-year-old nonunion with subsequent fatigue failure of Zickle device.

into five areas: loss of fixation, implant failure, nonunion, malunion, and sepsis.

LOSS OF FIXATION AND IMPLANT FAILURE

With current hip compression screws, implant failure most commonly occurs in osteopenic bone where the screw cuts out of the femoral head. It is important to obtain sufficient screw fixation of the plate to the shaft, but fixation of more than eight cortices distally is rarely necessary. Failure of fixation will manifest as progressive deformity and shortening of the leg or as an acute episode of snapping or popping followed by pain and

inability to bear weight (Fig. 45–28). Loss of fixation with intramedullary devices is related to not using a static interlocking construct, not evaluating the entry portal for comminution into the piriformis fossa (resulting in nail cutout proximally), or using implants without sufficient strength to stabilize the fracture for sufficient cycles of loading. With fractured plates and screws, in most series reoperation with repeated open reduction and reapplication of internal fixation, coupled with autogenous iliac bone graft, have achieved union. Aronoff et al.[4] recommend intramedullary nailing for failed plates and screws, as the trochanteric extension that may occur with type II subtrochanteric fractures usually heals first.

NONUNIONS

Nonunion of a subtrochanteric fracture usually is indicated by inability to resume full weight bearing in the usual three- to six-month period. Continued pain and warmth about the proximal thigh and pain with attempted weight bearing are clinical indicators of delayed union and nonunion, which are confirmed with radiographs and tomograms as necessary. Nonunion usually persists in the shaft portion of the fracture, actually converting the fracture to a type I injury, which is best treated with an intramedullary device in a static locking fashion. If open reduction is required, we believe autogenous iliac bone grafting is indicated. Nails may fail by implant failure and removal of the nail with repeat reaming and nailing with a larger implant yield a high success rate (Fig. 45–29). The question is whether or not the fracture should then be treated with dynamic locking or static locking. It has been our experience that static locking is preferable to resist rotational shear forces, which contribute to mechanical instability at the nonunion site.

MALUNION

The patient with a malunion usually complains of either shortness of the leg, a limp, or rotational deformity. The affected leg should be compared with the opposite side for evaluation of these deformities. Malunions relate to three aspects of reduction of the fracture. First, it is imperative that the neck shaft angle be restored; if not, the patient will have a Trendelenburg gait with abductor weakness from shortening of the muscle group. In plated fractures, a valgus osteotomy and repeat internal fixation with bone grafting is the treatment of choice. Varus deformity may occur if an intramedullary nail is used and the entry portal is too far lateral into the tip of the trochanter. However, such varus deformity is usually less than 10°, is frequently well tolerated by the patient, and does not require reoperation. Leg length discrepancy is a complex problem and is most likely to occur after a trochanteric fracture with extensive shaft comminution and extension into the diaphysis treated with a dynamic rather than a static locking nail construct. Because most current lengthening procedures in the adult are fraught with complications, avoidance is the best treatment for this problem. Careful attention must be paid preoperatively and intraoperatively to restore acceptable length. Occasionally, with locked intramedullary nailing, the injured limb is distracted and heals with excessive length. Malrotation may occur with either plated or intramedullary techniques if the surgeon is not alert to

this potential complication. Following guidelines for reduction and confirmation, including radiographic checks and matching of the linea aspera, will help prevent this complication. It is essential to compare leg lengths and also to confirm rotational alignment by comparing internal and external rotation ranges prior to awakening the patient after intramedullary nailing. This permits early correction of malalignment. If significant internal or external rotation deformities are detected late, reoperation with derotational osteotomy may be indicated. After medullary nailing, closed derotation osteotomy with a static interlocking nail is the treatment of choice.

SEPSIS

Infections generally are evident between the fourth and tenth postoperative days, usually by increasing pain and the usual signs of inflammation. Sterile aspiration of the operative site may be carried out to confirm infection. Bone scanning is rarely helpful for the diag-

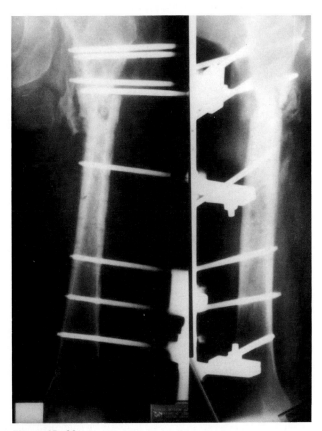

Figure 45–30

Deep sepsis and loss of fixation after fixation with blade plate device; septic nonunion was treated with debridement, irrigation, and stabilization with external fixation.

nosis of acute infection. Late infections are usually manifested as nonunions, in which sepsis is frequently occult. When evaluating a nonunion, we recommend biopsy of the site for anaerobic and aerobic cultures prior to revision surgery. Gallium scanning has been of limited use in diagnosing septic nonunion, and we prefer to rely on biopsy results. When any surgical revision is required for subtrochanteric complications, intraoperative cultures, both anaerobic and aerobic, should be taken. Sepsis in subtrochanteric fractures most commonly follows open reduction and internal fixation; with closed intramedullary nailing techniques, the risk of infection is significantly lowered. The use of prophylactic antibiotics also significantly decreases the possibility of postoperative sepsis. Acute postoperative infection is best managed by immediate surgery for drainage and debridement of all necrotic material. The wound should be left open for repeat debridements or closed over antibiotic beads. If fixation is stable, implants should be retained until the fracture has healed. If the implant is unstable, it should be removed and either traction or external fixation should be used during treatment of the infection; delayed bone grafting can then be performed to obtain union (Fig. 45–30). Prolonged antibiotic therapy, usually for six weeks, may be necessary in these difficult problems.

REFERENCES

1. Allis, O.H. Fracture in the upper third of the femur exclusive of the neck. Med News 59:585–589, 1891.
2. American Medical Association: Guide to the Evaluation of Permanent Impairment, Ed. 2. Chicago, AMA, 1984.
3. Andrew, T.A.; Thorogood, M. Subtrochanteric fracture after Garden screw fixation: A review of predisposing factors and management in nine cases. Injury 16:169–177, 1984.
4. Aronoff, P.M.; Davis, P.M. Jr.; Wickstrom, J.K.: Intramedullary nail fixation treatment of subtrochanteric fractures of the femur. J Trauma 11:637–650, 1971.
5. Asher, M.A.; Tipper, J.W.; Rockwood, C.A.; Zilber, S. Compression fixation of subtrochanteric fractures. Clin Orthop 117:202–208, 1976.
6. Bergman, G.D.; Winquist, R.A.; Mayo, K.A.; Hansen, S.T. Jr. Subtrochanteric fracture of the femur: Fixation using the Zickel nail. J Bone Joint Surg 69A:1032–1040, 1987.
7. Berman, A.T.; Metzger, P.C.; Bosacco, S.J.; et al. Treatment of the subtrochanteric fracture with the compression hip nail: A review of 138 consecutive cases. (Abstract) Orthop Trans 3:225–256, 1979.
8. Boyd, H.B.; Griffin, L.L. Classification and treatment of trochanteric fractures. Arch Surg. 58:853–866, 1949.
9. Boyd, H.B.; Lipiniski, S.W. Nonunion of trochanteric and subtrochanteric fractures. Surg Gynecol Obstet 104:463–470, 1957.
10. Brien, W.; Wiss, D.A.; Peter, K.; Merrett, P.O. Subtrochanteric fractures of the femur: Treatment with locked medullary nails. Presented at the 54th Annual Meeting of the American Academy of Orthopaedic Surgeons, San Francisco, January 25, 1987.
11. Browner, B. Personal communication, June 1989.
11A. Brumback, R.J.; Ellison, P.S. Jr.; Poka, A.; et al. Intramedullary nailing of open fractures of the femoral shaft. J Bone Joint Surg 71A:1324, 1989.
12. Brumback, R.J.; Lakatos, R.P.; Garbarino, J.L.; et al. Closed interlocking intramedullary nailing of subtrochanteric fractures. (Abstract) Orthop Trans 11:478, 1987.
13. Brumback, R.J.; Lakatos, R.P.; Poka, A.; Burgess, A.R. Risks of infection with reamed intramedullary femoral fixation in multiple trauma. (Abstract) Orthop Trans 11:490, 1987.
14. Brumback, R.J.; Reilly, J.P.; Poka, A.; et al. Intramedullary nailing of femoral shaft fractures. Part I. Decision-making errors with interlocking fixation. J Bone Joint Surg. 70A:1441–1452, 1988.
15. Brumback, R.J.; Uwagie-Ero, S.; Lakatos, R.P.; et al. Intramedullary nailing of femoral shaft fractures. Part II. Fracture-healing with static interlocking fixation. J Bone Joint Surg 70A:1453–1462, 1988.
16. Cech, H.; Sosna, A. Principles of the surgical treatment of subtrochanteric fractures. Orthop Clin North Am 5:651–662, 1974.
16A. Cole, J.D.; Browner, B.D.; Cotler, H.B.; et al. Initial experience with a second generation locking nail. Presented at the Fifth Annual Meeting of the Orthopaedic Trauma Association, Philadelphia, October 19–21, 1989.
17. Cuthbert, H.I.; Howat, T.W. The use of the Küntscher Y nail in the treatment of intertrochanteric and subtrochanteric fractures of the femur. Injury 8:135–142, 1974.
18. Davis, A.D.; Meyer, R.D.; Miller, M.E.; Killian, J.T. Closed Zickle nailing. Clin Orthop 201:138–146, 1985.
19. DeLee, J.C.; Clanton, T.O.; Rockwood, C.A. Jr. Closed treatment of subtrochanteric fractures of the femur in a modified cast-brace. J Bone Joint Surg 63A:773–779, 1982.
20. DiStefano, V.J.; Nixon, J.E.; Klein, K.S. Stable fixation of the difficult subtrochanteric fracture. J Trauma 12:1066–1070, 1972.
21. Dobozi, W.R.; Larson, B.J.; Zindrick, M.; et al. Flexible intramedullary nailing of subtrochanteric fractures of the femur. Clin Orthop 212:66–78, 1986.
22. Elabdien, B.S.Z.; Olerud, S.; Karlstrom, G. Subtrochanteric fractures: Classification and results of Ender nailing. Arch Orthop Trauma Surg 103:241–250, 1984.
23. Fielding, J.W.; Cochran, G.V.B.; Zickel, R.E. Biomechanical characteristics and surgical management of subtrochanteric fractures. Orthop Clin North Am 5:629–650, 1974.
24. Fielding, J.W.; Magliato, H.J. Subtrochanteric fractures. Surg Gynecol Obstet 122:555–560, 1966.
25. Frankel, V.H.; Burstein, A.H. Orthopaedic Biomechanics. Philadelphia, Lea & Febiger, 1970.
26. Froimson, A.L. Treatment of comminuted subtrochanteric fractures. Surg Gynecol Obstet 131:465–472, 1970.
27. Frost, H.M. The Laws of Bone Structure. Springfield, IL, Charles C Thomas, 1964.
28. Garbarino, J.L.; Brumback, R.J.; Poka, A.; Burgess, A.R. Closed interlocking intramedullary nailing of subtrochanteric fractures. Presented at the 54th Annual Meeting of the American Academy of Orthopaedic Surgeons, San Francisco, January 25, 1987.
29. Grosse, A.; Kempf, I.; Lafforgue, D. Le traitement des fracas, perte de substance osseouse et psuedoarthroses due femur et du tibia parl enclouage verrouille (a propos de 40 cas). Rev Chir Orthop 64 (suppl 2):33, 1978.
30. Gustilo, R.B. Management of Open Fractures and Their Complications. Philadelphia, W.B. Saunders, 1982.
31. Hanson, G.W.; Tullos, H.S. Subtrochanteric fractures of the

femur treated with nail plate devices: A retrospective study. Clin Orthop 131:191–194, 1978.

32. Heiple, K.G.; Brooks, D.B.; Sampson, B.L.; Burstein, A.H. A fluted intramedullary rod for subtrochanteric fractures. Biomechanical considerations and preliminary clinical results. J Bone Joint Surg 61A:730–737, 1979.

33. Hey-Groves, E.W. Ununited fractures, with special reference to gunshot injuries and the use of bone grafting. Br J Surg 203, 247, 1918–1919.

34. Hibbs, R.A. The management of the tendency of the upper fragment to tilt forward in fractures of the upper third of the femur. New York Med J 75:177–179, 1902.

35. Hogh, J. Sliding screw in the treatment of trochanteric fractures. Injury 14:141, 1982.

36. Jewett, E.L. New approach for subtrochanteric and upper femoral shaft fractures using a dual flange nail plate: Preliminary report. Am J Surg 81:186–188, 1951.

37. Johnson, K.D. Current techniques in the treatment of subtrochanteric fractures. Tech Orthop 3:14–24, 1988.

38. Jones, J.B. Screw fixation of the lesser trochanter. Clin Orthop 123:107, 1977.

39. Karr, R.K.; Schwab, J.P. Subtrochanteric fracture as a complication of proximal femoral pinning. Clin Orthop 194:214–217, 1985.

40. Keenan, M.A. Subtrochanteric fracture of the femur. (Abstract) Orthop Trans 4:359, 1980.

41. Kempf, I.; Grosse, A.; Beck, G. Closed locked intramedullary nailing. J Bone Joint Surg 67A:709–720, 1985.

42. Kinast, C.; Bolhofner, B.R.; Mast, J.W.; Ganz, R. Subtrochanteric fractures of the femur: Results of treatment with the 95-degree condylar blade plate. Clin Orthop 238:122–130, 1989.

43. Koch, J.C. The laws of bone architecture. Am J Anat 21:177–298, 1917.

44. Küntscher, G. Dauerbruch und Umbauzone. Bruns Beitrage Klin Chir 169:558, 1939.

45. Kyle, R.F.; Wright, T.M.; Burstein, A.H. Biomechanical analysis of the sliding characteristics of compression hip screws. J Bone Joint Surg 62A:1308–1314, 1980.

46. Levy, R.N.; Siegel, M.; Sedlin, E.D.; Siffert, R.S. Complications of Ender-pin fixation in basicervical, intertrochanteric, and subtrochanteric fractures of the hip. J Bone Joint Surg 65A:66–69, 1983.

47. Lhowe, D.W.; Hansen, S.T. Immediate nailing of open fractures of the femoral shaft. J Bone Joint Surg 70A:812–820, 1988.

48. Maatz, R.; Lentz, W.; Arens, W.; Beck, H., eds. Intramedullary Nailing and Other Intramedullary Osteosyntheses. Philadelphia, WB Saunders Co., 1986.

49. MacEachern, A.G.; Heyse-Moore, G.H.; Jones, R.N. Subtrochanteric fractures of the femur through the track of the lower Garden screw: Treatment with a Richards sliding screw. Injury 15:337–340, 1984.

50. Meggitt, B.F.; Juett, D.A.; Smith, J.D. Cast-bracing for fractures of the femoral shaft. J Bone Joint Surg 63B:12–23, 1981.

51. Mueller, M.E.; Allgower, M.; Schneider, R.; et al. Manual of Internal Fixation, Ed. 2. Berlin, Springer-Verlag, 1979.

52. Ovadia, D.N.; Chess, J.L. Intraoperative and postoperative subtrochanteric fracture of the femur associated with removal of the Zickle nail. J Bone Joint Surg 70A:239–243, 1988.

53. Pankovich, A.M.; Tarabishy, I.E. Ender nailing of intertrochanteric and subtrochanteric fractures of the femur. J Bone Joint Surg 62A:635–645, 1980.

54. Robey, L.R. Intertrochanteric and subtrochanteric fractures of the femur in the Negro. J Bone Joint Surg 38A:1301–1312, 1956.

55. Ruff, M.E.; Lubbers, L.M. Treatment of subtrochanteric fractures with a sliding screw-plate device. J Trauma 26:75–80, 1986.

56. Rybicki, E.F.; Simonen, F.A.; Weis, E.B. Jr. On the mathematical analysis of stress in the human femur. J Biomech 5:203–215, 1972.

57. Rydell, N.W. Forces acting on the femoral head prosthesis: A study on strain gauge supplied prostheses in living persons. Acta Orthop Scand 88 (suppl):1–132, 1972.

58. Sanders, R.; Regazzoni, P.; Routt, M.L. Jr. The treatment of subtrochanteric fractures of the femur using the dynamic condylar screw. Presented at American Academy of Orthopaedic Surgeons Annual Meeting, Atlanta, Georgia, February 4–9, 1988.

59. Sarmiento, A. Functional bracing of tibial and femoral shaft fractures. Clin Orthop 82:2–13, 1972.

60. Schatzker, J. Subtrochanteric fractures of the femur. In: Schatzker, J.; Tile, M., eds. The Rationale of Operative Fracture Care. Berlin, Springer-Verlag, 1987.

61. Scherfel, T. A new type of intramedullary nail for the internal fixation of subtrochanteric fractures of the femur. Int Orthop 8:255–261, 1985.

62. Seinsheimer, F. Subtrochanteric fractures of the femur. J Bone Joint Surg 60A:300–306, 1978.

63. Seinsheimer, F. Concerning the proper length of femoral side plates. J Trauma 21:42–45, 1981.

64. Seligson, D. Concepts in Intramedullary Nailing. Orlando, Grune and Stratton, 1985.

65. Shelton, M.L. Subtrochanteric fractures of the femur. Arch Surg 110:41–48, 1975.

66. Shifflett, M.W.; Bray, T.J. Subtrochanteric femur fractures treated by Zickle and Grosse-Kempf nailing. Presented at the 54th Annual Meeting of the American Academy of Orthopaedic Surgeons, San Francisco, January 25, 1987.

67. Stewart, M.J. Discussion of paper, "Classification, treatment and complicatons of the adult subtrochanteric fracture." J Trauma 4:481, 1964.

68. Taylor, J.C.; Russell, T.A.; LaVelle, D.G.; Calandruccio, R.A. Clinical results of 100 femoral shaft fractures treated with the Russell-Taylor interlocking nail system. (Abstract) Orthop Trans 11:491, 1987.

69. Teitge, R.A. Subtrochanteric fracture of the femur. J Bone Joint Surg 58A:282, 1976.

70. Templeton, T.; Saunders, E.A. A review of fractures in the proximal femur treated with the Zickle nail. Clin Orthop 141:213–216, 1979.

71. Tencer, A.F.; Calhoun, J.; Miller, B.B. Stiffness of subtrochanteric fracture of the femur stabilized using a Richards interlocking intramedullary rod or Richards AMBI. Orthop Biomech Lab Report #002. Memphis, Richards Medical Co, 1985.

72. Tencer, A.F.; Johnson, K.D.; Johnston, D.W.C.; Gill, K. A biomechanical comparison of various methods of stabilization of subtrochanteric fractures of the femur. J Orthop Res 2:297–305, 1984.

73. Thomas, W.G.; Villar, R.N. Subtrochanteric fractures: Zickle nail or nail plate? J Bone Joint Surg 68B:255–259, 1986.

74. Toridis, T.G. Stress analysis of the femur. J Biomech 2:163–174, 1969.

75. Trafton, P.G. Subtrochanteric-intertrochanteric femoral fractures. Orthop Clin North Am 18:59–71, 1987.

76. Velasco, R.U.; Comfort, T. Analysis of treatment problems in subtrochanteric fractures of the femur. J Trauma 18:513–522, 1978.

77. Waddell, J.P. Subtrochanteric fractures of the femur: A review of 130 patients. J Trauma 19:585–592, 1979.

78. Waddell, J.P. Sliding screw fixation for proximal femoral fractures. Orthop Clin North Am 11:607–622, 1980.
79. Watson, H.K.; Campbell, R.D.; Wade, P.A. Classification, treatment and complications of the adult subtrochanteric fracture. J Trauma 4:457–480, 1964.
80. Whatley, J.R.; Garland, D.E.; Whitecloud, T.; Wickstrom, J. Subtrochanteric fractures of the femur: Treatment with ASIF blade plate fixation. South Med J 17:1372–1375, 1978.
81. Wile, P.B.; Panjabi, M.M.; Southwick, W.O. Treatment of subtrochanteric fractures with a high-angle compression hip screw. Clin Orthop 175:72–78, 1983.
82. Yelton, C.; Low, W. Iatrogenic subtrochanteric fracture: A complication of Zickle nails. J Bone Joint Surg 68A:1237–1240, 1986.
83. Zickle, R.E. An intramedullary fixation device for the proximal part of the femur. J Bone Joint Surg 58A:866–872, 1976.
84. Zickle, R.E. A new fixation device for subtrochanteric fractures of the femur: Preliminary report. Clin Orthop 54:115–123, 1967.

Kenneth D. Johnson, M.D.

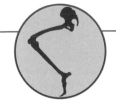

46

Femoral Shaft Fractures

A fracture of the shaft of the femur is a catastrophic event. This fracture is the result of severe, high-energy force that is strong enough to fracture the longest and strongest bone in the body. The injury is a serious injury that can result in up to two to three units of blood loss. The most common causes of such severe trauma are motor vehicle accidents, auto-pedestrian accidents, gunshot injuries, falls from great heights, and, increasingly, plane crashes. The fracture alone can cause complications that can be life-threatening. In many cases, the patient with a fracture of the shaft of the femur has additional severe violent trauma to other portions of the body that may require significant medical attention as well.[23] Therefore when dealing with a patient with a fracture of the shaft of the femur, many relevant topics must be discussed.

Because this bone is the longest and strongest bone in the body, it is a key factor in normal weight-bearing ambulation. The femur is subjected to very high stress in the activity of normal walking, which includes forces of axial loading, bending forces, and torsional forces.[85] The bone itself is surrounded by a large mass of muscle that, on contraction, adds even more force and stress to this large bone. Major joints of the hip and knee articulate on the proximal and distal end of this bone, and major fractures of the shaft can have a significant effect on either one of these joints as well.[271] Return of appropriate strength in this bone for full weight-bearing ambulation takes from three to six months. Most individuals are significantly unhappy with being incapacitated for this period of time. Current treatment modalities therefore are directed toward creating enough strength in the fractured femur to allow at least partial functional activity during the ongoing treatment process.

Many authors have written regarding treatment of femoral shaft fractures, and virtually every one is able to accomplish normal union with a fracture of this bone. Union itself appears not to be a significant problem. The more significant problem is to accomplish union consistently; allow the patient to be mobile at least to a chair and, commonly, to a car; restore normal length and alignment; and maintain a normal, functional range of motion in the hip and knee. Most authors state that the sum of hip and knee range of motion and flexion should total 160° before stair climbing, with one step for each lift of the leg allowed.[57]

Pathology

RELEVANT ANATOMY

The femur is a long, generally tubular bone that extends from the hip proximally to the knee distally.[252] This bone is not only the longest and strongest, but also the heaviest, bone in the body. A person's height can be measured from the length of the femur, as height is essentially four times the length of the femur. The femur consists of three major parts: the shaft, or diaphysis, and two ends—a proximal and distal end, or proximal and distal metaphysis. The proximal metaphysis consists of the head of the femur, the neck of the femur, and the greater and lesser trochanters. The distal femur consists of the distal metaphysis and knee joint.[302]

This chapter is devoted to the shaft, or diaphysis, of the femur, which extends from the level of the lesser trochanter to the flare of the condyles, or the level of the adductor tubercle. The femoral shaft is slightly bowed anteriorly and is narrowest at the midshaft.[302] Its cross section is approximately circular, except for a broad ridge of bone, the linea aspera (Latin, meaning "rough line"), running down the middle of the posterior surface of the femur. This broad, rough line is the attachment for many muscles, including the gluteus maximus, adductor magnus, adductor brevis, vastus lateralis, vastus medialis, vastus intermedius, and short head of the biceps.[189] Other muscular origins and insertions on the femur occur both proximally and distally (Fig. 46–1). Major muscles attach to the greater trochanter. These are rather large and extensive muscle attachments that tend to abduct the proximal fragment in areas of proximal fracture. The lesser trochanter is the attachment of another large, powerful muscle (the iliopsoas) that tends to flex and externally rotate the proximal femur with fractures in that area.[91] Although the iliopsoas is an internal rotator of the intact proximal femur through the hip joint, the change in axis of rotation associated with a proximal shaft fracture causes this muscle to act as an external rotator. The external rotation deformity that occurs is largely secondary to the fact that the lesser trochanter resides on the posterior aspect of the femur, and an anterior pull on this lesser trochanter causes flexion plus external rotation.

The complex anatomy of the proximal femur must be carefully considered if one wishes to perform intramedullary nailing of fractures.[189] The anterior bow of the femoral shaft has previously been mentioned. The femoral neck runs obliquely anterior from the proximal shaft of the femur and lies anterior to the long axis of the shaft. These anatomic facts significantly influence the mechanics of intramedullary nailing.

Major muscles insert on the distal femur as well (see Fig. 46–1C). The large adductor muscle mass attaching to the distal medial aspect of the femur tends to create an apex lateral angulation deformity in midshaft fractures. This apex lateral deformity can be distinctly accentuated by the force of longitudinal weight bearing, which has an axis of application medial to the shaft of the femur. These tremendous forces tending to create apex lateral angulation are counterbalanced by a large tension band of the fascia lata and lateral muscle mass. Finally, muscles originating on the distal femur are the medial and lateral heads of the gastrocnemius on the posterosuperior aspect of the femoral condyles (see Fig. 46–1C). These large muscles tend to create a flexion deformity in a distal fragment with a distal third fracture of the femur. These muscles can be counterbalanced by appropriate positioning of the knee and ankle.

Because of the extreme forces acting in various portions of the femur and because of its length, the major function of the femur is as a structure for standing and walking. The best overall design for strength, particularly with axial loading and bending, is a tubular structure, which best describes the femur. This tubular structure is reinforced posteriorly by the linea aspera, which counteracts the large anteroposterior bending forces that occur with flexion and extension of the knee and hip during weight-bearing ambulation. The intramedullary canal of the femur is essentially trumpet shaped, opening both proximally and distally.[252] Widening of the canal occurs to a lesser degree proximal to the isthmus than distal to the isthmus (Fig. 46–2).

The blood supply to the femur is a concern, as it is involved in femoral shaft fractures (Fig. 46–3). The blood supply in a long bone generally enters the bone both proximally and distally through arteries in the metaphysis that supply the metaphysis completely.[35,153] The femur has a single nutrient artery that penetrates the diaphyseal cortex in the area of the linea aspera. Nutrient arteries are branches of the profunda femoris artery. Generally only a single nutrient artery enters the femur in its proximal half; it is possible to have several nutrient arteries, but a single artery only is most common, as described by Lang.[153] The nutrient artery communicates with and forms medullary arteries in the intramedullary canal that extend proximally and distally through the medullary area of the bone.[218,219] These medullary arteries penetrate the endosteum of the bone to supply approximately two thirds of the width of the cortex of the diaphyseal bone. The medullary arteries communicate with the metaphyseal arteries proximally and distally. The metaphyseal arteries can supply the endosteum of the diaphyseal cortex through their communications proximally and distally if the nutrient artery is interrupted. Finally, periosteal arterioles enter the cortex from fascial attachments and normally supply the outer third of the cortex. They generally cannot penetrate the cortex any further or carry blood any deeper into the cortex. All venous drainage from the diaphyseal cortex is toward the periosteal surface. Interruption of the medullary blood supply, which supplies at least two thirds of the cortex of the femur, has been a concern of opponents of intramedullary nailing of the femoral shaft.[218-220] However, this medullary blood supply is reestablished over a six- to eight-week period if space for vascular ingrowth is available between the intramedullary nail and the cortex (e.g., within the shallow flutes of a Küntscher nail). Bone blood supply is modified during fracture healing to recruit arterial blood flow from surrounding local soft tissue to the healing callus.

The major arteries surrounding the femur are the superficial femoral artery and the profunda femoris artery (Fig. 46–4).[189] The profunda femoris artery branches off the main femoral artery just distal to the femoral head and runs distally along the posterior aspect of the femur. This artery sends a perforating

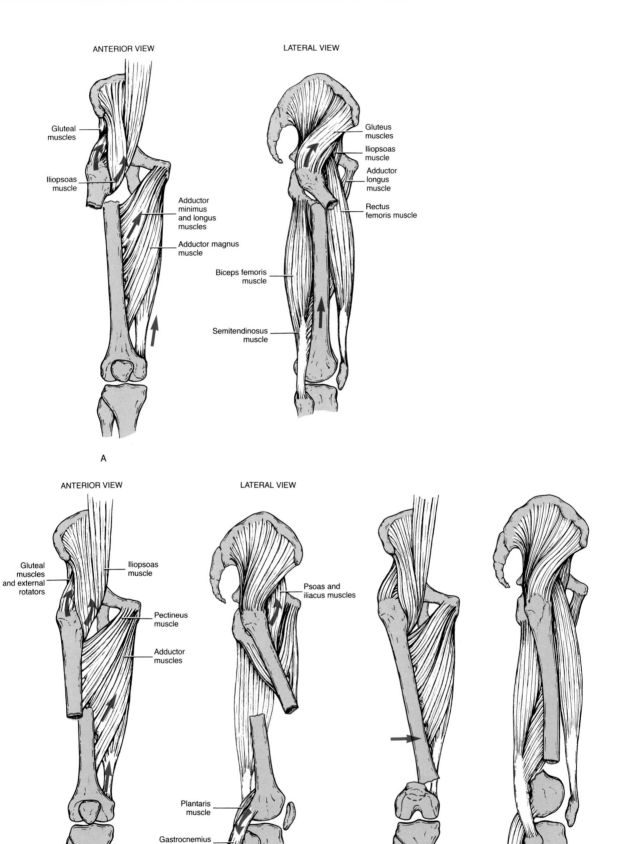

ANTERIOR VIEW   LATERAL VIEW

Gluteal
muscles

Iliopsoas
muscle

Adductor
minimus
and longus
muscles

Adductor magnus
muscle

Biceps femoris
muscle

Semitendinosus
muscle

Gluteus
muscles

Iliopsoas
muscle

Adductor
longus
muscle

Rectus
femoris muscle

A

ANTERIOR VIEW   LATERAL VIEW

Gluteal
muscles
and external
rotators

Iliopsoas
muscle

Pectineus
muscle

Adductor
muscles

Psoas and
iliacus muscles

Plantaris
muscle

Gastrocnemius
muscle

B   C

Figure 46–1

Typical deformities occurring with fractures at different levels as a result of muscle origins or insertions. *A*, Proximal, with proximal fragment flexed and externally rotated. *B*, Midshaft, with apex lateral angulation and shortening. *C*, Distal, with flexed distal fragment.

1527

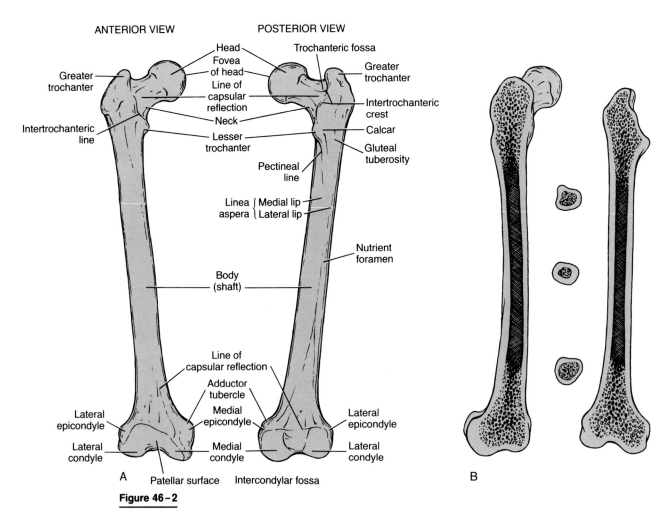

Figure 46-2

A, Femoral shaft with metaphysis, diaphysis, and isthmus. *B*, Shape of the intramedullary canal.

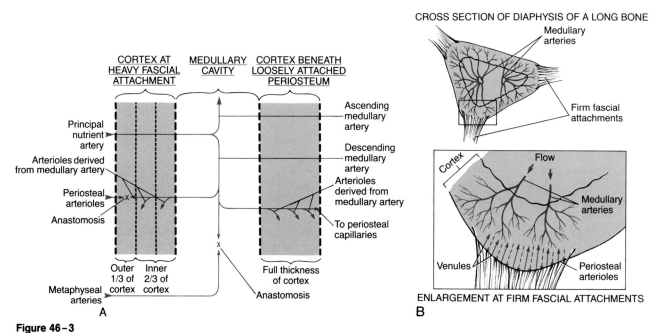

Figure 46-3

Blood supply to the femoral shaft. *A*, AP view. *B*, Cross section showing the linea aspera, intramedullary blood supply, and peripheral nerve position in the thigh.

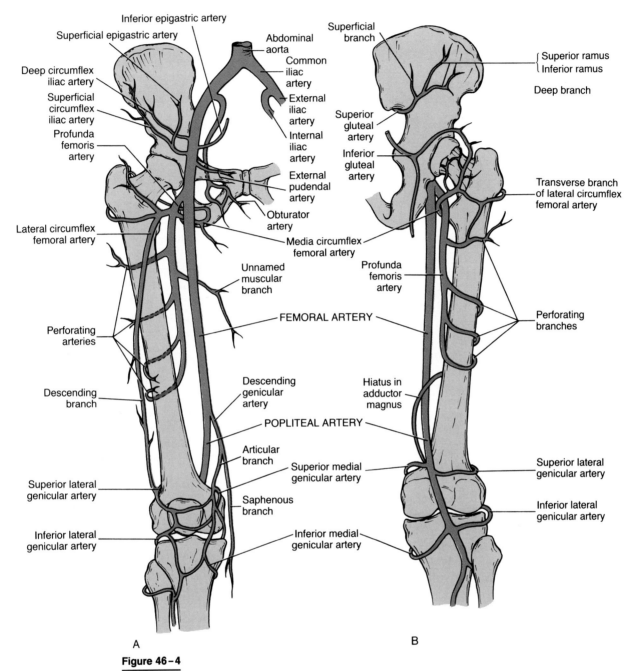

Figure 46-4

Blood supply to the thigh (AP, cross section). *A*, Superficial femoral. *B*, Profunda femoris.

branch to the proximal half of the femur as the nutrient artery to the femoral shaft. The profunda femoris artery also sends penetrating arteries through the intramuscular septum to supply major muscles that lie along the lateral side of the femur. These points of perforation through the intramuscular septum are points of potential injury to the profunda femoris arterial branches.

The femoral artery enters the thigh under the inguinal ligament and courses down the medial border of the thigh, where it turns lateral and posterior at the level of the adductor hiatus at the junction of the medial and distal third of the femur. At that point it becomes the popliteal artery and runs posteriorly down the calf. A major site of injury of the superficial femoral artery is at the adductor hiatus in the distal third of the femur, where it is tethered by soft tissue.

Finally, the sciatic nerve and femoral nerve are the major nerves coursing through the thigh adjacent to the femoral shaft. The femoral nerve enters the thigh under the inguinal ligament and supplies the quadriceps femoris muscles.[189] The sciatic nerve enters the thigh posteriorly under the piriformis muscle, which comes out of the pelvis to insert on the posterior aspect of the greater trochanter.[189] The sciatic nerve is well protected from the bone by muscle as it courses through the thigh. It is uncommonly injured with fractures of the femoral shaft, although it may be injured with fractures involving the pelvis or acetabulum because of the close proximity of the nerve to the posterior column of the pelvis.

Incidence

The incidence and the impact of femoral shaft fractures in the United States are defined by Grazier et al. based on data from 1970 to 1977.[101] Fractures of the femur, exclusive of hip fractures, occurred at a rate of one fracture per 10,000 people per year in the overall population. The injury was more common in those younger than 25 years and older than 65 years, with an incidence that approached three fractures per 10,000 persons. A fracture of the femur causes the patient restricted activity for 107 days on average, with 69 of those days spent restricted to the bed. An average loss of 30 days from work or school was reported as well. The average length of stay in the hospital was 25 days.

This injury is rather extreme, as a significant amount of energy must be applied to the thigh and femoral shaft to cause the fracture. Most authors feel that the incidence of femoral shaft fractures is increasing because of the increasing number of cars traveling at higher speeds, as well as the increasing number of recreational vehicles that expend high energy. Most series of femoral shaft fractures show a male preponderance, with an average of 25 to 30 years. The incidence of the injury is higher in major trauma centers that routinely care for victims of high-energy violent trauma such as motor vehicle, motorcycle, auto-pedestrian, and aircraft accidents.[12]

According to studies from England and Scandinavia, there is an increasing incidence of femoral shaft fractures in the elderly.[117,185,204] In contrast to femoral shaft fractures occurring in other populations, these fractures are commonly the result of low- to moderate-energy trauma. This increased incidence of fracture in the elderly is partly a result of the increased number of elderly persons in the general population but is slightly higher than would be expected as a result of a simple increase in elderly patients in the overall population. Thus perhaps elderly patients are becoming more active, predisposing this portion of the population to incidental trauma.

Mechanism of Injury

As stated, femoral shaft fractures are usually the result of major, violent trauma. These fractures occur most often in young adults, more commonly in young adult males, probably because those in this age group are more often involved in violent trauma associated with automobile accidents, motorcycle accidents, recreational vehicle accidents, and gunshot wounds. Recent advances in emergency medical services, patient identification, and transport have brought a larger number of severely injured patients to the hospital than ever before.[23,25,132,244] These patients are often resuscitated and survive injuries that would have been fatal in the past. This leaves the orthopedist with serious long-bone fractures that require treatment.

Gunshot fractures should be considered separately from those secondary to blunt trauma.[31,123] Low-velocity handgun and rifle injuries are treated as type I open fractures. High-velocity rifle injuries and close-range shotgun blasts should be considered type IIIB or IIIC open fractures (see Table 46–1).

The actual fracture pattern varies according to the line of force applied to the femur. Direct force applied perpendicular to the axis of the bone produces a transverse or short oblique fracture with local soft tissue trauma. Force applied to the femur in an axial direction risks injury to the hip or knee. Elderly patients tend to

Table 46–1.
Open Fracture Classification According to Gustilo et al.

Type I	An open fracture with a clean wound less than 1 cm long
Type II	An open fracture with a laceration more than 1 cm long without extensive soft tissue damage, flaps, or avulsions
Type IIIA	Adequate soft tissue coverage of a fractured bone despite extensive soft tissue laceration of flaps, or high-energy trauma regardless of the size of the wound
Type IIIB	Extensive soft tissue loss with periosteal stripping and bone exposure, usually associated with massive contamination
Type IIIC	Open fracture associated with arterial injury requiring repair

Source: Modified from Gustilo, R.B.; Anderson, J.T. Prevention of infection in the treatment of one thousand and twenty-five open fractures of long bones. J Bone Joint Surg 58A:453, 1976, and Gustilo, R.B.; Mendoza, R.M.; Williams, D.N. Problems in the management of type III (severe) open fractures: a new classification of type III open fractures. J Trauma 24:742, 1985.

sustain injury indirectly from a rotational force, which creates a long oblique or spiral fracture with minimal comminution. The amount of comminution at the fracture site tends to increase directly with the amount of energy absorbed by the femur at the time of fracture.

Anatomic and Functional Consequences of Injury

Femoral shaft fractures are a major insult to the patient's normal functional and physiologic status. A major absorption of energy within the femur is required to cause a simple femoral shaft fracture; absorption of excessive energy rapidly results in fracture comminution and the expenditure of energy that dissipates through the bone into the soft tissue, inflicting associated soft tissue damage. This damage may not be completely apparent from outward physical examination but can be anticipated from the comminution seen on radiographs. Loss of integrity of the femoral shaft places the patient immediately in a dependent position (i.e., he or she is left in bed with total dependence on others for normal function). Any attempt at motion in bed or any attempt to get out of bed will cause extreme pain, further blood loss and concurrent soft tissue trauma. It is accepted that a simple femoral shaft fracture can result in the loss of approximately two units of blood, or one fifth of the circulating blood volume.

Complications of femoral shaft fracture include those that are directly related to the fracture and those that are related to the specific fracture treatment modality. Complications directly related to the fracture include blood loss, total loss of independent functional activity, deterioration in pulmonary function (fat emboli, adult respiratory distress syndrome [ARDS]), and shock.[61,79,98,134,244,270] Any of these complications that are directly related to the fracture can be devastating to the multiply injured patient with other significant problems, such as head injury, chest injury, abdominal injury, or other fractures.[25,99,132] Most patients with a single, isolated femur fracture can generally tolerate the insult and survive with virtually any treatment of the femoral shaft fracture.[23,34]

Increasing evidence demonstrates that early stabilization of the femoral shaft fracture is a vital aspect in management of patients with multiple injuries.[23,25] Emergent fracture stabilization significantly decreases the incidence of pulmonary complications (ARDS, fat emboli, pneumonia, and total pulmonary failure). Fracture stabilization allows the patient to be mobilized out of the forced, supine position to an upright position, which immediately decreases the potential for the gut origin septic state described by Border.[25] Emergent fracture stabilization has been well documented to decrease medical and orthopedic complications in patients with complete or incomplete spinal cord lesions as well.[23,25,98,99,132,224–226,235,244] In addition to the proven clinical benefits of emergent fracture stabilization for femoral shaft fractures, the procedure significantly lowers the cost of health care to these patients.[132]

Complications directly related to individual treatment modalities include malunion, joint contracture of the hip or knee, heterotopic bone formation (myositis ossificans), loss of fixation, infection, and nonunion. As would be expected, certain treatment modalities are more prone to one complication than another, and these potential complications or the risk of them will be discussed with each treatment modality later on in this chapter.

As stated previously, once an individual sustains a femoral shaft fracture, he or she becomes immediately nonfunctional. The individual remains in this potential condition for a period of four to six months as the femoral shaft fracture heals. Open fractures and those fractures that are opened by the treating physician tend to be slower in healing. No treatment has been shown to speed healing of femoral shaft fractures (or of any other fracture), but certain treatment modalities allow patients to be more or less functional during the healing phase of the fracture. Most, if not all, femoral shaft fractures are currently treated surgically. Current practice emphasizes fracture stabilization that allows near-normal function of the lower extremity, with perhaps the exception of full weight-bearing ambulation during fracture healing. Any proposed new treatment modality for femoral shaft fractures must address the need to get the patient out of bed, upright, and functioning in a near-normal manner soon after injury.

Open femoral fractures and those that are opened by the treating physician carry an increased risk of infection, as well as of delayed union or nonunion. Nonunion can usually be related to opening the fracture site, lack of blood supply to the fracture, distraction of the fracture, or malnutrition. Fractures that are treated closed (i.e., the fracture site itself is not opened or exposed to the environment) have a virtually 100% rate of healing. Malunion consisting of shortening, malrotation, or angulation is more common with nonoperative treatment but can occur with any treatment modality. The physician must continually monitor fracture alignment to avoid malalignment in any plane.

Commonly Associated Injuries

As noted previously, peripheral nerve injuries associated with a femoral shaft fracture are rare. The sciatic nerve is well protected by muscle from the bone itself and requires extreme traumatic displacement of the fracture to allow injury directly to the nerve (Fig. 3B). The nerve is more commonly injured by direct, penetrating trauma (e.g., a gunshot wound or laceration) than it is by blunt trauma. Most neurologic injuries associated with femoral shaft fractures are the result of difficulties or problems with treatment rather than with the injury.

Vascular injuries associated with femoral shaft fractures are also uncommon. The literature indicates that these occur at a rate of approximately 2 per 100 fractures (2%).[66,68] Evidence implies that the incidence of occult injury to the femoral artery may actually be higher than previously thought.[16] Penetrating trauma in proximity to the femoral artery of sufficient energy to cause a fracture is an indicator for an arteriogram in *all* cases. If the patient has palpable peripheral pulses and a viable foot at the time of presentation, the arteriogram may be delayed until immediately following fracture stabilization. Blunt trauma causing a fracture of the distal fourth of the femoral shaft can tear the femoral artery at the level of the adductor canal, where it is tethered by local soft tissue structures. This injury may be an intimal tear, and the patient may have normal distal pulses. Complete occlusion of the artery with delayed distal ischemia may occur later.[215,239] Any question regarding an arterial injury with penetrating or blunt trauma should be resolved by arteriogram. This may be delayed (up to 24 hours) if distal pulses are present and the patient's peripheral vascular status can be closely monitored.

Specific treatment of arterial injuries is dependent on the severity of vascular compromise and the amount of time elapsed since injury. If distal pulses are present, indicating normal flow, the femoral shaft fracture should be stabilized initially and an arteriogram obtained following fracture stabilization. If arterial compromise is severe, as with complete laceration, arterial flow must be reestablished within 6 hours (Fig. 46–5).[13,89,247] The patient should be taken immediately to the surgical suite, where the artery is explored and a temporary shunt inserted by the vascular surgeon.[192,223] The femoral shaft fracture should then be stabilized by internal or external fixation.[221] This is followed by permanent arterial repair, all during a single operative procedure. Arterial repair is usually accomplished by interposition of a vein graft or by synthetic graft. When documented ischemia of the lower extremity has been present concomitant with a femoral shaft fracture, a four-compartment fasciotomy of the lower leg should always be performed early to prevent distal compartment syndrome in the calf resulting from the reperfusion of ischemic tissue.[68] This includes virtually all

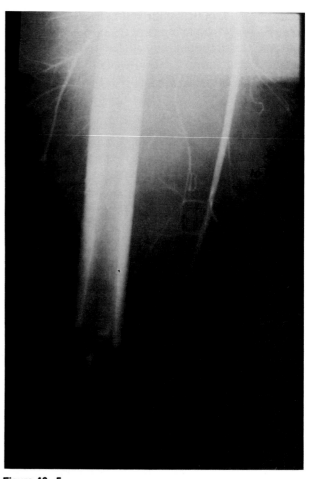

Figure 46–5

Arteriogram showing fracture of the distal one third of the femur with an associated femoral artery injury at the level of the fracture.

cases of acute femoral arterial repair. Whenever the femoral artery is repaired, any accompanying venous injury should be repaired as well, as this improves the early venous runoff. Sciatic nerve injuries in conjunction with arterial injury are generally caused by ischemia, contusion, or stretching and seldom require exploration or surgical repair.[89]

Open femoral shaft fractures are relatively common. In Winquist et al.'s classic study of femoral shaft fractures from Harborview Medical Center in Seattle, open fractures occurred in approximately 16.5% of the 520 femoral shaft fractures treated.[298] Of the 86 open fractures, 76 (88.4%) were type I open fractures (small skin wound with minimal or no stripping of soft tissue from bone). Eight (9.3%) were type II open fractures (moderate skin and muscle injury with wound contamination). Only two (2.3%) were type III open fractures (severe injury with devitalized skin, muscle, and neuromuscular structures that actually threaten the survival of the limb). Therefore, although open fracture is relatively common in the femur, this open injury tends to be rather mild as it presents to the outer skin because of the large soft tissue envelope surrounding the femur.[39,159] However, the deep soft tissue injury can be significant, in spite of the fact that the local skin has been violated only minimally. Type III open femoral shaft fractures are extremely severe injuries, and the femoral shaft fracture and soft tissue injury alone make this patient a multiply injured patient. The treatment of this particular injury pattern is the topic of another section of this chapter.

Several musculoskeletal injuries are frequently seen in conjunction with femoral shaft fractures. Injury to the proximal femur (femoral neck or intertrochanteric fracture), as well as hip dislocation, occurs uncommonly. Such injuries are more common in blunt trauma patients with multiple injuries.[15,20,240] The treating physician must continually be aware that injury may be present in the femur at more than one level. All femoral shaft fractures must be specifically evaluated with an anteroposterior (AP) radiograph of the pelvis and an internal rotation view of the femoral neck (Fig. 46–6). Failure to recognize a femoral neck fracture has been reported to occur in up to 30% of cases.[50,90,262,263] Failure to diagnose this severe injury and treat it appropriately can increase the risk of avas-

cular necrosis or nonunion of the femoral neck resulting in loss of hip function. Knee ligament injury has been reported to occur in association with femoral shaft fracture in 15% of cases.[262] Virtually all femoral shaft fractures result in an associated knee effusion, which is suggestive evidence of a major knee ligament injury.[206,248] It is difficult to evaluate the status of knee function and knee ligaments in the presence of an unstable fracture of the femoral shaft. Once fracture stability has been achieved by surgical treatment or fracture union, the knee ligament status must be evaluated and appropriately treated. Many of these knee ligament injuries require surgical attention. The most appropriate time for evaluation of the knee is on the operating room table immediately following femoral shaft fracture stabilization. Thus the operative permit obtained should include an examination under anesthesia and appropriate treatment as necessary for knee ligament injuries.

Ipsilateral fracture of the tibia occurs relatively commonly in conjunction with femoral shaft fracture. This injury pattern, the so-called "floating knee," is also common in the multiply injured patient.[20,170] Multiply injured patients with long-bone fractures have an approximately 50% incidence of ipsilateral femoral shaft and tibia fractures (Fig. 46–7).[132,137] This specific in-

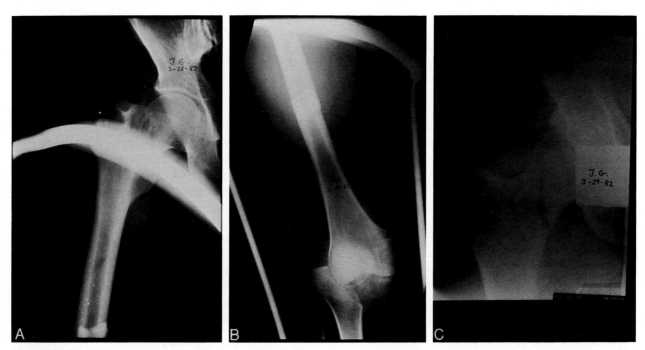

Figure 46–6

Fracture of the femur with femoral neck fracture. Notice the value of an internally rotated view of the femoral neck. *A*, AP radiograph of the proximal femur showing a transverse midshaft fracture of the femur. A Thomas splint ring obscures a view of the femoral neck. *B*, AP radiograph of the distal aspect of the same femur showing the femur fracture, as well as a fracture of the proximal tibia. *C*, In the operating room a radiograph is obtained with the hip in internal rotation. This view profiles the femoral neck and reveals a fracture.

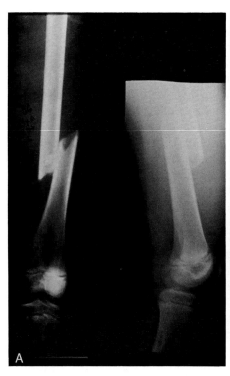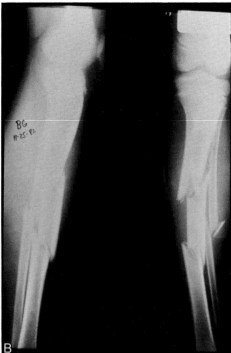

Figure 46–7

Fracture of the femoral shaft associated with fracture of the tibia, the "floating knee" lesion. *A*, AP and lateral radiographs of the femur and knee in a skeletally immature patient (13 years old) reveal a short oblique fracture of the femoral shaft. *B*, AP and lateral x-ray of the ipsilateral tibia in the same patient showing an unstable segmented tibia fracture.

jury combination requires stabilization of both femoral shaft and tibia fractures to optimize the functional outcome.[279] Failure to stabilize either the femur or the tibia results in loss of knee motion, which is generally unacceptable to most patients. All patients with an ipsilateral femoral shaft and tibial fracture should be approached as multiply injured patients because of the high frequency of injury to other body regions.[132]

The femoral shaft fracture is perhaps the most common orthopedic injury in a multiply injured patient, and virtually all major traumatic injuries can occur in association with a femoral shaft fracture.[23] It is not uncommon for patients with femoral shaft fractures to have associated traumatic injuries to the head, chest, spine, and abdomen. Therefore potential injuries to one or more of these major systems, many of which may be life-threatening, must be carefully explored and evaluated. Treatment of the associated injuries may have a significant effect on treatment of the femoral shaft fracture. This is true regarding both the timing of fracture stabilization and the specific technique utilized.

Classification

EVOLUTION

Basic surgical treatment is only minimally modified by a classification or extensive description of the fracture itself. Intramedullary nailing is the most commonly and widely accepted treatment for femoral shaft fractures. Classifying the fracture extensively does not change the fact that an intramedullary nail will be the best treatment. The classification scheme is somewhat helpful, however, in deciding whether to place a locked intramedullary nail with proximal or distal bolts or both.[53,138,145,298] Even this decision-making process should not be as complex as once thought, as both proximal and distal locking bolts are advisable in the majority of cases.[41,42] This issue is discussed in further detail later in the chapter.

It is important to distinguish open from closed fractures. Open fractures in the femur usually involve a more violent force. The open fracture requires immediate irrigation and debridement of the wound to counteract the greater potential for infection in these cases.[39,56] Because of the soft tissue stripping from the bone that occurs in open fractures, areas of cortical bone have a much greater tendency for necrosis, which can contribute to infectious complications.[227,275] Grading of open femoral shaft fractures using the Gustilo classification has prognostic value (Table 46–1).[9,105,106] As noted previously, type I and II open femoral shaft fractures have a minimal increase in complications when compared with closed fractures when treated by early irrigation and debridement, regardless of which treatment modality is chosen, including immediate intramedullary nailing.[39,159] On the other hand, type III open femoral shaft fractures—those with severe soft tissue damage, serious contamination, or arterial injury requiring repair — are major injuries that should be differentiated from type I and II open fractures in that their prognosis is significantly worse as to both the rate of infection and the rate of union. Type III open fractures should be specifically graded according to recommendations by Gustilo.[9,106] Type IIIA fractures have adequate soft tissue coverage of bone, despite extensive lacerations of flaps of soft tissue. Type IIIB fractures have extensive injury to the soft tissue, with periosteal stripping and exposure of bone. These fractures have appreciable contamination and require soft tissue coverage procedures that may include skin graft or flap coverage. A type IIIC fracture is associated with arterial injury that requires repair. Brumback and others have reported a significant difference in complications that increases from type IIIA to type IIIC.[39,127]

Classifications of femoral shaft fractures have tended to be rather simplistic. Fractures in the proximal femur that involve the metaphysis have been described as femoral neck fractures, intertrochanteric fractures, or subtrochanteric fractures. Subtrochanteric fractures have been defined and classified perhaps as much as any other fracture in orthopedic surgery.[91,305-307] Unfortunately most of the classification schemes for subtrochanteric fractures are quite confusing and have little relevance to current treatment modalities.

Subtrochanteric fractures are reviewed in detail in chapter 45. Earlier classifications of these injuries included the upper 5 cm of the femoral shaft (fractures that occur at the level of the lesser trochanter and 5 cm distal to it). With modern femoral shaft fracture treatment techniques, these injuries can be successfully treated in a manner similar to that for other diaphyseal fractures, so that there is little, if any, rationale for calling them subtrochanteric fractures.[131] Therefore this chapter covers femoral fractures that occur from the level of the lesser trochanter distally to the femoral condyles. Because fracture patterns do not always respect classification schemes, some transitional forms will be encountered. Fractures extending proximally only into the lesser trochanter can be treated as shaft fractures, with only minimal modification of surgical planning or technique. Fractures extending from the shaft into the greater trochanteric region are complex and difficult.[131] No "best" treatment is available for these injuries, and they demand careful analysis and individualized therapy, as discussed in chapter 45.

Previous classification schemes of femoral shaft fractures have included the location of the fracture (i.e., in the proximal, middle, or distal third of the shaft) and a description of the fracture based on its radiographic appearance.[186] This is a simple descriptive term for the fracture, such as "transverse," "short oblique," "lone

oblique," "butterfly fragment," "comminuted," or "segmental" (Fig. 46-8). Therefore a complete classification description would be "a transverse midshaft fracture of the femur" or "a short oblique fracture of the distal third of the femur." This classification scheme serves quite well for complete understanding of most femoral shaft fractures when the pattern and location of the fracture are given together (proximal third, middle third, distal third). It is simple and easy to understand, as it presents a graphic picture of the problem, with the exception of a more complete description of comminution.

A classification of comminution of femoral shaft fractures was described by Winquist and co-workers (Fig. 46-9).[297,298] This assigns comminuted fractures to one of five grades, with the numbers increasing with the degree of comminution. These fractures are caused by a high level of energy absorption in young, healthy bone. They have a high propensity to heal with shortening and malrotation if their degree of instability is not recognized and treated appropriately. A grade I comminuted fracture has a small butterfly fragment that is less than 25% of the width of the bone. A grade II comminuted fracture has a larger butterfly fragment of 50% or less of the width of the bone. These fractures (grade I and II) may be relatively stable in length and rotation, as there is good contact between the major proximal and distal fragments, if the fracture occurs away from the proximal or distal metaphyseal flare. Grade III comminuted fractures consist of a larger segment of comminution (greater than 50% of the width of the bone) with only a small spike of remaining proximal and distal fragments continuing in cortical contact. These fractures are always unstable in length and rotation. Grade IV comminuted fractures consist of segmental comminution with no bone contact between the major proximal and distal fragments. These fractures are always unstable in length and rotation. The final fracture grade (grade V) consists of segmental bone loss, which generally occurs in conjunction with an open fracture and is always an unstable fracture.

Fractures of the distal femoral metaphysis commonly involve the knee joint and are discussed in chapter 47. Treatment of these fractures is distinctly different from that of femoral shaft fractures. However, fractures in the distal third of the femur that have been termed "infraisthmal" may be classified as shaft fractures and treated in a similar manner with available treatment modalities.[37,222]

Two categories of femoral shaft fractures must be separated from those caused by significant trauma: pathologic fractures and fatigue fractures. Pathologic fractures occur with minimal trauma and can often be diagnosed prior to the occurrence of a displaced frac-

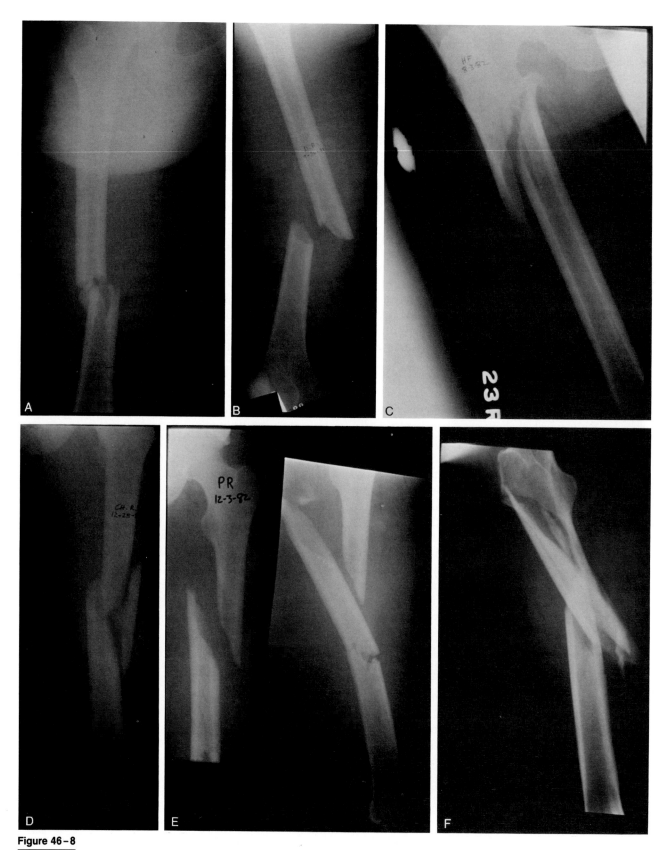

Figure 46-8

Descriptive terms used to characterize femoral shaft fractures. *A*, Transverse midshaft fracture. *B*, Short oblique fracture. *C*, Long oblique fracture. *D*, Butterfly (or wedge) fragment in midshaft femur fracture. *E*, Segmental fracture. *F*, Comminuted fracture.

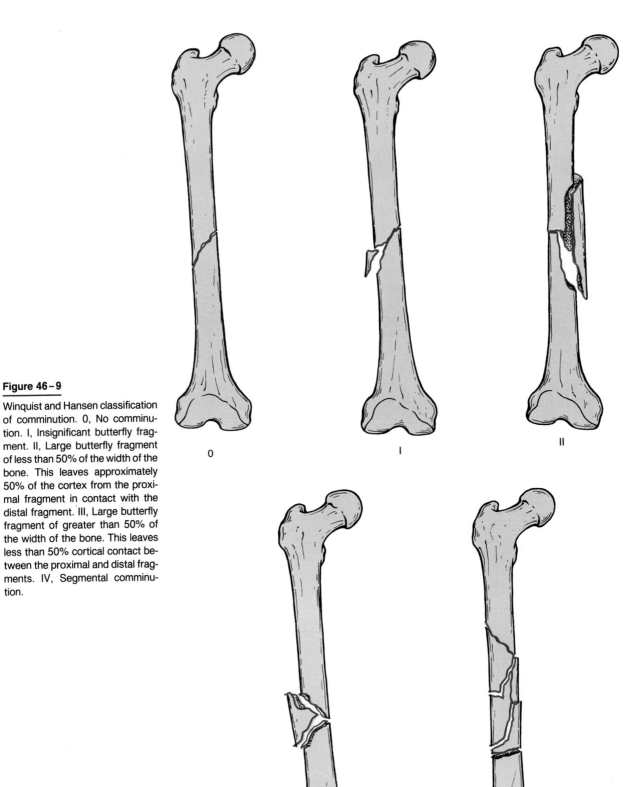

Figure 46–9

Winquist and Hansen classification of comminution. 0, No comminution. I, Insignificant butterfly fragment. II, Large butterfly fragment of less than 50% of the width of the bone. This leaves approximately 50% of the cortex from the proximal fragment in contact with the distal fragment. III, Large butterfly fragment of greater than 50% of the width of the bone. This leaves less than 50% cortical contact between the proximal and distal fragments. IV, Segmental comminution.

0

I

II

III

IV

II Butterfly with >50% circumferential contact
III Butterfly with <50% circumferential contact
IV Segmental comminution

1537

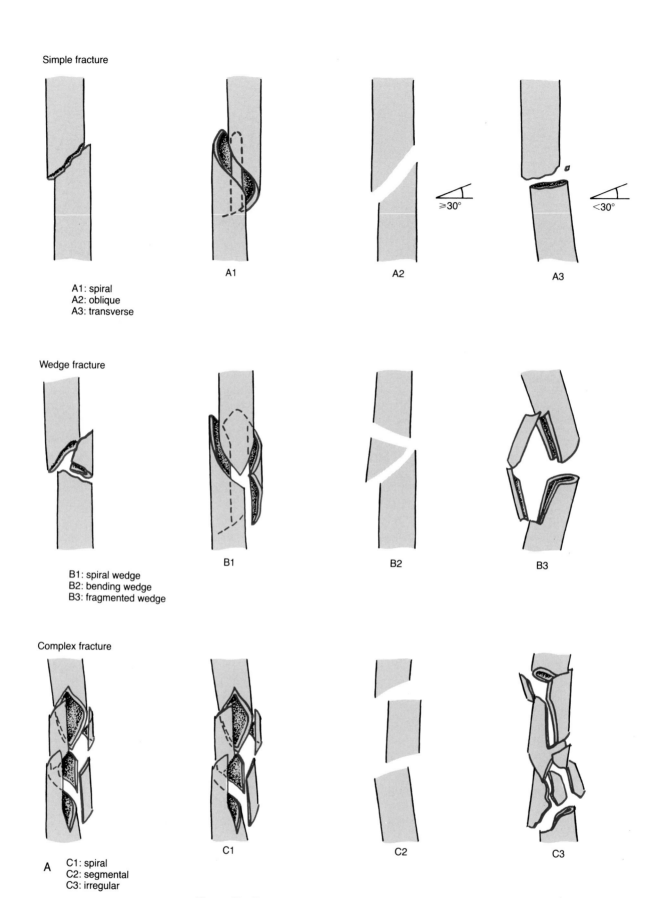

Simple fracture

A1: spiral
A2: oblique
A3: transverse

A1

A2

≥30°

A3

<30°

Wedge fracture

B1: spiral wedge
B2: bending wedge
B3: fragmented wedge

B1

B2

B3

Complex fracture

A   C1: spiral
C2: segmental
C3: irregular

C1

C2

C3

Figure 46–10

A, AO classification of femoral shaft fractures.

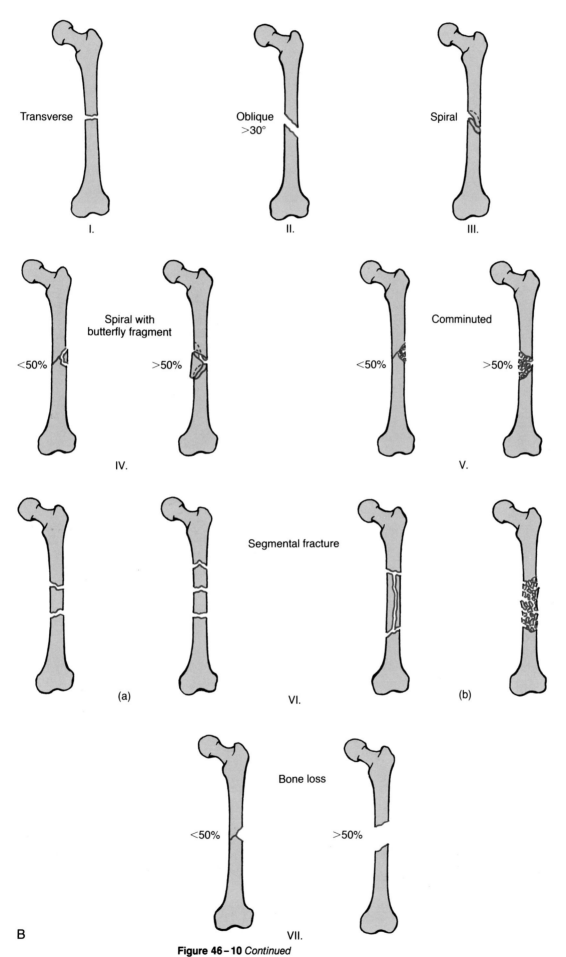

Transverse

I.

Oblique
>30°

II.

Spiral

III.

Spiral with
butterfly fragment

<50%   >50%

IV.

Comminuted

<50%   >50%

V.

Segmental fracture

(a)   VI.   (b)

Bone loss

<50%   >50%

VII.

B

Figure 46-10 *Continued*

B, OTA classification of femoral shaft fractures.

Illustration and legend continued on following page

LOCATION OF FRACTURE

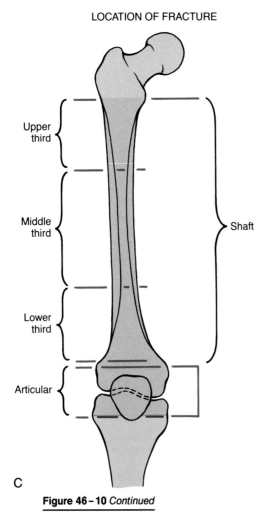

C

Figure 46 – 10 *Continued*

C, Descriptive terms for fracture location.

ture as a result of pain caused by microscopic infraction. Pathologic fractures caused by metastatic malignant tumors (with breast carcinoma being the most common) are common in the proximal femur.[107,114] Fractures caused by benign tumors can occur as well; these are more often primary lesions (solitary cyst, fibrous dysplasia, and enchondroma). Metabolic bone disease (Paget's disease, osteoporosis, and osteomalacia) can also cause pathologic fracture.[52] The femur is the most common bone fractured in patients with Paget's disease, and a significant deformity may be present within the affected femur that can render treatment difficult in these patients. Pathologic fractures are discussed in chapter 17.

Fractures caused by fatigue failure of bone can be a significant problem in the femur.[27] These may be asymptomatic until displaced fracture occurs.[175] They may actually be more common than metatarsal stress fractures in military recruits.[175] Exertional bone pain in

the thigh in a military recruit or long-distance runner should be treated with a high index of suspicion for fatigue fracture. Bone scans should be obtained, and if positive, the patient should be treated even in the presence of normal radiographs. Generally a period of rest is all that is required for treatment of most nondisplaced fatigue fractures of the femoral shaft, unless a lytic defect or lucent fracture line is present.

CURRENT CLASSIFICATION

Certain aspects of femoral shaft fractures are important in decision making regarding care for the patient and the fracture. A simple description of the level of the bone (proximal, middle, distal third) is important, as is a description of the fracture pattern, including the grade of comminution. Simple diaphyseal fracture classification schemes, offered by both the AO group (Müller) and the Orthopaedic Trauma Association (OTA), can be applied to femoral shaft fractures if a need to classify exists (Fig. 46 – 10).[104,186] These fractures can be understood in a matter of seconds from a simple review of the radiographs. Following classification of the fracture, it is important to classify the fracture as to the bone quality and patient age. Generally speaking, young patients have dense cortical bone. Elderly patients have brittle osteoporotic bone and a larger medullary canal.[185] The presence or absence of pathologic lesions, particularly in the elderly or middle-aged patient, is of significant concern. Whether the wound is open or closed should be determined, described, and classified as to grade of wound in all cases.[106,194,277] The fracture should be described as either an isolated injury or as part of a multiple-injury constellation. A multiply injured patient is described by injury severity scoring, and any patient with an injury severity score of 18 to 20 or more should be described as a multiply injured patient (Table 46 – 2). Following this, specific associated injuries that pertain to the femoral shaft fracture should be described. These would include an associated femoral neck fracture or vascular injury. Therefore, when describing a femoral shaft fracture, the following are important: whether the fracture is open or closed; whether the injury is isolated or one of multiple injuries; patient age; descriptive terminology including comminution of the fracture; level of the fracture; and finally, all significant or pertinent associated injuries. For example, the femoral fracture identified in Figure 46 – 11 would be classified as an isolated, closed, comminuted (Winquist grade IV) femoral shaft fracture in the middle third of the femur in a 30-year-old patient. This information includes all the important decision-making factors for this specific patient. If the patient has multiple injuries, the person

Table 46–2.

AIS Score	Injury
1	Minor
2	Moderate
3	Severe, not life-threatening
4	Severe, life-threatening
5	Critical, survival uncertain

Injury Severity Score (ISS)		
ISS Body Region	**AIS Score**	**Squared**
Head/neck	————	————
Face	————	————
Chest	————	————
ABD./pelvic contents	————	————
Extremities/pelvic girdle	————	————
External	————	————
ISS ———— (sum of squares of 3 most severe only)		

The Injury Severity Score (ISS) is an anatomically based system for grading injury severity for prediction of morbidity and mortality in patients with multiple injury combinations. Individual injuries are scored according to the Abbreviated Injury Scale (AIS) of the American Association for Automotive Medicine. (See Table 5–3.) Consistent ISS scoring requires that its precise definitions be followed. As described by Baker, the individual injuries are grouped into specified body regions. Only the most severe AIS for each region is considered. The ISS is calculated by adding the squares of the three highest regional AIS scores. It may not adequately represent the systemic challenge posed by multiple extremity injuries, since only the most severe contributes to the ISS.

American Association for Automotive Medicine: The Abbreviated Injury Scale (AIS), 1985 Revision. Des Plaines, IL, 1985.

Baker, S.P.; O'Neill, B.; Haddon, W.W., Jr. The injury severity score: a method for describing patients with multiple injuries and evaluating emergency care. J Trauma 14:187–196, 1974.

Copes, W.S.; Champion, H.R.; Sacco, W.J.; et al. The injury severity score revisited. J Trauma 28:69–77, 1988.

receiving the information needs to know the specific additional injuries. These factors have significant bearing on timing and treatment technique.

Diagnosis

The history of a potential femoral shaft fracture following presentation of the patient to the emergency department or to emergency medical personnel is often rather sparse. The patient will state, "I was in a car accident," or "My motorcycle crashed." The patient has little other information to provide. In many cases the patient is totally incapable of providing any information at all because of a closed head injury or some other extreme medical problem. Most historical information regarding the patient and circumstances of injury is obtained from the emergency medical personnel who deliver the patient to the medical facility. Important information that can be obtained from these personnel include the circumstances of the accident. Was this a rapid deceleration injury (as in a car striking a wall at high speed)? Did the accident occur in severe inclement weather? Did the accident involve a lake or river? A rapid deceleration injury suggests a potential diagnosis of aortic rupture, which may require an aortogram to confirm or

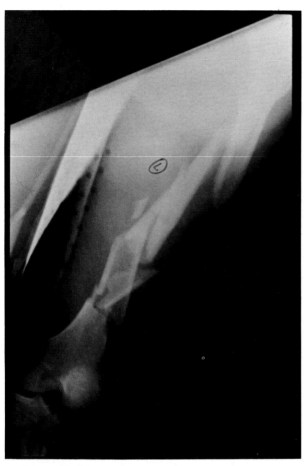

Figure 46–11

Comminuted midshaft femoral fracture (Winquist type IV).

history should be obtained from the patient and family as soon as possible.

The diagnosis of femoral shaft fracture is quite simple to make. Pain is extreme and excruciating, the limb is shortened, and marked deformity and instability are noted. In general, angulation is anterior and lateral. A large mass in the thigh may actually be a fracture fragment tenting the soft tissues. The patient is unable to move his or her hip, knee, or lower leg, generally because of extreme pain with any attempted motion. Although the diagnosis is made from the physical examination, radiographs are necessary to determine the optimal treatment modality. More significant physical findings are those caused by other injuries associated with femoral shaft fractures. The presence or absence of shock should be noted. Shock, which may have been present in the field, is a significant factor, and related information must be solicited from emergency medical personnel and recorded. Pain at the hip, back, or pelvis may indicate a complicating injury such as hip dislocation or hip fracture. These regions should be carefully evaluated. Knee effusion is often present with femoral shaft fracture and may be indicative of a significant knee ligament injury. It can be difficult to examine the knee until stabilization of the femur has taken place. The presence or absence of this effusion, along with localized tenderness involving the knee, should be duly noted in the record. Ligamentous stability must be determined by stress examination following stabilization of the femoral shaft fracture.

Of major importance in a femoral shaft fracture is the complete evaluation of nerve and vascular status at the time of presentation of the patient. Care should be taken to place the shaft fracture at rest with a temporary traction splint (Fig. 46–12). Following this, an immediate reevaluation is performed to determine neurologic and vascular status distal to the fracture. An attempt to perform this evaluation with the patient in an unstable situation and with a mobile femoral fracture can cause extreme pain and inability of the patient to cooperate for a thorough examination. However, the status of nerve or vessel function prior to splinting should be noted if possible. The most accurate examination, however, can be performed with gentle stabilization of the fracture by longitudinal traction. Partial reduction of the fracture through traction also allows the best evaluation of the vascular status by relieving any pressure or spasm the fracture itself may cause to local blood vessels. Symmetric palpable pulses in both bilateral feet generally indicate a lack of significant vascular injury. An absence of palpable pulses on the side of the fracture or asymmetric pulses should cause concern as to the vascular status of the fractured leg. Although distinct injury may or may not be present, a

disprove. Cold weather can cause hypothermia and associated metabolic problems. Water from certain lakes or rivers can contaminate an open femoral fracture with unusual organisms. Information such as whether the patient was pinned in a car for an extended duration of time and required a lengthy extrication is important to obtain. Gross neurologic function at the scene of the accident can also be reported historically by most trained emergency medical personnel and occasionally even by the lay public. Information regarding whether the individual was run over or simply struck by a vehicle may be available only from persons who were directly on the scene; these data can be crucial to treatment plans. Emergency medical personnel should be thoroughly questioned regarding the important aspects of the accident, as much valuable information can be obtained from them. Unless the patient is unusually alert, past medical history is difficult to obtain and generally has little bearing on the treatment modality chosen. Because drug allergies and other potentially serious medical conditions may be present, a complete

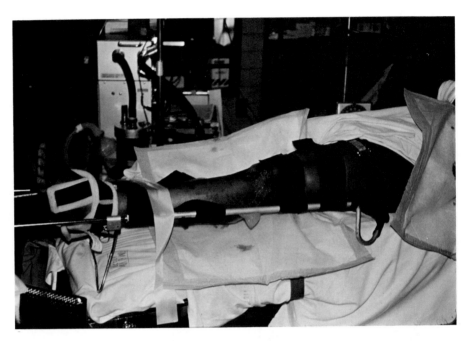

Figure 46–12

Patient in emergency department with Hare temporary traction splint in place to stabilize a femoral shaft fracture and aid in transport.

more thorough evaluation is then in order. Doppler pulse examination, with cuff pressure measurements if possible, is necessary in many patients with asymmetric pulses; such patients may need to be further evaluated by arteriography. Any question regarding the vascular status of the extremity should result in a prompt vascular surgical consultation to prevent major complications.

Neurologic evaluation should include the femoral nerve, which innervates the quadriceps musculature, as well as the peroneal and tibial branches of the sciatic nerve. As noted previously in this chapter, sciatic nerve injuries are relatively uncommon with femoral shaft fractures but have been reported. The neurologic status should be duly noted in the chart prior to undertaking any further treatment of the shaft fracture.

The soft tissue status of the thigh must be evaluated and recorded. The presence of abrasions, contusions, or hematomas should be documented. Degloving injuries of the skin must be noted and their extent evaluated and recorded. Open wounds should be thoroughly documented as to site on the thigh, as well as to size and surrounding tissue evaluation. They must be graded according to the grading schemes described by Gustilo or Tscherne.[106,194,275,277] The most appropriate evaluation of open wounds is done using a Polaroid camera at the time of presentation to the emergency department. This picture is added to the permanent hospital record. The open wounds are then covered with a sterile dressing that should not be removed until the patient is in the operating room for operative debridement. The photograph should be used to demonstrate the patient's wound to other members of the treatment team; a repeat inspection should not be made. Preoperative exposure of the wound repeated several times for wound inspection is associated with an increased risk of infection.[275]

RADIOGRAPHIC IMAGING

On patient presentation to the emergency department, it is usually apparent by physical evaluation that there is a femoral shaft fracture. These patients should all receive an AP radiographic evaluation of the pelvis at the time of presentation. This may be done as part of the patient's initial trauma evaluation and is generally done using a portable x-ray machine prior to sending a patient to the x-ray suite. This radiograph *must* be performed in addition to radiographs of the femur. Most x-ray cassettes in the United States will not allow the entire femur in an adult male to be recorded on one radiograph, thereby making the AP radiograph of the pelvis an even more crucial preliminary evaluation with femoral shaft fractures (Fig. 46–13). Other routine radiographs for multiply injured patients are a chest radiograph and a cervical spine trauma series, unless the patient is alert and completely asymptomatic. Complete evaluation of these plain radiographs obtained in the emergency department will document the fracture adequately to make definitive decisions regarding treatment. However, undisplaced proximal or distal fracture lines may be present but not noted on the immediate radiographic examination. Plain radiographs may not be clear in those femoral shaft fractures

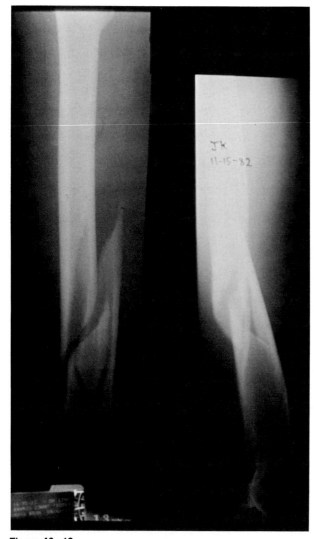

Figure 46 – 13

Radiograph of a femoral shaft fracture in an adult male that does not include the proximal femur.

that are secondary to fatigue or stress fracture or in those caused by pathologic lesion. Because of the poor quality of the radiograph (as a result of osteopenia), as well as the presence of the fracture through the potential pathologic lesion, these injuries may be difficult to define completely. In an elderly patient with a femoral shaft fracture, the presence of a potential pathologic lesion should be considered in the majority of cases.

Ipsilateral femoral neck and intertrochanteric fractures have reportedly been missed up to 30% of the time.[262,263] Generally the femoral neck fracture is missed because of failure to obtain an AP radiograph of the pelvis in the emergency department, because of an overlying foreign body such as a traction splint obscuring the fracture, or because of external rotation of the proximal femur, which obscures the fracture line on a

routine AP pelvis radiograph (Fig. 46 – 14). All surgically treated fractures of the femur require an internal rotation AP radiograph showing a profile of the femoral neck. This should be taken during anesthesia and may be done with image intensifier or by portable x-ray machine. However it is accomplished, the image should be obtained prior to completion of internal fixation of a femoral shaft fracture (Fig. 46 – 15). No femoral shaft fracture should undergo internal fixation without obtaining an AP radiograph of the pelvis. The internal rotation profile view of the femoral neck may be obtained on the fracture table with use of the C-arm image intensifier if closed intramedullary nailing is the surgical option chosen. If this is not the treatment modality chosen, then following surgical stabilization of any femoral shaft fracture, a plain internal rotation view profiling the femoral neck should be obtained during the anesthetic that is required for the surgery.

OTHER NECESSARY STUDIES

Any femoral shaft fracture that occurs from penetrating trauma (e.g., gunshot wound) with an entrance wound that is in proximity to a major vascular structure should have an arteriogram. This should be a mater of routine in all cases but may be delayed until after fracture stabilization if distal pulses are normal. If there is any question about differential pulses or circulatory disturbances in the foot, then the arteriogram is mandatory (Fig. 46 – 16) and should be obtained prior to fracture stabilization.

Those patients who appear with penetrating trauma in conjunction with a femoral shaft fracture and who have a cold, pulseless foot should undergo immediate exploration of the femoral artery at the level of the wound. Further definition of the injury by arteriogram will unacceptably delay vascular reconstruction and further jeopardize the limb.

One must remain aware of the possibility of femoral artery injury associated with distal third femoral shaft fractures. As previously noted in the section on anatomy, the femoral artery is tethered to soft tissue at the distal medial aspect of the thigh where the femoral artery exits the adductor canal (see Fig. 46 – 4). Because of this, if enough energy is applied to crease a distal third femoral shaft fracture, then there is significant potential for an arterial injury that will require reconstruction. All fractures that are distal to the midshaft of the femur should have careful evaluation of the vascular status of the limb. Any differential in pulse or change in pulse from one hour to the next should alert the treating physician to order an arteriogram to define the vascular anatomy. If the patient has normal pedal pulses on presentation, an arteriogram may be delayed until treatment of the femoral fracture has been accomplished. Careful consideration of the vascular status distal to the fracture should be given to all patients with fractures in the distal third of the femur. Any major concern should be evaluated by arteriography.

A report by Schwartz and co-workers has focused attention on a condition that was previously thought to be rare: thigh compartment syndrome.[242] The report, the largest in the world literature, noted thigh compartment syndrome in 1% of all femoral shaft fractures admitted at the authors' institution during a four-year study. Although the condition was rare in patients with uncomplicated, isolated, closed femoral shaft fractures,

10 of the 21 reported cases of thigh compartment syndrome occurred in multiply injured patients in conjunction with femoral shaft fracture. The syndrome developed most commonly in blunt trauma victims whose course was complicated by systemic hypotension and prolonged coagulopathy. The most common physical finding was a grossly swollen, tense thigh. In many cases the diagnosis was made following intramedullary nailing of the patient's femoral shaft fracture. At risk are multiply injured blunt trauma patients with prolonged systemic hypotension, a prolonged extrication from a vehicle, an extended period of hypothermia or exposure, or a history of external compres-

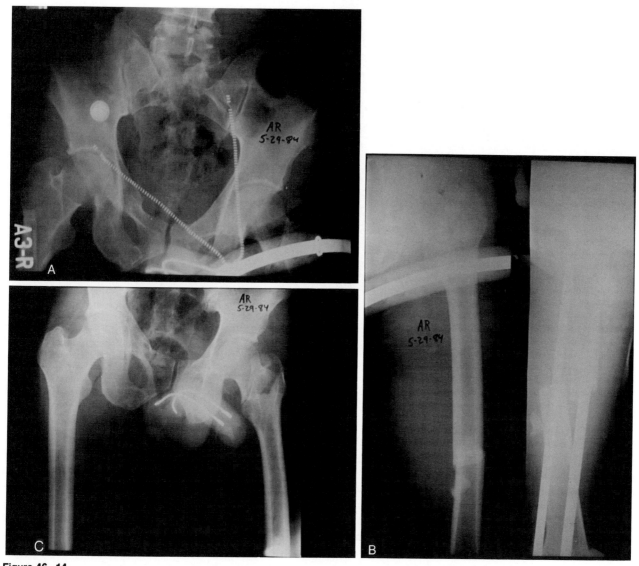

Figure 46–14

A, AP radiograph of the pelvis in a patient with a femoral shaft fracture. The splint obscures the view of the femoral neck. *B*, AP (left) and lateral (right) radiographs of the femur in the same patient, with a poor-quality radiograph of the hip and proximal femur. The Thomas splint obscures fracture detail. *C*, AP radiograph of the pelvis in the same patient with the Thomas splint removed, demonstrating femoral neck fracture.

Illustration and legend continued on following page

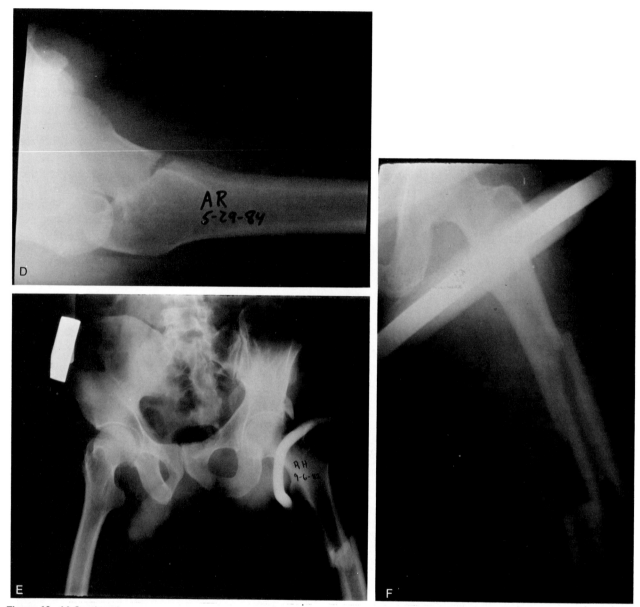

Figure 46-14 *Continued*

D, Lateral radiograph in the same patient, demonstrating femoral neck fracture. *E*, Similar AP radiograph of the pelvis in a patient with a femoral neck fracture. *F*, A proximal femur fracture may be hidden by the splint in this patient with a comminuted femoral shaft fracture.

sion of the thigh (including the use of the pneumatic anti-shock garment). The diagnosis is confirmed by intracompartmental pressure determinations. Intracompartmental pressures of more than 40 to 45 mm Hg in the thigh should be diagnostic of thigh compartment syndrome. In the Schwartz study, the average thigh compartment pressure in a patient with a thigh compartment syndrome was 49 mm Hg.[242] Eight patients (47%) died as a result of multiple injuries. In spite of prompt decompression and aggressive therapy, local wound problems, including infection and soft tissue necrosis requiring debridement and coverage, oc-

curred in more than 50% of patients who survived, indicating a high morbidity with this particular entity. The diagnosis of a thigh compartment syndrome should prompt an immediate decompressive fasciotomy.

Management

HISTORICAL REVIEW

Fracture of the femoral shaft has long been a catastrophic event that is limb-threatening and life-threat-

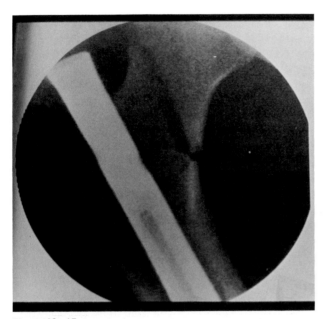

Figure 46-15

Permanent copy obtained from image intensifier during a surgical procedure to place an intermedullary nail in a femoral shaft fracture. The femoral neck fracture was not noted preoperatively but was seen intraoperatively with an internal rotation profile of the femoral neck.

ening. These injuries were virtually always treated with closed reduction and immobilization until 1940, when a distinct evolution in treatment began to take place.

Prior to the advent of radiography in the late 1890s, all treatment modalities for this injury centered on closed reduction, traction, manipulation, and gross anatomic realignment of the limb, accepting some deformity as inevitable. The limb was then immobilized using a variety of different materials, depending on availability. Some of the materials that have been used in various parts of the world to immobilize a fractured femur include plaster, wood or bamboo splints, fabric stiffened with wax, embalmer's fabric stiffened with gum, and others. Following the development of plaster of Paris–impregnated gauze in 1852 by Mathysen, this has been the material of choice, when available, to effect immobilization.[180,183]

With the advent of radiographs in the late 1890s, it became increasingly apparent that simple, gross reduction and immobilization of the fracture were not adequate for this injury. The healing thigh bone could be visualized deep within the sheath of surrounding muscles. Consecutive femur fractures reviewed at the Uni-

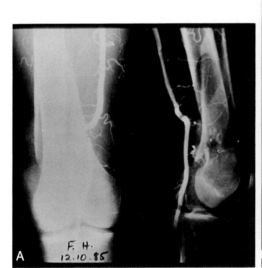
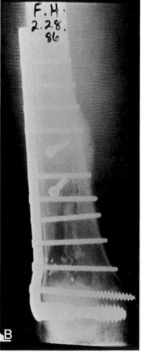
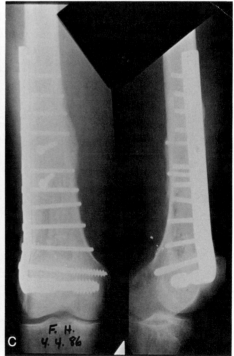

Figure 46-16

A, AP (left) and lateral (right) arteriograms demonstrating vascular injury in a patient with a gunshot fracture of the distal femur. The entrance wound is in proximity to the femoral artery. B, AP radiograph of the distal femur following arterial repair, internal fixation of the fracture, and autogenous bone grafting opposite the plate. C, AP (left) and lateral (right) radiographs four to five months later. Fracture healing is occurring normally, with periosteal callus formation as a result of the placement of bone graft.

versity of Pennsylvania were noted to result in an unsatisfactory result in 100% of the cases when treated with Buck's skin traction.[207]

In the early 1900s, efforts were directed toward finding better ways to apply longitudinal traction to the femur as a means of realigning it and maintaining length. Skeletal traction was developed and applied to femoral fractures by Steinmann and Kirschner, both of whom developed techniques using pins or wires inserted into the femur to apply stronger longitudinal traction.[183,257] Treatment with skeletal traction through a Steinmann pin or Kirschner wire has been used consistently in fracture treatment, particularly in the femur, since the early 1900s, with only minimal changes in the technique.

The Thomas splint, developed in the late 1800s by Hugh Owen Thomas in Great Britain, allowed for early ambulatory care of patients with femur fractures. It has been used for fractures of the femoral shaft since that time.[271] Only minimal modifications in the application of the splint have been made since Thomas's original innovation. The splint has been commonly used in conjunction with skeletal traction techniques and is used in many parts of the world (Fig. 46–17).

A major advance in the care of femoral shaft fractures occurred in 1940 with the first publication of Gerhardt Küntscher.[149,150,250] Although intramedullary nailing had been attempted sporadically in the care of long-bone fractures, it had never achieved generally accepted status. With his initial report in 1940 and the subsequent experience of Küntscher and other authors,

the trend began to change rapidly from nonoperative treatment of femoral shaft fractures to operative treatment of these fractures.[21,22,250] Excellent results in well-healed femurs and tibiae were noted in North America in 1945 when prisoners of war began returning from Germany. This triggered intense interest in the surgical treatment of femoral shaft fractures. Various surgical techniques were evaluated, including Küntscher's technique of closed reduction and intramedullary nailing.[22,30,47,78,79] Other methods were also evaluated in the United States and Europe, including open reduction and intramedullary nailing using various other designs of nails and open reduction and internal fixation with plate and screws.[28,30,87,129,241,259] As experience has been gained with various other forms of surgical treatment, including newer intramedullary nail designs and plates, most orthopedic surgeons have returned to Küntscher's original technique of closed reduction and intramedullary nailing using nails that are still quite similar to his original hollow cloverleaf cross-section nail (Fig. 46–18).[63,139,143–145,237,280]

Closed intramedullary nailing is the treatment of choice for virtually all femoral shaft fractures.[34,93,95,124,232,298] The origin and development of this technique should be directly credited to Gerhardt Küntscher.[148–150] A major development that has paralleled and allowed the development and use of the intramedullary nail is the improvement in portable fluoroscopy equipment and techniques. This has significantly increased the ease and safety of closed intramedullary nailing.

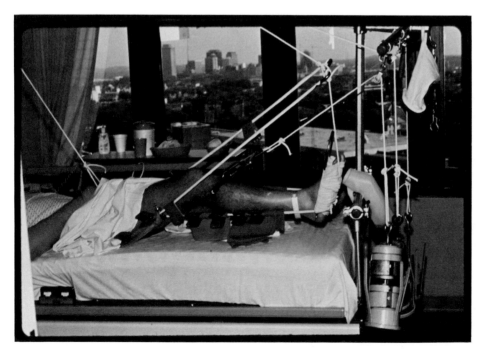

Figure 46–17

Thomas splint utilized with the Pearson attachment to apply skeletal traction and balanced suspension to a femoral shaft fracture.

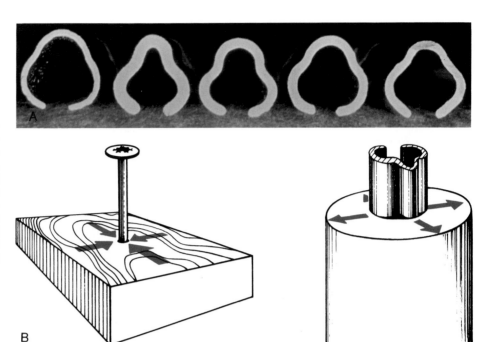

Figure 46-18

A, "Küntscher nails" from five different manufacturers, in cross section. Note differences in cross section and thickness of material. B, Küntscher's idea of the function of an intramedullary nail. Since bone is not as compliant as wood, he designed the nail as a slotted tube in hopes that it would be compressed and fit tightly into the medullary canal. This probably does not occur.

CURRENT MANAGEMENT

At present, the ideal treatment of a closed femoral shaft fracture is closed intramedullary nailing. This is true for all closed shaft fractures that occur from the level of the lesser trochanter to within 6 to 8 cm of the distal subchondral bone. It is true for both males and females and for patients ranging from early adolescents (10 to 12 years old) to the aged. It is a treatment modality that has proven to be perhaps as ideal a treatment modality as any in medicine.

Some decisions still remain to be made by the treating physician when dealing with unusual or concomitant fractures in the femur, most particularly proximal or distal metaphyseal fractures. The presence of fracture lines that extend into the metaphysis may modify decision making regarding femoral shaft fracture treatment. The presence or absence of an open wound, most particularly a severe contaminated open wound, may cause a change or modification in technique. Also, the presence or absence of severe comminution in the femoral shaft requires some extra attention to detail and perhaps some modification in the technique that might not otherwise have been considered.

Increasing reports in the orthopedic literature indicate that closed intramedullary nailing is the treatment of choice for femoral shaft fractures in adolescents as well as adults.[86,141,142,166,311,312] Young patients whose skeletal age is from 12 to 18 should be treated as adults when they have sustained a femoral shaft fracture. Difficulties with treating these patients in traction are quite similar to those encountered in adults. Basically these patients are too large to be easily cared for in a hip spica cast or any other means of immobilization. Physiologically their bone development is quite similar to an adult's, with the exception of the open distal femoral epiphysis, which in many cases is still contributing to longitudinal growth. The proximal femoral epiphysis, which extends from the capital femoral epiphysis down the lateral border of the femoral neck to include the greater trochanteric apophysis is well developed by age 12 (Fig. 46-19). The greater trochanter has generally completed its developmental growth. A potential growth arrest at this age interferes minimally with the development of the greater trochanter. The major concern about intramedullary nailing of femoral shaft fractures in patients of this age deals with the blood supply to the femoral head. Arterial blood enters the femoral head along the lateral border of the femoral neck from a complex of arterial anastomoses just medial to the greater trochanter. In spite of increasing numbers of adolescents whose femoral shaft fractures have been treated with intramedullary nailing, avascular necrosis of the capital femoral epiphysis has rarely been linked to this surgical procedure.[141]

Femoral shaft fractures in elderly patients are also managed best with closed intramedullary nailing.[185] Most large-diameter nails work well in the elderly patient because of the increased diameter of the intramedullary canal. Intramedullary nailing allows the elderly patient with a femoral shaft fracture to be upright virtually immediately in at least a sitting position if not in

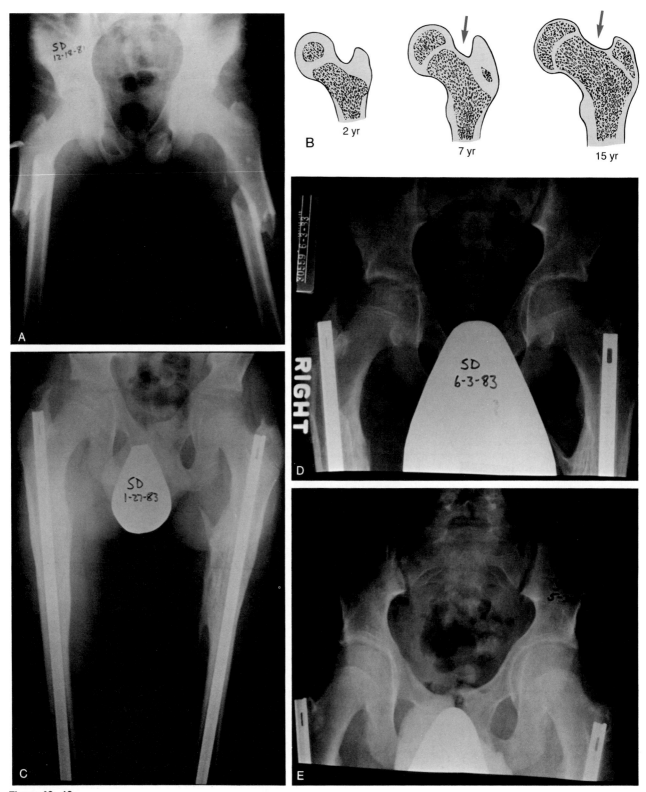

Figure 46–19

A, AP x-ray of the pelvis and proximal femur in a 10-year-old male with bilateral femoral shaft fractures and severe head injury. *B*, Drawing of a photomicrograph of proximal femoral epiphyseal development. *C*, AP x-ray of pelvis and femurs 1 year after intramedullary nailing and fracture healing. *D*, AP x-ray of pelvis 1.5 years after intramedullary nailing. *E*, AP x-ray of pelvis 35 years after intramedullary nailing and failure of attempted nail removal. Note overgrowth of left greater trochanter.

an ambulatory capacity. This has major therapeutic advantages to the elderly patient with multiple medical problems. Even the particularly large diameter of the intramedullary canal in elderly osteoporotic bone does not contraindicate intramedullary nailing. A large-diameter locked intramedullary nail with proximal and distal bolts will achieve adequate stability to allow the patient to at least be out of bed in a chair. The addition of distal bolts that expand and gain fixation to the nail rather than the bone may be of assistance in these cases.[278] Similar treatment can be used for intramedullary nailing in head-injured or spinal cord–injured patients.[14,94,95]

The degree and significance of comminution of the femoral shaft have been well described by Winquist and co-workers.[297,298] Classification of the severity of comminution aids in decision-making regarding the technique used for intramedullary nailing. Regardless of the extent of comminution at the fracture site, virtually all femoral shaft fractures can be treated with closed intramedullary nailing (see Fig. 46–10), but an interlocked nail is advisable, especially in fractures with higher grade comminution (grades II through V). Interlocking has been divided into *static* and *dynamic* types.

A static locked nail is an intramedullary nail with cross fixation using fixation through the nail both proximal and distal to the fracture. Cross fixation may be by means of bolts, pins, or blades placed through the femur and the nail. These devices fix the nail to the bone both above and below the fracture site (Fig. 46–20). This fixation controls length and rotation at the fracture site, which is not possible with routine intramedullary nailing. Locked intramedullary nailing has

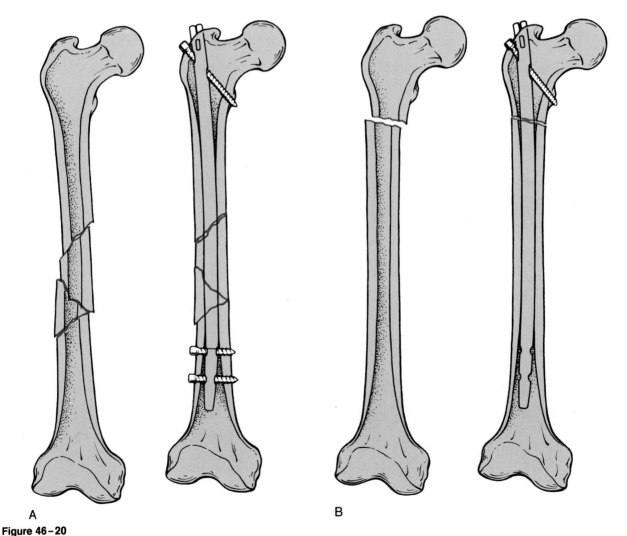

A   B

Figure 46–20

A, Static locked intramedullary nail fixed to both proximal and distal fragments. *B,* Dynamic locked intramedullary nail fixed to *either* the proximal (as shown) or distal fragment, but not to both.

extended the use of closed intramedullary nailing to virtually all femoral shaft fractures, regardless of the amount of comminution present. Only fractures with grade I comminution should be considered for anything less than a static locked nail. If more comminution occurs at the fracture site or there are longitudinal nondisplaced fissures in the bone, the patient should undergo static locked nailing.[41,42]

The term "dynamic locked nail" refers to an intramedullary nail that is fixed to the bone either proximal or distal to the fracture site but not both (Fig. 46-20). Dynamic locking improves purchase of the nail on the main fracture fragment to which it is interlocked but does not securely maintain length or rotation when there is comminution or limited fragment interdigitation. Control of the nonlocked fragment is provided only by interference fit of the nail within its medullary canal or by three- or four-point bending. It was originally felt that dynamic locking provided a more physiologic mechanical environment for fracture healing. However, experience has shown that sufficient fracture healing capability exists between statically locked fracture fragments so that callus formation is not retarded

when static locking is performed. Because failure to maintain alignment is a far more likely problem, static locking is generally preferred in most cases.

Segmental bone loss can occur with open femoral shaft fractures (Fig. 46-21).[313] These fractures may still be treated with a locked intramedullary nail (see section on open fractures). The major questions to be answered in these fractures are timing of bone grafting, type of fracture fixation, and whether to use a closed intramedullary bone graft as described by Chapman.[54] A minimally reamed or nonreamed (small-diameter) locked intramedullary nail may be placed in the open femur fracture for initial fracture stabilization. The patient is then returned to the operating room after the soft tissue injuries have been controlled for removal of this smaller, minimally reamed or nonreamed intramedullary nail. Closed intramedullary bone grafting using iliac crest bone graft is then performed, and the smaller diameter nail is replaced by a larger diameter static locked nail. Traction is necessary during this exchange to prevent femoral shortening.

Additional fractures in either the proximal metaphysis or distal metaphysis, in conjunction with a fem-

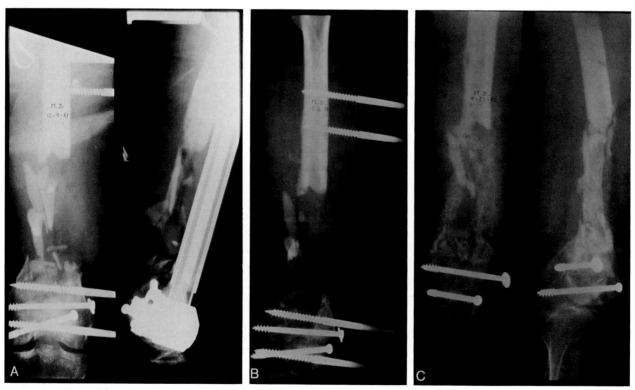

Figure 46-21

A, AP (left) and lateral (right) radiographs of an open distal femoral fracture with bone loss. Stabilization of intraarticular fractures was with lag screws for the articular components, and with a Wagner device for the shaft. B, Radiograph after autogenous bone grafting, when the wound was clean, closed, and dry. C, Following removal of external fixation, the patient was placed into a cast brace and allowed weight-bearing ambulation.

oral shaft fracture, may require distinct modification of the surgical technique of closed intramedullary nailing or selection of another treatment technique. Ipsilateral femoral neck or intertrochanteric fractures are difficult treatment problems and will be discussed in the section on special considerations. In many cases, with modification of the technique, a closed intramedullary nail may be selected, but in some instances the decision to use a plate on the femoral shaft fracture may be a reasonable alternative to the use of an intramedullary nail.

The presence of an open femoral shaft fracture requires due consideration and distinct changes in management. These are described in the next section.

OPEN FEMORAL SHAFT FRACTURES

Open femoral shaft fractures are categorized according to the Gustilo classification (Table 46–1).[106] As stated previously, because of the surrounding large muscle mass of the femur, a significant amount of energy absorption generally is required to create an open fracture of the femur.[194] Therefore even type I open femoral shaft fractures may be considered an extreme injury. Type IIIC open femoral shaft fractures are those that occur concomitantly with a major vascular injury that requires repair. These are severe injuries that are often limb- and life-threatening and generally occur in the presence of a significantly contaminated wound.

Because of the extreme amount of energy required to cause any open femoral fracture, these patients commonly have multiple associated injuries. A patient with an open fracture of the femur is considered to be a multiply injured patient and generally requires immediate fracture stabilization for this reason, as well as for the need to provide meticulous wound care.[56] Stabilization of open fractures has been shown to have many advantages.[173] Open femoral shaft fractures require individual consideration as to the appropriate mode of therapy. As stated in the previous section, intramedullary nailing of the femoral shaft is the treatment of choice for virtually all femoral shaft fractures, including open femoral shaft fractures.

Fortunately, severe open femoral shaft fractures (types IIIB and IIIC) are relatively uncommon occurrences. Brumback et al. described 469 fractures of the femur treated by intramedullary nailing over a 4½-year period.[39] Three hundred sixty-one (77%) were closed fractures, and 108 (23%) were open fractures. In this study from the Maryland Institute for Emergency Medical Services, more than half of these open femoral shaft fractures were type III open fractures (Table 46–1). The series seemed to be skewed toward more severe injuries. In another study by Lhowe and Hansen, 42 patients with open femoral shaft fractures and a 12-month follow-up were identified over a five-year period. Fifteen (36%) were type I, 19 (45%) were type II, and eight (19%) were type III.[159] This series appears to be more indicative of the severity of open fractures seen in most trauma institutions.

Open femoral shaft fractures require immediate formal irrigation and debridement in the operating room. This is true for all open femoral shaft fractures, including minimal type I open fractures with a wound that appears to be a small puncture. It is impossible to determine the degree of contamination of the sharp end of a bone that temporarily penetrates the skin and then recedes back into the wound. Treatment of the femoral shaft fracture following immediate irrigation and debridement remains somewhat controversial. Many authors, including Chapman, have advocated an initial period of traction (approximately ten days) to allow for soft tissue healing, after which time the patient should be returned to the operating room for closed intramedullary nailing.[55,56] Other authors, including Dabezies et al. and Hughes and Sauer, have advocated the use of an external fixation device, particularly for severe open femoral shaft fractures.[7,71,130] Increased attention has been given to immediate intramedullary nailing of open femoral shaft fractures (types II and III). Several reports are available in the literature regarding immediate intramedullary nailing of open femoral shaft fractures.[39,159] Lhowe and Hansen noted a 5% overall incidence of infection in the 42 patients treated with immediate intramedullary nailing in their series.[159] Brumback et al.[39] noted an overall infection rate of 3% in those patients treated with intramedullary nailing of open femoral shaft fractures. There was a 6% incidence of infection in type III open femoral shaft fractures; two of the three infected patients were treated with delayed intramedullary nailing. Templeman,[265a] reporting a combined series from Minneapolis and Sacramento, noted an overall infection rate of 1.5% in all open fractures treated by intramedullary nailing. The incidence of infection in type III open fractures was 4.8%. This series combined delayed intramedullary nailing with immediate intramedullary nailing. In all open femoral fractures, when delayed intramedullary nailing is compared with immediate intramedullary nailing, the incidence of infection is similar. Virtually all reported infections have occurred in type III open femoral fractures. Current recommendations from most authors on open femoral fractures are that types I and II open femoral fractures in either the isolated fracture or multiple injury patient can be appropriately treated by prompt irrigation and debridement, followed immediately by closed intramedullary nailing, all done on the day of injury. Multiply injured patients with a type III (A or B) open femoral shaft fracture should undergo irrigation and debridement, followed by immediate intramedullary nailing with an unreamed or minimally reamed (small-diameter) nail. Patients with a type III open fracture and no concomitant injuries should undergo immediate irrigation and debridement, followed by a brief (approximately ten-day) course of traction. Then they may be returned to the operating room for closed intramedullary nailing of the fracture following benign soft tissue healing. This is true for types IIIA and IIIB open femoral fractures. Type IIIC open fractures and those with severely contaminated wounds may be considered for application of external fixation accord-

ing to the individual patient's needs and the surgeon's experience.

Skeletal traction is not well tolerated by the patient who has sustained multiple injuries, which is often the case in the patient with an open fracture of the femoral shaft. Access to the wound is difficult, and the degree of soft tissue and bone instability makes this the least desirable of all treatment options. Skeletal traction can control length and rotation and occasionally may serve as a temporary means of stabilization in certain cases of isolated open fracture.

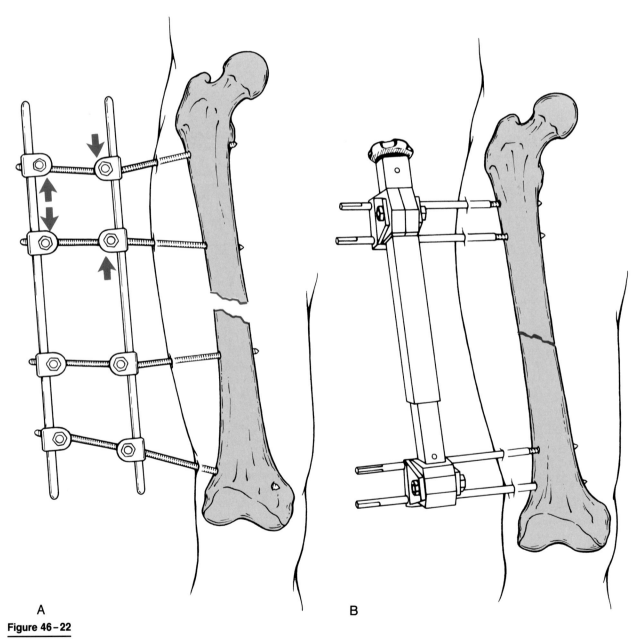

A   B

Figure 46-22

External fixation of the femur. A, Stacked lateral one-half pin frame (unilateral frame). B, Wagner external fixation. (Orthofix external fixator is applied with a similar construct using 6-mm pins.)

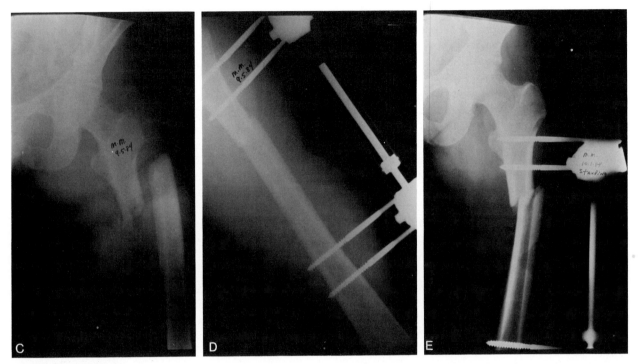

Figure 46-22 *Continued*

C, AP radiograph of the proximal femur in a patient with a type IIIC open fracture. *D,* AP radiograph following irrigation, debridement, and external fixation using the Wagner apparatus. *E,* AP radiograph of the femur with the patient standing, one month following *D,* demonstrating loss of alignment in external fixation.

Open reduction and internal fixation with a plate have been advocated for open fractures. However, increased rates of infection have been reported with this form of treatment.[26,164,228] This is thought to be the result of further devitalization of soft tissue and bone that often accompanies this technique.

Dabezies and associates[71] reported a series of open femoral shaft fractures treated with external fixation. They noted an incidence of soft tissue infection of 30%, consisting primarily of infected pin tracks. Loss of knee motion occurred in more than 50% of patients and in some was quite severe. Malunion or excessive angulation occurred in 15%. These results do not compare favorably with the use of immediate or delayed intramedullary nailing for open femoral shaft fractures. External fixation may play a role in treatment of patients with type IIIC fractures (those with a required vascular repair) or with a severely contaminated open fracture. When external fixation is indicated, every consideration should be given to the use of a stacked external fixation system applied laterally in a unilateral single plane configuration utilizing two parallel tubes or bars (Fig. 46-22), as opposed to the Wagner apparatus,[7] which is associated with a high incidence of malunion.[71] This allows pins to be configured in the femur in such a way as to improve mechanical stability and prevent potential malalignment problems.

PATHOLOGIC FRACTURES

Pathologic fractures are those produced by forces much less than required to disrupt normal bone. The femur is a common site for metastases of many malignancies and is also a relatively common site for benign bone tumors (fibrous dysplasia, solitary bone cyst, enchondroma). It is frequently involved in senile or postmenopausal osteoporosis. Each of these lesions can lead to pathologic fracture of the femoral shaft. Additionally the femur is a common location of fatigue fractures in individuals involved in high-level activity (e.g., military recruits and high-level athletes).[161,216,300] A prospective study by Milgrom et al. demonstrated that the femur is the most common site of fatigue fracture in military recruits.[175] These fatigue fractures of the femur can be asymptomatic. Asymptomatic fatigue fractures of the femur were diagnosed by bone scans in military recruits who had symptoms suggesting fatigue fracture in another area. Luchini and co-workers have shown that femoral fatigue fractures may displace.[161]

Exertional bone pain in a military recruit or a long-distance runner should be considered a fatigue fracture until proven otherwise. Bone scans should be obtained in all cases, and if they are positive, the patient should be treated, even when radiographs are normal. General first-line treatment is removal of the patient from the stressful activity (e.g., as marching in the case of a military recruit or running in the case of the long-distance runner). The use of crutches for weight bearing may be indicated as well. The idea is to protect and rest the femoral stress fracture and allow it to heal, hopefully preventing fracture displacement, which may require surgical stabilization.[216]

Malignant metastatic lesions tend to develop in the proximal metaphysis of the femur but can actually occur throughout its shaft (Fig. 46–23). Any patient with a femoral shaft fracture that occurs in the absence of major blunt or penetrating trauma should be thoroughly evaluated for a pathologic fracture. Patients with symptomatic lesions in their femur (pain with weight bearing) or those with lesions that appear to be greater than half the circumference of the bone should be considered for prophylactic stabilization of the femoral shaft prior to the onset of pathologic fracture. All too often patients are not referred to the orthopedic surgeon until after a femoral shaft fracture. Studies by Harrington,[114] Haberman,[107] and others have demonstrated that the morbidity created by internal fixation of an impending pathologic fracture of the femur is significantly less than the morbidity created by stabilization of the femur following pathologic fracture of the shaft. All pathologic fractures of the femoral shaft are best treated by intermedullary nailing if possible. In many cases, this may be done with an open technique to obtain a biopsy of the lesion. For pathologic lesions that involve the entire femur, including the shaft and proximal metaphysis, second-generation locked intramedullary nails are available that stabilize the entire femur essentially from the subchondral bone of the femoral head to the subchondral bone of the distal femur (see Fig. 46–23). For extensive pathologic lesions that involve a large portion of the proximal metaphysis and extend down into the diaphysis, consideration may also be given to prosthetic replacement of the proximal femur. However, this should be done only in rare instances.

The use of polymethylmethacrylate in addition to intramedullary nailing should be considered for pathologic fractures when the methylmethacrylate will add to the biomechanical stability of the surgical construct.[115] Methylmethacrylate is best used in conjunction with closed-section nails (Zickel nail, Russell-Taylor nail). When used with open-section nails (Küntscher nail, Grosse-Kempf nail, AO nail), the methylmethacrylate in a wet or doughy state often finds its way to the point of least resistance, which is the hollow center of the nail.

Benign pathologic fractures involving the femur are treated in a manner similar to that used for malignant pathologic fractures that involve the femur. In tumorous conditions, such as fibrous dysplasia or Paget's disease, that cause a significant deformity to occur in the femur, open or closed osteotomy of the femur may be required to assist in realignment of the femoral shaft prior to the placement of an intramedullary nail. Realignment adds to the mechanical stability of the femur, aids in ambulation, and may prevent further deformity from occurring. Benign lesions involving the femoral shaft that are symptomatic with ambulation or activity or involve more than half the circumference of the femoral shaft should be considered for prophylactic stabilization using an intramedullary nail. The femur is the most common bone fractured in patients with Paget's disease, and because of the significant deformity present and the extreme vascular nature of the bone, treatment of fractures that occur in conjunction with Paget's disease may be extremely difficult.[103]

Pathologic fractures are covered in greater detail in chapter 17.

Special Considerations

THE MULTIPLY INJURED PATIENT

The multiply injured patient is defined by injury severity scoring.[8] Such scoring is based on grading of the patient's anatomic injuries and is discussed in chapter 5. Injury severity scoring is a standard means of evaluating risks of morbidity and mortality in multiply injured patients and allows comparison of different treatments. A conventional definition of a multiply injured patient is one with an Injury Severity Score (ISS) of 18 or more (Table 46–2).[8] A closed femoral shaft fracture, a "major" injury as defined by this scoring system, contributes 9 points to the ISS. Therefore another "major" injury in any other system would make the patient a multiply injured patient.

Multiple retrospective studies have indicated a significant benefit in immediate stabilization (i.e., in the

---

Figure 46–23

A, Skull radiograph in a patient with metastatic breast carcinoma. *B,* AP radiograph of the pelvis in the same patient following a complaint of left hip pain. The patient was placed on crutches. *C,* AP radiograph of left femoral shaft. *D,* AP radiograph of right femoral shaft one month later at the onset of acute right leg failure.

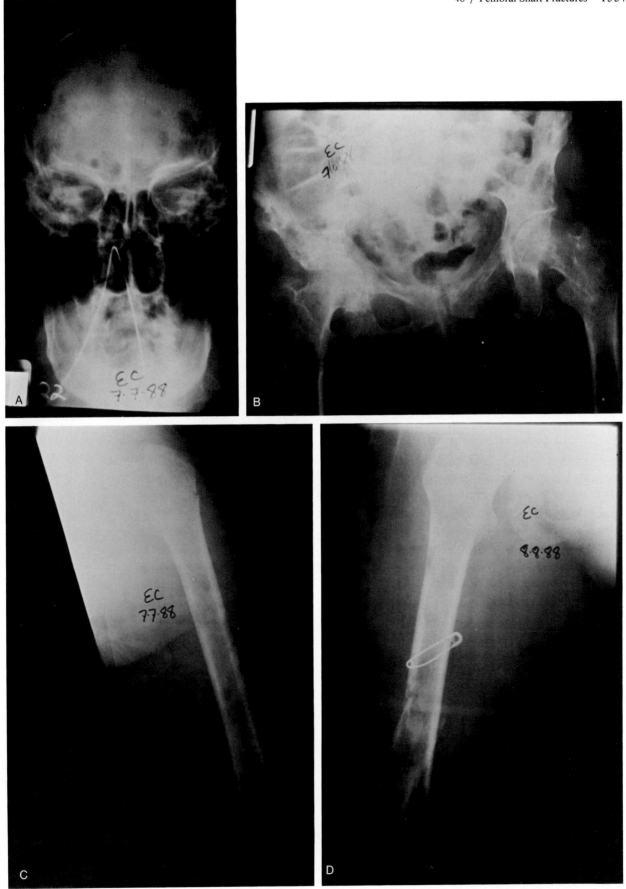

Illustration and legend continued on following page

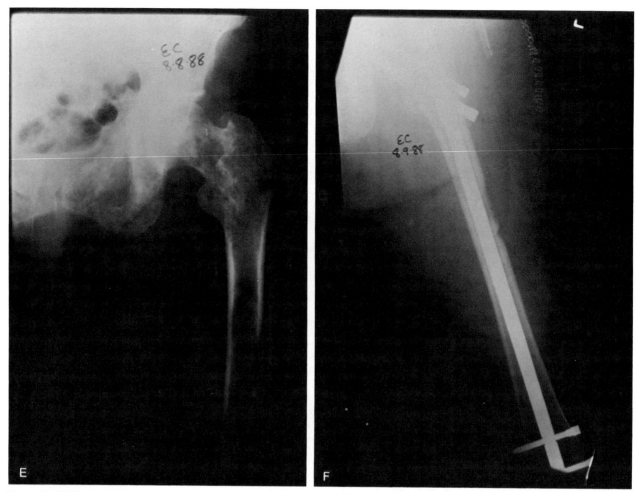

Figure 46–23 *Continued*

E, AP radiograph of left proximal femur and shaft taken at the same time as *D. F,* AP radiograph of the left femur following stabilization of the femur with a second-generation locked-in nail, which totally fills the intramedullary canal from hip to knee.

initial 24 hours after injury) of the femoral shaft fracture in caring for the multiply injured patient.[23,25,98,99,132,224–226,235,264] The reason for this is not known, but may be related to "decompression" of the femoral shaft, as well as to fracture stabilization.[270]

Immediate operative stabilization of long-bone fractures (which include the femur) has many advantages in the multiply injured patient, including early patient mobilization, improved long-term function, prevention of deep venous thrombosis and decubitus ulcer, improvement of nursing care, decrease in the need for analgesia, and marked improvement in pulmonary status. Good evidence supports the claim that early fracture stabilization significantly reduces the incidence of fat emboli and ARDS.[23,132] It can also decrease the frequency of posttraumatic sepsis and improve the overall mortality rate by getting patients upright and improving normal nutrition, thus reducing the dreaded

occurrence of multiple organ system failure and death from sepsis.[25] A study by Johnson et al. using injury severity scoring actually indicated that the more severely injured the patient was, the greater was the benefit of early fracture stabilization within the initial 24 hours following injury (Fig. 46–24 and Table 46–3).[132] The incidence of ARDS was essentially five times higher in patients with severe trauma (ISS > 40) whose fracture stabilization was delayed than in those patients who underwent immediate fracture stabilization. A prospective, randomized study by Bone and co-workers confirmed the findings of previous retrospective studies and conclusively demonstrated the beneficial effects of early fracture stabilization in the multiply injured patient with a femoral shaft fracture.[23] This study demonstrated statistically significant improvement in pulmonary function in the multiply injured patient, as well as a statistically significant decrease in

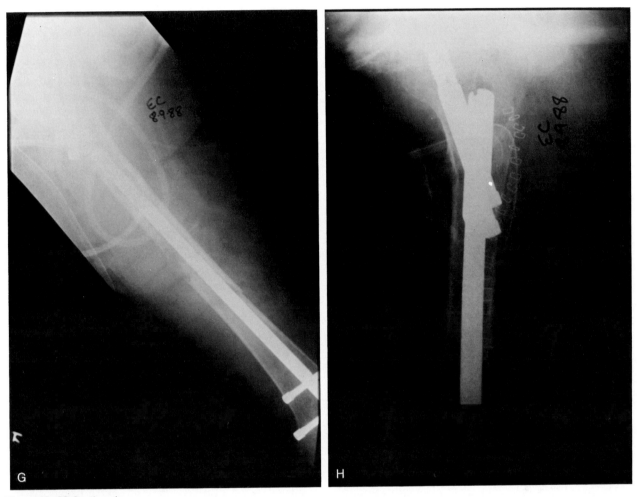

Figure 46–23 *Continued*

G, AP radiograph of the right femur after similar treatment. *H,* Lateral radiograph of the right proximal femur demonstrates correct placement of the proximal bolts.

hospital cost, with immediate stabilization of femoral shaft fractures in the multiply injured patient. The incidences of fat emboli, ARDS, pulmonary dysfunction, pneumonia, and abnormal blood gases were all significantly lowered by early femoral fracture stabilization. Early fracture stabilization in the patient with an isolated femoral shaft fracture also improved pulmonary function and lowered hospital costs, but this did not reach statistical significance in the patient with an isolated femur fracture (ISS < 18). Therefore multiply injured patients with femoral shaft fractures should undergo immediate stabilization of the femoral shaft fracture in the initial 24 hours following injury if this capability exists in the treating institution. If this treatment option does not exist in the treating institution, the patient should be rapidly stabilized and promptly transferred according to accepted transfer protocols to an institution where this treatment is available.[65]

THE "FLOATING KNEE"

The term "floating knee" lesion (i.e., fracture of the femur with an ipsilateral fracture of the tibia) was originally coined by McBryde in 1965.[20,170] This concomitant injury has a high association with the multiply injured patient. McBryde noticed a strikingly high complication rate of this lesion, with an incidence of 60% to 70% permanent disability in his patients. He felt that the difference in the rate of complications was a result of multiple factors, including the high energy absorption necessary to create the injury pattern, inability to mobilize the patient, and the multiply injured status of the patient. In a retrospective study of multiply injured patients with long-bone fractures, this injury was noted to occur in about 50% of patients.[132] Many of the patients with this combination injury have other life-threatening injuries. The mortality rate in

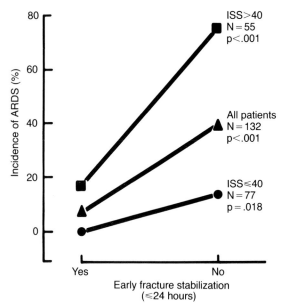

Figure 46-24

Graph showing the statistical significance (denoted by the slope of the lines) of early fracture stabilization in injured patients. Note that the more severely injured the patient, the more significant early fracture stabilization is in the prevention of adult respiratory distress syndrome.

patients with floating knees has been reported to vary from 5% to 15%, indicating the severe nature of this lesion.

Recent studies of ipsilateral fractures of the tibia and femur have recommended surgical stabilization of both fractures in the initial treatment period.[137,279] A high complication rate has been noted in patients who

Table 46-3.

Different Outcomes With and Without Early Fracture Fixation

	Early Fracture Fixation		
	Yes	No	Total
Number of patients	83	49*	132
Mean age (years)	30.7	30.6	30.6
Mean ISS	38.2	38	38.1
ARDS	6	19	25
Major systemic infection	4	12	16
Major orthopedic infection	17	4	21
Mortality (patients)	2	6	8
Mean ICU time (days)	4.9	11.1	7.2
Mean intubation time (days)	4.9	11.1	6.8
Mean hospital stay (days)	31.6	38.3	34.1

* Includes seven patients treated conservatively with no operative stabilization of major fractures.

have had one of the two concomitant fractures treated nonoperatively. These complications include death, fat emboli, healing problems, and decreased range of motion of the joints, all of which can be prevented by immediate fracture stabilization of both the femur and the tibia. Veith et al. in 1984 recommended immediate stabilization of both the femur and the tibia.[279] In their study they noted pulmonary embolization and fat emboli to be a major problem in patients who had a delay in fracture stabilization, particularly of the femoral shaft. A decrease in knee range of motion was noted when only the femur was stabilized.

In fracture stabilization of patients with floating knees, the tibia is generally splinted and the femoral shaft treated first with closed intramedullary nailing. Debridement and irrigation of an open wound are essential prior to fixation. Following stabilization of the femoral shaft fracture, attention is turned to stabilization of the tibia fracture.

IPSILATERAL FEMORAL NECK AND FEMORAL SHAFT FRACTURES

All studies dealing with ipsilateral hip and femoral shaft fractures have noted a high association of this injury pattern with the multiply injured patient.[15,50,77,90,96,262,263,304] Most of these studies have recommended early operative stabilization of both fractures. One author noted a 25% incidence of significant pulmonary complications when this injury pattern was treated nonoperatively in traction.[263] Diagnosis appears to be a crucial factor, as authors reporting on the subject have stated that in 30% of such cases, the diagnosis of hip fracture was either missed or delayed during the initial evaluation.[262,263] A delayed or missed diagnosis means that the higher priority fracture, the hip fracture, is treated secondarily or by means that are less than ideal. The most common hip fracture dealt with in this injury pattern is a femoral neck fracture; less common is an intertrochanteric fracture.

All orthopedic surgeons are familiar with the morbidity of femoral neck fractures. Even with ideal treatment, nonunion and avascular necrosis of the femoral head can be major complications, with incidence rates of 10% and 30%, respectively.[262,263] Because delayed treatment for femoral neck fractures increases the risk of avascular necrosis, the timely diagnosis of this injury is crucial. It should be emphasized that treatment of the femoral neck fracture should always take precedence over treatment of the femoral shaft fracture. This is because the options for salvage of complications after femoral neck fractures are limited, compared with available treatments of malunion or nonunion of femoral shaft fractures.

As previously stated, every patient with a femoral shaft fracture should have a thorough evaluation of the femoral head and neck with the hip in internal rotation. Most AP radiographs of the pelvis obtained in the emergency room are inadequate to reveal the most common fracture pattern of the femoral neck with this concomitant injury (see Fig. 46–15). AP radiographs of the pelvis in patients with a femoral shaft fracture almost always show an externally rotated view of the femoral neck, which does not profile the femoral neck. Many femoral neck fractures that occur in conjunction with a femoral shaft fracture are nondisplaced, with a longitudinal shear fracture pattern that begins proximally and laterally in the femoral neck and runs longitudinally down it to end there distally and medially. Whether nondisplaced or minimally displaced, they always require surgical stabilization to prevent the immediate displacement that will occur following attempts to mobilize the patient after closed intramedullary nailing of the femoral shaft (Fig. 46–25). Orthopedic surgeons who deal operatively with femoral shaft fractures must also be prepared to deal with the previously undiagnosed ipsilateral femoral neck fracture diagnosed in the operating room with the patient anesthetized.

Many treatment modalities have been described for treatment of the ipsilateral femoral shaft and femoral neck fracture. The treating orthopedic surgeon must possess great confidence in his or her treatment plan for this complex combination injury. The femoral neck fracture should take precedence over the femoral shaft fracture and should always be treated with an accurate anatomic reduction and stable internal fixation. Stable internal fixation of this fracture may consist of as little as two parallel cancellous screws. A technique for ideal stabilization of the femoral neck fracture described by Swiontkowski et al. uses parallel compression screws inserted into the femoral head followed by retrograde nailing of the femoral shaft fracture with a short intramedullary nail, beginning at either the intracondylar notch or at the medial femoral condyle (Fig. 46–26).[262,263] This technique, although successful for the authors, has not been widely accepted because of its degree of technical difficulty.

This combination injury may be one of the few instances in which plating of the femoral shaft fracture is acceptable. The surgeon who is most comfortable with parallel compression screws in the femoral neck as treatment for the femoral neck fracture may not feel confident in his or her ability to place an intramedullary nail down the femoral shaft without encountering the screws previously placed into the femoral neck. In that case, it is acceptable to open the femoral shaft fracture and apply a lateral compression plate (Fig. 46–27). Autogenous cancellous bone graft should be placed on the medial side of the femoral shaft opposite the plate. This treatment modality is recommended when this problem is diagnosed prior to operative intervention, and when experience and equipment to perform closed intramedullary nailing are not present or are not available within a reasonable distance and patient transfer is not an option.

For surgeons experienced in modern closed intramedullary nailing techniques, closed reduction of both the femoral neck and femoral shaft fracture is the most acceptable alternative. This can be performed with closed reduction of the femoral neck fracture, followed by temporary stabilization with parallel pins placed from anterior on the femoral shaft obliquely down into the posterior aspect of the femoral head (Fig. 46–28).[44] Two parallel pins will stabilize the femoral neck fracture and allow routine intramedullary nailing of the femoral shaft fracture to take place. Following intramedullary nailing of the femoral shaft fracture with either a routine or locked intramedullary nail, these parallel pins can be replaced with compression lag screws. Cannulated lag screw systems (6.5- to 7.0-mm diameter) make this technique easier to perform. After prior drilling and tapping over the pins, they are replaced by cannulated lag screws. Two or three parallel screws placed anterior to the intramedullary nail are adequate to handle the femoral neck fracture. Occasionally a screw may be placed posterior to the intramedullary nail. The femoral shaft fracture can be treated with a routine locked intramedullary nail in most instances. It should be stressed that these parallel screws placed up the femoral neck are not within the nail but are separate cancellous bone screws placed outside the nail. Compression or impaction can then occur along the parallel screws. When using this technique, one may wish to use a slightly smaller diameter nail and start the nail slightly more posterior to the usual position.

Recent developments with locked intramedullary nails have produced a second-generation locked intramedullary nail that may be used to treat the ipsilateral femoral shaft and neck fracture with a single implant (Fig. 46–29). These devices require closed reduction and provisional stabilization of the femoral neck with pins placed into it in a manner similar to that described previously. At that point, the intramedullary canal is addressed and reamed, and an intramedullary nail is placed down the femoral canal. Using a targeting device firmly attached to the proximal aspect of the nail, two parallel screws are then inserted through the nail and into the femoral head. The implant system is designed to allow telescoping of the screws with compression of the femoral neck fracture. Following placement

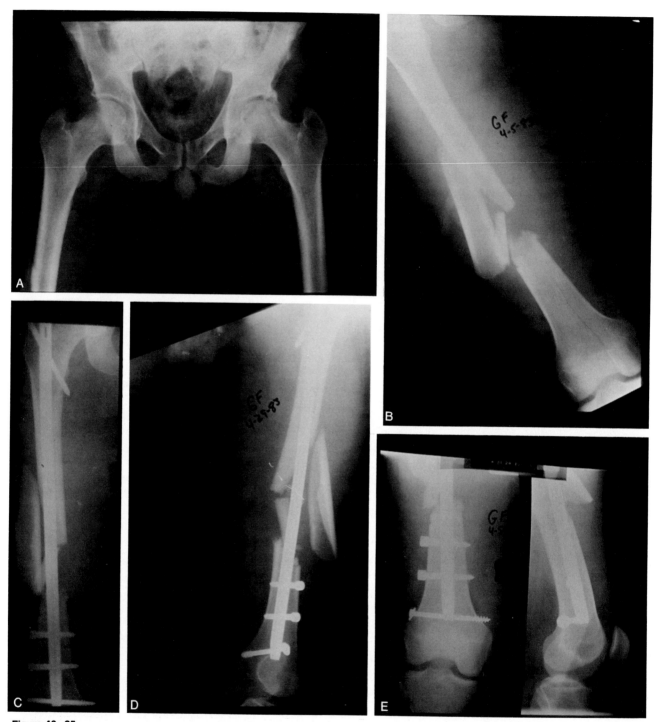

Figure 46-25

A, AP radiograph of the pelvis taken on the day of injury in a patient with a comminuted right femoral shaft fracture. *B,* AP radiograph of the right femur in the same patient. Note fracture extension into the knee. *C,* AP radiograph of the femur following stabilization of the femoral shaft and distal femur. *D,* Lateral radiograph of the femur demonstrating fracture stabilization. *E,* AP (left) and lateral (right) radiographs of the distal femur. *F,* The patient returned to the clinic three weeks after discharge with right hip pain. He had been ambulating, non-weight bearing, on crutches. *G,* Three cancellous screws were placed anterior to the nail. *H,* Uneventful healing of femoral neck fracture ten months later. *I,* Another patient's intraoperative radiograph from the image intensifier. The awl is beginning a starting hole for intramedullary nailing of the femoral shaft fracture. Note the previously undiagnosed femoral neck fracture.

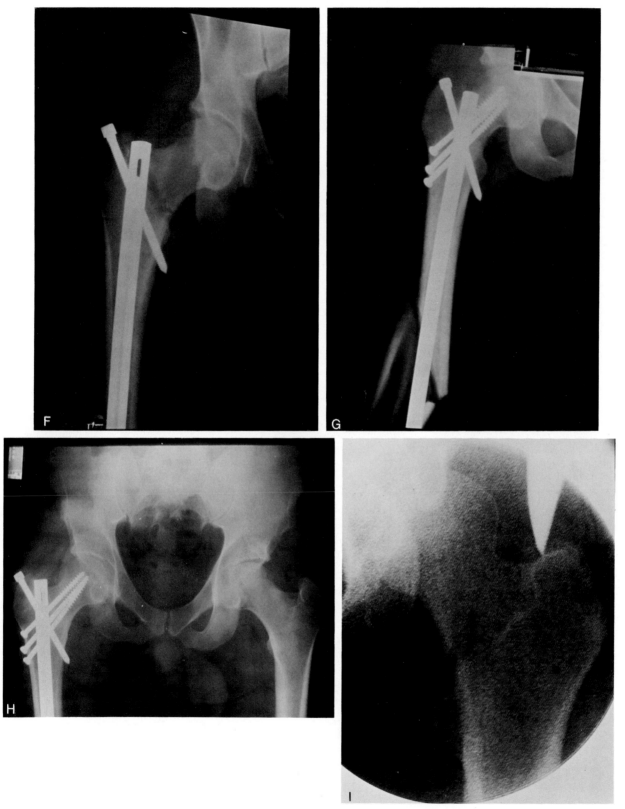

Figure 46–25 *Continued*

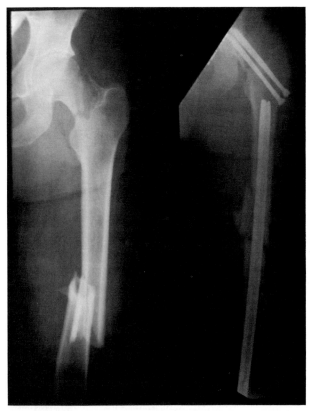

Figure 46–26

Multiple screws used to fix a displaced femoral neck fracture. An intramedullary nail is placed retrograde from the medial femoral condyle. (From Swiontkowski, M.F.; Hansen, S.T.; Kellam, J.T. J Bone Joint Surg 66A:260–268, 1984).

of the two parallel screws into the femoral head through the nail, the provisional pin stabilization is removed. These nails also have provision for distal locking screws so that the nail acts like a locked intramedullary nail for the femoral shaft fracture. This implant system is complicated, and reduction and nailing of two concomitant fractures in one bone with one piece of hardware are technically complex. The technique is not recommended for those without experience with the hardware. It should also be noted that there is as yet little long-term experience with this surgical technique, although preliminary reports indicate good results.[103,125]

Another technique that has been reported for treatment of ipsilateral shaft and hip fractures is closed reduction of both fractures and retrograde nailing using flexible nails (Ender nails). This technique may be considered when the proximal fracture is an intertrochanteric fracture. However, it is difficult and prone to failure if attempted for associated neck and shaft fractures. Although Ender nails should never be used to fix both femoral neck *and* femoral shaft fractures, they can satisfactorily stabilize some femoral shaft fractures after

multiple screws have been used to fix an associated femoral neck injury.

IPSILATERAL FEMORAL SHAFT AND INTERTROCHANTERIC FRACTURES

Concomitant ipslateral femoral shaft and intertrochanteric fractures are some of the most challenging injury patterns for orthopedic surgeons. This combination also is common in multiply injured patients. This severe injury pattern, like other femoral shaft fractures in the multiply injured patient, should be treated with immediate internal fixation to allow early mobilization. Therefore each fracture surgeon should have a predetermined treatment modality available for this particular combination injury. Although the intertrochanteric fracture does not have the severe complications and morbidity found with the femoral neck fracture, inadequate treatment of this fracture can lead to a crippling malalignment problem. Thus, although the morbidity is perhaps less with this particular combination injury, it can be more technically demanding for the surgeon.

Currently there are two acceptable methods of treatment for this injury pattern. The most common acceptable treatment is open reduction and internal fixation of the intertrochanteric fracture using a compression hip screw or other fixed-angle device, with an extra long side plate that will allow rigid stabilization of the femoral shaft fracture with one implant (Fig. 46–30). This implant should allow at least four screws ("eight cortices") distal to the femoral shaft fracture. This may necessitate an extremely long side plate that may not be available in the armamentarium of equipment and implants available in the treating hospital. Attempting an open reduction and stabilization of two unstable fractures in the same bone is difficult and can be a taxing experience. Unfortunately as well, open reduction and internal fixation of both of these fractures requires extensive dissection of virtually the entire thigh, necessitating extra blood loss and prolonged operative times. It is advisable to bone graft the femoral shaft fracture with autogenous cancellous bone placed on the medial side of the femur opposite the plate; this may be delayed if necessary.

Again, the second-generation locked intramedullary nails that allow fixation through the intramedullary nail into the femoral head and neck provide an alternative for stabilization of this femoral fracture combination (Fig. 46–31). The technique employed should include open reduction and provisional stabilization of the proximal femoral fracture, either with provisional pin or screw fixation or with bone clamp fixation, to restore normal anatomy to the proximal femur. Closed

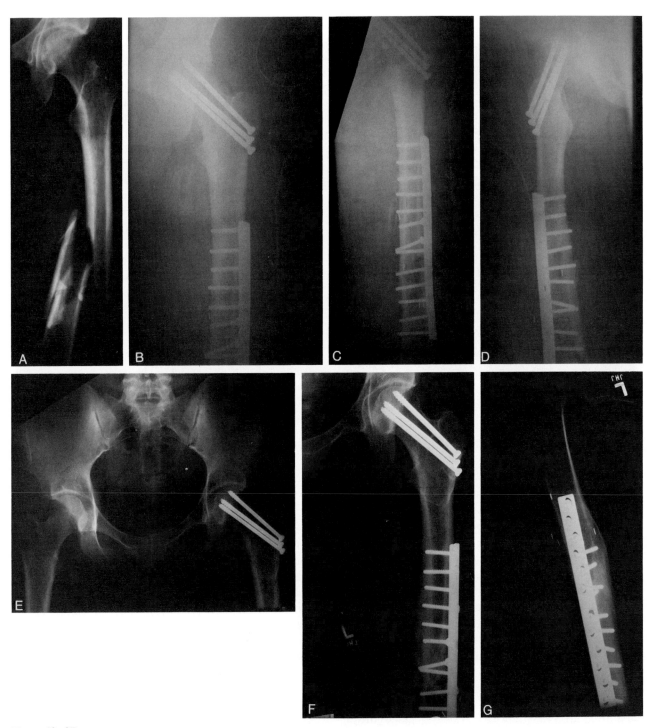

Figure 46–27

A, Comminuted fracture of the femoral shaft with associated fracture of the ipsilateral femoral neck (displaced). *B,* Postoperative radiograph showing multiple screws used to reduce and stabilize the femoral neck fracture following plate application to the femoral shaft. *C,* AP radiograph of femoral shaft fracture. *D,* Postoperative lateral radiograph of femoral shaft and neck fractures. *E,* AP radiograph of the pelvis three years after injury with healed femoral neck fracture. *F,* AP radiograph of the femur three years after injury. *G,* Lateral radiograph of the femur three years after injury.

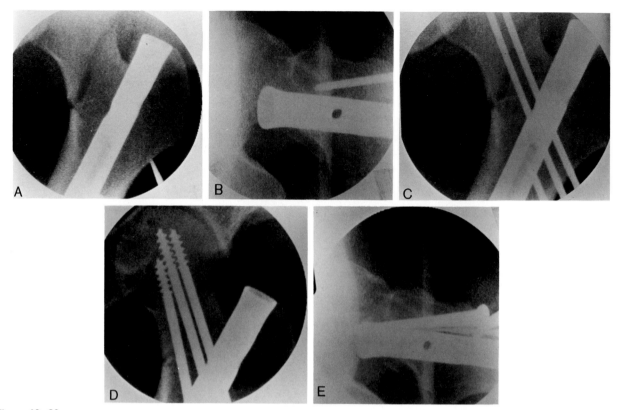

Figure 46-28

Operative stabilization of a femoral neck fracture with multiple screws following adequate reduction. This may be performed following intramedullary nailing. The screws should be anterior to the nail. *A*, AP radiograph obtained from the intensifier intraoperatively. The nail has been placed, the femoral neck fracture has been reduced, and the drill shows the position for screw placement. *B*, Lateral radiograph obtained from the image intensifier at the same time. Note that the fracture is reduced and the drill starts are anterior on the femur, angling slightly posterior into the femoral head. *C*, AP radiograph showing pins or drill bits placed across the femoral neck fracture in a parallel manner. *D*, AP radiograph showing cancellous screws that have replaced the pins or drill bits. Some compression has been placed on the fracture. *E*, Lateral radiograph demonstrating screw placement anterior to the intramedullary nail.

intramedullary nailing of the femoral shaft fracture should then take place with the intramedullary nail portion of the device. Following placement of the intramedullary nail, two parallel screws are placed through it into the femoral head and neck using the drill guide, which is firmly attached to the proximal part of the nail. Care must be taken to ensure that both screws are placed directly up the femoral neck and into the femoral head and not anteriorly or posteriorly out of the neck. Following stabilization of the intertrochanteric fracture, the provisional fixation is removed. As stated previously, these intramedullary nails permit distal locking as well, so that the femoral shaft fracture may be treated by a locked intramedullary nail if comminution is a problem. It must be reiterated that this is a complex technique that should not be undertaken by an individual inexperienced with closed intramedullary nailing. Closed reduction of both the unstable proximal intertrochanteric fracture and the fracture of

the shaft is virtually impossible to accomplish on a consistent basis. Therefore the recommendation is to first perform an open reduction and provisional stabilization of the unstable proximal fracture to allow accurate introduction of the nail into the femur. The parallel screws placed through the intramedullary nail into the femoral head and neck are not rigidly fixed to the nail and will allow some compression or impaction of the intertrochanteric fracture. The advantage of this device is that it does not require open reduction and internal fixation of the femoral shaft fracture. Therefore extensive dissection in the thigh is unnecessary and blood loss is kept to a minimum. Ideal stabilization of both the intertrochanteric and the shaft fractures is possible if the procedure is meticulously performed. The patient must be supine on the fracture table to allow visualization of the femoral head and neck with the image intensifier.

This combination injury may also be managed by

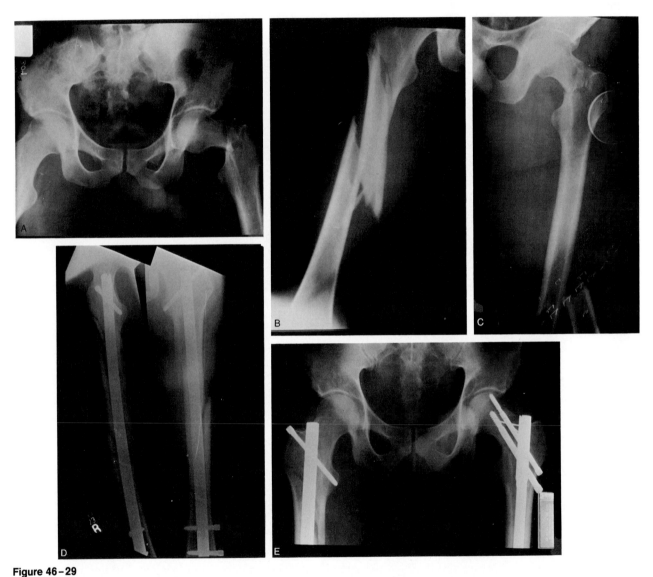

Figure 46–29

Femoral neck and shaft fracture treated with a second-generation locked intramedullary nail. *A*, AP radiograph of the pelvis in a trauma patient taken on the day of the injury. Note the displaced left femoral neck fracture. *B*, AP radiograph of the right femur in the same patient. *C*, AP radiograph of the left femur in the same patient on the day of the injury. *D*, Postoperative AP radiograph of the pelvis showing placement of a second-generation locked nail in the left femur with anatomic reduction of femoral neck fracture. A routine locked nail was used in the right femur. *E*, AP (left) and lateral (right) radiographs of the right femur taken postoperatively.

Illustration and legend continued on following page

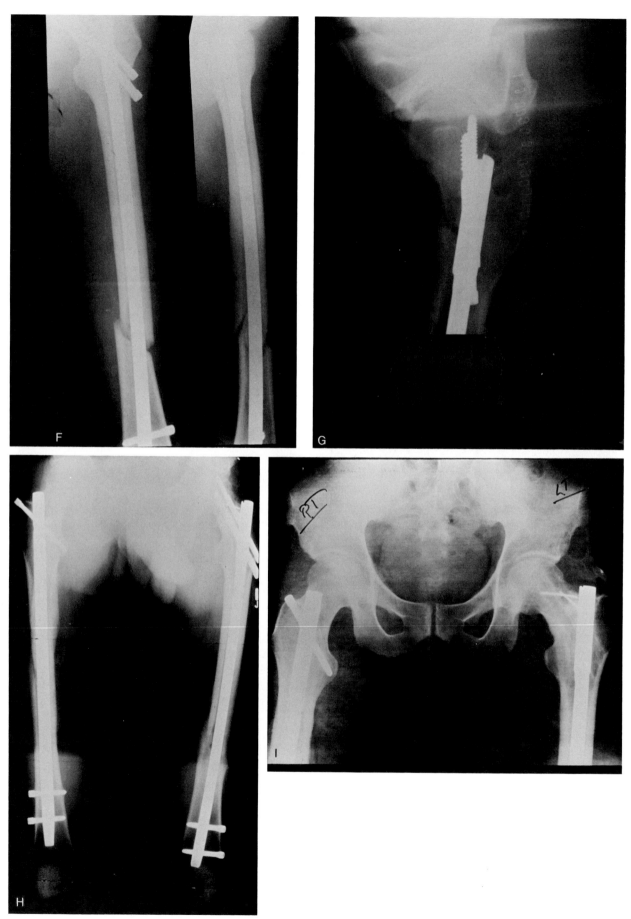

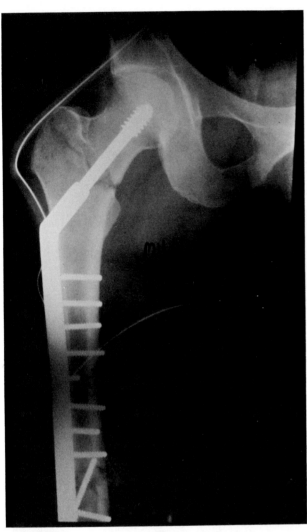

Figure 46-30

Fixation of ipsilateral femoral shaft and intertrochanteric fractures using a compression hip screw with long side plate.

danger of shortening. It avoids the soft tissue stripping necessary with plate fixation. The patient is positioned supine on the fracture table. The technique of Ender nail insertion is described later in the chapter.

The previously mentioned treatment modalities are indicated for treatment of the multiply injured patient with an ipsilateral femoral shaft and intertrochanteric fracture. Occasionally this injury pattern may appear as an isolated injury in a patient without other orthopedic or medical problems. In this case, it may be acceptable to perform routine open reduction and internal fixation of the intertrochanteric fracture with a compression hip screw, which has become standard in North America. The femoral shaft fracture can then be treated with either traction or open reduction and internal fixation with a secondary laterally placed compression plate. Treatment in traction generally requires approximately four to six weeks of balanced suspension or roller traction followed by six to ten weeks of casting using a spica cast or cast brace. The use of traction for these extended periods of time is not acceptable in the multiply injured patient with additional orthopedic or other major system problems.

SUBTROCHANTERIC FRACTURES

Subtrochanteric fractures were first distinguished because of their high risk of complications when treated with fixed-angle nail-plate implants such as the Jewett nail.[274] Given our present-day techniques for femoral fracture fixation, historical classifications of subtrochanteric fractures are no longer relevant.[131] (See chapter 45.) As stated previously, femoral shaft fractures extend from the level of the lesser trochanter to within 6 to 8 cm of the distal articular surface. This leaves little, if any, of the femur to be described as subtrochanteric, since fractures at the lesser trochanter and above are "intertrochanteric." This approach to subtrochanteric fractures is based on the concept that all fractures in the shaft at the level of or distal to the lesser trochanter are best managed by closed intramedullary nailing. Fractures with comminution that extend up to the lesser trochanter can be managed with routine locked intramedullary nailing, utilizing most first-generation locked intramedullary nails. This has been performed widely across North America with reported results that

compression hip screw fixation of the intertrochanteric fracture followed by retrograde Ender nailing of the femoral shaft fracture. The Ender nails are inserted from medial and lateral distal ports and passed proximally. It is usually possible to insert the nails past the screws of the plate on the proximal femur with little difficulty. The technique is best for stable femoral shaft fractures that are transverse or short oblique and in no

Figure 46-29 *Continued*

F, AP (left) and lateral (right) radiographs of the left femur taken postoperatively. *G*, Lateral radiograph of the left proximal femur taken postoperatively. *H*, AP radiograph of the left and right femur four months after injury. *I*, AP radiograph of the pelvis following symptomatic bolt removal from the left proximal femur at nine months after injury, with solidly healed femoral neck fracture. There is a small amount of ectopic bone formation proximal to the nail. The patient functions normally.

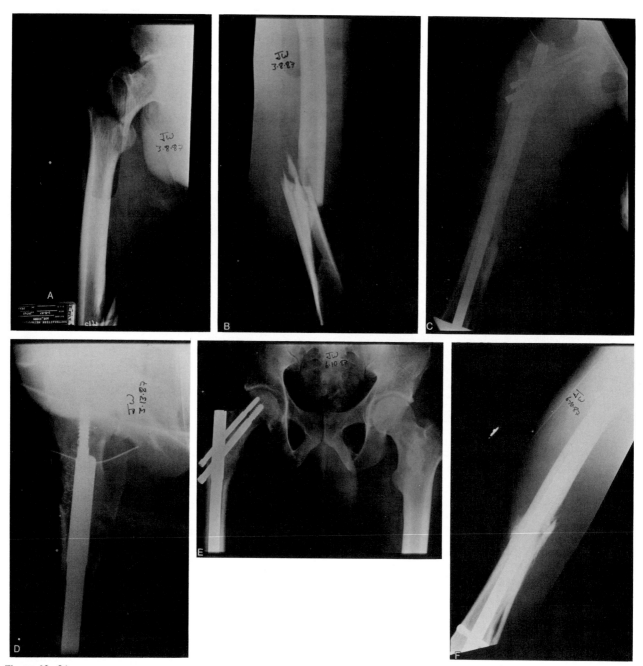

Figure 46–31

Ipsilateral femoral shaft and intertrochanteric fractures fixed with a second-generation locked intramedullary nail. *A,* AP radiograph of the proximal femur taken on the day of injury. *B,* Lateral radiograph of the femoral shaft taken on the day of injury. *C,* AP radiograph of the proximal femur and shaft taken postoperatively. *D,* Lateral radiograph of the proximal femur taken postoperatively. *E,* AP radiograph of the pelvis three months after injury demonstrating healing of the intertrochanteric fracture. *F,* AP radiograph of the femoral shaft three months after injury showing progressive healing of the femoral shaft.

are better than those for any other treatment modality available for these fractures.[19,131,266] Therefore the zone of "subtrochanteric fractures" is much restricted today, as most fractures that would previously have been termed "subtrochanteric" are commonly treated as any routine femoral shaft fracture might be. Results can also be expected to be similar to those for femoral shaft fractures.

However, one exception to the preceding statements does exist. A fracture in the proximal shaft of the femur that extends proximally into the area of the trochanters, especially the greater trochanter (Fig. 46–32), may be called a subtrochanteric fracture with greater trochanteric extension, or perhaps an intertrochanteric fracture with diaphyseal extension.[274] This is a difficult fracture to treat. Currently it is usually treated with open reduction and internal fixation using a compression hip screw device or a fixed-angle blade plate.[233] Either device should have a side plate long enough to allow adequate fixation to the distal shaft (Fig. 46–33). All fractures treated in this manner should have autogenous cancellous bone placed along the medial aspect of the femur on the opposite side of the plate. This surgical technique is demanding and

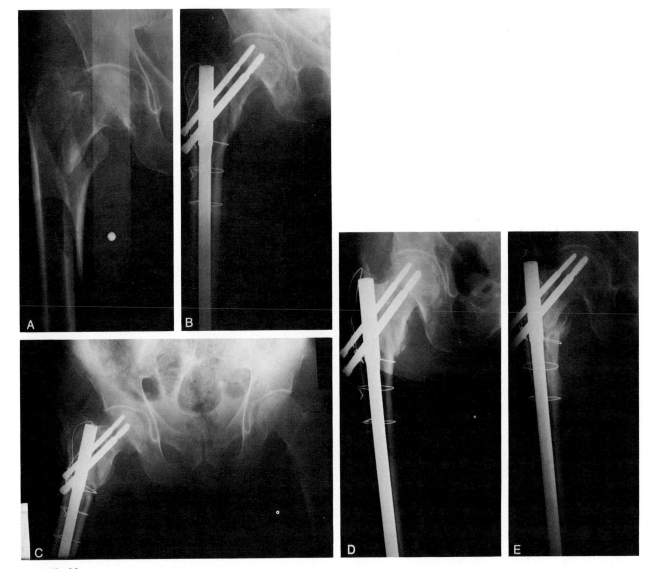

Figure 46–32

A, AP radiograph of the proximal femur in a 60-year-old male with a complex proximal femur fracture. B, Immediate postoperative radiograph showing open reduction, internal fixation with a second-generation locked nail plus cerclage wires and tension, and a wire around the greater trochanter. C, AP radiograph of the pelvis with a near-lateral view of the right proximal femur taken immediately postoperatively. D, Notice that the proximal bolts have backed out and the fracture is setting. E, Radiograph taken at eight months after injury showing a healed fracture.

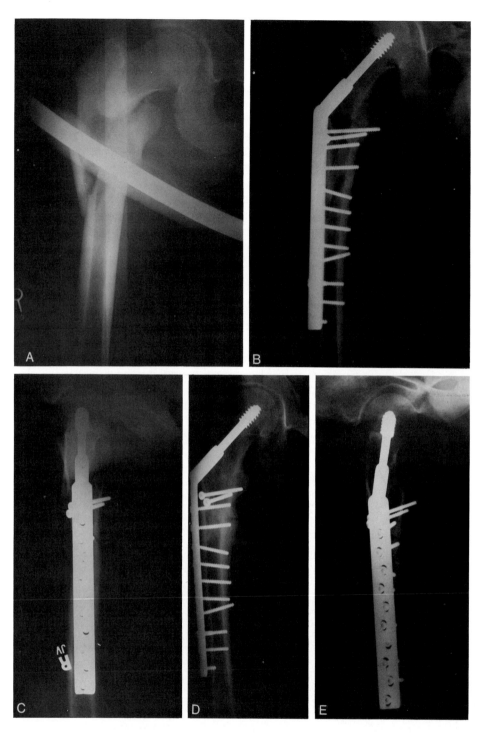

Figure 46–33

Complex proximal femur fracture with subtrochanteric comminution and extension into the greater trochanter. *A*, AP radiograph of the proximal femur taken on the day of injury. *B*, Immediate postoperative AP radiograph of the proximal femur following open reduction and internal fixation with a compression hip screw and long side plate. *C*, Postoperative radiograph of the proximal femur. *D*, AP radiograph of the proximal femur taken six months after injury showing a healed fracture. *E*, Lateral radiograph of the proximal femur six months after injury.

requires extensive dissection of the entire fracture for anatomic reduction and stabilization.

A technically challenging alternative to the use of an eccentrically placed side plate on these difficult femoral fractures is the use of a second-generation cephalomedullary locked intramedullary nail.[19,121,127] With longitudinal traction applied to the patient in the supine position, closed intramedullary nailing of the femoral shaft fracture can be performed without extensive dissection of the diaphysis. Occasionally, open reduction and temporary stabilization of the most proximal fracture fragments are necessary to allow accurate introduction of the nail into the femur. Loose fragments of the greater trochanter may require fixation by means of a tension band wire (see Fig. 46–32). This type of stabilization has been of value, in that the operative time and blood loss are significantly less. Stabilization secure enough to allow immediate immobilization of the patient is possible with this technique. All comminuted proximal shaft fractures treated with this device should have static locked nailing performed to prevent rotational instability.

IPSILATERAL FEMORAL SHAFT AND DISTAL METAPHYSEAL FRACTURES

Ipsilateral femoral shaft and distal metaphyseal fractures are a relatively rare combination, with little reported experience in the literature. Fracture of the distal femoral metaphysis involving intraarticular comminution of the distal femur with significant displacement can be corrected only by open reduction and stable internal fixation of the distal femur with a plate. Virtually no other treatment results in an outcome acceptable to patient and physician. Following that, the shaft fracture proximal to the distal femur can be fixed either with an extension of the plate used to fix the distal femur or with a separate plate placed on the lateral shaft of the femur. Again, an autogenous cancellous bone graft placed on the medial aspect of the femoral shaft opposite the plate is recommended.

It is not uncommon to see nondisplaced fracture lines that extend from the fracture of the femoral shaft longitudinally down the femur into the distal femoral metaphysis. Many times these fracture lines are minimally displaced or nondisplaced and require little or no surgical manipulation to achieve an accurate and stable reduction. These fractures can be adequately stabilized with percutaneous insertion of interfragmentary lag screws to control the intraarticular fracture.

Cannulated lag screws are also helpful. These screws can be placed either anterior or posterior to the path of the nail or distal to the final resting position of the nail. Following application of the percutaneous interfragmentary lag screws, the femoral shaft fracture is fixed with closed intramedullary nailing using a locked intramedullary nail as indicated by the individual fracture pattern (Fig. 46–34). This has been a useful technique in the multiply injured patient. Some caution must be expressed, however. Most of these femoral shaft fractures are in the distal third, often in the low distal third, of the femur, where many times there are only borderline indications for the use of the locked intramedullary nail. When a locked intramedullary nail is placed into these distal third fractures and full weight bearing is allowed early (prior to six weeks) or a small-diameter (12- to 13-mm) nail is used, a fatigue fracture of the distal part of the nail may occur (Fig. 46–35).[45] Therefore when dealing with these complex distal third femoral fractures, it is best to use a larger diameter (14-mm) nail if possible and to keep the patient absolutely non–weight bearing for a period of six to eight weeks, or at

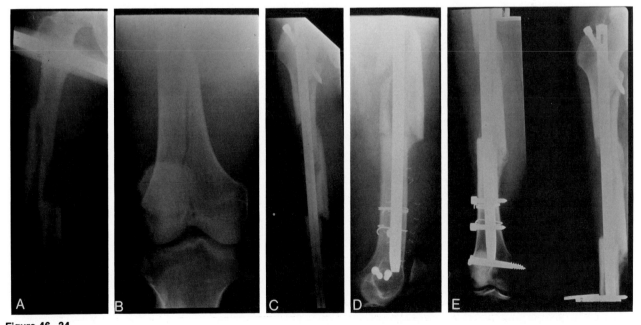

Figure 46–34

Comminuted femoral shaft fracture with intraarticular extension into the distal femur stabilized with screws and a locked intramedullary nail. *A*, AP radiograph of the femoral shaft on the day of injury. *B*, AP radiograph of the distal femur on the day of injury. *C*, AP radiograph of the femoral shaft following surgical stabilization with a static locked intramedullary nail. *D*, Lateral radiograph of the distal femur following surgical stabilization. *E*, AP radiographs of distal and proximal femur at four months following injury with progressive fracture healing.

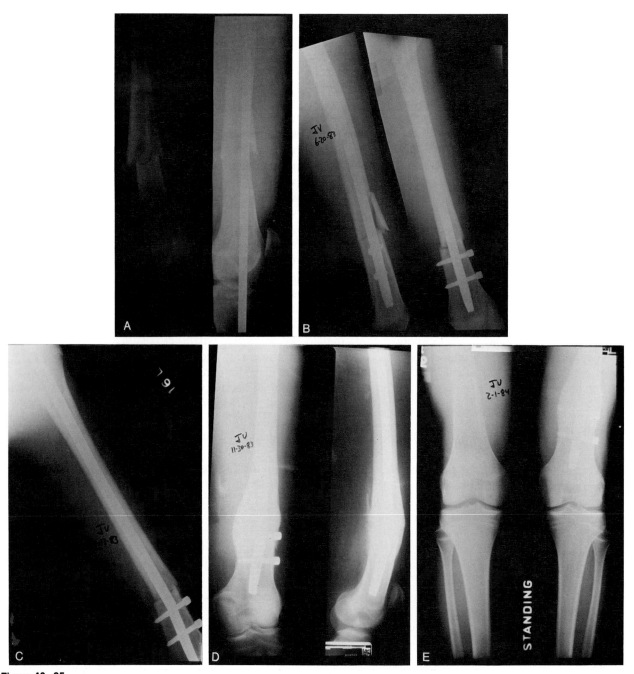

Figure 46-35

Fracture of an intramedullary nail used to stabilize a distal one-third femoral shaft fracture. *A*, AP (left) and lateral (right) radiographs of a distal one-third femoral shaft fracture in a 16-year-old skeletally immature patient. *B*, Stabilization with a locked intramedullary nail. Note that the distal bolts are within 1 to 2 cm of the fracture. The nail is 12 mm in diameter. *C*, The nail is broken at four weeks after injury with the patient fully weight bearing. *D*, Healed distal femur fracture five months after injury with deformity. *E*, AP radiograph of the knees at eight months after injury.

least until early callus formation has been adequately determined on follow-up radiologic evaluation. The use of these precautions will lead to satisfying results with this method.

FEMORAL SHAFT FRACTURE WITH ARTERIAL INJURY

Arterial injury with a femoral shaft fracture may present in several different ways. Increasingly, femoral shaft fracture is seen secondary to acute, penetrating trauma, usually a gunshot wound. These gunshot wounds can cause fracture of the femur, as well as arterial or neurologic injury. When the gunshot wound is in proximity to the major femoral vessels as they course through the thigh, arteriograms should *always* be performed, even if peripheral pulses are present in the foot. If peripheral pulses are not present in the foot and the patient arrives with a cold, pulseless, and (often) insensate foot, then the patient should be taken immediately to the operating room by a combined orthopedic and vascular surgery team. The femoral artery should be explored in the area of the penetrating wound and a temporary vascular shunt applied. Following revascularization of the leg by means of a temporary shunt, the orthopedic surgeon should stabilize the femoral shaft fracture. In many cases, the most rapid means of stabilization of the femoral shaft fracture is either by application of external fixation or by application of a lateral compression plate. In most instances, patient positioning for the application of an intramedullary nail and for vascular repair are not compatible. Therefore intramedullary nailing is not the best alternative for most fractures with vascular injuries caused by penetrating trauma. Following stabilization of the femoral shaft fracture, the vascular injury may be permanently repaired by means of a vein graft or by whatever repair is best indicated for the lesion.

Although treatment of a femoral shaft fracture with traction in the presence of an arterial repair has been reported in the literature, this treatment modality is not advisable.[68] It is difficult to control the amount of longitudinal traction and motion of the femoral shaft at the fracture site, both of which can significantly endanger the arterial repair.[89] It is also difficult and dangerous to allow any sort of patient mobility in this instance. Therefore stabilization of the femoral shaft is indicated for fractures associated with arterial injuries.

Vascular injury associated with femoral shaft fracture is a relatively rare occurrence in civilian medical practice. The injury is even more rare when associated with blunt trauma and has been estimated to occur at a rate of approximately 1 in 1000.[89,215] However, vascular injuries associated with penetrating trauma (gunshot injuries) are far more common. In the military practice of medicine and in certain urban trauma centers, gunshot femoral shaft fractures are relatively frequent.

If the mechanism of injury is blunt trauma, the vascular injury tends to be in the area of the popliteal space and is associated with a fracture of the distal third of the femur. These injuries are secondary to tethering of the femoral artery at the adductor hiatus.[126] Injury to the femoral artery in any other area is uncommon with blunt trauma. The major concern in the patient with blunt trauma is the possible presence of an intimal flap tear of the artery.[24,215,231,239] Such a patient may have a normal arterial examination in the emergency room with near symmetric peripheral pulses, but in the presence of a distal third femoral shaft fracture, the vascular status of the lower extremity should be reevaluated frequently during the initial 24 to 48 hours for vascular deterioration. A high-quality arteriogram is advisable if there is any suspicion of vascular compromise. The arteriogram may demonstrate an intimal defect or subsequent occlusion of the artery as a result of the flap tear in the intima and secondary thrombosis. Arteriography is the best means to delineate arterial injury and should be performed whenever possible. In the case of blunt trauma, any evidence of diminished blood supply in the distal limb in conjunction with a distal third femoral shaft fracture should immediately direct the treating physician to the need for an arteriogram, unless there is already limb-threatening ischemia, in which case exploration and revascularization take precedence over arteriography.

Following complete interruption of flow in the femoral artery there is a time interval of only 6 to 8 hours after which permanent necrotic changes in muscle occur.[68] Therefore the vascular injury must be identified, if present, at the earliest point in time and definitive treatment instituted. If the arteriogram will delay surgical reestablishment of blood flow beyond this 6- to 8-hour range, then immediate arterial exploration should be performed.

Connolly et al., reporting on a series of 14 patients, suggested that it was not always necessary to perform internal fixation of the fracture at the time of arterial repair.[68] This was a retrospective series in which six patients were treated with skeletal traction in conjunction with their arterial repair. Various forms of internal fixation were also employed; fasciotomy was performed only sporadically. No statistical conclusion about the best mode of treatment of the femoral shaft fracture could be determined. Connolly et al. did point out that the key determinants of extremity survival were the successful restoration of peripheral blood flow, length of delay prior to repair (8-hour maximum), amount of associated soft tissue damage, and the presence or absence of infection. They also pointed out the need for fasciotomy in all cases. However, they also stated that skeletal traction could be effective in fracture management in the presence of a vascular injury requiring repair. Most trauma surgeons would refute this.

Current recommendations for treatment of vascular injury associated with a femoral shaft fracture are well outlined.[89,221] All patients with vascular injury or suspected vascular injury are thoroughly evaluated, including a thorough physical examination, Doppler arterial pressure evaluation, and an arteriogram (if time allows). In cases of delay in diagnosis or in patients with penetrating injury, direct exploration of the vessels should be performed. Immediate stabilization of the femoral shaft fracture should be performed in conjunction with the vascular repair. Soft tissues are best treated by stable skeletal fixation, which will maximize conditions for vascular repair and decrease the threat of infection.

Under ideal circumstances the sequence of events should be the following. The vascular surgeon should restore peripheral blood flow by means of a temporary shunt. This requires shunting of both the arterial supply and the venous flow.[192,223] Definitive fracture stabilization is then carried out. The choice of fracture stabilization belongs to the orthopedic surgeon and may be one of several options. Following femoral fracture stabilization, the vascular surgeon then restores peripheral blood flow by means of either direct repair or a vein graft. Fasciotomies of the lower leg should *always* be performed in these cases where vascular repair occurs in conjunction with femoral shaft fractures. Stable fracture fixation allows easier care of both the local wound and the open fasciotomy incisions following arterial repair.

Options for surgical stabilization of the femoral shaft fracture include internal fixation using plates and screws; closed intramedullary nailing; external fixation; or the Zickel supracondylar device. The exact choice of fixation depends a great deal on the fracture pattern, the surgeon's experience, the specific approach used for the vascular repair, and cooperation of the vascular surgeon. In cases of intimal flap tear with good distal perfusion (and thus less urgency for repairing the arterial injury), the femoral shaft fracture can be treated by whatever means are most appropriate. Generally this is an intramedullary nail with static locking. However, in cases of acute ischemia, this is generally not possible. In many cases the region of the buttock where insertion of the nail is necessary is not prepped. Therefore options for fracture stabilization are restricted to those that can be locally applied into the

surgically prepared wound, such as plate fixation or external fixation.

An anteromedial approach to the vascular injury is usually best. Therefore the orthopedic surgeon is left with applying some device through an anteromedial approach or using a separate incision laterally to apply a plate. This may create two long incisions with the resultant extensive blood loss and soft tissue dissection necessary for both. A plate can be applied medially to the femur through the incision used for the vascular repair. This is not a commonly used approach to the femur but is acceptable in this particular situation. Unfortunately, the biggest problem with plate fixation in this instance is removal of the plate, which may be necessary in the future. If plate removal is necessary, scarring around the arterial repair may complicate this procedure.

External fixation can be rapidly applied through separate lateral stab incisions. Holding the fracture reduced through the medial incision for vascular repair, anatomic alignment can be obtained and an external fixator applied by means of four pins placed laterally through the soft tissue. Although this form of stabilization is not the most ideal, it will allow delivery of local care to the wound, as well as patient mobilization during the time necessary for maturation of the vascular repair (two to three weeks). At the end of this time, consideration can be given to transferring the patient from external fixation to some form of stable internal fixation if indicated.

Our choice for stabilization of the femoral shaft fracture in the setting of vascular injury is the Zickel supracondylar device.[308,309] This device is particularly appropriate when dealing with a transverse or short oblique fracture of the distal third of the femur that is minimally comminuted (Winquist grade II or less). Fortunately, this makes up the majority of cases involving blunt trauma. The Zickel device consists of two separate, distally locked, sledge-shaped intramedullary implants. These are inserted through entry portals in both the medial and lateral femoral condyles. The device comes in three different sizes or widths, with a similar length for each size. Reduction of the fracture is easily obtained through the medial incision for vascular repair (Fig. 46–36). The medial implant can easily be applied through the anteromedial incision utilizing an entry portal in the medial femoral condyle. The only extra incision that is necessary is a small 2- to 3-cm incision directly over the lateral femoral condyle. This is done for entrance of the lateral implant. With stable fracture patterns, this device gives stable internal fixation that will allow for local wound care and patient mobilization when using intramedullary fixation at the level of the fracture site. The biggest drawback to the

Figure 46–36

Distal one-third fracture of the femur with vascular repair and insertion of Zickel supracondylar device. *A*, Acute fracture of the distal third of the femur with arterial injury documented by arteriogram. *B*, Following operative arterial repair, the Zickel supracondylar device is inserted through the large medial incision used for arterial repair and a small (2- to 3-cm) lateral incision. Intraoperative arteriogram documenting patent vascular repair following hardware insertion. *C*, Postoperative femoral arteriogram documenting revascularization. *D*, Healing distal femoral shaft fracture at four months after injury.

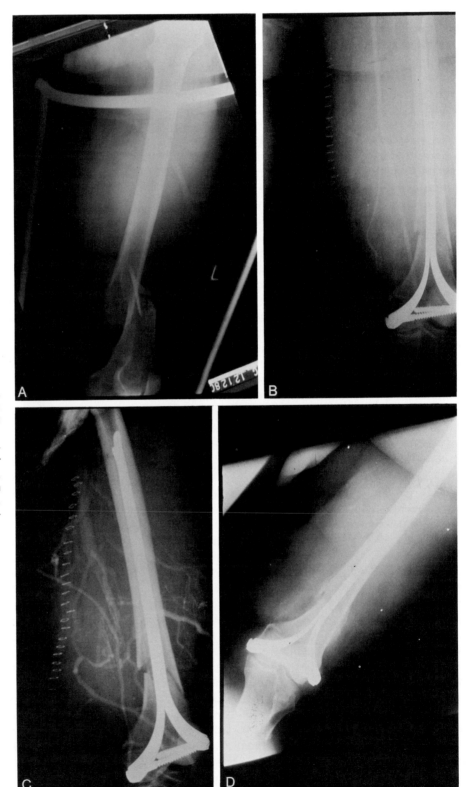

use of the Zickel supracondylar device is that it will not control length when excessive comminution is present at the fracture site. In this situation, significant shortening can occur. The device is also not useful for fractures above the level of the midshaft of the femur. However, this particular device can be inserted in the fracture patterns described in approximately 30 minutes during the vascular repair and is thus the quickest and most reliable means of fracture stabilization in this particular setting.

The presence or absence of infection is the crucial late determinant of a successful arterial repair.[68] Infection, rather than osteomyelitis and nonunion, is the major cause of late disruption of the vascular repair. A stable femoral shaft will allow local wound care and patient mobility, adequate debridement of necrotic tissue, and the performance of a fasciotomy to prevent occurrence of further dead tissue. These three factors assist in decreasing the incidence of infection following arterial repair. Prophylactic broad-spectrum antibiotics begun preoperatively and continued for 24 to 48 hours postoperatively are routinely used with surgical treatment of combined femoral fractures and arterial injuries. Redebridement of these wounds is often necessary, so that in addition to open management (with protection of the vascular anastomoses against dessication) a return to the operating room should be planned for 24 to 48 hours after the initial procedure, with repeated procedures until an entirely viable wound can be closed as soon as safely possible.

VENOUS THROMBOEMBOLISM

Venous thromboembolism, although commonly discussed as a possibility in association with femoral shaft fracture care, is a relatively uncommon occurrence. This may be because thromboembolic disease is less common in a younger patient population. It is, however, becoming increasingly apparent that late pulmonary emboli following femoral shaft fracture can be a problem.[23] In general, pulmonary emboli occur in a patient who has been immobilized in traction for even brief periods of time (48 hours or more). The basic question is the need for prophylactic treatment to prevent potential venous thromboembolism from occurring. This is seldom indicated in the presence of a fresh femoral shaft fracture, as anticoagulation can significantly complicate the acute fracture.[51] The safest prophylaxis against venous thromboembolism is muscle activity and patient mobilization, both of which are accomplished by early fracture stabilization and institution of vigorous physical therapy for motor activity in the affected extremity. The use of sequential pneumatic compression stockings or static compression stockings may be indicated in patients older than 40 years. Anticoagulation should be carefully selected for those extremely high-risk patients older than 40 who are obese, have a prior history of thromboembolic disease, or have other medical problems. Anticoagulant therapy should be instituted generally only after completion of all potential surgical procedures on the patient with a femoral shaft fracture.

TIMING OF STABILIZATION

Reports from the 1960s and 1970s recommended that intramedullary nailing of isolated femoral shaft fractures is best performed approximately three to seven days after injury.[108,109,291] Prior to surgery, the patient is observed for complications, particularly fat embolism. Many articles have indicated that there is an additional advantage to postponing a surgical procedure for 10 to 14 days, as delaying internal fixation can enhance union.[53,84,154,198,293] Smith in 1964 reported a series of femoral fractures that were stabilized between 7 and 21 days following injury, a time when active fracture repair is taking place.[251] He noted that fractures fixed then seemed to heal more quickly. This was thought to be caused by the addition of cancellous bone fragments produced by reaming to an active or ongoing repair process in the organizing fracture hematoma. He concluded that the optimum time for operation was between the tenth and fourteenth day. We cannot refute the accuracy of these statements. However, this stimulus to more rapid union does not result in a functional improvement in patient care. Following stable intramedullary fixation of femoral shaft fractures, the patient cannot detect exactly when fracture union occurs. After four to six weeks following intramedullary nailing, the patient's functional status changes very little. Therefore the actual timing of fracture stabilization should be dependent on factors that will provide maximum patient benefit. In general, union is routinely anticipated within three to four months following closed intramedullary nailing. If union occurs sooner, there is no additional functional benefit.

In the multiply injured patient (ISS > 18), immediate stabilization of the femoral shaft fracture within the initial 24 hours is essential.[8,23,264] Unless the patient is hemodynamically unstable and any further blood loss will be life threatening, the orthopedic surgeon should insist that the femoral shaft fracture be stabilized acutely. This will lead to improved patient mobility, which will allow improved care of other system injuries. Immediate stabilization will decrease the incidence of pulmonary complications and systemic infection and significantly decrease the mortality rate in multiply injured patients. Additionally, by offering the best treatment for the femoral shaft fracture, it avoids the chronic disability that is often associated with less than ideal treatment of the femoral shaft fracture. This may occur if the patient develops significant respiratory distress syndrome or multiple organ system failure because of a delay in fracture stabilization.

Isolated femoral shaft fractures (ISS < 18) should be cared for at the most convenient time.[8,23] In many in-stitutions, this may be in the initial 24 hours after injury. If this is significantly inconvenient and the patient has been documented to be in no pulmonary distress, the surgical procedure can be delayed for two to five days. However, it is incumbent on the treating physician to prove that the patient is in no respiratory distress prior to making this decision. To provide this information, an arterial blood gas determination

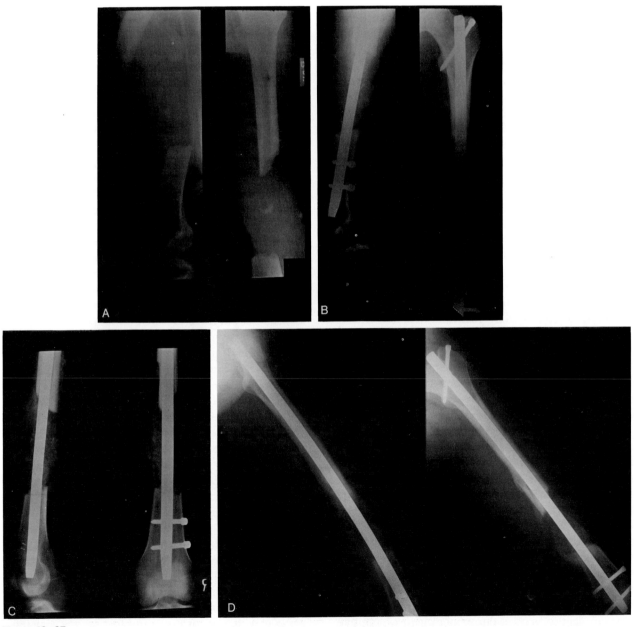

Figure 46–37

Intramedullary bone grafting of femoral shaft fracture. A, AP (left) and lateral (right) radiographs of the femoral shaft showing segmental bone loss measuring 8 cm. The patient was in traction during wound care. B, Following wound stabilization with a dry, clean, and closed wound, intramedullary bone grafting with autogenous cancellous bone was performed. The fracture was stabilized with an intramedullary locked nail. C, AP (left) and lateral (right) radiographs of the distal femur demonstrating placement of the bone graft. D, Early consolidation of the bone graft at four months after grafting.

should be obtained in the emergency department, using room air, prior to making this decision. This should be repeated at 12- to 24-hour intervals for approximately 48 hours to confirm that the patient is in no significant pulmonary distress. A pulse oximeter may be used to provide similar information. In the young trauma patient who is relatively healthy prior to injury, clinical fat emboli syndrome or other forms of pulmonary compromise cannot be detected without some evaluation of the patient's oxygenation status.[270] This can only be provided by arterial blood gas determination or by pulse oximeter. There may be no significant benefit in performing intramedullary nailing of these isolated femoral shaft fractures within the initial 24 hours unless pulmonary compromise is apparent. However, delaying the surgical procedure longer than necessary cannot be demonstrated to have any functional benefit and simply increases the patient's length of stay in the hospital, thereby increasing the patient's cost. Success rates (as measured by fracture healing or patient function) following surgical stabilization done acutely or delayed for a few days are essentially the same.

BONE GRAFTING

With closed, reamed intramedullary nailing, even the most comminuted femoral shaft fracture does not require bone grafting. Local reamings deposited within the fracture hematoma during intramedullary nailing stimulate healing. Therefore routine bone grafting of nailed femoral fractures is not indicated. However, in the presence of significant bone loss or in the case of internal fixation by means of a plate, additional autogenous cancellous bone graft should be performed. The timing of this bone graft should be carefully considered.

In the patient with an open femur fracture and significant bone loss, any bone grafting should be delayed until benign soft tissue healing has occurred in the thigh (this may take as long as four to six weeks). Generally the femur has been temporarily stabilized with a small intramedullary nail (10- to 12-mm) or an external fixator. Following benign and mature soft tissue healing in the thigh, the femoral shaft can be bone grafted using the closed intramedullary bone grafting technique described by Chapman (Fig. 46–37).[54] This requires removal of a previously placed small intramedullary nail or perhaps the removal of an external fixator that has been in place for a short period of time (less than two weeks). Closed intramedullary bone grafting is followed by insertion of a reamed nail of larger diameter (12- to 14-mm).

All plates applied to the femoral diaphysis, including the subtrochanteric area or supracondylar area, should be protected with autogenous cancellous bone grafting. The graft is placed along the fracture opposite the plate, thus promoting callus formation opposite the plate. This protects the plate from failure by resisting cyclic bending as soon as it consolidates. Rigid internal fixation heals by primary bone formation without periosteal callus. Primary bone healing is less strong than periosteal callus formation and requires protection for long periods of time (one to two years) before equal bone strength is achieved. Any delay in bone healing or premature plate removal prior to complete maturation of union will risk hardware failure (plate breakage, screw breakage, or screw loosening). External fixation of femoral shaft fractures should be carried out in a manner similar to plate fixation.

Individual Treatment Modalities

Current treatment modalities available for femoral shaft fractures include (1) skeletal traction followed by cast brace application, (2) roller traction, (3) external fixation, (4) application of a compression plate with bone grafting, (5) flexible intramedullary nailing, and (6) closed intramedullary nailing.

SKELETAL TRACTION

Skeletal traction is historically the longest-standing treatment of femoral shaft fractures in modern times.[11,48,165,208,260] In an attempt to return the lower leg to its normal alignment, application of longitudinal traction and then immobilization of the fracture with splints alongside the leg has been applied to these fractures since the time of the ancient Egyptians and Hippocrates. Skin traction has played only a minimal role in the development of traction as a major treatment modality. Currently, skin traction is used for adults only as temporary immobilization to allow patient transport. An example of this would be emergency splints, such as the Hare traction splint, for patient transport (see Fig. 46–12). This device allows countertraction in the area of the groin and immobilization of the extremity with longitudinal metal bars passing medial and lateral to the limb. The limb is attached to the metal bars using elastic Velcro closing straps. Traction is applied to the foot and ankle using nonelastic Velcro straps applied to the foot and ankle and attached to a windlass type traction apparatus for the foot. Skin traction simply cannot allow enough pull longitudinally over a long enough period of time to reduce the femoral shaft fracture without causing major complications such as skin sores or compartment syndromes.

Skeletal traction is perhaps the most common

method of treatment of femoral shaft fractures throughout the world. Many physicians use a period of skeletal traction prior to closed intramedullary nailing. Virtually any closed or open femoral shaft fracture is amenable to this mode of therapy, but it is generally reserved for less sophisticated medical communities and third-world nations where modern facilities and modern surgical care are not available to the treating physician.[133,134]

Technique

A skeletal traction pin is applied either to the distal femur or the proximal tibia. The size of the traction pin varies according to the method or reason for use of the traction. If traction is being used as the primary treatment modality, a pin threaded in the bone is recommended, because it tends not to slip back and forth through the bone. However, if temporary traction is planned for the femoral shaft fracture, a large, smooth Steinmann pin (3/16-in) can be applied. It is stronger and tends not to bend when traction is applied to the pin in the operating room. A large, smooth or threaded Steinmann pin is attached to traction ropes using a Steinmann pin bow. Smaller diameter pins (wires) are

attached with a Kirschner wire bow, which applies tension to the wire so that it does not bend when traction is applied. Placing the pin or wire under tension allows the smaller diameter to be used (Fig. 46-38).

The correct place for the skeletal traction pin has been debated. From a rational and mechanical standpoint, the distal femur is perhaps the best location. Thus longitudinal traction then, does not put extra stress on potentially damaged knee ligaments. This position allows a more direct pull of traction, as well as better correction of alignment. However, placement of the traction pin in the distal femur risks problems with knee stiffness and potential infection. The potential for infection includes direct innoculation of the suprapatellar pouch, as well as infection of an operative procedure such as closed intramedullary nailing that may be carried out in the future. Currently, because of the short time that patients are in traction and because of advances made in techniques of pin application and antibiotics, there is little reason that a skeletal traction pin should not be applied to the distal femur other than the minimal risk of injury to local vessels and nerves or to the distal femoral growth plate in immature patients.

The skeletal traction pin should be applied at the level of the adductor tubercle, and if intramedullary

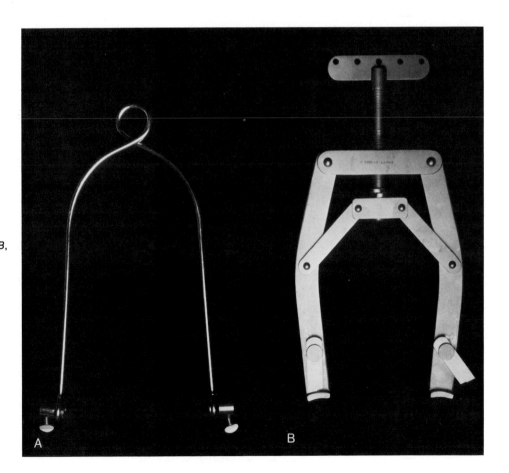

Figure 46-38

A, Steinmann pin holder. *B*, Kirschner wire bow.

nailing is planned in the future, it should be placed into the anterior third of the distal femoral shaft. This will allow a nail to pass posterior to the skeletal traction pin without requiring removal of the pin during nail insertion. A two-pin technique of skeletal traction — with a pin in the distal femur, as well as a pin in the tibia — was described by Stewart and co-workers for improved control of distal femur fractures[258] (see chapter 47).

In spite of the mechanical benefits of distal femoral traction, however, the most frequently used site for application of skeletal traction to the femoral shaft is the proximal tibia. This site is subcutaneous and provides easy access without threat of damage to neurologic or vascular structures at the time of pin application. This makes pin insertion convenient. The major drawback of this site is the fact that significant forces are applied to the femur through the knee ligaments. Although most normal knee ligaments can tolerate a considerable amount of longitudinal traction, even small amounts of traction to damaged knee ligaments can be harmful. Unfortunately, with most femoral shaft fractures knee effusions and potential knee ligament injuries are difficult to evaluate early, therefore making application of proximal tibial traction less than ideal. In spite of the theoretic problems, there have been no published reports of further damage to ligamentous structures about the knee related to skeletal traction pins in the proximal tibia.

Other methods of application of longitudinal traction include the use of an os calcis pin or perhaps a distal tibial pin. These forms of traction are in far less common use and are generally used only secondarily.

The major problem noted with the treatment of skeletal traction is malalignment. The most common malalignment is a varus (internal rotation) deformity of the distal fragment. This has been well described and explained in the literature.[188] In the supine patient, forces about the proximal aspect of the femur favor abduction and external rotation of the proximal fragment. By pulling on the distal fragment, the pull of the adductor magnus favors internal rotation of the distal fragment, as well as a varus or adducted position of the distal fragment. If this deformity is not carefully observed and corrected during the application of traction, union will occur with the leg in this malaligned position. As with all manipulative or traction methods of fracture reduction, the distal fragment should be carefully aligned with the proximal fragment, as the proximal fragment is not controlled by traction. This can be achieved by careful positioning of the skeletal traction pin within the bone, as well as by carefully directing the application of force to the pin itself.

Insertion of a skeletal traction pin is a surgical procedure and therefore should be done under sterile conditions with sterile equipment and instruments. The procedure can be accomplished under local anesthesia, as the skin and periosteum of the bone are the only structures with sensory input. The surgeon must remember that both medial and lateral aspects of the skin and bone should be treated with the anesthetic to avoid excessive pain. In spite of the insertion of local anesthetic, some pain is still experienced because of pressure differentials within the bone itself. This is transitory. Insertion of a skeletal traction pin alone should rarely be considered an indication for general anesthesia.

Perhaps more significant than the line of insertion of the skeletal traction pin is the suspension technique used to connect the traction pin to the weights.[48] This aspect of skeletal traction is most onerous for the treating physician. Much time must be spent in considering and reevaluating at least once daily the suspension system in use. The most versatile and commonly used system is the application of balanced suspension through a modified Thomas splint with a Pearson attachment (Fig. 46–39). This system uses a modified Thomas ring (only a half ring is used proximally) and splint, with a second device, the Pearson attachment, fixed to the splint. This attachment provides some flexion at the knee. The most comfortable position is with the knee flexed 15° to 20°. This position also reduces muscular forces, particularly that of the gastrocnemius, which allows the limb to be more easily realigned by the use of longitudinal traction. Flexion of the knee with longitudinal skeletal traction for femoral shaft fractures has been an important modification in application of traction to femoral shaft fractures. It aids in alignment and avoids decreased knee motion secondary to arthrofibrosis. Methods of skeletal traction that allow active knee motion have also been described and have proven to be beneficial.[209] These methods require considerable sophistication in their application and are seldom used routinely.

Use of skeletal traction for a femoral shaft fracture need not be a complex undertaking. Balanced suspension can also be applied to femoral shaft fractures without modified Thompson splints with Pearson attachments. Utilizing the skeletal traction pin itself, a traction bow, pulleys, ropes, stockinette, and routine plaster of Paris, skeletal traction can be applied to virtually all femoral shaft fractures. These materials are in common use throughout the world for treatment of all fractures. Balanced suspension can be created by applying a cast to the lower leg, a skeletal traction pin to the distal or proximal tibia, and stockinette slings to the proximal femur and distal tibia (see Fig. 46–39B).

The 90-90 method of application of skeletal traction and suspension is also useful for alignment of femoral

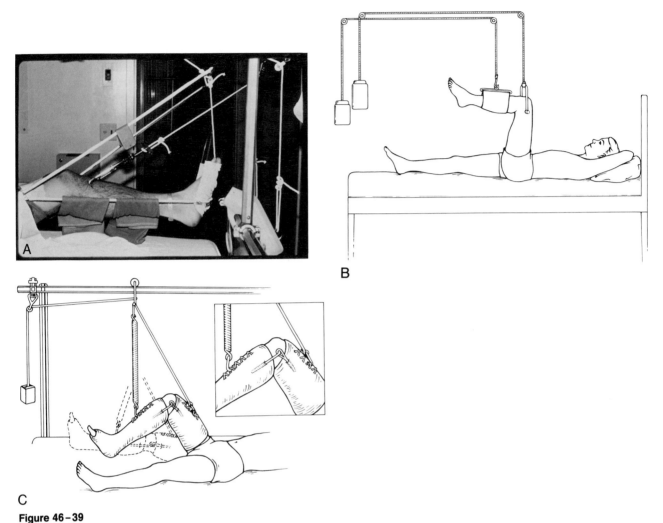

Figure 46-39

A, Skeletal traction applied to a femoral shaft fracture through a tibial pin utilizing balanced suspension with a Thomas splint and Pearson attachment. *B,* 90-90 skeletal traction. *C,* Roller traction.

shaft fractures (see Fig. 46-39*C*). It is especially beneficial where major soft tissue lesions exist in the buttock or posterior thigh. Body weight applies countertraction, and alignment is achieved through the natural tendency of the distal fragment to line up with the proximal fragment with this method of traction. The knee is flexed at 90°, as is the hip. This amount of knee flexion is a cause of mild knee stiffness, which can generally be overcome following fracture union. The greatest drawback is the patient's need to remain relatively immobile in the supine position in the bed. This can be a major problem with multiply injured patients, as indicated previously. The application of 90-90 traction also requires little in the way of sophisticated equipment.

Although skeletal traction is still in common use, there are many problems that lead more sophisticated medical communities away from the technique. These problems include inability to mobilize the patient, malalignment, decreased knee motion, the cost of medical care as a result of greater time in the hospital, and patient inconvenience.[49,79,134,260,285] As has been previously stated, the ability to mobilize patients with femoral shaft fractures, particularly those who have other significant injuries, is absolutely crucial to overall patient well being. This is simply not possible when skeletal traction is chosen as a means of treatment for a femoral shaft fracture. Diagnostic techniques such as computed tomographic (CT) scanning, magnetic resonance imaging (MRI), ultrasound, and others that may be necessary for evaluation of other medical problems are difficult to accomplish with this method of treatment. Limb length inequality (shortening) and rotational and angulatory malalignment problems have all been associated with this method of therapy.[49,134,285] The severity of these problems is inversely related to the amount of time and concern directed by the treating physician to the patient during the course of traction.

Skeletal traction requires that the patient be hospitalized for at least four to six weeks for appropriate treatment. The patient spends four to six weeks in traction, at which time he or she is transferred to either a spica cast or a cast brace. Following application of the cast or cast brace, the patient requires up to a week of therapy to reach a level of independence necessary for discharge. This will total six to eight weeks of hospitalization. The cost of medical care in the United States is directly related to the number of days spent in the hospital. Therefore this method can be costly to the patient and third-party insurance carrier. Finally, patients in the United States today dislike being admitted to the hospital at all, and with this method they are absolutely confined to the bed during their stay, which is additionally unpleasant. This is uncomfortable and makes the patient relatively dependent on nursing care and family members for even the most intimate of needs (food, hygiene, fellowship). For these reasons, this treatment, although time-honored, is steadily decreasing in popularity throughout the world. However, there likely will always be a need for application of skeletal traction to femoral shaft fractures, even if it is only a temporary procedure.

All forms of traction applied to femoral shaft fractures have certain features in common.[11,79,168,169,208] These include the necessity for marked attention to detail on a daily basis by the treating physician. The treating physician must take great care to evaluate the suspension and make sure that it is lined up appropriately and is being applied without complications. These complications can include pin track infections; skin breakdown, either on the buttock or in association with the suspension device; lack of ideal alignment because of inappropriate traction or inappropriately suspended traction; and other medical problems (e.g., fat embolism, pneumonia). The overall outcome of treatment with traction is directly related to the attention paid by the treating physician to the patient.

Radiographic evaluation of the femoral shaft fracture in traction is most crucial to the method. During the initial seven to ten days, the fracture must be radiographed frequently. Alignment must be achieved by ten days, or great difficulty occurs in achieving appropriate alignment because of early callus formation. Radiographs must be ordered on a timely basis, and quality radiographs that are consistent and reproducible must be obtained. The x-ray technician must be experienced, and the x-ray beam must be directed perpendicular to the femoral shaft. X-ray technicians instead commonly direct the x-ray beam perpendicular to the bed or floor, as is common practice in the radiology

suite. This will not allow an appropriate evaluation of alignment with a patient in traction. Ropes, other extremities, casts, hinges, hooks, loops, and other objects also interfere with radiographs taken of patients in traction. This is a most crucial portion of the application of traction to the femoral shaft fracture, and the treating surgeon becomes absolutely dependent on the quality of service provided by the radiology department. This may add another source of frustration in the use of traction for definitive treatment of femoral shaft fractures.

Cast Brace

The cast brace was developed basically as an alternative to the spica cast commonly applied to a femoral shaft fracture following four to six weeks of traction.[67,110,152,157,171,174,177,182,184,250] Application of skeletal traction for a prolonged period of time followed by immobilization of the femoral shaft and knee in a spica cast led to significant difficulties with overall patient care, knee motion, and mobility. The cast brace was developed to provide functional knee and hip motion following a period of traction. It provided enough control of some fractures to reduce the time in traction and hospital. It was initially felt to be so successful that it came to be applied at an earlier and earlier point in time following a period of skeletal traction. In some cases the cast brace has been applied as early as one to two weeks following application of skeletal traction. A variation of the cast brace is used with roller traction to achieve traction plus functional knee motion even while in traction. The cast brace is most successful following an appropriate period of skeletal traction. The time in skeletal traction should be long enough to allow good early callus formation. This is best indicated by a pain-free fracture, as well as by evidence of callus formation on radiographic evaluation. This will allow some stability to the fracture site during application of the cast brace.

As shown by Mooney and others, the cast brace initially can carry up to 50% of the load applied in normal weight bearing.[182,184] This rapidly decreases to 10% to 20% of the load applied in normal weight bearing as soft tissue atrophy occurs under the cast.

The cast brace is generally applied using a quadrilateral socket proximally, which allows for a good rotational fit to the proximal (thigh) portion of the cast (Fig. 46–40). The socket may also transfer force from the leg to the pelvis in a manner similar to that of an above-knee amputation prosthesis. Knee hinges are of a polycentric design and must be carefully applied to the appropriate center of knee motion. This is a crucial aspect of the application of the cast brace and must be per-

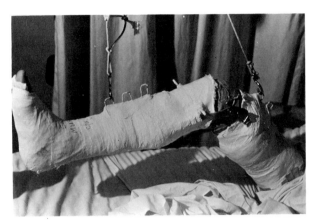

Figure 46–40

Cast brace applied to the femoral shaft following a period of traction. This particular cast brace is applied in conjunction with the use of roller traction.

formed by an experienced individual. Polyethylene knee hinges have been described with cast braces, as well as with roller traction; however, they may not adequately transfer stress in the longitudinal manner, although they do allow good knee flexion and duplicate a polycentric hinge quite well in that regard. A metal polycentric hinge appropriately applied allows the best form of knee motion, as well as longitudinal stress transfer from the foot and lower leg to the thigh. The hinge is applied to the lower leg by means of a routine below-knee cast with the foot and ankle in a neutral position.

The cast brace is most successful for distal femoral shaft fractures and less so for more proximal fractures.[183] The method is inappropriate for proximal shaft fractures, as the cast achieves essentially no control of the fracture in anteroposterior or mediolateral bending. If a cast brace is used for fractures in the proximal half of the shaft, suspension of the cast brace by means of a belt and pelvic band should be considered.[75] Malalignment in proximal shaft fractures is extremely difficult to prevent with a cast brace.

Small amounts of malalignment and angulation (1° to 3°) can be corrected by wedging of the plaster cast. Use of a cast brace, as with other methods of traction application, requires acceptance of a certain amount of shortening (1 cm). This small amount of shortening is only marginally acceptable to patients in the United States. The shortening does allow for good early callus formation, and the femoral shaft fracture can be expected to be solidly united at a period of four to five months following the fracture.

The cast brace is designed to maintain position that has been achieved and stabilized by means of traction. The cast brace is not intended to correct length or an-

gulation problems that are present in traction. It is appropriate only for fractures that are stable and have early callus formation.

ROLLER TRACTION

Perhaps the most sophisticated and best system for application of traction to femoral shaft fractures is that of roller traction, originally designed by Neufeld (see Fig. 46–39D).[38,157,169,181] This system is said to flow according to patient movements, is found to be quite comfortable, and allows the patient to be out of bed at an earlier time than standard skeletal traction would allow. The technique applies traction through casts or splints incorporating a skeletal traction pin in the proximal tibia. The leg, thus supported, is suspended from a wheel on an overhead track and distal traction is applied to the rolling wheel. Although many variations of the technique exist, it generally involves a cast brace with a series of wire loops incorporated along the anterior aspect of the thigh and proximal lower leg. The cast brace is usually hinged at the knee by means of a flexible hinge device made of polyethylene. The lower leg is suspended from the overhead device by means of a large spring, and longitudinal traction is applied to the femur by means of a hook attached to one of the loops incorporated into the cast along the anterior aspect of the thigh. Fifteen to 25 pounds traction can be applied, and by flexing and extending the knee through the cast brace device while traction is applied, dynamic function of the lower extremity can be achieved. This is obviously beneficial for joint function at the knee and allows normal muscle function to occur in the thigh and calf.

Following early fracture stabilization by callus formation (usually after two to four weeks in traction), the patient can begin non–weight-bearing ambulation with crutches. This is relatively easy to accomplish by detaching the hooks from the loops in the suspension apparatus. Radiographs are obtained with the patient out of traction. If shortening or malalignment occurs following a brief period out of traction, the patient is placed back in traction for another week. Patients can disassemble the device themselves and put themselves back in the traction system after a little coaching. Traction is discontinued once ambulation is pain free and the patient's limb has not demonstrated a capacity for shortening or malalignment after 24 hours out of traction.

This system has proven to be a most versatile and functional method of traction for femoral shaft fractures. It is more physiologic than other means of skeletal traction, is less invasive, and can perhaps decrease the average time spent in the hospital. However, it requires more sophisticated medical equipment and experience to achieve the ideal result than does skeletal traction. It also requires that the patient be virtually supine in bed for a period of two to three weeks, which has detrimental effects on the patient similar to those of other forms of traction. In spite of the benefits of this method over other methods of traction, its drawbacks when compared with early fracture stabilization by means of surgery also make it a less common mode of treatment. Malunion is a common complication.[134]

EXTERNAL FIXATION

External fixation has also been described for treatment of femoral shaft fractures.[7,14,100,167] It may be considered a method of applying fixed skeletal traction.[167] External fixation is a method of fracture care that allows excellent treatment of soft tissues while avoiding the additional surgical trauma of inserting a large foreign body implant into the area of the fracture wound. For the femur, this treatment is best restricted to severe open fractures with extensive contamination of the wound and the fracture site, infected nonunions of femoral shaft fractures, and perhaps those femoral shaft fractures associated with a vascular injury. Its drawbacks include pin site problems, interference with quadriceps and knee motion, and limited ability to maintain fracture alignment until healing is secure. Therefore it should be restricted to situations in which other treatments are even riskier. Considerable improvement in the methodology of external fixation for femoral shaft fractures has occurred since the 1980s.

External fixation, as originally described ay authors such as Anderson and Hoffman, frequently utilized multiplanar fixation of the fracture.[2,70,122] These systems were at a distinct disadvantage when treating femoral shaft fractures, unlike their use in tibial shaft fractures. That is, it was necessary to penetrate the anterior aspect of the thigh with pins to achieve appropriate stabilization of a femoral shaft fracture. This resulted in significant problems of scarring and decreased knee motion, in addition to pin track infection caused by excessive soft tissue movement about the pin. Alternative methods of application of external fixation,

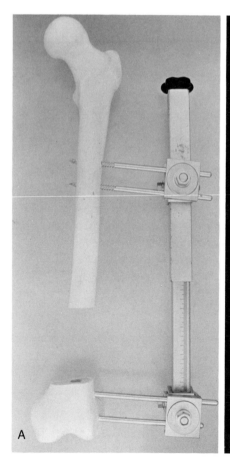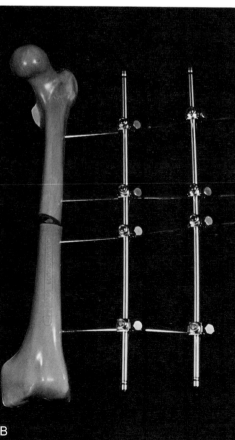

Figure 46–41

External fixation that may be applied to a femoral shaft. A, Wagner leg-lengthening device (6-mm pins). B, Stacked half-pin unilateral frame (5-mm pins).

such as application of the Wagner leg lengthening device, have resulted in improved results (Fig. 46–41*A*).[71,73,100,130,167,246,283] The Wagner device is applied utilizing pin fixation in a single plane. Four pins are inserted from lateral to medial and attached to a lateral outrigger device that can be locked into a rigid form that will allow reasonable length and stability to be achieved. Dabezies et al. have described the use of this form of external fixator for open femoral shaft fractures.[71] Their results with the method indicate a high incidence of malalignment (2%), pin track infection (20%), and loss of knee motion (45%).

The Wagner external fixator employs two 6-mm pins in single clamps proximally and distally. This leaves a relatively large span of femoral shaft without a fixation pin to stabilize it. Unfortunately, this can lead to malalignment problems because of lack of stability. Ideal pin placement for external fixation of a long bone has been described by Behrens and others as using two pins in each major fragment, one close to the fracture site in intact bone and the other well removed from the fracture.[18] Neither the Wagner external fixator nor the Hoffman external fixator will allow for this type of pin placement.

External fixation of a femoral shaft fracture is best achieved with a single-plane half-pin device applied by a lateral approach. This usually provides good fracture control with minimal impact on soft tissue management. Large pins (5- or 6-mm) should be applied in each fragment (proximal and distal) near the fracture site and as far from the fracture site as reasonable. These large pins should be connected by means of a clamp to a rigid connecting rod. Two rigid connecting rods stacked on the pins allow better stabilization of the femoral shaft fracture (see Fig. 46–41*B*). A device applied in this manner will decrease malalignment complications with femoral shaft fractures.[7] Because of the mobile muscles that continually slide over the pins with normal knee motion, pin track infection and loss of knee motion continue to be problems when external fixation is used for a femoral shaft fracture. Meticulous pin care and avoidance of the use of pins in thickly muscled areas may decrease this incidence somewhat, but a 10% to 15% pin track infection rate should be expected with application of external fixation to a femoral shaft fracture.

External fixation is far from the ideal method of care for most femoral shaft fractures. Because of malalignment and pin track infection problems, the use of this technique should be restricted to type III open femoral shaft fractures with extensive contamination of soft tissues, infected femoral shaft fractures, and infected nonunions of the femoral shaft.[7,100,230] It can also be used as a temporizing device that will rapidly stabilize a femoral fracture in certain life- or limb-threatening circumstances.[187] External fixation can be applied to a femoral shaft fracture in approximately 20 to 30 minutes when the fracture site is open. This can be beneficial for extremely ill patients, such as a multiply injured patient who is near death with a thigh compartment syndrome or a patient with femoral arterial injury that requires rapid fracture stabilization during revascularization. Following revascularization or return to reasonable health of the patient, the device can be removed and replaced with more appropriate internal fixation of the femoral shaft fracture.

Surgical Technique*

The external fixator is applied with the femoral shaft fracture held reduced. The most proximal and distal pins are first inserted parallel to each other. The pin sites are predrilled with a 3.5-mm drill bit using a double drill sleeve with a trocar. Appropriate length 5-mm pins are selected and inserted by hand through the outside sleeve. If possible, the pin placement should be under or posterior to the vastus lateralis muscle. This may be possible if the wound is open, and this will avoid penetration of the muscle belly. Unfortunately, this may not always be possible. Following insertion of the most proximal and distal pins, two connecting rods with four clamps each are connected to the pins using the most proximal and distal clamps on the rods. Then the pins that are near the fracture site in each main fragment are placed by predrilling through the middle pairs of clamps using the drill sleeve placed through both clamps. Each pin is then inserted through the clamps. The pins are placed at least 1 cm away from obvious fracture lines but as close as reasonable to the fracture site. This allows the pins in each main fragment to be as widely spaced as possible. The rods are attached proximally and distally first to ensure that the middle pins will fit through both of the more constrained middle clamps. Following insertion of the pins into the femur through the clamps, the connecting rods are clamped onto all four pins. To prevent pin track infection, all pin sites are carefully released so that the skin is not tented up over the external fixation pins. This leaves a stacked (two rods), half-pin frame.[18]

External fixation is not indicated in the majority of femoral shaft fractures and is seldom used for closed fractures.[100,230] It is often best to remove a femoral external fixator before complete fracture consolidation

---

* The surgical technique described here refers to use of the AO/ASIF tubular external fixator.[7,18]

occurs. External fixation devices act as distracting devices that will tend to discourage fracture union. Dynamization of external fixation in the femoral shaft is not recommended. Because of the extreme forces applied across the femur, it is much more difficult to control alignment when clamps are loosened, thereby making dynamic compression at the fracture site more difficult to achieve than in tibial shaft fractures. Most often it is necessary to transfer from the use of an external fixator to some more commonly applied internal fixation device or use a cast brace to achieve final union in a femoral shaft fracture. This transfer from external fixation to another form of treatment can be complex and difficult and may jeopardize alignment. It is also associated with an increased risk of infection because of contamination of the bone by the pins. In summary, this technique should be applied only to those fractures associated with the most complex soft tissue problems.

Pins in plaster is another form of external fixation.[243] The pins-in-plaster method of treating complex femoral shaft fractures has become obsolete with more modern techniques of external and internal fixation. This form of treatment for femoral shaft fractures is not recommended when more modern techniques are available.

COMPRESSION PLATING

Compression plating is a well-described technique for treatment of femoral shaft fractures.[10,59,93,193,253,254,272] Although only sporadic and incomplete reports of plate fixation of femoral shaft fractures are available in the literature, the technique gained popularity in the 1960s following publication of the AO method.[186,282] The AO group designed a large compression plate for specific use in femoral shaft fractures (Fig. 46–42A). They also designed larger screws (4.5-mm) with larger core diameters that are essentially twice as strong as screws used previously in orthopedic surgery. This justified the application of a compression plate to femoral shaft fractures. However, reported results have not supported the initial enthusiasm for this technique.[164,235] In spite of the design changes, a plate on the femoral shaft is at a distinct disadvantage when compared with an intramedullary nail. The plate is placed eccentrically on the femoral shaft. The line of application of the weight-bearing force is approximately 1 to 2 cm more distant from the force of application with plate fixation of the femur than with an intramedullary nail. This places more stress on the plate than on the intramedullary nail, as the bending moment experienced by the plate or nail is directly related to the force of application and the distance of the implant from the force of application (see Fig. 46–42B).

By design a plate is also a weight-absorbing device.[183] Stress applied to the femur passes directly up the femoral shaft and bypasses the femur by means of absorption of stress through the distal screws into the plate and back into the femur through proximal screws (see Fig. 46–42C). Intramedullary nails are, in general, weight-sharing devices that share stress with the femoral shaft as fracture healing occurs. Because plates are stress-absorbing devices, stress shielding and localized osteoporosis occur under the plate, with a potentially increased risk of refracture of the femoral shaft following removal of a plate, even long after fracture union. Refracture has occurred up to 39 months following plate removal.[83]

Plate application to the femoral shaft, by necessity, requires an open surgical procedure, with at least some devascularization of the femoral shaft occurring at the time of plate application. Furthermore, the entire fracture hematoma must be evacuated to allow adequate visualization of the fracture site as needed to achieve the anatomic realignment of the femoral shaft that is required for plate fixation. Both devitalization of the shaft and evacuation of the fracture hematoma predispose plated fractures to delayed healing. The combination of the plate's mechanical disadvantage and the delay in fracture healing risks fixation failure, such as plate or screw breakage or loosening, prior to fracture healing.[26,164,228,235]

In spite of the disadvantages of compression plates, there are indications for the use of plates in femoral shaft fractures. Therefore the orthopedic trauma surgeon should be familiar with techniques of proper application of plates to femoral shaft fractures.[59,118,119,160] Acceptable results have been achieved by surgeons experienced in the correct technique of application of plates to the femoral shaft fracture.[59] Many of the unacceptable results achieved with plate application to the femoral shaft have been related to poor technique and improper indications for the operative procedure.[282] Indications for the use of compression plating

---

Figure 46–42

Plate application to femoral shaft fracture. *A*, Broad DC plate with 4.5-mm screws. Preoperative, early, and later views demonstrating fixation and medial bone graft. *B*, Drawing of plate vs. nail fixation of femoral shaft. A plate situated lateral to the weight-bearing axis of the femur is subjected to a larger bending moment (= f × d) than an intramedullary nail. *C*, The plate prevents loading of the underlying fracture. See text.

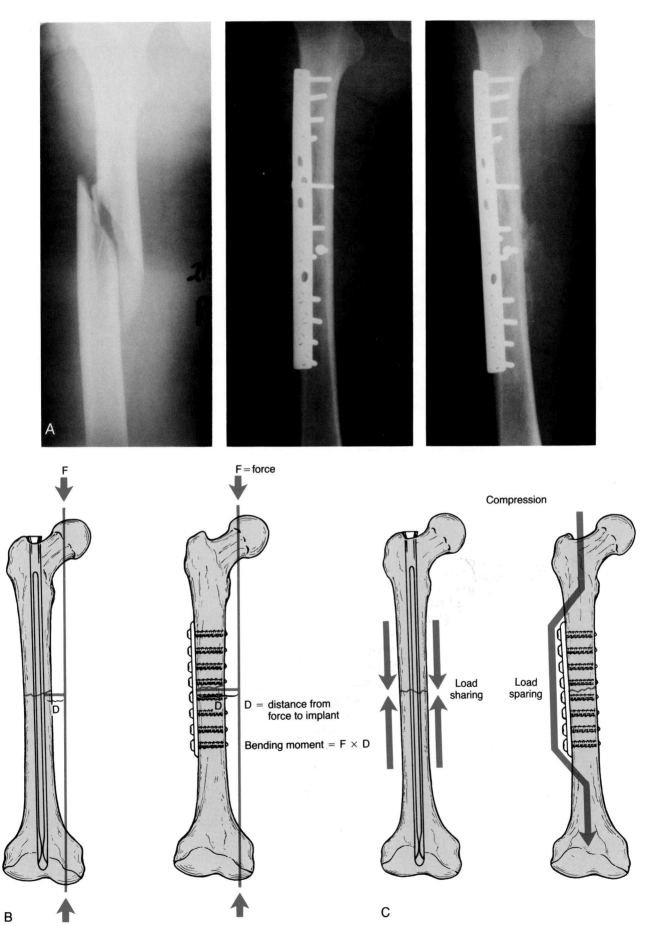

A

F

F = force

D

D = distance from force to implant

Bending moment = F × D

Compression

Load sharing

Load sparing

B

C

1589

for femoral shaft fracture are ipsilateral fractures of the femoral shaft associated with fractures of the proximal or distal femur, femoral shaft fractures that occur in conjunction with a major arterial injury requiring repair, or occasionally a severe open femoral shaft fracture in which no further exposure is required to gain secure plate fixation.

Ipsilateral femoral shaft and concomitant proximal femoral metaphyseal injury is a most difficult problem to face. Use of a single method for treatment of both fractures is fraught with many technical difficulties. The proximal metaphyseal fracture of the femur should take precedence over the femoral shaft fracture. The treatment chosen should be the one that is most appropriate for the proximal metaphyseal fracture instead of the one that is best for the femoral shaft fracture. A similar situation may occur in the instance of a comminuted interarticular distal femur fracture with a concomitant femoral shaft fracture.

The association of a major arterial injury requiring vascular repair with a femoral shaft fracture can also be a difficult undertaking. A compression plate may allow the appropriate fracture stabilization necessary to achieve a successful outcome of the vascular repair. If the vascular surgeon has exposed the femoral artery through an extensile medial approach, the orthopedic surgeon may choose to apply a medial compression plate to the femoral shaft fracture without exposing the lateral portion of the femur.

A severe open femoral shaft fracture in a severely compromised patient may be another indication for use of a compression plate. Such a fracture requires irrigation and debridement in the operating rom. If the patient is a multiply traumatized patient with life-threatening injuries, the surgeon may not have the time to move the patient to a fracture table after irrigation and debridement for closed intramedullary nailing. Orthopedic surgeons with extensive experience in plate application may choose in this situation to apply a plate to such a femoral shaft fracture following thorough irrigation and debridement rather than perform closed or open intramedullary nailing. The most expedient treatment of the femoral shaft fracture should take precedence in a severely compromised patient with a major open femoral shaft fracture. External fixation is another option, but it has its own drawbacks, as previously discussed.

The most significant improvement in the use of plate application to femoral shaft fractures is the ability to achieve fracture stabilization without absolute anatomic reduction of all fracture fragments by utilizing a femoral distractor or the technique of distraction at the fracture site.[11,119,167a] Reports of plate application to femoral shaft fractures utilizing a femoral distractor

and avoiding absolute anatomic reduction indicate improved results. The femoral distractor will allow correction of length and alignment. The plate can then be applied with the femur correctly aligned in length, rotation, and angulation. With plate fixation that includes eight to nine cortices in each major fragment, the fracture can be stabilized. All fracture fragments need not be anatomically reduced and fixed with interfragmentary compression. In the past, absolute anatomic reduction with interfragmentary compression of fragments has led to excessive bone devitalization and increased length of time to union. By achieving length and alignment utilizing a distractor or plate-tensioning device, the plate can be applied without devitalization of bone fragments. Fracture union then occurs with periosteal callous formation rather than primary bone union, and overall results are improved.

Plates may be replaced by intramedullary nails. This can be accomplished after enough time has passed to allow for revascularization of the femoral cortex (generally six to eight weeks). Therefore application of a compression plate to the femoral shaft may be considered a temporary technique for early fracture stabilization that can then be exchanged for more permanent fracture stabilization, such as an intramedullary nail.

Intramedullary nailing of femoral shaft fractures has not become commonplace in certain settings because of lack of equipment and experienced surgeons. Individuals practicing in such an environment may wish to use compression plate fixation as their method of treatment for femoral shaft fractures. Generally, less capital equipment and experience are required throughout the hospital for use of plate fixation of femoral fractures, as compared with closed intramedullary nailing techniques. In this situation, surgeons should consider the use of a femoral distractor or plate-tensioning device and should avoid absolute anatomic reduction and rigid fixation of all fracture fragments. If correct alignment is achieved and an adequate length of plate is used without excessive soft tissue stripping, risks of failure are reduced. The routine use of autogenous cancellous bone graft placed on the medial aspect of the femur also will improve overall results and is recommended with plate application.

Surgical Technique

The patient is positioned either supine with a roll under the buttock or in the lateral decubitus position. The leg, as well as the ipsilateral iliac crest, is prepped to allow for the harvest of an autogenous cancellous bone graft. A straight lateral incision, which will include exposure of the majority of the lateral thigh from the distal metaphysis to the proximal metaphysis, is utilized. The fascia lata is split the length of the incision, giving access to the vastus lateralis, which is dissected from the intermuscular septum and elevated anteriorly. Care is taken to identify all vessels that perforate the septum. These are securely ligated. Elevation of the vastus lateralis provides access to the fracture site. Soft tissue dissection of bone fragments should be limited as much as possible. A femoral distractor can then be applied to the femoral shaft by means of a single pin placed anteriorly into the proximal fragment and one placed anteriorly into the distal fragment. These are either 5-mm Schanz screws or the special fixation screws that are provided with the femoral distractor. The femoral distractor then is applied to these bicortical pins, and the femur is distracted to length. This requires little stripping of soft tissue from bone. When the shortening at the fracture site has been slightly overcorrected, final adjustments in fracture alignment can be accomplished utilizing a dental pick, and the distractor is then adjusted to optimize interfragmentary apposition. Anatomic reduction of most bone fragments requires absolute exposure and the use of large bone reduction clamps, all of which devitalize bone fragments. Large butterfly fragments may be secured anatomically to the shaft without excessive devitalization. However, smaller fragments, by necessity, are completely devitalized by anatomic reduction. The linea aspera provides a guide to rotational alignment.

A broad dynamic compression plate is used for the femoral shaft. This plate is distinctly larger than other available plates. The appropriate length plate is determined, ensuring that eight to ten intact cortices are available in both proximal and distal fragments. Only minimal contouring of the plate is necessary, as the lateral shaft of the femur is essentially a straight line. If the plate extends onto the proximal or distal metaphysis, some contouring may be necessary. In this case, a large plate bender should be available, as well as appropriate templates to define the exact contour required for the plate (see Fig. 46–42D). The plate is then applied directly to the lateral aspect of the femur with the posterior border of the plate parallel to the linea aspera along the posterior border of the femoral shaft. Autogenous cancellous bone grafting is recommended opposite the plate. This is absolutely necessary when the medial cortex is deficient (Fig. 46–43). Only large butterfly fragments are anatomically reduced and fixed with interfragmentary compression.

An image intensifier may help to define overall alignment when using a femoral distractor; this requires a radiolucent operating room table. Initially open wounds are left open, and thick sterile dressings are applied. Otherwise the skin wound is closed over a suction drain, and sterile dressings are applied. No ex-

ternal support is generally required following application of a plate to the femoral shaft. The leg is best positioned with the knee flexed on a Böhler-Braun frame or by application of a continuous passive motion (CPM) machine to achieve hip and knee motion. Normal hip and knee motion are essential to an ideal outcome. A stiff joint proximal or distal to the plate transfers increased stress to the stabilized fracture. Delayed attempts to mobilize the stiff joint add additional stress to the plated fracture and increase the risk of failure.

After plate fixation of a femoral shaft fracture, weight-bearing must be delayed until the bone has healed. Premature weight-bearing risks hardware failure. Repeated radiographs are necessary every four to six weeks until healing is certain. Oblique views may be informative. Failure to unite will require bone grafting, revision of fixation, or both. Significant resistance exercises to restore strength and endurance to lower extremity muscles must similarly be delayed.

Plates on the femoral shaft should not be removed prior to two years postoperatively. If earlier plate removal is necessary, consideration may be given to supporting the femur with an intramedullary nail or an orthosis to prevent refracture. Refracture following plate removal has been a significant problem[164,245] and has been noted to occur even up to one year following plate removal.[83] Obviously, if refracture occurs in a femoral shaft, the patient is immediately back to his or her preoperative functional state, and repeat internal fixation is then necessary.

FLEXIBLE INTRAMEDULLARY NAILING

The use of flexible intramedullary nails to fix femoral shaft fractures has been described by Rush, who used the rods he designed.[236] These were redesigned and made popular by Ender and Simon-Widener in Austria.[82] The technique has been championed in the United States by Pankovitch.[199-203] The majority of flexible intramedullary nails in use in North America are those designed by Ender. These nails were originally introduced to North America for fixation of intertrochanteric fractures. The use of these nails for unstable intertrochanteric fractures has proven to be less than ideal, because they fail to control external rotation and shortening. However, the implants have gained some popularity in the United States for treatment of more stable long-bone fractures, including both the subtrochanteric region and the distal third.[37,81,178]

Use of flexible intramedullary nails for treatment of femoral shaft fractures is generally restricted to stable fracture patterns in young adults and adolescents, certain pathologic lesions, occasional open fractures, and

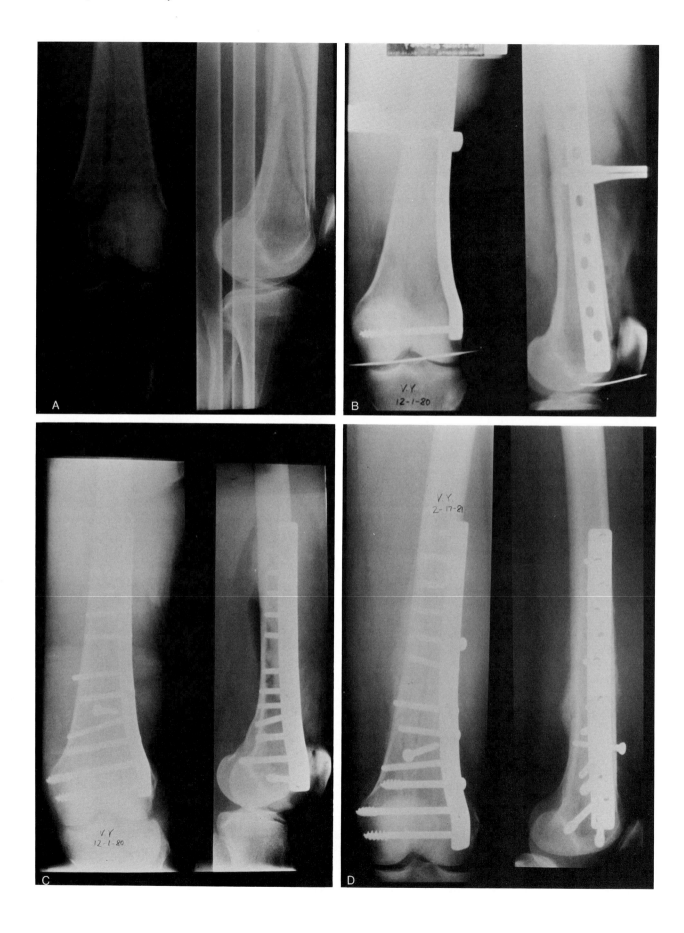

certain difficult fractures associated with metallic implants, such as uncemented joint prostheses.[81,86,166] Perry and Pankovitch have extended the technique to some unstable fracture patterns by simply adding locking screws applied through the eye of the Ender nails to avoid nail migration and shortening.[21] In spite of this, even Pankovitch concedes that difficult comminuted and unstable fractures will result in shortening and malrotation with the simple use of Ender nails.[20] He recommends adjunctive fixation in these fractures with cerclage wiring, unicortical plating, nail locking, or, occasionally, traction. Both cerclage wiring and unicortical plating require complete exposure of the fracture site for reduction and alignment of fracture fragments. This can lead to infection and fracture healing problems like those seen with plate fixation. The combination of cerclage wires with intramedullary nailing has led to an unacceptable incidence of delayed union and infection in reported series.[134,204,276]

Ender nails should not be used in severely osteoporotic bone in elderly patients. Fracture fixation, both proximally and distally, is too difficult to secure in these cases. The entry portal sites are easily comminuted by the awl, and the intramedullary canal is often so wide that it requires stacking with multiple nails, sometimes as many as six to nine.

Timing of surgical treatment with flexible intramedullary nails is similar to that of other forms of femoral shaft fracture fixation. Ender nails are inserted through distal portals in so-called retrograde nailing. The use of both medial and lateral distal portals is important. The 4.0-mm and 4.5-mm diameter Ender nails with a "C" configuration are selected. A wide variety of length of nails is necessary for the procedure. Nails are inserted simultaneously from both medial and lateral portals and cross each other twice in the medullary canal, gaining a secure fixation within the shaft of the femur (Fig. 46–44). It is important to attempt to get at least one nail into the femoral neck and one nail into the area of the greater trochanter. For unstable fracture patterns or for prevention of nail migration distally out of the femur, fixation of the nails with wires or 3.5-mm screws is recommended through the eyes in the nails. The wires are passed through the distal femur to connect the eyes of the medial nails with those of the lateral nails, thereby preventing nail migration.

Surgical Technique

Closed flexible intramedullary nailing is performed with the patient in the supine position on a fracture table and under general or spinal anesthesia.[200] Nails are inserted in the retrograde direction from distal portals. Traction is applied by means of a boot if the patient is operated on less than 48 hours after fracture. Skeletal traction is thus usually not required and may interfere with nail insertion if a traction pin is close to the knee. Image intensification is necessary for visualization of the starting position of the nails, as well as for fracture reduction and nail length selection. Rotational malalignment can be avoided if the patella is internally rotated 10° to 15° from midposition by rotation of the foot. Fracture realignment is rehearsed under image intensification prior to prepping the leg, and the techniques necessary to manually reduce the fracture are repeated during insertion of the nails.

The leg is prepped and draped to above the hip. The nailing is performed by two surgeons, one positioned on each side of the knee. Straight medial and lateral skin incisions are made extending 5 to 6 cm in length. The incision begins at the level of the knee joint and is carried proximally. Laterally, the vastus lateralis is dissected from the intramuscular septum to reach the distal shaft of the femur. Medially, dissection is carried posterior to the vastus medialis, which is retracted anteriorly. Holes are made using a drill bit in the posteromedial and posterolateral aspects of the femoral cortex at a level 2 to 3 cm proximal to the superior pole of the patella. The holes are enlarged with an awl or rongeur to permit the entrance of one or two Ender nails. The entry portals must be large enough to accommodate the planned number of nails. The portals are enlarged proximally, limiting their anteroposterior diameter to twice that of the nails. If intramedullary nailing is being performed in a skeletally immature patient, care must be taken to avoid the distal femoral physis at the time of creation of entry portals.

The length of the nails is determined by placement of

Figure 46-43

Plate application to a femoral fracture with a bone graft and periosteal callus formation. *A*, AP (left) and lateral (right) radiographs of the distal femur shaft showing a long oblique fracture extending into the distal metaphyseal bone. *B*, Intraoperative AP (left) and lateral (right) radiographs demonstrating a large plate that was carefully contoured to apply close to the distal femur. *C*, Postoperative AP (left) and lateral (right) radiographs of complete fracture stabilization. Bone graft has been placed opposite the plate. *D*, Follow-up radiograph three months after injury showing progressive healing. Note periosteal bone forming opposite the plate as a result of application of a cancellous bone graft. A blade plate or condylar compression screw might have improved purchase on the distal segment.

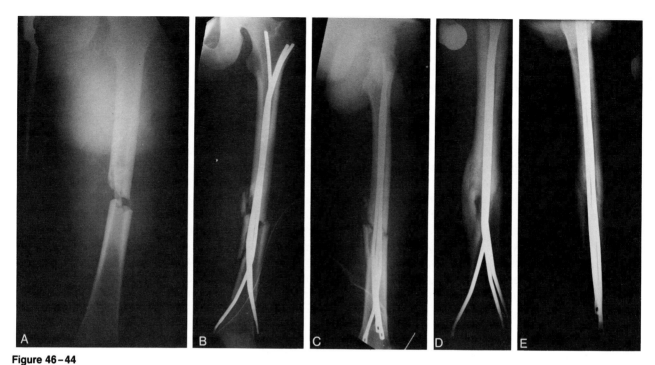

Figure 46–44

Femoral shaft fracture fixed with flexible intramedullary nails. *A*, Midshaft femoral shaft fracture in traction awaiting surgical stabilization. *B*, Postoperative AP radiograph following stabilization with 4.5-mm Ender nails. Two nails were inserted through a lateral portal and one nail through a medial portal. *C*, Postoperative lateral radiograph following Ender nail fixation. *D* AP radiograph six months postoperatively showing complete fracture healing. *E*, Lateral radiograph.

a nail along the anterior surface of the thigh on top of drapes. The distal point of the nail must rest at the level of the drill holes. The proximal point of the nail must be in the area of the femoral neck or tip of the greater trochanter. The Ender nails are then gently driven proximally across the fracture site, simultaneously holding the fracture reduced. After crossing the fracture site, the first nail may be rotated to realign the fracture fragments and facilitate passage of the second nail. Traction is released at this point, and the nails are driven proximally so that the tips reach a point proximal to the lesser trochanter. An attempt should be made to place one nail into the femoral neck and at least one other nail into the greater trochanter. In many instances additional intramedullary nails may be inserted through larger medial and lateral cortex portals to fill the intramedullary canal. This gains further fracture stability and prevents nail migration. If severe bicortical comminution is present, the traction should not be released prior to final impaction of nails or, in some cases, prior to the application of a cast brace to prevent excessive shortening.

At this point the nails are impacted into the femoral neck and the area of the greater trochanter. Attempts are made to lock the nails distally by means of 3.5-mm screws or cables passed through the eyes of each Ender

nail, engaging the other Ender nail. Perry[214] has described the use of titanium cable or 18-gauge stainless steel wires threaded through the eye of the medial nails, passed through the femur from medial to lateral portal, and then passed through the eye of the lateral nails. Cable that has been swaged on a trocar needle is utilized, or wire may be passed through a large spinal needle placed across the distal femur. Again, when nailing skeletally immature patients, care must be taken not to violate the capital femoral epiphysis, greater trochanteric apophysis, or distal femoral epiphysis. Care must also be taken not to perforate the femoral head or neck. Non–weight-bearing status of the patient is maintained until callus formation is apparent on radiographs, at which time the patient is allowed to bear 20 to 30 pounds of weight. The patient is further advanced to full weight bearing based on subsequent clinical and radiographic evidence of healing.

In Pankovitch et al.'s paper regarding closed Ender nailing of femoral shaft fractures, three types of major intraoperative problems were reported[199,202]: problems with insertion of the nails, problems with passage of the nails across the fracture site, and problems with positioning of the nails in the proximal femur. Surgeons interested in performing closed flexible nailing of femoral shaft fractures should review this experience to avoid many of the problems and pitfalls associated with this technique. Malrotation must be prevented by proper reduction of fracture fragments at the time of surgery. It is essential to check rotational alignment after nails are driven across the fracture site. Intraoperative fractures can occur at the entry portals as longitudinal cortical splits that extend proximally. A supracondylar fracture in the femur can occur if an entry portal is made too large and the bone is osteoporotic. Selection of correct length nails is essential to gain secure purchase in the upper femur.

Postoperative complications include distal migration of nails, which can occur because of telescoping of the fracture or distal portals that are too large or because the medullary canal is wide and has not been stacked completely with nails.[81,178] Distal locking of the nails with screws or wires is effective in preventing such distal migration. Nonunion and infection are other complications that have been seen postoperatively. These two complications following flexible intramedullary nailing have incidence rates similar to those following more rigid intramedullary nails (i.e., approximately a 1.0% incidence of either nonunion or infection). Shortening and malrotation are perhaps the major complications caused by the use of these flexible nails. These problems occur more commonly in comminuted or unstable fracture patterns. Biomechanical studies of various methods of stabilization have indicated that Ender nails do not control length of unstable femoral shaft fractures nearly as well as the more rigid locked nails.[135,268]

Hardware removal is recommended when nailing adolescent femoral shaft fractures. Removal is performed six to nine months following injury, provided there is clinical and radiographic evidence of healing. This is necessary, because with growth, the entry portals become diaphyseal, making nail removal increasingly difficult.

INTRAMEDULLARY NAILING

Intramedullary nailing is the best treatment available for the vast majority of femoral shaft fractures.[22,63,148–150,291,298] Indications for intramedullary fixation of fractures of the femoral shaft have been expanded with the use of locked intramedullary nails to include virtually all fractures in the femoral shaft.[1,32,296,298] With new nail designs that allow secure fixation in both the proximal and distal femur, it has become possible to nail virtually any fracture of the femoral shaft.[40,62,129,139,144,273] These intramedullary nails are biomechanically stable because of their large diameter (12- to 17-mm) and thick wall (1.5- to 2.0-mm). They can be inserted as load-sharing devices that transfer at least some of the stress of weight bearing to the bone. Beginning in 1940, when Küntscher first reported his experience with an intramedullary nail for a fractured femur, the device has been modified and changed to achieve the current designs.[148,150] Many of Küntscher's original concepts are still recognizable in modern intramedullary nail designs. Image intensification in the operating room has allowed the technique of closed intramedullary nailing to flourish. This technique allows the nail to be inserted into the medullary canal distant from the fracture site, and with image intensification guiding the three-dimensional reduction of the fracture, the nail is driven across it and securely positioned in both proximal and distal fragments.

The original Küntscher nail design was appropriate only for the nailing of relatively stable fracture patterns.[238] Malrotation and shortening of unstable fracture patterns plagued the technique until the introduction of locked intramedullary nails to the United States in 1981.[74,76,280,281,297] Since that time, several new designs of locked intramedullary nails have become available in North America.[1,40,133,139,144,145,237,289] Virtually any one of the current locked nail systems available in the United States will do a good job with a wide variety of femoral shaft fractures. Only minor differences in surgical instrumentation and ease of insertion exist among these nail systems. Intramedullary nail designs continue to improve, with nails now available that will allow fixation of combinations of femoral shaft and proximal femoral fractures, as well as the most complex of femoral shaft fractures. Instrumentation also continues to improve significantly.

The indications for intramedullary fixation of fractures of the femoral shaft include a femoral shaft fracture from the level of the lesser trochanter to within 6 to 8 cm of the articular surface of the distal femur. As stated in the section on open fractures of the femur, type I and type II open femoral shaft fractures appear to pose no contraindication to closed intramedullary nailing, provided the initial debridement has been adequate. Type III open femoral shaft fractures require further consideration regarding the use of immediate nailing or delayed nailing following a period of wound care and traction. This decision is generally made according to overall patient status. If the patient is severely injured and would gain significant benefit by immediate fracture stabilization and mobilization, closed intramedullary nailing should be considered. However, if the patient has an isolated injury, consideration should be given to immediate irrigation and debridement, followed by wound closure and delayed intramedullary nailing after 10 to 14 days. Recent smaller diameter nail designs may allow the use of a relatively strong, though unreamed, locked intramedullary nail for the femur. This nail would provide the benefits of a larger reamed nail and allow stabilization by locking, but with minimal or no reaming, which devitalizes fragments of bone and predisposes open fractures to infection. Preliminary research has indicated that the use of these unreamed intramedullary nails may indeed preserve some of the blood supply that is lost during reaming of the medullary canal.[64]

Prior to development of unreamed, locked intramedullary femoral nails, most modern intramedullary nail systems for stabilization of femoral shaft fracture required reaming of the intramedullary canal. Reaming allows insertion of larger diameter nails (12- to 16-mm) that allow stable fixation of the femoral shaft.[108] These large diameter nails effectively prevent bending and loss of fixation of the fracture site, even with the application of significant amounts of stress, including weight-bearing ambulation.[12] They are also of large enough diameter that drill holes for locking bolts can be placed through the nail both proximally and distally without significantly weakening the implant.

Reaming the medullary canal does damage the endosteal blood supply of the femoral shaft.[72] The endosteal blood supply provides vascularity to the inner third of the cortex of the femoral shaft.[140] Rhinelander and others have demonstrated that as long as space remains within the intramedullary canal after insertion of the intramedullary nail, this bone is revascularized by six to eight weeks following reaming of the intramedullary canal.[218-220] Certainly, reaming of the intramedullary canal has demonstrated no major drawbacks as applied to closed fractures of the femur and in fact may actually aid in fracture healing by deposition of many small bone fragments within the fracture hematoma. A major concern with loss of the endosteal blood supply has been in intramedullary nailing of open fractures or intramedullary nailing of fractures that require open surgical manipulation of the fracture fragments. In these instances loss of periosteal as well as endosteal blood supply may predispose the fracture to delayed healing and a higher rate of infection. This concern has been borne out in reported clinical series.[102,162,163] Other series on open fractures have demonstrated that type I and type II open fractures can be safely nailed early with no significant increase in complications.[39,159]

Any surgeon contemplating closed intramedullary nailing of femoral shaft fractures should have locked intramedullary nails available in his or her institution. Unlocked intramedullary nails, such as the Küntscher nail, Sampson nail, Schneider nail, Hansen-Street nail, and the original AO intramedullary nail, are of historic interest only.[111,241,259,288] These nails may still find some utility in fixation of stable femoral shaft fracture patterns (transverse or short oblique midshaft fractures). Their versatility is significantly limited, however, and will not allow the surgeon the full benefit of intramedullary nailing techniques. Therefore the technique of insertion of intramedullary nails will be described as it pertains to locked intramedullary nails. Similar techniques may be used for any of the aforementioned nails, with omission of the locking steps, if sufficient fracture stability is present. When in doubt, it is better to lock both proximally and distally.[41]

Timing of surgical treatment of femoral shaft fractures has been previously discussed in this chapter. The multiply injured patient with significant other injuries should undergo nailing within the initial 24 hours following injury. This allows appropriate patient mobilization and patient care and markedly improves the patient's overall pulmonary status. Intramedullary nailing of the isolated femoral fracture should also be performed at the earliest possible date but is a less urgent priority.

Appropriate radiographs should be obtained prior to beginning the surgical procedure. These include full-length AP and lateral radiographs of the femur, as well as an AP radiograph of the pelvis and AP and lateral radiographs of the knee. Full-length radiographs of the intact femur are quite helpful in determining the length as well as the diameter of the nail to be used during the surgical procedure. A 10% to 15% magnification occurs with routine radiographs taken at a tube-to-plate distance of 1 m. The width of the medullary canal and the length of the normal femur from the tip of the trochanter to the epiphyseal scar, the proximal pole of the patella, or posterior condylar line can be measured using the Küntscher ossimeter (the ossimeter contains a scale that allows for 10% magnification) (Fig. 46–45). In cases of severe comminution or large butterfly fragments, there is a distinct inability to determine correct femoral length from the pattern of the fractured femur. For such cases, radiographs of the intact normal femur are absolutely necessary to measure the appropriate length of nail. The patient's uninjured extremity should be measured preoperatively from the tip of the trochanter to a reproducible point on the distal femur. A length of nail is selected that would fit from the tip of the trochanter to the old epiphyseal scar, proximal pole of the patella, adductor tubercle, or whatever point is measured. A nail of that length is inserted and locked in the predetermined proximal and distal locations. The diameter of nail to be used can be determined from the width of the femoral canal on the radiogram using the Küntscher ossimeter, or from the diameter of reamers during nailing. Generally speaking, intramedullary

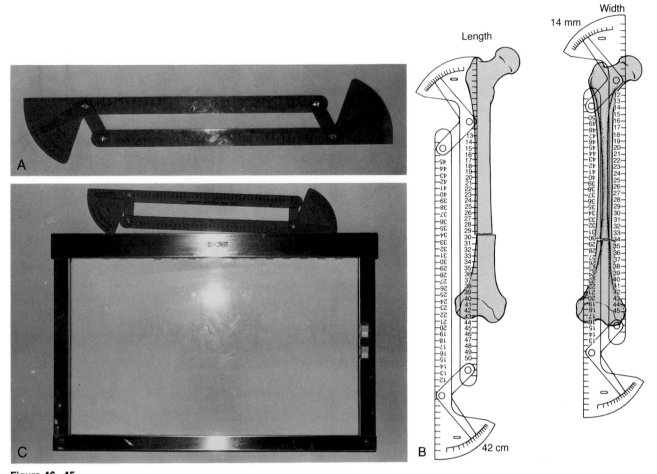

Figure 46–45

Küntscher ossimeter used to measure femoral length and the width of the intramedullary canal. *B*, Drawing of Küntscher ossimeter. *C*, Viewbox.

nails of diameter 12 to 14 mm are adequate in females, and those 13 to 15 mm in diameter are adequate in most males. Care should be taken preoperatively to evaluate the patient's proximal and distal femur, looking for fractures of the femoral neck or distal femur. In many cases there is minimally displaced or nondisplaced comminution of the femoral shaft that may only be apparent on careful scrutiny of the preoperative radiographs. In fractures that appear to be stable, the presence of nondisplaced fracture lines should persuade the surgeon to use a static locked nail (proximally and distally locked) instead of a dynamic locked nail.[32,53,133] This decision may be made preoperatively but may require modification if comminution increases intraoperatively. It is increasngly felt that static locked nails should be used in virtually all femoral shaft fractures, unless the surgeon has a specific reason to use a dynamic locked nail.[41] They do not interfere with healing and do not usually require dynamization. There is no protection against displacement of previously nondisplaced fracture fragments and eventual

shortening by telescoping at the fracture site with a dynamic locked nail. This has been shown by Brumback to be a potential problem that must be carefully evaluated.[41] It must be remembered that unlocked nails can be unstable in rotation and may require protection to prevent malrotation postoperatively.[135,136,268,269] This may only be necessary for a few days, until the patient achieves interdigitation of fracture fragments with full weight bearing and has adequate return of quadriceps strength to control rotation with his or her own musculature (i.e., patient may perform a straight leg raise). This control of rotation may be accomplished with a simple derotation boot used postoperatively (Fig. 46–46). Alternatively, one can use a waist-to-ankle "minispica" cast with the knee flexed enough to prevent rotation.

Intramedullary nailing of the femur is performed utilizing a closed technique and is thereby often known as "closed intramedullary nailing."[290] This means that the fracture site itself is not opened for surgical manipulation.[290] The incision utilized to insert a nail is placed

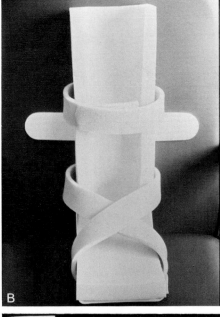

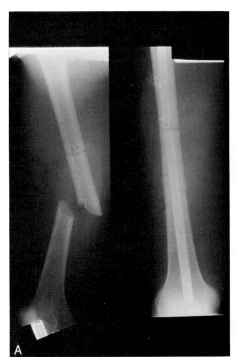

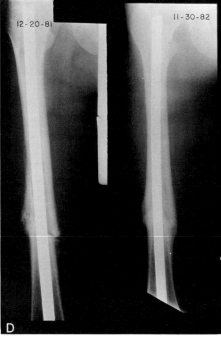

Figure 46–46

A, Midshaft femoral shaft fracture fixed with "routine" intramedullary nailing utilizing a Küntscher nail without locking bolts. B, Foot brace to prevent malrotation following nonlocked intramedullary nailing. C, The derotation foot is used for three to five days until the patient has good quadriceps strength and is fully weight bearing on crutches. This causes fracture interdigitation to occur. D, Radiographs show fracture healing at three months (left) and one year (right).

distant from the fracture site. Most recent series report results using the closed technique.[34,217,232] If only a minimal incision is used at the fracture site for simple fracture reduction only, results may be similar to those reported with the closed technique.[156,229] This may be necessary if an image intensifier is not available or the patient is very sick. However, major surgical dissection at the fracture site for insertion of cerclage wires or retrograde reaming will lead to a significantly increased rate of complications. There is usually little reason to open the fracture site during intramedullary nailing, if

modern equipment is available to the surgeon. The surgical procedure can be performed just as quickly and often more reliably utilizing the closed technique. With the use of current locked-nail systems, further fracture dissection is seldom, if ever, necessary for supplementary fixation.[92,134,276]

Intramedullary Nail Biomechanics

The intramedullary nail is inserted proximally and passed through the medullary nail. Any mismatch in

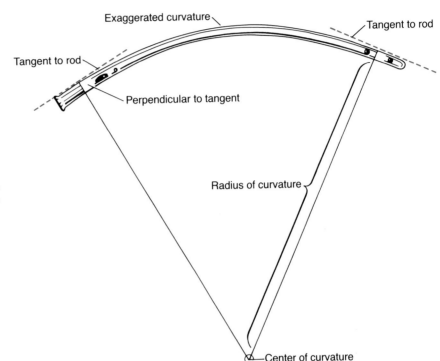

Figure 46–47

Illustration demonstrating how the radius of curvature of an intramedullary nail is measured.

curvatures between the femoral canal and the nail dictates the amount of the bending, which occurs primarily in the nail to allow conformity of the two curvatures so that the nail can pass through the canal.

Harper and Carson[113] measured the radii of curvatures of 14 femurs, which averaged 114.4 cm; nails available ranged in curvature from 132 cm to 405 cm. A larger sample by Zuber et al.[312a] of 100 femurs confirmed the values obtained by Harper and Carson, reporting an average radius of curvature of 109 cm (Fig. 46–47). Both groups concluded that significant bending of the nail is necessary in available nails in order for them to fit into the femoral canal.

In addition to the mismatch in curvature, the location of the entrance hole for the nail can affect the actual shape the nail assumes as it is inserted. By retrograde insertion of the flexible guide pin, a region of anatomic exit points has been defined in the medullary canal of the proximal femur. In general, these are localized to a region at the base of the femoral neck adjacent to the greater trochanter and anterior to the pyriformis recess.[113]

A third consideration in the biomechanics of insertion is the stiffness of the intramedullary nail in bending. Lower bending stiffnesses are associated with nails of thinner cross section and those with open sections (slotted) as compared with those that are unslotted. An example of this was reported by Tencer et al.,[268] who tested five commercially available intramedullary nails of the same nominal size for bending and torsion. The cross sections of these nails are shown in Figure 46–48.

These three aspects—mismatch in curvature, a non-anatomic starting point, and varying stiffness—govern the performance of the nail during and after insertion of the implant. To demonstrate this effect, the force required to insert various implants into the same femur was explored.[136,272] The axial force of insertion was directly related to the bending moment that must be generated for the implant to conform to the shape of the femur.

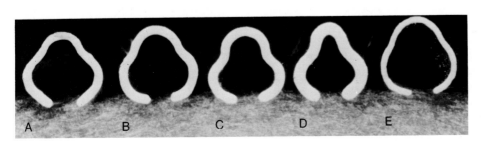

Figure 46–48

Cross sections of intramedullary nails of the same nominal diameter from five different manufacturers. Note the different thicknesses and different cross sections. (From Johnson K.D.; Tencer, A.F.; Sherman, M.C. J Orthop Trauma 1:3, 1987.)

Figure 46–49A demonstrates different force profiles for a fixed location of insertion (i.e., starting hole position). The force profiles can be related to the nail cross sections and their bending rigidities, respectively. Distinctly different force profiles are not unexpected for nails of the same diameter, given the variation in design characteristics of the nails. The axial force as full insertion is achieved provides a measure of the anatomic conformance of the implant to the curvature of the femur. If the conformance is good, the ending insertion force should be low. The peak force, occurring in general around an insertion depth of 30 cm, is caused by significant bending of the nail to conform to the shape of the medullary canal; this force varies with implant stiffness. Nail type B, though less stiff than nail type D, requires more force to insert, presumably because of more mismatch of curvatures, and maintains this high force requirement even when fully inserted. Nail type D, on the other hand, requires significant force to insert because it has the greatest flexural rigidity, but this drops to nearly zero near full insertion because of shape conformance.

The consequences of high insertion forces resulting from large bending deflections can be significant. As the distal tip of the nail penetrates the canal, the nail must bend to pass through the canal. Bending of the nail is produced by large contact forces acting at the tip of the nail where it engages the cortical wall of the canal.

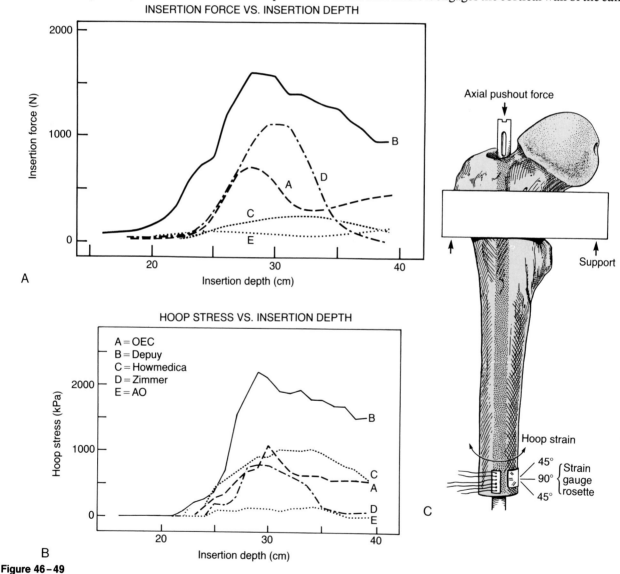

Figure 46–49

A, Axial force of insertion vs. depth of insertion for five different intramedullary nails of 15-mm nominal diameter inserted through the same starting hole in the same femur. See text. B, Hoop stresses in the distal end of a proximal fracture component vs. insertion depths for five different intramedullary nails inserted in the same femur. C, Drawing demonstrating the method of measuring hoop stress during insertion of the nail. Note the rosette strain gauge, which measures stress in several planes.

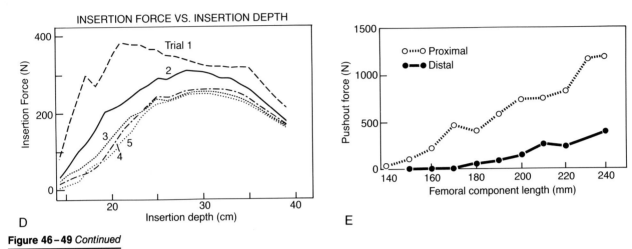

Figure 46–49 *Continued*

D, Pushout insertion force of an intramedullary nail vs. length of the fracture component for a given nail type and proximal starting hole location. Repeated insertion of the nail tends to act similarly to overreaming and lowers the axial force of the insertion. *E,* Pushout or insertion force of an intramedullary nail vs. length of the fracture component for a given nail type and proximal starting hole location. (*A, B, D,* and *E* from Johnson, K.D.; Tencer, A.F.; Sherman, M.C. J Orthop Trauma 1:5,7, 1987.)

These forces, acting on the cortical bone, tend to create distortion of its circumferential shape, leading to circumferential or hoop stresses. If these stresses become excessively large, cracking of the distal end of the proximal fracture component can occur.

The hoop stresses in the circumference of the distal end of a proximal fracture component have been measured as part of the same experiment in which the insertion forces were determined (see Fig. 46–49*C*).[136,272] The results, shown in Figure 49–49*B*, indicate a trend similar to that of the insertion forces of Figure 46–49*A*. That is, the greater the insertion force, the larger the peak hoop stresses.

Large hoop stresses can lead to significant clinical complications, namely bursting of the proximal femoral component during insertion of the intramedullary nail. In addition to the rigidity and shape of the nail, several other factors can affect the hoop stresses generated during insertion. Overreaming the canal tends to decrease the bending in the nail and hence lowers the axial force of insertion and the hoop stresses (see Fig. 46–49*D*).[3] Eccentric reaming (i.e., thinning the anterior cortex in the midshaft region) significantly increases the potential for femoral bursting. Another important variable is the length of the femoral segment into which the implant is inserted. In the proximal part of the femur (see Fig. 46–49*E*) the insertion force decreases as the segment shortens (i.e., the fracture becomes more proximally located). At a length of about 140 mm, the insertion force goes to zero. This is because the intramedullary nail does not need to bend to conform to the shape of the canal at this short length. This result gives some indication as to when proximal locking of the nail is advisable. If the insertion force is significantly higher than the expected axial force caused by body weight, then proximal nail locking is probably not required. One should note, however, that the average force caused by body weight (about 700 N) is never exceeded in the distal femoral components that are not locked (see Fig. 46–49*E*), and the insertion force drops quickly as the distal component length shortens (i.e., the fracture becomes more distally located). Therefore distal locking of the nail may be necessary in all cases.

Another important aspect is the location of the starting hole in the proximal femur. In an attempt to conform nails to the curvature of the medullary canal, Harper and Carson[113] showed that anatomic starting positions would occur in the region just medial to the greater trochanter. Studies similar to those described previously were performed to determine the effect of starting hole location on insertion force and hoop stress.[136,272] In this case, one nail type was selected, and the starting hole locations were altered in a number of femurs. As shown in Figure 46–50, offsetting the starting hole anterior to the midline of the femur increased the hoop stresses, whereas posterior positioning decreased these stresses and the potential for bursting. This result is not unexpected, as the bow of the femur is anterior and the distal and proximal ends of the axis of curvature lie more posterior. Forcing the nail into the femur from an anterior starting position tends to create significant distortion of the nail, as demonstrated in Figure 46–51, in which casts of the interior shape of the medullary canal were made in three femurs with different starting hole locations.

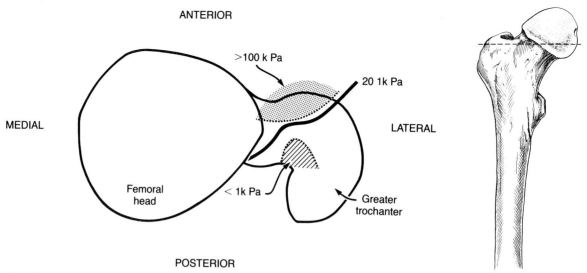

Figure 46-50

Zones of similar hoop stress values from different starting hole positions in the proximal femur. (From Johnson, K.D.; Tencer, A.F.; Sherman, M.C. J Orthop Trauma 1:7, 1987.)

In summary, insertion of an intramedullary nail requires bending of the implant to conform to the shape of the femoral canal. The insertion force is a measure of the frictional resistance to passage of the nail along the internal cortex, which increases as bending of the nail

occurs. Increased bending of the nail also results in greater hoop stresses in the femoral cortex, which can result in bursting of the femur. A number of geometric and mechanical parameters affect the insertion procedure and the resultant stresses generated. These include

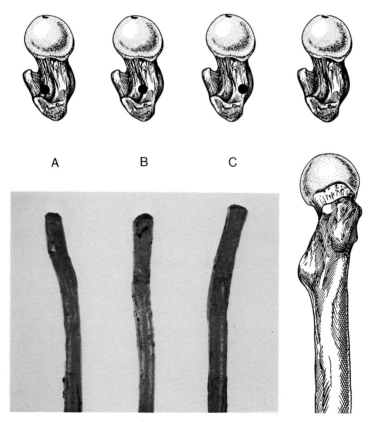

A   B   C

Figure 46-51

Internal shapes of the medullary canal corresponding to different starting hole positions in the proximal femur. A, Posterior. B, Neutral. C, Anterior. (From Johnson, K.D.; Tencer, A.F.; Sherman, M.C. J Orthop Trauma 1:4, 1987.)

the rigidity of the nail and its curvature, the curvature of the femur, the position of the starting hole, the length of the femoral component, and the reamed diameter of the canal (Fig. 46–52).

Mechanical Stability of Femurs Fixed with Intramedullary Nails

The purpose of implanting an intramedullary nail is to provide sufficient stability to the fracture site so that load bearing can be tolerated and fracture site motion minimized. In the best case, it is hoped that the implant-bone construct can support the full loads of ambulation with negligible displacement of the fracture. This requirement also brings into question the optimum stiffness of an implant, to avoid the extremes of excessive stress-shielding and inadequate fracture control. Optimum implant stiffness will be discussed in the following section. This section reviews a number of studies which define the mechanical stability of an intramedullary nail/femur construct.

A study was performed to determine the potential of a number of different methods in common use for stabilization of subtrochanteric fractures of the femur with and without cortical contact. The devices included the angle blade plate, the compression hip screw, Ender nails, and various interlocking intramedullary (IM) nails.[267] In torsional testing of constructs (Fig. 46–53A, B), of these various devices implanted in cadaver femurs, the stiffest was found to be the closed-section (unslotted) Russell-Taylor IM nail, regaining just over 50% of the stiffness of the intact femur with cortical contact. This was followed by the screw- and blade plate–fixed femurs. The open-section interlocking nails and the Ender pins could not produce a construct more than about 3% as stiff as the intact femur. In anteroposterior bending, all the IM nails, whether open- or closed-section, were capable of producing constructs more than 75% as rigid as the intact femur, with the closed-section nail again the stiffest at about 100% that of the intact femur (see Fig. 46–53C).

Axial loading to failure, in which a physiologic offset load was applied to the femoral head with supporting reaction loads through the femoral condyles, indicated that the Russell-Taylor and Grose-Kempf IM nails could support about 400% of average body weight (70 kg) without cortical contact between the fracture components. The Klemm-Schellman IM nail failed at slightly lower loads, and all the others failed at considerably lower loads (between 100% and 200% of body weight) (see Fig. 46–53D). Three modes of failure of interlocking nails in subtrochanteric fracture fixation were noted: bending of the nail at the site of the fracture, splitting of the intertrochanteric region of the femur, and protrusion of the proximal end of the nail and its interlocking screw through the bone in the trochanteric region of the femur.

Some other studies have addressed the fixation of femoral fractures at other sites. In a study of intramedullary devices used to fix worst-case femoral shaft fractures with 8-cm defects, Johnson et al.[135] showed that femurs fixed with the three IM nails tested were similar in torsional stiffness and axial load to failure, and the stiffnesses were not significantly different from those of constructs with subtrochanteric fractures, except in anteroposterior bending (see Fig. 46–53C). The lower values in A-P bending can be explained by the much larger segment of femur that was removed (8 cm midshaft versus 3 cm subtrochanteric).

Further insight into the problems of low torsional stiffness of femur–locked nail constructs was provided by McKellop et al.[172] They showed, for a variety of IM nails, that the axial load applied was an important variable in determining the torque required to reach a particular relative angle of rotation between the proximal and distal fracture components. As seen in Figure 53, the torsional stiffnesses of all constructs, in which the model was a subtrochanteric 3-cm segmental defect, increased significantly once the axial load was increased from 150 N to 1000 N. They attributed this effect to increased bending of the nail in the intramedullary canal creating greater frictional contact with the cortical bone of the medullary canal.

Some comments on the effect of the cross-locking screws are appropriate. As stated above (see Fig. 46–49E), the insertion force varies with the length of the fracture component for the distal end. Because the maximum supportable axial force is quite low (about 350 N or 50% of body weight), even in the best case, distal locking is important to prevent axial slip and subsequent shortening. The distal bolts also improve the torsional performance of the locked nail in two ways. First, the torsional stiffness is significantly increased. Second, the "spring back" effect is improved. "Spring back" is defined as the residual deformation remaining once an applied torque has been removed.[151] It can be interpreted as the angular difference between the points where the torque angle curves cross the horizontal axis. These points define the remaining deformation after the load has been released. It is evident that this spring back, which is caused by slipping of the nail in rotation with respect to the femur, is reduced with the distal locking bolts in place.

Another study of distal locking of femoral components addressed the difference in performance between one- and two-screw placement.[97] The results were quantified as a measured anteroposterior toggle at a

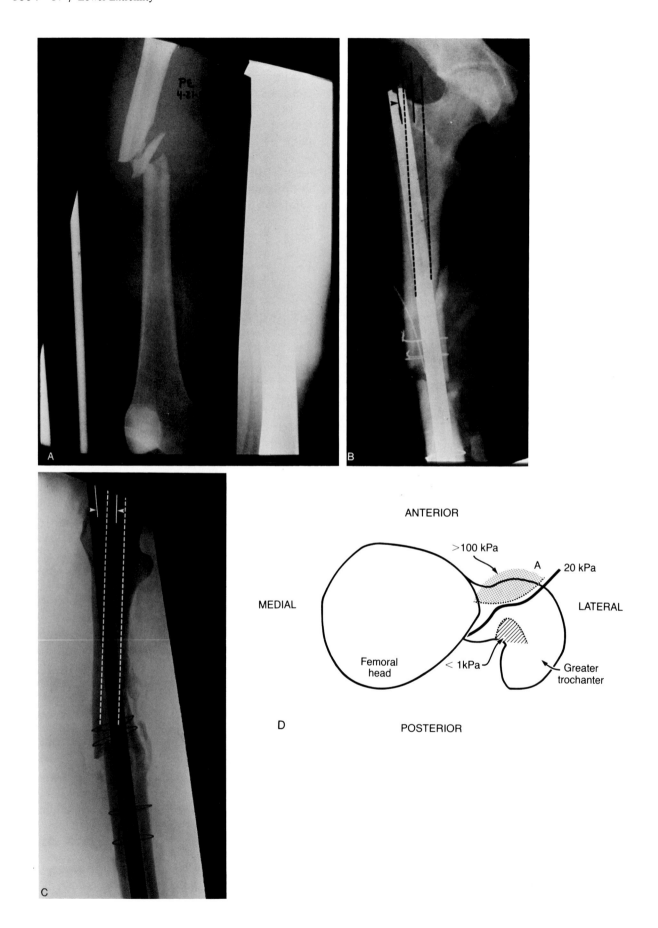

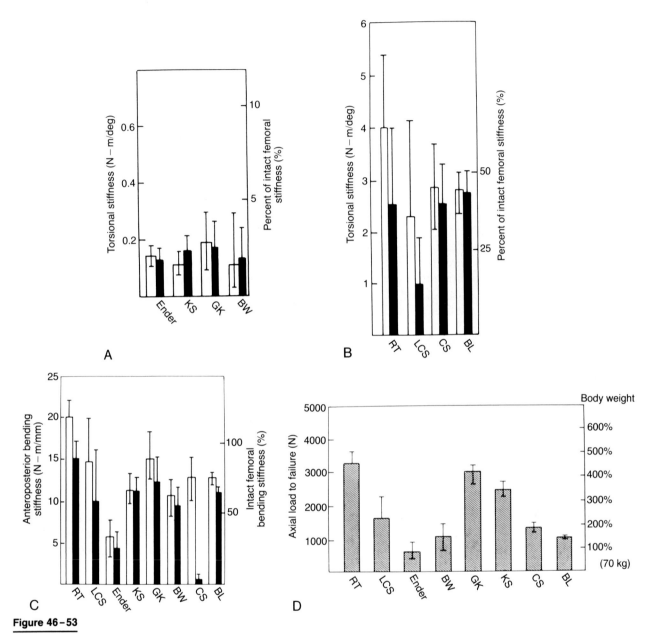

Figure 46–53

Relative stability produced by various implant/bone constructs in torsion. *A*, Torsional stiffness of certain intramedullary devices (Ender nails [4.5 mm × 4]; KS, Klemm-Schellinon nail; GK, Grosse-Kempf nail; BW, Brooker-Wills nail). Note the comparison to intact femoral stiffness, less than 5%. Dark bar is 8-cm segmental defect, and white bar is 3-cm segmental defect. *B*, Torsional stiffness of other internal fixation devices for femoral shaft fractures (RT, Russell-Taylor nail; LCS, locked compression hip screw; CS, unlocked compression hip screw; BL, blade plate device). Note the comparison to intact femoral stiffness, generally less than 25%. *C*, Anteroposterior bending stiffness of devices used to fix femoral shaft fractures. Note that bolt-locked nails (RT, GK, KS) provide greater than 300% body weight, *D*.

Figure 46–52

A, AP radiograph of a fracture of the femoral shaft. Mild comminution is present (Winquist type II or III). *B*, Postoperative AP radiograph demonstrating significant comminution following intramedullary nailing with a lateral starting positon. *C*, Postoperative lateral radiograph demonstrating a severely abnormal anterior starting position, which is the cause of postoperative comminution. The distal fragment is comminuted as a result of driving the nail across an unreduced fracture. *D*, Plot of a cross section of the proximal femur. Note A, which shows an abnormal position in an area of high loop stress that causes the comminution.

fixed distance from the proximal end of the nail for a fixed applied load. These authors showed that toggle increased as the distal component was shortened and was significantly affected by the use of one instead of two screws, especially in shorter components.

In summary, femoral constructs consisting of experimental fractures fixed with a variety of locked nails have been found to achieve high values of stability in A-P bending (at least 75% of the intact femur) and to offset axial loading (about four times body weight). In torsion, the closed-section locked nail (unslotted) can produce constructs about 50% as stiff as the intact femur, whereas all the open-section (slotted) implants generate stiffnesses about 3% that of the intact femur. Axial loading significantly increases the torsional stiffness of the constructs, even without cortical contact. The distal locking screws are important in increasing the torsional stiffness of the construct and reducing residual displacement after removal of a loading torque. Furthermore, two distal screws are recommended for any distal fracture component having a length less than 60% of that from the distal end of the femur to the isthmus, to avoid excessive toggle of the fracture component on the nail.

The Effect of Interlocking Nail Rigidity on Fracture Healing

Although it is well accepted that the use of locked intramedullary nails is the treatment of choice for femoral shaft fractures, questions remain as to the relative efficacy of, for example, a stiff closed-section (unslotted) nail compared with a more flexible slotted (e.g., Küntscher nail. Questions as to the time frame for dynamization (i.e., removal of the distal locking bolts) have not been completely answered.

A study was performed by Molster et al.[179] in rats to determine the effect of rotational stiffness on fracture healing with the use of intramedullary nails. Three groups of rats had their experimentally created femoral fracture fixed with IM nails, the first group without locking, the second with distal locking only, and the third group with both distal and proximal locking of the nail to the femur. The relative rotational stiffnesses, compared with the intact femur, were 28.4%, 36.8%, and 38%, respectively. Although all groups reached the same bending strength at 25 weeks, the most rotationally stiff group had significantly greater strength at earlier times.

A study comparing the efficacy of slotted and closed-section (unslotted) IM nails in healing midshaft transverse osteotomies in dogs was performed by Woodard et al.[301] In the study, 9-mm locking nails of open or closed section were used. Biomechanical testing showed that although the bending rigidities were equivalent, the torsional rigidities of slotted and unslotted nail-femur constructs were 41.8% and 11.7% of those of intact femurs, respectively. The basic difference in healing between the two implants was greater callus formation with the torsionally more flexible implant.

Biomechanical studies have provided insight into the function and performance of intramedullary nails for femoral fractures. A number of general conclusions can be made:

1. An appropriately sized femoral IM nail should have a radius of curvature of about 109 cm best to match the anterior bow of most human femurs.

2. A number of parameters can interact to result in bursting of the femur during insertion of the nail. These include mismatch in curvature of the nail and femur, high stiffness in bending, and poor location of the starting hole.

3. The anatomic starting position for the IM nail is just medial to the greater trochanter and anterior to the pyriformis recess. Moving anterior to the midline of the femur significantly increases the potential for bursting the femur during insertion of the nail.

4. Other factors can decrease the force of insertion of the IM nail in the femur. These include overreaming, shortening the axial length of the fracture component, and using a nail of lower bending rigidity.

5. IM nail–fixed femoral shaft fractures with locking bolts can be expected to be about 75% as rigid as the intact femur in bending and can support about 400% of normal body weight (70 kg).

6. Slotted IM nail–femur constructs are only about 3% as rigid as the intact femur in torsion, whereas an unslotted (closed) section implant produces constructs about 50% as rigid.

7. The distal locking bolts increase the torsional rigidity and maximum axial load capacity of the construct and reduce the potential for shortening and the residual deformation on release of a torsional load. Two distal bolts reduce the toggle of the nail in the femoral shaft.

8. Use of a more rigid locking nail in torsion tends to produce fractures that heal with less callus formation.

Surgical Technique

The patient is brought to the operating room in a bed or on an emergency room gurney with preliminary traction in place (this may be skin traction with a Hare splint). Intramedullary nailing of the femoral shaft is best performed under general anesthesia. Most patients cannot withstand the pain produced by the positioning necessary for spinal anesthetic. Induction of general anesthesia is performed with the patient in bed or on the gurney. The patient is then transferred to the fracture table and placed in either the lateral or supine position. With an appropriate fracture table, either position allows excellent radiographic evaluation of the femoral shaft using the C-arm image intensifier. However, evaluation of the femoral head and neck in the lateral view on the image intensifier is difficult with the patient in the lateral position. This particular evaluation may not be necessary for insertion of a routine locked intramedullary nail but is essential for insertion of locked nails with proximal bolts that extend into the femoral head and neck.

The supine position is more versatile than the lateral (Fig. 46–54A). One advantage is that it is more "physiologic" for the multiply injured patient. Ventilation of the lungs is easier, and all lung fields are equally expanded using volume or pressure ventilators. Multiply injured patients with potential cervical spine or thoracolumbar spine injuries, bilateral femoral fractures, or other significant medical problems are more safely handled in the supine position. Correct rotational alignment of a femoral shaft fracture is easier to appraise with the patient in the supine position, when compared with the lateral. Fracture reduction is easier to accomplish in the supine position as well. The major drawback to positioning the patient supine on the fracture table is that access to the greater trochanter entry portal is difficult. Some adduction of the leg may be helpful. Obese patients require a large extensile incision to obtain access to the greater trochanter. This is because of the excessive accumulation of soft tissue that

protrudes in an outward or lateral direction. Guide pins, reamers, and nails are used in a direct line with the intramedullary canal. This may also be directly through excessive soft tissue, which must therefore be incised.

The lateral position for closed intramedullary nailing of femoral shaft fractures has been well described in North American literature (Fig. 46–54B). It is the favored position for closed intramedullary nailing at Seattle's Harborview Medical Center, the origin of many articles on this surgical technique.[108,109,296–298,313] The position is nonphysiologic and puts significant stress on the recumbent (dependent) leg. The lung on the recumbent side is difficult to ventilate and tends to accumulate fluid. Anesthesiologists may find complete ventilation of the entire lung difficult. Patients with potential cervical or thoracolumbar spine fractures should not be considered for the lateral decubitus position for intramedullary nailing, as the lateral position may deform such injuries and harm the spinal cord. Care must be taken to avoid positioning the knee significantly lower than the level of the hip. This tends to adduct the hip, as well as tighten the iliotibial band, which then places an angulatory force on the fracture site, positioning it with an apex medial angulation (valgus). To prevent this valgus sag, it is best to position the knee at approximately the level of the hip (i.e., with the femur essentially horizontal to the floor) when the lateral position is used. The correct alignment of the femur in rotation is somewhat difficult to ascertain as well. It is more difficult to attempt to align the foot,

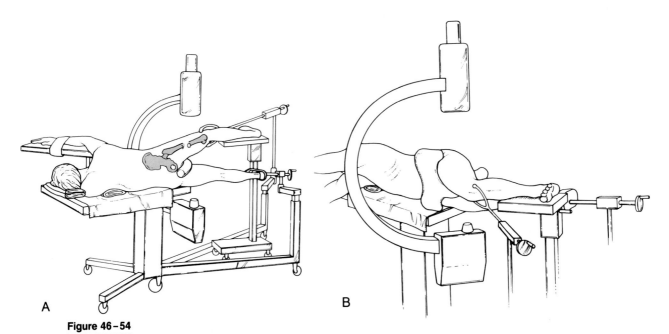

Figure 46–54

Patient position for closed intramedullary nailing with concomitant position of the image intensifier. *A*, Supine. *B*, Lateral.

knee, and hip in the correct rotational alignment because of the difficulty in evaluating these landmarks in the lateral position. It has been recommended that the patient's skin folds be observed, and if abnormal rotation in the skin folds is noted, this should then be corrected in order to prevent malrotation when using a lateral position. However, we find the correct alignment of skin folds an elusive factor to evaluate.

A most important drawback of the lateral position is that a lateral image of the femoral head and neck is nearly impossible to achieve on the image intensifier. This makes insertion of intramedullary nails or other devices that require positioning of the implant into the femoral head and neck extremely difficult, if not impossible, to perform accurately.

After the patient is placed on the fracture table, the image intensifier is brought up to the patient. The image intensifier is positioned on the opposite side of the table from the operating surgeon. Using the image intensifier with the patient unprepped, a reduction of the femoral shaft fracture is achieved. The forces applied to reduce the fracture are noted so that they may be reproduced during the operative procedure. A variety of reduction aids are available. Fracture tables with radiolucent rings that apply force and counterforce, various lengths of crutches, lead-lined gloves, as well as devices to apply local pressure and counter-pressure during the operative procedure (e.g., medium to large Richardson retractors), can all help reduce the fracture (Fig. 46–55). Following the identification of forces necessary to obtain a reduction, the fractured leg is prepped from below the knee to above the iliac crest. It is generally only necessary to drape the lateral aspect of the thigh, leaving the remainder of the thigh unsterile to allow for assistance with reduction techniques. Following preparation and draping, a surgical incision is then made extending from approximately 2 to 3 cm distal to the greater trochanter in a longitudinal line extending over the greater trochanter and running for approximately 6 to 8 cm proximal to the trochanter (total incision = 8 to 11 cm). In general the incision is made in a line parallel to the plane of the femoral shaft but may take a slightly posterior line. Dissection is carried down through skin and subcutaneous tissue. The gluteus maximus and fascia lata are identified and split the length of the incision. Following splitting of the gluteus maximus, a layer of fatty tissue is identified. On entering this fatty tissue, a finger may be used to palpate the

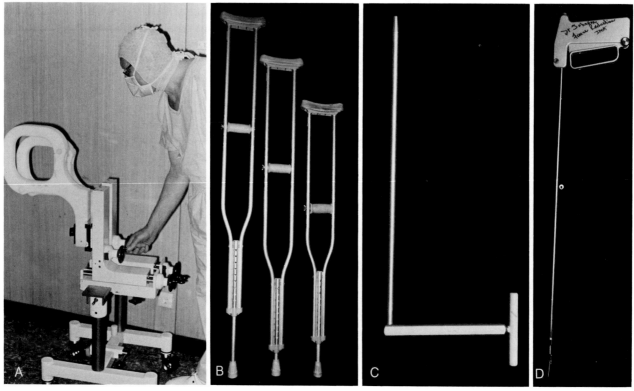

Figure 46–55

Reduction aids that may be utilized in fracture reduction intraoperatively. *A,* Radiolucent repositioning rings to be used with fracture table. *B,* Various lengths of crutches. *C,* Intramedullary reduction tool. Its cannulated shaft slides over bulb-tipped guide wire. *D,* Intramedullary reduction tool. Squeezing the pistol grip angulates the point to facilitate reduction.

tip of the greater trochanter and the pyriformis fossa. Self-retaining retractors are then used to retract the gluteus maximus muscle. This will give good access to the greater trochanter and pyriformis fossa.

The starting point for an intramedullary nail in the femur has been controverial. The correct starting point is directly in line with the intramedullary canal on a point identified on both the AP and lateral images on the image intensifier.[136,269] It can be identified with a guide wire for a cannulated drill bit or a cannulated reamer. It is best hammered into the chosen entry site, as soft tissues tend to force a drill laterally. The insertion point for the guide wire is just medial to the most prominent point of the greater trochanter and slightly posterior to it. Following identification of this point, the wire is inserted a short distance. The correct starting point is outside the capsule of the hip.[147] Position and alignment of the wire are then verified on both the AP and lateral images on the image intensifier. The wire is repositioned until it is in a direct line with the intramedullary canal on both the AP and lateral radiographs (Fig. 46–56). It is then advanced to approximately the level of the lesser trochanter. A cannulated drill bit or reamer is next advanced over the wire. The best device for this task has been the center core reamer of the triple reamer for a compression hip screw. It is widely available, easy to find, easy to use, and cost effective. The reamer creates an excellent initial aperture for intramedullary nailing. It may still be necessary to break through metaphyseal bone in the proximal femur to enter the intramedullary canal. This can be simply done with sharp T-handled reamers (Fig. 46–57) introduced into the previously drilled starting hole. Following drilling and expansion of the starting hole, the instruments are removed and exchanged for a 3-mm bulb-tipped guide with a short bend near the tip. This guide rod is generally placed within a cannulated T-handled chuck that can be tightened and loosened by hand (see Fig. 46–57A). This allows the chuck to slide up and down the guide rod to aid in positioning. This "reaming guide wire" is introduced into the starting hole that has been created. The bulb-tipped reaming guide is then placed to the level of the fracture. This is verified under the image intensifier. The maneuver used to reduce the fracture previously is then repeated if necessary, and the bulb-tipped guide is directed across the fracture site. Rotation of the bent tip of the guide is useful when passing the bulb-tipped guide across the fracture site and reducing the fracture.

In proximal fractures or in those cases where an experienced unscrubbed assistant is not available, the use of a small-diameter cannulated intramedullary nail or other long cannulated handle may be of assistance in aiding fracture reduction and passage of the bulb-tipped guide (see Fig. 46–57C). The guide is generally 8 to 10 mm in diameter, and most physicians find that an old Küntscher nail 9 mm by approximately 48 to 50 cm long is quite sufficient to achieve this task. This may require reaming of the proximal fragment over the bulb-tipped guide to approximately a 9-mm diameter using the end-cutting reamer. The small-diameter nail or maneuvering device is then placed over the bulb-tipped guide. This gives excellent control of the proximal fragment, which is often flexed and abducted. By simply elevating the nail or maneuvering device, the proximal fragment can be lined up with the distal fragment.

Following placement of the bulb-tipped reaming guide across the fracture site, absolute verification of this placement of the guide across the fracture site must be obtained utilizing the image intensifier in both the AP and mediolateral planes. The guide is then introduced distally to a reproducible point in the distal femur. Some surgeons define this point to be the level of the proximal pole of the patella, the old distal femoral epiphyseal scar, or the notable curve of the posterior condyles that can be viewed on the AP radiograph or image intensifier (Fig. 46–58). The fracture is then carefully reduced, and appropriate traction is applied to maintain the reduction but not overdistract the fracture. Another guide wire of length equal to the 3-mm bulb-tipped reaming guide may be used to measure the length of the medullary canal by subtracting the length of the exposed portion of the reaming guide. One end of the second wire is placed at the tip of the greater trochanter, and it is held against the protruding reaming guide. The excess length of the second wire is measured with a ruler or one of the nails available in the sterile set (see Fig. 46–57D). The resulting length may need adjustment depending on fracture alignment or any difference between the position of the tip of the reaming guide and that desired for the end of the nail.

Following verification of nail length, the bulb-tipped guide is then impacted as well as possible into the distal femur to avoid pulling it out during reaming of the intramedullary canal. Reaming generally commences with an end-cutting reamer, which may be any diameter from 5 to 9 mm. An end-cutting reamer is used to smooth and open the intramedullary canal. Reaming then proceeds from the end-cutting reamer to side-cutting reamers. The reaming is performed in sequentially increasing diameters by approximately 0.5- to 1.0-mm increments. Once reaming commences in dense cortical bone, which can be identified by increased purchase and slower progress of the reamer, one should not advance by more than 0.5 mm at any one time. The canal is reamed 1 to 2 mm larger than the size of the selected nail. With locked intramedullary nailing, it is easier to

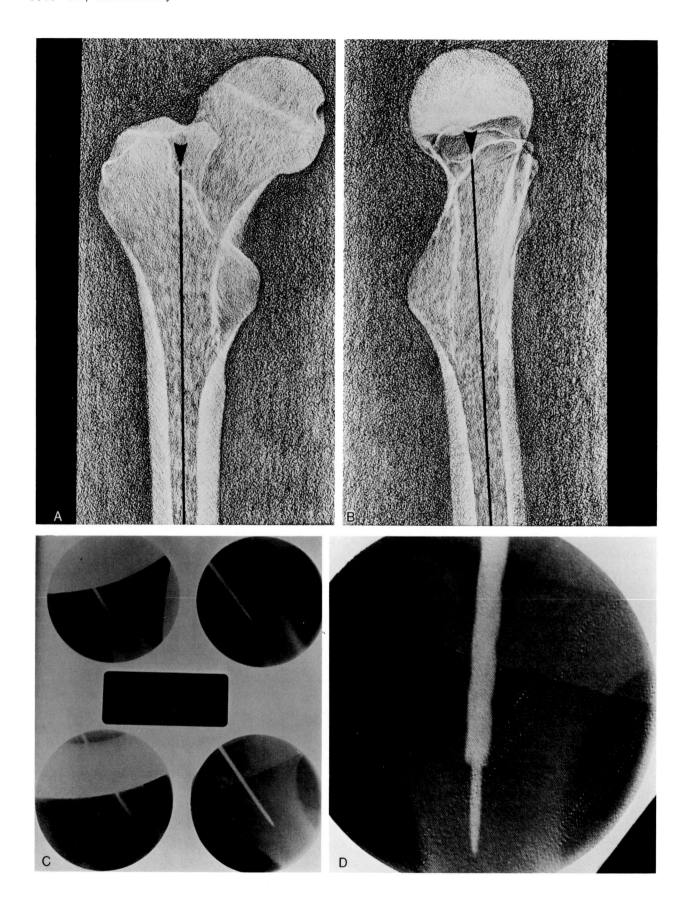

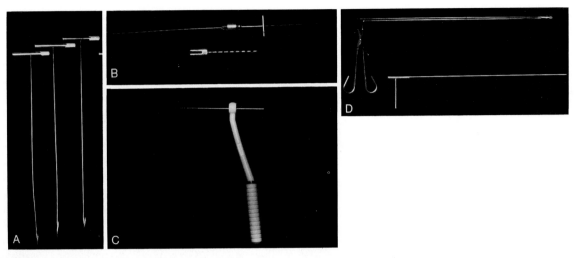

Figure 46–57

Equipment that is of assistance with closed intramedullary nailing. A, T-handled reamers with sharp points. B, Adjustable T-handle on bulb tipped guide wire with slotted mallet. C, Radiolucent pin holder for starting distal interlocking holes. D, Intramedullary grasper (top), and sharp-tipped pseudoarthrosis chisel (bottom).

overream the intramedullary canal, which allows insertion of the nail without force, because of the ability to perform static locking.

During reaming of the medullary canal, care must be taken to avoid pulling the bulb-tipped guide back across the fracture site as the reamer is extracted. This can be a problem with distal third femoral shaft fractures and may require verification that the bulb-tipped guide remains across the fracture site using the image intensifier after each pass of the reamer. Reaming is necessary through the small-diameter isthmus of the intramedullary and is not necessary in the distal femur, as the femur flares into the trumpet shape of the metaphysis. If the reamer is carried down all the way on the angled bulb-tipped guide, it will encounter the angle on the bulb-tipped guide, and this will impact the bulb-tipped guide into the reamer. This necessitates removal of the guide with the reamer. Therefore once active reaming of the canal is complete with the pass of each reamer, no further reaming is necessary. After a few operative procedures it becomes quite apparent when the reamer is actually reaming cortical bone.

When reaming comminuted fractures, it may be necessary to turn the reamer off when the reamer head reaches the level of comminution. The reamer can then be simply pushed across the length of comminution

while off and then turned on again when intact femoral intramedullary canal is reentered. Reaming significantly comminuted fractures tends to spin isolated fracture fragments, stripping them from any soft tissue attachments that they may have. Generally, reaming can be performed easily in segmental fractures that have a complete intact segment. These segments remain firmly attached to the linea aspera posteriorly and tend not to rotate.

Selection of the diameter of the intramedullary nail to be used in the intramedullary canal is relatively simple. The preoperative radiograph can be measured using an ossimeter to select the correct diameter nail (see Fig. 46–45). Using the magnification side of the ossimeter, the diameter selected is approximately 2 mm larger than the measured width of the intramedullary canal. During the operative procedure, when reaming of the cortical bone commences, the nail selected should be approximately 2 mm larger than this. When locked intramedullary nails are in use, appropriate strength is available with even the smaller diameter nails (12- to 13-mm). Most average-sized females do well with an intramedullary nail of 12 to 13 mm in diameter. Most adult males do well with an intramedullary nail of 13 to 14 mm in diameter. Larger diameter nails than this are used only for extremely large intra-

Figure 46–56

Correct starting point, determined intraoperatively, for insertion of the intramedullary nail. The Kirschner wire is then overdrilled with a cannulated drill, smoothly creating an accurate starting position. A, AP view as seen on the image intensifier. B, Lateral view as seen on the image intensifier. C, Kirschner wire is inserted into the proximal femur in the correct starting position. D, The Kirschner wire is then overdrilled with a cannulated drill or a center-core reamer from a compression hip screw.

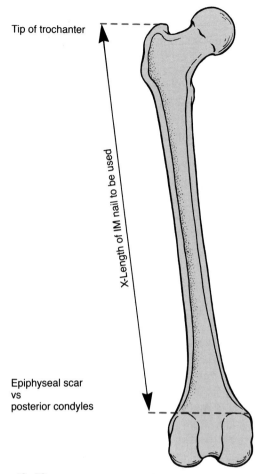

Tip of trochanter

X-Length of IM nail to be used

Epiphyseal scar
vs
posterior condyles

Figure 46–58

Reproducible points on the proximal and distal femur that may be
seen on radiographs and identified on C-arm image intensification.

medullary canals in elderly or excessively large patients. Nails smaller than 12 mm in diameter may not
be available in most routine locked-nail systems.
Smaller diameter nails are available through certain
manufacturers and may be necessary for closed intramedullary nailing of young patients (10 to 13 years of
age) or small females. It must be remembered that significantly decreasing the diameter of the nail will definitely weaken the nail when holes are drilled in the
proximal and distal aspect of the nail for placement of
locking bolts or blades. Therefore nails smaller than 10
mm should have a closed-section, thicker wall to increase the strength of the nail.

Following reaming, the 3-mm bulb-tipped reaming
guide is exchanged for a 4-mm nail-driving guide. This
is done by sliding a plastic exchange tube over the bulb-
tipped reaming guide and exchanging the 3-mm guide
for the 4-mm guide through the plastic exchange tube.
Insertion of the intramedullary nail is then performed.
The nail previously selected is mounted on the nail-

driving device for insertion into the intramedullary
canal. Care must be taken to ascertain that the appropriate nail is placed into the femur. The surgeon must
verify the exact length and diameter, as well as whether
the nail is for a right or left femur. The anterior bow of
the nail should match that of the femur into which it is
inserted. Most systems have a nail-driving device that is
attached to the proximal femur and is actually the
proximal targeting device as well. After application of
the nail-driving proximal targeting device, the nail is
inserted into the intramedullary canal over the 4-mm
nail-driving guide. The nail is easily introduced into the
proximal aspect of the intramedullary canal and may
actually be driven to the level of the fracture site or the
level of the isthmus without use of a hammer or mallet.
If static locked nailing is to be performed, reaming can
be done to allow insertion of the intramedullary nail by
hand. Incarceration of an intramedullary nail during
driving of the nail should never be allowed. The nail is
then driven to the level of the fracture site. Using the
image intensifier, the fracture site is anatomically reduced, and the nail is then carefully driven across an
absolutely reduced fracture site. Small offsets of the
cortex may become a problem with driving of the nail.
If the tip of the nail impacts the distal cortex, it will
comminute the distal fragment or further extend fracture lines. Following documentation of the passage of
the intramedullary nail across the fracture site, longitudinal traction may be released to allow impaction of the
fracture site as necessary. The nail is then driven carefully down to the level of the distal femur previously
identified by marking of the appropriate-length nail.
Once the nail is distinctly past the fracture site, the
4-mm nail-driving guide may be removed. The image
intensifier can be used to verify the position of the tip of
the nail in the distal femur. The AP image is used to
verify that the nail is appropriately placed within the
femur proximally.

During insertion of the intramedullary nail, particularly when the supine position is utilized, care must be
taken to avoid external rotation of the nail. Gravity
tends to pull the driving or targeting device down,
thereby externally rotating the nail. Care must be taken
to maintain the driving or targeting device parallel to
the shaft of the femur, and this may require a slight
internal rotation force during the driving of the nail.
Nails that are inserted significantly externally rotated
will make application of distal locking bolts extremely
difficult. It may be necessary to place these bolts from
anterior to posterior rather than lateral to medial if
excessive rotation of the nail is allowed during insertion.

The proximal end of the nail is positioned at the level
of the tip of the greater trochanter for virtually all nail

systems currently available in North America. If the nail system in use requires the exchange of a nail-driving guide for a proximal targeting device in the proximal end of the nail, this exchange should take place prior to complete insertion of the femoral nail. Once the nail is buried within the soft tissue, exchange of devices on the proximal end of the nail is difficult, particularly when the patient is in the supine position.

Once the nail is completely inserted within the femoral canal and its position verified by image intensification both proximally and distally, insertion of locking bolts may be performed. Insertion of locking bolts to intramedullary nail systems is performed by a variety of methods. Most proximal femoral locking bolts are placed by using a proximal targeting device that is firmly attached to the proximal end of the nail. These are accurate when the proximal targeting device is firmly attached to the proximal aspect of the nail, generally utilizing threaded attachment systems. When the proximal targeting device is not firmly attached to the proximal end of the nail by this type of system, or when the appropriate drill guides are not utilized, it is possible to miss the hole in the nail.

Proximal locking bolts are placed by indenting the cortex with a sharp awl, predrilling with an appropriate size drill bit through the drill guide, determining length using a depth gauge, and then placing the proximal locking bolt. Depth gauges for interlocking nail systems are notoriously inaccurate. The image intensifier is of great assistance when attempting to measure the bolt length needed for placement across an intramedullary nail.

Proximal locking bolts are usually inserted first, followed by the distal bolts. In certain intramedullary nailing systems, it may be possible to insert distal locking bolts first and then further impact the fracture site using the proximal slap hammer device, which is firmly attached to the proximal end of the nail through the proximal targeting device. This can be helpful when significant distraction of the fracture site has occurred during driving of the nail. It must be pointed out that only certain nail systems provide this method of impaction following placement of distal locking bolts. Following impaction of the fracture site, proximal locking bolts are then inserted.

Certain nail systems also provide two different styles of bolts. Fully threaded proximal locking bolts are designed to be threaded through the intramedullary nail. The same system may also have distal locking bolts that are not completely threaded. The surgeon must be extremely careful not to mistakenly put nonthreaded distal locking bolts into the proximal aspect of the femur when utilizing this system. If the distal locking bolts are not threaded and the proximal hole in the intramedul-

lary nail is threaded, the distal locking bolts will not go through the nail. In fact, the unthreaded bolt will obliterate the threads within the proximal aspect of the nail and will then not allow subsequent insertion of the normal fully threaded proximal locking bolt. This may then require removal of the intramedullary nail and insertion of a completely new nail or drilling out of the proximal hole of the nail to a larger diameter. Drilling the threads out will allow insertion of a nonthreaded bolt through the nail. However, if the surgeon takes care to ascertain that the appropriate bolt is inserted into the proximal or distal femur as intended, these frustrating complications will be avoided.

Insertion of distal locking bolts usually follows the insertion of proximal locking bolts, with the exception of the situation dicussed previously. The decision as to whether to place proximal or distal locking bolts, or both, should be made *prior* to undertaking the surgical procedure. As pointed out by Brumback et al., most intramedullary nails placed into femoral shaft fractures should be placed in the static locking mode unless there is a specific reason not to place both proximal and distal locking bolts or mechanisms.[41] This circumstance may include the simple transverse or short oblique fracture through the isthmus. Absence of further fracture comminution should be verified intraoperatively. This is also true for stable proximal or distal shaft fractures that have excellent cortical contact between the two main fragments and only require the application of either proximal or distal locking bolts to avoid rotational malalignment.

A variety of targeting devices are available for inserting distal locking bolts. These may be complex or simple, depending on the system and intention of the surgeon. Each individual locking nail system provides at least one or two different ways to insert distal locking bolts. Specific information as to the exact use of a distal targeting device should be provided by the manufacturer of the nail system or targeting device. In general, most experienced surgeons use the freehand method of insertion of distal locking bolts. This method, which is applicable to any hospital at any point in time, will be described in detail.

DISTAL INTERLOCKING

Following insertion of the intramedullary nail and proximal locking bolt, attention is turned to the distal femur. The femur is positioned in such a manner as to allow good positioning of the image intensifier perpendicular to the distal aspect of the femur (Fig. 46–59A). This may require abducting the hip somewhat if the patient is supine. The image intensifier is positioned perpendicular to the distal aspect of the femur. Abso-

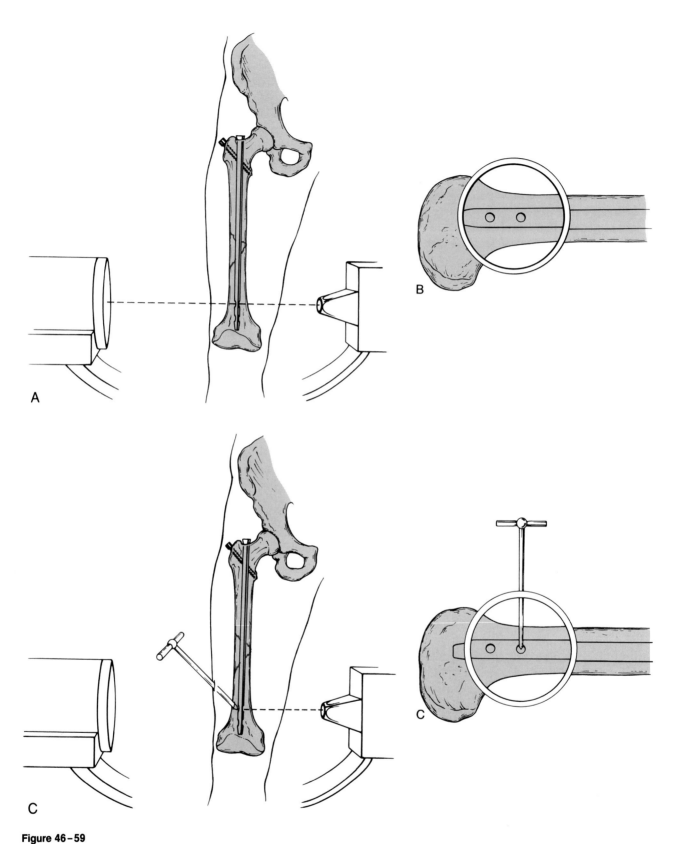

Figure 46–59

Freehand method of insertion of distal bolts. *A*, Position of leg and image intensifier. *B*, Absolutely round holes on C-arm. *C*, Awl used to mark level of incision (two views).

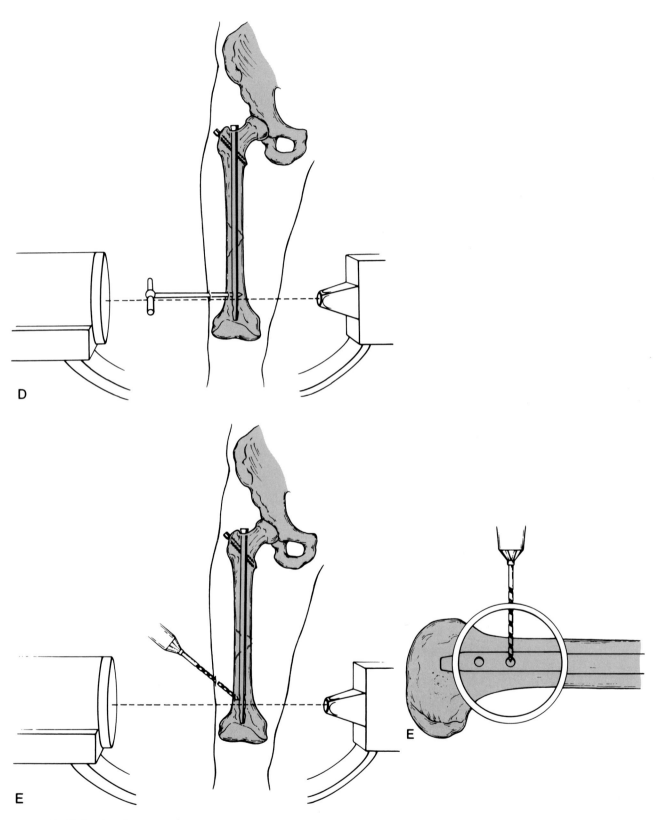

Figure 46–59 *Continued*

D, Awl used to indent near cortex, parallel to beam of image. *E*, Drill used to create hole for bolt (two views).

Illustration and legend continued on following page

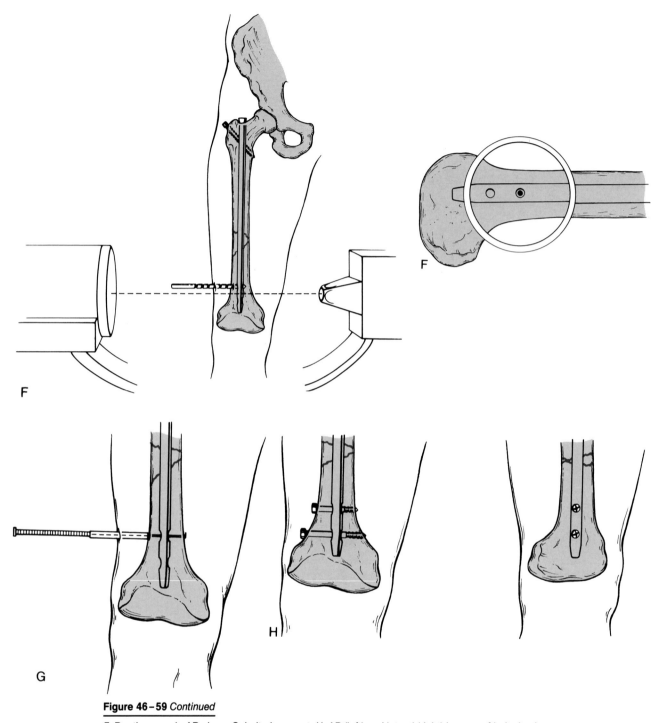

Figure 46–59 *Continued*

F, Depth gauge in AP plane. *G*, bolt placement. *H*, AP (left) and lateral (right) images of bolts in place.

lutely round holes *must* be identified on the monitor of the image intensifier (see Fig. 46–59*B*). Once absolutely round holes are identified, care can be taken to magnify or cone down on one or the other of the distal holes. The image intensifier is positioned to allow adequate room between the image intensifier and the thigh to manipulate the instruments. An awl or other marking device can be used to identify the appropriate position for a stab incision in the distal femur (see Fig. 46–59*C*). A stab incision approximately 1 to 2 cm in length is then made in the distal femur. This stab incision should be carried directly down through the soft tissue to the shaft of the femur. A sharp awl is then placed through the stab incision directly down on the lateral cortex of the femur. It is better when the awl is longer, allowing the surgeon to keep his or her hands out of the x-ray field. Lead-lined gloves are available that will attenuate the image intensifier radiation by 15% to 20%. By keeping his or her hands out of the beam of the image intensifier, the surgeon receives little radiation to the hands.[158] Once the awl is positioned directly on the lateral cortex in the middle of the hole identified on the image intensifier beam, the awl is then brought to a position parallel to the image intensifier beam (see Fig. 46–59D). The parallel orientation of the awl can be verified by the operating surgeon and an assistant. The image intensifier is not in use during this positioning of the awl. Care is taken to avoid allowing the awl point to slip on the femur during this positioning. The sharp point of the awl is then used to indent or, in most cases, penetrate the lateral cortex of the femur, creating a hole or indentation that will allow a drill bit to gain access to the femur without slipping or sliding on the wet bone. Most drill bits in use for locked intramedullary nailing tend to be dull and will slide on the surface of wet bone. Therefore it is imperative to create this indentation or penetration. If the awl is used to penetrate the lateral cortex, subsequent overdrilling of the near cortex is not necessary. The awl is then exchanged for the drill bit and drill. The drill bit is placed into the indentation made in the lateral cortex. This can be verified using the image intensifier. The drill bit is also placed parallel to the image intensifier beam and verified by the surgeon and an assistant (Fig. 46–59E). Once again, the image intensifier is not turned on during this process. The drill is then turned on, and the drill bit is placed through the hole in the intramedullary nail and across the far cortex of the femur. Once the far cortex of the femur has been drilled, the drill is removed from the drill bit, and the image intensifier is used to verify placement of the drill bit through the hole in the nail. After drilling one hole in the distal femur, attention is turned to the second hole in the distal femur. A similar procedure is used to drill a hole across the femur in the second hole. In obese individuals, it may be necessary to connect the two stab incisions for the two holes necessary for locking of the distal femur. This simply allows better visualization and retraction of soft tissue with only a minor increase in visible scarring.

Following drilling of the two transverse holes through the nail and through the femur, the image intensifier is then rotated to the anteroposterior view. The image is centered on the distal femur and on the two distal holes. The depth gauge is then used to measure the appropriate length for the screw or bolt necessary for each hole in the distal femur (see Fig. 46–59F). Once again, use of the depth gauge in the lateral position is notoriously inaccurate, and the image intensifier

is useful in identifying the appropriate length bolt necessary. Following length discernment, the two transverse locking bolts are then placed across the distal femur.

Once placed, appropriate length and positioning of the bolts are verified in both AP and lateral planes (see Fig. 46–59G). Bolts that are visualized on the lateral view are not placed across the femoral nail. Neither the bolt nor the hole in the nail should be visualized on a true lateral view of the implant. Correct placement of both proximal and distal locking bolts should be verified, as it is much easier to identify and exchange inappropriately placed bolts during the initial operative procedure than to identify that the bolts are inappropriately placed after the patient has recovered from the anesthesia, thus requiring another surgical procedure.[40]

All wounds are thoroughly irrigated with normal saline and closed in layers. A small-diameter suction drain ($\frac{1}{8}$-in) is generally placed into the proximal wound and left for 24 to 48 hours. Sterile dressings are applied.

Hard copy radiographs of the femoral shaft fracture are then obtained in the operating room prior to awakening the patient from general anesthesia. Appropriate images can be obtained from the image intensifier if a disc recorder and camera are available on the image intensifier. Unfortunately, these show only small areas of the femur. Full-length radiographs of the femur, both AP and lateral to include the proximal femur, should be obtained in the operating room to verify correct placement of the nail and reduction of the fracture. If examination or radiographs are not acceptable, the patient remains under anesthesia, and correction of specific problems can be performed. The patient is then allowed to awaken from the general anesthetic and taken to the recovery room.

Aftercare

Patients are generally fairly comfortable following insertion of an intramedullary nail into the femur. Emphasis is placed postoperatively on muscle strengthening in the thigh, as well as on range of motion of the knee.[190,191] This is best done with physical therapy.[128,303] A CPM device may aid in early return of motion. However, by three to six months after injury, all patients have a near-normal range of motion regardless of whether this range of motion has been emphasized.[191] More is gained by specific work on muscle strengthening, which will aid the patient in control of his or her leg during ambulation.[176,255] Patients are up ambulating within 24 to 48 hours of their injury using crutches or a walker. Flatfoot weight bearing can be allowed after insertion of all intramedullary nails into the femur. This is defined as enough weight to allow the foot to be placed in a plantigrade position (generally 15 to 20 pounds). If the patient has a stable fracture that has had insertion of a dynamic locked nail, full weight-bearing ambulation may be allowed immediately post-operatively. Protection from malrotation is necessary in these patients until full weight bearing is achieved and adequate control of the lower extremity is accomplished with appropriate muscle strengthening.

The patient is discharged from the hospital when he or she is able to perform a straight leg raise with the fractured femur elevated off the bed and held there for a brief period of time. This indicates good quadriceps function and good control of the leg. Knee flexion should be approximately 70° prior to discharge from the hospital.

If the patient receives adequate instruction as to muscle strengthening and knee range-of-motion exercises in the hospital, then physical therapy on an outpatient basis is seldom necessary. The patient is expected to perform these activities at home. The patient is then seen in orthopedic follow-up at varying intervals. The patient is initially seen at two weeks postoperatively, at which time sutures or staples are removed. Radiographs are seldom necessary at this point in time, unless the patient relates some specific incident requiring radiographic evaluation or feels inordinate pain or the surgeon notices some abnormality. Following this visit, the patient is seen at six weeks postoperatively, at which time full-length AP and lateral radiographs of the femur are necessary. The radiology department in the surgeon's office or in the hospital should be instructed on how to perform full-length radiographs of the femur. This should include the proximal aspect of the femur, as well as the distal intraarticular aspect, on the same cassette. Early callus formation is generally present at six weeks after injury, and the patient may begin partial weight bearing with up to 50% of body weight. By six weeks postoperatively, the patient should have a range of motion in the knee from full extension to flexion of 90° to 100°. The patient is then seen at three months postoperatively, at which time full-length AP and lateral radiographs of the femur are again obtained. The fracture may be united at this time, as evidenced by periosteal bridging callus. The patient is then begun on full weight bearing and weaned from the use of crutches. The patient should have near-normal range of motion of the knee (from 0° to 120° to 135°). At this point, the patient may begin complaining of pain or irritation over the proximal or distal locking bolt heads on the lateral aspect of the proximal or distal femur. If excessively long distal bolts were used that protrude into soft tissue for a centimeter or more, these

bolt tips may interfere with knee motion by irritation of the vastus medialis. The patient is seen at six-week intervals until absolute fracture union has been obtained and verified radiographically. The patient is then seen at six months and one year following injury.

If the patient is not demonstrating normal periosteal bridging callus formation at three months after injury, then he or she is seen at more frequent intervals, generally four to six weeks. All femoral shaft fractures, whether dynamically or statically locked, should be united by four to five months after injury. By three months after surgery, excellent periosteal bridging callus should be apparent. If this is not the case, the patient must be followed more closely. Occasionally, consideration is given to changing the patient from a static locking mode to a dynamic locking mode to allow further fracture impaction. The decision as to whether to perform this procedure is somewhat difficult to make. Conversion from static locking to dynamic locking ("dynamization") is unnecessary for routine femoral shaft fracture healing. If delayed healing or absent healing is present on the radiograph at four to five months after injury, consideration may be given to converting a static locked nail to a dynamic locked nail that may then encourage union. This decision requires a femoral shaft that will not substantially shorten when these bolts are removed. This means that when the femur is allowed to impact, there is adequate cortical contact to prevent telescoping and shortening or at least appropriate periosteal bridging callus that will likewise prevent shortening. This may be difficult to determine. Malrotation is seldom a problem when bolts are removed at this point in time following conversion of a static locked nail to a dynamic locked nail. Generally, dynamization, if it is to take place, is performed at four to six months postoperative. If by some chance the patient was nailed with an excessively long bolt (1 cm or more too long), these bolts may be removed at an earlier point in time (two to three months postoperatively) to allow some shortening to occur. Shortening and impaction of the fracture site can occur until absolute fracture healing has been noted to take place.

Excessive pain over the proximal or distal bolt heads may necessitate their removal. These bolts are best removed following absolute verification of fracture healing. Once verification of fracture healing has been made, they may be removed with impunity. This can be done under local anesthesia in the office in a slender, compliant patient but more commonly requires a short general anesthetic on an outpatient basis. The outpatient facility must be aware of and have available the appropriate-size bolt or screw remover in order to perform this procedure.

In general, with the use of locked nails, it is much more common to have to remove annoying proximal or distal locking bolts than to remove the intramedullary nail itself. An appropriately placed nail that ends at the level of the greater trochanter is seldom an annoyance to the patient. It will not interfere with hip or knee range of motion, and patients can seldom feel it. However, this is certainly not the case for the locking bolts. Removal of the intramedullary nail is recommended only in patients who are symptomatic or in younger patients, perhaps younger than 18 to 20 years. Refracture of the femoral shaft is an extremely rare occurrence following verification of fracture healing with an intramedullary nail.

Skeletally immature patients who appear to have remaining growth in their greater trochanter or proximal femur should be considered for early removal of their intramedullary nail. Nail removal should be performed within six to nine months postoperatively and following verification of fracture healing. If removal is postponed for more than one year postoperatively, difficulty may be experienced, in attempting to remove the nail, because the proximal femur will have overgrown the nail, making access difficult.

Following any femoral shaft fracture the patient will require significant rehabilitation to return to prefracture status.[190] This rehabilitative period should continue for one year following fracture. During the phase of fracture healing (three to five months after injury), emphasis is given to muscle strengthening to control the leg, as well as to return of normal range of motion. Thus by the time fracture healing has occurred, the patient should have a near-normal range of motion in the knee with good leg control and reasonable quadriceps muscle function. Following fracture healing, the patient is instructed to increase activity and muscle strengthening. Generally, by simply returning the patient to a normal physical status, he or she can increase muscle strength and function for the next six months and by one year following fracture be back to the preinjury status. This is true following intramedullary nailing of a femoral shaft fracture, but return to preinjury status is somewhat delayed following internal fixation using a plate.

Complications

In general, femoral shaft fractures are handled in a routine manner, and the complication rate is extremely low. In approximately 99% of all femoral fracture patients, a solidly united bone can be expected with near-normal function. Unfortunately, a significant number of complications can occur in spite of this. Most of these complications are directly related to initial management of the fracture or to difficulties related to the type of fracture management selected.

REFRACTURE

Refracture of a femoral shaft fracture that has been reported to be healed is a most devastating complication.[33,116,245,261] The incidence of refracture is difficult to evaluate and is distinctly dependent on the initial management of the femoral shaft fracture. A 9% to 15% incidence of refracture was reported in the 1940s and 1950s.[116,261] Most of these patients were treated with traction and plating. The potential problem of refracture following plating has been previously discussed in the section on plating.

Refracture is more likely to occur when minimal or insufficient fracture callus occurs at the fracture site. Management systems that allow an incremental increase of stress to occur at the level of the fracture site until functional stresses have been achieved generally result in a lower rate of refracture. Living bone that is well vascularized will respond by increasing strength and modifying orientation of fibers according to the mechanical stresses applied to it. In general, those fractures with a generous proportion of periosteal callus formation are the least prone to refracture. Those fractures with a small amount of callus formation, such as that seen after rigid internal fixation and "primary bone healing," are the most prone to refracture.[195,210,211]

Refracture following internal fixation of the skeleton is a major problem. This has significant bearing on the timing of hardware removal from the femur and whether that may predispose the patient to refracture or stress fracture of the femoral shaft. If refracture does occur following internal fixation, repeat internal fixation is generally in order. Rigid skeletal fixation that does not allow the transference of stress to the fracture site will also not allow adequate periosteal callus formation with subsequent remodeling of callus to enable hardware to be removed prior to two or more years following internal fixation. Those internal fixation devices that apply rigid skeletal fixation and also cause decreased local blood supply to the fracture by stripping of local periosteal soft tissues are more prone to refracture. Therefore plates and screws that rigidly fix the fracture, when appropriately applied, are the most prone to refracture following hardware removal.[33,83,164,234] Plate-fixed fractures are intended to heal with primary bone formation (minimal periosteal callus formation and simply do not develop the broad periosteal callus necessary to provide adequate fracture stability during the lengthy remodeling process.[210] The surgical procedure to apply the plate also causes some devascularization of bone, which takes a significant time to revascularize. The screw site can be a source of stress concentration in bone, particularly in high-risk athletes.[46]

The controversy over what predisposes plates to refracture centers around whether the stress absorption by the plates and screws aborts stress concentration at the fracture site and the associated remodeling or whether the phenomenon is vascular in nature, having to do with loss of vascularity at the fracture site at the time of plating, with subsequent inadequate revascularization at the fracture site postoperatively. Inadequate revascularization will lead to inability to fully remodel the bone and strengthen it with appropriately applied stress. In a series reported by Magerl et al. involving plate fixation of diaphyseal femoral fractures, the authors noted two cases of refracture following plate removal, for a 3% incidence of this complication.[164] Rüedi and Luscher, in a similar study of plate fixation of comminuted femoral fractures, noted two instances of fracture of the femur associated with plate fixation, for a 1% incidence using dynamic compression plates.[234] Refracture of the femoral shaft following closed fixation or closed intramedullary nailing of femoral fractures is extremely rare, and it is difficult to find even one example of this particular complication in the literature.[33,116]

Eriksson and Frankel have noted the significant problem that stress concentrated in bone can be following plate fixation or screw fixation of lower extremity long bones.[83] In a questionnaire distributed to orthopedic departments in Sweden, 40 refractures were reported, of which 23 could be analyzed. Refracture in these instances occurred even up to 12 months following hardware removal, but the majority occurred within two to six months of hardware removal. Most refractures occurred with what the authors felt were subcritical fracture forces. Most occurred through screw holes that remained evident even to the time of refracture. Radiographs were of no use in identifying whether the screw hole had been filled with enough subperiosteal bone to have lost its weakening effect. Thus, because fractures through screw holes had been documented up to 11 months following screw removal, it was concluded that heavy contact sports involving direct blows or torsional forces delivered to the area of the screw hole could result in refracture with less than the force required to cause the original fracture. These authors recommended alternative methods to plate or screw fixation in high-performance athletes.

Refracture of the femoral shaft following closed treatment has an incidence rate as high as 6%.[33,116,245] Following open treatment methods the refracture rate is 1% to 3% and significantly less when using intramedullary nails. Removal of an intramedullary device, if necessary, can be recommended at one year following radiographic evidence of fracture consolidation. Plate removal from the femoral shaft may be considered at two years following radiographic evidence of consolidation of the fracture site. If there is major concern about the potential for refracture, consideration may be given to insertion of an intramedullary device following plate removal.

HARDWARE FAILURE

Failure of a fracture fixation device is a relatively common complication of internal fixation of femoral shaft fractures. However, with improved understanding of the function of these internal fixation devices, this complication is becoming increasingly less common. Magerl et al. reported seven bent or broken plates in their study on plate osteosynthesis in femoral shaft fractures, an incidence of 10%.[164] Rüedi and Luscher noted nine cases of bent or broken plates in their series, an incidence of 7%.[234] Older plate designs cannot be recommended for femoral shaft fractures because of their insufficient strength and inability to tolerate normal weight-bearing stress. Plates are placed eccentrically on the femoral shaft, which predisposes them to significant bending stresses, even with minimal motion by the patient. The technique to apply the plate may require significant soft tissue stripping and devascularization of the bone, thereby impeding fracture healing. This predisposes the plate to fatigue fracture. If internal fixation with a plate is considered for a femoral shaft fracture, attention must be paid to the technique principles outlined by the Swiss AO group for application of a plate.[6,186,212,213,253] Consideration must also be given to cancellous bone grafting of the femoral shaft opposite the plate.

Failure of intramedullary nail fixation of femoral shaft fractures has also been reported.[17,69,287,310] Bucholz et al. reported that fractures in the distal femur tend to be more commonly associated with breakage of an intramedullary nail than do fractures elsewhere in the shaft (see Fig. 46–35).[45] They recommended that when treating the distal third femoral shaft fracture with an intramedullary nail, an attempt should be made to place a larger diameter nail and avoid full weight bearing until the fracture has radiographic evidence of early union. A large series by Franklin and co-workers reported on 60 broken intramedullary nails.[88] These nails were of a very broad variety, including hollow nails with an open cloverleaf cross section, as well as nails that were welded or joined proximally from an open section to a closed section. In their series they noted multiple factors involved in nail breakage. Similar to Bucholz et al.'s study, they noted that the distal interlocking holes created a major stress concentration within the nail, predisposing locked nails with distal holes to breakage, particularly when placed in distal third femoral shaft fractures. A proximal weld in the nail also predisposed the nail to breakage. They reported that the design of the nail is a major factor in the frequency of nail breakage.

Interestingly, the AO group has followed a series of 560,000 AO nails.[17] They noted that partial cracking had occurred at the weld site in the proximal aspect of the nail in about 25% of nails. Complete breakage of the nail developed in only 67 of these intramedullary nails, even when a proximal weld had been used, an extremely low incidence (0.01%) of hardware failure.

Recent design and manufacturing changes in intramedullary nails have significantly decreased the incidence of implant breakage. Most intramedullary nails with a cloverleaf or hollow design are manufactured by gun drilling, and most no longer have proximal welds. Some manufacturers have closed the cross section of the nail, making it a cylinder rather than a cloverleaf with a slot. Other manufacturers have significantly decreased the width of the open slot and designed it so that even the slot does not predispose the nail to breakage, but actually relieves stress. The anteriorly placed slot has been removed and replaced with a posteriorly placed slot in most nail designs. With appropriate nail insertion techniques and application of recently designed intramedullary nails, the incidence of implant failure should be relatively uncommon.

Franklin et al. reported several different techniques that may be utilized for removing broken intramedullary nails.[88] They recommended several forms of hooks that reach down through the cannulated portion of the intramedullary nail, hooking the nail at the distal end. These long hooklike devices can then retrieve the nail by backing it out retrograde. The authors noted that solid section nails are significantly more difficult to remove when broken. It is of note that a solid-section nail, the Zickel subtrochanteric nail or the fluted femoral rod, has been associated with a significant incidence of refracture of the femoral shaft following nail removal.[197,256] This has been determined by Ovadia and Chess to be a distinctly separate fracture from that originally treated with the Zickel device.[197] For this reason, the Zickel cephalomedullary nail is no longer recommended for young trauma patients who may require removal of the intramedullary device.

Probably the more significant complication with intramedullary nailing is the incidence of prominent, symptomatic hardware.[36,40,53,76,298] With the original Küntscher nail, this occurred frequently by the nail backing out through its insertion site in the proximal femur and becoming prominent in the buttocks. The routine Küntscher nail was noted to be rotationally unstable, and with weight-bearing ambulation the nail could back out by impaction at the fracture site, or simple rotation of the femur could cause it to twist out through the insertion site or occasionally migrate distally toward the knee.[74] When using Küntscher intramedullary nails, this was a relatively frequent phenomenon, although it caused minimal long-term difficulty with fracture healing. It did require removal of the intramedullary nail in most instances following fracture union. With the recent use of locked intramedullary nails, this complication is extremely uncommon. Simple application of a proximal cross-locking bolt will prevent the intramedullary nail from backing out. However, a cross-locking bolt placed directly on the lateral aspect of the greater trochanter can be quite symptomatic in some patients. Most authors will note a significant incidence of greater trochanteric bursitis and other problems related to the proximal cross-locking bolt. These symptoms have very little effect on fracture healing but commonly lead to the necessity of bolt removal following fracture union. Proximal bolt removal can be performed alone or in conjunction with removal of the intramedullary device itself. Removal of the bolts is not recommended until fracture union has been achieved.

The distal cross-locking bolts can also be a source of irritation for the patient. These bolts have a large head that can interfere with the normal excursion of the iliotibial band, creating a symptomatic adventitial bursitis. This generally necessitates removal of the distal cross-locking bolts. In our experience, removal of distal cross-locking bolts is necessary more often because of symptoms directly related to these bolts than because of the need for dynamization or increased corticalization of callus. Removal of these bolts can be safely performed after fracture consolidation is apparent on routine follow-up radiographs. This should occur generally within four to six months following surgery. Nails with distal locking by means of blades also have significant problems related to insertion and removal.[40]

An interesting complication that is a source of consternation to an occasional orthopedic surgeon is the bent intramedullary nail (Fig. 46–60). This has most often been associated with the use of a Küntscher intramedullary nail or the original AO intramedullary nail. This complication generally occurs prior to fracture consolidation and should only occur because of significant stress overload at the fracture site. Most often, the force applied to the femur is similar to the force that caused the original fracture. Most current locked-nail

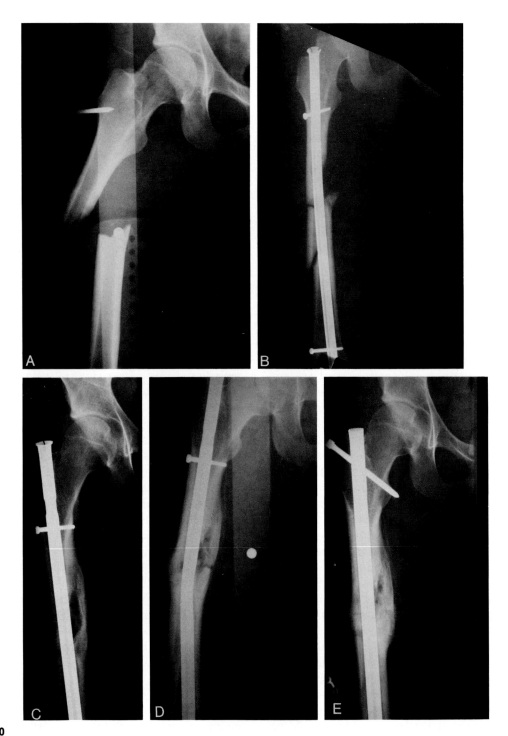

Figure 46-60

Bent intramedullary nail. *A*, AP x-ray of the proximal femur, demonstrating displaced oblique fracture sustained in a motor vehicle accident. Fracture is closed. *B*, AP x-ray of proximal femur 2 weeks following static locked intramedullary nailing with slotted nail. *C*, AP x-ray of the proximal femur demonstrating fracture healing at 10 months postsurgery. Static locked nail is still in place. *D*, AP x-ray of the proximal femur reveals refracture of the femur and a bent intramedullary nail following a second motor vehicle accident 11 months following the first. *E*, AP x-ray shows solid healing 5 months following the removal and renailing of the bent nail (no special technique was required for removal).

devices will absorb a considerable amount of stress without bending, but these original intramedullary devices will not. In many instances, the bending or twisting of the nail is associated with significant additional comminution at the fracture site and shortening of the femur. This poses a significant problem for the orthopedic surgeon as to how to remove the intramedullary device and realign and restabilize the femur. The best solution to this problem is to place the patient under general anesthesia and straighten the intramedullary nail out by closed manipulation. Generally, the intramedullary nail can be straightened out sufficiently to remove it without serious difficulty. Very little bending force is necessary to deform these original intramedullary devices. Following removal of the bent nail, our recommendation is to ream the intramedullary canal and place a larger diameter statically locked intramedullary nail. Fracture union will generally occur in a routine manner following the restoration of length and alignment to the femoral shaft.

NEUROLOGIC COMPLICATIONS

Nerve injury is relatively uncommon in conjunction with femoral shaft fractures because of the large soft tissue muscular envelope surrounding the femoral shaft and vital structures. The most common nerve injury associated with a femoral shaft fracture is a peroneal nerve palsy. In Winquist et al.'s series of 520 femoral shaft fractures, they noted six patients in whom an initial peroneal palsy was apparent at the time of patient presentation to the emergency treatment facility.[298] They also had four patients in whom a peroneal palsy was related to the surgical procedure. In these instances inadequate distraction of the fracture occurred before closed intramedullary nailing, which necessitated strong traction during the operative procedure. Complete recovery occurred in three of the four patients. Patients in their series were routinely positioned in the lateral position on the fracture table, and great care was taken during patient positioning to prevent stretch to the sciatic and peroneal nerves. In general, when a patient is positioned on the table, the extremity to be operated on is flexed at the hip and the knee is kept straight. This position stretches the sciatic nerve. If strong traction is necessary for fracture reduction, a distal femoral skeletal traction pin should be inserted, and the knee should be bent to relax the sciatic nerve. Peroneal nerve palsy can also occur as a result of prolonged and poorly managed traction with the leg in external rotation. This can place pressure on the peroneal nerve at the area at the head of the fibula and result in a peroneal nerve palsy. This is increasingly less common with the decreased use of preoperative traction.

When patients are positioned supine on a fracture table for internal fixation using an intramedullary nail, another nerve injury can occur. If extensive traction is applied, the perineal post can place excessive pressure on the pudendal nerve. This will result in a pudendal nerve palsy, which leads in a male to decreased or absent sensation on the head of the penis and in a female to a similar lack of sensation over the labia. Needless to say, this can be a distressing complication. The exact incidence of this complication is somewhat difficult to define in the literature on closed intramedullary nailing. Most surgeons who perform this procedure in the supine position on the fracture table are distinctly aware of its potential. This dreaded complication can be avoided by the use of appropriate preoperative traction that will distract the femoral shaft fracture, thereby avoiding excessive traction intraoperatively. The perineal countertraction post should also be well padded to prevent this complication.

VASCULAR COMPLICATIONS

Vascular injury associated with femoral shaft fracture has been previously discussed (see Venous Thromboembolism). Most of these injuries occur at the time of trauma and only seldom at the time of treatment. Most can be diagnosed by careful preoperative evaluation of the patient. The fracture most prone to vascular injury is the displaced distal third fracture of the femoral shaft. Late vascular problems, such as false aneurysm, arteriovenous fistula formation, or injury to the intima with resultant late thrombosis, are relatively uncommon.[36,80] Great care should be taken with penetrating trauma (e.g., gunshot injuries) to carefully explore or study wounds that are near vascular structures. The development of arteriovenous fistula following insertion of closed intramedullary nails has occurred but is extremely rare (Fig. 46–61). Pulsatile masses that occur in conjunction with the insertion of intramedullary nails or percutaneous cross-locking bolts require arteriography. Care should be taken to avoid aspiration or puncturing of these pulsatile masses because of the significant bleeding that may occur.

THROMBOEMBOLIC DISORDERS

An area of concern following intramedullary nailing is potential pulmonary embolism. These deep venous thromboses and complications have not been reported or identified to any large degree in the literature. In Winquist et al.'s series on 520 femoral shaft fractures, they noted nine patients with a pulmonary embolism.[298] Eight of these patients had multiple injuries, and the ninth patient, who actually died from the em-

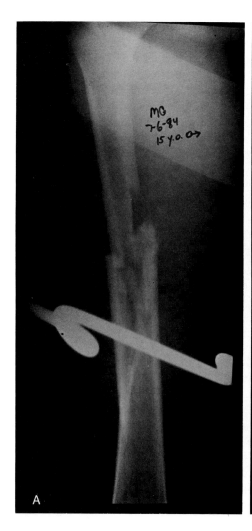
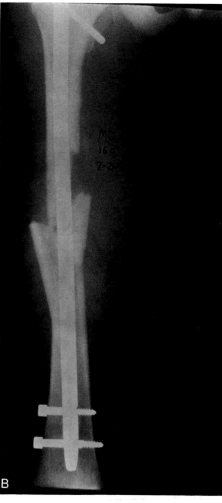

Figure 46–61

Arteriovenous fistula following closed intramedullary nailing. *A,* AP radiograph of comminuted femoral neck fracture in 15-year-old patient. *B,* Postoperative AP radiograph.

bolism, had an isolated femoral shaft fracture. No statement is made as to the timing of the fracture fixation in these cases. In a study of early versus delayed stabilization of femoral fractures, pulmonary embolus was noted in four cases of 178 patients.[23] Three of these occurred following late stabilization of femoral shaft fractures, and two occurred in instances of isolated femoral fractures with delayed stabilization. It becomes increasingly apparent that thromboembolism can be a problem in the femoral shaft fracture. Most authors agree that the most reliable defense against thromboembolism is muscle activity and mobilization. This is best achieved by early fracture stabilization and patient mobilization. The complication is much more common in patients older than 40 than in younger patients and is much more common in patients with additional lower extremity or pelvic problems than in other patients placed on bed rest. Currently there is no official recommendation for prophylaxis of thromboembolism following femoral shaft fracture. The use of compression stockings and patient mobilization are perhaps the best preventions.

COMPARTMENT SYNDROME

Compartment syndrome of the thigh is a rare phenomenon. The study by Schwartz and co-workers represents the world's largest experience with this entity.[242] They reported on 21 acute compartment syndromes of the thigh in 17 patients. Ten were associated with an ipsilateral femoral fracture, and five of these femoral fractures were open fractures. In five patients the syndrome followed closed intramedullary nailing of the femur. The entity is more common in multiply injured patients.

The predisposing risk factors for developing thigh compartment syndrome include, most importantly, multiple injuries. The addition of systemic hypotension, external compression of the thigh, a history of the use of the pneumatic anti-shock garment, coagulop-

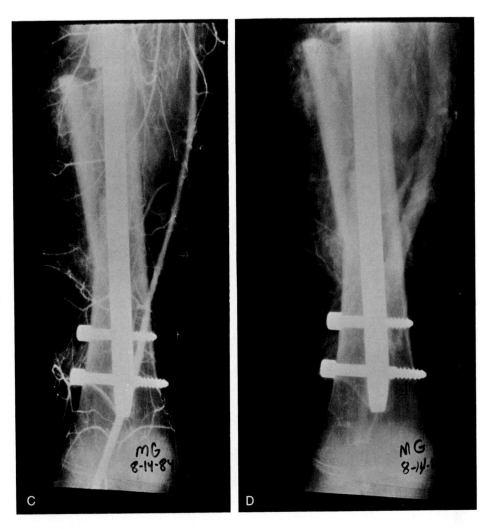

Figure 46–61 *Continued*

C, Arteriogram showing arteriovenous fistula. *D,* Another view of arteriovenous fistula, which required resection. Notice early filling of large femoral vein.

athy, vascular injury, or any trauma to the thigh with or without a fracture of the femur should lead to suspicion of potential thigh compartment syndrome. In 13 of the 21 patients studied in this series, another compartment syndrome developed in addition to the thigh. All 13 had a compartment syndrome of the ipsilateral leg. Treatment of a thigh compartment syndrome includes definitive diagnosis, which is done by direct pressure measurement. The critical threshold for fasciotomy used in the Schwartz et al.'s series was a pressure of greater than 40 mm Hg. The exact critical threshold necessitating fasciotomy has been a point of contention, and certainly the patient's overall status should be considered when attempting to rule out the diagnosis of thigh compartment syndrome. This diagnosis carried with it an extreme morbidity in the series mentioned. Eight patients (47%) died as a result of multiple injuries. Six of the nine patients (ten compartment syndromes) who survived developed infection at the site of fasciotomy. These patients at follow-up examination

revealed significant morbidity, including sensory deficit and motor weakness of the lower extremity. Thus compartment syndrome of the thigh is a significant complication in the multiply injured patient and should be considered whenever a significant blunt injury to the thigh has been sustained.

NONUNION

In most large series of femoral shaft fractures treated with closed intramedullary nailing, the nonunion rate is less than 1%.[49,298] The diagnosis of nonunion of the femoral shaft can usually be traced to lack of blood supply at the fracture site caused either by an open fracture or by open reduction and surgical manipulation at the fracture site.[134] Other potential causes of nonunion include inadequate stabilization of the fracture site postoperatively, wound infection, or prolonged distraction.[28,265]

Delayed union is similar to nonunion and is seen

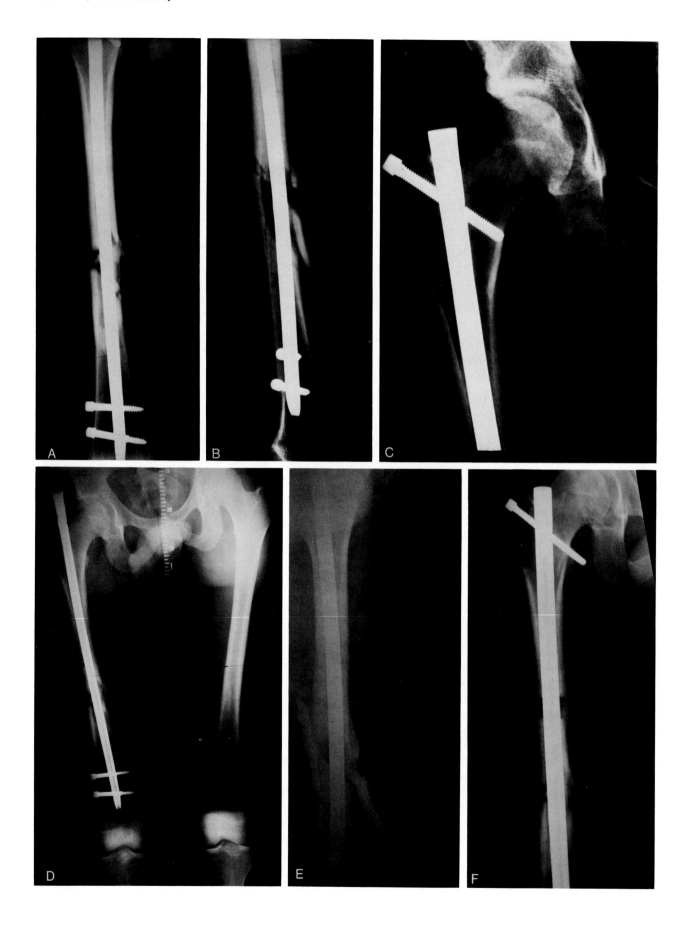

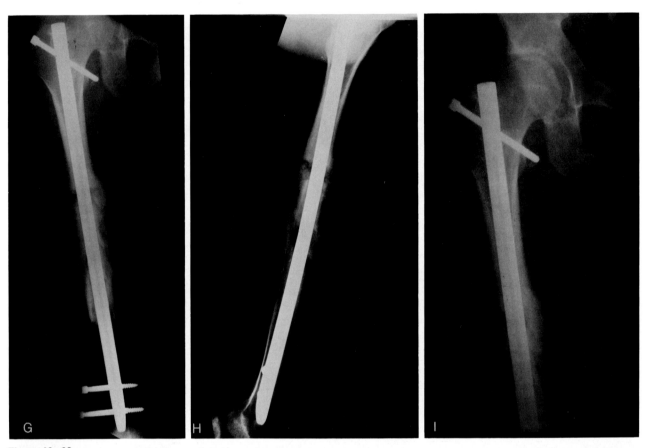

Figure 46-62

Premature removal of distal and proximal bolts in the presence of a length-unstable delayed union allowed shortening and necessitated reoperation. *A*, AP radiograph following static locked nailing of comminuted femoral shaft fracture. *B*, Postoperative lateral radiograph demonstrating stable fixation. *C*, AP radiograph of the proximal femur following intramedullary nail fixation. *D*, AP radiograph of both femurs following dynamization by removal of proximal bolt at six weeks following intramedullary nailing. Note shortening of the intramedullary nail. *E*, Lateral radiograph of the femur following bolt removal demonstrates significant shortening. *F*, Radiograph after femoral osteotomy to restore length at four months following fracture. *G*, AP radiograph demonstrating subsequent fracture healing at three months following osteotomy. *H*, Lateral radiograph demonstrating progressive fracture healing three months following osteotomy. *I*, AP radiograph demonstrating healed femoral fracture one year following injury and eight months following osteotomy.

slightly more commonly. This problem is more frequent in the patient with multiple fractures or other major sources of nitrogen loss such as a burn or open wounds. If a static locked nail has been used and the femur has been distracted somewhat, healing may be delayed. If the fracture has regained its length and rotational stability, this problem can be simply treated by removal of static locking bolts from the proximal or distal aspect of the nail, allowing impaction to occur at the fracture site, which will generally encourage union. Care should be taken, however, with a static locked nail in a fracture with delayed union regarding continued length instability following bolt removal. Removal of proximal or distal locking bolts may allow the inadequately healed fracture to shorten considerably prior to the occurrence of a solid union (Fig. 46-62). In these particular cases, consideration should be given to bone grafting of the femoral shaft fracture, followed by dynamization of the nail at three to four months after bone grafting. This may prevent excessive shortening in the length-unstable femur with a delayed union.

In the absence of infection, treatment of a femoral shaft nonunion is straightforward. The use of an intramedullary nail appears to be the treatment of choice.[29,60,112,155,265,286] If an intramedullary nail is in place, simple exchange nailing will generally encourage fracture healing. The intramedullary nail is removed, and the intramedullary canal is reamed to allow insertion of a nail at least 2 mm larger. This allows fracture healing to occur with the least morbidity. If malalignment or failed hardware exists in conjunction with the femoral shaft nonunion, it may be necessary to open the fracture site for realignment or hardware removal followed by closed intramedullary nailing. If this is the case, consideration should be given to autogenous cancellous bone grafting at the time of surgical treatment of the nonunion. A simple exchange nailing does not require bone grafting. Cultures should always be obtained from the medullary reamings, because of the possibility of an occult infection.

Treatment of a nonunion in the presence of infection is a significantly more complicated undertaking.[146] The nonunion may be treated by simple exchange nailing as mentioned previously, as long as the acute infection is decompressed.[143] This may allow fracture healing as long as the acute infection remains decompressed and continues to drain. In many cases, the fracture must be debrided and necrotic bone removed from the fracture site. This will generally leave a large bone defect, and application of an external fixation device and open cancellous bone grafting may be necessary to allow union to occur.[7] Infected nonunion of the femoral shaft is an extremely complex complication that requires considerable consultation and preoperative planning to obtain a successful outcome.

There is virtually no place for the use of electrical stimulation in the treatment of nonunion or delayed union of the femoral shaft. Significant difficulty must be overcome in delivering the electrical impulse to the nonunion site through the large muscles in the thigh, and only minimal success has been reported in the case of femoral nonunions.

MALUNION

Malunion following femoral shaft fracture has been discussed extensively in the literature. Malunion can occur from shortening (>1 cm), malrotation ($>10°$), angulatory deformity ($>15°$), or any combination thereof.[134] Closed treatment of femoral shaft fractures (traction plus bracing) will generally lead to malalignment problems with shortening of at least 1 cm.[134,181,183] Treatment in traction followed by a cast brace virtually requires shortening for uncomplicated fracture healing. This must be accepted prior to beginning treatment with this method. Shortening of 1 cm is quite acceptable in most femoral shaft fractures, but shortening of greater than 2 cm is unacceptable. Malalignment generally occurs in the AP plane, with apex anterior angulation occurring most frequently (Fig. 46–63).[134] Rotational malalignment and angulatory alignment in the AP plane are less common with closed treatment and casting of femoral shaft fractures. These malalignment problems are easier to evaluate and easier to adjust with this treatment method, thus making this complication less likely to occur. In a series of comminuted femoral shaft fractures treated with roller traction and a cast brace, angulation of greater than 10°

occurred in 62% of patients, and shortening of greater than 1 cm occurred in 78% of patients, with the average being 1.7 cm.[134] The average hospital stay to achieve this result was 31 days. While most femoral shaft fractures heal when treated with closed reduction using traction followed by casting, the majority have a malalignment problem that is a major annoyance to the patient. Correction of these malalignment problems will require a major operative procedure consisting of a femoral osteotomy, the use of internal or external fixation and potential bone grafting, as well as several months of therapy after bone healing to achieve an acceptable outcome.

With closed intramedullary nailing of femoral shaft fractures, malalignment problems in rotation are more common than those in angulation. In Winquist and Hansen's series of 520 femoral shaft fractures treated by intramedullary nailing, external rotation deformity and shortening were the most commonly encountered malalignment problems.[298] Shortening (>1 cm) occurred in 9% of patients and external rotation ($>10°$) in 8% of patients. It must be remembered that the majority of patients in this series were treated with a routine Küntscher nail without proximal or distal locking bolts. This series consisted of patients treated prior to 1980 and includes no locked intramedullary nails. The authors reported that routine Küntscher nails are not indicated for most comminuted femoral shaft fractures (Winquist types II through V).[297] This amount of comminution requires the use of a static locked intramedullary nail to prevent excessive shortening. Similarly, external rotation malunion must be prevented when utilizing a dynamic or unlocked intramedullary nail for a femoral shaft fracture. Winquist and Hansen reported that external rotation deformities can occur because of placement of the intramedullary nail with the leg externally rotated.[108,109,298] They also reported that malalignment may occur postoperatively, because the unrestrained lower limb tends to fall into external rotation without good motor function. With unlocked intramedullary nails, instability at the fracture site that may be caused by the fracture pattern or by an inadvertent fall can also create malalignment problems. As with shortening, external rotational malalignment can be prevented with the use of static locked intramedullary nails, particularly in distal third femoral shaft fractures.

When an unlocked intramedullary nail or a dynamic locked intramedullary nail is used, care must be taken to protect the patient from the externally rotated position that is most comfortable for them postoperatively. A derotation boot should be applied in all such cases. This derotation boot is generally necessary for approximately three to five days postoperatively, until the pa-

Figure 46–63

Femoral shaft fracture treated closed with traction and bracing. This resulted in apex anterior angulation of 40°. *A*, AP (left) and lateral (right) radiographs after injury. *B*, In roller traction. *C*, Continued treatment of femoral shaft fracture in a fracture brace demonstrating progressive apex anterior angulation. *D*, AP (left) and lateral (right) radiographs showing fracture healing at more than 1 year and demonstrating significant apex anterior angulation.

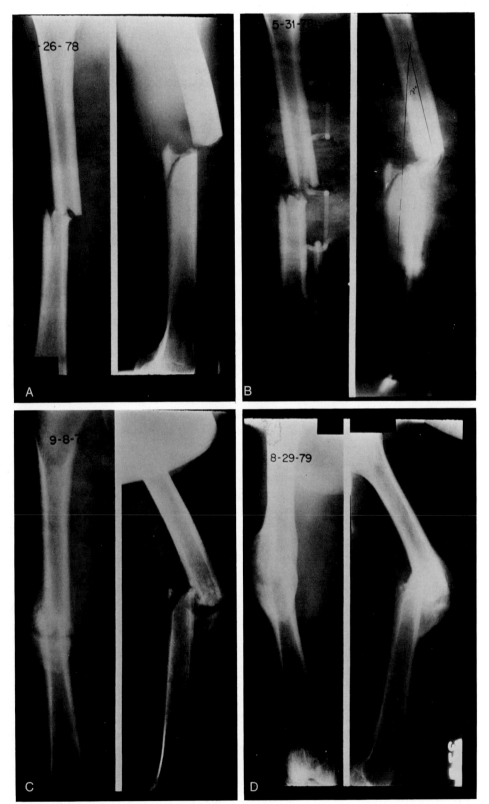

tient has enough quadriceps function to be able to do a straight leg raise and is weight bearing with crutches, causing some interdigitation of the fracture at the fracture site.

With the current use of locked intramedullary nails, malrotation generally occurs at the time of surgery, with the fracture being locked into malalignment.[133] The patient will heal in that amount of malalignment unless the problem is noted and corrected at the time of original surgery or soon thereafter. Patients can compensate reasonably well for mild internal rotation deformities but tolerate poorly any excessive external rotation deformity. Thus care must be taken to position the femur in the appropriate rotational alignment at the time of surgery when applying a static locked nail.

Correction of a rotational malalignment following fracture union can be accomplished by performing a closed intramedullary osteotomy.[295] This osteotomy should be performed away from the fracture callus, as the saw cuts a circle and will not cut through excessive periosteal callus. Following closed femoral osteotomy, fixation of the femur in the correct rotational alignment is accomplished with a static locked nail.

With the increased use of locked intramedullary nails, shortening is becoming less of a problem. Comminuted femoral shaft fractures are fixed at their position of union at the time of surgery with a static locked intramedullary nail. In many Winquist grade III and IV comminuted fractures the appropriate length measurement is often difficult to determine at the time of surgery.[133] In these cases, backup decision making regarding femoral length should be made. This may include getting a full-length radiograph of the uninvolved femur and measuring from the tip of the trochanter to a reproducible mark on the distal femur. Taking into account 10% to 15% magnification, the appropriate length nail is then measured and used at the time of surgery. A similar method is accomplished by laying an estimated appropriate-length nail alongside the femur and obtaining a radiograph of the intact femur and normal nail length. Another, less accurate method is physical measurement from the tip of the trochanter to the midpoint of the lateral femoral condyle clinically. If these appropriate measures are not taken preoperatively, it is difficult to ascertain correct femoral length at the time of surgery.

Locked intramedullary nails, particularly those that are placed for treatment of significantly comminuted fractures, tend to cause excessive lengthening rather than shortening.[36,133,138,299,313] Care must be taken at the time of surgery to determine the correct length and to position the fractured femur to within 1 cm of the length of the uninvolved femoral shaft. When bilateral shaft fractures occur, nails of similar length are placed

in both femora. Patients will not tolerate excessive lengthening of the extremity; even 1 cm of excess is noticeable to the patient and is a source of displeasure. Occasionally, excessive length obtained at the time of surgery can be improved by early removal of static locking bolts. If the limb is 1 to 2 cm too long, the removal of static locking bolts at 8 to 12 weeks postoperatively with encouragement of full weight-bearing ambulation will cause the femoral shaft to shorten through the healing callus. Unfortunately, this is not an accurate way to correct length deformity and is inconsistent at best. Most comminuted femoral shaft fractures have the potential for shortening of some degree for up to three months, and occasionally four to five months, following insertion of a static locked intramedullary nail.

Angulatory deformity following intramedullary nailing has also been reported for femoral fractures. This was noted to occur in approximately 1.5% of patients following an intramedullary nailing in Winquist et al.'s series.[298] In their experience, this angulatory deformity tended to occur in distal third femoral shaft fractures that were nailed with the patient in the lateral position. In this case, inadequate support of the thigh, inadequate reduction of the fracture, or a tight iliotibial band allowed the fracture to be nailed in a valgus position (apex medial angulation). Thus orthopedic surgeons should avoid a valgus position at the fracture site when performing closed intramedullary nailing in distal third femoral shaft fractures. This can be done by femoral nailing in the supine position, adequate support of the thigh when the patient is in the lateral position, or positioning the femoral shaft parallel to the floor to avoid tightness of the iliotibial band. The incidence of this is decreasing in current practice because of surgeon awareness.

Angulatory malalignment also occurs when proximal femoral shaft fractures (those that used to be termed "subtrochanteric fractures") are treated with an intramedullary nail. These fractures tend to be positioned in excessive flexion and abduction. If the surgeon is not careful, the tendency is to obtain an anterior and lateral starting position of the intramedullary nail. If this position is obtained, a fracture will heal in a varus (apex lateral) alignment (Fig. 46–64). Generally speaking, angulatory deformity that is not excessive (neck shift angle of 110° to 120°), is not a clinical problem. The fracture will generally proceed to solid union, and no untoward effect may be noted. This deformity can be avoided, however, with careful attention to detail at the time of the surgical procedure, attempting to obtain, even though difficult, the correct starting position for the intramedullary nail.[135] Angulatory deformity in the lateral plane (apex anterior or

Figure 46–64

A, AP radiograph of comminuted femoral shaft and lesser trochanter fractures. *B*, AP radiograph taken postoperatively. A slightly lateral starting position was used for a static locked intramedullary nail. *C*, Fracture healing demonstrating a significant decrease in normal neck-shaft angle because of the lateral starting position. This is seldom a major problem, although slight femoral shortening occurs. *D*, AP radiograph following intramedullary nail removal showing a varus neck-shaft angle.

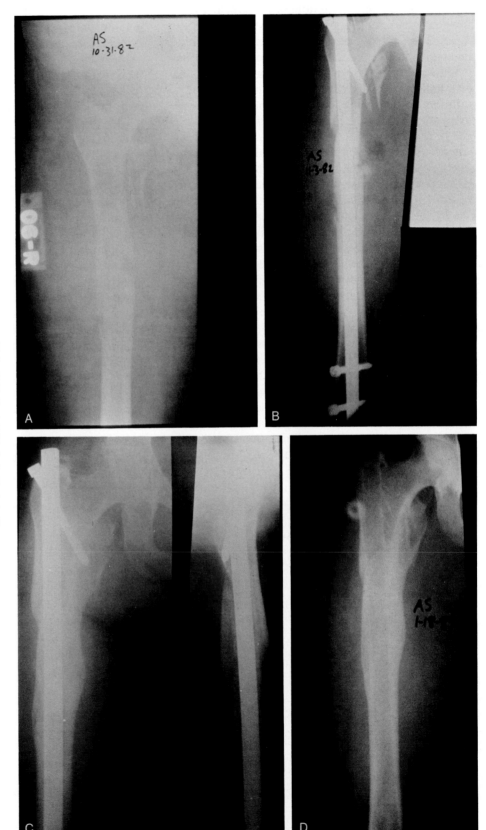

posterior) is relatively uncommon with use of an intramedullary nail. Even if this type of deformity does occur, it is seldom a clinical problem. In summary, angulatory deformities with femoral shaft fractures are increasingly less common than the originally noted 1.5% incidence of Winquist et al.[298]

HETEROTOPIC OSSIFICATION

Heterotopic ossification is a complication of variable severity following intramedullary nailing of the femoral shaft. It is not uncommon for small amounts of heterotopic ossification to occur routinely over the proximal end of the nail (Fig. 46–65). This creates a bony cap over the nail that is seldom a clinical problem. On rare occasions, this heterotopic ossification is so large that it interferes with hip motion. Recommended treatment for this complication is simply to allow the femoral shaft fracture to heal solidly and the heterotopic ossification to mature. When the femoral shaft fracture is solidly united and no change has occurred in the heterotopic ossification over the proximal end of the femur for three to six months, the intramedullary nail is removed from the femur, and the heterotopic ossification existing over the proximal end of the nail in the area of the gluteus maximus is surgically excised. If the ossification is mature, that is, no new bone has been formed over a period of three months, the bone can be surgically removed without its recurrence. This should

only be necessary if the heterotopic ossification is causing clinical symptoms such as pain or limitation of motion. Generally, excision of symptomatic heterotopic ossification and hardware removal can be timed such that these are performed simultaneously, perhaps 18 months following the original accident. Although these bony caps over the intramedullary nail are relatively common, it is also relatively uncommon for them to significantly interfere with patient function. Most of the time this problem is simply ignored, and the patient notes no serious setback to overall condition.

The exact cause of heterotopic ossification in the area of the gluteus maximus following intramedullary nailing is obscure. There may also be local damage to muscle that allows metastatic calcification to occur in the muscle. Perhaps the cause of this phenomenon is the deposition of bone fragments from the reamed intramedullary canal that are not fully washed from the wound following the surgical procedure. However, a trial of pulsed lavage irrigation of the nailing wound showed no reduction in heterotopic bone.[42a]

INFECTION

Infection is the complication dreaded by all fracture surgeons. A bone infection following a fracture is a serious complication that has far-reaching effects so-

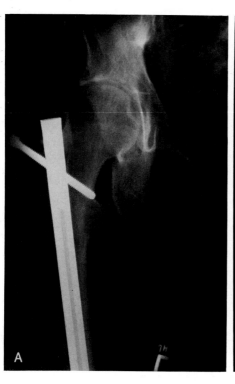
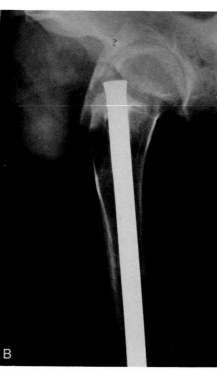

Figure 46–65

A, Heterotopic ossification of the proximal femur. Heterotopic bone formation has occurred at the proximal end of the nail. B, Lateral radiograph of the proximal femur demonstrating heterotopic bone formation.

cially and economically. The potential for infecting a closed fracture by using operative intervention when such a fracture has historically always been treated closed with fair results is, perhaps more than anything else, what has caused femoral fracture fixation to be accepted slowly. With current femoral shaft fracture management regimens, we now have a good understanding for what the potential infection rate actually should be. In Winquist et al.'s classic article dealing with 520 femoral shaft fractures, their infection rate was 0.9%[298] Christie and co-workers dealt with 120 femoral fractures and noted no infections.[62] In a study comparing closed treatment of femoral shaft fractures with open reduction and internal fixation and also closed intramedullary nailing, there were no infections in the closed treatment group and the closed intramedullary nailing group, but there was a 13% infection rate with open reduction followed by intramedullary nailing.[134] Open reduction and internal fixation utilizing plate fixation, on the other hand, carry a 1% to 7% infection rate.[26,59,160,164,234,254]

Causes of acute postoperative infection following intramedullary nailing include prolonged operating time, excessive devascularization or stripping of bone fragments, inappropriate internal fixation, and serious problems with postoperative management. Wiss et al., in a study of comminuted femoral shaft fractures treated with a locked intramedullary nail, noted no instances of deep wound infection or osteomyelitis.[299] This series of 112 nailings dealt wth some of the most difficult comminuted femoral shaft fractures and actually included 32 open fractures (six grade I, five grade II, four grade III, and 17 gunshot fractures).

Open femoral shaft fractures have been a major concern for orthopedic trauma surgeons. This injury is associated with multiply injured patients, and therefore surgeons should have such patients stabilized immediately. As stated many places previously the best fracture stabilization for femoral shaft fractures is an intramedullary nail. Reports dealing with intramedullary nailing of open fractures indicated that the infection rate with type I and II open fractures treated with immediate intramedullary nailing is similar to that for closed fractures. In most series dealing with this subject the infection rate associated with delayed intramedullary nailing was equal to that associated with immediate intramedullary nailing.[39,55,159,298] The infection rate with immediate intramedullary nailing of open femoral shaft fractures types I and II appears to be in the 1% to 2% range. On the other hand, intramedullary nailing of type III open femoral shaft fractures has a significantly higher infection rate (4% to 5%).[39,55,159]

Treatment of an infected femoral shaft fracture requires fracture stability.[102,105,162,163,205] In most cases this is achieved by leaving the original device in place.[205] Local irrigation and debridement is performed, with excision of all necrotic bone and soft tissue. Adequate drainage of the infected fracture site should be assured. Broad-spectrum antibiotics are provided parenterally initially, followed by culture-specific antibiotics. It must be kept in mind that antibiotics play only a small role in the treatment of an infected fracture. The primary goal should be to achieve fracture union first, and then clear up the local infection secondarily. Stable hardware such as an intramedullary nail should remain in place.[105,205,294] If the local infection cannot be controlled with local irrigation and debridement, if the fixation device is unstable, or if the patient becomes systemically ill, consideration should be given to removal of the intramedullary nail or other fracture fixation device.[294] At this point another fracture fixation device (i.e., a larger intramedullary nail or external fixation), may provide improved stability. However, alternative methods are necessary only in rare instances. Following clearing of the local infection, the wound may be closed by delayed primary closure, skin grafting, or local flaps. If the bone debridement has left a gap at the fracture site, consideration should be given to autogenous cancellous bone grafting. This procedure should not be considered until the fracture site has a clean, closed wound.

Following fracture healing, in the presence of infection, the surgical implant is removed. This should be considered the final treatment necessary for an infected fracture or infected hardware. At the time of hardware removal, radical debridement of local soft tissue is performed. The infected medullary canal is overreamed 1 to 2 mm to remove infected granulation tissue surrounding the nail. It may be necessary to open the intramedullary canal in the distal femoral metaphysis with a drill hole in the medial femoral condyle. This improves irrigation and debridement of the medullary canal. In the case of an infected locked intramedullary nail, the distal bolt holes may be enlarged or connected to provide this communication with the intramedullary canal. Pulse lavage irrigating systems are used to thoroughly irrigate the intramedullary canal, and suction drains are placed into the canal. Parenteral antibiotics are provided following hardware removal for a period of three to five days, and culture-specific antibiotics, either intravenous or oral, may be provided at home for a total course of two to three weeks.

Following such a regimen, it is uncommon to have long-term cases of chronic osteomyelitis or drainage following a femoral shaft fracture. In general, if one can obtain fracture union, chronic ostomyelitis and amputation are rare. It is of note that implant removal followed by radical irrigation and debridement should be routinely performed after fracture union. This is the most definitive step in treatment of an infected femoral shaft fracture.

MISCELLANEOUS COMPLICATIONS

Several miscellaneous complications have been noted to occur in femoral shaft fractures. The majority of these complications occur intraoperatively but are not noted during the procedures, and therefore become complications. Such things as femoral neck fractures, extension of fracture lines or creation of excessive comminution, bolts that miss the femoral nail, and broken hardware, among others, are all aspects of treatment that can be avoided.[36,45,61,88] If one is to perform closed intramedullary nailing of a femoral shaft fracture, then, as previously noted in this chapter, it is incumbent on the surgeon to determine the integrity of the femoral neck. A femoral neck fracture that occurs at the time of operative procedure is very uncommon, and most can be related to undiagnosed femoral neck fractures that occurred at the time of the accident. These may be nondisplaced. The use of a large, dull awl to create a starting hole for intramedullary nailing is to be condemned. Awls that become dull after several intramedullary nailing procedures will create a femoral neck fracture when they are pounded on with a mallet. A correct starting position can be identified by means of a K wire and overdrilled by means of a cannulated drill bit or the center core of the reamer for a compression hip screw. If this is not available, a *sharp* awl must be used to expand the starting hole or even a regular drill bit. Treatment of a femoral neck fracture noted at the time of surgery has already been discussed.

A correct starting position that is directly in line with the intramedullary canal is important to avoid comminuting the femur at the fracture. Utilization of an anterior starting hole with a curved, stiff intramedullary nail risks comminution because of excessive hoop stress in the proximal segment.[136] Correct understanding of the mechanics of the surgical procedure is absolutely necessary.

The use of locking bolts of the wrong length can easily be prevented by careful attention to detail. Each bolt must be verified with the image intensifier. This should be done in the operating room with the patient on the fracture table. There is little reason to return the patient to the operating room to exchange inappropriately placed locking bolts; this complication should be apparent at the time of surgery.

Finally, permanent-copy radiographs should be obtained in the operating room prior to awakening the patient from general anesthesia. This will ensure that any major changes in hardware already implanted in the operating room can be performed under the same general anesthetic, thereby avoiding returning the patient to the operating room for a second general anesthesia to revise the surgical procedure. This recommendation cannot be emphasized enough.

REFERENCES

1. Acker, J.; Murphy, C.; D'Ambrosia, R. Treatment of fractures of the femur with the Gorsse-Kempf rod. Orthopaedics 8:1393–1401, 1985.
2. Adrey, J., ed. Hoffman's External Anchorage Coupled in Frame Arrangement: Biomechanical Survey of the Leg Fracture, Ed. 2. Paris, Gaed, 1971.
3. Allen, W.C.; Piotrowski, G.; Burstein, A.H.; Frankel, V.H. Biomechanical principles of intramedullary fixation. Clin Orthop 60:13–20, 1968.
4. Allen, W.; Heiple, K.; Burstein, A. A fluted femoral intramedullary rod: Biomechanical analysis and preliminary clinical results. J Bone Joint Surg 60A:506–515, 1978.
5. Allgöwer, M.; Ehrsam, R.; Ganz, R.; et al. Clinical experience with a new compression plate "DCP." Acta Orthop Scand 36(suppl.):277–279, 1969.
6. Allgöwer, M.; Kinzl, L.; Matter, P.; et al. The Dynamic Compression Plate. New York, Springer-Verlag, 1977.
7. Alonzo, J.; Geissler, W.; Hughes, J.L. External fixation of femoral fractures. Indications and limitations. Clin Orthop 241:83–88, 1989.
8. American Association of Automotive Medicine. Abbreviated Injury Scale, 1985 Revision. Arlington Heights, IL, AAAM, 1985.
9. Anderson, J.T.; Gustilo, R.B. Immediate internal fixation in open fractures. Orthop Clin 11:569, 1980.
10. Anderson, L.D. Compression plate fixation and the effect of different types of internal fixation on fracture healing. J Bone Joint Surg 47A:191–208, 1965.
11. Anderson, R.L. Conservative treatment of fractures of the femur. J Bone Joint Surg 49A:1371–1375, 1967.
12. Arneson, T.J.; Melton, L.J. III; Lewallen, D.G.; O'Fallon, W.M. Epidemiology of diaphyseal and distal femoral fractures in Rochester, Minnesota, 1965–1984. Clin Orthop 234:188–194, 1988.
13. Ashworth, E.M.; Dalsing, M.C.; Glover, J.L.; Reilly, M.K. Lower extremity vascular trauma: A comprehensive, aggressive approach. J Trauma 28:329, 1988.
14. Baird, R.A.; Kreitenberg, A; Eltoria, I. External fixation of femoral shaft fractures in spinal cord injury patients. J Parapleg 24:183–190, 1986.
15. Barquet, A.; Fernandez, A.; Leon, H. Simultaneous ipsilateral trochanteric and femoral shaft fracture. Acta Orthop Scand 15:36–39, 1985.
16. Barr, H,; Santer, G.J.; Stephenson, I.M. Occult femoral artery injury in relation to fracture of the femoral shaft. J Cardiovasc Surg 28:193–195, 1987.
17. Beaupré, G.S.; Schneider, E.; Perren, S.M. Stress analysis of a partially slotted intramedullary nail. J Orthop Res 2:369–376, 1984.
18. Behrens, F.; Jones, R.E.; Weats, P.C.; Fischer, D.A.; External skeletal fixation. In: Murray, D.G., ed. AAOS Instructional Course Lectures, Vol. 30. St. Louis, C.V. Mosby, 1981, p. 112.
19. Bergman, G.D.; Winquist, R.A.; Mayo, K.A.; Hansen, S.T. Jr. Subtrochanteric fracture of the femur: Fixation using the Zickel nail. J Bone Joint Surg 69A:1032–1040, 1987.

20. Blake, R; McBryde, A. Jr. The floating knee: Ipsilateral fractures of the tibia and femur. South Med J 68:13–16, 1975.

21. Böhler, J. Results in medullary nailing of ninety-five fresh fractures of the femur. J Bone Joint Surg 33A:670–678, 1951.

22. Böhler, J. Closed intramedullary nailing of the femur. Clin Orthop 60:51–67, 1968.

23. Bone, L.B.; Johnson, K.D.; Weigelt, J.; Scheinberg, R. Early versus delayed stabilization of femoral fractures: A prospective randomized study. J Bone Joint Surg 71A:336–340, 1989.

24. Bonney G. Thrombosis of the femoral artery complicating fracture of the femur. Treatment by endarterectomy. J Bone Joint Surg 45B:344–345, 1963.

25. Border, J.R.; LaDuca, J.; Seibel, R. Priorities in the management of the patient with polytrauma. Prog Surg 14:84–120, 1975.

26. Böstman, O.; Varjonen, L.; Vainionpää, S.; et al. Incidence of local complications after intramedullary nailing and after plate fixation of femoral shaft fractures. J Trauma 29:639–645, 1989.

27. Branch, H.E. March fractures of the femur. J Bone Joint Surg 26:387–391, 1944.

28. Brav, E.A. Further evaluation of the use of intramedullary nailing in the treatment of gunshot fractures of the extremities. J Bone Joint Surg 39A:513–520, 1957.

29. Brav, E.A. The use of intramedullary nailing for nonunion of the femur. Clin Orthop 60:69–75, 1968.

30. Brav, E.A.; Jeffress, V.H. Fractures of the femoral shaft. A clinical comparison of treatment by traction suspension and intramedullary nailing. Am J Surg 84:16–25, 1952.

31. Brav, E.A.; Jeffress, V.H. Modified intramedullary nailing in recent gunshot fractures of the femoral shaft. J Bone Joint Surg 35A:141–152, 1953.

32. Bray, T.J. Indications for locked intramedullary nailing. Tech Orthop 3:9–13, 1988.

33. Breederveld, R.S.; Patka, P.; van Mourick, J. Refractures of the femoral shaft. Neth J Surg 37:114–116, 1985.

34. Breen, T.F. Jr.; Jones, G.S.; Seligson, D. Fractures of the femoral shaft in a regional hospital setting. J Trauma 23:483–487, 1983.

35. Brookes, M.; Elkin, A.C.; Harrison, R.G.; Heald, C.B. A new concept of capillary circulation in bone cortex—some clinical applications. Lancet 1:1078–1081, 1961.

36. Browner, B.D. Pitfalls, errors, and complications in the use of locking Küntscher nails. Clin Orthop 212:192–208, 1986.

37. Browner, B.D.; Burgess, A.R.; Robertson, R.J.; et al. Immediate closed antegrade Ender nailing of femoral fractures in polytrauma patients. J Trauma 24:921–925, 1984.

38. Browner, B.D.; Kenzora, J.E.; Edwards, C.C. The use of modified Neufeld traction in the management of femoral fractures in polytrauma. J Trauma 21(9):779–787, 1981.

39. Brumback, R.J.; Ellison, P.S.; Poka, A.; et al. Intramedullary nailing of open fractures of femoral shaft. J Bone Joint Surg 71A:1324–1330,1989.

40. Brumback,R.J.; Handal, J.A.; Poka, A.; et al. Radiograph analysis of the Brooker-Wills interlocking nail in the treatment of comminuted femoral fractures. J Orthop Trauma 1:120–129, 1987.

41. Brumback, R.J.; Reilly, J.P.; Poka, A.; et al. Intramedullary nailing of femoral shaft fractures. Part I: Decisions-making errors with interlocking fixation. J Bone Joint Surg 70A:1441–1452, 1988.

42. Brumback,R.J.; Uwagie-Ero, S.; Lakatos, R.P.; et al. Intramedullary nailing of femoral shaft fractures. Part II: Fracture-healing with static interlocking fixation. J Bone Joint Surg 70A:1453–1462, 1988.

42a. Brumback, R.J.; Wells, D.; Lakatos, R.P.; et al. Heterotopic ossification about the hip after intramedullary nailing for femoral fractures. Presented to the 6th Annual Meeting of the Orthopaedic Trauma Association, Toronto, Ontario, November 9, 1990.

43. Brunner, C.F.; Weber, B.G. Besondere Osteosynthesetechniken. Berlin, Springer-Verlag, 1981.

44. Bucholz, R.W.; Rathjen, K. Concomitant ipsilateral fractures of the hip and femur treated with interlocking nails. Orthopedics 8:1402–1406, 1985.

45. Bucholz, R.W.; Ross. S.E.; Lawrence, K.L. Fatigue fracture of the interlocking nail in the treatment of fractures of the distal part of the femoral shaft. J Bone Joint Surg 69A:1391–1399, 1987.

46. Burstein, A.H.; Currey, J.; Frankel, V.H.; et al. Bone strength—the effect of screw holes. J Bone Joint Surg 54A:1143–1156, 1972.

47. Burwell, H.N. Internal fixation in the treatment of fractures of the femoral shaft. Injury 2:235, 1971.

48. Buxton, R.A. The use of Perkins' traction in the treatment of femoral shaft fractures. J Bone Joint Surg 63B:362–366, 1981.

49. Carr, C.R.; Wingo, C.H. Fractures of the femoral diaphysis. A retrospective study of the results and costs of treatment by intramedullary nailing and by traction and a spica cast. J Bone Joint Surg 55A:690–700, 1973.

50. Casey, J.J.; Chapman M.W. Ipsilateral concomitant fractures of the hip and femoral shaft. J Bone Joint Surg 61A:503–509, 1979.

51. Castle, M.E.; Orinion, E.A. Prophylactic anticoagulation in fractures. J Bone Joint Surg 52A:521–528, 1970.

52. Chalmers, J. Subtrochanteric fractures in osteomalacia. J Bone Joint Surg 52B:509–513, 1970.

53. Chandler, R.W. Limitations of conventional nailing.Orthopedics 8:1354–1355, 1985.

54. Chapman, M.W. Closed intramedullary bone grafting and nailing of segmental defects of the femur. J Bone Joint Surg 62A:1004–1008, 1980.

55. Chapman, M.W. The role of intramedullary fixation in open fractures. Clin Orthop 212:26–34, 1986.

56. Chapman, M.W.; Mahoney, M. The role of early internal fixation in the management of open fractures. Clin Orthop 138:120, 1979.

57. Charnley, J. Knee movement following fractures of the femoral shaft. J Bone Joint Surg 29:679–686, 1947.

58. Charnley, J.; Guindy, A. Delayed operation in the open reduction of fractures of the long bones. J Bone Joint Surg 43B:664–671, 1961.

59. Cheng, J.C.Y.; Tse, P.Y.T.; Chow, Y.Y.N. The place of the dynamic compression plate in femoral shaft fractures. Injury 16:529–534, 1985.

60. Christensen, N.O. Küntscher intramedullary reaming and nail fixation for non-union of fracture of the femur and the tibia. J Bone Joint Surg 55B:312–318, 1973.

61. Christie, J; Court-Brown, C. Femoral neck fracture during closed medullary nailing: Brief report. J Bone Joint Surg 70B:670, 1988.

62. Christie, J.; Court-Brown, C.; Kinninmouth, A.W.G.; Howie, C.R. Intramedullary locking nails in the management of femoral shaft fractures. J Bone Joint Surg 70B:206–210, 1988.

63. Clawson, D.K.; Smith, R.F.; Hansen, S.T. Closed intramedullary nailing of the femur. J Bone Joint Surg 53A:681–692, 1971.

64. Cole, J.D. Personal communication, 1989.

65. Committee on Trauma, American College of Surgeons. Re-

sources for Optimal Care of the Injured Patient. Chicago, American College of Surgeons, 1990, p. 61.

66. Cone, J.B. Vascular injury associated with fracture-dislocations of the lower extremity. Clin Orthop 243:30–35, 1989.

67. Connolly, J.; King, P. Closed reduction and immediate cast-brace ambulation in the treatment of femoral fractures. J Bone Joint Surg 55A:1559–1580, 1973

68. Connolly, J.F.; Whittaker, D.; Williams, E. Femoral and tibial fractures combined with injuries to the femoral or popliteal artery: A review of the literature and analysis of 14 cases. J Bone Joint Surg 53A:56–68, 1971.

69. Cook, S.D.; Barrack, R.L.; Renz, E.; et al. Retrieval and analysis of intramedullary rods: A follow-up study. Clin Orthop 191:269–273, 1984.

70. Coppola, A.J. Jr.; Anzel, S.H. Use of the Hoffmann external fixator in the treatment of femoral fractures. Clin Orthop 180:78–82, 1983.

71. Dabezies, E.J.; D'Ambrosia, R.; Shoji, H.; et al. Fractures of the femoral shaft treated by external fixation with the Wagner device. J Bone Joint Surg 66A:360–364, 1984.

72. Danckwardt-Lilliestrom, G. Reaming of medullary cavity and its effect on diaphyseal bone: Fluorochromic, microangiographic and histologic study on the rabbit tibia and dog femur. Acta Orthop Scand 50(suppl.):128, 1969.

73. Debasitani, B.; Aldegheri, R.; Renzo-Brivio, L. The treatment of fractures with a dynamic axial fixator. J Bone Joint Surg 66B:538–545, 1984.

74. de Belder, K.R.J. Distal migration of the femoral intramedullary nail. Report of seven cases. J Bone Joint Surg 50B:324–333, 1968.

75. DeLee, J.C.; Clanton, T.O.; Rockwood, C.A. Closed treatment of subtrochanteric fractures of the femur in a modified cast-brace, J Bone Joint Surg 63A:773–779, 1981

76. Dencker, H. Errors in technique and complications specific to intramedullary nailing. A study based on 459 nailed femoral shaft fractures. Acta Orthop Scand 35:164–169, 1964.

77. Dencker, H. Femoral shaft fracture and fracture of the neck of the same femur. Acta Chir Scand 129:597–605, 1965.

78. Dencker, H. Is the length of hospitalization for patients with femoral shaft fractures shortened by intramedullary nailing? Acta Orthop Scand 35:67–73, 1964.

79. Dencker, H. Shaft fractures of the femur: A comparative study of the results of various methods of treatment in 1,003 cases. Acta Chir Scand 130:173–184, 1965.

80. Dickson, J.W. False aneurysm after intramedullary nailing of the femur. J Bone Joint Surg 50B:144–145, 1968.

81. Dobozi, W.R.; Larson, B.J.; Zindrick, M. et al. Flexible intramedullary nailing of subtrochanteric fractures of the femur: A multi-center analysis. Clin Orthop 212:68–78, 1986.

82. Ender, J.; Simon-Weidner, R. Fixierung trochanterer frakturen mit elastischen kondylennaegeln. Acta Chir Austr 1:40, 1970.

83. Eriksson, E; Frankel, V.H. Stress risers in bone. Letter to the Editor. Clin Orthop 193:310–312, 1985.

84. Eriksson, E.; Wallin, C. Immediate or delayed Küntscher-rodding of femoral shaft fractures. Orthopaedics 9:201–204, 1986.

85. Evans, F.G.; Pedersen, H.E.; Lissner,H.R. The role of tensile stress in the mechanism of femoral fractures. J Bone Joint Surg 33A:485–501, 1951.

86. Fein, L.H.; Pankovitch, A.M.; Spero, C.M.; Baruch, H.M. Closed flexible intramedullary nailing of adolescent femoral shaft fractures. J Orthop Trauma 3:133–141, 1989.

87. Fisk, G.R. The fractured femoral shaft—new approach to the problem. Lancet 1:659, 1944.

88. Franklin, J.L.; Winquist, R.A.; Benirsche, S.K.; Hansen, S.T. Broken intramedullary nails. J Bone Joint Surg 70A:1463–1471, 1988.

89. Fried, G.; Salerno, T.; Burke, D.; et al. Management of the extremity with combined neurovascular and musculoskeletal trauma. J Trauma 18:481–485, 1978.

90. Friedman, R.J.; Wyman, E.T. Ipsilateral hip and femoral shaft fractures. Clin Orthop 208:188–194, 1986.

91. Froimson, A.I. Treatment of comminuted subtrochanteric fractures of the femur. Surg Gynecol Obstet 131:465–472, 1970.

92. Funk, F.J.; Wells, R.E.; Street, D.M. Supplementary fixation of femoral fractures. Clin Orthop 60:41–49, 1968.

93. Gant, G.C.; Shaftan, G.W.; Herbsman, H. Experience with the ASIF compression plate in the management of femoral shaft fractures. J Trauma 10:458–471, 1970.

94. Garland, D.E.; Rieser, T.V.; Singer, D.I. Treatment of femoral shaft fractures associated with acute spinal cord injuries. Clin Orthop 197:191–195, 1985.

95. Garland, D.E.; Rothi, B.; Waters, R.L. Femoral fractures in head injured adults. Clin Orthop 156:219–225, 1982.

96. Geissler, W.B.; Savoie, F.H.; Culpepper, R.D.; Hughes, J.L. Operative management of ipsilateral fractures of the hip and femur. J Orthop Trauma 2:297–302, 1989.

97. Gleis, G.E.; Frederick, L.D.; Johnson, J.R. Biomechanical stability of distally blocked femoral fractures: Is one screw enough? Tech Orthop 3:608, 1988.

99. Goris, R.J.A.; Gimbrére, J.S.F.; van Niekerk, J.L.M.; et al. Early osteosynthesis and prophylactic mechanical ventilation in the multitrauma patient. J Trauma 22:895–903, 1982.

100. Gottschalk, F.A.; Graham, A.J.; Morein, G. The management of severely comminuted fractures of the femoral shaft using the external fixator. Injury 16:377–381, 1985.

101. Grazier, K.L.; Holbrook, T.L.; Kelsey, J.L.; Stauffer, R.N. The Frequency of Occurrence, Impact, and Cost of Selected Musculoskeletal Conditions in the United States. Chicago, AAOS, 1984, pp. 73–135.

102. Green, S.A.; Larson, M.J.: Moore, T.J. Chronic sepsis following intramedullary nailing of femoral fractures. J Trauma 27:52–57, 1987.

103. Grundy, M. Fractures of the femur in Paget's disease of bone—their etiology and treatment. J Bone Joint Surg 52B:252–262, 1970.

104. Gustilo, R. The Classification Manual. St. Louis, Mosby Year Book, 1990.

105. Gustilo, R.B. Management of infected fractures. In: Gustilo, R.B., ed. Management of Open Fractures and Their Complications. Philadelphia, W.B. Saunders, 1982, pp. 133–157.

106. Gustilo, R.B.; Mendoza, R.M.; Williams, D.N. Problems in the management of type III (severe) open fractures: A new classification of type III open fractures. J Trauma 24:742–746, 1984.

107. Haberman, E.T. The pathology and treatment of metastatic disease of the femur. Clin Orthop 169:70–82, 1982.

108. Hansen, S.T.; Winquist, R. Closed intramedullary nailing of the femur: Küntscher technique with reaming. Clin Orthop 138:56–61, 1979.

109. Hansen, S.T.; Winquist, R.A. Closed intramedullary nailing of fractures of the femoral shaft. Part II. Technical considerations. AAOS Instr Course Lect 27:90, 1978.

110. Hardy, A.E. The treatment of femoral fractures by cast-brace application and early ambulation: A prospective review of one hundred and six patients. J Bone Joint Surg 65A:56–65, 1983.

111. Harper, M.C. Fractures of the femur treated by open and closed intramedullary nailing using the fluted rod. J Bone Joint Surg 67A:699–708, 1985.

112. Harper, M.C. Ununited fractures of the femur stabilized with the fluted rod. Clin Orthop 190:273–278, 1984.

113. Harper, M.C.; Carson, W.L. Curvature of the femur and the proximal entry point for an intramedullary rod. Clin Orthop 220:155–161, 1987.

114. Harrington, K.D. Impending pathologic fractures from metastatic malignancy: Evaluation and management. In: Anderson, L.D., ed. AAOS Instructional Course Lectures, Vol. 35. Louis, C.V. Mosby, 1986, p. 357.

115. Harrington, K.D.; Sim, F.H.; Enis, J.E.; et al. Methylmethacrylate as an adjunct in internal fixation of pathologic fractures. J Bone Joint Surg 58A:1047–1055, 1976.

116. Hartmann, E.R.; Brav, E.A. The problem of refracture in fractures of the femoral shaft. J Bone Joint Surg 36A:1071–1079, 1954.

117. Hedlund, R.; Lindgren, U. Epidemiology of diaphyseal femoral fracture. Acta Orthop Scand 57:423–427, 1986.

118. Heitemeyer, U.; Heirholzer, A.G.; Terhorst, J. Der stellenwert der ueberbrueckenden plattenosteosynthese bei mehrfragmentbruchschaedigungen des femur im klinischen vergleich. Unfallchirurg 89:533–538, 1986.

119. Heitemeyer, U.; Kemper, F.; Hierholzer, G.; Haines, J. Severely comminuted femoral shaft fractures: Treatment by bridging plate osteosynthesis. Arch Orthop Trauma Surg 106:327–330, 1987.

120. Henry, S.; Seligson, D. Ipsilateral femoral neck-shaft fractures: A comparison of therapeutic devices. Orthop Trans 14:276, 1990.

121. Henry, S.L.; Williams, M.; Seligson, D. The Williams interlocking Y nail for fixation of proximal femoral fractures. Tech Orthop 3:25–32, 1988.

122. Hoffman, R. Osteotaxis, osteosynthese externe por fiches et rotules. Acta Chir Scand 107:72, 1954.

123. Hollman, M.W.; Horowitz, M. Femoral fractures secondary to low velocity missiles: Treatment with delayed intramedullary fixation. J Orthop Trauma 4:64–69, 1990.

124. Hooper, G.J.; Lyon, D.W. Closed unlocked nailing for comminuted femoral fractures. J Bone Joint Surg 70B:619–622, 1988.

125. Cole, J.D.; Browner, B.D.; Cottler, H.B.; et al. Initial experience with a second generation locking nail. Orthop Trans 14:269, 1990.

126. Hoover, N.W. Injuries of the popliteal artery associated with fractures and dislocation. Surg Clin North Am 41:1099–1112, 1961.

127. Huckstep, R.L. The Huckstep intramedullary compression nail: Indications, technique, and results. Clin Orthop 212:48–61, 1986.

128. Huckstep, R.L. Early mobilization and rehabilitation in orthopedic surgery and fractures. Aust J Surg 47:344, 1977.

129. Huckstep, R.L. Rigid intramedullary fixation of femoral shaft fractures with compression. J Bone Joint Surg 54B:204, 1972.

130. Hughes, J.L.; Sauer, B.W. Wagner apparatus: A protable traction device. In: Seligson, D.; Pope, M., ed. Concepts in External Fixation. New York, Grune and Stratton, 1982.

131. Johnson K.D. Current techniques in the treatment of subtrochanteric fractures. Tech Ortho 3:14–24, 1988.

132. Johnson, K.D.; Cadambi, A.; Seibert, G.B. Incidence of adult respiratory distress syndrome in patients with multiple musculoskeletal injuries: Effect of early operative stabilization of fractures. J Trauma 25:375–384, 1985.

133. Johnson, K.D.; Greenberg, M. Comminuted femoral shaft fractures. Orthop Clin North Am 18:133–147, 1987.

134. Johnson, K.D.; Johnston, D.W.C.; Parker, B. Comminuted femoral-shaft fractures: Treatment by roller traction, cerclage wires and intramedullary nail, or an interlocking intramedullary nail. J Bone Joint Surg 66A:1222–1235, 1984.

135. Johnson, K.D.; Tencer, A.F.; Blumenthal, S.; et al. Biomechanical performance of locked intramedullary nail systems in comminuted femoral shaft fractures. Clin Orthop 206:151–161, 1986.

136. Johnson, K.D.; Tencer, A.F.; Sherman, M.C. Biomechanical factors affecting fracture stability and femoral bursting in closed intramedullary nailing of femoral shaft fractures, with illustrative case presentations. J Orthop Trauma 1:1–11, 1987.

137. Karlström, G.; Olerud, S. Ipsilateral fracture of the femur and tibia. J Bone Joint Surg 59A:240–243, 1977.

138. Kellam, J.F. Early results of the Sunnybrook experience with locked intramedullary nailing. Orthopedics 8:133–147, 1985.

139. Kempf, I.; Grosse, A.; Beck, G. Closed interlocking intramedullary nailing. Its application to comminuted fractures of the femur. J Bone Joint Surg 67A:709–720, 1985.

140. Kessler, S.B.; Hallfeldt, K.K.J.; Perren, S.M.; Schweiber, L. The effects of reaming and intramedullary nailing on fracture healing. Clin Orthop 212:18–25, 1986.

141. Kirby, M.R.; Winquist, R.A. Femoral shaft fractures in adolescents: A comparison between traction plus cast treatment and closed intramedullary nailing. J Pediatr Orthop 1:193–197, 1981.

142. Kissell, E.U.; Miller, M.E.; Closed Ender nailing of femur fractures in older children. J Trauma 29:1585–1588, 1989.

143. Klemm, K. Die stabilisierung infizierter pseudarthrosen mit verriegelungsnagel. Langenbecks Arch Chir 334:559–561, 1973.

144. Klemm, K.W.; Börner, M. Interlocking nailing of complex fractures of the femur and tibia. Clin Orthop 212:89–100, 1986.

145. Klemm, K.; Schellman, W.D. Dynamische und statische verriegelung des marknagels. Monatsschr Unfallheilk 75:568–575, 1972.

146. Kostuik, J.P.; Harrington, I.J. Treatment of infected ununited femoral shaft fractures. Clin Orthop 108:90, 1975.

147. Kristiansen, T.; Seligson, D.; Blakeslee, M. Hip arthrograms following femoral intramedullary nailing. Unfallheikunde 87:129–131, 1984.

148. Küntscher, G. Intramedullary surgical technique and its place in orthopaedic surgery. J Bone Joint Surg 47A:809–818, 1965.

149. Küntscher, G. Practice of Intramedullary Nailing. Springfield, IL, Charles C Thomas, 1967.

150. Küntscher, G. The intramedullary nailing of fractures. Clin Orthop 60:5–12, 1968.

151. Kyle, R.F. Biomechanics of intramedullary fracture fixation. Orthopedics 8:1356–1359, 1985.

152. LaFollett, A.; Griffith, T.; Roach, J.; Albertson, C. Management of femoral shaft fractures and cast brace with immediate ambulation. AAOS Scientific Exhibit, San Francisco, 1979.

153. Laing, P.G. The blood supply of the femoral shaft: Anatomical study. J Bone Joint Surg 35B:462–466, 1953.

154. Lam, S.J. The place of delayed internal fixation in the treatment of fractures of the long bones. J Bone Joint Surg 46B:393–397, 1964.

155. Laurent, L.E.; Lagenskiold, A. Osteosynthesis with a thick medullary nail in non-union of long bones. Acta Orthop Scand 38:341–350, 1967.

156. Leighton, R.K.; Waddell, J.P.; Kellam, J.F.; Orrell, K.G. Open

versus closed intramedullary nailing of femoral shaft fractures. J Trauma 26:923–926, 1986.

157. Lesin, B.; Mooney, V.; Ashby, M. Cast bracing of fractures of the femur: A preliminary report of a modified device. J Bone Joint Surg 59A:917–923, 1977.

158. Levin, P.E.; Schoen, R.W. Jr.; Browner, B.D. Radiation exposure to the surgeon during closed interlocking intramedullary nailing. J Bone Joint Surg 69A:761–766, 1987.

159. Lhowe, D.W.; Hansen, S.T. Immediate nailing of open fractures of the femoral shaft. J Bone Joint Surg 70A:812–820, 1988.

160. Loomer, R.L.: Meek, R.; DeSommer, F. Plating of femoral shaft fractures: The Vancouver experience. J Trauma 20:1038–1042, 1980.

161. Luchini, M.A.; Sarokhan, A.J.; Micheli, L.J. Acute displaced femoral shaft fractures in long-distance runners: Two case reports. J Bone Joint Surg 65A:689–691, 1983.

162. MacAusland, W.R. Treatment of sepsis after intramedullary nailing of fractures of femur. Clin Orthop 60:87–94, 1968.

163. MacAusland, W.R. Jr.; Eaton, R.G. The management of sepsis following intramedullary fixation for fractures of the femur. J Bone Joint Surg 45A:1643–1650, 1963.

164. Magerl, F.; Wyss, A.; Brunner, C.; et al. Plate osteosynthesis of femoral shaft fractures in adults: A follow-up study. Clin Orthop 138:62–73, 1979.

165. Mahorner, H.R.; Bradburn, M. Fractures of the femur—report of 308 cases. Surg Gynecol Obstet 62:1066–1079, 1936.

166. Mann, D.C.; Weddington, J.; Davenport, K. Closed Ender nailing of femoral shaft fractures in adolescents. J Pediatr Orthop 6:651–655, 1986.

167. Marsh, C.H.; Reagan, M.W. Late positional correction of uniting femoral fractures using the Wagner external fixator. Injury 17:248–250, 1986.

167a. Mast, J.; Jakob, R.; Ganz, R. Planning and Reduction Technique in Fracture Surgery. New York, Springer-Verlag, 1989.

168. Mathews, S.S. A simple wire pin skeletal traction apparatus. J Bone Joint Surg 13:595–597, 1931.

169. Mays, J.; Neufeld, A.J. Skeletal traction methods. Clin Orthop 102:141–151, 1975.

170. McBryde, A.M. Jr.; Blake, R. The floating knee-ipsilateral fractures of the femur and tibia. Proceedings of the American Academy of Orthopaedic Surgeons. J Bone Joint Surg 56A:1309, 1974.

171. McIvor, J.B.; Ross, P.; Landry, G.; Davis, L.A. Treatment of femoral fractures with the cast brace. Can J Surg 27:592–594, 1984.

172. McKellop, H.; Ebramzadeh, E.; Fortune, J.; et al. Stability of subtrochanteric fractures fixed with intramedullary rods. In: Transactions of the 13th Meeting of the Society for Biomaterials. 1987, p. 101.

173. McNeur, J.C. The management of open skeletal trauma with particular reference to internal fixation. J Bone Joint Surg 52B:54–60, 1970.

174. Meggitt, B.F.; Juett, D.A.; Derek-Smith, S.J. Cast bracing for fractures of the femoral shaft; A biomechanical and clinical study. J Bone Joint Surg 63B:12–23, 1981.

175. Milgrom, C.; Giladi, M.; Stein, M.; et al. Stress fractures in military recruits, A prospective study showing an unusually high incidence. J Bone Joint Surg 67B:732–735, 1985.

176. Mira, A.J.; Markley, K.; Greer, R.B. III. A critical analysis of quadriceps function after femoral shaft fracture in adults. J Bone Joint Surg 62A:61–67, 1980.

177. Moll, J. The cast-brace walking treatment of open and closed femoral fractures. South Med J 66:345–352, 1973.

178. Mollica, Q.; Gangitano, R.; Longo, G. Elastic intramedullary nailing in shaft fractures of the femur and tibia. Orthopaedics 9:1065–1077, 1986.

179. Mølster, A.O.; Gjerdot, N.R.; Alho, A. Effect of rotational instability on the healing of femoral osteotomies in rats. Orthop Trans 8:305, 1984.

180. Monro, J.K. The history of plaster-of-Paris in the treatment of fractures. Br J Surg 23:257, 1935.

181. Montgomery, S.; Mooney, V. Femur fractures: Treatment with roller traction and early ambulation. Clin Orthop 156:196–201, 1981.

182. Mooney, V. Cast bracing. Clin Orthop 102:159–166, 1974.

183. Mooney, V.; Claudi, B. Fractures of the shaft of the femur. In: Fractures. Rockwood, C.A. Jr.; Green, D.P., eds. Philadelphia, J.B. Lippincott, 1975, p. 1093.

184. Mooney, V.; Nickel, V.L.; Harvey, J.P.; Snelson, R. Cast-brace treatment for fractures of the distal part of the femur. J Bone Joint Surg 52A: 1563–1578, 1970.

185. Moran, C.G.; Gibson, M.J.; Cross, A.T. Intramedullary locking nails for femoral shaft fractures in elderly patients. J Bone Joint Surg 72B:19–22, 1990.

186. Müller, M.E.; Allgöwer, M.; Schneider, R.; Willenegger, H. Manual of Internal Fixation, 3rd ed. New York, Springer-Verlag, 1991.

187. Murphy, C.P.; d'Ambrosia, R.D.; Dabezies, E.J.; et al. Complex femur fractures: Treatment with the Wagner external fixation device or the Grosse-Kempf interlocking nail. J Trauma 28:1553–1561, 1988.

188. Neer, C.S.II; Grantham, S.A.; Shelton, M. Supracondylar fracture of the adult femur. A study of 110 cases. J Bone Joint Surg 49A:591–613, 1967.

189. Netter, F. Atlas of Human Anatomy. Summit, NJ, Ciba-Geigy Corp., pp. 458–476.

190. Nichols, P.J.R. Rehabilitation after fractures of the shaft of the femur. J Bone Joint Surg 45B:96–102, 1963.

191. Nicoll, E.A. Quadricepsplasty. J Bone Joint Surg 45B:483–490, 1963.

192. Nunley, J.A.; Koman, L.A.; Urbaniak, J.R. Arterial shunting as an adjunct to major limb revascularization. Ann Surg 193:271, 1981.

193. O'Beirne, J.; O'Connell, R.J.; White, J.M.; Flynn, M. Fractures of the femur treated by femoral plating using the anterolateral approach. Injury 17:387–390, 1986.

194. Oestern, H.J.; Tscherne, H. Pathophysiology and classification of soft-tissue injuries associated with fractures. In: Tscherne, H.; Gotzen, L., eds. Fractures With Soft Tissue Injuries. New York, Springer-Verlag, 1984, pp. 1–9.

195. Olerud, S.; Danckwardt-Lilliestrom, G. Fracture healing in compression osteosynthesis in the dog. J Bone Joint Surg 50B:844–851, 1968.

196. Onkey, R.G.; Brannan, J.J. The anterior thigh syndrome. J Bone Joint Surg 47A:855–856, 1965.

197. Ovadia, D.N.; Chess, J.L. Intraoperative and postoperative subtrochanteric fracture of the femur associated with removal of the Zickel nail. J Bone Joint Surg 70A:239–243, 1988.

198. Pahud, B.; Vasey, H. Delayed internal fixation of femoral shaft fractures—is there an advantage. J Bone Joint Surg 69B:391–394, 1987.

199. Pankovich, A.M. Adjunctive fixation in flexible intramedullary nailing of femoral fractures. A study of twenty-six cases. Clin Orthop 157:301–309, 1981.

200. Pankovitch, A.M. Flexible intramedullary nailing of femoral shaft fractures. AAOS Instr Course Lect 36:324–338,1987.

201. Pankovitch, A.M. Flexible intramedullary nailing of long bone fractures: A review. J Orthop Trauma 1:78–95, 1987.

202. Pankovich, A.M.; Goldflies, M.L.; Pearson, R.L. Closed Ender

nailing of femoral shaft fractures. J Bone Joint Surg 61A:222–232, 1979.

203. Pankovitch, A.M.; Tarabishy, I.E. Ender nailing of intertrochanteric and subtrochanteric fractures of the femur. Complications, failures, and errors. J Bone Joint Surg 62A:635–645, 1986.

204. Partridge, A.J.; Evans, P.E.L. The treatment of fractures of the shaft of the femur using nylon cerclage. J Bone Joint Surg 64B:910–914, 1982.

205. Patzakis, M.J.; Wilkins, J.; Wiss, D.A. Infection following intramedullary nailing of long bones: Diagnosis and management. Clin Orthop 212:182–191, 1986.

206. Pedersen, H.E.; Serra, J.B. Injury to the collateral ligaments of the knee associated with femoral shaft fractures. Clin Orthop 60:119–121, 1968.

207. Peltier, L.F. The impact of Roentgen's discovery upon the treatment of fractures. Surgery 33:579–586, 1953.

208. Peltier, L.F. A brief history of traction. J Bone Joint Surg 50A:1603–1615, 1968.

209. Perkins, G. Fractures and Dislocations. London, The Athlone Press, 1958.

210. Perren, S.M. Physical and biologic aspects of fracture healing with special reference to internal fixation. Clin Orthop 138:175–196, 1979.

211. Perren, S.M.; Huggler, A.; Russenberger, M.; et al. The reaction of cortical bone to compression. Acta Orthop Scand 36(suppl.):125, 1969.

212. Perren, S.M.; Huggler, A.; Russenberger, M.; A method of measuring the change in compression applied to living cortical bone. Acta Orthop Scand 36(suppl.):125, 1969.

213. Perren, S.M.; Russenberger, M.; Steinemann, S.; et al. A dynamic compression plate. Acta Orthop Scand 36(suppl.):125, 1969.

214. Perry, C.R.; Pankovich, A.M.; Cohn, S.L. Locked flexible intramedullary nails in treatment of unstable femoral fractures. J Orthop Trauma 1:130–140, 1987.

214a. Phillips, T.F.; Contreras, D.M. Current Concepts Review. Timing of operative treatment of fractures in patients who have multiple injuries. J Bone Joint Surg 72A:784–788, 1990.

215. Porter, M.F. Delayed arterial occlusion in limb injuries. A report of three cases. J Bone Joint Surg 50B:138–140, 1968.

216. Provost, R.A.; Morris, J.M. Fatigue fracture of the femoral shaft. J Bone Joint Surg 51A:487–498, 1969.

217. Rascher, J.J.; Nahigan, S.H.; Macys, J.R.; Brown, J.E. Closed nailing of femoral shaft fractures. J Bone Joint Surg 54A:534–544, 1972.

218. Rhinelander, F.W. Effects of medullary nailing of the normal blood supply of the diaphyseal cortex. AAOS Instr Course Lect 22:161–187, 1973.

219. Rhinelander, F.W. The normal microcirculation of diaphyseal cortex and its response to fracture. J Bone Joint Surg 50A:784–800, 1968.

220. Rhinelander, F.W.; Phillips, R.S.; Steel, W.M.; Beer, J.C. Microangiography in bone healing. II. Displaced closed fractures. J Bone Joint Surg 50A:643–662, 1968.

221. Rich, N.M.; Metz, C.W.; Hutton, J.E. Jr. Internal vs. external fixation of fractures with concomitant vascular injuries. J Trauma 11:463, 1971.

222. Richards, R.R.; Waddell, J.P.; Sullivan, T.R.; et al. Infra-isthmal fractures of the femur: A review of 82 cases. J Trauma 24:735–741, 1984.

223. Richardson, J.B.; Jurkovich, G.J.; Walker, G.T.; Bone, E.G. A temporary arteriovenous shunt (Scribner) in the management of traumatic venous injuries of the lower extremity. J Trauma 26:503, 1986.

224. Riska, E.B.; Myllynen, P. Fat embolism in patients with multiple injuries. J Trauma 22:891–894, 1982.

225. Riska, E.B.; von Bonsdorff, H.; Hakkinen, S.; et al. Prevention of fat embolism by early internal fixation of fracture in patients with multiple injuries. Injury 8:110, 1976.

226. Riska, E.B.; von Bonsdorff, H.; Hakkinen, S.; et al. Primary operative fixation of long bone fractures in patients with multiple injuries. J Trauma 17:111–121, 1977.

227. Rittman, W.W.; Schibli, M.; Matter, P.; Allgöwer, M. Open fractures: Long term results in 200 consecutive cases. Clin Orthop 138:132, 1979.

228. Roberts, J.B. Management of fracture and fracture complications of the femoral shaft using the ASIF compression plate. J Trauma 17:20–28, 1977.

229. Rokkanen, P.; Slates, P.; Vankka, E. Closed or open intramedullary nailing of femoral shaft fractures? A comparison of conservatively treated cases. J Bone Joint Surg 51B:313–323, 1969.

230. Rööser, B.; Benston, S.; Herrlin, K.; Onnerfält, R. External fixation of femoral fractures: Experience with 15 cases. J Orthop Trauma 4:70–74, 1990.

231. Roper, B.A.; Provan, J.L. Late thrombosis of the femoral artery complicating fracture of the femur. J Bone Joint Surg 47B:510–513, 1965.

232. Rothwell, A.G. Closed Küntscher nailing for comminuted femoral shaft fractures. J Bone Joint Surg 64B:12–16, 1982.

233. Ruff, M.E.; Lubbers, L.M. Treatment of subtrochanteric fractures with a sliding screw plate device. J Trauma 26:75–80, 1986.

234. Rüedi, T.; Luscher, N. Results after internal fixation of comminuted fractures of the femoral shaft with DC plates. Clin Orthop 138:74, 1979.

235. Rüedi, T.; Wolff, G. Vermeidung posttraumatischer komplikationen durch frühe versorgung van polytraumatisierten mit frakturen des bewegungs. Helv Chir Acta 42:507–12, 1975.

236. Rush, L.V. Dynamic intramedullary fracture-fixation of the femur. Reflections on the use of the round rod after thirty years. Clin Orthop 60:21–27, 1968.

237. Russell, T.; Taylor, J. Interlocking intramedullary nailing of the femur: Current concepts. Semin Orthop 1:217–231, 1986.

238. Sage, F.P. The second decade of experience with the Küntscher medullary nail in the femur. Clin Orthop 60:77–85, 1968.

239. Saletta, J.D.; Freeark, R.J. The partially severed artery. Arch Surg 97:198–205, 1968.

239a. Sanders, R.; Regazzoni, P. Treatment of subtrochanteric femur fractures using the dynamic condylar screw. J Orthop Trauma 3:206–213, 1989.

240. Schatzker, J.; Barrington, T.W. Fractures of the femoral neck associated with fractures of the same femoral shaft. Can J Surg 11:297, 1968.

241. Schneider, H.W. Use of the four-flanged self-cutting intramedullary nail for fixation of femoral fractures. Clin Orthop 60:29–39, 1968.

242. Schwartz, J.T.; Brumback, R.J.; Lakatos, R.; et al. Acute compartment syndrome of the thigh: A spectrum of injury. J Bone Joint Surg 71A:392–400, 1989.

243. Scudese, V.A. Femoral shaft fractures, percutaneous multiple pin fixation, thigh cylinder plaster cast and early weight bearing. Clin Orthop 77:164–178, 1971.

244. Seibel, R.; LaDuca, J.; Hassett, J.M.; et al. Blunt multiple trauma (ISS-36), femur traction, and the pulmonary failure-septic state. Ann. Surg 202:283–295, 1985.

245. Seimon, L.P. Refracture of the shaft of the femur. J Bone Joint Surg 46B:32–39, 1964.

246. Seligson, D.; Kristiansen, T.K. Use of the Wagner apparatus in

complicated fractures of the distal femur. J Trauma 18:795–789, 1978.

247. Shah, D.M.; Corson, J.D.; Karmody, A.M.; et al. Optimal management of tibial arterial trauma. J Trauma 28:228, 1968.

248. Shelton, M.L.; Neer, C.S. II; Grantham, S.A. Occult knee ligament ruptures associated with fractures. J Trauma 11:853, 1971.

249. Smith, D.G. The development of fracture bracing. Resident papers, Rancho Los Amigos Hospital, Downey, CA, 1969.

250. Smith, H. Medullary fixation of the femur. Radiology 61:194–199, 1953.

251. Smith, J.E.M. The results of early and delayed internal fixation of fractures of the shaft of the femur. J Bone Joint Surg 46B:28–31, 1964.

252. Sofield, H.A. Anatomy of medullary canals. AAOS Instr Course Lect 8:8, 1951.

253. Solheim, K.; Vaage, S. Operative treatment of femoral fractures with the AO method. Injury 4:54–60, 1972.

254. Sprenger, T.F. Fractures of the shaft of the femur treated with a single A.O. plate. South Med J 76:471–474, 1983.

255. Stappaerts, K.H.; Broos, P.; Willcox, T.; et al. Factors determining quadriceps recovery following femoral shaft fractures. Unfallchirurg 89:121–126, 1986.

256. Star, A.M.; Whittaker, R.P.; Shuster, H.M.; et al. Difficulties during removal of fluted femoral intramedullary rods. J Bone Joint Surg 71A:341–344, 1989.

257. Steinmann, F.R. Eine neue extensions methode in der frakturenbehandlung. Zentralbe Chir 34:938–942, 1907.

258. Stewart, M.J.; Sisk, T.O.; Wallace, S.L. Fractures of the distal third of the femur. J Bone Joint Surg 48A:787–807, 1966.

259. Street, D.M. One hundred fractures of the femur treated by means of the diamond-shaped medullary nail. J Bone Joint Surg 33A:659–669, 1951.

260. Stryker, W.S.; Russell, M.E.; West, H.D. Comparison of the results of operative and nonoperative treatment of diaphyseal fractures of the femur at the Naval Hospital, San Diego, over a five-year period. J Bone Joint Surg 52A:815, 1970.

261. Stuck, W.G.; Frebe, A.A. Complications of treatment of fractures of the shaft of the femur. South Surg 14:735–754, 1948.

262. Swiontkowski, M.F. Ipsilateral femoral shaft and hip fractures Orthop Clin North Am 18:73–84, 1987.

263. Swiontkowski, M.F.; Hansen, S.T.; Kellam, J.T. Ipsilateral fractures of the femoral neck and shaft. A treatment protocol. J Bone Joint Surg 66A:260–268, 1984.

264. Talucci, R.C.; Manning, J.; Lampard, S.; et al. Early intramedullary nailing of femoral shaft fractures: The cause of fat embolism syndrome. Am J Surg 146:107–111, 1983.

265. Taylor, L.W. Principles of treatment of fractures and nonunion of the shaft of the femur. J Bone Joint Surg 45A:191–198, 1963.

265a. Templeman, D.; Sweeney, C.; Chapman, M.W.; et al. Critical analysis of the management of open femur fractures at two regional trauma centers. Orthop Trans 14:675, 1990.

266. Templeton, T.S.; Saunders, E.A. A review of fractures in the proximal femur treated with the Zickel nail. Clin Orthop 141:213–216, 1979.

267. Tencer, A.F.; Johnson, K.D.; Johnston, D.W.C.; Gill, K. A biomechanical comparison of various methods of stabilization of subtrochanteric fractures of the femur. J Orthop Res 2:297–305, 1984.

268. Tencer, A.F.; Johnson, K.D.; Sherman, M.C. Biomechanical considerations in intramedullary nailing of femoral shaft fractures. Tech Orthop 3:1–5, 1988.

269. Tencer, A.F.; Sherman, M.C.; Johnson, K.D. Intramedullary rod fixation of femur fractures: Parameters affecting fracture

stability and bursting during insertion. J Biomech Eng 107:104–111, 1985.

270. ten-Duis, H.J.; Nijsten, M.W.; Klasen, H.J.; Binnendi, J.K.B. Fat embolism in patient with an isolated fracture of the femoral shaft. J Trauma 28:383–390, 1988.

271. Thomas, H.O. Disease of the Hip, Knee and Ankle Joints. Liverpool, England, T. Dobb and Co., 1875.

272. Thompson, F.; O'Beirne, J.; Gallagher, J.; et al. Fractures of the femoral shaft treated by plating. Injury 16:535–538, 1985.

273. Thorenson, B.O.; Alho, A.; Ekeland, A.; et al. Interlocking intramedullary nailing in femoral shaft fractures. A report of forty-eight cases. J Bone Joint Surg 67A:1313–1320, 1985.

274. Trafton, P.G. Subtrochanteric-intertrochanteric femoral fractures. Orthop Clin North Am 18:59–71, 1987.

275. Tscherne, H. The management of open fractures. In: Tscherne, H.; Gotzen, L., eds. Fractures With Soft Tissue Injuries. New York, Springer-Verlag, 1984, pp. 10–32.

276. Tscherne, H.; Haas, N.; Krettek, C. Intramedullary nailing combined with cerclage wiring in the treatment of fractures of the femoral shaft. Clin Orthop 212:62–67, 1986.

277. Tscherne, H.; Rojczyk, M. The treatment of closed fractures with soft tissue injuries. In: Tscherne, H.; Gotzen, L., eds. Fractures With Soft Tissue Injuries. New York, Springer-Verlag, 1984, pp. 39–45.

278. Vécsei, V. Expansion bolts: An accessory for interlocking nailing. Tech Orthop 3:94–98, 1988.

279. Veith, R.G.; Winquist, R.A.; Hansen, S.T. Jr. Ipsilateral fractures of the femur and tibia: A report of fifty-seven consecutive cases. J Bone Joint Surg 66A:991–1002, 1984.

280. Vesely, D.G. Technique for use of the single and double split diamond nail for fractures of the femur. Clin Orthop 60:95–97, 1968.

281. Vesely, D.G. The single and double split diamond femoral intramedullary nail. Clin Orthop 92:235–238, 1973.

282. Wade, P.A. ASIF compression has a problem. J Trauma 10:513–518, 1970.

283. Wagner, H. Technik und indikation der operativen verkuerzung und verlaengerung von ober-und unterschenkel. Orthopedics 1:59, 1972.

284. Watson-Jones, R. Fractures and Joint Injuries, Vol. 2, Ed. 4. Baltimore, Williams and Wilkins, 1960.

285. Webb, L.; Gristina, A.; Fowler, H.L. Unstable femoral shaft fractures: A comparison of interlocking nailing versus traction and casting methods. J Orthop Trauma 1:10–12, 1988.

286. Webb, L.X.; Winquist, R.A.; Hansen, S.T. Intramedullary nailing and reaming for delayed union or nonunion of the femoral shaft. A report of 105 consecutive cases. Clin Orthop 212:133–141, 1986.

287. Weinstein, A.M.; Clemow, A.J.T.; Starkebaum, W.; et al. Retrieval and analysis of intramedullary rods. J Bone Joint Surg 63A:1443–1448, 1981.

288. Weller, S.; Kuner, E.; Schweikert, H. Medullary nailing according to Swiss study group principles. Clin Orthop 138:45, 1979.

289. White, G.M.; Healy, W.L.; Brumback, R.J.; et al. The treatment of fractures of the femoral shaft with Brooker-Wills distal locking intramedullary nail. J Bone Joint Surg 68A:865–876, 1986.

290. Whittaker, R.P.; Heppenstall, B.; Menkowitz, E.; et al. Comparison of open vs. closed rodding of femurs utilizing a Sampson rod. J Trauma 22:461–468, 1982.

291. Wickstrom, J.; Corban, M.S. Intramedullary fixation for fractures of the femoral shaft. J Trauma 7:551, 1967.

292. Wickstrom, J.; Corban, M.S.; Vise, G.T. Jr. Complications following intramedullary fixation of 325 fractured femurs. Clin Orthop 60:103–113, 1968.

293. Wilber, M.C.; Evans, E.B. Fractures of the femoral shaft treated surgically: Comparative results of early and delayed operative stabilization. J Bone Joint Surg 60A:489–491, 1978.

294. Wilson, J.N. The management of infection after Küntscher nailing of the femur. J Bone Joint Surg 48B:112–116, 1966.

295. Winquist, R.A. Closed intramedullary osteotomies of the femur. Clin Orthop 212:155–164, 1986.

296. Winquist, R.; Hansen, S.T. Segmental fracture of the femur treated by closed intramedullary nailing. J Bone Joint Surg 60A:934–939, 1978.

297. Winquist, R.A.; Hansen, S.T. Comminuted fractures of the femoral shaft treated by intramedullary nailing. Orthop Clin North Am 11:633–648, 1980.

298. Winquist, R.A.; Hansen, S.T. Jr.; Clawson, D.K. Closed intramedullary nailing of femoral fractures: A report of five hundred and twenty cases. J Bone Joint Surg 66A:529–539, 1984.

299. Wiss, D.; Fleming, C.; Matta, J.; Clark, D. Comminuted and rotationally unstable fractures of the femur treated with an interlocking nail. Clin Orthop 212:35–47, 1986.

300. Wolfe, H.R.I.; Robertson, J.M. Fatigue fracture of femur and tibia. Lancet 2:11–13, 1945.

301. Woodard, P.L.; Self, J.; Calhoun, J.; et al. The effect of implant axial and torsional stiffness on fracture healing. J Orthop Trauma 1:331–340, 1988.

302. Yoshioka, Y.; Siu, D.; Cooke, T.D.V. The anatomy and functional axes of the femur. J Bone Joint Surg 69A:873–880, 1987.

303. Young, R.H. Prophylaxis and treatment of the stiff knee following fracture of the femur. Proc R Soc Med 35:716, 1942.

304. Zettas, J.P.; Zettas, P. Ipsilateral fractures of the femoral neck and shaft. Clin Orthop 160:63–73, 1981.

305. Zickel, R.E. A new fixation device for subtrochanteric fractures of the femur. A preliminary report. Clin Orthop 54:115–123, 1967.

306. Zickel, R.E. An intramedullary fixation device for the proximal part of the femur. J Bone Joint Surg 58A:866, 1976.

307. Zickel, R.E. Fractures of the adult femur excluding the femoral head and neck: A review and evaluation of current therapy. Clin Orthop 147:93–114, 1980.

308. Zickel, R.E.; Fietti, V.G. Jr.; Lawsing, J.F. III; Cochran, G.V.B. A new intramedullary fixation device for the distal third of the femur. Clin Orthop. 125:185–191, 1977.

309. Zickel, R.E.; Hobeika, P.; Robbins, D.S. Zickel supracondylar nails for fractures of the distal end of the femur. Clin Orthop 212:79–88, 1986.

310. Zimmerman, K.W.; Klasen, H.J. Mechanical failure of intramedullary nails after fracture union. J Bone Joint Surg 65B:274–275, 1983.

311. Ziv, I.; Blackburn, N.; Rang, M. Femoral intramedullary nailing in the growing child. J Trauma 24:432–434, 1984.

312. Ziv, I.; Rang, M. Treatment of femoral fracture in the child with head injury. J Bone Joint Surg 65B:276–278, 1983.

312a. Zuber, K.; Schneider, E.; Eulenberger, J.; Perren, S.M. Form und dimension der markhole menschlicher femora im hinblick auf die passung von marknagelimplantaten. Unfallchirurg 91:314–319, 1988.

313. Zuckerman, J.; Veith, R.; Johnson, K.; et al. Treatment of unstable femoral shaft fractures with closed interlocking intramedullary nailing. J Orthop Trauma 1:209–218, 1987.

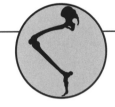

David L. Helfet, M.D.

47

Fractures of the Distal Femur

Pathology

RELEVANT ANATOMY

The anatomic area referred to by the term "distal femur" traditionally encompasses the lower third of the femur. This zone in the literature varies greatly between the distal 7.6 cm and the distal 15 cm of the femur. This chapter deals only with fractures that involve the supracondylar (metaphyseal) or intracondylar (epiphyseal) areas of the distal femur. Distal femoral fractures that are purely diaphyseal are discussed in chapter 46.

Bone

The supracondylar (metaphyseal) area of the distal femur is the transition zone between the distal diaphysis and the femoral articular condyles (Fig. 47–1A). At the diaphyseal-metaphyseal junction, the metaphysis flares, especially on the medial side, to provide a platform for the broad condylar weight-bearing surface of the knee joint. Anteriorly between these two condyles is the smooth articular depression for the patella and the trochlea, and posteriorly between the two condyles is the intercondyloid notch. Medially a readily identifiable landmark is the adductor tubercle at the maximum point of flare of the metaphysis. Both condyles have epicondyles on their outer surfaces.

Of surgical importance, the shaft of the femur in the sagittal view is aligned to the anterior half of the condyles, leaving the posterior half of both condyles posterior relative to the proximal femoral shaft. Also the condyles are wider posteriorly than anteriorly. A transverse cut through the condyles will show a trapezoid with a 25° decrease in the width, from posterior to anterior, on the medial side.

Muscle

Anteriorly the extensor compartment contains the quadriceps femoris, the single largest muscle in the body. It consists of four heads: the rectus femoris more superficially and, in the deeper layer from lateral to medial, the vastus lateralis, vastus intermedius, and vastus medialis. The anterior extensor compartment is separated from the posterior compartment by the lateral and medial intermuscular septa. These provide important landmarks for both the lateral and medial approaches to the knee joint. Of major significance on the medial side is the superficial femoral artery, which runs down the thigh between the extensor and adductor compartments. The artery passes into the popliteal fossa approximately 10 cm above the knee joint by passing through the adductor magnus muscle. It obviously must be identified and avoided in medial approaches to the distal femur.

The powerful muscles of the distal thigh produce characteristic bony deformities with fractures. The muscle pull of the quadriceps and posterior hamstrings produce shortening of the femur. As the shaft overrides anteriorly and the gastrocnemius muscles pull posteriorly, the condyles are displaced and angulated posteriorly (Fig. 47–1B). When the condyles are separated by the fracture, rotational malalignments are common because of the unrestrained pull of the gastrocnemius muscles and the anterior overriding of the shaft.

Alignment

The anatomic axis of the shaft of the femur is different from the weight-bearing, or mechanical, axis (Fig. 47–2). The latter passes through the head of the femur and the middle of the knee joint. Generally, the weight-bearing, or mechanical, femoral axis subtends an angle

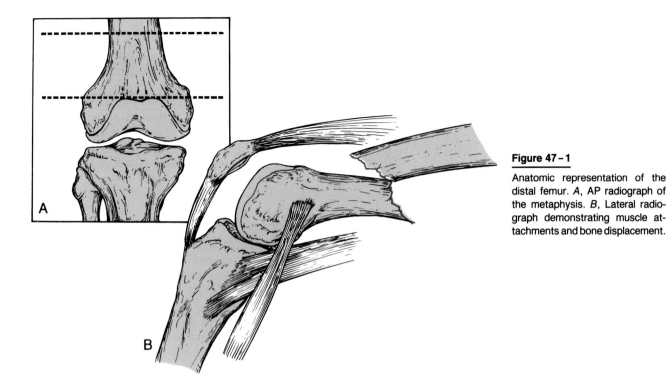

Figure 47–1

Anatomic representation of the distal femur. *A*, AP radiograph of the metaphysis. *B*, Lateral radiograph demonstrating muscle attachments and bone displacement.

of 3° from the vertical. The anatomic femoral axis has a valgus angulation of 7° to 11° (average 9°) relative to the vertical axis. Normally the knee joint axis is parallel to the ground. With an anatomic femoral axis of 9°, it will subtend an 81° lateral and 99° medial angle relative to the knee joint axis. For each patient it is important to determine the normal valgus angle from the opposite femur. Then at the time of surgical reconstruction, the correct femoral valgus angulation (anatomic axis) can be re-created and the knee joint kept parallel to the ground.

INCIDENCE

Fractures of the distal femur have been reported to account for between 4%[25] and 7%[39] of all femoral fractures. This corresponds, in Sweden, to an annual incidence of 51 per million inhabitants older than 16 years.[25] If fractures of the hip are excluded, 31% of femoral fractures involve the distal femur.[2] With the modern trends of high-energy life-styles combined with increased longevity, this incidence is probably increasing.

Distal femur fractures seem to occur predominantly in two patient populations: the young, especially male, following high-energy trauma, and the elderly, especially female, following a low-energy injury. In one series from Sweden, up to 84% of distal femur fractures occurred in patients older than 50 years.[25] In a Roches-

ter, Minnesota, study, of patients 65 years or older, 84% of the femoral fractures occurred in women. The conclusion of this epidemiologic study was that the "incidence rates for distal femoral fractures do indeed rise exponentially with age and are greater among elderly women than men."[2]

In the elderly group, it would appear that most of the injuries occur following "moderate" trauma, such as falls on the flexed knee. It is not surprising that two thirds of the fractures caused by moderate trauma were "preceded by prior age-related fractures (hip, proximal humerus, distal forearm, pelvis or vertebra) or with roentgenographic evidence of generalized osteopenia."[2]

In the younger group, distal femur fractures occur following high-energy trauma. These fractures are often open, comminuted, and most probably the result of direct loading on the flexed knee. The majority are caused by vehicular accidents, including motorcycles, but they can also be caused by industrial accidents or falls from heights. Most of these patients are younger than 35 years of age, with a definite male predominance.

Surprisingly, there is often equivalent comminution in the supracondylar region in both these groups. However, younger patients experiencing high-energy trauma have a greater incidence of additional intraarticular disruption and/or segmental or more proximal shaft comminution.[45]

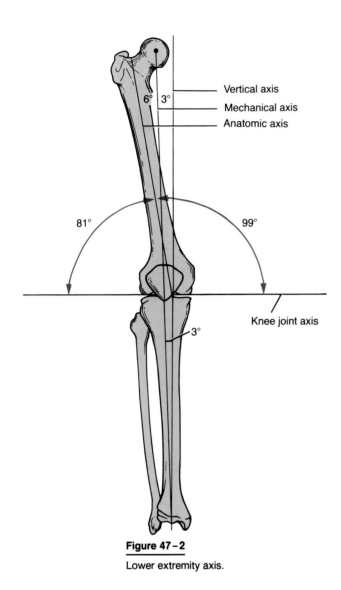

Figure 47–2

Lower extremity axis.

Vertical axis
Mechanical axis
Anatomic axis
Knee joint axis

ANATOMIC AND FUNCTIONAL CONSEQUENCES OF THE INJURY

Fractures in the supracondylar area characteristically deform with femoral shortening and posterior angulation and displacement of the distal fragment. In the more severe fractures, when there is intercondylar involvement, rotational malalignment of the condyles relative to each other is common as a result of their respective muscle attachments.

Even with significant supracondylar comminution and displacement of the distal fragment, axial alignment can often be regained with traction, but this is hard to maintain. Conversely, when there is intercondylar involvement and malrotation of the condyles, reduction is almost impossible by traction alone and is often difficult even with surgery. The aims of treatment must be to restore length, rotation, and axial alignment and the anatomic reconstitution of the articular surface in order to avoid long-term morbidity associated with these fractures. Length and rotation can usually be restored by traction alone, but restoration of the axial alignment of the knee joint relative to the femoral anatomic axis often requires additional measures, including surgical intervention. Disruption of the articular surface with malrotation or malalignment of the condyles requires anatomic reduction and usually mandates an operative procedure.

COMMONLY ASSOCIATED INJURIES

High-energy fractures of the distal femur, especially in young patients, are often only one of a spectrum of multiple injuries sustained by the individual. The whole patient has to be carefully evaluated by a multidisciplinary team approach (see chapter 5). This section will address only the common associated injuries in the involved lower extremity.

The most common mechanism for distal femur fracture is the flexed knee that sustains direct trauma, especially an impact against the dashboard of a moving vehicle. The position of the leg at the time of the injury will determine the presence and type of injury. Care must be taken to exclude concomitant acetabular fractures, hip dislocations, femoral neck fractures, and associated femoral shaft fractures.

Significant soft tissue injuries of the knee are often associated with distal femoral fractures. Associated ligamentous disruptions of the knee joint have been reported in approximately 20% of these fractures.[55] These are hard to diagnose until the distal femur has been stabilized, as both the clinical exam and stress radiographs require stability above the knee to provide useful information.

In the polytraumatized individual, associated injuries to the tibia occur not uncommonly with distal femoral fractures. Associated tibial plateau fractures occur following a predominantly varus or valgus force. Careful evaluation of the plateau is necessary and often requires tomograms. Associated tibial shaft fractures, often comminuted or open, mandate aggressive treatment of both injuries to avoid the morbidity associated with the "floating knee" syndrome.

The femoral artery in the adductor canal is in close proximity to the medial cortex of the distal femur and passes through to the posterior compartment only 10 cm above the knee joint. With high-energy or open injuries to the distal femur, the artery is at significant risk of injury. With associated ligament disruptions of the knee (especially a posterior dislocation), the popliteal artery is at risk of injury—up to 40% in some series.[17,23,29,48] Arterial injuries must be aggressively sought. Arteriography or immediate surgical exploration is mandatory if there is any suspicion on history or clinical exam.

CLASSIFICATION

One of the original and more simple classification schemes for supracondylar/intracondylar femur fractures was that of Neer et al.[35] (Fig. 47–3), which subdivided the intracondylar fractures into the following categories:

I. Minimal displacement
II. Displacement of the condyles: (A) medial, (B) lateral
III. Concomitant supracondylar and shaft fractures

This classification system is very basic and does not provide the surgeon with much clinical and prognostic information.

Seinsheimer classified fractures of the distal $3\frac{1}{2}$ inches of the femur into four basic types (Fig. 47–4)[46]:

I. Nondisplaced fractures—any fracture with less than 2 mm of displacement of fractured fragments.

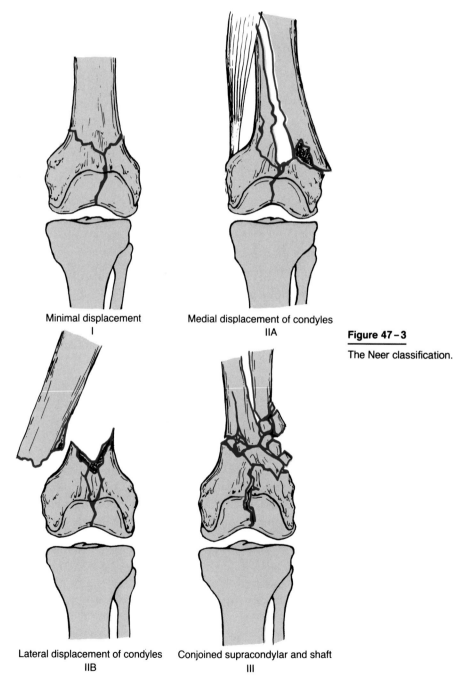

Minimal displacement
I

Medial displacement of condyles
IIA

Lateral displacement of condyles
IIB

Conjoined supracondylar and shaft
III

Figure 47–3

The Neer classification.

Type II

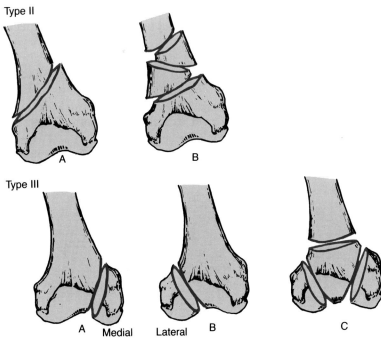

Type III

A Medial   Lateral   B   C

Figure 47–4

The Sensheimer classification.
Type I—undisplaced—is omitted.

Type IV

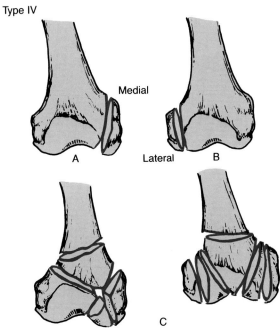

Medial

A   Lateral   B

C

II. Fractures involving only the distal metaphysis, without extension into the intracondylar region:
   A. Two-part fractures.
   B. Comminuted fractures.
III. Fractures involving the intercondylar notch in which one or both condyles are separate fragments:
   A. The medial condyle is a separate fragment; the lateral condyle remains attached to the femoral shaft.

   B. The lateral condyle is a separate fragment; medial condyle is intact.
   C. Both condyles are separated from the femoral shaft and from each other.
IV. Fractures extending through the articular surface of the femoral condyles:
   A. A fracture through the medial condyle (two parts are comminuted).
   B. A fracture through the lateral condyle (two parts are comminuted).

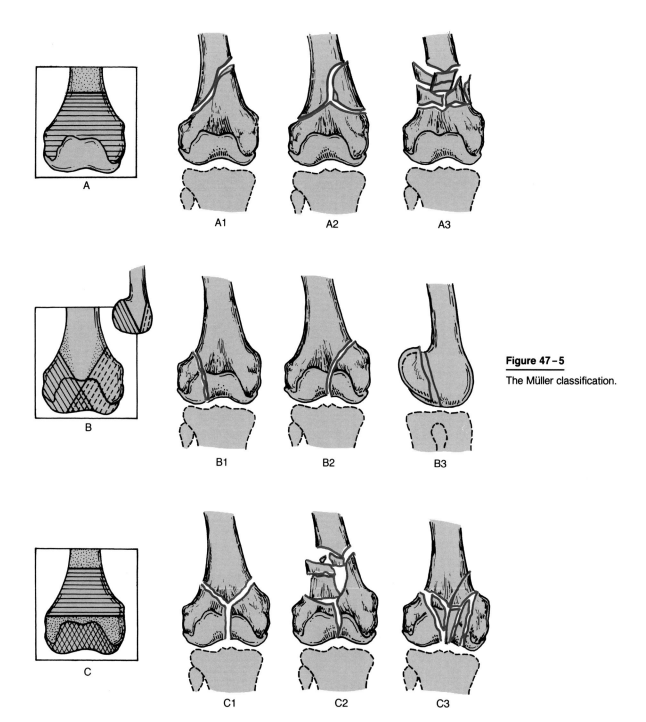

Figure 47–5
The Müller classification.

C. More complex and comminuted fractures in which a fracture involves one femoral condyle and the intercondylar notch, both femoral condyles, or all three. This usually involves a comminuted fracture across the metaphysis as well.

Seinsheimer found that patients with type I nondisplaced fractures and type II simple, two-part supracondylar fractures all had preexisting pathologic osteopo-

rosis prior to their injury. At the other end of the spectrum, patients with type IV fractures involving the articular surface were the youngest patients, and all fractures resulted from high-energy trauma. Additionally, type IIB fractures with comminution in the supracondylar region sustained higher energy trauma and were more severe than IIA type fractures; predictably, their end result was not as good. There was also a significant difference between the patients with the IIIA or

IIIB unicondylar fractures compared to the bicondylar type IIIC fractures. The average age of patients with IIIA and IIIB fractures was 63 years, compared with only 52 years for patients with the type IIIC. Obviously, the type IIIC fractures were more complicated, and the prognosis and results were not as good.

The Swiss Arbeitsgemeinschaft für Osteosystheses fragen (AO) Group, through the AO Documentation Centre, has collated its vast experience and has documentation on thousands of these fractures. Müller et al.[33] in an updated AO classification system for fractures of the distal femur, separate the fractures into three main groups (Fig. 47–5)[34]:

Type A: Extraarticular
Type B: Unicondylar
Type C: Bicondylar

The three groups are further subdivided into three subgroups. Type A fractures (extraarticular): simple, two-part supracondylar fractures are type AI; metaphyseal wedge fractures, type AII; and comminuted supracondylar, type AIII. The type B fractures (unicondylar) are subdivided into lateral condyle sagittal, type BI; medial condyle sagittal, type BII; and coronal, type BIII. Type C (bicondylar) fractures are subdivided into noncomminuted supracondylar (T or Y), type CI; supracondylar comminution, type CII; and supracondylar or intercondylar comminution, type CIII. In progressing from A to C, the severity of the fracture increases, and the prognosis for a good result decreases. This is also true for the progression from I to III in each subgroup.

For a classification system to have clinical significance it must be able to do the following:

1. Allow for adequate documentation of all fractures so that a common language is possible when discussing these injuries.

2. Be simple enough that it is "user friendly."

3. Help the surgeon in clinical decision making so that the correct treatment option can be selected for a particular fracture.

4. Provide prognostic information detailing the results that can be expected for a particular fracture depending on the treatment option selected.

The Müller updated classification system meets these criteria and will be used for fracture classification and description for the remainder of this chapter.

Diagnosis

HISTORY AND PHYSICAL EXAMINATION

A careful evaluation of the whole patient and also of the involved lower extremity is mandatory, especially in the polytraumatized, often obtunded patient. This must include careful scrutiny of the hip joint above and the knee and leg below the fracture. If there is any concern about vascularity to the lower extremity, compartment pressure can be monitored, and Doppler popliteal and distal pulse pressures can be obtained. If there is still concern following these procedures, an urgent arteriogram is indicated. Although rare, if there is tense swelling of the thigh, the presence of an undetected thigh compartment syndrome also must be ruled out by compartment pressure monitoring.

Grossly open and contaminated wounds are easily identifiable. However, when the injury results from direct trauma there are often skin abrasions that must be differentiated from open fracture wounds of the soft tissues. The examination will generally reveal swelling of the knee and supracondylar area, often obvious deformity, and marked tenderness on palpation. Manipulation of the extremity, if tolerated by the patient, will demonstrate motion and crepitance at the fracture site. However, this is cruel and unnecessary if immediate radiographs are available.

RADIOGRAPHIC EVALUATIONS

Routine anteroposterior (AP) and lateral radiographs of the knee and supracondylar region are standard. When the fractures are comminuted or displaced, an exact classification of the fracture is often difficult to make. In order to better identify the particular fracture anatomy, radiographs, both AP and lateral, in the emergency room with manual traction applied to the lower extremity will often allow a much clearer picture of the fracture morphology (Fig. 47–6A,C). If there is intracondylar involvement, 45° oblique radiographs will also help delineate the extent of the injury. This is especially so if there is comminution or additional tibial plateau injuries. Stress radiographs to identify ligamentous disruptions of the knee or associated tibial plateau fractures are generally not indicated until the distal femoral injury is stabilized. Tomograms or computed tomography (CT) scans are indicated to further delineate significant intraarticular involvement or displacement. They may also be useful for isolated chondral or osteochondral lesions.

As with all orthopedic injuries, it is necessary to rule out additional injuries of the "joint above and joint below." There is a significant incidence of ipsilateral fractures to the femur, especially in high-energy vehicular trauma. An adequate AP view of the pelvis, and AP and lateral views of the hip and whole femur are indicated in all these fractures.

Unless there is a frank dislocation of the knee joint associated with the distal femoral fracture, radiographic evaluation of the knee joint has not proved as

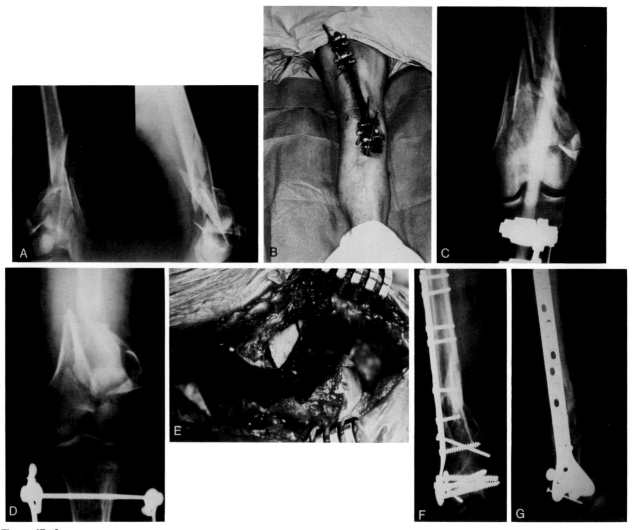

Figure 47–6

Grade I open comminuted C3 fracture of the right distal femur in an 81-year-old woman. *A*, AP (left) and lateral (right) radiographs. *B*, Clinical picture in the external fixator after irrigation and debridement. The proximal pin is close to the fracture. *C*, AP radiograph in the external fixator. *D*, AP radiograph in traction after removal of external fixator and prior to open reduction and internal fixation to allow pin tract healing. *E*, Clinical picture at surgery demonstrating condylar comminution, including a coronal fracture of the lateral condyle. *F,G*, AP and lateral radiographs, respectively, at nine months follow-up with healing despite marked comminution (residual valgus deformity, 5°).

reliable as a careful examination in evaluating the extent of the ligamentous and soft tissue injury. New techniques, especially magnetic resonance imaging (MRI), might prove useful in ascertaining preoperatively whether concomitant injuries to the knee joint ligamentous or meniscal tissue are present.

Comparison radiographs of the normal or uninvolved opposite extremity will help the surgeon with preoperative planning. These should include an AP view of the whole femur to determine the valgus alignment and AP and lateral views of the distal femur to allow superimposition of the fracture fragments on the "normal" template (see section on preoperative planning).

Arteriography is indicated when there is an associated frank dislocation of the knee joint, as there is a reported approximately 40% incidence of arterial injuries with knee dislocations.[17,23,29,48] An absent or diminished pulse (determined clinically or by Doppler assessment in the emergency room), when compared with the normal lower extremity, is also an indication for immediate arteriography or vascular exploration.

Management

Previously, the treatment of choice for the management of femoral fractures, including the supracondylar type, was traction and subsequent mobilization in cast braces. The traction technique employed was either a single pin in the tibial tuberosity[24,26,50] or a two-pin system with an additional pin through the supracondylar fragment.[19,31,60] Reduction was then obtained with traction and, if necessary, manipulation under anesthesia. Traction was maintained for 6 to 12 weeks, followed by mobilization in a cast brace. However, most investigators discussed femoral fractures as a whole and did not differentiate the supracondylar fractures into a separate group. Mahorner and Bradburn reported in 1933 on their results with skeletal traction.[26] Thirty-one fractures involved the distal femur; of all the fractures in their series, these had the poorest results. In 1937, Tees listed the problems associated with traction management of supracondylar femur fractures, specifically the inability to control the distal fragment and its tendency to remain flexed.[52] Because of this, a number of investigators recommended the two-pin technique to control the supracondylar fragment.[19,31,60] Watson-Jones, in 1955, disagreed, believing that the risk of perforation of the femoral artery was too high. He recommended standard proximal tibial skeletal traction only, using knee flexion to control the supracondylar fragment.[56]

In 1935, Lorenz Böhler recommended a Braun splint, placed posteriorly at the level of the fracture rather than the knee, to help control the supracondylar fragment.[5] He subsequently reported a 100% success rate in controlling posterior angulation of the supracondylar fragment in 100 of his own cases.[6] This technique was also subsequently advocated by both Smillie[50] and Charnley.[11] The remaining primary problem encountered in the conservative treatment of distal femur fractures is the inability to adequately control the displaced intraarticular fragments either with manipulation or traction. In addition, prolonged traction across the knee joint often results in significant knee stiffness in addition to the generalized patient problems associated with prolonged hospitalization and bed rest.

Little was written in the early literature on the results of open reduction and internal fixation. In the 1940s the use of the Blount plate was advocated by a number of authors who reported satisfactory results with this technique.[1,54] Open reduction and internal fixation were recommended as the standard of care for supracondylar fractures by White and Russin in 1956.[59] However, they reported 25% poor results in their series. Wertzberger and Peltier recommended open reduction and internal fixation for those supracondylar fractures that were comminuted or unstable.[58] They used Rush pins in 16 of their 45 cases and felt that this provided better fixation, thus allowing more rapid mobilization.

Two classic articles came out within a year of each other in the North American literature in the 1960s. Stewart et al., from the Campbell Clinic, reported in 1966 on a 20-year review of 442 fractures of the distal femur.[51] Of the 213 patients followed for one year or longer, 144 were treated by closed methods, and 69 were treated by open reduction with internal metallic fixation or some type of bone graft. Sixty-seven percent of those treated by closed methods had an excellent or good results, compared with 54% who had good or excellent results in the operative treated group. The poor results in the operative treated patients were caused by infections, poor surgical technique, or homeopathic fixation. In others, treatment with internal fixation failed because it was mechanically impossible to stabilize the multiple fragments. The authors concluded as follows:

The additional trauma of surgery and the proximity of metallic implants to the joint predisposed to excessive reaction and subsequent adhesions. Even though one obtains an excellent roentgenographic result with solid union, final function may be quite poor. No doubt a few surgeons have mastered the technique of operative correction and internal fixation with Blount plates, Rush pins, screws and wire loops, but they are in the minority. Therefore, it is our belief that conservatism should be taught and practiced more universally. Treat the patient, not the x-ray.

Neer et al., in 1967, reported on 110 supracondylar fractures treated at New York Orthopedic Hospital over a 24-year period.[35] They proposed a three-part classification system (discussed earlier) and also a rating system for evaluation based on a functional and anatomic assessment. Ninety percent of those treated by closed methods had satisfactory results, compared with only 52% in the open treated group. However, it must be appreciated that in their rating system, they felt patients were "satisfied" as long as they had strong extensor power and could flex the knee 70°! These are obviously unacceptable criteria for a satisfactory result in the 1990s. In their summary they stated that "no category of fracture at this level seemed well suited for internal fixation, and sufficient fixation to eliminate the need for external support or to shorten convalescence was rarely attained." In fact, almost all their surgically treated patients had prolonged postoperative immobilization because of the inadequacy of the fixation techniques used at that time. In conclusion, Neer et al. felt operative intervention should be limited to the debridement of open fractures or the internal fixation of a fracture with an associated problem such as an arterial injury.

These two papers definitely prejudiced the North American orthopedic community against internal fixation during the 1960s and 1970s. As a result, more advanced techniques of closed treatment were proposed in the early 1970s by Connolly and Dehne[14] and Mooney.[32] In order to shorten traction time and allow earlier ambulation and knee motion, they recommended the use of early cast bracing for femoral shaft and supracondylar fractures.

In 1958, the Swiss AO Group was formed, commencing a new era of fracture care. Their desire was to restore full function to the limb and the patient and to avoid "the fracture disease" associated with prolonged immobilization.[33] They recommended the principles of anatomic reduction of the fracture fragments, preservation of the blood supply, stable internal fixation, and early active pain-free mobilization. It was not until 1970 that the AO published its first results on the treatment of supracondylar femur fractures according to these principles. Wenzl et al. reported on 112 patients, 73.5% of whom had good or excellent results.[57] These results were far superior for open reduction than the 52% satisfactory results reported by Neer et al., even though Wenzl et al.'s criteria for excellent and good were much more stringent.

Schatzker et al. reported on 71 fractures of the distal femur, 32 of which were treated with open reduction and internal fixation.[43] They were able to achieve good or excellent results in 75% of those fractures treated with the AO method as compared with only 32% in the conservatively treated group. They concluded "if normal function or near normal function is to be achieved . . . then unquestionably, if correctly employed, open reduction internal fixation ensures a very high rate of success." However, they did emphasize that they were not advocating open reduction and internal fixation for all patients. For fractures that were undisplaced or were easily reduced, especially in the elderly, immediate mobilization in weight-bearing functional braces was the treatment of choice. They also cautioned against internal fixation in the severely osteoporotic patient. Schatzker and Lambert in 1979 reviewed an additional 35 patients with supracondylar distal femoral fractures treated by open reduction and internal fixation; only 49% had good or excellent results.[44] When they analyzed the 17 cases treated in accordance with the principles of rigid internal fixation as promoted by the AO Group, 71% had good to excellent results. In the 18 patients treated with the AO implants but not AO technique, the results were horrendous, with only 21% having a good to excellent outcome. On critical review of these latter 18 patients, most were elderly with severe comminution; however, surgical technical error was the common denominator contributing to the poor results. The most common errors included the following:

1. Incomplete reduction
2. Failure to achieve interfragmentary compression with lag screws
3. Failure to use autogenous cancellous bone graft to fill defects or comminution
4. Ineffective use of acrylic cement to supplement screw fixation in osteoporotic bone
5. Use of blade plates that were either too long or too far from the joint

Schatzker et al. recommended that elderly patients with thin osteoporotic bone and comminuted fractures "are better treated by such methods as closed reduction and early cast bracing, than an attempt at operative reduction." In such patients the only clear indication for open reduction and internal fixation is an intraarticular fracture in which adequate joint congruity cannot be restored by manipulation. In conclusion they stated:

Rigid fixation is difficult to achieve with osteoporotic bone because of the degree of comminution and the poor holding power of the bone. The mere use of the appropriate implant does not assure rigid fixation. Failure to meticulously observe all the details of the method of rigid fixation, resulted in a high complication rate with failures. These factors must be considered in evaluating criteria for surgical treatment.[43]

Slatis et al. reported in 1971 on 21 "severe" fractures of the lower end of the femur that were treated with open reduction using the AO method.[49] In the 16 patients available for more than one year follow-up, 83% had good to excellent results. Slatis et al. recommended the technique as "reliable," but stated that it "should be restricted to fractures of considerable severity and to selected cases among patients with multiple injuries." Olerud, in 1972, reviewed 15 patients with complex articular fractures of the distal femur.[37] He reported 92% good to excellent results with the use of the angled blade plate but concluded that satisfactory osteosynthesis of fractures of this type is a difficult procedure and should not be attempted without experience with the technique.

In 1974, Chiron et al. reviewed 137 patients with fractures of the distal femur who underwent stable internal fixation with the 95° condylar blade plate.[12] Seventy-two percent of patients fulfilled their criteria for good to excellent results (i.e., 135° of motion and only mild swelling on prolonged weight bearing). In 1982, Mize et al. reported on 30 supracondylar and intracondylar fractures of the femur that were reduced and stabilized with the AO technique.[30] They reported good to excellent results in 80% of patients and also recommended the use of an extensile surgical exposure with elevation of tibial tuberosity to facilitate exposure of the condyles for the more complex fractures with intraarticular comminution. Healy et al., in 1983, reviewed 98 distal femoral fractures to compare open and closed treatment methods.[20] Thirty-eight of the 47 fractures treated by open methods had good functional results. However, only 18 of 51 fractures treated by closed methods had good functional results. Of significance in this review was that age, with an increasing degree of osteoporosis, did not adversely affect their operative results. They concluded that fractures of the distal femur, except in more simple cases, are best managed by open treatment methods.

From all recent reports, it would appear that better functional results can be obtained in all but the most simple fracture types with open reduction and internal fixation. However, the improved outcome seems to depend on the use of improved fixation devices, meticulous surgical technique, and adherence to the principles of the AO Group: anatomic reduction, stable internal fixation, preservation of tissue vascularity, and early mobilization.

In the 1970s and 1980s the wave of enthusiasm for open reduction and internal fixation was not limited to AO techniques. In an attempt to find alternate procedures that were less technically demanding but produced the same results, numerous fixation devices were popularized. Zickel et al. reported in 1977 on the use of the supracondylar Zickel device.[62] This consisted of tapered rods inserted through the medial and lateral femoral condyles into the medullary canal and anchored distally with transverse condylar screws. This early report dealt with 17 patients, 82% of whom had satisfactory healing and functional results. They concluded that the device is ideally suited for the transverse supracondylar fractures. However, it was also used in oblique and "T" intracondylar distal femur fractures, but additional fixation was required in four such fractures intraoperatively. Postoperatively 55% of the patients required casting or cast bracing. In 1986, Zickel et al. reported on an additional 67 cases treated with this device.[63] Ninety-eight percent of the fracture group healed, but functional results were poor in the T and Y intracondylar fracture group: only 48% achieved greater than 90° knee motion.

Shelbourne and Brueckmann reported in 1982 on the use of Rush pin fixation in the management of 98 supracondylar and intracondylar fractures of the femur.[47] They reported 84% excellent and good results, stressing the importance of proper surgical techniques. Rush pins alone were used for noncomminuted fractures, but in the more comminuted supracondylar fractures, they advocated additional cerclage wiring, with minimal soft tissue stripping from the fracture fragments. In summary, they felt that the correct use of Rush pins for supracondylar fractures provided the ad-

vantages of both closed and open techniques without their respective disadvantages. They recommended the Rush pin technique for any adult patient with a supracondylar or intracondylar fracture of the femur: "no fracture was considered too comminuted, no patient was considered too old and no femur was deemed too osteoporotic for this method of treatment." Giles et al. reported in 1982 on the use of a supracondylar lag screw and side plate for fixation of 26 supracondylar/intracondylar fractures of the distal femur.[16] They felt that "the advantages of this device over others, are that the lag screw supplies not only interfragmentary compression across the intracondylar fractured surfaces, but also better purchase in osteopenic bone," allowing earlier aggressive restoration of knee motion and muscle power. In their series there were no nonunions and no infections, and their average postoperative range of motion was 120°, which compared very favorably with other reported series of similar fractures. In conclusion, they felt that "meticulous open reduction and stable internal fixation of supracondylar fractures with supracondylar plate and lag screw, combined with autogenous bone grafting in patients with severe comminution, provide an excellent opportunity to secure bone union and restore limb alignment, joint congruity and range of motion." Similar excellent results with the use of this device have been reported by Hall,[18] Pritchett,[38] Regazzoni et al.,[39] and Sanders et al.[41]

Brown and D'Arcy reported on the use of a nail plate with an adapted additional medial compression plate to provide stable fixation on both sides of the femoral condyles.[8] They recommended this technique to obtain better fixation in the elderly osteoporotic patient; in their series, all but one patient obtained knee flexion better than 55°, and the average time to walking was only four weeks.

The use of bone cement as an adjunct to stable internal fixation in osteoporotic femurs for supracondylar fractures was advocated by Benum in 1977.[4] He reviewed 14 patients with an average age of 75 years. Eight-six percent (12 patients) healed uneventfully, despite early mobilization. The two failures were the result of technical error in the application of the plate and not of loosening of the screw from the bone cement.

Sanders et al. reported on the use of double plate fixation for complicated, comminuted, intraarticular fractures of the distal femur; union was obtained in all patients.[42]

ASSESSMENT FOR SURGERY

In assessing any patient for surgery, it is important to assess not only the "personality" of the fracture, but also the personality of the patient. Many of the supracondylar/intracondylar fractures occur in younger patients as a result of high-energy trauma and are often associated with multisystem injuries. Careful assessment of the patient using a team approach is necessary, whether this consists of members of general and other surgical disciplines (for the polytraumatized patient) or members of the internal medicine disciplines (for the elderly or geriatric patient). Consultation with these colleagues will optimize preparation and timing if surgical intervention is indicated. Patient factors in deciding between operative and nonoperative treatment must include age, activity level, medical condition, hemodynamic status, the presence of infection, ipsilateral or contralateral injuries, the etiology of the injury (high or low velocity), and the "personality" of the distal femoral fracture itself. However, deciding that both the patient and the fracture are candidates for surgery is not sufficient. It is important that the potential surgeon honestly assess his or her own expertise in the management of these difficult problems. This should include a clear understanding of the pathomechanics and morphology of the fracture, necessary practical experience, equipment, and knowledgeable operating personnel and assistants. In further assessing the personality of the fracture itself, it is essential to appreciate the following objectives of the operative management of periarticular fractures:

1. Anatomic reconstitution of the articular surface
2. Reduction of the metaphyseal component of the fracture to the diaphysis, with restoration of normal axial alignment, length, and rotation
3. Stable internal fixation
4. Early motion and functional rehabilitation of the limb

Schatzker and Lambert have shown that the mere use of an optimal implant alone is not sufficient to guarantee a good result with these difficult fractures.[44] If the preceding objectives cannot be obtained by surgical intervention, either because of the complexity of the fracture or because of the lack of equipment or skill of the surgical team, then conservative treatment is preferable to the complications of poor surgery followed by prolonged immobilization.

INDICATIONS FOR SURGERY

Absolute Indications

Displaced Intraarticular Fractures

In displaced intraarticular fractures, joint congruity cannot be restored by closed methods. These fractures include unicondylar and bicondylar fractures.

Unicondylar Fractures (Type B). Because of the pull of the gastrocnemius muscle, most unicondylar fractures are displaced by posterior rotation of the condyle relative to the knee joint axis. As a result, there is joint incongruity, and anatomic reduction is mandatory to prevent long-term axial malalignment and posttraumatic arthritis. These are exceptionally difficult to reduce by closed means and in most cases require open reduction and anatomic reconstitution. Of particular importance is the BIII or coronal fracture (Hoffa), where the only soft tissue attachment is the posterior capsule, which behaves like a large loose fragment in the joint. Traction and closed means will have no effect on the reduction of this fracture, and surgical intervention is necessary.

Bicondylar Fractures (Type C). The predominant deforming force on the condyles is the gastrocnemius muscles, which cause posterior angulation and rotation. This is compounded by the shortening and anterior displacement of the shaft caused by the unrestrained pull of the quadriceps and hamstring muscles. Traction, if performed early, can generally correct the shortening, but in most cases, even flexion of the knee will not correct the rotational displacement of the condyles relative to each other. If joint congruity cannot be restored by closed means, the only viable option is surgery. Only in this way can an accurate anatomic reduction of the articular surface be accomplished.

Open Fractures

All open fractures require aggressive surgical debridement. The controversial issue concerns whether open reduction and internal fixation should be performed at that time. Most would agree that joint congruity should be restored immediately. This can be accomplished in most cases by limited internal fixation of the condyles. Whether stable internal fixation of the condyles to the shaft should be performed primarily, however, remains controversial. Experimental and clinical evidence suggests that the rate of sepsis can be decreased by stabilizing the bony skeleton and hence the surrounding soft tissues.[28] Experience and clinical judgment is required, as each of these injuries must be individualized by assessing the whole patient, the associated injury, the energy and type of fracture involved, the degree of contamination of the soft tissue injury, the adequacy of the debridement, and the ability of the surgery to stabilize the bony skeleton without further devascularization of the already compromised bone and soft tissue. In grade I and most grade II soft tissue injuries, after adequate debridement of all contaminated and devitalized bone and soft tissue, stabilization of the reduced condyles to the shaft can be performed in a standard fashion. However, it is essential to leave the injury wound open and return the patient to the operating room within 48 hours for redebridement repeatedly until the soft tissues can be safely closed. The most difficult problems are the grade III fractures, which are often associated with high-energy bone and soft tissue injury and significant contamination. Absolute and aggressive debridement of all contaminated and devitalized soft tissues and bone is mandatory. Copious irrigation should be performed with 9 to 12 L of irrigating solution, followed by restitution of the articular condyles with minimal internal fixation. At this stage, the treating surgeon has two options: (1) stable internal fixation of the condyles to the shaft, and (2) stabilization of the bony skeleton and the soft tissues by applying an external fixator across the knee joint (probably a safer option). The latter will allow immediate stabilization of the bone and soft tissues and permit adequate access, debridement, and care of the wounds. Eventual control of the soft tissues is obtained by either delayed primary closure of the wound or some additional soft tissue procedure for wound coverage. Once there is adequate control of the soft tissue, delayed internal fixation restoring the condyles to the shaft can be performed.

Associated Vascular Compromise

Injury to the superficial femoral artery in the adductor canal or popliteal artery in the popliteal fossa associated with a distal femoral fracture is a true orthopedic limb-threatening emergency. If reconstitution of blood flow to the distal extremity is not accomplished within 6 hours of the injury, the chance for successful limb salvage decreases exponentially with greater delay. Timing of the vascular repair relative to the stable fixation of the fracture is critical. Optimally, the wound should be debrided, if open, and the rapid but stable internal fixation performed prior to the vascular repair. If the vascular repair is done prior to bony stabilization, manipulation of the extremity and fracture fragments can disrupt the repair. If the debridement and skeletal stabilization will require a delay of more than 6 hours following the injury, Johansen et al. have recommended using a temporary arterial shunt to restore flow. This will afford sufficient time for adequate debridement and skeletal stabilization without compromising salvage of the extremity.[21]

Ipsilateral Fractures of the Tibial Shaft

An ipsilateral fracture of the tibia associated with femoral fractures is a well-described injury complex — "the floating knee." The best method of restoring knee motion and function in these severe injuries is by surgical fixation of both sides of the knee joint.

Ipsilateral Fractures of the Tibial Plateau

Ipsilateral fractures of the tibial plateau with an associated distal femoral fracture should be addressed like any complex intraarticular fracture (i.e., with anatomic reduction of the articular surface and stable internal fixation, allowing early functional mobilization).

Bilateral Femoral Fractures

Patients with bilateral femoral fractures do not tolerate traction well. Nursing care is extremely difficult, and functional rehabilitation is decidedly impaired. As a result, open reduction and internal fixation are indicated to allow patient mobilization.

The Polytraumatized Patient

The severely injured patient with multisystem involvement and an associated femur fracture is at significant risk of mortality and prolonged morbidity. Bone[7] has conclusively shown that stabilization of the femoral shaft within the first 24 hours decreases not only the mortality but also the significant morbidity. The incidence of multisystem organ failure and adult respiratory distress syndrome (ARDS), number of respirator and intensive care unit (ICU) days, and sepsis were all decreased by the immediate stabilization of the femoral shaft fracture. Conversely, traction and prolonged bed rest in patients with high Injury Severity Scores and multisystem trauma had a significant detrimental effect on mortality rate and long-term morbidity. In the polytraumatized patient, the same indications for early femoral shaft fracture stabilization and patient mobilization also apply to fractures of the distal femur.

Patients with distal femur fractures and associated head injuries represent a selected group of the polytrauma patient population. When there is coma or a decreased level of consciousness, often with associated spasticity, reduction is difficult to maintain with traction or closed means. Also, the avoidance of skin breakdown and joint contractures is particularly difficult. Early open reduction and internal fixation will facilitate nursing care and allow easier maintenance of skeletal alignment.

Patients with significant burns in addition to their femoral fractures require skilled nursing, frequent immersion in tubs, and multiple dressing changes. Treatment with closed methods and traction severely compromises the management of burns which are potentially life threatening. Once again, operative stabilization prior to burn colonization is the treatment of choice.

Pathologic Fractures

In pathologic fractures, especially with bone loss, healing cannot be expected to occur with treatment by closed means and prolonged immobilization. Surgical options will depend not only on the type of tumor (primary or metastatic) but also on the many patient factors, including medical status, life expectancy, and functional demands. Decision making will have to be individualized. Open reduction and internal fixation of pathologic distal femoral fractures is technically demanding, often requiring multiple forms of internal fixation and additional stabilization with methylmethacrylate.

Associated Ligamentous Disruption of the Knee Joint

Fractures of the distal femur with associated knee ligament disruptions require a stable distal femoral platform, not only for the repair or augmentation of ligaments, but also to allow functional aftercare and rehabilitation. This can only be accomplished by initial open reduction and internal fixation of the distal femur fracture.

Extraarticular Fractures in Which Reduction Cannot be Obtained or Maintained

Supracondylar extraarticular fractures that are displaced or markedly comminuted and in which axial alignment length or rotation cannot be restored or maintained by traditional closed means require open reduction and internal fixation.

Relative Indications

Patients in whom axial alignment, rotation, and length can be obtained or maintained by closed means are considered relative candidates for operative stabilization if they prefer to avoid the prolonged immobilization associated with closed treatment methods. However, the patient must be made aware of the risks and benefits of all treatment options.

Recent reports also indicate that elderly patients are candidates for operative intervention in the management of distal femur fractures.[20,36,39,41,42,44,47,63] However, the decision as to operative versus closed treatments must be based on the personality of both the patient and the fracture, as discussed previously. Stable fixation can often be obtained, especially if the surgeon is aware of all available techniques in the armamentarium, including the use of methylmethacrylate. Careful assessment of the degree of osteopenia and the amount of comminution is necessary to avoid operative intervention that is inadequate, necessitating prolonged traction or immobilization postoperatively. However, if stable fixation is achieved, the adverse effects of prolonged immobilization, especially in the elderly, can be avoided.

Contraindications

In the polytraumatized patient, orthopedic "tunnel vision" must be avoided. Consultation with the general surgery team leader is necessary to optimize the care of not only the orthopedic injury, but also the patient as a whole. If the patient is hemodynamically labile, is septic, or has severely contaminated soft tissues that cannot be debrided or are inadequately debrided, surgical stabilization of the orthopedic injury is contraindicated until these problems can be resolved.

Medical conditions, especially in the elderly, in which the anesthetic and operative risks are potentially life threatening (e.g., as in an associated myocardial infarction), are obvious contraindications to surgical intervention for return of function to a limb.

Massive comminution of the fracture or very severe osteopenia (e.g., a paralyzed limb) should be considered contraindications, as the chances of obtaining stable fixation from operative intervention are not very good. These fractures are probably better treated by closed methods.

It is mandatory that the surgeon evaluate the complexity of the injury, and make an honest appraisal of his or her experience, the ability of the team to deal with such technically demanding fractures, and the facilities available. If any of these factors are found to be lacking, the patient is best served by treatment with closed methods.

Principles of Surgical Treatment

PREOPERATIVE PLANNING

Preoperative planning is essential to help the surgeon anticipate the potential problems associated with the operative fixation of all fractures, especially the more complex periarticular fractures. This lesson was brought home during my fellowship with Professor Maurice Müller in Bern. Even though a founder of the AO school and with more than 30 years experience in the treatment of complex fractures, Dr. Müller drew his own preoperative plan prior to surgery on every case. This philosophy has subsequently been expanded by Mast et al. in an excellent treatise on planning and reduction techniques.[27]

The planning technique is relatively simple and can usually be accomplished within 10 minutes (Fig. 47–7). Tracings are made on tracing paper of the uninvolved or opposite femur, both in the AP and the lateral plane. These are then turned over to form templates for the involved extremity. Tracings are made of all the fracture fragments on the involved side, both in the AP and the lateral plane. These fragments are individually reduced and drawn in different colors on the tracing of the normal femur. This will demonstrate the amount of comminution and whether bone defects are present. At this stage, the planned internal fixation can be drawn from transparent templates that are obtainable from Synthes, USA (Paoli, Pennsylvania). By using the templates, the need for and position of temporary fixation with Kirschner wires, the optimal location and angle for lag screws, the type and size of plates required, the angle of the screws in the plate (to avoid fracture lines on the opposite side), the necessity for bone graft based on comminution or defect, and the need for adjunctive fixation (e.g., methylmethacrylate) can be determined. On the final drawing showing the reduction of the fracture lines and the composite fixation, a "surgical tactic" that lists the steps of the procedure "by the numbers" should also be developed.

The advantages of careful preoperative planning cannot be sufficiently stressed. It allows the surgeon to study the fracture more carefully and understand its particular morphology and what will be required to obtain reduction. This ensures that all equipment and implants required for the procedure will be available in the operating room, thus avoiding having to compromise the fixation. The delays of intraoperative indecision and the waiting for instruments and implants, which often prolong open wound time, will decrease, as will the infection rate. By comparing the postoperative result with the preoperative plan, the surgeon has a readily available method to assess results and to help with quality control.

Timing of Surgery

The operative management of fractures of the distal femur, particularly when comminuted or intraarticular, is very demanding. Surgery should not be undertaken, especially at night, without adequate preoperative evaluation and the availability of an experienced team, including assistants, nurses, and the necessary equipment. In certain situations, however, immediate emergency surgery is indicated (i.e., open fractures or fractures with vascular impairment).

Optimally, it is preferable to undertake this kind of procedure following careful evaluation of the patient and the fracture and good preoperative planning, thus assuring that the required equipment is available and the desired end result can be achieved. Surgery should be performed within the first 24 to 48 hours after the injury. In patients with a high Injury Severity Score, stabilization of the femur within the first 24 hours of the injury has definitely been shown to decrease the significant morbidity associated with these multiple injuries. However, the condition of the patient and asso-

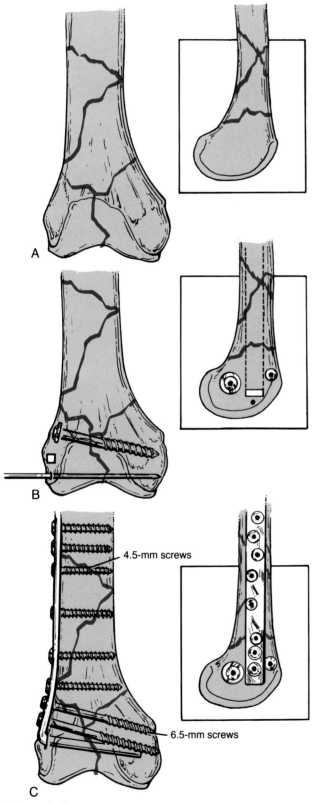

Figure 47–7

Preoperative planning. *A,* The fracture lines reduced. *B,* Position for insertion of lag screws, summation Kirschner wire, and the 95° condylar blade. *C,* Final plan with the fracture reduced and position and fixation of all hardware.

4.5-mm screws

6.5-mm screws

ciated injuries might prohibit surgery during this optimal period. In open fractures, discretion is necessary to determine whether and what type of internal fixation is indicated at the time of the initial debridement.

Successful management of the soft tissue envelope is the key to avoiding the major complications associated with surgical intervention and internal fixation. Decision making as to the timing of definitive internal fixation and the optimal management of the soft tissues is one of the hardest aspects to teach in the treatment of these fractures. The surgeon must use his or her own experience, good clinical judgment, and, if necessary, consultation with others in order to optimize this timing. Delay of definitive stabilization for three weeks or more makes the surgery much more difficult. The limb often remains malreduced and shortened, early callus forms, and the fracture lines lose their clear demarcation, especially in the cancellous bone. This makes exposure and reduction technically more demanding.

If surgery is to be delayed more than a few hours, the limb should be treated as if closed treatment were being used definitively. A tibial traction pin should be inserted at least 10 cm below the tibial tubercle to avoid the potential operative field. The patient is then placed in balanced suspended traction in a Thomas splint, with a Pearson attachment flexed at approximately 20° to 30°. The weight of the traction should be sufficient to correct length (generally between 15 and 30 pounds). This will greatly facilitate future manipulation of the fracture fragments at the time of surgical reduction, allowing the use of indirect techniques with less exposure and soft tissue stripping at the time of stable internal fixation.

PRINCIPLES OF SURGICAL TECHNIQUE

Principles of surgical treatment include the following:
1. Careful handling of soft tissues.
2. Indirect reduction techniques to preserve as much vascularity as possible to the fracture fragments.
3. Anatomic reduction of the articular surface and restoration of limb axial alignment, rotation, and length.
4. Stable internal fixation, with bone grafting of defects where vascularity is impaired or where there is significant comminution.
5. Early active functional rehabilitation of the patient and the limb.

Treatment Options

EARLY FRACTURE BRACING/CAST BRACING

Impacted supracondylar fractures that do not have intracondylar extension can, in most cases, be reliably stabilized immediately in a knee immobilizer con-

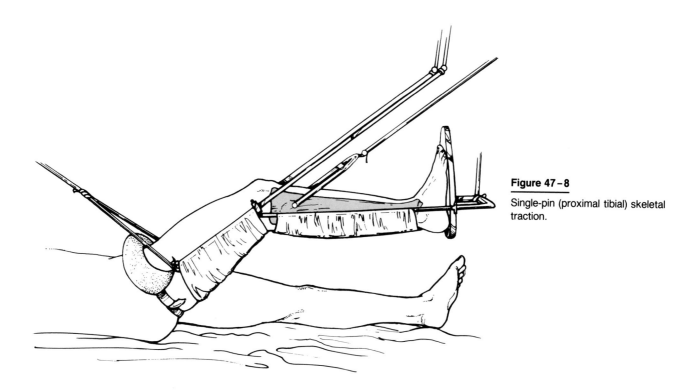

Figure 47-8

Single-pin (proximal tibial) skeletal traction.

verted to a fracture brace/cast brace once pain and swelling have decreased. Care must be taken to monitor progress until union, as the powerful muscles of the thigh can easily cause angulation or displacement. It is probably wiser to start treatment with the patient in skeleton traction to allow the swelling to decrease and the fracture to become "sticky," making for a better cast/brace application and less likelihood of displacement in the future.

TRACTION

Traction can be used for the treatment of Müller type AII and AIII supracondylar femur fractures as long as it is possible to restore limb axial alignment, rotation, and length. Commonly, this is skeletal traction with one pin placed 10 cm below the tibial tubercle and the leg maintained in a Thomas splint with a Pearson attachment at the level of the fracture flexed about 20° to 30° (Fig. 47–8). This requires immobilization of the patient and maintenance of the traction from 2 to 12 weeks, depending on the fracture. Manipulation can be performed under anesthesia to obtain reduction if traction alone is not successful. In the present era of diagnosis-related groups (DRGs), low-risk anesthesia, and better surgical implants and techniques, most surgeons would opt for surgical stabilization and early active mobilization. However, medical complications, the age of the patient, the functional demands of the patient, and local factors such as excessive comminution

or the inability to adequately control soft tissue injury make the option of traction more favorable. Occasionally, the use of two-pin traction, with the second pin through the femoral condyles, may provide a better configuration with which to obtain a more favorable reduction (Fig. 47–9). However, this technique adds significant risks to traction treatment (i.e., the potential for vascular impairment from the pin insertion and also intraarticular and fracture sepsis if the condylar pin develops a pin track infection).

Prolonged joint immobilization with traction will result in intraarticular adhesions and fibrosis and scarring of the quadriceps musculature. Thus active flexion and extension of the knee, even in traction, must be encouraged as soon as pain tolerance will allow. Excessive or prolonged traction is obviously detrimental to the functional rehabilitation of the patient and the extremity. As such, Connolly,[13] Mooney,[32] and others[31a,39a] have advocated the use of early cast bracing for the management of femoral and supracondylar fractures. In most cases, traction can be converted to cast brace treatment at three to eight weeks even without radiographic evidence of early healing.

DELAYED CAST BRACING

The main indication for cast bracing is in a delayed fashion, as a subsequent stage of treatment. The patient has been treated with traction, traditionally for from 6 to 12 weeks, and when there are sufficient signs of early

Figure 47–9

Double-pin (proximal tibial and distal femoral) skeletal traction.

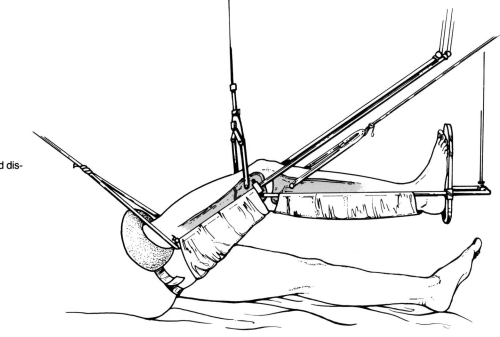

healing, a cast brace is applied. Connolly,[13] Mooney,[32] and others have reported that earlier progression from traction to cast bracing (i.e., at two to three weeks) prevents the sequelae of prolonged traction immobilization and gives good results. This requires experience, not only an understanding of the pathomechanics of the fracture but also a knowledge of the technique of successful cast brace application. Optimally, patients should be administered a general anesthetic or an intravenous (IV) sedative. When applying the cast brace, the knee should be extended with 20° of external rotation and slight valgus angulation of the leg. Knee extension will counteract the posterior displacement and angulation of the condyles. The external rotation and valgus force counteracts the common varus deformity seen after prolonged traction. The stability of the cast brace is greatly enhanced by careful molding around the femoral condyles distally and by sufficient proximal control above the fracture site. A longer thigh and a more slender habitus improve the control provided by a long-leg fracture brace. Although plaster is easier to mold, fiberglass cast material is lighter and more durable. Combining the two is an often helpful compromise.

SURGERY

Surgical Exposure

The patient is placed supine on a fluoroscopy table, a tourniquet is applied to the proximal thigh, and the ipsilateral iliac crest and the whole lower extremity below the tourniquet are prepped in a sterile fashion. (If there is proximal extension of the fracture above the supracondylar area, the whole lower extremity, including the thigh, must be draped free. Then, if necessary, a sterile tourniquet can be used.)

The majority of fractures of the distal femur can be approached through a single lateral incision (Fig. 47-10). The incision is made directly lateral in the thigh and through the midpoint of the lateral condyle distally, staying anterior to the proximal insertion of the lateral collateral ligament. Proximally the incision is extended as necessary for diaphyseal involvement of the supracondylar fracture. The distal incision can be extended, curving from the knee joint axis gently anteriorly to the lateral border of the tibial tubercle, when there is associated intracondylar fracture involvement. The fascia lata is incised in line with the skin incision and its fibers. Distally it is often necessary to incise the anterior fibers of the iliotibial tract, and the incision is then carried down through the capsule and synovium on the lateral aspect of the lateral femoral condyle. Care must be taken to identify the superior lateral geniculate

artery, which often requires ligation, and to avoid damage distally to the lateral meniscus. By placing a blunt Hohmann retractor across the joint and over the medial femoral condyle and retracting gently, easy visualization of the articular surfaces of the medial and lateral femoral condyle can be obtained. This is necessary even in type A supracondylar femur fractures in order to insert the Kirschner guide wires prior to stable fixation. To expose the distal femoral shaft, the vastus lateralis muscle must be reflected off the lateral intermuscular septum. Care must be taken to identify and ligate perforating vessels. It is only necessary to expose enough of the lateral cortex to apply the plate. Avoid any additional unnecessary soft tissue stripping or the careless insertion of anterior or posterior retractors.

Occasionally in the type CIII distal femur fractures, when there is intercondylar comminution, more extensive exposure is necessary in order to increase the intra-articular exposure. Mize et al. recommended accomplishing this with a tibial tubercle osteotomy.[30] The distal incision is extended inferiorly and medially, exposing the tibial tuberosity. A 3.2-mm drill hole is made in the middle of the tibial tuberosity from anterior to posterior tibial cortex. The depth is measured, and the near cortex is tapped with the 6.5-mm tap. Using a fine oscillating saw, the tibial tuberosity is osteotomized with a piece of bone approximately 1.5 × 3 × 0.5 cm. Because the tibial tuberosity bone block and infrapatellar tendon are reflected proximally, it is necessary to detach the fat pad from the tibia. This provides exposure of the whole articular distal end of the femur. If further medial exposure is necessary, the supracondylar synovium can be incised, and then the whole quadriceps mechanism can be reflected proximally and medially. This will provide enough exposure if an additional medial plating is indicated. At closure, the tibial tubercle bone block is replaced into its bed and fixed with the appropriate length 6.5-mm cancellous screw.

An alternate method for an extensive exposure of the distal femoral articular surface is a Z infrapatellar tenotomy. This technique, however, requires not only repair of the infrapatellar tendon, but also protection of the repair with an anterior wire tension band from the patella to the tibial tubercle.

Occasionally a medial exposure to the distal femur is indicated, primarily for the open reduction and internal fixation of type BII unicondylar medial femoral condyle fractures. However, it is also used in conjunction with lateral exposure when double plating of the distal femur is indicated for severe supracondylar comminution or bone defects requiring additional medial stabilization or for complex combined supracondylar

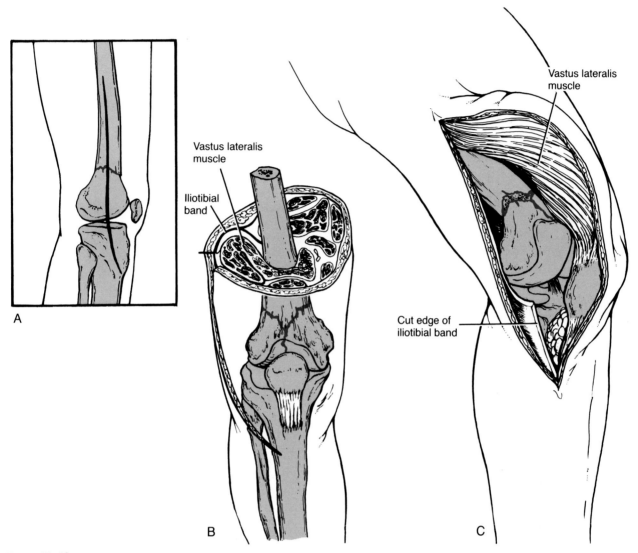

Figure 47–10

Lateral exposure of the distal femur. *A*, Lateral skin incision. *B*, Demonstration of the lateral incision for femoral exposure posterior to the vastus lateralis and anterior to the intermuscular septum. *C*, Extensive exposure is possible, but care must be taken not to strip the soft tissues unnecessarily.

and intracondylar type CIII distal femur fractures. The incision is straight medial just anterior to the adductor tubercle and mid medial in the thigh. The deep fascia is incised in the same line as the skin incision. The vastus medialis is reflected anteriorly off the adductor magnus, exposing the distal medial shaft of the femur. Care must be taken to identify the superior medial geniculate artery; often this has to be ligated. The incision must remain anterior to the proximal insertion of the superficial medial collateral ligament on the adductor tubercle. For complete exposure of the medial femoral condyle, the medial patellar retinaculum and capsule are incised, taking care to avoid damage to medial meniscus. The major risk with medial exposure is damage to the femoral artery and vein as they pierce the adductor magnus one handbreadth above the knee joint to enter the popliteal space.

Of the three extensile exposures available and just described, the most widely used is the tibial tubercle osteotomy. However, a recent review by Sanders et al. suggests an additional medial incision, which has the lowest morbidity and requires the least additional soft tissue dissection and stripping.[42]

Fracture Reduction and Stabilization

Because of the diversity of fracture types encountered in the distal femur, it is necessary to discuss first the basic techniques available for reduction and stabilization and then specific applications for each fracture type.

95° Condylar Blade Plate

For illustrative purposes the fracture type CI is selected (T or Y supracondylar fracture with intracondylar extension). The incision is the standard lateral as described. The initial step must be anatomic reduction of the condyles, both the distal articular surface and the patellar femoral groove. This is provisionally secured with temporary 2.0-mm Kirschner wire fixation from lateral to medial.

The next step is the insertion of the 95° condylar blade plate (Fig. 47–11). The length of the blade and side plate are determined by the preoperative planning, as described previously. The position for insertion of the blade plate is 1.5 cm to 2 cm from the inferior articular surface and in the middle third of the anterior half of the sagittal diameter of the condyles at their widest point (Fig. 47–12). This can be determined by palpating the posterior edge of the lateral femoral condyle while visualizing the anterior margin. At its broadest point, the distance is divided in two. Divide the anterior half of this distance in three; the middle third is

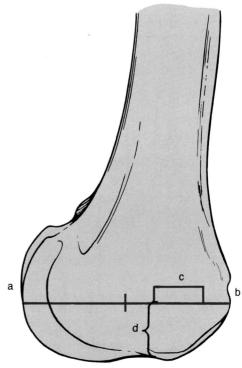

Figure 47–12

Position for insertion of the 95° condylar blade plate in the lateral cortex of the distal femur. *a* to *b*, Longest sagittal diameter on the lateral femoral condyle. *c*, Middle third of the anterior half. *d*, 1.5 to 2 cm proximal to the articular surface.

the location for the insertion of the blade and should be marked with the cautery. This must be determined exactly in order to correctly realign the condyles and articular surface with the femoral shaft. The blade must be inserted in line with the longest sagittal diameter, so that the plate, which is perpendicular, correctly restores the relationship between condyles and shaft and lies along the shaft, on the lateral view, rather than with its proximal end too anteriorly or posteriorly.

Next is the lag screw fixation of the condyles to each other. This is generally accomplished with 6.5-mm cancellous screws, one anteriorly and one posteriorly. Only by the prior marking of the place for the insertion of the seating chisel can the lag screws be assured to not interfere with the subsequent insertion of the 95° condylar blade plate. Both 6.5-mm cancellous screws should be inserted slightly proximally to the level of insertion of the blade plate (see Fig. 47–7). The anterior screw is inserted in a slightly anterior to posterior direction from lateral to medial, just inferiorly laterally to the most anterior aspect of the patellar femoral group. This anterior 6.5-mm cancellous screw should be inserted without a washer to assure that it does not interfere with the patellofemoral mechanism. The posterior screw is also inserted slightly proximally to the

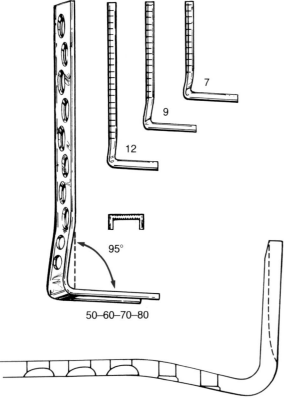

Figure 47–11

The 95° condylar blade plate. Blade lengths range from 50 to 80 mm; plate lengths, from 92 mm (5 holes) to 299 mm (18 holes).

insertion of the blade and just anterior to the proximal insertion of the lateral collateral ligament. It should be inserted in a slightly posterior to anterior direction to avoid penetrating the intracondylar notch and should be inserted with a washer. It is important that both screws act as lag screws (i.e., their threads must all be on the far side of the fracture and neither should penetrate the medial cortex), or long-term pain and disability can result from interference with medial structures with knee movement.

Once the condyles are anatomically reduced and internally fixed, it is then necessary to realign the condyles, the articular surface of the distal femur, to the femoral shaft. This is done by inserting the blade plate correctly into the condyles and then using it to reduce and stabilize the fracture. Two temporary Kirschner wires are placed as guides for the insertion of the seating chisel of the 95° condylar blade plate (Fig. 47–13). Kirschner wire no. 1 is inserted across the knee joint parallel to the inferior aspect of the medial and lateral condyles (i.e., the knee joint axis). Kirschner wire no. 2 is inserted anteriorly across the patellofemoral joint, sloping from anterior to posterior parallel to the condyles in the coronal plane (Fig. 47–14). The definitive Kirschner wire no. 3 is inserted approximately 1 cm proximal to the inferior aspect of the knee joint, just inferior to the area marked out on the lateral condyle for insertion of the seating chisel (see Fig. 47–13). Kirschner wire no. 3 must be parallel to both Kirschner

wires no. 1 and no. 2 and represents the definitive guide for insertion of the 95° condylar blade plate. It must therefore be parallel to Kirschner wire no. 1 in the frontal plane (see Fig. 47–13) and Kirschner wire no. 2 in the coronal plane (see Fig. 47–14). If inexperienced with this technique, it is a good idea to check the position of Kirschner wire no. 3, parallel to the knee joint axis in the frontal plane, with fluoroscopy. In fractures without supracondylar comminution, the position of the summation Kirschner wire no. 3 can also be checked with the condylar guide, which represents a mirror image of the condylar plate (Fig. 47–15). The provisional guide wires no. 1 and no. 2 are then removed.

In young patients with dense trabecular cancellous bone, it is necessary to predrill the condylar tract for the seating chisel. If this is not done, impaction of the seating chisel into the condyles can require tremendous force and as a result may disrupt the lag screw fixation of the condyles. Predrilling is easily accomplished by using a 4.5-mm drill bit and the appropriate triple guide. This triple guide is applied on the lateral condyle parallel to the summation Kirschner wire no. 3. Three 4.5-mm channels can be drilled out from lateral to medial in the previously marked window for insertion of the chisel. If uncertain, this can be checked on the fluoroscopy. The window in the lateral cortex is then expanded by using the router in the three 4.5-mm drill holes. To seat the condylar plate flush to the lateral

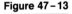

Figure 47–13

Position for insertion of alignment and summation Kirschner wires. Kirschner wire 1: inferiorly along the femoral condyles; Kirschner wire 2: anteriorly along the femoral condyles; and Kirschner wire 3 (summation): parallel to both 1 and 2 and inferior to the window for blade plate insertion.

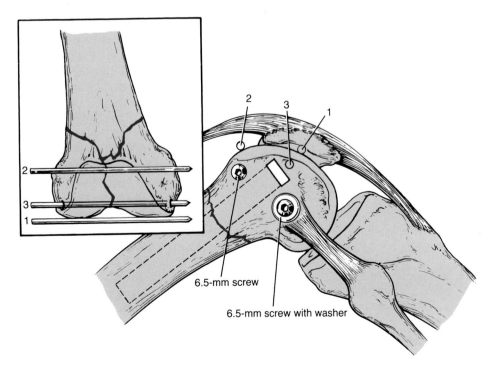

6.5-mm screw

6.5-mm screw with washer

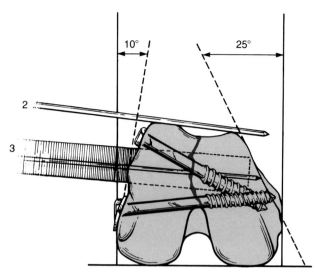

Figure 47-14

Coronal view of the distal femur demonstrating trapezoidal shape, the angle for the lag screws, and the position for the insertion of the chisel.

cortex in young patients, it is useful to bevel the proximal lip of the lateral window with an osteotome, removing approximately 0.5 cm of bone.

The seating chisel is assembled with the seating chisel guide. This allows assessment of flexion and extension in the sagittal plane as the chisel is inserted into the condyles. The seating chisel is then inserted into the

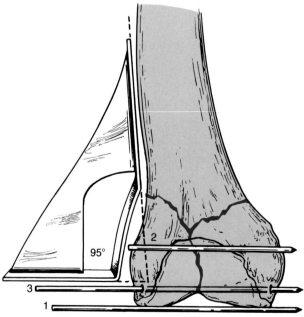

Figure 47-15

Use of the condylar guide for checking position of summation Kirschner wire 3.

condylar fragment, maintaining it parallel to Kirschner wire no. 3 both in the frontal and coronal planes, and assuring the correct rotation in the sagittal plane. The blade must remain parallel with the longest sagittal diameter of the condyles, as rotation will angulate the fracture on the lateral view. In young individuals with good bone, it is helpful to insert the chisel approximately 1 cm at a time and then back it out a few millimeters before continuing. This will greatly facilitate the ability to subsequently remove the seating chisel once fully inserted. Again, if inexperienced with this technique, the use of fluoroscopy will reassure the surgeon of the correct position for the seating chisel. The seating chisel is inserted to the predetermined depth. It should be appreciated that the distal femur is a trapezoid, with a 25° angle on the medial side from posterior to anterior (see Fig. 47-14); care must be taken not to penetrate the medial condylar cortex with the seating chisel. The 95° condylar blade plate is then inserted along the prepared tract in the femoral condyles and impacted to lie flush with the lateral cortex.

The shaft of the femur and fracture fragments (*if* present) are then reduced to the stabilized condylar fragment and held on the side plate with a Verbrugge clamp. Prior to placing the fracture under axial compression, it is necessary to stabilize the fixation of the condylar plate in the condyles. This is accomplished by the insertion of one or two 6.5-mm cancellous lag screws through the distal plate holes into the condylar fragment. This will not only enhance the rotational stability of the condylar fragment but also prevent lateral excursion of the blade with the application of axial compression. The latter is then accomplished by use of the tension device. (Occasionally, with no bony defect and an anatomic reduction, this can be accomplished by the use of loaded screws in the dynamic compression plate.) If at all possible, a lag screw should be inserted across the supracondylar fracture through the plate. This greatly enhances the stability of the fixation. When there is a bone defect or lack of cortical contact after fracture reduction, axial compression cannot be achieved without causing shortening.

The 95° angle condylar blade plate is indicated for most supracondylar and bicondylar distal femur fractures. However, it requires excellent purchase in the distal condyles to be efficacious. Distal fixation is achieved (1) by the contact of the broad surface of the blade and (2) by the addition of the distal cancellous lag screws through the plate into the condyles. In very low transcondylar fractures, especially in the elderly, distal fixation using the condylar blade plate will be inadequate, and an alternate method such as use of a condylar buttress plate might be indicated. If there is marked comminution of the lateral condyle or of the intercondylar area, adequate fixation distally of the blade will not be possible. This again is an indication for an alternate implant such as the condylar buttress plate.

Condylar Compression Screw and Side Plate

The condylar compression screw system has basically the same design as the 95° condylar blade plate, but the blade has been replaced by a cannulated compression screw system (Fig. 47 – 16). A significant advantage of the dynamic condylar screw over the 95° blade plate is the additional compression provided by the large condylar screw across the condyles. Technically this may be an easier device to use, as most surgeons are familiar with cannulated compression screw systems for the fixation of intertrochanteric hip fractures. It is easier to insert into the condyles than is the 95° blade plate for the following reasons:

1. It is a cannulated screw system inserted over a guide wire.

2. By using a power-driven triple reamer, which allows precutting of the path of the condylar screw, it eliminates the problems encountered in hammering the chisel into the condyles.

3. It eliminates the necessity to control flexion and extension in the sagittal plane when inserting the condylar screw, as this can be corrected by rotation of the screw and side plate.

The operative technique for the insertion of the dynamic condylar screw differs from that of the 95° blade plate only in the technique for insertion of the condylar screw. Again, three Kirschner wires are inserted. Kirschner wire no. 1 is inserted parallel to the knee joint axis, and Kirschner wire no. 2 is inserted parallel to the anterior patellofemoral articulation. The location on the lateral femoral condyle for insertion of the dynamic condylar screw differs slightly from that of the 95° blade plate, being approximately 2 cm from the inferior articular surface and at the junction of the anterior and middle thirds of the longest sagittal diameter of the lateral femoral condyle (Fig. 47 – 17). (This is just proximal to the posterior edge of the window for insertion of the 95° blade plate (see Fig. 47 – 12). The third guide wire becomes the definitive guide for the cannulated screw system. This 230-mm guide wire with a threaded tip is inserted into the premarked area on the lateral cortex parallel to both Kirschner wires 1 and 2 (Fig. 47 – 18). The condylar compression screw angle

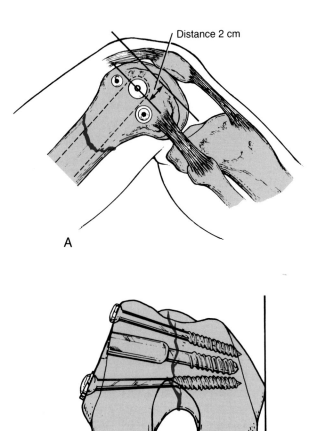

Distance 2 cm

A

B

Figure 47 – 17

Position for insertion of the condylar compression screw. *A,* Lateral view: junction of the anterior and middle thirds, 2 cm from the articular surface. *B,* Coronal view.

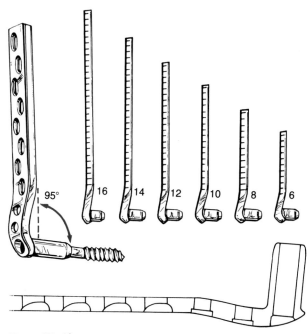

95°   16   14   12   10   8   6

Figure 47 – 16

The condylar compression screw system. The 95° angled side plate slides over a cannulated lag screw. Lag screw lengths range from 50 to 75 mm. Side plates (6 to 16 holes), from 113.5 mm to 273.5 mm.

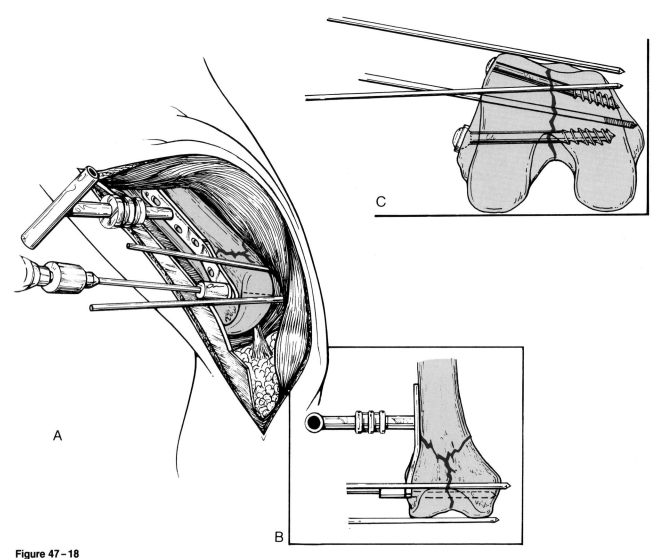

Figure 47–18

Technique for insertion of a threaded summation guide wire for placement of a condylar screw. *A*, Position for the condylar compression screw guide. *B*, AP view. *C*, Coronal view.

guide may be helpful when there is no supracondylar comminution. This angle guide is a mirror image of the side plate and is held against the lateral cortex with a T-handle chuck. Again, guide wire no. 3 is the definitive guide for the cannulated condylar screw system and must be inserted parallel to both Kirschner wires no. 1 and no. 2 so that it is parallel to the articular surface on the AP view and angled posteriorly to avoid the patellar articulation. This process is greatly facilitated, as in hip fracture surgery, by the use of fluoroscopy. The threaded guide wire should be inserted until the tip is felt to just penetrate the medial cortex (here fluoroscopy may be deceiving, as the posterior femoral condyles are broader than the anterior ones, especially on the medial side) (Fig. 47–19). A reverse calibrated

measuring device is placed over the guide wire to allow direct measurement of the length. The triple cannulated reamer is set for the desired length, which should be 10 mm less than the measurement to prevent penetration of the medial cortex. The channel is power reamed over the guide wire; again, this can be checked with fluoroscopy. In young patients with firm trabecular cancellous bone, a cannulated tap with a short centering sleeve is used. The cannulated compression screw of the correct length is connected to the T handle and wrench and inserted over the guide wire with the long centering sleeve (Fig. 47–20). It is inserted until the zero mark on the wrench is visible flush with the lateral cortex, and the handle of the inserter is parallel with the femoral shaft. In the elderly patient with po-

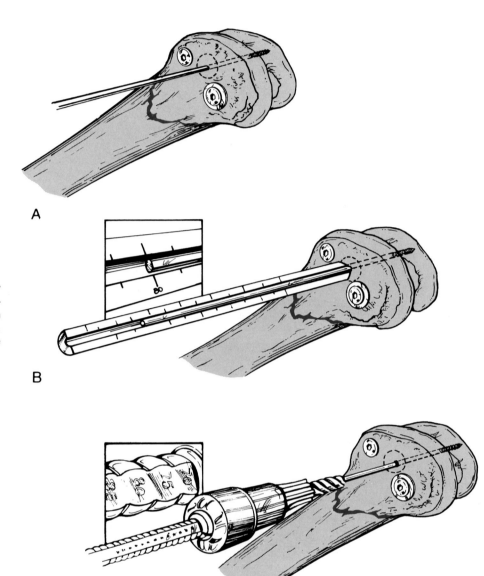

Figure 47–19

Technique for condylar screw measurement of length and cannulated reaming. *A*, Final position of threaded summation guide wire. *B*, Measurement of length. *C*, Use of the triple-cannulated reamer.

A

B

C

rotic bone, the condylar screw can be inserted an extra 5 mm beyond the prereamed channel to obtain better fixation. The appropriate length side plate is then slid over the condylar screw and keyed to align with the proximal femur in the sagittal plane. The remainder of the technique is similar to that described for the 95° angle blade plate.

Condylar Buttress Plate

The condylar buttress plate was designed to allow multiple lag screw fixation of complex condylar fractures. It consists of a broad compression side plate and a bifurcated precontoured distal portion to fit the lateral surface of the femoral condyle (Fig. 47–21). The posterior projection is broader and longer than the anterior in order to fit the larger posterior aspect of the femoral condyle, thus necessitating different plates for the right and left. It allows insertion of six interfragmentary lag screws through the distal portion of the plate for fixation of the condyles. However, this device is not a fixed angle device and therefore does not maintain correct axial alignment of the joint axis. It should be used only when the fracture morphology does not allow the use of either the 95° angle plate or the condylar screw. Its primary indications are (1) very low transcondylar fractures or comminuted fractures of the lateral or medial condyles in which stable fixation with a fixed angle device is not possible; and (2) coronal or very comminuted articular fractures in which screw fixation of the condyles precludes insertion of a fixed angle device.

The condylar buttress plate should be part of the armamentarium available for the fixation of all distal

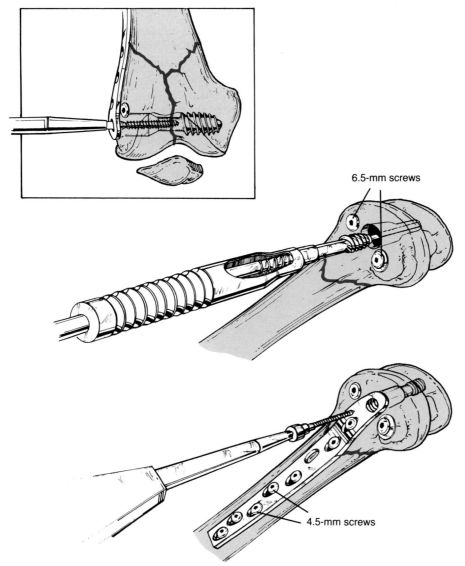

Figure 47–20

Technique for insertion of the condylar lag screw and side plate. *A*, Insertion of the condylar lag screw to desired length. *B*, Insertion of the set screw after side plate fixation. *C*, AP view showing condylar screw threads engaging the medial fragment only to ensure that it compresses the fracture as a lag screw.

6.5-mm screws

4.5-mm screws

femur fractures, even the most simple, in case intraoperative complications make the use of one of the fixed angle devices impossible. The most common mistake is to lag the condyles to the condylar buttress plate in a valgus position. This should be carefully checked intraoperatively with radiographs or fluoroscopy.

Since the condylar buttress plate is not a fixed angle device, it cannot guarantee axial alignment, especially in the frontal plane. This is especially problematic when there is comminution in the supracondylar region. One of the major long-term deforming forces on fixation of fractures of the distal femur remains the tendency for the condyles to drift into varus angulation. This is a problem especially with the use of the condylar buttress plate, as the individual lag screws are not fixed to the plate and can shift their angulation relative to it. This is much more likely to happen when

there is supracondylar comminution or bone loss. To avoid the tendency of the fracture to drift into varus angulation in these cases, a medial buttressing plate and bone graft for long-term medial support are indicated.[42] This can readily be accomplished following the lateral fixation through a separate small medial incision.

Intramedullary Nail Fixation

Interlocking Intramedullary Reamed Nail. It is now possible to stabilize supracondylar femur fractures with an interlocking intramedullary reamed nail. It is essential to obtain two interlocking screws in the distal fragment, and most authors recommend that the fracture be at least 10 cm from the joint line. Careful evaluation of the intracondylar area is necessary to assure that there is no undetected intracondylar fracture line. This

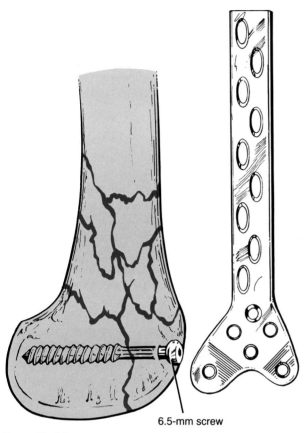

6.5-mm screw

Figure 47–21

The condylar buttress plate must be used when sagittally directed lag screws are required to fix coronal fracture planes.

procedure is much more technically demanding than standard femoral shaft intramedullary nailing and requires a great deal of experience with intramedullary nailing of femoral fractures. Intraoperatively, attention must be directed to maintaining axial alignment, length, and rotation. This is especially important when the procedure is done on a fracture table with the patient in the lateral decubitus position, as the tendency is then to fix the distal fragment in an externally rotated and valgus position. If at all possible, the supine position using a distal femoral traction pin is preferable for distal femoral fractures, and specific attention must be paid to maintaining alignment with nail insertion. Bucholz et al. have reported on nail breakage in distal femur fractures, especially through the distal interlocking screw holes.[10] The majority occurred after intramedullary nailing with interlocking was used for distal femur fractures. Thus they cautioned about its use when there was significant comminution or for very low fractures.

Supracondylar Zickle Fixation System. Zickle et al. described, in 1977, a new intramedullary system for the fixation of supracondylar femur fractures.[62] It consists of medial and lateral 11-inch proximal tapered intramedullary rods, both allowing a distal cross-condylar compression screw that locks into the nail. The medial and lateral appliances differ only in the angle of the distal cross-screw tunnel, the lateral at 90° to the longitudinal axis and the medial at 75°. The two preshaped rods are inserted through the medial and lateral femoral condyles by separate medial and lateral incisions into the proximal femoral medullary canal. The cross-compression screws are then inserted into the distal condylar ends anchoring the rods, providing, if necessary, additional fixation for intercondylar fractures. Zickle et al. stated that the device was "ideally suited for transverse supracondylar fractures," but felt that it was also able to stabilize "oblique, 'T', and high fractures."[62] (See Fig. 46–34.) Its use is primarily indicated for elderly osteopenic patients in whom screw fixation would be suboptimal.

Rush Pin Fixation. Rush[40] and Shelbourne and Brueckmann[47] reported on the use of medial and lateral Rush nails for the stabilization of supracondylar and intracondylar fractures of the distal femur. Even though this technique has often been condemned for not providing adequate fixation, the authors felt that this was mainly the result of improper technique. In order for this technique to be efficacious, the fracture has to be reduced using closed methods prior to the insertion of Rush rods. A 2.5-cm incision is made over each condyle and a 4.8-mm awl, using image intensification, is inserted into the condyle just proximal to the medial or lateral articular margin. Two 4.8-mm Rush pins of sufficient length are appropriately contoured and then inserted distally across the fracture into the femoral diaphysis until they contact the opposite inner cortex of the femur. This should be confirmed with fluoroscopy. The "sled runner" tip of the rod is positioned so that it will glide along the femoral cortex, and the rods are then tapped in alternately. This technique may, however, require additional fixation with cerclage wires when there is significant obliquity or comminution of the fracture.

Ender Nails. Another implant available for the stabilization of supracondylar femur fractures is the use of flexible Ender nails. The technique for the insertion of medial and lateral Ender nails is similar to that for inserting Rush rods. However, fracture reduction has to be accomplished prior to the insertion of the nails. An advantage of Ender nails over Rush rods is their ability to obtain additional fixation in the condyles by the insertion of 3.5-mm screws through the distal eyelets of the rods. Browner et al. have also described antegrade (proximal to distal) Ender nailing for some supracondylar femur fractures.[9]

Further details of the techniques, indications, complications, and results of the use of intramedullary fixation for femur and supracondylar femur fractures can be obtained from chapter 46.

External Fixation

The external fixator is used in the management of fractures of the distal femur not to treat the bony injury, but rather to treat the soft tissues. In patients with significant open, contaminated wounds or burns, or in those who are septic, the use of a temporary external fixator across the knee joint will allow adequate access and management of the soft tissues. It will also facilitate nursing care and patient mobilization.

The proximal 4.5-mm half pins are placed laterally in the femoral shaft and the distal 4.5-mm half pins are placed anteriorly in the tibial shaft. Care must be taken to make sure the pins are sufficiently proximal and distal so that even if they become infected, they will not compromise later surgical exposure of the distal femur.

Using bar-to-bar connectors, it is then possible to connect the proximal and distal pins across the knee joint. This system will allow adequate temporary stabilization of the supracondylar component and the knee joint. However, if there is articular condyle displacement, limited articular surface reconstruction and lag screw fixation, in addition to the external fixation, are probably indicated, and should be done as early as possible in the care of the patient. Screws for this purpose should be placed in a way that will not interfere with future definitive internal fixation, as described previously.

Specific Techniques and Recommendations for Open Reduction and Internal Fixation of Various Fracture Types

Because of the tremendous diversity of fractures encountered in the distal femur, specific techniques are required for their stabilization. The fracture types will be discussed according to the Müller classification. The fixation described will be that recommended and used by the author.

TYPE A FRACTURES

The extraarticular distal femur fractures are subdivided into type A1 (noncomminuted), type A2 (metaphyseal wedge) fractures, and type A3 (comminuted) fractures. These are best stabilized with a fixed angle device, either the 95° condylar blade plate or the dynamic condylar screw. In type A1 fractures, temporary reduc-

tion of the supracondylar component can be obtained by the use of crossed Kirschner wires. In types A2 and A3 fractures, it is important to preserve the vascularity of all the fracture fragments. To accomplish the supracondylar reduction and fixation without unnecessary devascularization, the indirect techniques proposed by Mast et al. should be used.[27] The condylar fragment is stabilized and the 95° blade plate or condylar screw is inserted as previously described. Additional lag screws are required in the distal plate holes to stabilize the implant to the condylar fragment. If there is only a small malreduction or limited comminution in the supracondylar region, distraction for fracture reduction can be obtained by using the tension device in the reversed mode. The tension device is fixed to the femoral shaft with a 4.5-mm cortical screw, just proximal to the proximal tip of the side plate. The hook on the tension device is reversed and inserted under the proximal end of the side plate in a notch designed for this purpose. With the wrench the fracture can then be distracted by pushing the fixed angle plate with the attached condyles distally. Distraction and reduction can be checked on fluoroscopy. If necessary, individual large fragments can be teased into reduction on the medial side with the use of a dental pick or small instrument. Again, care must be taken to avoid unnecessary soft tissue stripping. Once this has been accomplished, lag screw fixation of these fragments can be obtained through the plate. The tension device is then reversed, the hook is placed into the proximal hole of the side plate, and axial compression is applied across the fracture prior to the insertion of the proximal plate screws (Fig. 47–22).

With more significant comminution, as in the severe type A3 supracondylar fracture, the reversed tension device does not provide enough distraction to allow an atraumatic reduction of the fragments. The AO femoral distractor is an excellent device for this purpose and should be used because of the tremendous mechanical advantage it allows, not only for distraction but also in maintaining axial alignment and rotational control of the distal fragment, precluding the necessity of exposing the multiple supracondylar fragments to obtain reduction (Fig. 47–23). One of the distractor bolts or a 5-mm Schanz screw is inserted into one of the distal two holes of the plate. A second bolt or 4.5-mm Schanz screw is inserted into the femur well proximal to the plate. Prior to the insertion of these two bolts, it is advisable to correct rotational alignment. The bolts or Schanz screws for the distractor must be inserted parallel to each other in the frontal plane to maintain axial alignment. By turning the adjusting nut on the femoral distractor, the supracondylar fracture can be distracted to restore axial length and alignment. Fracture reduc-

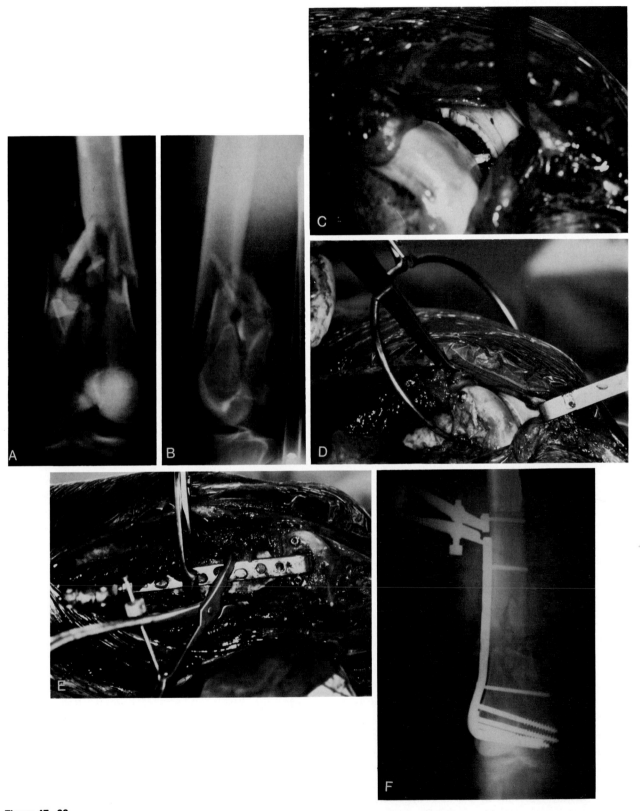

Figure 47–22

Closed supracondylar comminuted C2 fracture of the right distal femur in a 23-year-old man. *A,B,* AP and lateral radiographs, respectively. *C,* Intraoperative clinical picture showing the intracondylar fracture. *D,* Intracondylar fracture reduced with a clamp and stabilized with two 6.5-mm cancellous screws. *E,* Restoration of the condyles to the shaft with a 95° condylar blade device and fracture reduction with bone clamps (no anteromedial supracondylar soft tissue stripping). *F,* AP radiograph after axial compression of the indirectly reduced supracondylar comminuted fractures with the eccentric compression device.

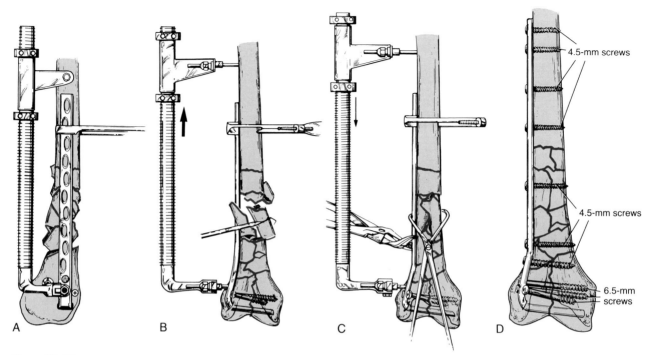

Figure 47–23

Technique for use of the femoral distractor for indirect fracture reduction after plate fixation distally. *A*, Insertion of Schanz screws proximal and distal (the latter through the plate). *B*, Distraction applied for fracture reduction. The fracture fragments are teased into place with a dental pick, avoiding unnecessary soft tissue stripping. *C*, Compression with the femoral distractor to provide axial loading when the fracture has sufficient bony support, using bone reduction clamps as indicated. *D*, Final construct after indirect fracture reduction, screw stabilization of the plate proximally, and judicious lag screw fixation of the fracture as indicated.

tion is facilitated by overdistraction and by visualizing the fracture on the fluoroscopy. Commonly, the fracture fragments will reduce according to the principle of "ligamentotaxis" by applying tension to the soft tissue attachments. As with the use of the reversed tension device, a dental pick can be used to gently tease in major fragments on the medial side, avoiding unnecessary soft tissue stripping. Atraumatic bone clamps are applied if necessary, followed by lag screw fixation of the larger comminuted fragments to each other or to the plate. If there is cortical contact, the distraction can be released, axial compression can be applied proximally with the tension device, and the proximal plate can be fixed to the shaft with 4.5-mm cortical screws. However, if the comminution is severe or there is a bone defect in the supracondylar region, then following distraction of the fracture and restoration of axial alignment, rotation, and length, the proximal plate is held to the femoral shaft with a Verbrugge clamp and fixed with 4.5-mm cortical screws without addressing the comminuted supracondylar area. The surgeon then has to assess the medial stability. Lack of medial cortical contact as a result of severe comminution or a bone defect will cause the fixed angle device on the lateral side to cycle and fall into varus angulation. If such is the

case, additional medial support with a T plate through a limited medial exposure is indicated. (Adjunctive medial bone grafting is also indicated; see section on bone grafting.)

TYPE B FRACTURES (UNICONDYLAR)

Type B1 and B2 Fractures

The type B1 or B2 distal femur fracture is a unicondylar fracture of either the lateral or medial condyle. The fracture is exposed through a small medial or lateral incision. The condyle must be anatomically reduced and held temporarily with Kirschner wires. In young patients with firm cancellous bone, stable fixation can be accomplished with the use of 6.5-mm cancellous screws (32-mm threads) and washers. However, in elderly patients with osteoporotic bone, additional fixation is required. The use of a T buttress plate allowing cancellous screw fixation through the distal two holes is preferred. Similarly, an "antiglide" or buttress plate is indicated when the condylar fracture line extends into the proximal metaphysis/diaphysis, to counteract the potential for sheer and proximal fracture migration. A well-contoured T buttress plate with 6.5-mm cancellous lag screws distally, 4.5-mm cortical screws proximally, and lag screws across the fracture line is required.

Type B3 Fractures

The type B3 unicondylar distal femur fracture is a coronal fracture through the femoral condyle (Hoffa fracture). Again, a small medial or lateral incision is necessary to expose the articular condyle. Anatomic reduction of the articular surface is mandatory; this is temporarily stabilized with Kirschner wires. Permanent stable fixation is accomplished with lag screws in the anterior/posterior direction at a right angle to the plane of the fracture. The screws should be inserted as far laterally or medially as possible to avoid the articular cartilage. The size of the fragments determines the size of the screw. For larger fragments, 6.5-mm cancellous screw with 16-mm threads should be used, whereas 4-mm cancellous screws are used for smaller fragments. If, because of the particular fracture morphology, it is necessary to insert the screws through the articular cartilage, the screw heads should be countersunk.

Osteochondral Fractures

Osteochondral fractures of the femoral condyles are not uncommon. Sometimes it is hard to differentiate those caused by osteochondritis dessicans from those caused by an acute traumatic episode. If the fracture occurs in the patellofemoral articulation or in the weight-bearing region of the femoral condyles, or if it is large enough, it should be anatomically reduced and stabilized. Diagnosis and the techniques for operative evaluation and stabilization (arthroscopically or open) of these fractures will be addressed in chapter 49.

TYPE C FRACTURES

Type C fractures are bicondylar supracondylar femur fractures.

Type C1 and C2 Fractures

Type C1 and C2 fractures are bicondylar supracondylar fractures in which there is no intracondylar comminution (Fig. 47–24). Type C2 is complicated by additional supracondylar comminution (Fig. 47–25). The implant of choice is a fixed angle device, either the 95° angle blade plate or the condylar compression screw. Of prime importance is anatomic reconstruction of the vertical component of the intracondylar fracture and, thus, the articular surface. This is accomplished temporarily with provisional K-wire fixation and then defini-

tively using 6.5-mm lag screws as described in the technique for use of the 95° angle blade plate (see Fig. 47–22). Once the condyles are reconstituted to one fragment, the fracture pattern is converted to type A2 or A3, depending on the presence of supracondylar comminution (Fig. 47–26). The stabilization of the condyles to the shaft will then be identical to that previously described for the type A2 or A3 supracondylar fractures.

Type C3 Fractures

The most complex and difficult of all the distal femur fractures is the type C3 fracture, which has both supracondylar and intercondylar comminution. This often necessitates either a more extensile lateral approach with an osteotomy of the tibial tubercle or bilateral approaches to adequately view the femoral condyles from below. The first step is anatomic reconstruction of the articular surface. This is not always possible because of articular damage, impaction, or severe comminution. However, if possible this should be accomplished provisionally with Kirschner wires. Definitive fixation of the articular fragments is then accomplished with lag screws. Optimally, these should be inserted through the nonarticular portions of the joint. If this is not possible, all attempts should be made to avoid inserting the screws through the weight-bearing area of the joint surface, and the screw heads should be countersunk below the level of the articular cartilage.

When there is significant comminution between the condyles, it is important not to narrow the intercondylar distance and hence the femoral articulation with either the tibia or the patella. In this situation, intercondylar screws across the area of the comminution should be inserted as "position screws" and not lag screws. A corticocancellous iliac crest bone graft can also be fashioned to fill the defect and thus allow increased stability and possibly lag screw fixation across the condyles. The use of a 95° angled blade plate or a condylar compression screw is optimal. If correctly inserted it will not only restore axial alignment but also, by virtue of its fixed angle, provide better long-term stability. However, in low supracondylar fractures and where there is significant intracondylar comminution or bone loss of the condyles, it may not be possible to obtain stability of the blade or the condylar screw. Additionally, in fractures with significant comminution, especially in the coronal plane, condylar lag screw fixation may preclude the ability to insert a fixed angle device. In these instances the implant of choice is the condylar buttress plate, which allows multiple lag screw fixation into the condyles (see Fig. 47–21). Although

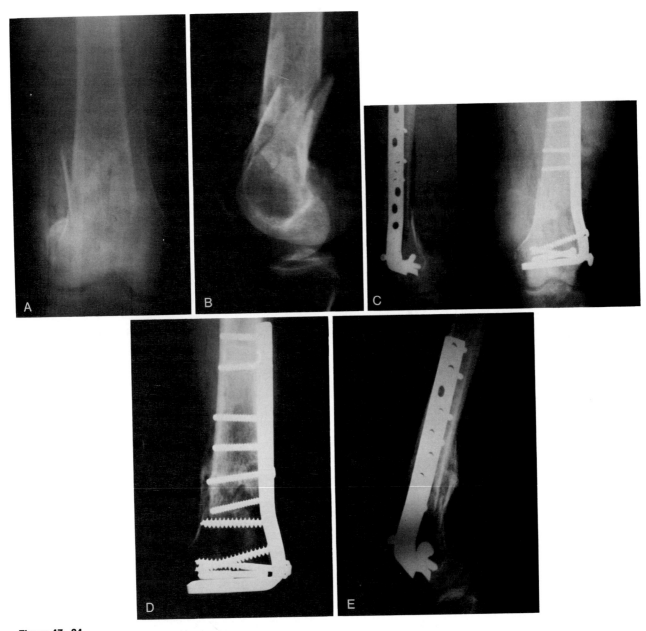

Figure 47–24

Supracondylar-intracondylar (C1) fracture of the distal femur in a 60-year-old woman with marked osteopenia. *A,B,* AP and lateral radiographs, respectively, of the distal femur. *C,* Intraoperative AP and lateral radiographs following distal condylar lag screw fixation and 95° condylar blade plate stabilization of the condyles to the shaft. *D,E,* AP and lateral radiographs, respectively, of the distal femur at four months follow-up. The fracture had healed, and the patient was fully weight bearing.

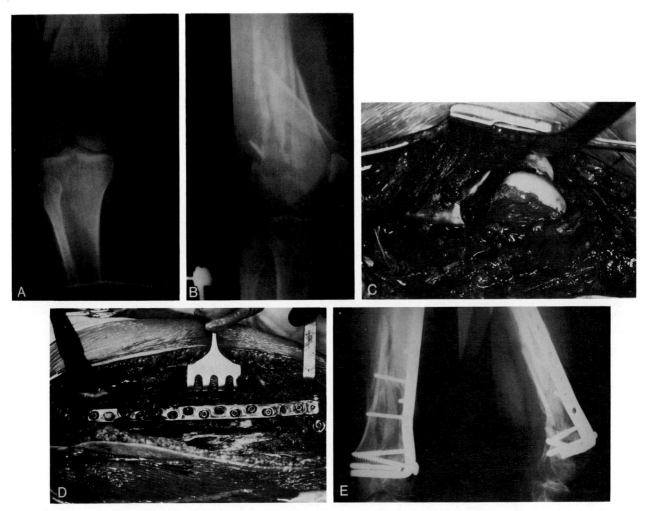

Figure 47-25

A comminuted supracondylar-intercondylar (C2) fracture of the right distal femur in a 32-year-old woman. AP (*A*) and lateral (*B*) radiographs of the distal femur in skeletal traction taken at the time of transfer. *C,D,* Intraoperative clinical photographs demonstrating the supracondylar/intercondylar distal femur fracture and subsequent indirect stabilization with 6.5-mm cancellous condylar lag screws and a 95° condylar blade plate and with no anteromedial soft tissue stripping. *E,* AP (left) and lateral (right) distal femur radiographs at 5 months follow-up demonstrating complete healing (2-mm intercondylar step).

the condylar buttress plate is an excellent salvage device for more complicated fractures, it poses significant inherent problems. Axial alignment is more difficult to obtain, and cyclic loading into varus angulation is common. Intraoperative fluoroscopy or radiographs are necessary to confirm the alignment; often additional medial support to prevent long-term varus malalignment is indicated. Subsequent restoration of the condyles to the shaft is as previously described for the type A3 comminuted supracondylar fracture.

BONE GRAFTING

All patients undergoing open reduction and internal fixation of distal femur fractures should have the ipsilateral iliac crest prepped and draped in a sterile fashion in case adjunctive bone grafting is necessary. In comminuted supracondylar fractures, either in the elderly or in the young following high-energy trauma, and in fractures in which adequate medial stability cannot be obtained at the time of fracture reduction and stabilization, primary medial autogenous cancellous bone grafting is indicated. In fractures in which there is significant bone devascularization, such as high-energy or open fractures, bone grafting is also indicated. However, the timing of this should depend on the condition and control of the soft tissues. When in doubt, delay bone grafting after severe soft tissue injuries. In fractures necessitating additional medial plating (i.e., where there is significant instability or bone defect), bone grafting is also indicated. The liberal use of autogenous cancellous bone graft in supracondylar femoral

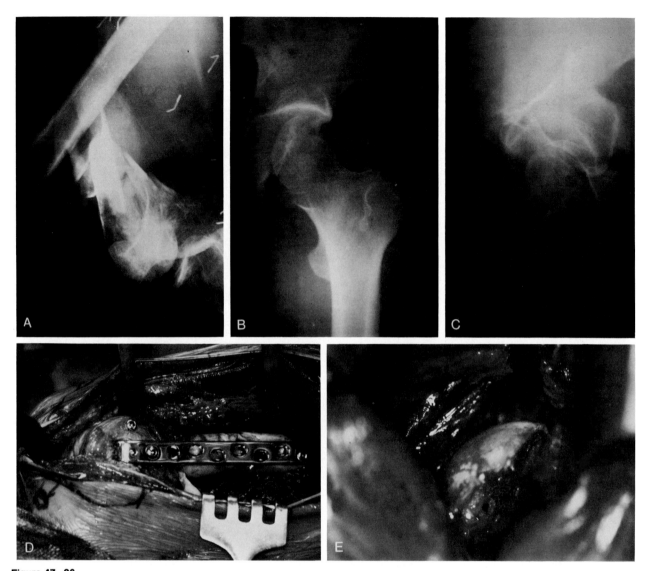

Figure 47–26

Grade III comminuted supracondylar/intercondylar (C2) left distal femur fracture and ipsilateral posterior fracture-dislocation (Pipkin) of the hip in a 40-year-old male. *A*, Oblique radiograph of the distal femur. *B,C*, AP and lateral radiographs, respectively, of the hip. *D*, Intraoperative photograph following irrigation and debridement and open reduction and internal fixation of the distal femur fracture with primary lag screw condylar fixation and a 95° condylar blade plate. *E*, Intraoperative photograph of the hip showing a Pipkin fracture of the femoral head. An anterior approach was used. *F*, AP radiograph of the distal femur at three months follow-up when the patient was rescheduled for medial autogenous cancellous bone graft. *G,H*, AP and lateral radiographs, respectively, of the distal femur at 11 months follow-up with complete healing and the patient fully weight bearing. *I*, AP (left) and lateral (right) radiographs of the hip at six months follow-up with healing of the fracture-dislocation following primary reduction and 6.5-mm cancellous lag screw fixation.

fractures with bone loss, severe comminution, or bony devascularization will help win the ever-present race between implant failure and bone healing.

The intercondylar portion of the distal femur is well vascularized and nonunions are very rare. The only indication for intercondylar bone grafting is for significant comminution or bone defects, especially between the condyles. By fashioning a well-contoured cortico-cancellous graft, the defect can be spanned, allowing compression fixation between the condyles and increasing the stability of the construct.

ADJUNCTIVE FIXATION TECHNIQUES

In elderly patients with severe osteoporosis, the holding power of screws is often inadequate to provide stable fixation. Screw fixation can be greatly enhanced by the use of methylmethacrylate. It is advisable to maintain

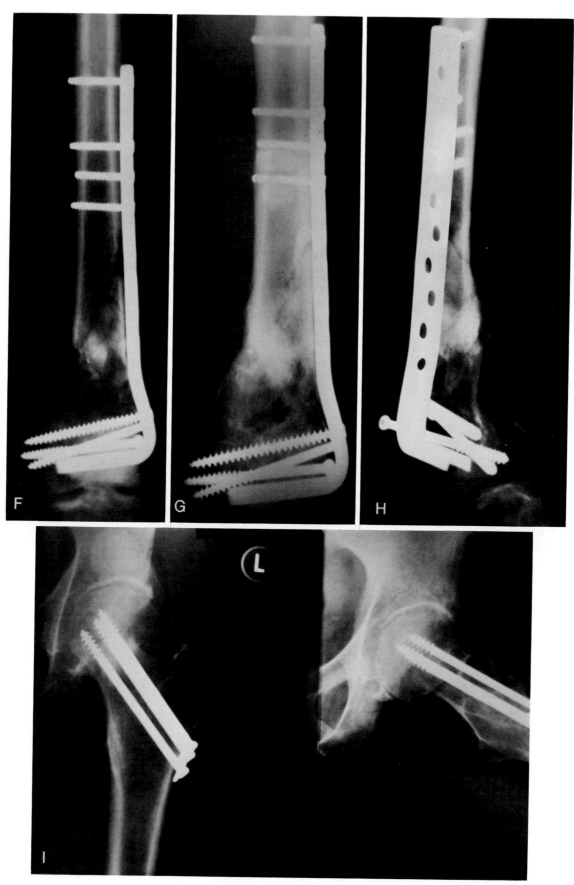

Figure 47–26 *Continued*

both the methylmethacrylate powder and the liquid methylmethacrylate refrigerated prior to use to slow down the polymerization process. The questionable screws are removed, and the precooled methylmethacrylate is mixed and, while liquid, poured into a 30-mm plastic syringe. It is then injected into the screw holes under pressure. (To facilitate this process, it is useful to widen the tip of the syringe with a 3.5-mm drill bit.) The screws are then inserted into their respective holes but are not tightened fully. Once the cement hardens, the screws are tightened the final few turns. This technique will greatly enhance the stability of the screw-bone interface and provide more stable fixation. Care must be taken to avoid extravasation of the methylmethacrylate into the fracture site, as in this location it may interfere with fracture healing. Additionally, if the distal cortex of a screw hole is intraarticular, the insertion of methylmethacrylate under pressure is contraindicated to avoid extravasation of the cement into the joint.

The use of additional cerclage wire fixation might be indicated in elderly patients with osteoporotic bone. To avoid devascularization of the fracture, its use should not be indiscriminate, but occasionally one or two cerclage wires in the supracondylar area may help restore reasonable fragment alignment and thus provide greater stability.

Follow-up Care and Rehabilitation

Postoperatively, the patient is placed into a soft bulky dressing from groin to toes. Müller et al.[33] recommended immobilization of the knee at 90° of flexion on a Böhler-Braun frame for three to four days. Following the work by Salter et al.,[15] it became apparent that immediate continuous passive motion not only enhances cartilage healing but also helped prevent quadriceps contractures, decreased swelling, and enhanced early knee motion. Use of the continuous passive motion (CPM) machine immediately postoperatively is tolerated better by the patient if the joint is injected prior to wound closure with 20 ml of 0.5% bupivacaine with epinephrine (1 : 200,000). The continued passive motion is maintained full time until ambulation is commenced on the third to fourth postoperative day and thereafter only intermittently while in bed. In conjunction with the CPM, the patient is started on active exercises of the quadriceps and hamstring musculature on postoperative day two. Gait training on days three to five progresses from the use of the parallel bars to a walker or crutches, with weight bearing as determined by the stability of the fixation intraoperatively. If stable fixation has been achieved, the patient can begin immediate minimal weight bearing (20 lbs); alternatively, toe-touch gait is indicated. Active physical therapy and limited weight bearing with crutches or a walker is continued until there is clinical and radiographic evidence of fracture healing. At this point (usually two to three months postoperatively), the patient progressively increases weight bearing and resistance exercises until solid union at about four to six months.

The necessity for additional support is determined by the presence of additional or associated injuries and the type of reduction and the stability of fixation obtained at the time of surgery. In patients who have associated ligamentous disruptions of the knee, functional bracing or cast bracing is indicated to control motion in the allowable range, yet allow early active mobilization of the knee. However, the primary indication for additional external support is in the patient with tenuous internal fixation. Only the surgeon, at the end of the procedure, can honestly determine the efficacy of the fixation. If there is any suspicion concerning the adequacy of the fixation, the holding power of the bone, or the stability of the construct, external protection must be employed to avoid loss of fixation, malunion, or nonunion prior to bone healing. However, as with all periarticular fractures, early active motion must be encouraged to promote restoration of joint motion and function. The judicious use of functional or cast braces lends external support while still allowing active rehabilitation. In the patient with markedly unstable fixation, postoperative skeletal traction will provide the best control and stability for fracture healing. The patient should be encouraged, even in traction, to start early, active (although limited) functional rehabilitation of the knee.

Complications

INFECTION

The major complication of operative intervention in the management of distal femoral fractures is infection. In the older literature, especially that of the 1960s, the postoperative infection rate was approximately 20%.[35,51] In more recent literature the infection rate from the operative stabilization of these demanding fractures has ranged from zero to approximately 7%.[12,16,20,22,30,41,44] Factors that predispose to infection include (1) high-energy injuries, especially when there is significant bony devascularization; (2) open fractures; (3) extensive surgical dissection that further compromises bony vascularity; (4) an inexperienced operating team with prolonged open wound time; and (5) inadequate fixation. Acceptable rates of postoperative infection can be obtained with meticulous surgical technique, gentle handling and preservation of the soft tissues, the use of prophylactic antibiotics, and adequate, rigid, bony stabilization with external or internal fixation. Optimal timing of surgery is essential, especially with open wounds or major injuries to the soft tissues. Additionally, open wounds should not be primarily closed but should be returned to the operating room for serial redebridement until delayed primary closure or additional soft tissue procedures can be safely performed. By strict adherence to these principles, the benefits of stable internal fixation and early mobilization will produce better functional results and outweigh the risks of infection (1% to 2% incidence is acceptable).

The presence of a postoperative infection mandates aggressive management. The patient must be returned emergently to the operating room for irrigation and debridement. As long as the internal fixation is sound and adequate, it should not be removed. If there is a large soft tissue defect, antibiotic-impregnated cement beads will not only leach antibiotic locally in the hematoma but also act as a soft tissue spacer. Repeated irrigation and debridement is performed until bone cultures indicate the infection is controlled. Intravenous antibiotic coverage is recommended for up to six weeks if bone cultures are positive.

NONUNION

Nonunion of fractures of the distal third of the femur have been reported to occur regardless of the treatment modality used. The incidence varies greatly in the literature, but some of the early larger series reported a greater than 10% nonunion rate with open reduction and internal fixation.[35] More recent series indicate a nonunion rate of zero to 4% with open reduction and internal fixation.[12,16,20,22,30,39,41,44,53,61] The nonunions invariably occur in the supracondylar region and not in the very vascular intercondylar region. Factors predisposing to nonunions include (1) bone loss or defect; (2) high-energy injuries, especially in fractures that are open or comminuted with significant soft tissue stripping and loss of bony vascularity; (3) inability of the surgical team to obtain adequate bony fixation; (4) failure to augment healing in comminuted fractures with autogenous bone graft; and (5) the presence of a wound infection.

Nonunions of the distal femur are extremely difficult management problems, and the best treatment is prophylaxis. In long-standing nonunions the knee joint will become stiff, and most of the motion that is present will occur through pseudarthrosis. Successful management requires addressing both the stable fixation of the

nonunion and restoration of knee movement in one stage. Early mobilization postoperatively will increase the vascularity to the area and decrease the lever arm on the fixation of the nonunion. Nonunion fixation in the supracondylar region, if the fractures are high supracondylar, can be accomplished with a locked intramedullary nail. Most supracondylar nonunions, however, are not amenable to this form of treatment and will require internal fixation with a fixed angle device and side plate. The addition of lag screws significantly increases the stability across the nonunion site. If the nonunion is hypertrophic, stable fixation and thus restoration of mechanical stability is all that is required. If the nonunion is atrophic, then, in addition to mechanical stability, the biologic potential of the bone to heal must be restored by decortication and bone grafting for all such injuries (Fig. 47–27). If there is a bone defect or the distal fragment is small and osteopenic, adequate fixation with a fixed angle device might not be possible. Then both medial and lateral buttress plating might be indicated. If fixation cannot be achieved in the distal femur, Beall et al. have recommended the use of a Küntscher intramedullary rod driven across the knee joint as a salvage procedure.[3]

MALUNION

Malunion following the treatment of fractures of the distal femur is more common with conservative than with operative treatment. The major problems are malrotation, shortening, and axial malalignment. If conservative treatment with traction or bracing cannot maintain length, rotation, or axial alignment, then open reduction and internal fixation should be considered.

Following open reduction and internal fixation, when there is significant supracondylar comminution, even though anatomic reduction might be obtained, there is a tendency for the distal femoral fixation to cycle and fail, producing a varus malunion.[42] To avoid this complication, supplementary medial bone grafting or plating is indicated. An additional problem with open reduction and internal fixation is fixation of the distal fragment in either too much extension or too much flexion. This occurs when the distal fragment is small and it is hard to determine, at the time of surgical reconstruction, the correct flexion or extension alignment. When using fixed angle devices from the lateral side of the distal femur, unless these are absolutely parallel to the knee joint AP axis, varus or valgus deformities will result. To avoid these potential malalignment problems with internal fixation, adequate preoperative planning is essential. Determining normal anatomy from the opposite uninvolved side, choosing the exact

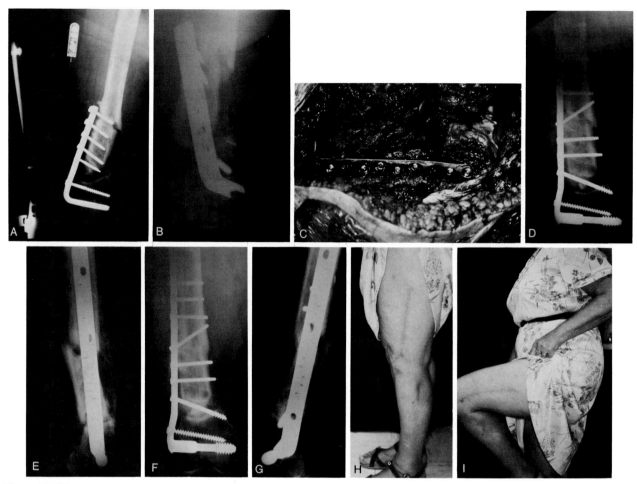

Figure 47–27

A 50-year-old woman had blade plate fixation of the right distal femur two years previously and implantable electrical stimulation for nonunion nine months previously. She had a fall with a resulting acute fracture at the plate-bone junction and metaphyseal nonunion of the right distal femur. *A,B,* AP and lateral radiographs, respectively, of the right distal femur. *C,* Intraoperative photograph after condylar screw and side plate fixation of both the nonunion and the acute distal femur fracture. Complete arthrolysis and soft tissue release of the right knee joint were also performed. *D,E,*Postoperative AP and lateral radiographs, respectively, following condylar screw, side plate, and lag screw fixation, with autogenous iliac crest bone graft of the nonunion and acute fracture. *F,G,* AP and lateral radiographs, respectively, at seven months follow-up with complete healing of both the nonunion and acute fracture. *H,I,* Clinical follow-up photographs demonstrating restoration of functional range of motion.

location for the fixation device, and obtaining adequate intraoperative radiographs to assure that the preoperative plan is followed all help avoid malalignment.

When intramedullary nails are used for distal femoral and supracondylar fractures, especially with the patient on a fracture table in the lateral decubitus position, there is a tendency to nail the distal fragment in valgus angulation with excessive malrotation. Appreciation and avoidance of this potential problem is essential at the time of the nailing.

Once malunion of the distal femur is established, the degree and planes of deformity must be exactly determined. This requires adequate AP and lateral radio-graphs of the involved and the contralateral side and appreciation of both displacement and angulation in all planes. Shortening must also be determined and scanograms may be indicated for this. Rotational malalignment is best determined clinically or, if necessary, with CT scanning. Correction of malunion is accomplished with a supracondylar osteotomy. The type of osteotomy will be determined by the deformity present.

Rarely, there is an associated intercondylar malunion with deformity of the articular surface. This might require tomograms or a CT scan to determine the exact degree of the deformity. This significantly complicates the osteotomy, as an intraarticular osteotomy is required to correct this additional deformity.

LOSS OF FIXATION

One of the major complications following open reduction and internal fixation of the distal femur, is loss of bony fixation. Factors predisposing to the loss of fixation include (1) increased comminution; (2) increased age and osteopenia; (3) low transcondylar and comminuted intracondylar fractures in which distal fixation is hard to achieve; (4) poor patient compliance with loading and weight bearing before healing; and (5) infection. Optimally, early mobilization is preferred following open reduction and internal fixation, initially with continuous passive motion and subsequently with active and active-assisted physical therapy. However, the surgeon has to determine at the time of surgery the degree of bony fixation achieved. If the quality of the bone or the fracture type prohibits stable or adequate fixation, mobilization should be delayed, and supplementary procedures such as bone grafting or double plating are required. Once there is evidence of progressive loss of fixation, the surgeon has to decide whether by decreasing mobilization or weight bearing, union can still be achieved without loss of function. If not, then repeat open reduction and stabilization are indicated. The addition of a biologic stimulator, such as a bone graft, is also useful in this scenario to speed union before fixation is lost.

Whenever loss of fixation occurs, infection must be definitely excluded as a cause. Careful clinical evaluation, a white blood cell count with a differential, a sedimentation rate, and aspiration under fluoroscopy are probably all indicated.

CONTRACTURES/DECREASED KNEE MOTION

Following treatment of fractures of the distal femur, it is quite common to have some loss of motion. However, it is important to obtain a functional range of motion (i.e., full extension and at least 110° of flexion). If there is limitation of range of motion, the cause must be determined. Possibilities include (1) malreduction of the articular surface, either patellofemoral or tibiofemoral; (2) intraarticular hardware; (3) intraarticular joint adhesions; (4) ligamentous or capsular contractures; (5) quadriceps or hamstring scarring; and (6) posttraumatic arthritis.

Once the cause of the loss of motion is determined, then a decision can be made as to whether there is an option for improvement. If there is malreduction of the articular surface or intraarticular hardware, the only chance of restoring function is repeat surgery to correct the deformity or remove the hardware. Intraarticular adhesions and periarticular and muscular contractures initially should be treated with aggressive physical therapy. If this fails, then manipulation under anesthesia, arthrotomy and lysis of adhesions, and progressive capsular, ligamentous, and muscular releases may be indicated. Severe quadriceps contractures are particularly vexing problems to treat especially if the muscle is scarred to the supracondylar region of the distal femur. If the limitation of motion is significant, then quadriceps release from the underlying bone may be indicated. If there is intramuscular quadriceps contracture and scarring, then a quadriceps V-Y advancement or other type of lengthening procedure may be indicated. For joint stiffness following any of these procedures, the patient should be placed in a continuous passive motion machine and started on a very aggressive rehabilitation program.

If significant posttraumatic arthrosis or arthritis develops in the joint with pain and limitation of motion, it should be treated initially with antiinflammatory agents and physical therapy procedures to decrease the inflammation and increase the motion. If these measures prove unsuccessful, arthroscopic evaluation of the articular surface may be indicated. If significant long-term pain, decreased function, and disability ensue, then salvage procedures such as arthrodesis or arthroplasty may be indicated.

REFERENCES

1. Altenberg. A.R.; Shorkey, R.L. Blade-plate fixation in nonunion and in complicated fractures of the supracondylar region of the femur. J Bone Joint Surg 31A:312–316, 1949.
2. Arneson, T.J.; Melton, L.J. III; Lewallen, D.G.; O'Fallon, W.M. Epidemiology of diaphyseal and distal femoral fractures in Rochester, Minnesota, 1965–1984. Clin Orthop 234:188–194, 1988.
3. Beall, M.S.; Nebel, E.; Bailey, R. Transarticular fixation in the treatment of non-union of supracondylar fractures of the femur: A salvage procedure. J Bone Joint Surg 61A:1018–1023, 1979.
4. Benum, P. The use of bone cement as an adjunct to internal fixation of supracondylar fractures of osteoporotic femurs. Acta Orthop Scand 48:52–56, 1977.
5. Böhler, L. The Treatment of Fractures, Ed. 4. Bristol, England. Wright, 1935.
6. Böhler, L. Treatment of Fractures. New York, Grune and Stratton, 1956.
7. Bone, L.T. The management of fractures in the patient with multiple trauma. J Bone Joint Surg 68A:945–949, 1986.
8. Brown, A.; D'Arcy, J.C. Internal fixation for supracondylar fractures of the femur in the elderly patient. J Bone Joint Surg 53Br:420–424, 1971.

9. Browner, B.D.; Burgess, A.R.; Robertson, R.J.; el al. Immediate closed antegrade Ender nailing of femoral fractures in polytrauma patients. J Trauma 24(11):921–927, 1984.

10. Bucholz, R.W.; Ross, S.E.; Lawrence, K.L. Fatigue fracture of the interlocking nail in the treatment of fractures of the distal part of the femoral shaft. J Bone Joint Surg 69A:1391–1399, 1987.

11. Charnley, J. The Closed Treatment of Common Fractures, Ed. 3. Edinburgh, E. & S. Livingstone, 1961.

12. Chiron, H.S.; Casey, P. Fractures of the distal third of the femur treated by internal fixation. Clin Orthop 100:160–170, 1974.

13. Connolly, J.F. Closed management of distal femoral fractures. Instr Course Lect 36:428–437, 1987.

14. Connolly, J.F.; Dehne, E. Closed reduction and early cast-brace ambulation in the treatment of femoral fractures. J Bone Joint Surg 55A:1581–1599, 1973.

15. Driscoll, S.W.; Keeley, F.W.; Salter, R.B. The chondrogenic potential of free autogenous periosteal grafts for biological resurfacing of major full-thickness defects in joint surfaces under the influence of continuous passive motion. J Bone Joint Surg 68A:1017–1034, 1986.

16. Giles, J.B.; DeLee, J.C.; Heckman, J.D.; Keever, J.E. Supracondylar-intercondylar fractures of the femur treated with a supracondylar plate and lag screw. J Bone Joint Surg 64A:864–870, 1982.

17. Green, N.E.; Allen, F.L. Vascular injuries associated with dislocation of the knee. J Bone Joint Surg 59A:236–239, 1977.

18. Hall, M.F. Two-plane fixation of acute supracondylar and intracondylar fractures of the femur. South Med J 71(12):1474–1479, 1978.

19. Hampton, O.P. Wounds of the extremities in military surgery. St. Louis, C. V. Mosby, 1951.

20. Healy, W.L.; Brooker, A.F. Jr. Distal femoral fractures. Comparison of open and closed methods of treatment. Clin Orthop 174:166–171, 1983.

21. Johansen, K.; Bandyk, D.; Thiele, B.; Hansen, S.T. Temporary intraluminal shunts: Resolution of a management dilemma in complex vascular injuries. J Trauma 22:395–402, 1982.

22. Johnson, K.D.; Hicken, G. Distal femoral fractures. Orthop Clin North Am 18(1):115–131, 1987.

23. Kennedy, J.C. Complete dislocation of the knee joint. J Bone Joint Surg 45A:889–904, 1963.

24. Kirschner, M. Ueber nagelextension. Beitr Klin Chir 64:266–279, 1909.

25. Kolmert, L.; Wulff, K. Epidemiology and treatment of distal femoral fractures in adults. Acta Orthop Scand 53(6):957–962, 1982.

26. Mahorner, H.R.; Bradburn, M. Fractures of the femur. Report of 308 cases. Surg Gynecol Obstet 56:1066–1079, 1933.

27. Mast, J.; Jakob, R.; Ganz, R. Planning and Reduction Techniques in Fracture Surgery. New York, Springer-Verlag, 1989.

28. Matter, P.; Rittman, W. The Open Fracture. Bern, Huber, 1978.

29. Meyers, M.H.; Moore, T.M.; Harvey, J.P. Traumatic dislocation of the knee joint. J Bone Joint Surg 57A:430–433,1975.

30. Mize, R.D.; Bucholz, R.W.; Grogan, D.P. Surgical treatment of displaced, comminuted fractures of the distal end of the femur. J Bone Joint Surg 64A:871–879, 1982.

31. Modlin, J. Double skeletal traction in battle fractures of the lower femur. Bull US Army Med Dept 4:119–120, 1945.

31a. Moll, J. The cast brace walking treatment of open and closed femur fractures. South Med J 66:345–352, 1973.

32. Mooney, V. Fractures of the distal femur. Instr Course Lect 36:427,1987.

33. Müller, M.E.; Allgower, M.; Schneider, R.; Willenegger, H. Manual of Internal Fixation, Ed. 2. New York, Springer-Verlag, 1979.

34. Müller, M.E.; Nazarian, S.; Koch, P. Classification AO des Fractures. New York, Springer-Verlag, 1987.

35. Neer, C.S. II; Grantham, S.A.; Shelton, M.L. Supracondylar fracture of the adult femur. J Bone Joint Surg 49A:591–613, 1967.

36. Nielsen, B. F.; Petersen, V.S.; Varmarken, J.E. Fracture of the femur after knee arthroplasty. Acta Orthop Scand 59(2):155–157, 1988.

37. Olerud, S. Operative treatment of supracondylar-condylar fractures of the femur. Technique and results in fifteen cases. J Bone Joint Surg 54A:1015-1032, 1972.

38. Pritchett, J.W. Supracondylar fractures of the femur. Clin Orthop 184:173–177, 1984.

39. Regazzoni, P.; Leutenegger, A.; Ruedi, T.; Staehelin, F. Erste erfahrungen mit der dynamischen kondylenschraube (dcs) bei distalen femurfrakturen. Helv Chir Acta 53:61–64, 1986.

39a. Rockwood, C.A. Jr.; Ryan, V.L.; Richards, J.A. Experience with quadrilateral cast brace. [Abstr.] J Bone Joint Surg 55A:421, 1973.

40. Rush, L.V. Dynamic intramedullary fracture fixation of the femur. Clin Orthop 60:21–27, 1968.

41. Sanders, R.; Regazzoni, P.; Reudi, T. Treatment of supracondylar-intraarticular fractures of the femur using the dynamic condylar screw. J Orthop Trauma 3(3):214–222, 1989.

42. Sanders, R.W.; Swiontkowski, M.; Rosen, H.; Helfet, D. Complex fractures and malunions of the distal femur: results of treatment with double plates. J Bone Joint Surg, 73A: 341–346, 1991.

43. Schatzker, J.; Horne, G.; Waddell, J. The Toronto experience with the supracondylar fracture of the femur, 1966–72. Injury 6(2):113–128, 1975.

44. Schatzker, J.; Lambert, D.C. Supracondylar fractures of the femur. Clin Orthop 138:77–83, 1979.

45. Schatzker, J.; Tile, M. The Rationale of Operative Fracture Care. New York, Springer-Verlag, 1987.

46. Seinsheimer, F. Fractures of the distal femur. Clin Orthop 153:169–179, 1980.

47. Shelbourne, K.D.; Brueckmann, F.R. Rush-pin fixation of supracondylar and intercondylar fractures of the femur. J Bone Joint Surg 64A:161–169, 1982.

48. Sisto, D.J.; Warren, R.F. Complete knee dislocation. Clin Orthop 198:94–101, 1985.

49. Slatis, P.; Ryoppy, S.; Huttinen, V. AO osteosynthesis of fractures of the distal third of the femur. Acta Orthop Scand 42:162–172, 1971.

50. Smillie, I.S. Injuries of the Knee Joint, Ed. 4. Baltimore, Williams and Wilkins, 1971, pp. 246–259.

50a. Steinman, F.R. Eine neue Extensionsmethode in der Frakturenbehandlung. Zentralbl Chir 34:398–442, 1907.

51. Stewart, M.J.; Sisk, T.D.; Wallace, S.L. Fractures of the distal third of the femur. J Bone Joint Surg 48A(4):784–807, 1966.

52. Tees, J.D. Fracture of the lower end of the femur. Am J Surg 38:656–659, 1937.

53. Tscherne, H.; Trentz, O. Recent injuries of the femoral condyles (author's transl). Langenbecks Arch Chir 345:396–401, 1977.

54. Unmansky, A.L. Blade-plate internal fixation for fracture of the distal end of the femur. Bull Hosp Joint Dis 9(1):18–21, 1948.

55. Walling, A.K.; Seradge, H.; Spiegel, P.G. Injuries to the knee ligaments with fractures of the femur. J Bone Joint Surg 64A:1324–1327, 1982.

56. Watson Jones, R. Fractures and Joint Injuries, Ed. 4. Baltimore, Williams and Wilkins, 1956.

57. Wenzl, H.; Casey, P.A.; Herbert, P.; Belin, J. Die operative behandlung der distalen Femurfraktur. AO Bull Dec 1970.
58. Wertzberger, J.J.; Peltier, L.F. Supracondylar fractures. Kansas Med Soc 68:328–332, 1967.
59. White, E.H.; Russin, L.A. Supracondylar fractures of the femur treated by internal fixation with immediate knee motion. Am J Surg 22:801–820, 1956.
60. Wiggins, H.E. Vertical traction in open fractures of the femur. US Armed Forces Med J 4:1633–1636, 1953.

61. Zickle, R.E. Nonunions of fractures of the proximal and distal thirds of the shaft of the femur. Instr Course Lect 37:173–179, 1988.
62. Zickle, R.E.; Fietti, V.G. Jr.; Lawsing, J.F. III; Cochran, G.V. A new intramedullary fixation device for the distal third of the femur. Clin Orthop 125:185–191, 1977.
63. Zickle, R.E.; Hobeika, P.; Robbins, D.S. Zickle supracondylar nails for fractures of the distal end of the femur. Clin Orthop 212:79–88, 1986.

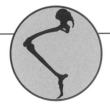

Patella Fractures and Extensor Mechanism Injuries

Historical Background

Before the beginning of the twentieth century, the treatment of patella fractures was extremely controversial. Nonoperative methods, usually extension splinting and rest, were most commonly employed. Results were poor, bony union was rare, and permanent disability was expected.[24] As improvements in surgical asepsis occurred, two operative solutions to the problem emerged: arthrotomy with open wiring and patellectomy. Heineck reviewed 1100 cases of patella fractures and advised operative treatment over extension splinting for the following reasons: improved fracture reduction, maintenance of reduction until union, reestablishment of soft tissue continuity, and restoration of the functional integrity of the knee joint.[39] Open reduction and wire fixation subsequently became the treatment of choice for patella fractures.

Although reduction in simple transverse fractures was made possible by an open procedure, stable fixation remained difficult. Various materials, including silver, aluminum, and copper wire; chromic suture; kangaroo tendon; cancellous bone pegs; Achilles tendon; and fascial strips were tried.[41] In 1936, Blodgett and Fairchild reported on 35 cases of patella fractures treated with open reduction and wire suture; less than 50% had good results. They then reported on the use of partial or, in certain cases, total excision of the patella for fractures and described excellent clinical results.[7] A year earlier, Thompson had also recommended partial excision of the patella.[82] That same year, Brooke published a revolutionary paper on the treatment of patella fractures by total excision.[13] Quoting embryologic data

to support the vestigial nature of the patella, his functional studies showed that postpatellectomy limbs were stronger than their normal counterparts. Patellectomy was immediately and enthusiastically received.[24,32,35,36,41]

This initial enthusiasm was tempered by many experimental and long-term clinical studies that disproved these claims.[14,21,23,28,38,45,46,53,55,59,71,81,85,89,90,92] Cohn[21] and Bruce and Walmsley[14] both studied patellectomized rabbits and found degenerative changes on the femoral condyles. They suggested that this could occur in humans as well. Haxton and others presented biomechanical evidence that the patella served a necessary purpose in the extensor mechanism.[23,38,46,53,85,89] In long-term clinical studies evaluating total patellectomy patients, variable results were also found.[23,28,45,55,59,81,90,92] These studies revealed poor patient satisfaction, decreased quadriceps power, prolonged recovery time, and significant changes in the activities of daily living.[28,71,81,92]

In the early 1950s, Pauwels reported on the treatment of patella fractures using the anterior tension band principle.[62] This was subsequently advocated by the Arbeitsgemeinschaft für Osteosynthesefragen/Association for the Study of Internal Fixation (AO/ASIF) group as the treatment of choice for transverse patellar fractures.[62] Weber et al. compared the tension band principle with cerclage and interosseous wire suture in cadavers.[88] They found that modified anterior tension band wiring with a retinacular repair gave the most stable fixation of the transversely fractured patella. Additionally, this was the only construct that allowed early active range of motion of the knee.[88] Other authors subsequently confirmed this fact clinically.[8,9,43,50]

1685

Presently, three forms of operative treatment survive: various forms of fixation, usually with tension band wiring; partial patellectomy; and total patellectomy. Definitive indications for each procedure are related to the type of fracture encountered. Good results can be expected with proper treatment.

Anatomy

SKELETAL ANATOMY

The patella lies deep to the fascia lata and tendinous fibers of the rectus femoris (Fig. 48–1). It is flat, roughly oval in shape, and comes to a rounded point, known as the apex, on its anteroinferior margin. Its proximal part is called the basis.[10]

The articular surface is divided into seven facets by several ridges (Fig. 48–1). A major vertical ridge separates the medial from the lateral facets, while a second vertical ridge near the medial border isolates a narrow strip known as the odd facet. In addition, two transverse ridges create superior, intermediate, and inferior facets.[10,69]

Wiberg classified patellae into three types based on the size of the medial and lateral facets.[91] In type I, the medial and lateral facets are approximately equal, whereas in types II and III the medial facets are progressively smaller than the lateral. Baumgartl described a fourth type, the "Jägerhut patella," where the medial facet is lacking altogether.[5] These facets have importance with respect to the functional anatomy of the patellofemoral joint (see section on extensor apparatus biomechanics).

SOFT TISSUE ANATOMY

Quadriceps Mechanism

The quadriceps muscle complex is composed of four separate muscles: the rectus femoris, the vastus medialis, the vastus lateralis, and the vastus intermedius (Fig. 48–2). Classically, the quadriceps tendon is described as trilaminar in structure, inserting onto the patella with the rectus superficial, the vasti in the middle, and the intermedius deep.[53] The actual arrangement is more complex as a result of blending of the tendons as they insert on the patella.[69]

The rectus femoris is a long fusiform muscle that assumes the central and superficial position in the quadriceps structure.[69] The fibers angle 7° to 10° medially in the frontal plane relative to the shaft of the femur.[53]

The vastus medialis divides into two parts. The more proximal fibers are known as the vastus medialis longus

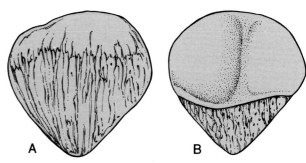

Figure 48–1

A, Superficial aspect of the patella, with extensive soft tissue attachments indicated by roughened surface. B, Articular surface of the patella (see text). Note the extraarticular distal pole occupying a significant portion of the bone's length.

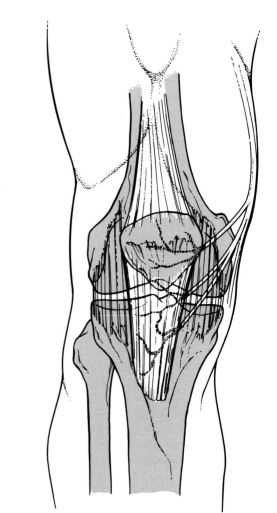

Figure 48–2

Soft tissue attachments of the patella. Major components of the extensor mechanism include the quadriceps tendon proximally and the patellar ligament (tendon) distally. The medial and lateral retinacula help position the patella and can provide active knee extension if they remain intact after a patellar fracture without significant displacement.

and enter the patella at an angle of 15° to 18°. The more distal fibers, the vastus medialis obliquus, enter the patella at an angle of 50° to 55°.[53] The fibers of each group are divided by fascia into separate fascicles. Innervation of the vastus medialis obliquus is by a separate branch of the femoral nerve.[53,69]

The fibers of the vastus lateralis approach the patella at an angle of approximately 30°, terminating more proximally than do the fibers of the vastus medialis. The most medial fibers insert into the supralateral edge of the patella, with the more lateral fibers traveling laterally past the patella. These fibers contribute to the lateral retinaculum and at their lateral extreme fuse with the iliotibial tract.

The vastus intermedius lies in a plane deep to the other three elements of the quadriceps. Most of the fibers insert directly into the superior aspect of the patella. Deep to the major components of the quadriceps lies the articularis genu. This muscle is highly variable in occurrence and arises from the anterior aspect of the supracondylar portion of the femur. It inserts on the joint capsule at the suprapatellar pouch.

Patellar Retinaculum

The deep investing fascial layer of the thigh is known as the fascia lata. As it spreads over the anterior surface of the knee, its medial and lateral extensions combine with aponeurotic fibers from both the vastus medialis and vastus lateralis to form the patellar retinaculum, which inserts directly into the proximal tibia (Fig. 48–2). The patellofemoral ligaments, deep transverse fibers that are palpable thickenings of the joint capsule connecting the patella with the femoral epicondyles, complete the retinaculum.[10,69] In addition, the lateral aspect of the vastus lateralis and the iliotibial tract both contribute to the thicker lateral patellar retinaculum. Together the patellar retinaculum and the iliotibial band serve as "the auxiliary extensors of the knee."[10]

Patellar Tendon

Derived primarily from the fibers of the rectus femoris, the patellar tendon is flat and strong and inserts onto the tibial tubercle. Its average length is slightly less than 5 cm. The fascial expansions of the iliotibial tract and the patella retinaculum blend into the patellar tendon as it inserts onto the anterior surface of the tibia.

ARTERIAL BLOOD SUPPLY

The anterior surface of the patella is covered with an extraosseous arterial ring derived mainly from branches of the geniculate arteries (Fig. 48–3).[22] The

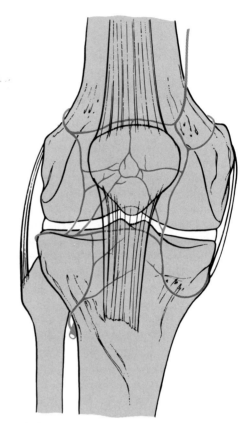

Figure 48–3

Blood supply of the patella. Note the extraosseous arterial anastomotic ring, which receives inflow from branches of each of the genicular arteries. (From Scapinelli R. J Bone Joint Surg 49B:563–570, 1967.)

intraosseous blood supply of the patella is supplied by two systems of vessels, both derived from this extraosseous vascular ring: the midpatellar vessels, which penetrate the middle third of the anterior surface of the patella, and the polar vessels, which enter the patella at its apex.[3,70]

Extensor Apparatus Biomechanics

The principal function of the extensor mechanism of the knee in humans is to maintain the erect position. Ambulation, rising from a chair, and ascending or descending stairs are examples of this ability to overcome gravity. The biomechanical principles necessary for this to occur should be understood to treat extensor mechanism injuries rationally.

A *moment* is a force that produces rotation about an axis. It is equal to the product of a force and the perpendicular distance from the line of action of that force to the axis of rotation. This perpendicular distance is the *moment arm*.[73] The force necessary for knee extension *(torque)* is directly dependent on the perpendicular distance between the patellar tendon and the knee flexion axis (moment arm) (Fig. 48–4A).[46]

Twice as much torque is needed to extend the knee the final 15° than to bring it from a fully flexed position to 15°.[53] To do this, the knee requires a moment arm that increases during extension so that it can maintain a constant level of torque. The patella provides this mechanical advantage by two separate mechanisms: linking and displacement.[46]

As the knee begins extension from the fully flexed position, the patella functions primarily as a link between the quadriceps and the patellar tendon. This allows for torque generation from the quadriceps muscle to the tibia.[46] Maximal forces across the quadriceps tendon have been recorded at 3200 N, whereas those across the patellar tendon are 2800 N.[42] These values are between four and five times standard body weight of 700 N. For young, physically trained men, these forces can reach up to 6000 N.[42]

Typically, the linking function occurs in the more flexed positions. At 135° of flexion the patella slips into the intercondylar notch. The patellar facets of the femur exhibit an extensive contact area with both the patella and the broad posterior surface of the quadriceps tendon. Load bearing shifts to a combination of the patellofemoral and the tendofemoral areas, with the latter being the greater of the two after 90° of flexion.[33] Without patellofemoral contact, the moment

arm is small (Fig. 48–4B).[33] From 135° to 45° of flexion, the odd facet engages the femur. It is the only part of the patella that fails to meet the true patellar facets of the femur and the only part to articulate with the true tibial surface of the medial femoral condyle of the femur.[33]

From 45° of flexion to full extension, the patella is the only component of the extensor mechanism to contact the femur. It acts to displace the quadriceps tendon–patellar tendon linkage away from the axis of knee rotation. This increases the effective moment arm of the quadriceps mechanism and contributes the additional 60% of torque that is needed to gain the last 15° of knee extension.[53] This second action, therefore, creates a mechanical advantage analogous to that of a pulley.[46,89]

By displacing the tendon away from the axis of rotation, a greater excursion of the quadriceps is required for a given range of motion.[89] Theoretically, when performing a patellectomy, a quadriceps shortening or tubercle elevation procedure may be performed to take this into account.

Diagnosis

HISTORY AND PHYSICAL EXAMINATION

Fractures of the patella are diagnosed by obtaining a history of the injury, performing a thorough physical examination, and acquiring the appropriate radiographic studies. The completion of these investigations should result in a final diagnosis that includes fracture type, the presence or absence of retinacular disruption, a description of the wound, if any, and the presence of any associated injuries.

The history usually describes a fall from a height, a near fall, a direct blow to the patella, or a combination of these. Correlation with the mechanism of injury allows the physician to anticipate the fracture pattern. If the patient presents with an open wound, the history should include questions regarding the location of the accident (e.g., at home, in the water, or on a farm).

The physical exam should include an evaluation of the skin, noting contusions, abrasions, blisters (if treatment has been delayed), and the presence of an open fracture or open joint injury. If a displaced patella fracture is present, the physical examination will reveal a visible or palpable defect between the fragments. A significant hemarthrosis usually develops secondary to the fracture. If a palpable bony defect is present with little or no effusion, a large retinacular tear should be expected.

Knee extension is then evaluated. A tense hemarthrosis will make this part of the examination ex-

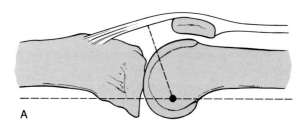

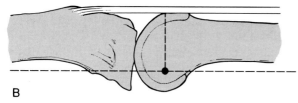

Figure 48–4

The mechanical role of the patella. *A,* The patella increases the moment arm of the extensor mechanism (i.e., the distance between the vector of applied force and the knee's instant center of rotation). *B,* After patellectomy, this moment is decreased, and thus extensor force is effectively diminished. (Redrawn from Kaufer, H. J Bone Joint Surg 53A:1551–1560, 1971.)

tremely painful for the patient. Arthrocentesis with injection of lidocaine or bupivacaine into the joint is often helpful. The patient's ability to extend the knee does not rule out a patella fracture and may simply mean that the patellar retinaculum is intact. The inability to extend the knee, however, suggests that a discontinuity in the extensor mechanism exists. In a patellar fracture this implies a tear of both the medial and the lateral quadriceps expansion.[10,57,74]

Occasionally a laceration exists in proximity to a patella fracture. This may represent an open fracture or an open joint injury. Because both are surgical emergencies, it becomes imperative to diagnose these early. A simple means of evaluation is the saline load test. A large-bore needle (18-gauge or higher) and a 50-ml syringe are used to perform a joint aspiration. A significant amount of bloody fluid may be removed, usually resulting in relief of pain. The needle is left in place while the syringe is removed and filled with saline. This is then injected into the knee joint. Any communication between the fracture or joint and the outside environment will become obvious if the saline exits the wound.

After a history and physical examination are obtained, radiographic evaluation is performed. Once a diagnosis is made, the knee is splinted in a position of comfort (usually slight flexion), iced, and elevated. If the patient requires immediate transfer to the operating room or intensive care unit, portable radiographs will suffice.

RADIOGRAPHIC EVALUATION

The radiographic evaluation of the patella includes standard and specialized radiographic techniques, tomography, computed tomography, and bone scanning. When time permits, standard radiographic evaluation of the uninvolved knee should be obtained. This affords the physician a comparison view for evaluation and allows for any preoperative planning that might be necessary.

Standard Views

Anteroposterior

The normal anteroposterior radiograph is taken with the patient standing, but this is impossible in the patient with an acute fracture. Instead, the film must be taken with the cassette underneath the knee of a supine patient. The extremity should be aligned so that the patella points straight up. This is especially important

in the patient with an ipsilateral femoral shaft fracture. If the patient has a large hemarthrosis creating moderate knee flexion, the x-ray beam must be angled accordingly. Because the possibility of occult concomitant ipsilateral leg injuries exists, the largest cassette possible (14″ × 17″) should be employed.

Evaluation of the anteroposterior radiograph requires analysis of several factors (Fig. 48–5). Patella position should be assessed; the patella should lie in the midline of the femoral sulcus. In addition, patellar height should be examined; the inferior pole of the patella is normally located just above a line drawn across the distal profile of the femoral condyles (see Fig. 48–7A).

At times mistaken for a patellar fracture, a bi- or tripartite patella is a developmental residual from a variation in which the patella arises from two or more ossification centers that fail to fuse (Fig. 48–6). This usually is a bilateral finding. The most common type is the bipartite. This exhibits a bony mass located in the upper outer quadrant of the patella. It is separated from the main patellar mass by opposing smooth bony surfaces. The condition is usually asymptomatic and requires no treatment, but it can cause confusion when there has been a history of injury to the knee area.[57] In these cases, a radiograph of the opposite patella should be obtained. Invariably a similar pattern will be found, thus making the diagnosis. True unilateral bipartite patella is very rare and may represent an old marginal patella fracture.[25]

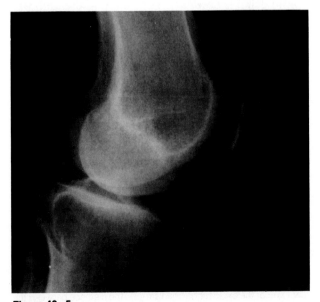

Figure 48–5

Lateral radiograph of the normal patella. (From Resnick, D.; Niwayama, G. Diagnosis of Bone and Joint Disorders, 2nd ed. Philadelphia, W.B. Saunders, 1988.)

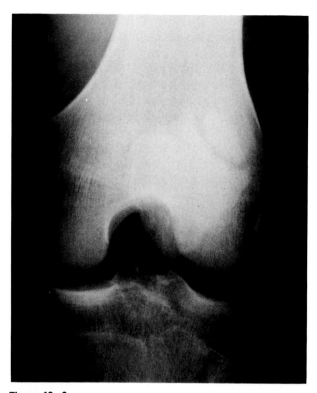

Figure 48-6

Radiograph of bipartite patella demonstrating characteristic proximal lateral ossification center with curved, well-demarcated lucent zone of separation.

Lateral

Although the lateral radiograph is easy to obtain, attention to detail is necessary, as rotation of the limb will negate the benefits of this view. The proximal tibia must be seen to exclude patellar ligament ruptures or avulsions (see Fig. 48-5). This view of the knee will present a transverse or comminuted patellar fracture rather dramatically. Unfortunately, however, this may prevent the examiner's discovery of subtler findings.

In patients with a patella fracture, additional injury to the patella tendon may occur. This can best be evaluated with a comparison radiograph of the other limb. This and other indicators of abnormal patellotibial relationships are shown in Figure 48-7. In the normal subject, the most reliable method for the assessment of patellar height is the method of Insall et al.[16,44] This technique employs the ratio of greatest diagonal patella length to patella tendon length. In the normal subject this ratio is 1.0. A ratio of less than 1.0 suggests a high-riding patella (patella alta) or patellar tendon rupture. Up to 20% variance is normal.

Tangential

Tangential or axial ("sunrise," "sunset," or "skyline") views of the patella are primarily used in the analysis of patellofemoral disorders (Fig. 48-8). In fractures of the patella, these studies aid the surgeon in the diagnosis of longitudinal (i.e., marginal or vertical) fractures and osteochondral defects.

The three most common views are those of Hughston, Laurin, and Merchant.[16,58] Although all give approximately the same information with respect to patellofemoral congruence, the views of Hughston and Laurin are impractical in the trauma setting. The former requires that the patient be prone, whereas the latter requires patient participation.

Merchant, in 1974, described a method of obtaining an axial view of the patella (Fig. 48-8A).[58] The patient is placed supine on the x-ray table with the knees flexed 45° over the end. The knees are elevated slightly to keep the femurs horizontal and parallel with the table surface. An x-ray beam is angled 30° from the horizontal. The cassette is then placed about one foot below the knees and perpendicular to the x-ray beam. This method is simple, easily reproducible by x-ray technicians, and able to obtain accurate radiographs in the patient with a painful partially flexed knee secondary to hemarthrosis (Fig. 48-8B).

Tomography

The principal use of tomography in the evaluation of bony injuries about the knee is in the detection of occult fractures. Apple et al. recommended tomography over bone scanning in these cases, especially for stress fractures and in elderly patients with osteopenia and hemarthrosis.[2] In their series, routine radiographs were negative in all cases; 71% of the fractures were identified with tomography, compared with only 30% using bone scans. Tomography also may be of benefit in the evaluation of a patellar nonunion or malunion.[87]

Computed Tomography

Although theoretically of benefit to the diagnostician, computed tomography (CT) scanning is rarely employed for evaluation of an isolated patella fracture. It is usually performed as an incidental study during the evaluation of distal femoral or proximal tibial fractures. The information presented rarely adds to that obtained with more conventional techniques. CT may aid the surgeon in the evaluation of articular incongruity in cases of nonunion, malunion, and patellofemoral alignment disorders (Fig. 48-9).

Bone Scanning

Scintigraphic examinations with technetium-labeled phosphate compounds are helpful in the diagnosis of stress fractures, although our preference would be to

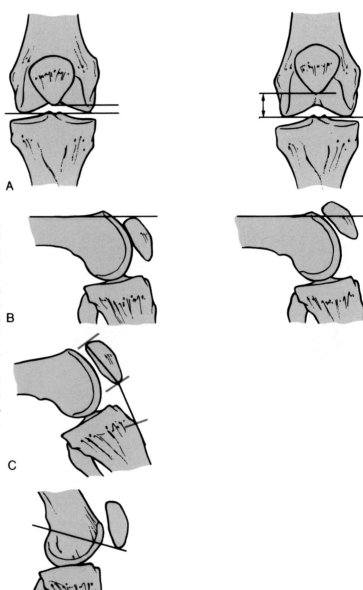

Figure 48–7

Radiographic indicators of an abnormal patellotibial relationship. An excessive distance between the distal pole of the patella and the tibial tubercule may represent disruption of the patellar ligament or chronic patella alta. *A*, On the AP view, the distal pole of the patella lies no more than 20 mm above the plane of the femoral condyles. *B*, When the knee is flexed 90°, the proximal pole of the patella should lie posterior to the anterior surface of the femoral shaft. *C*, On a lateral radiograph, the length of the patellar ligament (from the distal pole of the patella to the tibial tubercule) approximates that of the patella. If the ratio of patella to patellar ligament is less than 0.8, then the patella is excessively high. *D*, Blumensaat's line, the plane of the residual distal femoral physeal scar, normally projects near the distal pole of the patella (see Figure 48–5). (Redrawn from Resneck, D.; Niwayama, G. Diagnosis of Bone and Joint Disorders, 2nd ed. Philadelphia, W.B. Saunders, 1988.)

obtain plain tomograms. The bone scan may also be useful with indium-labeled leukocytes or gallium scanning in the assessment of patellar osteomyelitis.

Fracture Classification

There are three major categories of patellar fractures: transverse, stellate, and vertical. Transverse fractures that are proximal (basal) or distal (apical) are termed *polar*. Because these usually extraarticular disruptions of the quadriceps pose different therapeutic challenges, they are classified separately (Fig. 48–10).[10,54] Wide variations within each fracture pattern have prevented the creation of a useful classification scheme.[8,10,74] Because of this difficulty, most authors have reviewed long-term results according to treatment rather than fracture type.[8,10,11,19,54,65,74,82]

For the purposes of this chapter, existing classification schemes were combined for better understanding (Table 48–1).[8,10,54,82] Although the terms "stellate" and "comminuted" are interchangeable in much of the published literature, to avoid confusion when speaking of a comminuted transverse fracture, a stellate patellar fracture is one created by a direct blow resulting in varying degrees of patellar comminution.

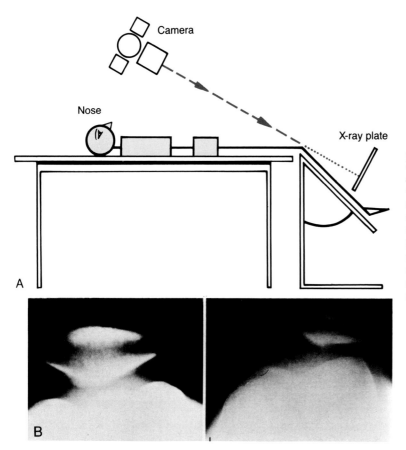

Figure 48–8

A, Merchant's tangential view of the patella is made with the knee flexed 45° and the radiograph exposed as shown (see text). B, A "skyline" type radiograph exposed in this fashion. It demonstrates the patellofemoral relationship, which may be made incongruent by quadriceps contraction. The image on the left is normal; that on the right shows lateral subluxation. (B, from Resnick, D.; Niwayama, G. Diagnosis of Bone and Joint Disorders, 2nd ed. Philadelphia, W.B. Saunders, 1988.)

NONDISPLACED FRACTURES

Stellate

Stellate fractures of the patella are the result of a direct compressive blow that forces the bone against the fem-

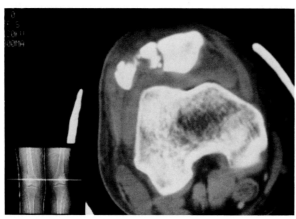

Figure 48–9

Computerized tomography scan of a fractured patella. Note the extent of comminution as well as the secondary sagittal fracture and the resulting articular incongruity.

oral condyles. Damage to the articular cartilage of the femoral condyles and the creation of osteochondral fragments may occur and must be ruled out.[15] Typically, well over half (65%) of these fractures are nondisplaced.[10] In these fractures the blow is insufficient to tear the patellar retinaculum, and active extension of the knee is therefore possible. Displacement between fragments is, by definition, less than 3 mm and between the articular surfaces, less than 2 mm. Unless an osteochondral fragment exists requiring arthrotomy or arthroscopy, nonoperative therapy is indicated (Fig. 48–11).

Transverse

Transverse fractures of the patella are the result of a tensile stress applied to the extensor mechanism. Typically, 35% or more of all transverse patellar fractures are nondisplaced.[1,10] Damage to both the femoral and patellar articular surface is minimal,[71] and usually the force is insufficient to tear the medial and lateral patellar retinaculum.[10,34,57,71,74] As a result, the patient retains the ability to extend the knee. In addition, the intact soft tissue envelope maintains patellar align-

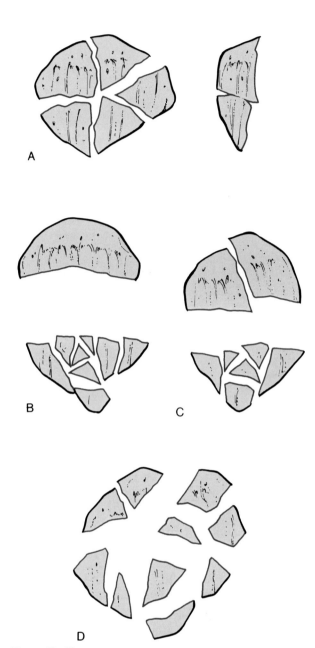

Figure 48–10

Examples of patellar fractures. *A*, Undisplaced fractures may have any degree of comminution, but fragments are displaced no more than 3 mm. The articular surface as seen on the lateral view should not have a step-off of more than 2 mm. *B*, Displaced transverse fracture with comminution of apical pole. *C*, Displaced transverse fracture with comminution of both apical and basilar poles. *D*, Highly comminuted, highly displaced fracture.

Table 48–1.

Fracture Classification

A. Nondisplaced Fractures
  1. Stellate
  2. Transverse
  3. Vertical
B. Displaced Fractures
  1. Noncomminuted
    a. Transverse (central)
    b. Polar
      1. Apical
      2. Basal
  2. Comminuted
    a. Stellate
    b. Transverse
    c. Polar
    d. Highly comminuted, highly displaced

---

ment; typically less than 3 mm of fragment diastasis and 2 mm of articular incongruity exist. If these conditions are met, nonoperative treatment is suggested (Fig. 48–10).

Vertical

Vertical fractures (marginal or longitudinal fractures), contrary to earlier reports, are a common type of patellar fracture, with a combined incidence of 22% (384/1707) in several large series.[6,11,25] The fracture may be caused by different mechanisms. Dowd stated that direct compression of the patella in a slightly hyperflexed knee created this fracture.[25] In Bostrom's series, lateral avulsions accounted for more than 75% of all vertical fractures.[11] Bony separation is most commonly found at the junction of the middle and lateral thirds of the patella; less commonly, a medial pole avulsion occurs.[6]

Clinically, the patient presents with a somewhat painful knee and a mild effusion. Full extension of the joint is possible, because the patellar retinaculum is intact.[6,11,25] A diastasis of greater than 3 mm is most unusual.[10,11] The fracture may be missed on standard radiographs; axial views are usually necessary to make the diagnosis.[6,11] If the defect is seen on the anteroposterior radiograph, it may be easily mistaken for a bipartite patella, and radiographs of the opposite limb should be obtained. Because there is minimal displacement of the fracture fragments and the patellar retinaculum remains intact, these fractures are best treated nonoperatively.

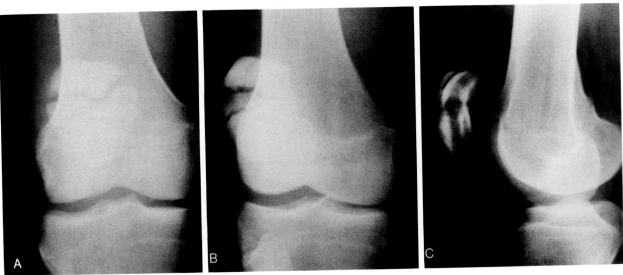

Figure 48–11

A nondisplaced stellate fracture of the patella. Radiographic projections are (A) AP, (B) oblique, and (C) lateral.

DISPLACED FRACTURES

Noncomminuted

Transverse/Midpatellar

Displaced fractures account for slightly more than half (52%) of all noncomminuted transverse fractures of the patella. The diagnosis is made in a patient with loss of active extension of the knee (after aspiration), a separation of greater than 3 mm between fracture fragments, or an articular step of greater than 2 mm.[8–10,57,74] These findings suggest retinacular disruption and joint incongruity. Either finding warrants an operative repair (Fig. 48–12).

Some patients may present with a gap of 4 to 5 mm between fracture fragments but can extend their leg actively. McMaster warned of nonunion in these patients when treated conservatively.[57] Boström, in reviewing the results of his and other large published series, however, concluded that active extension implied retinacular continuity and could heal satisfactorily without surgery.[10] I concur with his advice.

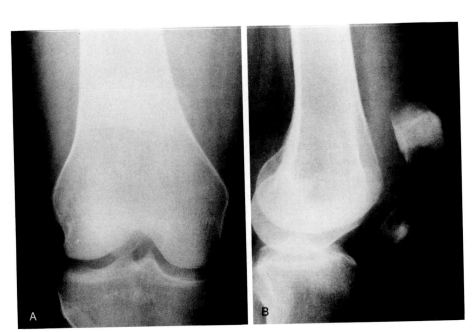

Figure 48–12

A displaced transverse fracture of the patella. A, AP radiograph. B, Lateral radiograph.

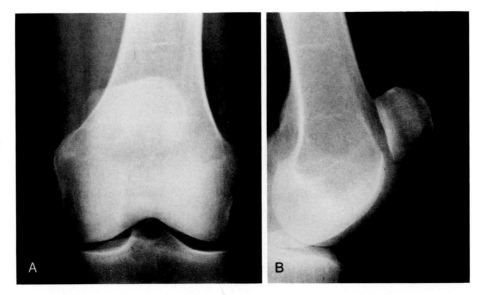

Figure 48 – 13

Displaced distal polar fracture of the patella. *A*, AP radiograph. *B*, Lateral radiograph.

Polar

Polar fractures of the patella are transverse fractures occurring either proximal or distal to the patella equator and taking varying amounts of bone. Proximal, or basal pole, fractures imply an avulsion of the quadriceps mechanism from the patella. The amount of accompanying retinacular rupture will determine the patient's ability to extend the leg. Displacement is extremely rare and accounts for less than 4% in several large series.[10]

Distal, or apical, fractures are bony avulsions of the proximal patellar tendon (Fig. 48 – 13). These fractures, occurring toward the distal margin of the retinaculum, are almost invariably associated with a loss of knee extension. As a result, displacement in apical fractures is almost three times as common (11.5%) as in basal injuries.[10]

Comminuted

Stellate

A result of direct compression, comminuted stellate fractures usually exhibit displacement with varying degrees of comminution.[15] Although the patellar retinaculum is intact, operative intervention is indicated because of existing articular incongruity (Fig. 48 – 14).

Transverse/Polar

These comminuted fractures exhibit varying degrees of comminution of one major patella fragment. Upper

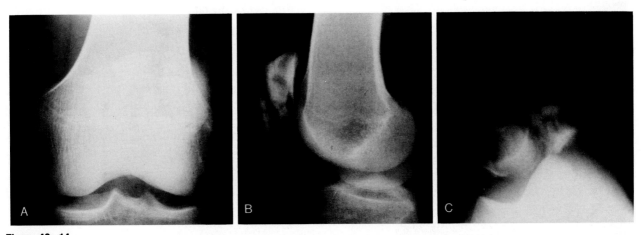

Figure 48 – 14

Displaced stellate fracture of the patella. *A*, AP view; the fracture is difficult to see. *B*, Lateral view; the fracture is apparent, but displacement appears to be only moderate. *C*, Skyline radiograph clearly indicates displacement and incongruity of articular surfaces.

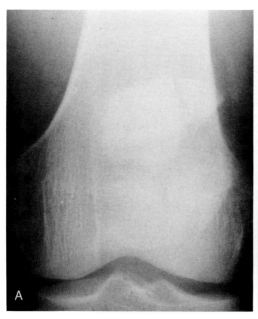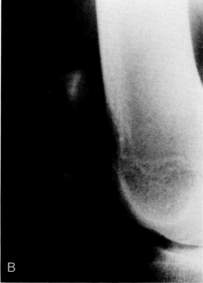

Figure 48–15

Comminuted transverse fracture of patella. *A*, AP view; the details of fracture configuration are hard to see. The main displaced transverse component and secondary vertical fracture lines are evident. *B*, Lateral view; displacement is more obvious, but comminution is less apparent.

fragment comminution usually presents with one or two additional fracture lines that are minimally displaced. Lower fragment comminution is usually more severe and may be accompanied by upper pole comminution.[8,10] Comminution is much more prevalent in the lower pole than in the upper pole.

Highly Comminuted, Highly Displaced

Highly comminuted and displaced fractures consist of transverse fractures with massive comminution secondary to compression or stellate fractures with massive diastasis secondary to a violent quadriceps contraction (Fig. 48–15). All major fragments are separated by more than 6 mm, and sagittal splits are often present as well. These fractures frequently present as open injuries and can occur with supracondylar femur fractures.

Treatment

The management of patella fractures is based on the pattern of injury encountered. Treatment options include nonoperative treatment, tension band wiring, partial patellectomy, partial patellectomy combined with tension band wiring, and total patellectomy. These are performed with careful reconstruction of the extensor mechanism and of the patellar joint surface whenever possible. Figure 48–16 outlines this chapter's proposed algorithm for the management of patella fractures. Specific details of fixation may need to be modified to accommodate a given fracture pattern.

NONOPERATIVE TREATMENT

Indications for nonoperative management include transverse, stellate, and vertical nondisplaced closed patellar fractures. Treatment consists of extension splinting for four to six weeks.[10,34,57,71,74] If plaster is used, care should be taken to extend the cast from just above the ankle to the groin (not the middle of the thigh). If the patient is elderly or has varicose veins, an Unna's boot is applied to the foot and ankle prior to casting to minimize swelling.[74]

Immediate weight bearing as tolerated is permitted. Isometric quadriceps exercises and straight leg raises are encouraged several days postoperatively.[10,34,57] After radiographic evidence of consolidation, usually at four weeks, the plaster may be removed, and progressive active (not passive) flexion and strengthening exercises are begun.

In reliable patients, I prefer the use of an off-the-shelf hinged knee brace. This is lightweight and easily adjustable and permits controlled motion of the knee joint. The knee hinge is locked in extension during ambulation but may be opened to permit controlled motion during the convalescent period. This may be advantageous for elderly patients.

OPERATIVE TREATMENT

Open Fractures

Open patellar fractures are surgical emergencies. Awareness of the possibilities of osteomyelitis or septic arthritis is necessary. Irrigation with debridement and

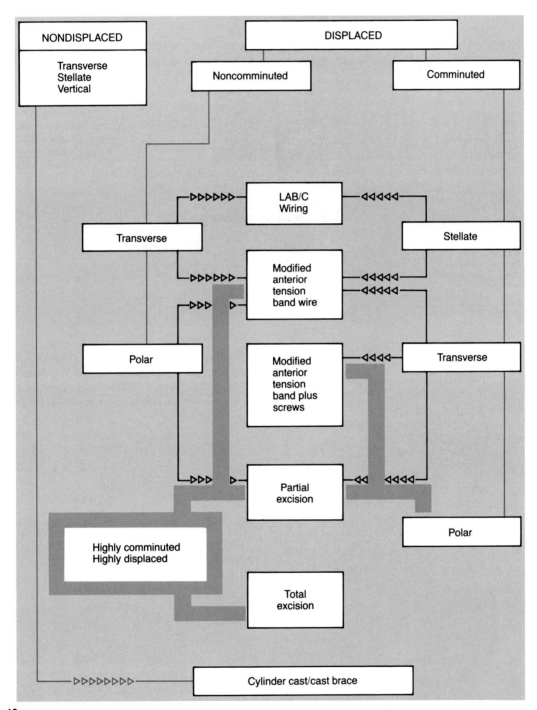

Figure 48–16

Displacement and fracture pattern both guide choice of treatment with which to obtain the two primary goals of quadriceps mechanism continuity and a stable anatomic reduction of the patellar articular surface. Nondisplaced fractures are managed nonoperatively. Displaced articular fractures are repaired, if possible, using tension band wiring techniques with or without screws or interosseous wiring. Polar avulsion fractures may be excised, but a secure reattachment of the quadriceps or patellar tendon is required. If comminution prevents satisfactory repair, total patellectomy may be the only option to restore the quadriceps.

stable fixation remain the principles of treatment. Devitalized fragments should not be saved, and heroic efforts at salvage are not indicated. Fixation should be performed with a minimum of soft tissue stripping and must be stable. Subsequent redebridements will be necessary, and closure may require skin grafts, muscle flaps, or free tissue transfer.

Preoperative Planning

Before embarking on surgical repair of the patella, an operative plan should be firmly established. This requires a radiographic evaluation of the normal oppo-

site patella. Using tracing paper or clear x-ray film, outline the normal patella. The fracture fragments are then superimposed onto this outline in both the anteroposterior and the lateral planes. This in effect "reduces" the fracture. Attention is then turned to fixation, be it wires, screws, partial excision, or a combination of modalities. These should be drawn onto the plan and numbered in sequence. Finally, contingency plans, as well as the necessary equipment, should be listed. The surgeon should be aware that the superimposition of the patella on the femur makes this exercise difficult at times. It therefore requires optimum radiographic technique.

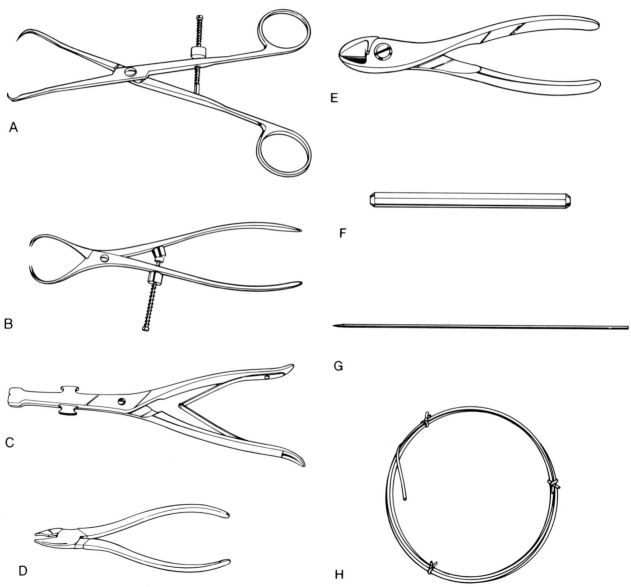

Figure 48–17

Instruments and implants helpful for fixation of patella fractures include pointed reduction forceps for large bones (*A*), patella forceps (*B*), wire tightener (*C*), wire-bending pliers (*D*), wire cutter (*E*) for Kirschner wires, wire bender/impactor (*F*), Kirschner wire (*G*), and malleable wire of at least 1 mm diameter (*H*).

Preoperative planning allows the surgeon to think through the operative procedure and become acquainted with the "personality of the fracture." In addition, equipment requirements will be known beforehand, thus assuring a smooth intraoperative course. When this plan is adhered to, the postoperative film will appear remarkably similar to the preoperative plan.

Equipment

A wire set incorporating Kirschner wires, 1.2 mm (18-gauge) and 1 mm (19-gauge) wire on spools, wire holders, wire tighteners, wire pliers, and a wire passer is necessary, along with a power drill and a wire driver (Fig. 48–17). A small fragment instrument and implant set and Weber (large pointed) bone reduction forceps are also useful. A special patella clamp is an invaluable device, as the Weber clamps often rotate. Angiocatheters (14- or 16-gauge) are helpful for passing wire. A large fragment set should always be available. Large osteochondral fragments will require minifragment screws or Herbert screws, and for small fragments, absorbable Vicryl pins (Ethipins) should be available.

Setup

The patient is placed in the supine position, and a tourniquet located high on the thigh is used. Trapping of the quadriceps may cause difficulty with repositioning of the patella when the tourniquet is inflated. To avoid this, the knee should be carefully flexed beyond 90° to bring the quadriceps and proximal patella fragment down before inflating the tourniquet. In patients with complete retinacular disruption and a very high-riding proximal patellar fragment, a sterile tourniquet can be inflated after the patella has been brought down by using an Esmarch's bandage wrapped in a proximal to distal direction.[17]

Incisions

Although any knee incision can be used, a transverse, midline longitudinal, or lateral parapatellar incision is preferred (Fig. 48–18). In patients with severe retinacular disruption, a transverse incision parallels this disruption and minimizes the development of flaps.[54,62] In more comminuted fractures, a midline longitudinal or lateral parapatellar incision is necessary, especially if concomitant injuries suggest the possibility of a joint replacement in the future. These latter incisions also avoid damage to the saphenous branch of the femoral nerve medially.[1]

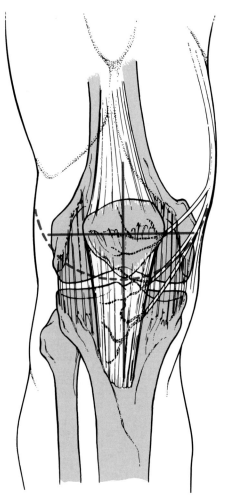

Figure 48–18

Incisions for exposure and treatment of patellar fractures. Either a longitudinal or a transverse approach may be used. Sufficient exposure to see and effectively repair medial and lateral retinacular tears is important. Superficial dissection should be avoided to preserve thickness and viability of the skin flaps.

Operative Techniques

All displaced fractures of the patella require operative intervention. As previously mentioned, the techniques employed are based on the fracture pattern and concomitant injuries (Table 48–2).

Tension Band Wiring

Modified Anterior Tension Band Wiring. For displaced noncomminuted two-part transverse patellar fractures, open reduction and internal fixation using the modified anterior tension band technique is the treatment of choice (Fig. 48–19).

A midline longitudinal incision is made through the skin and overlying bursa. The fracture edges are exposed and cleaned completely of debris and clot, with

Table 48-2.

Treatment of Patella Fractures

Patella Fracture Type	Treatment
A. Nondisplaced fractures	1. Cylinder cast
1. Transverse	
2. Stellate	
3. Vertical	
B. Displaced fractures	
1. Noncomminuted	
a. Transverse	1. Modified anterior tension band wiring
b. Polar	1. Partial patellectomy
1. Apical	2. Modified anterior tension band wiring
2. Basal	
2. Comminuted	
a. Stellate	1. Modified anterior tension band wiring
	2. Longitudinal anterior tension band plus cerclage
b. Transverse	1. Independent lag screws plus modified anterior tension band wiring
	2. Longitudinal anterior tension band wiring
	3. Partial patellectomy
c. Polar	1. Partial patellectomy
d. Highly comminuted, highly displaced	1. Modified anterior tension band wiring
	2. Longitudinal anterior tension band wiring (LAB)
	3. Partial patellectomy
	4. Total patellectomy

care taken not to devitalize the fragments. The knee joint is then irrigated to remove any loose fragments.

A preliminary reduction is then performed to evaluate the proper position of the fragments. The reduction is then taken down and the proximal fragment is flexed 90°. Using a 2-mm drill bit, a hole is drilled through the proximal fragment in a retrograde manner. This hole should start within the fracture line, approximately 5 mm from the anterior surface of the patella and at the junction of a line separating the patella into thirds. The drill bit is then exchanged for a 1.6-mm Kirschner wire that is pushed proximally until it is flush with the fracture edge. A second hole (parallel to the first and at the junction of a line separating the patella into thirds) is drilled. Its drill bit is exchanged with a K-wire in a similar manner. The fracture is then reduced and held with Weber or patellar reduction forceps. The wires are then sequentially removed, and the holes drilled distally with a 2.0-mm drill bit up to, but not through, the distal cortex. A prebent 1.6-mm K-wire is then inserted

into the drill hole and hammered through the far cortex. Next a 1.2-mm (18-gauge) wire is placed underneath the upper hooks and the lower protruding pin tips. The wire is loosely tightened with a wire tightener. The reduction is checked by extending the knee and palpating the undersurface of the patella with a finger. If a finger cannot be easily inserted through the retinacular tear (or if none exists), the retinaculum should be longitudinally incised to permit this. If articular congruity is satisfactory, the wire should then be twisted tightly with a wire tightener and buried. The K-wires are twisted so that the bend is facing backward and buried into the patella. The excess distal ends of the K-wires are then cut off distally.

Although certain authors recommend crossing the tension band wire, in my experience this reduces the area of patella that can be compressed and often leads to an unstable osteosynthesis. A prefabricated cerclage loop (AO type) is also not recommended for use as a tension band wire, as in my experience this can come undone with early motion. The retinaculum is then sutured closed with figure-of-eight 0 Vicryl interrupted sutures, and the wound is closed in layers over a drain.

Longitudinal Anterior Band plus Cerclage (LAB/C) Wiring. Minimally displaced stellate fractures requiring operative intervention may not present with a single fragment large enough to permit a modified anterior tension band technique. In these cases either the K-wire should be angled appropriately or the Longitudinal Anterior Band plus Cerclage (LAB/C) wiring technique of Lotke and Ecker may be employed (Fig. 48-20).[54]

The patella is approached, and the fragments are cleaned as described in the section on modified anterior tension band wiring. Two parallel Beath-Steinman pins (with holes in the distal tip), are drilled 1 cm from the patellar edges through the aligned patella fragments in an antegrade manner. A 22-gauge wire is then inserted into both drill bit holes, and both pins are removed proximally. The distal loop is brought anteriorly, and one free proximal end is passed through this anterior loop. It is then tied to the other proximal end and tightened. This results in a strong and secure combination of anterior band and interosseous wiring techniques. Heavier-gauge wire may be safer for fixation — e.g., 18-gauge wire passed with the aid of a large angiocatheter placed over the K-wire and held in place when it is withdrawn.

If marked comminution is present, an initial cerclage wire should be placed around the circumference of the patella. This can easily be done with a wire passer or a 16- or 14-gauge angiocatheter inserted immediately next to the patella. The LAB/C wiring is then per-

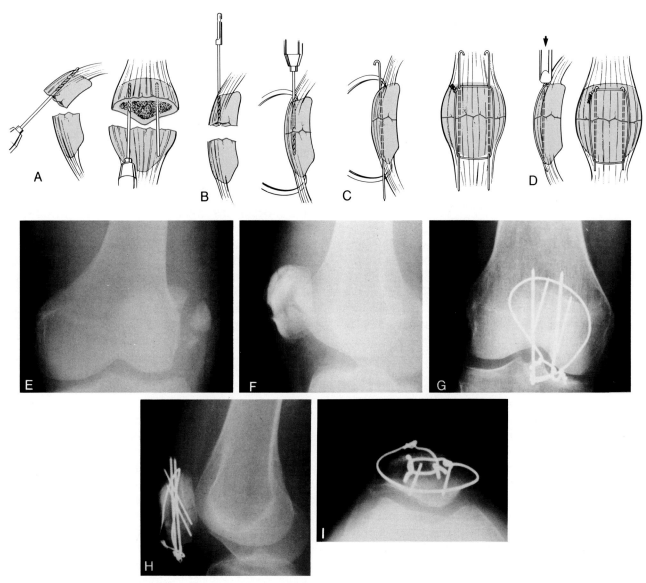

Figure 48–19

Modified AO tension band technique for patella fracture fixation (see text). *A,* Retrograde drilling of proximal fragment. K-wires mark the proximal ends of the holes during reduction. *B,* Reduction, clamping, and antegrade partial drilling of distal fragment. K-wires with prebent proximal ends are then hammered through the remaining bone of the distal pole. *C,* With a large-bore needle, the 1.2-mm tension band wire is placed deep to the proximal and distal ends of the K-wires immediately adjacent to the patella through the stout soft tissue attachments of the quadriceps tendon and patellar ligament. Medially and laterally, the tension band wire lies anterior to the patella and is not usually crossed. It is tightened and twisted securely, and the "pigtail" end is bent flush with the bone surface. A twist or a square knot is reliable. The AO bent wire fastening technique is not secure enough for definitive fixation. *D,* The prebent proximal ends of the K-wires are driven into the proximal pole, and the distal ends are trimmed if necessary. *E,F,* AP and lateral radiographs showing a displaced comminuted patellar fracture. *G,* AP radiograph after fixation. Note technique modifications for fixation of comminuted fragments: supplementary K-wires, distal-to-proximal K-wire insertion, and a distally crossed tension band wire, which was tightened with medial and lateral twists to equalize tension. *H,I,* Lateral and skyline views show anatomic reduction and anterior placement of the tension band wire.

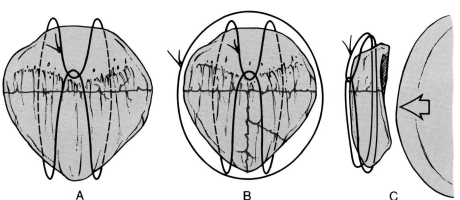

Figure 48-20

Longitudinal anterior band (LAB) technique for interfragmentary wire loop fixation of patella fractures. *A*, For transverse fractures, the two ends of a wire loop are passed through longitudinal drill holes in the patella. One of these is then passed through the loop made by the middle of the wire distally. Next the ends are pulled tight and twisted to provide a taut anterior tension band. *B*, Lateral view. *C*, If there is significant comminution, fixation is aided by first placing a cerclage wire around the patella to trap the comminuted fragments and then drilling and applying the LAB wire as above. (Redrawn from Lotke, P.A., Ecker, M.L. Clin Orthop 158:180–184, 1981.)

formed. The retinaculum is sutured closed with figure-of-eight 0 Vicryl interrupted sutures, and the wound is closed in layers over a drain.

Independent Lag Screws plus Modified Anterior Tension Band Wiring. Transverse fractures may present with one or two additional fracture lines in the main fragments, separating the main fragments into halves or thirds. These secondary fracture lines are usually not displaced but may become so after operative intervention is attempted. The general principles of internal fixation of fractures should be employed (i.e., to make many fragments into two main fragments and then unite these two into one). This can usually be accomplished by independent lag screws placed in a horizontal direction, followed by a modified anterior tension band wiring technique. The size of the screw should fit the size of the bone (i.e., 3.5 cortical screws will usually suffice, except in large adult males, in whom 4.5 screws should be used) (Fig. 48–21). If the fragment is comminuted at the point of screw entry, a washer is employed. Frequently a fragment has or develops a sagittal split during the insertion of the lag screw, separating the anterior cortex from the main chondral surface of that fragment. If this cannot be salvaged by repositioning the screw, LAB/C wiring or excision of the fragment should be considered.

Partial Patellectomy

Not infrequently, patellar fractures exhibit significant comminution of one pole. This may constitute a small or larger portion of the patella. At times, an indirect reduction using a modified anterior tension band or LAB/C wiring technique will be effective. If these techniques are not possible, the time-honored method of partial patellectomy should be employed (Fig. 48–22).[1,19,62,83]

Approach the patella and expose the fracture as previously described. All large, stable, distal fragments should be retained, and all small, comminuted fragments should be excised. All loose strands of the torn quadriceps expansion are removed. If one large distal fragment is present, it may be lagged into position with screws after a reduction has been secured. Care must be taken not to angle this fragment or patellofemoral arthritis will develop. This can be simplified by placing a bolster underneath the ankle to extend the knee (Fig. 48–21*C*).

Because of the powerful tension developed in the quadriceps mechanism, there is significant stress on the repair, which must be protected. This can be accomplished by using a crossed tension band either through the quadriceps insertion or proximal patella and through the proximal tibia by a variety of means (Fig. 48–23). I prefer wire passed directly through the bone, as it is less bulky and easier to remove. Mersilene tape or fascia also may be employed.

If only small fragments remain, the following technique is used. Reflect the anterior periosteum on the proximal fragment approximately 5 mm and, with a rongeur, make a transverse groove in the proximal fragment within the fracture line itself. Then drill three pairs of holes into the anterior cortex so that the drill exits into the fracture line. Excise all bone (except the flecks of bony insertion) from the patellar tendon. Using heavy Mersilene, Ethibond, or equivalent sutures, the proximal patellar tendon is pulled up into the trough of the proximal fragment. The knee should be hyperextended while the suture is tied. A tension band should be added to neutralize stresses on the repair. The retinaculum is then sutured closed with figure-of-eight 0 Vicryl interrupted sutures, and the wound is closed in layers over a drain.

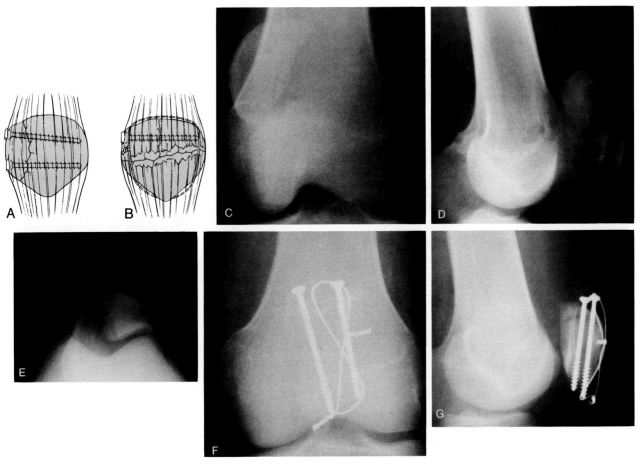

Figure 48–21

AO lag screw plus tension band technique. *A*, Small-fragment screws can be used alone to fix vertical components or comminuted portions of the patella. *B*, These should be supplemented with a tension band wire for fixation of displaced transverse fractures, as screws alone may not withstand the significant forces developed by the quadriceps mechanism. *C* through *E*, AP, lateral, and skyline radiographs, respectively, showing a displaced oblique (functionally transverse) patella fracture. *F,G*, Postoperative AP and lateral radiographs show use of 4.0 cancellous lag screws supplemented by an anterior tension band wire. The wire is crossed in this case to maintain its position anterior to the fracture.

Total Patellectomy

For highly displaced, highly comminuted fractures, an attempt at reconstruction should be made before a total patellectomy is performed. Several authors have stressed the retention of even one fragment to maintain a lever arm.[26,74,82,83] A combination of partial patellectomy and modified anterior tension band or LAB/C wiring is usually tried before total excision is performed. Although many techniques exist, those presented as follows are the most favorably reviewed in the literature.

Because total patellectomy is often a salvage procedure, the surgeon may find various skin incisions and retinacular remnants. Once the decision for total extirpation has been made, all fragments of bone and shredded tendon are removed sharply, but leaving as much tendinous expansion as possible. The critical feature of

a total patellectomy is the tendinous repair. Because the quadriceps tendon is effectively lengthened by the removal of bone, this slack should be taken up by imbrication (i.e., in a purse string repair) or an extensor lag will result.

If insufficient tendon exists for a primary repair, several options are available. These can be separated into two categories: quadriceps turndown procedures and fascial or tendinous weaving. The former technique is used when the prepatellar soft tissue is absent, whereas the latter is reserved for those injuries with destroyed quadriceps tendon as well.

The most common quadriceps turndown technique is the inverted V- plasty of Shorbe and Dobson.[75] After the patella has been excised, the quadriceps tendon is exposed for approximately 3 inches (Fig. 48–24). A full-thickness incision is then made into the quadriceps tendon in the shape of a V, with the apex located 2.5

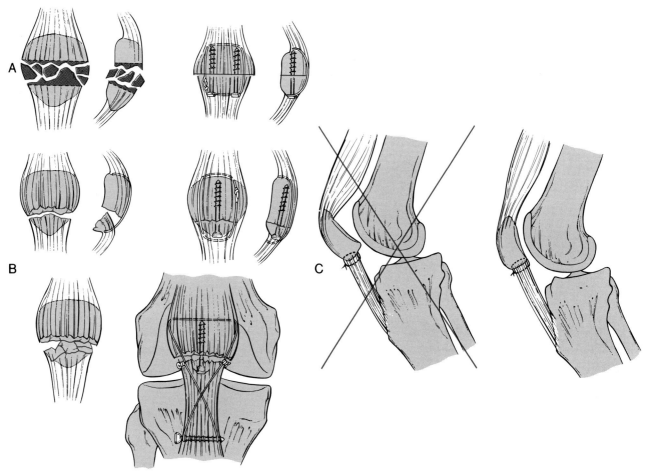

Figure 48-22

Techniques of partial patellectomy. *A*, Extensive comminution of the central portion may be excised, with fixation of proximal-to-distal poles using screws or K-wires and a tension band. The results of this technique are not well documented. *B*, A small (usually extraarticular) bony fragment may aid reattachment of the patellar ligament distally. Screws, K-wires, or sutures may be used, but they should always be protected with a tension band, either limited to the patella if the distal pole fragment is sufficient or from the patella to the tibial tubercule if it is not. *C*, When suturing the patellar ligament into a defect in the distal pole of the patella, it is essential not to attach it too anteriorly, as this will result in malalignment of the patella (*left*), the distal articular surface being forced too far posteriorly. The example on the right shows proper reattachment of the patellar ligament. A tension band from the patella to the tibia should protect this repair.

inches proximal to the former proximal patella edge. The limbs of the incisions extend distally for 2 inches such that one-fourth to one-half inch of tendon is continuous with the retinaculum. The corners may be reinforced with suture if necessary. The apex is then folded down and inserted through the proximal portion of the patellar tendon and sutured down. The quadriceps tendon should then be closed and all edges repaired. This repair is simple to perform, yet has the advantage of being strong enough to allow early motion.

Should a large defect be present involving the quadriceps tendon, a free fascial or tendinous strip is woven into the tendinous remnants after the method of Gallie and Lemesurier.[31] First, clean all excess tendinous shreds from the wound. Extend the knee with padding

under the ankle and measure the defect. This length should be doubled and 2 inches added to obtain the ideal length of fascial graft. Make a separate lateral incision or extend the wound and obtain a strip of fascia lata or iliotibial band of the appropriate length and 1 to 1.5 cm in width. The strip of fascia is then rolled into a cylinder along its long axis and sutured to itself. It is then woven through the remaining quadriceps tendon or muscle, sewn to itself, and passed through the patellar tendon, tacking it down after the slack is taken out. The graft should be of sufficient length to sew one end down to the other. Finally, all edges are firmly sutured down. If the defect requires an exceptionally long strip, plantaris tendon can be used.

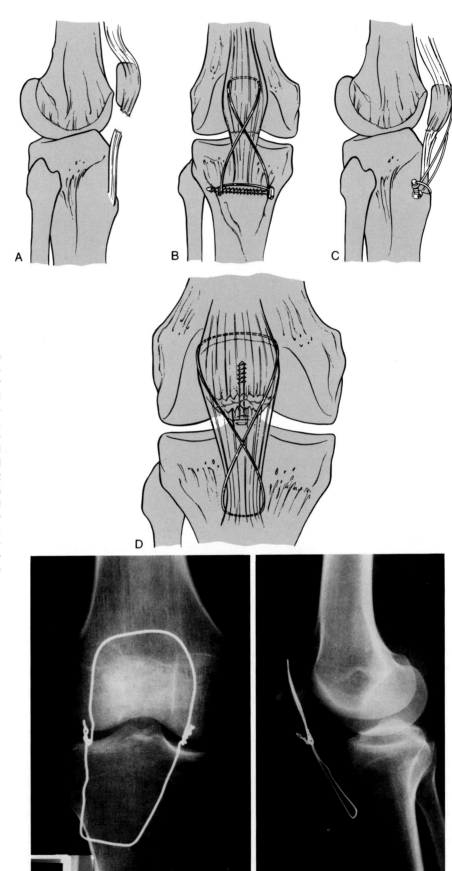

Figure 48–23

A tension band wire technique should be used to protect the patellar ligament reattachment after distal pole fracture fixation, partial patellectomy, or repair of a ruptured patellar ligament (*A*). *B,C,* The 1.0- or 1.2-mm wire can be attached to a screw through the tibial tubercule. *D,* It can be placed through the quadriceps tendon just proximal to the patella or through a drill hole in the patella and through a drill hole distally. *E,F,* AP and lateral radiographs, respectively, showing tension band wire protecting the reattached patellar ligament after distal partial patellectomy.

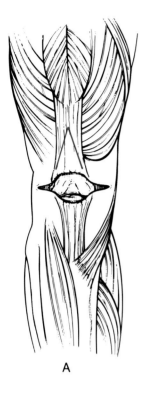
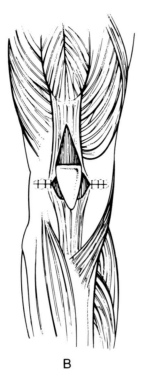
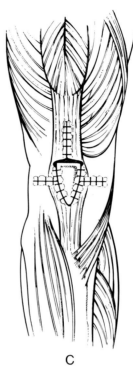

A   B   C

Figure 48-24

Inverted V-plasty technique of Shorbe and Dobson for repair of a patellectomy defect. *A*, The patella is resected, leaving a transverse defect in the quadriceps mechanism. The retinacular rents are first repaired. *B*, If a defect remains centrally, an inverted, distally based V-shaped flap of quadriceps tendon is turned distally as shown. *C*, The flap is sutured in place to cover and reinforce the defect.

Postoperative Management

For all stable osteosyntheses, the patient may begin using a continuous passive motion machine to tolerance immediately postoperatively. In my experience, this decreases pain and stiffness. On the first postoperative day the patient can be out of bed with the leg elevated, and quadriceps isometric exercises are begun. Drains are usually removed after 48 hours. The patient is then placed in a removable knee brace and permitted to ambulate with weight bearing as tolerated with the knee locked in extension. The hinges may be loosened for active range-of-motion exercises. These exercises should not be employed until the wound is well healed, usually at three weeks. Active extension and straight leg raising exercises may be begun as early as one week postoperatively. Progressive resistance exercises are employed when there is radiographic evidence of healing, usually at six weeks. The patient is then weaned from the brace and by three months postoperatively should have a healed fracture and strong quadriceps. Sports and vigorous work may be resumed after rehabilitation is complete, usually $4\frac{1}{2}$ to 6 months.

For unstable osteosyntheses, the repair must be protected. Ideally, a knee brace with locking hinges will permit controlled motion. The hinges are set to allow full extension. Flexion to the degree possible during intraoperative assessment of the repair is permitted, primarily for cartilage nutrition. The brace should be worn at all times, and active flexion exercises should not begin until the fracture has healed. Isometric quadriceps extension exercises should begin at two weeks. Weight bearing should be progressive, with full weight bearing determined by pain. The patient should be made aware of possible knee stiffness. When the fracture has healed radiographically and is clinically stable, attempts at rehabilitation are begun to improve flexion range and strength of all muscle groups.

Implant removal occurs after healing has taken place. K-wires are extracted if they are painful and protruding, but early loosening (before six weeks) may require revision surgery. Asymptomatic implants may be retained indefinitely. Wires used to protect tendon repairs should be left in place for a minimum of three to six months.

RESULTS

Standardization of results in the treatment of patella fractures does not exist. Most authors base outcome on subjective complaints of pain, limitations in activities of daily living, change in job status, and ambulation.[11,28,74] Böstman et al. developed the most complete evaluation of clinical results to date (Table 48-3).[8] This table, however, like most reports in the literature, does not evaluate radiographic findings. Radiographic criteria would include osteoarthritis, fibrous union or

Table 48–3.

Clinical Grading Scale

Clinical Grading Scale/Variable	Score
A. Range of motion (ROM)	
a. Full extension, ROM > 120°	6
b. Full extension, ROM 90°–120°	3
c. Loss of full extension, ROM < 90°	0
B. Pain	
a. None or minimal on exertion	6
b. Moderate on exertion	3
c. In daily activities	0
C. Work	
a. Original job	4
b. Different job	2
c. Cannot work	0
D. Atrophy (10 cm proximal patella)	
a. < 12 mm	4
b. 12–25 mm	2
c. > 25 mm	0
E. Aids	
a. None	4
b. Cane part-time	2
c. Cane full-time	0
F. Effusion	
a. None	2
b. Reported to be present	1
c. Present	0
G. Giving way	
a. No	2
b. Sometimes	1
c. All the time	0
H. Stair climbing	
a. Normal	2
b. Difficult	1
c. Disabling	0

Excellent = 30–28 points; Good = 20–27 points; Failure = < 20 points.

Source: Modified from Böstman, O., et al. Injury 13:196–202, 1981.

Table 48–4.

Combined Results of Various Forms of Operative Treatment in the Literature

Treatment	Results			Total No.
	Excellent	*Good*	*Fair*	
ORIF	135 (37%)	129 (36%)	97 (27%)	361
Partial excision	32 (23%)	67 (49%)	39 (28%)	138
Total excision	62 (28%)	96 (44%)	61 (28%)	219
Totals	229	292	197	718

findings of other large series in that the failure rate from nonoperatively treated nondisplaced patellar fractures was < 5%.[11]

Operative Treatment

Results of operative repair are based on the type of fracture present and the technique employed (Table 48–5). Modified anterior tension band wiring has given the best results in the literature to date, with 57% excellent and 29% good results (Table 48–6).[8,9,43,50,88] Unfortunately, many studies are vague in reporting results, and those reporting this technique are small in number. Analysis of combined data shows tension band wiring to be superior to simple cerclage clinically. Additionally, Weber et al. have shown this to be true biomechanically (Table 48–6).[88] Modified wiring techniques can also be effective. In Lotke and Ecker's report on LAB/C wiring, 16 cases were presented; 13 (81%) had excellent results.[54]

Partial Patellectomy

Partial patellectomy may give functional results comparable to those for open reduction and internal fixation (ORIF), but comparison is difficult, because the fractures patterns treated by these techniques are different.[9,10,50,54,83] Sutton et al. showed that the only deficit with partial excision of at least one third of the patella is an 18° loss of motion.[81] In studies by Böstman et al. and Boström, Mishra, Nummi, and Seligo, a near normal outcome occurred when large fragments of patella were kept and articular congruity was maintained.[9,10,59,65,74] Small fragments without soft tissue, sagittally split fragments, and those missing cartilage were excised. These authors found that saving these fragments did not improve function and even compromised it. Retention of one or two large fragments, however, improved quadriceps function.[9,10,33,46,50,83,89]

nonunion, the presence of osteochondral fragments, and the degree of articular step-off on radiograph.[8,15,74] This lack of standardization allows only broad generalizations to be made (Table 48–4).

Nonoperative Treatment

Nonoperative treatment for nondisplaced fractures has a uniformly good outcome.[10,57,71,78] This implies a full range of motion and no arthrosis, weakness, or pain (see Table 48–3). In Boström's series of 422 patellar fractures, 219 were treated nonoperatively and were available for follow-up.[11] All cases initially had less than 4 mm of articular incongruity; 54% (118/219) had excellent results, and 44% (97/219) had good results. There were only two failures. His results agree with the

Table 48-5.

Results of Operative Repair in Patellar Fractures

			Results		
Author	Year	ORIF	Excellent	Good	Fair
Seligo[74]	1971	35	10	18	7
Nummi[65]	1971	66	3	18	45
Boström[10]	1972	75	19	42	14
Böstman et al.[9]	1983	48	17	21	10
Ma et al.[54a]	1984	107	77	20	10
Levack et al.[50]	1985	30	9	10	11
Total		361	135 (37%)	129 (36%)	97 (27%)

		Partial	Results		
Author	Year	Excision	Excellent	Good	Fair
Seligo[74]	1971	3	0	1	2
Nummi[65]	1971	68	14	28	26
Boström[10]	1972	28	8	15	5
Böstman et al.[9]	1983	35	8	22	5
Mishra[59]	1972	4	2	1	1
Total		138	32 (23%)	67 (49%)	39 (28%)

		Total	Results		
Author	Year	Excision	Excellent	Good	Fair
Seligo[74]	1971	44	14	25	5
Nummi[65]	1971	13	0	5	8
Boström[10]	1972	5	0	1	4
Böstman et al.[9]	1983	10	0	3	7
Levack et al.[50]	1985	34	20	7	7
Wilkinson[92]	1977	31	7	12	12
Mishra[59]	1972	26	3	15	8
Einola et al.[28]	1976	28	6	18	4
Jakobsen et al.[45]	1985	28	12	10	6
Total		219	62 (28%)	96 (44%)	61 (28%)

Total Patellectomy

Total patellectomy has resulted in varying degrees of success. Before the 1970s, poor reconstructive results justified total patellectomy.[13,24,32,35,36,41] Authors compared operative repair using a single cerclage wire with total excision. Although many stated that good clinical results were expected, more recent studies have questioned this conclusion (Table 48-5).[8,10,50,71]

Sutton et al. evaluated quadriceps strength, activities of daily living, and functional ability in patients who had undergone either partial or total patellectomy.[81] The opposite normal knee was the control. Both groups had an average loss of 18° range of motion. A 49% reduction in strength of the extensor mechanism was present in the total excision group. This was the result of loss of the lever arm produced by loss of the patella. Instability was greater in this group, with the patellectomized knee losing almost 50% of excursion in stance phase flexion. This was the result of the patellar tendon's sinking into the intercondylar notch. Clinically this presented as insufficiency and inability to support the loaded knee in stair climbing. Biomechanical studies on cadaver knees performed by Watkins et al., Wendt and Johnson, and others all showed that total patellectomy resulted in a loss of tibial torque and, therefore, strength.[42,46,85,89]

Sørensen noted that the quadriceps did not improve in strength after patellectomy.[78] All patients complained of frequent giving way and difficulty running and walking down stairs. He concluded that none of his operative reconstructions would have fared better with a total excision of the patella and thus justified attempt at salvage. Wilkinson evaluated 31 cases 4.5 to 13 years after total excision.[92] In this study, less than one fourth of patients had an excellent result. He also noted that maximal recovery took up to three years. Einola et al. were able to follow 28 patients for an average of 7.5

Table 48-6.

Comparison of Anterior Tension Band vs. Cerclage Wiring

		Results of Anterior Tension Band			Results of Cerclage Wiring		
Author	No. Patients	Excellent	Good	Poor	Excellent	Good	Poor
Böstman et al.[9]	29	9	3	2	6	6	3
Boström[10]	75	—	—	—	19	42	14
Levack et al.[50]	30	7	5	2	2	5	9
Seligo[74]	31	—	—	—	10	14	7
Ma et al.[54a]	81	—	—	—	59	15	7
Nummi[65]	66	—	—	—	3	18	45
Totals	312	16 (57%)	8 (29%)	4 (14%)	99 (35%)	100 (35%)	85 (30%)

years after total excision.[28] Good results were seen in only six patients. The predominant complaint was weakness and pain on movement and exertion. The most common finding was quadriceps atrophy. Quadriceps power was within 75% of the normal knee in only seven cases. He concluded that saving as much patella as possible was advisable. Scott reported that only 6% (4/71) of patients were happy with their long-term outcome after patellectomy.[71] Ninety percent had aching in the joint, and 60% complained of weakness. Quadriceps wasting was a constant finding.

Present recommendations therefore, are to retain as much patella as possible.[8,9,10,26,43,50,62,82,83] Total patellectomy is reserved for those fractures that are so comminuted that repair is futile. This plan will offer the patient the best possible knee function for the longest period. How much patella should be saved? No definitive answer exists. It is my opinion that as little as 25% of the patella (i.e., one quadrant) may be retained with a subsequently good outcome. I have never found a patella so comminuted that one fragment could not be salvaged with repair. If no articular congruity exists, however, excision is the only option.

Complications

INFECTION

Superficial wound infections should be treated by standard protocol based on the degree of soft tissue involvement. Osteomyelitis is aggressively treated with resection of all sequestra and dead tissue. Irrigation and debridement of the knee must be repeated every 48 to 72 hours until the joint is free of necrotic tissue to prevent septic arthritis. Daily bedside aspirations are not indicated. The patient should be placed on six weeks of culture-specific intravenous antibiotics. Once the deep bone infection is under control, an attempt should be made to salvage any remaining patella using individualized and modified wiring techniques. If this is not possible, total patellectomy may be required.

BREAKAGE OF WIRES, LOSS OF FIXATION, AND REFRACTURE

After osteosynthesis, especially with early motion, the tension band may break. It is unusual for this to occur before healing of the patella. If the fracture is healed, the wire, pins, or screws may be removed if they become symptomatic.

Loss of fixation during the healing phase will require revision if the fragments separate more than 3 to 4 mm or the articular surface develops an incongruity of greater than 3 mm. Before returning to the operating room, a radiograph should be obtained in full extension. If the reduction has improved, the patient may benefit from six weeks of extension splinting. Usually isometric exercises will continue to separate the fragments, however, and unless the patient refuses, revision should be undertaken.

Refracture should be treated as a fresh fracture according to the principles previously described (i.e., nondisplaced fractures are treated nonoperatively, and displaced fractures are treated operatively).

DELAYED UNION AND MALUNION

Delayed union, once a routine result, is extremely uncommon. If identified, a period of decreased motion is begun, as often the fracture will then spontaneously unite. Weber and Cech could find only three cases of patellar pseudarthrosis in their large series of nonunions.[87] All healed with revision surgery utilizing established fracture fixation methods. If it is an old nonunion with 4 to 5 inches of separation, reconstruction should be attempted. Quadriceps shortening will make this repair difficult, and a formal quadricepsplasty may be required. Care must be taken to obtain the correct length, or disability will continue. If chondromalacia exists, consideration should be given to performing a total patellectomy and fascial reconstruction according to Gallie and Lemesurier.[31]

LOSS OF KNEE MOTION

The advent of tension band wiring has permitted early range of motion, and a functional range of motion can be expected in most cases. If flexion is still decreased several months postoperatively, intensive physiotherapy is begun. If this does not suffice, a manipulation under anesthesia should be contemplated. Care must be exercised in patients requiring manipulation and who have had patellectomies, as a rupture of the repair may occur. Recently a report has been published of a boutonnière deformity resulting after manipulation of a longitudinally repaired extensor retinaculum.[64] If manipulation fails, consideration is given to arthroscopic lysis of intraarticular adhesions. A quadricepsplasty is utilized only in exceptional cases, usually when no improvement is seen after 9 to 12 months. This is most often the case after concomitant injury to the distal femur has resulted in binding down of the quadriceps mechanism.

Occasionally after total patellectomy, the extensor mechanism is too long, which may result in a loss of full extension. The patient presents with a sensation of instability and giving way.[78] In this rare case, consideration is given to a Maquet procedure to bring the patella tendon forward and increase its mechanical advantage.

This has been described by Kaufer in excellent biomechanical studies.[46] Reports of clinical results using a Maquet procedure for this purpose are nonexistent. I would caution against using too large a bone block because of subsequent skin breakdown and pain. Other authors suggest reefing the extensor mechanism, but this runs the risk of rerupture.[75]

OSTEOARTHRITIS AND PATELLAR ENLARGEMENT

Although Bruce and Walmsley[14] and Cohn[21] showed that osteoarthritis occurred in rabbits after patellectomy, this has never been borne out in long-term studies of postpatellectomy human knees.[1,10,15,28,45,59,81,92] Additionally, articular incongruity causing osteoarthritis has also not been shown in long-term studies.[10,78]

Two situations have been shown to increase the incidence of osteoarthritis. Patellar enlargement, a result of exuberant bone formation during the healing of comminuted fractures, has been shown unequivocally to cause patellofemoral arthritis. A total patellectomy should be entertained if this has developed.

The second situation that will cause osteoarthritis is posterior rotation of the distal pole of the patella after a too anterior reattachment of the patellar ligament in distal pole patellectomy.[26,74] Care must be taken during repair to avoid this (see section on partial patellectomy and Fig. 48–22C).

TENDON RUPTURE AFTER TOTAL PATELLECTOMY

Rarely, the extensor mechanism will rupture after total patellectomy, usually at the proximal edge of the patellar tendon.[29] This should be repaired by the variety of techniques suggested in the following section on extensor mechanism injuries.

Extensor Mechanism Injuries

A patient that presents with posttraumatic loss of knee extension and negative results on radiograph should be suspected of having a quadriceps or a patellar tendon rupture. The tendon may rupture from a tension tear, direct sharp or blunt trauma, metabolic abnormalities, collagen disease, repeated microtrauma, or repeated injections.[60] In elderly patients, fatty degeneration and tendon scarring are the predisposing cause.[72]

QUADRICEPS RUPTURE

Rupture of the quadriceps occurs primarily in the rectus tendon, usually 0 to 2 cm from the superior pole of the patella.[72,76] The diagnosis may be missed if the patient has little pain or effusion.[67] Physical examination will reveal a palpable defect proximal to the superior pole of the patella.[67] In addition, extension against gravity must be assessed. If there is a palpable defect in the quadriceps tendon but active, full extension is maintained, the tear is incomplete. A partial tear such as this does not require operative repair.[72]

If the ability to extend the knee is completely lost, both the tendon and the retinaculum are torn. the patient will have difficulty climbing stairs, and the knee will buckle with ambulation.[67] Operative repair will be required.[76] Furthermore, if a complete quadriceps rupture is not treated acutely, the quadriceps may ride as far as 5 cm proximally on the femur and then bind down.[72] For this reason, a repair should be done as quickly as possible.

Acute Ruptures

Most authors agree that an end-to-end repair produces excellent results in acute quadriceps tendon ruptures.[49,60,76,77,84] In Miskew et al.'s series, 90% of cases had an excellent outcome.[60] Similarly, Larsen and Lund considered results in 15 of 18 cases (83%) to be excellent[49] while Vainionpää et al. had only one failure in 12 cases.[84] The largest series in the literature is that of Siwek and Rao, who reported on 36 cases of rupture. They found that all 30 patients with an immediate end-to-end repair had excellent or good results with a knee range of motion of 0° to 120°.[77] Complicating primary end-to-end repairs is the difficulty in neutralizing forces across the repair. A review of the literature revealed only five cases in which a stress-relieving wire was used to protect this repair.[49,77,79,84] Several authors reported on the use of a 5-mm Dacron graft to protect the primary repair.[52,60] Levy et al., using this technique, permitted early motion without the use of a cast postoperatively, but weight bearing was delayed for six weeks.[52] Most published series used a local reinforcement flap as suggested by Scuderi, followed by six weeks in an extension cast.[49,67,72,76,77,84]

Scuderi Repair

In the Scuderi repair (Fig. 48–25), the edges of the torn quadriceps are freshened and then pulled together so that a slightly overlapping repair is performed. A distally based, partial-thickness triangular flap of quadriceps tendon is then turned down over the suture line to protect the repair. This flap is an isosceles triangle,

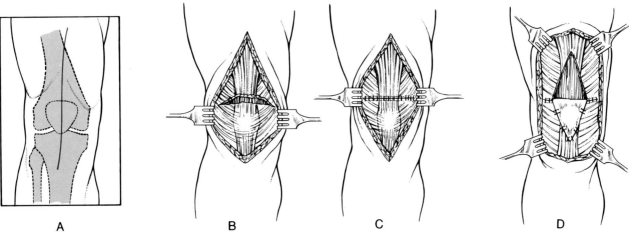

Figure 48-25

Scuderi repair of a ruptured quadriceps tendon. *A*, The defect is exposed through a midline longitudinal incision. *B*, Fasciocutanous flaps are developed to reveal the defect. *C*, Interrupted nonabsorbable stout mattress sutures repair the tendon. These may be directed to the patella centrally. *D*, An inverted, partial-thickness, distally based V-shaped flap is used to reinforce the repair. (Redrawn from Scuderi, C. Am J Surg 95:626-635, 1958.)

3 inches along each side and 2 inches at the base. Alternatively, a variation using the middle third of the patellar tendon may be employed.[18] In this case, the tendon is freed distally, folded proximally, and sewn down. The patient is then placed in a cylinder cast for six weeks.

Chronic Ruptures

In patients with quadriceps ruptures older than two weeks, muscle retraction of as much as 5 cm with adherence of the quadriceps muscle to the femur is common.[72,77] The delay in treatment may require quadriceps lengthening, tendon or muscle transfers, or a combination of these modalities as discussed in the sections that follow.[18,40,66,72,77]

Codivilla V-Y Lengthening

For a Codivilla V-Y lengthening procedure (Fig. 48-26), a standard midline or lateral incision is made, and all soft tissue adhesions are freed from the quadriceps tendon and muscle. The quadriceps muscle is then freed from the femur, using elevators if necessary to break all scars. The knee should be in extension with a roll under the heel. The old tear is located, and the ends are freshened. The gap is then measured. A full-thickness, distally based, V-shaped incision is then made in the quadriceps tendon. Partial-thickness incisions in the vasti may be necessary to aid stretching. The original quadriceps defect is then repaired. The V may be turned distally to reinforce the repair in the method of Scuderi. The proximal defect in the quadriceps tendon

Figure 48-26

The Codivilla V-Y plasty repair for neglected ruptures of the quadriceps tendon. *A*, A distally based V of quadriceps tendon is developed proximal to the defect. *B*, As much of the defect as possible is closed using nonabsorbable stout mattress sutures medially and laterally in the retinacula. *C*, The flap is turned distally and sutured in place over the defect in the quadriceps tendon, restoring central continuity. As much as possible of the defect left by the V is then closed from proximal to distal.

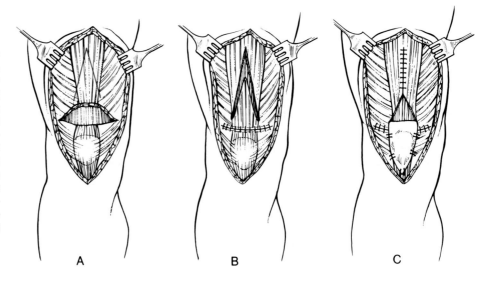

is then repaired in a side-to-side manner. A cylinder cast is employed for six weeks.

Myoplasties and Tendon Transfers

When quadriceps retraction and adhesions make standard techniques impossible (as in neglected tears), neither the Scuderi technique nor the Codivilla V-Y lengthening may be sufficient. In these complex longstanding cases, an aponeurotic vastus lateralis strip 2 to 5 cm thick may be used. This strip is left proximally based and swung medially. The remaining vastus lateralis and medialis are then closed around it. The patient is kept in a cylinder cast for six weeks.[66]

In cases where large defects occur, as in major wounds of the anterior knee, no quadriceps, patella, or patellar ligament may exist. The sartorius can be employed as a rotational flap to cover the area.[40] The tendon is freed distally and inserted into the tibial tubercle region. The advantage of this transfer over the semitendinosus transfer is muscle bulk. Postoperatively, the patient is placed into a cylinder cast for six weeks.

Postoperative Rehabilitation

In all cases, the patient is able to walk several weeks postoperatively in the cylinder cast. Isometric quadriceps setting exercises are not begun until after the cast is removed (six weeks). Controlled motion to 45°, isometric exercises, and straight leg raises are then begun. One month later, range of motion may be increased to 115°, and strengthening exercises are begun. The third month should be spent returning the limb to its preinjury status. The patient should expect a near normal outcome at six months postoperatively.

PATELLAR TENDON RUPTURES

Acute Ruptures

Acute patellar tendon ruptures result in an inability to extend the knee actively. Over time, a neglected tear will permit quadriceps retraction with subsequent contracture. An immediate repair, combined with a wire to relieve stress from the suture line, is the standard treatment for these injuries.[49,56,62,77,86] Although many authors place their patients into a cylinder cast for six weeks postoperatively, the original purpose of the pullout wire as described by McLaughlin and Francis[56] was to allow early knee motion.[62,86]

Repair

For repair of acute ruptures, apply a toe-to-groin Esmarch's bandage and then pull down the proximal end. This will bring down the patella. Inflate the tourniquet and remove the bandage. This prevents getting the quadriceps stuck under the tourniquet.[17] A standard midline longitudinal incision is used. The tendon ends are freshened, and if bony avulsion has occurred, several drill holes should be made in bone to allow for strong fixation. Care should be taken in determining the length of the repair, as studies have shown an incidence of patellofemoral incongruence when this is incorrect.[49]

An 18-gauge wire should be placed closely along the medial, superior, and lateral borders of the patella. It may be attached to the tibia, (posterior and slightly distal to the tubercle) via a drill hole, a bolt, or a screw (see Fig. 48–23). In the latter two cases, a pull-out wire may be added for removal of the 18-gauge wire in the office. After the wire has been tightened, an end-to-end repair with heavy suture is performed. The torn retinaculum should be repaired as well. The repair is then tested in flexion in the operating room, and any loose sutures are repaired. Standard closure over a suction drain is then performed.

Several authors have used fabric material (i.e., Dacron graft or Mersilene tape) for repair, reinforcement, or both.[49,51,52,60] Levin presented a case with a 5-cm gap.[51] Drill holes were made in the patella and tibia, and Dacron vascular graft was used to reconstruct the tendon, pulling the graft tight for tension. At 15 months the repair was still good. Levy et al. used Dacron in place of wire with good results, thus obviating the need for subsequent wire removal.[52] Miskew et al. used 5-mm Mersilene tape as suture to augment the primary repair.[60] If the tendon was avulsed from the proximal patella, holes were drilled into the distal patella. If the tendon was avulsed distally, holes were drilled into the tibia. They reported ten cases with good results.

Chronic Ruptures

Reconstructions months and years later prove unsatisfactory because of difficulty overcoming contracture and adhesions. Similar to repair of the quadriceps mechanism, reconstruction of tendon ruptures can be separated into quadriceps lengthening, tendon transfers, the use of fascial or synthetic grafts, or a combination of these techniques.

Tendon Transfers

For late repairs with large patellar tendon defects, first free the quadriceps from the femur (Fig. 48–27). A Kirschner wire and traction bow are then placed into the patella, and traction is applied. When lateral radiographs show the patella to be correctly positioned, make two drill holes into the patella and one oblique drill hole into the tibia. Release the semitendinosus and

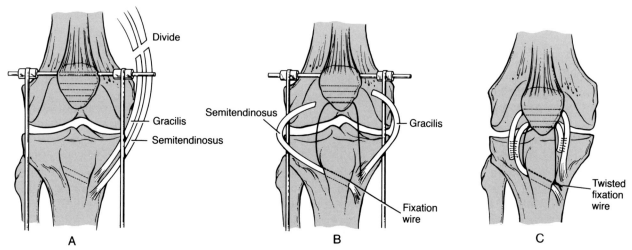

Figure 48–27

Late reconstruction of the patellar ligament using the semitendinosus and gracillis tendons (after Ecker). *A*, The patella is brought down with traction, and the semitendinosus and gracillis tendons are cut as far proximally as possible. *B*, These are routed as shown through drill holes in the patella. Note also the use of a tension band wire through both patella and tibia. *C*, The tendons are sutured distally and the wire secured with appropriate tension. (Modified from Ecker, M.L., et al. J Bone Joint Surg 61A:884–886, 1979.)

semimembranosus tendons proximally. Route the tendons through the tibial hole; then run each tendon into the patella from opposite sides. Pass a pull-out wire through the tibial tubercle region, pull down on the pin, tighten the wire, and then suture the tendons together. A cylinder cast is worn for six weeks.[27,47]

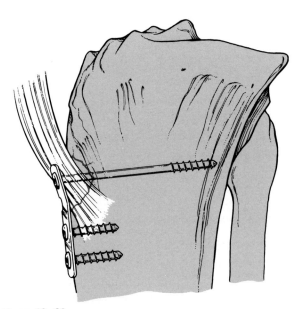

Figure 48–28

Repair of an avulsion fracture of the tibial tubercule can be made more secure with a small plate. The plate acts as a tension band to stabilize the head of a lag screw through the avulsed fragment.

TIBIAL TUBERCLE AVULSIONS

Repair of tibial tubercle avulsions, a variant of patellar tendon avulsions, should incorporate bony reconstruction with 3.5- or 4.5-mm lag screws and a stress-relieving wire, if possible, to guarantee accurate tendinous length and patellar tracking. Anchorage may be improved with a small plate (Fig. 48–28). If the tubercle is comminuted and the fragments are too small for screw fixation, drill holes placed distal and posterior to the avulsion site in the tibia should be employed. Fixation should then proceed as with tendon avulsions.

ACUTE PATELLAR DISLOCATIONS

Although recurrent patellar subluxations are a common cause of knee injury, an acute traumatic patellar dislocation is a rare event. These most commonly present as lateral dislocations, but intraarticular and superior dislocations may occasionally occur.

Lateral Dislocations

The mechanism of lateral patellar dislocation is forced internal rotation of the femur on an externally rotated and planted tibia, with the knee flexed. Tension in the quadriceps pulls the patella laterally. If the medial retinaculum tears, the patella dislocates over the edge of the lateral femoral condyle. This results in shearing between the medial inferior edge of the patella and the lateral femoral condyle.[61] Osteochondral fractures in these areas strongly suggest a lateral patellar dislocation, with the former having an incidence of 5%.[61,68]

Diagnosis

The patient with an unreduced lateral patellar dislocation will present with a large lateral mass, hemarthrosis, medial retinacular pain, and an inability to flex the knee. An attempt should be made to reduce the patella on evaluation to decrease the patient's discomfort. Standard radiographs are then taken, including a tangential view to rule out osteochondral fractures.[61] If the bony portion of the osteochondral fragment is small, the lesion may be missed on radiographs.[4] For this reason, as well as for comfort, an arthrocentesis is performed. If blood from the hemarthrosis contains fat globules on aspiration, then an osteochondral fracture should be considered.[4,61,68]

If the patella is already reduced, the diagnosis of an acute traumatic dislocation will be made more difficult, as medial joint pain and an effusion may be the only findings. This is an important diagnosis to make, because osteochondral fractures must be ruled out. Common symptoms associated with osteochondral fragments include blocking, locking, giving way, and tenderness to palpation on the medial side of knee that is not meniscal or ligamentous in origin.[61]

Treatment

Treatment of an acute lateral patellar dislocation consists of reduction and extension casting for three to six weeks. Cofield and Bryan evaluated 50 cases treated conservatively in extension casts with a follow-up period of five years or until operative reconstruction was needed. Patient age, sex, the mechanism of injury, and the length of time spent in a cast had no effect on outcome.[20] Although one third of their patients were considered treatment failures, they concluded that initial surgery for acute patellar dislocations was not warranted except in those cases with displaced intraarticular fractures exclusive of the medial border.[20] I agree with these findings.

Larsen and Lauridsen studied the incidence of redislocation after conservative treatment of 79 acute patellar dislocations.[48] Treatment included a cylinder cast in 22 patients and an elastic wrap in 57 patients. The clinical results and the tendency to redislocate were independent of the treatment method used. The risk of redislocation was statistically significantly less in patients older than 20 years at the time of the first episode of dislocation. The authors stressed initial conservative treatment and quadriceps strengthening exercises, with realignment procedures considered only if redislocation occurs.

In Morscher's series of 34 osteochondral fractures of the knee, the fracture was caused by an acute lateral dislocation of the patella in 21 of the 34 fractures (62%).[61] Sixteen were found on the medial edge of the patella, one on the lateral femoral condyle, and four on both surfaces. Operative treatment was chosen in all cases.

Currently, I recommend conservative treatment with a cast or brace in extension for ambulation for three weeks. Flexion can then be progressively increased until the patient feels comfortable, usually in another three weeks. If an osteochondral fragment is suspected, a diagnostic arthroscopy is recommended, and if a fragment is present, an operative repair or excision is warranted.

Intraarticular Dislocations

Although rare, intraarticular or horizontal dislocations of the patella usually occur in adolescent boys.[63] In these dislocations, the patella is violently ripped off the quadriceps tendon and rotated around its horizontal axis such that the proximal patella becomes stuck within the intercondylar notch. The knee is slightly flexed, and the quadriceps tendon is intact.[12,30,63,80] Treatment consists of closed manipulation under anesthesia and extension casting for six weeks with quadriceps exercises. Healing is usually uneventful.[12,30,63,80,93]

Superior Dislocations

Four cases of superior patella dislocation exist in the literature.[37,93] The injury occurs in an older population and results from hyperextension of the knee with the patella locked on a femoral osteophyte. Gentle manipulation in the emergency room is all that is usually required.[37,93]

REFERENCES

1. Andrews, J.R.; Hughston, J.C. Treatment of patellar fractures by partial patellectomy. South Med J 70(7):809–813, 1977.
2. Apple, J.S.; Martinez, S.; Allen, N.B.; et al. Occult fractures of the knee: Tomographic evaluation. Radiology 148:383–387, 1983.
3. Arnoczky, S.P. Blood supply to the anterior cruciate ligament and supporting structures. Orthop Clin North Am 16(1):15–28, 1985.
4. Ashby, M.E.; Shields, C.L.; Karmy, J.R. Diagnosis of osteochondral fractures in acute traumatic patellar-dislocations using air arthrography. J Trauma 15(11):1032–1033, 1975.
5. Baumgartl, F. Das Kniegelenk. Berlin, Springer-Verlag, 1964.
6. Black, J.K.; Conners, J.J. Vertical fractures of the patella. South Med J 62:76–77, 1969.
7. Blodgett, W.E.; Fairchild, R.D. Fractures of the patella. JAMA 20.:2121–2125, 1936.
8. Böstman, O.; Kiviluoto, O.; Nirhamo, J. Comminuted displaced fractures of the patella. Injury 13:196–202, 1981.

9. Böstman, O.; Kiviluoto, O.; Santavirta, S.; et al. Fractures of the patella treated by operation. Arch Orthop Trauma Surg 102:78–81, 1983.

10. Boström, A. Fracture of the patella. Acta Orthop Scand 143(suppl):1–80, 1972.

11. Boström, A. Longitudinal fractures of the patella. Reconstr Surg Traumatol 14:136–146, 1974.

12. Brady, T.A.; Russell, D. Interarticular horizontal dislocation of the patella. J Bone Joint Surg 47A(7):1393–1396, 1965.

13. Brooke, R. The treatment of fractured patella by excision. A study of morphology and function. Br J Surg 24:733–747, 1936.

14. Bruce, J.; Walmsley, R. Excision of the patella. J Bone Joint Surg 24:311–325, 1942.

15. Cargill, A.O'R. The long-term effect on the tibiofemoral compartment of the knee joint of comminuted fractures of the patella. Injury 6(4):309–312, 1975.

16. Carson, W. G.; James, S.L.; Larson, R.L.; et al. Patellofemoral disorders: Physical and radiographic evaluation, part II: Radiographic examination. Clin Orthop 185:178–186, 1984.

17. Chari, P.R.; Kishore, R.G.; Satyanarayana, M.V. Repair of the quadriceps apparatus following patellectomy in recent fractures of the patella: A new technique with results. Aust N Z J Surg 48(1):99–103, 1978.

18. Chekofsky, K.M.; Spero, C.R.; Scott, W.N. A method of repair of late quadriceps rupture. Clin Orthop 147:190–191, 1980.

19. Chiroff, R.T. A new technique for the treatment of comminuted, transverse fractures of the patella. Surg Gynecol Obstet 145:909–912, 1977.

20. Cofield, R.H.; Bryan, R.S. Acute dislocation of the patella: Results of conservative treatment. J Trauma 17(7):526–531, 1977.

21. Cohn, B.N.E. Total and partial patellectomy. Surg Gynecol Obstet 79:526–536, 1944.

22. Crock, H.V. The arterial supply and venous drainage of the bones of the human knee joint. Anat Rec 144:199–218, 1962.

23. Depalma, A.F., Flynn, J.J. Joint changes following experimental partial and total patellectomy. J Bone Joint Surg 40A(2):395–413, 1958.

24. Dobbie, R.P.; Ryerson, S. The treatment of fractured patella by excision. Am J Surg 55:339–373, 1942.

25. Dowd, G.S.E. Marginal fractures of the patella. Injury 14:287–291, 1982.

26. Duthie, H.L.; Hutchinson, J.R. The results of partial and total excision of the patella. J Bone Joint Surg 40B(1):75–81, 1958.

27. Ecker, M.L.; Lotke, P.A.; Glazer, R.M. Late reconstruction of the patellar tendon. J Bone Joint Surg 61A(6):884–886, 1979.

28. Einola, S.; Aho, A.J.; Kallio, P. Patellectomy after fracture. Acta Orthop Scand 47:441–447, 1976.

29. Evans, P.D.; Pritchard, G.A.; Jenkins, D.H.R. Carbon fibre used in the late reconstruction of rupture of the extensor mechanism of the knee. Injury 18:57–60, 1987.

30. Feneley, R.C.L. Intra-articular dislocation of the patella. J Bone Joint Surg 50B(3):653–655, 1968.

31. Gallie, W.E.; Lemesurier, A.B. The late repair of fractures of the patella and of rupture of the ligamentum patellae and quadriceps tendon. J Bone Joint Surg 9:48–54, 1927.

32. Geckler, E.O.; Queranta, A.V. Patellectomy for degenerative arthritis of the knee—late results. J Bone Joint Surg 44A:1109, 1962.

33. Goodfellow, J.; Hungerford, D.S.; Zindel, M. Patello-femoral joint mechanics and pathology: 1. Functional anatomy of the patello-femoral joint. J Bone Joint Surg 58B(3):287–299, 1976.

34. Griswold, A.S. Fractures of the patella. Clin Orthop 4:44–56, 1954.

35. Haggart, G.E. Surgical treatment of degenerative arthritis of the knee joint. J Bone Joint Surg 22:717, 1940.

36. Halliburton, R.A.; Sullivan, C.R. The patella in degenerative joint diseases. Arch Surg 77:677–683, 1958.

37. Hanspal, R.S. Superior dislocation of the patella. Injury 16:487–488, 1985.

38. Haxton, H. The function of the patella and the effects of its excision. Surg Gynecol Obstet 80:389–395, 1945.

39. Heineck, A.P. The modern operative treatment of fractures of the patella. Surg Gynecol Obstet 9:177–248, 1909.

40. Hess, P.; Reinders, J. Transposition of the sartorius muscle for reconstruction of the extensor apparatus of the knee. J Trauma 26(1):90–91, 1986.

41. Horwitz, T.; Lambert, R.C. Patellectomy in the military service. A report of 19 cases. Surg Gynecol Obstet 82:423–426, 1946.

42. Huberti, H.H.; Hayes, W.C.; Stone, J.L.; Shybut, G.T. Force ratios in the quadriceps tendon and the ligamentum patellae. J Orthop Res 2:49–54, 1984.

43. Hung, L.K.; Chan, K.M.; Chow, Y.N.; Leung, P.C. Fractured patella: Operative treatment using the tension band principle. Injury 16:343–347, 1985.

44. Insall, J.; Goldberg, V.; Salvati, E. Recurrent dislocation and the high riding patella. Clin Orthop 88:67–69, 1972.

45. Jakobsen, J.; Christensen, K.S.; Rasmussen, O.S. Patellectomy—a 20 year follow-up. Acta Orthop Scand 56:430–432, 1985.

46. Kaufer, H. Mechanical function of the patella. J Bone Joint Surg 53-A(8):1551–1560, 1971.

47. Kelikian, H.; Riashi, E.; Gleason, J. Restoration of quadriceps function in neglected tears of the patellar tendon. Surg Gynecol Obstet 104:200–204, 1957.

48. Larsen, E.; Lauridsen, F. Conservative treatment of patellar dislocations. Clin Orthop 171:131–136, 1982.

49. Larsen, E.; Lund, P.M. Ruptures of the extensor mechanism of the knee joint. Clin Orthop 213:150–153, 1986.

50. Levack, B.; Flannagan, J.P.; Hobbs, S. Results of surgical treatment of patellar fractures. J Bone Joint Surg 67B(2):416–419, 1985.

51. Levin, P. Reconstruction of the patellar tendon using a Dacron graft. Clin Orthop 118:70–72, 1976.

52. Levy, M.; Goldstein, J.; Rosner, M. A method of repair for quadriceps tendon or patellar ligament ruptures without cast immobilization. Clin Orthop 218:297–301, 1987.

53. Lieb, F.J.; Perry, J. Quadriceps function. J Bone Joint Surg 50A(8):1535–1548, 1968.

54. Lotke, P.A.; Ecker, M.L. Transverse fractures of the patella. Clin Orthop 158:180–184, 1981.

54a. Ma, Y.Z.; Zheng, Y.F.; Qu, K.F.; et al. Treatment of fractures of the patella with percutaneous suture. Clin Orthop 191:235–241, 1984.

55. Macausland, W.R. Total excision of the patella for fracture. Am J Surg 72(4):510–516, 1946.

56. McLaughlin, H.L.; Francis, K.C. Operative repair of injuries to the quadriceps extensor mechanism. Am J Surg 91:651–653, 1956.

57. McMaster, P.E. Fractures of the patella. Clin Orthop 4:24–43, 1954.

58. Merchant, A.C.; Mercer, R.L.; Jacobsen, R.H.; Cool, R.T. Roentgenographic analysis of patellofemoral congruence. J Bone Joint Surg 56A(7):1391–1396, 1974.

59. Mishra, U.S. Late results of patellectomy in fractured patella. Acta Orthop Scand 43:256–263, 1972.

60. Miskew, D.B.W.; Pearson, R.L.; Pankovich, A.M. Mersilene strip suture in repair of disruptions of the quadriceps and patellar tendons. J Trauma 20(10):867–872, 1980.

61. Morscher, E. Cartilage-bone lesions of the knee joint following injury. Reconstr Surg Traumatol 12:2–26, 1971.

62. Muller, M.E.; Allgower, M.; Schneider, R.; Willinegger, H. Man-

ual of Internal Fixation. Techniques Recommended by the AO Group. Berlin, Springer-Verlag, 1979, pp. 248–253.

63. Murakami, Y. Intra-articular dislocation of the patella. Clin Orthop 171:137–139, 1982.

64. Noble, H.B.; Hajek, M.R. Boutonniere-type deformity of the knee following patellectomy and manipulations. J Bone Joint Surg 66A:137–138, 1984.

65. Nummi, J. Operative treatment of patella fractures. Acta Orthop Scand 42:437–438, 1971.

66. Oni, O.O.A.; Ahmad, S.H. The vastus lateralis derived flap for repair of neglected rupture of the quadriceps femoris tendon. Surg Gynecol Obstet 161:385–387, 1985.

67. Ramsey, R.H.; Muller, G.E. Quadriceps tendon rupture: A diagnostic trap. Clin Orthop 70:161–164, 1970.

68. Rees, D.; Thompson, S.K. Osteochondral fractures of the patella. J R Coll Surg Edinb 30(2):88–90, 1985.

69. Reider, B.; Marshall, J.L.; Koslin, B.; et al. The anterior aspect of the knee joint. J Bone Joint Surg 63A(3):351–356, 1981.

70. Scapinelli, R. Blood supply of the human patella. J Bone Joint Surg 49B(3):563–570, 1967.

71. Scott, J.C. Fractures of the patella. J Bone Joint Surg 31B(1):76–81, 1949.

72. Scuderi, C. Ruptures of the quadriceps tendon. Am J Surg 95:626–635, 1958.

73. Sears, F.W.; Zemansky, M.W. University Physics. Reading, MA, Addison-Wesley, 1970, pp. 30–31.

74. Seligo, W. Fractures of the patella. Reconstr Surg Traumatol 12:84–102, 1971.

75. Shorbe, H.B.; Dobson, C.H. Patellectomy. J Bone Joint Surg 40A(6):1281–1284, 1958.

76. Siwek, K.W.; Rao, J.P. Bilateral simultaneous rupture of the quadriceps tendon. Clin Orthop 131:252–254, 1978.

77. Siwek, K.W.; Rao, J.P. Ruptures of the extensor mechanism of the knee joint. J Bone Joint Surg 63A(6):932–937, 1981.

78. Sørensen, K.H. The late prognosis after fracture of the patella. Acta Orthop Scand 34:198–212, 1964.

79. Stern, R.E.; Harwin, S.F. Spontaneous and simultaneous rupture of both quadriceps tendons. Clin Orthop 147:188–189, 1980.

80. Stover, C.N. Interarticular dislocation of the patella. JAMA 200(11):966, 1967.

81. Sutton, F.S.; Thompson, C.H.; Lipke, J.; Kettlekamp, D.B. The effect of patellectomy on knee function. J Bone Joint Surg 58A(4):537–540, 1976.

82. Thompson, J.E.M. Comminuted fractures of the patella. J Bone Joint Surg 17A(2):431–434, 1935.

83. Thompson, J.E.M. Fracture of the patella treated by removal of the loose fragments and plastic repair of the tendon. Surg Gynecol Obstet 74:860–866, 1942.

84. Vainionpä, S.; Böstman, O.; Patiala, H.; Rokkanen, P. Rupture of the quadriceps tendon. Acta Orthop Scand 56:433–435, 1985.

85. Watkins, M.P.; Harris, B.A.; Wender, S.; et al. Effect of patellectomy on the function of the quadriceps and hamstrings. J Bone Joint Surg 65A(3):390–395, 1983.

86. Webb, L.X.; Toby, E.B. Bilateral rupture of the patellar tendon in an otherwise healthy male patient following minor trauma. J Trauma 26(11):1045–1048, 1986.

87. Weber, B.G.; Cech, O. Pseudarthrosis. New York, Grune and Stratton, 1976, pp. 224–225.

88. Weber, M.J.; Janecki, C.J.; McLeod, P.; et al. Efficacy of various forms of fixation of transverse fractures of the patella. J Bone Joint Surg 62A(2):215–220, 1980.

89. Wendt, P.P.; Johnson, R.P. A study of quadriceps excursion, torque, and the effect of patellectomy on cadaver knees. J Bone Joint Surg 67A(5):726–732, 1985.

90. West, F.E. End results of patellectomy. J Bone Joint Surg 44A(6):1089–1108, 1962.

91. Wiberg, G. Roentgenographic and anatomic studies on the patellofemoral joint. Acta Orthop Scand 12:319–410, 1941.

92. Wilkinson, J. Fracture of the patella treated by total excision. J Bone Joint Surg 59B(3):352–354, 1977.

93. Wimsatt, M.H.; Carey, E.J. Superior dislocation of the patella. J Trauma 17(1):77–80, 1977.

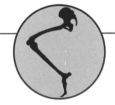

David Leffers, M.D.

49

Dislocations and Soft Tissue Injuries of the Knee

*T*he knee is the largest and arguably the most complex joint in the body. Its bony geometry with dissimilar articulating surfaces offers little inherent stability. The components of the soft tissue envelope of the knee, including the primary static capsuloligamentous and meniscal restraints and the dynamic secondary musculotendinous units, work in concert to stabilize the knee and allow multidirectional motion. Not simply a hinge joint, the knee has six degrees of freedom, with flexion-extension, internal-external rotation, and abduction-adduction ranges.

Injury to the knee is common and can result from varying levels of energy. Knee injury is the most frequent cause of disability related to sports activity. In the polytrauma setting, knee injury is often occult and unrecognized and frequently causes prolonged morbidity. Unlike fracture assessment, the acutely injured knee often lacks radiographic clues to diagnosis, and a premium is placed on knowledge of functional anatomy, hands-on examination, diagnostic acumen, and appropriate ancillary tests. A correct diagnosis allows implementation of appropriate treatment according to the nature of injury, patient-related variables, and the abilities of the medical team.

Knee injuries can be divided into broad diagnostic categories including injuries to the extensor mechanism, ligamentous structures, menisci, articular surfaces, and musculotendinous structures and fractures. It is the intention of this chapter to introduce an approach to the acutely injured knee with a discussion of the examination and recognition of symptom complexes, the use of appropriate ancillary diagnostic tests, and a treatment philosophy for soft tissue injury. Emphasis will be placed on diagnosis and conceptual treatment algorithms. Paralleling the advances in functional treatment of fractures, there has been a welcome and aggressive trend toward early, stable soft tissue repair in acute knee injury, minimizing joint immobility and promoting early return of function.

Diagnostic Approach to the Injured Knee

The type of knee injury can often be inferred from a proper history. The diagnostic approach (Fig. 49–1) should begin with establishing the magnitude and direction of forces applied to the knee (Fig. 49–2). The forces may vary from high-velocity vehicular accidents to noncontact sports injuries. The application of the force can be direct, such as contact of the anterior knee on the dashboard in a motor vehicle accident, or indirect, such as rotational forces applied through the leg with dissipation of forces through the knee ligaments, causing injury.[8] A combination of forces can also occur, exemplified by a valgus rotational injury sustained by a football player struck from the outside on his planted leg. An accurate knowledge of the magnitude and direction of forces applied and the position of the knee at impact, coupled with an understanding of anatomy, often leads to a suspected diagnosis or pattern of injury prior to physical examination. In polytraumatized patients, particularly those with long-bone lower extremity fractures, the possibility of traumatic soft tissue injury of the knee must be expected rather than excluded.

In isolated injury to the knee, important factors to determine in the history are the ability to ambulate

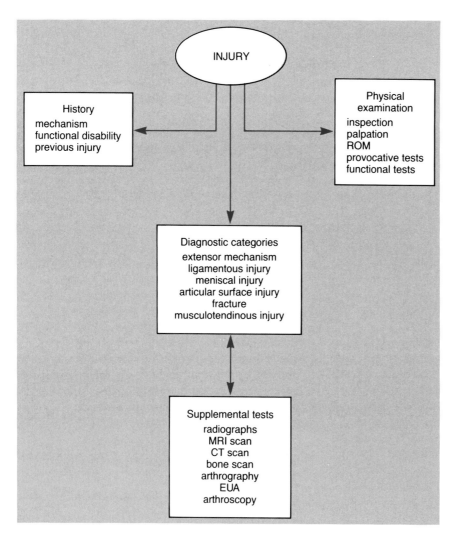

Figure 49-1

Diagnostic approach to the injured knee. ROM = range of motion. EUA = examination under anesthesia.

following injury, the rapidity of onset or presence of swelling, whether audible tearing or popping was heard, and whether an initial deformity reduced spontaneously or in response to manipulation. The presence of acute hemarthrosis following knee injury has been shown conclusively to be an indicator of significant intraarticular injury.[1,2,9] In 75% to 80% of cases, this means a tear of the anterior cruciate ligament. Other causes of hemarthrosis are meniscal tears, osteochondral fractures, and patellar dislocation.

Hemarthrosis is a sign, not a diagnosis. When present, a systematic approach must be taken to arrive at a pathoanatomic diagnosis and should include careful clinical examination and radiographs. On occasion, supplemental studies include stress radiographs, tomograms, and magnetic resonance imaging (MRI) scans.

The clinical exam should be performed in a relaxed setting. For unilateral knee injuries, it is wise to examine the uninvolved knee for range of motion and inherent stability. This gives the examiner a baseline for comparison and often allays patient apprehension. Inspection is quick to note areas of ecchymosis or swelling. Topographic anatomic structures are palpated, with emphasis on ligament origin and insertion sites, medial and lateral joint lines, and the extensor mechanism. Volitional range of motion is requested, and its presence and arc are recorded against passive measurements. Discrepancies in active and passive motion are usually secondary to pain but may reflect extensor mechanism disruption. Restriction of passive motion may implicate muscle spasm, effusion, or internal derangement.

Hemarthrosis usually incites protective muscle spasm and makes adequate ligamentous examination difficult. Aspiration of the hemarthrosis and installation into the joint of 10 to 15 ml of a local anesthetic may afford relaxation and improve diagnostic accuracy, particularly with collateral ligamentous injury. The sensitivity of clinical examination for isolated anterior cruciate ligament tears, however, has been shown

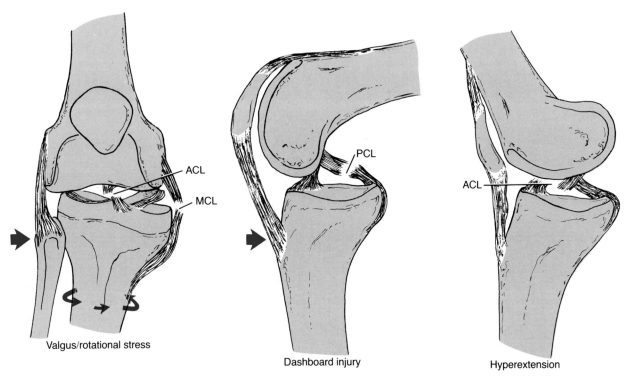

Valgus/rotational stress

Dashboard injury

Hyperextension

Figure 49-2

Common mechanisms of knee injury. ACL = Anterior cruciate ligament; MCL = medial cruciate ligament; PCL = posterior cruciate ligament.

to be unsatisfactory.[9] Diagnostic accuracy is improved significantly with examination under anesthesia (EUA). EUA is recommended when clinical examination and supportive studies do not yield a diagnosis. EUA coupled with diagnostic arthroscopy is now the standard by which other investigative studies must be measured. The treatment rendered a particular injury certainly may differ according to many patient variables, but arrival at an accurate diagnosis should not.

INVESTIGATIVE AIDS

Radiographs should be obtained for all acute knee injuries. The standard trauma series includes anteroposterior (AP), lateral, oblique, and patellar tangential views. Alignment, soft tissue detail, and presence or absence of bony injury should be discerned. Ligamentous injury may be associated with avulsion fractures. The lateral capsular sign implicates an anterior cruciate ligament tear. Osteochondral fractures may be apparent. Patellar dislocations are frequently accompanied by a fracture of the odd facet medially. All radiographic clues are valuable in making a diagnosis and planning appropriate treatment.

Stress radiographs have not been shown to increase diagnostic accuracy over EUA and arthroscopy. Their use may aid in grading isolated collateral ligamentous

injuries, in assessing the stability of nondisplaced avulsion fractures, and in differentiating skeletal vs. ligamentous instability in skeletally immature patients.

A ligament laxity exam should include anterior and posterior translational tests for the cruciate ligaments, fixed-fulcrum varus and valgus tests for the collateral ligaments, and special tests for combined or rotational instabilities.

For the anterior cruciate ligament, the Lachman test (Fig. 49-3) is performed with the knee in approximately 20° of flexion, the distal femur stabilized by the examiner's upper hand, and an anterior force applied to the posterior aspect of the upper tibia by the lower hand.[12] Anterior translation of the tibia on the femur is estimated in millimeters, and the status of the end point is noted. The Lachman test is more sensitive than the classic anterior drawer test performed at 90° of flexion and is certainly more comfortable for the patient in the acute setting. The status of the posterior cruciate ligament can also be ascertained in moderate flexion with reversal of the direction of tibial force. Posterior sag of the proximal tibia with the hip and knee flexed at 90° is pathognomonic for posterior cruciate instability. Varus and valgus stress tests for the lateral and medial collateral ligaments, respectively, are performed in full extension and at 20° to 30° of flexion. Again, estimates are made in terms of millimeters of laxity and end

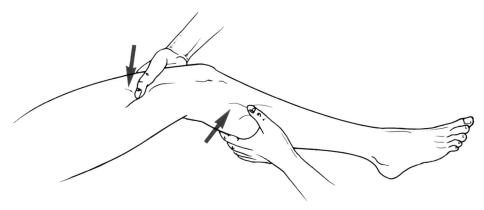

Figure 49-3

The Lachman test for anterior cruciate instability. See text.

point. Ligament tears are conventionally graded from I to III. A grade I injury is indicated by a painful stress examination with at most minimal instability. A grade II injury is a more significant incomplete ligament tear, with obvious laxity, but a definite endpoint. A grade III injury is a complete tear, with no apparent end. Instability in extension implies a complete (grade III) tear of the collateral ligament and its associated posterior quadrant capsular mechanism and probable posterior cruciate sprain to a variable degree. Stability in extension generally excludes significant capsular and posterior cruciate injury.[3,4] Rotational instability of the knee signifies abnormal excursion of the tibial condyle in relation to the femur and theoretically can occur in four quadrants: anteromedial, anterolateral, posteromedial, and posterolateral. Combined rotational instabilities can also exist. As its name implies, rotational instability involves a shift in the center of rotation (cruciate ligament injury) and loss of secondary capsular restraint. Anteromedial instability is documented by excessive displacement during an anterior drawer test with the leg in internal rotation. Tests for anterolateral laxity (pivot shift, Slocum, jerk, Losee, and flexion-rotation drawer) have as a common denominator a valgus load with extension or flexion either to reproduce or reduce tibial subluxation.[6,11,12] Posterolateral instability can be shown by a reverse pivot shift or external rotation recurvatum test performed by lifting the leg by the great toe. The quantification of rotational instability is highly subjective and is best determined by comparing the injured with the uninjured knee.

The use of ligament arthrometers is increasing.

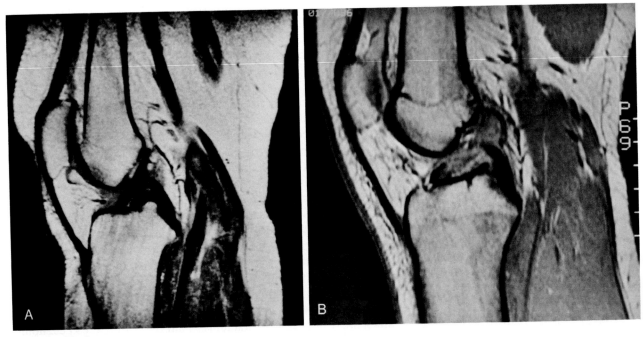

Figure 49-4

A, Normal MR scan of the anterior and posterior cruciate ligaments. *B,* MR scan showing acute anterior cruciate ligament disruption.

These are in large part educational and research tools to supply objective data for highly subjective clinical laxity examinations for anterior or posterior instability. However, there is no universally accepted arthrometer or standardization among different devices. Their use is most valuable in private practice when making side-to-side comparisons and in longitudinal evaluations following injury and treatment. It should be remembered that the loads applied in clinical laxity tests are nonphysiologic and must be correlated with functional patient evaluation.

Tomograms of the acutely injured knee are largely reserved for evaluation of intraarticular fractures involving weight-bearing surfaces and for localization of the origin of osteochondral fractures when this is not evident from plain films.

The use of magnetic resonance imaging (MRI) in the evaluation of acute knee injuries is evolving.[5,7,10] The sensitivity and specificity of MRI for the menisci and cruciate ligaments is greater than 90% when correlated with arthroscopy (Fig. 49–4). It is also noninvasive and eliminates exposure to ionizing radiation; thus it has largely supplanted knee arthrography. However, MRI should not be used to supplant careful clinical examination and plain radiographs. Its benefit in an acute knee injury may lie in excluding meniscal tears in isolated ligament injuries, particularly of the collateral ligaments, which can otherwise be treated successfully by nonoperative means. MRI poorly delineates cartilaginous defects, chondromalacia, and loose bodies other than osteochondral bodies. MRI can also be used to forge a preoperative plan in accordance with meniscal tear size, type, and location as to probability of repair vs. excision.

With meniscal tears, changes in signal intensity vary from focal intrameniscal degeneration (grade I) (Fig. 49–5) to clear-cut linear communications with an articular surface (grade III). The former condition is generally treated nonoperatively and the latter with surgical excision or repair. MRI should certainly be considered a valuable adjunct in the diagnostic armamentarium but should be used in a thoughtful and purposeful manner.

The indications for arthrography in acute knee injury are limited, and MRI is a superior study without patient risk. In suspected penetrating knee injury, however, arthrography or a saline load test may confirm extravasation. The latter is a sterile injection to distend the joint while examining for leakage through the open wound.

Arteriograms are indicated in suspected vascular injury or insufficiency following knee trauma. It is mandatory following knee dislocation, if pedal pulses are present, to rule out intimal injury. When vascular in-

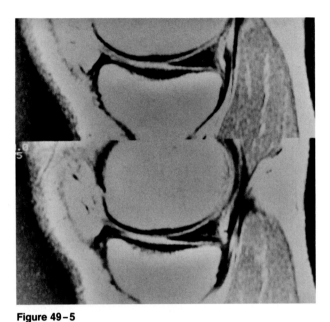

Figure 49–5

MR scan showing intrameniscal degeneration (light zone within wedge-shaped meniscus cross-section).

jury is clinically present, arteriography should not delay operative restoration of flow for more than 6 hours after injury.

Knee Injury in Polytrauma Patients

Knee injury should be suspected in any patient with lower extremity long-bone fracture, polytrauma, or head injury.[17] The acute management of a knee injury in these circumstances is a low priority (unless associated with vascular injury). If unrecognized, however, knee injury is often the source of long-term functional disability after fracture union. For polytrauma patients, resuscitation and skeleton stabilization allow patient mobilization. Knee injury can be addressed when optimal patient conditions allow, preferably within ten days of injury but often satisfactorily as late as three weeks following trauma. Pending surgical repair, the injured knee can be immobilized in appropriate splints or braces without disrupting mobilization.

With a long-bone fracture, an ipsilateral knee injury should be suspected in the presence of ecchymosis, tenderness, or swelling about the knee.[13] In any lower extremity, fracture or dislocation radiographs should include the knee. With skeletal instability, it is often impossible to obtain an adequate examination for ligamentous competency. If skeletal stabilization of the long-bone fracture is planned, EUA of the knee should immediately follow.[14] Ligamentous injury may be treated primarily or with delayed repair, depending on the overall condition of the patient and the surgical team. Temporary skeletal stabilization with a transfixion pin through the distal femur or proximal tibia can be used preoperatively to allow stress evaluation of the knee. In suspected gross knee ligamentous disruption, traction across the knee through a tibial pin should be avoided. In patients with a floating knee and ipsilateral femoral and tibial fractures, rigid skeletal fixation of at least the femur should be obtained, followed by examination of the knee under anesthesia (Fig. 49–6).[16]

Management of vascular injuries about the knee is

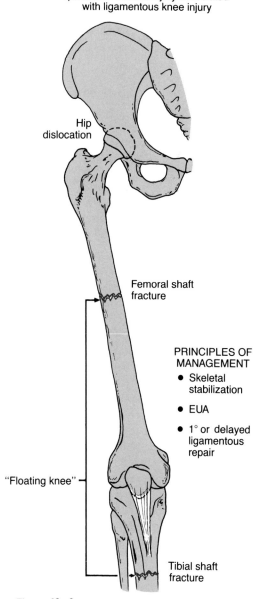

Ipisilateral skeletal injury associated with ligamentous knee injury

Hip dislocation

Femoral shaft fracture

PRINCIPLES OF MANAGEMENT
• Skeletal stabilization
• EUA
• 1° or delayed ligamentous repair

"Floating knee"

Tibial shaft fracture

Figure 49–6

Fractures associated with ligamentous knee injury.

emergent and should follow patient resuscitation immediately if limb-threatening ischemia is present. If the popliteal artery is occluded, rapid restoration of perfusion is urgent to avoid amputation. Timing and technique of skeletal stabilization must be determined by close consultation between vascular and orthopedic surgeons. A temporary arterial shunt and/or rapid application of an external fixator may facilitate limb salvage. In the absence of ischemia, preliminary fracture stabilization may simplify arterial repair.

Neurologic injury is generally an axonotmesis, except in cases of penetrating trauma. Acute repair is generally not indicated, and exploration is deferred unless it is part of a planned surgical approach. In soft tissue injuries, the principles of debridement apply, with removal of devitalized tissue, irrigation, capsular closure to prevent cartilage desiccation, and appropriate soft tissue coverage.

Appropriate suspicion must be maintained to rule out knee ligament injury adjacent to a fracture of the femur or tibia. Prospective studies of presumably isolated femoral and tibial shaft fractures have shown the incidence of associated knee ligament injury to be 33%[18] and 22%,[15] respectively, although many injuries are relatively mild.

Open Knee Injuries

The knee is the most commonly involved joint incurring penetrating or open injury (Fig. 49–7). Joint penetration can be direct from without, such as gunshot or stab wounds, or from extension into the knee through open periarticular fractures. Knee dislocations are open in 20% to 30% of cases. Proper recognition and treatment of periarticular soft tissue injury, associated capsuloligamentous damage, and intraarticular pathology is requisite to restore joint function.

CLASSIFICATION

Patzakis and co-workers classified open joint injuries into those with fractures, those without fracture, and gunshot wounds.[20] In their review of 140 cases, however, the parameter most closely correlating with poor outcome and wound infection was the degree of soft tissue injury about the open joint. Collins and Temple have recently proposed a grading system based principally on the periarticular soft tissue injury. Class I injury is a singular laceration without extensive soft tissue injury.[19] Class II includes single or multiple lacerations with extensive soft tissue injury or loss. Class III comprises open joints from extension of open periarticular

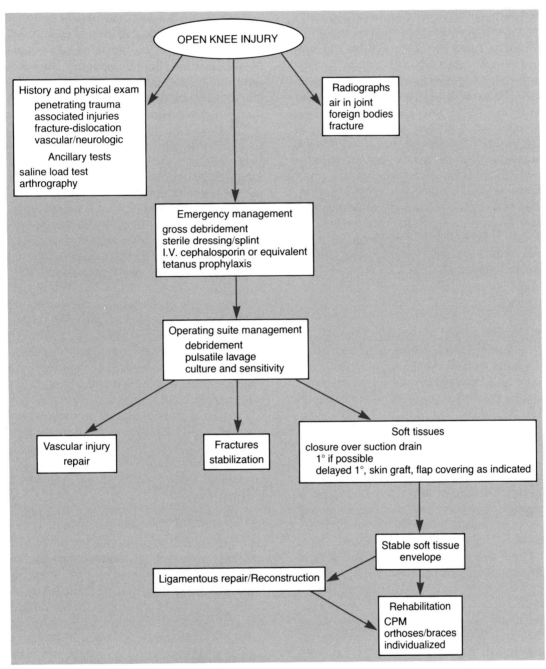

Figure 49-7

Treatment algorithm for an open knee injury.

fractures. Each class is subdivided according to the degree of articular injury and meniscoligamentous disruption. Class IV injuries are open dislocations with nerve or vascular injury requiring repair. This classification system is more useful than that of Patzakis et al., as it comprises injury grading of both the soft tissue component, which influences early outcome, and the articular surface, which bears long-term prognostic significance.

DIAGNOSIS

Open knee injuries range from visible communication with the joint to a quite imperceptible puncture wound. Particularly with penetrating trauma to the anterior knee in a position of flexion, the skin and joint capsule wounds may not be superimposed because of the excursion of the quadriceps mechanism during knee extension. Passive flexion of the knee will often elucidate the staggered nature of the wound and may produce a characteristic sucking sound. Radiographs should be obtained on all suspected open knee injuries; the presence of air in the joint confirms the diagnosis. A saline load test can be performed in certain cases to note extravasation. This is helpful when skin and capsular disruptions are at different levels. Under sterile conditions, 30 to 50 ml of nonbacteriostatic saline can be injected intraarticularly through nonviolated skin, noting drainage through open wounds. Arthrograms are of limited value but can aid in ruling out an intraarticular foreign body. Xerograms can detect nonradiopaque foreign bodies such as palm fronds or unleaded glass. Probing of a wound should probably be discouraged, as it is an unreliable test, may introduce additional contaminated material into the joint, and is often painful to the patient.

TREATMENT

The mainstays of treatment of open knee injuries are antibiotics, thorough wound debridement and irrigation, and capsular closure. Antibiotic administration should be considered therapeutic and not prophylactic, as the wound is contaminated. Sterile dressings should be applied in the emergency department following removal of any grossly apparent and accessible foreign material. Tetanus prophylaxis should be given if indicated, and a broad-spectrum cephalosporin or equivalent started intravenously. Antibiotics are continued for 48 to 72 hours. Extended use is indicated for positive wound cultures until clinical parameters are acceptable for cessation. Debridement of devitalized soft tissue followed by pulsatile saline lavage of the joint is next carried out. We usually take aerobic and anaerobic wound cultures following debridement. Primary skin closure for clean lacerations, regardless of length, is appropriate. Delayed primary closure, split-thickness skin grafts, soft tissue rotation flaps, or other measures may be required depending on the wound severity. If extensive soft tissue loss is present, the knee should be packed open, with redebridement and coverage as rapidly as clinically acceptable to avoid articular cartilage desiccation. The treatment of articular surface injury should generally proceed as if it were a closed joint injury. This includes operative fixation of periarticular and intraarticular fractures. The management of an associated ligamentous injury is probably best deferred until a stable joint milieu is obtained following wound closure. This limits further acute insult to the knee from the soft tissue dissection or secondary incisions often necessary for ligamentous repair. Exceptions are isolated ligamentous injuries in open wounds resulting from direct laceration, and ligaments avulsed in continuity with their bony attachment.

If possible, capsular closure should be done over suction tubes. The use of suction-irrigation systems has been questioned by Patzakis et al. as a possible source of iatrogenic joint contamination.[20] The benefit of mechanical fluid lavage is unknown but probably negligible. The risks present in using closed irrigation systems are infection and the disturbance of cartilage matrix by prolonged exposure to irrigating fluids. The validity of a positive effluent culture also must be questioned. It is suggested that suction tubes be removed after 24 to 48 hours. If drainage remains copious or is of ill nature, then repeat debridement is indicated.

The role of arthroscopy in open knee injuries is limited, but it is valuable in selected cases. It is of primary benefit in foreign body perforations, such as gunshot or pellet injuries, when the soft tissue injury is small (often the size of a normal arthroscopic portal), thus limiting fluid extravasation. Arthroscopic debridement, irrigation, removal of loose and foreign bodies, and documentation and treatment of articular surface injury can be accomplished. The arthroscope can also be used in a "dry" fashion through an open injury or accessory portal to visualize areas in the knee not readily accessible from the primary wound, perhaps limiting the need for extension of surgical incisions.

The ease of an arthroscopic procedure should not be allowed to cloud judgment. If adequate debridement has not been, or will not be, obtained by arthroscopy, then open arthrotomy should be carried out. The difference in short-term morbidity is indeed secondary to ultimate outcome.

A special consideration in open knee injuries is vascular disruption. The vascular injury and its ramifications assume first priority, followed by treatment of the joint injury using the aforementioned guidelines.

Rehabilitation following an open knee injury is in large part dictated by the soft tissue injury. After successful closure and removal of drains, controlled passive and active motion can be instituted. Early passive motion is helpful in preventing arthrofibrosis and has a beneficial effect on cartilage metabolism. The rapidity and intensity of exercise and therapeutic modalities are based on articular and capsuloligamentous integrity. In cases where soft tissue injury has been extensive, requiring multiple operative procedures for joint closure and coverage or treatment necessitating joint immobilization, early manipulation under anesthesia and arthroscopic lysis of adhesions should be considered.

Traumatic Dislocation of the Knee

Traumatic dislocation of the knee (Fig. 49–8) is relatively uncommon but is limb-threatening because of

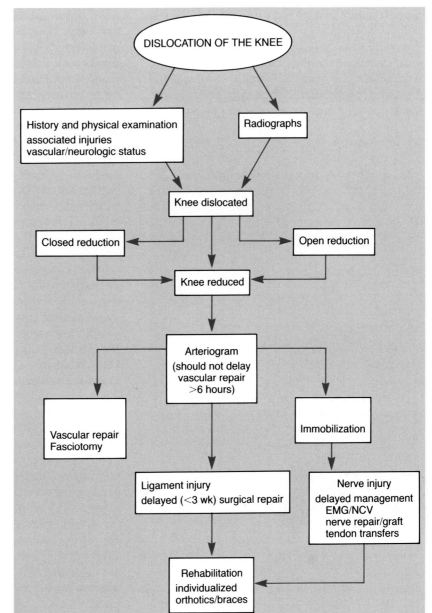

Figure 49-8

Treatment algorithm for dislocation of the knee.

the possibility of vascular disruption in the popliteal fossa and therefore is considered an orthopedic emergency.

CLASSIFICATION

Vehicular accidents are the most common cause of dislocation of the knee and signify high-energy trauma. Dislocation of the knee has also occurred from falls and in sports, these often being caused by rotational forces of lower energy.[29] The classification of knee dislocations is based on the relationship of the tibia to the femur and the resultant forces incurred. An anterior dislocation occurs most often from a posterior-directed force on the anterior thigh with the foot planted, causing hyperextension and, as shown by Kennedy, sequential disruption of the posterior capsule, posterior cruciate, and anterior cruciate ligaments.[22] In cadaver specimens, tearing of the popliteal artery occurred, on the average, at 50° of hyperextension. Posterior dislocation typically results from the "dashboard injury" in which the flexed knee has a posteriorly directed force applied to the anterior tibia (Fig. 49-9). A lateral dislocation (Fig. 49-10) occurs from a valgus stress with the tibia fixed and the thigh adducted. Medial dislocation of the knee can result from a varus force to the thigh but often has a rotational component. Rotational dislocations can occur in any quadrant of the knee, with the

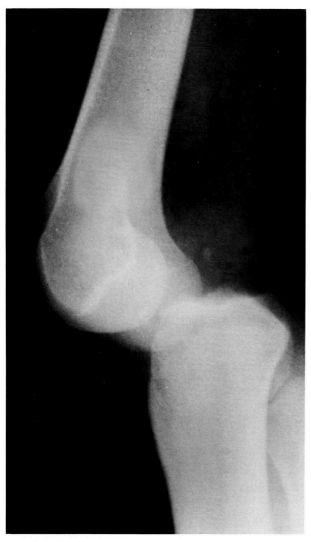

Figure 49-9

Posterior dislocation of the knee from a dashboard injury.

posterolateral quadrant being the most common (Fig. 49-11). Anterior and posterior dislocations account for 50% to 75% of all dislocations. As a result of high-energy trauma, 20% to 30% of dislocations are open injuries.[22-24,27,28,30]

DIAGNOSIS

Dislocation of the knee is probably underdiagnosed for several reasons. Spontaneous reduction and realignment of the limb at the scene of the accident are often possible because of the severe soft tissue injury that facilitates reduction. Secondary to the extreme capsular disruption there is generally absence of tense hemarthrosis, and overt signs of knee injury may be absent, particularly in the patient with associated skeletal instability or multiple trauma. A clue to the presence of a reduced knee dislocation is coexistent varus or valgus instability in full extension, implicating tears of both the anterior cruciate and posterior cruciate ligaments. Exaggerated hyperextension or recurvatum also implicates combined cruciate and posterior capsular disruption. Diffuse tenderness about the knee, absence of hemarthrosis, and the presence of popliteal ecchymosis may also be presenting signs. Vascular insufficiency following closed knee injury suggests severe instability. An associated peroneal nerve deficit is also suggestive of knee dislocation. The principal test for instability is an adequate examination of the ligaments, which may often require examination following skeletal stabilization in those with ipsilateral long-bone fractures. This documentation is mandatory for appropriate diagnosis, classification, and treatment. With gross ligamentous disruption, diagnostic arthroscopy is a relative contraindication because of possible fluid extravasation resulting in increased soft tissue compartment pressures. Thorough clinical examination may include radiographs, stress films, and MRI scans. Plain radiographs of the knee should be obtained to look for possible avulsion fractures, which are clues to ligamentous injury. Injuries associated with knee dislocation include fractures of the patella, tibial spine, tibial plateau, and fibular head and a variety of intraarticular fractures. In those patients with avulsion fractures or tibial plateau fractures, stress films can be used if necessary to differentiate skeletal vs. ligamentous instability. MRI can be used to identify meniscal injury preoperatively and to define the pathoanatomy of ligament injury (midsubstance vs. avulsion tears). It may also be of benefit in those patients who are not operative candidates for knee repair and for whom the pattern of ligamentous and meniscal injury can be established and appropriate immobilization and therapy can be instituted.

REDUCTION

When faced with a dislocated knee, documentation of the neurovascular status of the limb is mandatory. Closed reduction of the dislocated knee can generally be accomplished in the emergency suite with appropriate analgesia. For anterior dislocation, reduction is carried out with traction of the limb and elevation of the distal femur. Posterior dislocation is reduced with traction on the tibia coupled with extension and lifting of the proximal tibia in an anterior direction. The principle in reduction is to not direct any force against the popliteal fossa where compromised vascularity may be present. Medial and lateral dislocations are reduced by longitudinal traction and appropriate translation of the

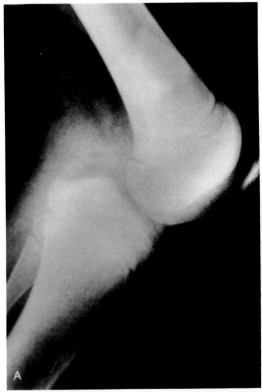

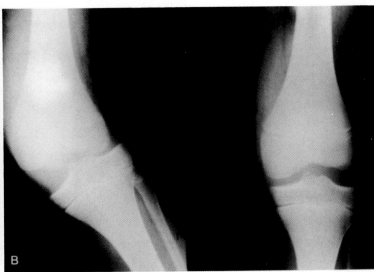

Figure 49–10

A, Posterior dislocations in skeletally immature male. *B,* Gross valgus instability in extension. Note the absence of physeal injury.

femur and tibia. Rotational injuries are reduced by traction and appropriate derotation of the tibia. The posterolateral dislocation has been called the "irreducible dislocation." With this type of injury clinically there will often be a "dimple sign" on the medial joint line as a result of medial capsular and collateral ligament invagination with a buttonhole of the medial femoral condyle through the soft tissue rent.[25] For a dislocation that is irreducible by the preceding means, emergent reduction attempted under general anesthesia is necessary, and on rare occasions open reduction may be required. It is important to document the neurologic and vascular status prior to and following any attempt at reduction. Following reduction, the knee should be immobilized in 20° to 30° of flexion, pending further evaluation. No circular plaster or constricting dressing should be applied.

VASCULAR INJURY

The sinister reputation of knee dislocation comes from the possible presence of vascular injury. Injury to the popliteal artery occurs in 25% to 30% of all dislocations but is more common (approximately 40%) in the most common dislocations, anterior and posterior, because of the tethering of the popliteal artery at its entrance to

the fossa at the adductor hiatus and at its exit by the soleal arch. With significant tibial displacement, the artery is at risk because of this proximal and distal fixation. Important tenets in regard to vascular injury at this level are (1) the collateral circulation about the knee is inadequate to maintain limb viability if popliteal artery disruption is present; and (2) the presence of pedal pulses does not exclude vascular injury. The majority of patients with vascular deficiency prior to reduction will continue to have ischemia following reduction. Green and Allen reported only 5 of 56 absent pulses restored following closed reduction of a knee dislocation.[21] Thus if vascular insufficiency is present distal to a knee dislocation, an arterial injury is present until proven otherwise. Diminished pulses must not be ascribed to "vascular spasm." The importance of recognizing vascular injury was documented in wartime experience, which showed that without vascular repair or with popliteal artery ligation or repair 8 hours after injury, the amputation rate was 86%. With recognition of vascular injury and appropriate repair within 8 hours from the time of injury, an 80% salvage rate was obtained. An arteriogram is mandatory after reduction of a knee dislocation, if perfusion seems satisfactory (Fig. 49–12). An intimal tear may be present and precipitate a thrombus and subsequent arterial occlusion.

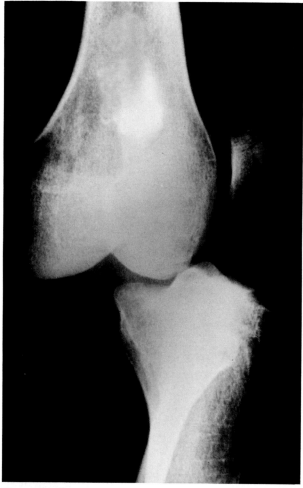

Figure 49-11

Posterolateral dislocation of the knee caused by a short fall and rotational stress.

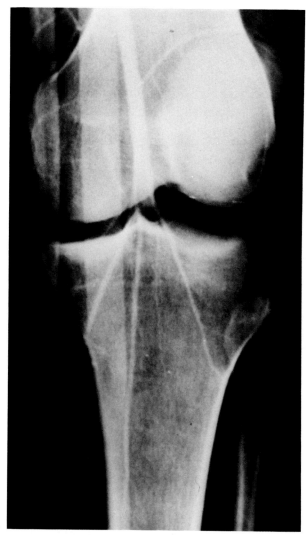

Figure 49-12

Arteriogram demonstrating popliteal artery disruption.

However, if after reduction vascular insufficiency is present on clinical or Doppler examination, then surgical exploration and restoration of flow are urgent and should not be delayed to obtain an arteriogram. If necessary, an arteriogram can be performed in the surgical suite prior to exploration. Time is of the essence, and because of the high probability of popliteal fossa localization, arteriography adds little to confirmation or surgical planning in the isolated knee dislocation with vascular injury. After repair of the popliteal artery a complete four-compartment fasciotomy is almost always the best protection against reperfusion swelling and compartment syndrome.

NEUROLOGIC INJURY

The incidence of peroneal nerve injury has been reported as ranging from 14% to 35%.[26] This usually is an axonotmesis over a broad area of injury and carries with it a poor prognosis. Primary exploration with repair or grafting has not been effective and is not recommended. Secondary exploration at three months for complete injury with nerve grafting also has produced poor functional results. Resultant muscular deficiencies usually require bracing or tendon transfers to normalize foot posture and gait.

TREATMENT

The treatment of the ligamentous injuries resulting from knee dislocation has been the subject of some debate.[24,30] The majority currently favor operative repair of all ligamentous injuries followed by early mobilization and functional bracing to promote optimal results. In dislocation, the majority of knees will have a combined anterior and posterior cruciate ligament disruption associated with variable collateral ligament, capsular, and meniscal tears. The timing of ligamentous repair is dependent on the condition of both patient and limb. Priority of repair is vascular repair, skeletal stabilization, and lastly, ligamentous repair. If vascular repair is undertaken, ligamentous repair can be delayed up to two to three weeks following injury, pending vascular stabilization and soft tissue healing. The surgical approach should be predicated on an accurate ligamentous exam and on the instability pattern, but most can be approached by lateral or medial arthrotomies. Because of the significant capsular and ligamentous disruption, exposure is generally not a problem, making primary repair often easier than when undertaken for an isolated ligamentous injury.

Sequential repair of the capsule, menisci, and cruciate and collateral ligament tears is undertaken. Appropriate drill holes for sutures of capsular and cruciate repairs are best made first while exposure is maximal, then subsequent sutures are placed and tagged, beginning posteriorly and working outward. Meniscal injury is addressed, with repair of peripheral tears or detachments and excision of avascular or complex tears. Capsular sutures are then secured, followed by the meniscal and cruciate ligatures. Collateral ligaments are repaired by the appropriate suture or ligament fixation system. With stable soft tissue repair, it is generally unnecessary to maintain reduction with transarticular pins. A hinged postoperative brace affords initial immobilization, wound access, and early controlled range of motion. Immobilization in 45° of flexion is a compromise position for anterior and posterior cruciate ligament repairs. The rapidity of graduated mobilization depends on the adequacy of repair, but it is desirable to regain full passive motion six to eight weeks following surgery. Protected weight bearing can begin at approximately four to six weeks.

Anterior Cruciate Ligament Injury

There is no doubt as to the importance of the anterior cruciate ligament in the overall kinematics and stability of the knee.[31,34,37,43] There is disagreement, however, as to the appropriate treatment of the anterior cruciate ligament injury (Fig. 49–13).[41] One would certainly like to offer the best possible treatment for any given anatomic injury to restore its function. The difficulty in decision making with anterior cruciate ligament injury lies in the many variables that influence the degree of functional loss and in the variable expression of this functional loss from individual to individual. The two main subgroups of variables are those related to the pathoanatomy of injury and patient-related variables. Anterior cruciate ligament sprain can be an incomplete or complete lesion, isolated or associated with other ligamentous or meniscal injury, and acute or chronic in nature. Patient-related variables include the age, activity level, and phenotype of the individual.[40] Anterior cruciate injury has variable expressivity, and the decision as to whether to treat an individual with nonoperative or operative measures must include an analysis of these variables in order to make an appropriate treatment decision. A knowledge of these variables and how they impact on operative and nonoperative treatment is important.

An accurate diagnosis is the foundation for treatment of any injury. The classic history of anterior cruciate ligament sprain is a decelerating, hyperextension or twisting injury to the knee, often associated with a pop, immediate functional loss, rapid onset of swelling, and pain.

If acute swelling and muscle spasm preclude an accurate physical diagnosis, aspiration of the knee and instillation of local anesthetic may facilitate examination. Plain radiographs of the knee should be taken in all cases of acute injury to inspect for bony avulsions or fractures. In the acute setting, when a diagnosis is suspected but not confirmed, EUA may be warranted. This allows for complete muscle relaxation and evaluation of knee stability in all planes and comparison with the opposite knee. The degree of instability is quite subjective, varies according to the experience of the examiner, and should always be compared with that of the opposite knee. Instrumented knee ligament–testing devices are more objective in quantifying anterior instability and may be useful. The presence of rotational instability (pivot shift) correlates highly with functional disability in the high-demand knee.[49,51] The role of arthroscopy in the diagnosis and management of acute knee injuries is well documented. The type of anterior cruciate ligament injury can be determined based on inspection and palpation. The status of the menisci and chondral surfaces can also be ascertained, and this may directly impact the type of treatment deemed optimal. Again, the key to appropriate management is an exact diagnosis. Once the pathoanatomy is known, other variables can be examined. The patient variables also play a significant role in this decision. A young, athletically active patient involved in a high-demand sport would be a more likely candidate for arthroscopy and subsequent surgical intervention than an older, recreationally active individual involved in low-demand activities.[33,47] In terms of knee strain, high-demand sports include contact sports and those involved with jumping, twisting, and deceleratory forces (e.g., football, soccer, basketball, and wrestling).

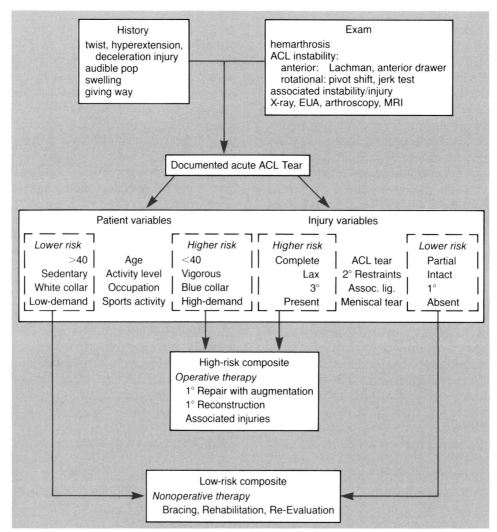

Figure 49-13

Treatment algorithm for an acute anterior ligament tear.

Less demanding sports include racquet sports, skiing, and running. The level of athletic competition also is a significant factor.[49] The physician might suggest a change from a high-demand to a low-demand sport for the recreationally competitive athlete that would not be acceptable to an elite athlete or professional.[39,51] Expected time loss from work also is important when discussing various treatment options with the patient. As a result of financial concerns, a patient may not wish to undergo an operative procedure that would limit employability. An individual may not want the "best knee possible" if it is going to require a significant time loss from work, but the active, competitive athlete who wishes to maintain that performance level without compromise will likely request and deserve surgical intervention. In those cases treated nonoperatively, it has been shown that with rehabilitative exercises, functional bracing, and activity modification there is a rea-sonable chance to have a successful outcome in terms of functional stability.[50,51] This is particularly true for isolated partial injuries of the anterior cruciate liga-ment.[42] In these less active individuals, associated in-traarticular injury could be treated arthroscopically and a similar pathway followed with rehabilitation, bracing, and activity modification.[35] In competitive athletes or laborers, treatment of any existing intraar-ticular injury, as well as surgical treatment of the ante-rior cruciate ligament to restore its anatomic function, is desirable.[33–36,38,47,48] Whether this is an operative re-pair, with or without augmentation, or a reconstructive procedure is largely dependent on the preferences and experience of the treating physician. Isolated primary repair of the anterior cruciate ligament has been shown to be less effective than repair with augmentation.[32,45,46] Acute, intraarticular reconstruction is gaining support following technical improvements in isometric placement and fixation of substitutes. There are currently no significant long-term follow-up studies to determine the treatment of choice in anterior cruciate ligament surgery. Of paramount importance in a surgical approach are a successful rehabilitation program and utmost patient compliance.[50]

It must be remembered that isolated injury to the anterior cruciate ligament is not a static injury. The syndrome of the anterior cruciate–insufficient knee is well documented.[31,34,38,44] Recurrent episodes of giving way place intact menisci at risk of tearing, and the strain on secondary restraints also increases and may worsen functional disability.[51] In cases of anterior cruciate ligament injury and associated reparable meniscal lesions, repair of the menisci alone in the face of cruciate instability often leads to failure. If meniscal repair is undertaken, it is recommended that the anterior cruciate ligament also be addressed surgically for joint stabilization. If the patient does not wish to undertake this option, then the meniscal lesion should be treated accordingly with appropriate resection.

In terms of therapy, appropriate muscle reeducation and strengthening generally should include all muscle groups that act about the knee. Emphasis is placed on rehabilitation of the hamstrings, which are anterior cruciate ligament agonists. One must not forget, however, maximum strengthening in the quadriceps musculature and gastrocnemius complex. Institution of rehabilitation generally follows restoration of motion and absence of pain in both nonoperative and operatively treated patients. Full range of motion should be the goal. Flexion contracture produces excessive patellofemoral compression and is a primary source of pain in those who do not regain full extension. There is evidence to suggest that the older, less physically active individual can respond to this program favorably. Patient understanding and compliance is the key factor in the success or failure of such a program. It also must be understood that rehabilitation must be followed by maintenance exercise. The use of functional knee braces in the anterior cruciate–deficient knee is an ongoing topic of discussion and research, but these are generally utilized to increase the margin of safety in both operatively and conservatively managed patients. They are more helpful in controlling one-plane anterior instability than rotational instability. It is important to let the patient know that a brace is not a substitute for vigorous and conscientious muscle strengthening and proprioceptive training. In certain individuals operative treatment is recognized as the treatment of choice. Anterior cruciate ligament disruptions associated with recognizable injury to secondary restraints or other complete ligamentous injury are best treated with appropriate operative intervention and stabilization. Knees with combined acute ligamentous injuries and multiplane instability have poor functional outcome if treated nonoperatively. These knees have limited functional reserve when treated conservatively. Also injuries associated with displaced bony avulsion fractures are best stabilized surgically and when treated in this fashion often will yield the best results because of bone-to-bone healing and a structurally intact ligament.

In summary, treatment options offered to a patient are predicated on an accurate anatomic diagnosis of both the type of anterior cruciate ligament injury and associated intraarticular and other ligamentous injuries. Once these are defined, a treatment plan can be offered, with attendant risks and benefits based on the patient's age, employment, level and type of sports participation, and ability and willingness to adapt this participation according to functional impairment, if present.

Posterior Cruciate Injury

The primary function of the posterior cruciate ligament is to prevent posterior translation of the tibia on the femur. It also plays a role as a central axis in controlling and imparting rotational stability to the knee.[57] It is less commonly injured and more often passes unrecognized than does injury to its counterpart, the anterior cruciate ligament.

Injury most often occurs from trauma to the anterior aspect of the proximal tibia with the knee flexed, as in a fall or dashboard injury. It can also be torn during extreme hyperextension or rotational or varus/valgus stress. Posterior cruciate injury may be isolated or associated with other capsuloligamentous injury. In the acute setting, pain may significantly decrease the accuracy of the ligamentous exam, and evaluation under anesthesia may be necessary.

The clinical findings with isolated injury may be subtle because of its posterior position, frequent lack of swelling or ecchymosis, and uncommon history of a pop or tearing sensation. This injury will frequently be diagnosed as a sprain and treated symptomatically. It is not uncommon to detect posterior instability on routine screening of athletes in whom no functional deficit has been present. In one-plane posterior instability, secondary restraints at the posterior corners prevent rotational instability.[56] Diagnostic tests for isolated posterior cruciate instability are the posterior sag and posterior drawer signs. A decrease in posterior drawer with the tibia in internal rotation implies some functional restraint in the posterior cruciate (a grade I or II tear) or integrity of the posterior meniscofemoral ligaments.[53] Radiographs of the knee should be obtained in an acute injury to rule out avulsion fracture. This most commonly occurs at the tibial insertion and is more frequent than avulsion fractures of the anterior cruciate, particularly in skeletally mature patients. Biomechanically this may be a result of the posterior cruciate's larger size, broader area of bony insertion, and the lack of bony impingement from the intercondylar notch. Grade III instability (grossly positive posterior sag or drawer) with avulsion fracture of the posterior cruciate is an indication for primary repair, as bone-to-bone fixation can be achieved, and an excellent result can be expected. Literature reviews generally support nonoperative treatment of the isolated posterior cruciate tear.[54,55,59,60] Individuals who maximize quadriceps strength, the agonist of the posterior cruciate ligament, experience the best outcome. It has been shown in a case study of a professional athlete that the conditioned quadriceps contracts earlier in the gait cycle, dynamically limiting posterior tibial translation.[53] The onset of medial compartment degenerative changes has not been statistically proven in the isolated posterior unstable knee.

The key in evaluating posterior cruciate injury is to search for and identify associated capsuloligamentous injury. Combined posterior and collateral or capsular tears impart multiplane and rotational instability, lead to functional disability, and have a positive correlation with medial compartment arthrosis.[53] Combined injury also jeopardizes the popliteal vessels more frequently, and as a result, clinical evaluation is mandatory.

Clinical laxity tests for combined injuries attempt to detect one-plane collateral and associated rotational instabilities. Collateral instability in extension implicates complete tear of the primary collateral restraint and associated capsular structures and probable cruciate injury. With loss of posterior cruciate function, additional laxity of the posterolateral corner increases external tibial rotation and rollback, demonstrated by the reverse pivot shift[58] and external rotation recurvatum tests.[57]

Primary surgical repair or augmentation is recommended for combined posterior cruciate and associated ligamentous injuries. Medial arthrosis has been reported in 48% of *functionally unstable* posterior cruciate–deficient knees and increases with the chronicity of injury.

Medial Collateral Ligament Injury

The medial collateral ligament is the primary medial stabilizer of the knee and is generally depicted as having a superficial fan-shaped component and a deeper capsular complex consisting of the meniscofemoral and meniscotibial ligaments.[64] The fan-shaped superficial ligament has, by design, anterior fibers that are most taut in flexion and posterior fibers that are most taut in extension. Secondary static restraints to valgus stress include the cruciate ligaments. Medial collateral ligament injury is most often caused by a valgus stress produced by trauma to the lateral aspect of the knee with the foot planted. Sprain to the medial collateral is the most common of knee ligamentous injuries. Recognition is by appropriate history, tenderness along the course of its orientation, and the presence of medial swelling and possibly ecchymosis. Valgus stress testing in extension and at 30° of flexion should be performed and compared with the opposite knee. Instability in extension indicates complete injury to the medial collateral ligament as well as posterior and medial capsular involvement and possibly posterior cruciate injury. Medial stability in extension does not exclude third-degree or complete rupture. At 30° of flexion, the restraining force of the capsular complex is removed.

The treatment of medial collateral ligament injuries of isolated nature is symptomatic and functional with the use of controlled-motion, hinged bracing to prevent valgus stress. Onset of motion is dictated largely by patient comfort. For complete grade III injuries, fixed hinges at 30° to 45° of flexion for two to four weeks can be used to allow for decreases in swelling and pain; then motion is begun. Once satisfactory painless range of motion has been restored, appropriate muscle rehabilitation and proprioceptive training can begin. The results from isolated medial collateral ligament injury treated nonoperatively are quite good.[61–63] With complete injuries, there often is a resultant clinical laxity by examination but little functional loss. The use of prophylactic knee bracing to prevent knee ligament injury has been the subject of a number of reviews, with mixed conclusions as to their efficacy. Reasons for failure of laterally hinged braces include alternation of knee axis of rotation, preload in tension of the medial collateral ligament, and improper fit. However, in a controlled prospective study, the incidence, but not the severity, of medial collateral ligament injury was reduced by bracing.[64]

Combined ligamentous injury, particularly that to the medial collateral–anterior cruciate ligament complex, generally warrants surgical intervention, as multiplane instability is present. This is particularly true for the young, active, athletic individual. In combined injuries as well as complete grade III medial collateral disruptions, the presence of meniscal injury must be excluded, as this may compromise treatment if present. MRI or arthroscopy is appropriate for this purpose. One must be concerned with capsular disruption and the use of arthroscopy because of extravasation of fluid.

Lateral Collateral Ligament Injury

The lateral collateral ligament is a cordlike structure running from the fibular head to the lateral femoral condyle.[71] It is readily palpable with the knee placed in a figure of 4 position. Its function is to resist tensile stress when varus force is applied to the knee, and it is aided on the lateral side, particularly in extension, by the iliotibial tract. Other secondary restraints include the arcuate ligament and popliteus muscle, which combine with the fibular collateral ligament to form the arcuate complex at the posterolateral corner of the knee.[70] Isolated injury to the lateral collateral ligament is unusual and may signify high-energy trauma. An example is the wind-swept or sideswipe knee injury with contralateral injury to the medial structures of the opposite knee. With lateral collateral ligament injury the peroneal nerve should be checked during the physical examination. Testing for varus instability should be performed in full extension and at relaxed flexion, with similar implications of capsular and possible cruciate disruption if instability is present in extension.[69,70] Isolated grade III injury to the lateral collateral ligament (varus laxity without endpoint in full extension) is unusual and is more often associated with combined cruciate and secondary restraint tears.[67] Avulsion fractures (lateral capsular sign) are indicators of significant soft tissue injury.[72]

Isolated injury to the posterolateral corner (arcuate complex) results from trauma to the anterior medial aspect of the extended knee, noted clinically by varus instability at 30° of flexion and a positive posterolateral drawer sign.[66] The cruciate ligaments are generally spared. Isolated injury to the lateral collateral ligament, particularly incomplete lesions, can be treated nonoperatively with limited bracing and rehabilitation, but grade III injuries warrant primary surgical intervention. Functional problems in laterally unstable knees may be more common than with isolated medial collateral injury as a result of the normal varus thrust and tensile forces on the lateral side of the knee with ambulation. Chronic lateral collateral ligament insufficiency is more apt to require late surgical intervention because of this functional deficit.

Principles of Ligament Surgery

The general function of ligaments is to resist tensile or joint distraction forces. This function can be lost through injury and affected by treatment. The goal in the treatment of ligamentous injury to the knee is to restore functional stability and normal kinematics. The biology of ligament injury and repair must be considered in the decision-making process. At the cellular level, ligaments undergo a continuum of events in response to injury. The stages of inflammation (injury to 48 hours), proliferation (48 hours to six weeks), remodeling and maturation (up to 12 months or more) can be altered favorably or unfavorably by surgical intervention,[73] type and length of immobilization, and rehabilitation.

Nonsurgical treatment is generally indicated for grade I and grade II collateral ligament injuries and isolated grade III injuries to these same structures. Isolated injuries to the anterior or posterior cruciate ligaments are variable in their presentation and instability pattern. The variables involved in treatment of these injuries have been discussed previously. Operative repair is indicated in ligamentous avulsion fractures and combined collateral, cruciate, and capsular ligamentous tears.

Repair of ligamentous injury involves one of three scenarios: (1) end-to-end ligament anastomosis; (2) ligament-to-bone fixation; and (3) bone-to-bone fixation. End-to-end ligament anastomosis is probably unnecessary for midsubstance tears of the collateral ligaments. Proponents of repair cite realignment of soft tissue with gap closure and reduction of scar during the proliferative phase as yielding better ultimate tensile strength.[74,75] However, in medial collateral ligament injury models treated nonoperatively, ultimate tensile strength was improved over those treated by operative repair, and additional tissue morbidity of surgical exposure was avoided.[76] Clinical experience substantiates this approach.

End-to-end suture fixation can be used in primary cruciate repairs when supplemented by intraarticular augmentation. Multiple loop sutures,[76,77] Bunnell sutures, and a locked-loop suture technique have been described to coapt ligament ends.[77] A heavy, nonabsorbable suture is recommended (Fig. 49–14). When brought out through drill holes, sutures should not be tied over a bone bridge, as they are at risk of cutting through the bone and thereby decreasing knot tension. An effective way to anchor sutures through bone is to secure the knot around the smooth proximal shank of a bone screw. The screw acts as a fixation post, and tension can be increased by angling the screw away from the direction of the suture line, securing the knot prior to final seating of the screw.

Ligament-to-bone fixation affords the best opportunity to restore anatomy, isometry, and tension in ligament repair. Soft tissue fixation techniques have been studied by Robertson et al.[78] The use of staples was inadequate in terms of pull-out strength and amount of tissue necrosis beneath the implant. Best results were

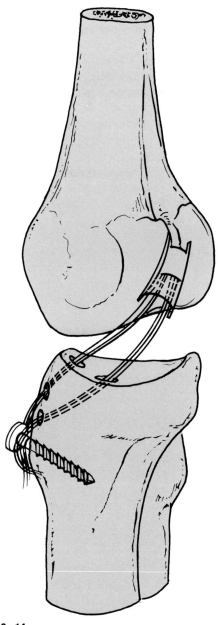

Figure 49–14

Ligament fixation to bone. This technique uses multiple nonabsorbable sutures placed through drill holes. The knot is sutured around the smooth shank of a bone screw acting as a fixation post.

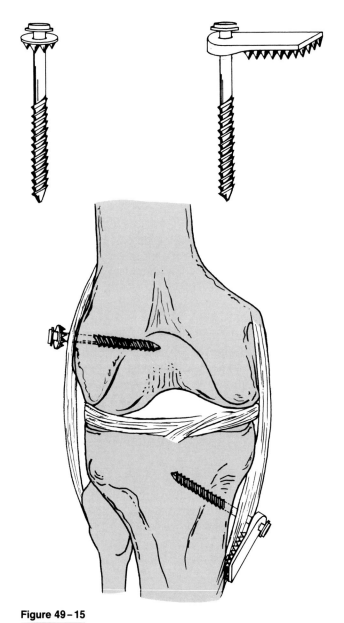

Figure 49–15

Ligament fixation to bone using a spiked washer and spiked soft tissue plate. The spiked design gives firm fixation and allows microcirculation beneath the implant.

obtained with the use of a screw with a spiked plastic washer or with a spiked ligament plate (Fig. 49–15). The spiked design allows microcirculation beneath the washer or plate and multiple fixation sites. Strength was improved by placing the screw through the tissue rather than in an adjacent position where only partial capture may occur.

Bone-to-bone fixation in ligamentous avulsion fractures can be secured, depending on size, with lag screws or tension band wires. Secure bone-to-bone fixation allows early motion and is the ideal scenario for ligament repair.

The purpose of secure soft tissue fixation is to allow controlled passive motion following repair. The effects of immobilization[79] (loss of collagen fiber orientation, increased stiffness, and subchondral resorption at the ligament-bone interface) can be countered with mobilization and graduated tensile stress application to the repaired ligament.

Meniscal Injury

The menisci of the knee are vital to knee function and longevity. Although the menisci were once considered vestigial structures, preservation of the menisci is now believed to be of paramount importance. They transmit up to 50% of the force across the knee, aid in shock absorption, and provide joint stability, particularly in ligament-deficient knees.[90,94] Their absence has been shown to lead to degenerative joint changes, as the loss of the load-sharing and shock-absorption functions effectively increases load per unit area on the articular surfaces.[86,89,96]

Meniscal tears (Fig. 49–16) are generally caused by a combination of axial loading and rotational forces, shearing the meniscus between the femoral and tibial condyles. Traumatic tears are usually associated with a known insult to the knee and may be isolated or associated with ligamentous or articular surface injury. Traumatic tears generally occur in the younger, active individual. Degenerative tears reflect cumulative stress

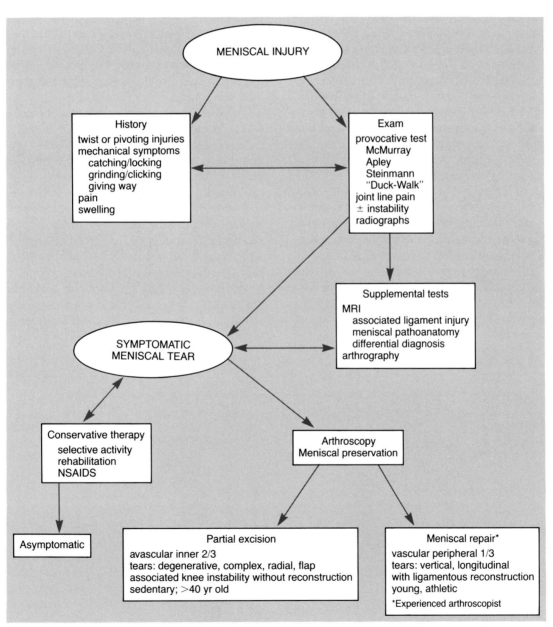

Figure 49–16

Treatment algorithm for meniscal injuries.

and correlate with the presence of associated chondromalacia. Symptoms produced by a meniscal tear are generally mechanical in nature: locking, catching, grinding, and giving way are common complaints. The frequency and severity of the symptoms vary according to the size and mobility of the meniscal tear. Pain and swelling are also variable. The body of the meniscus is aneural, and pain is generally produced by abnormal traction on the meniscocapsular junction or meniscofemoral ligaments (which are enervated), by the abnormal stress distribution created, or by localized inflammation.[84]

Clinical diagnosis is aided by provocative meniscal impingement tests (e.g., McMurray, Apley, and Steinmann) that attempt to produce pain or a mechanical event, such as a click or pop, by applying an axial load and rotational stress to the knee. An excellent functional test is the ability to "duck walk," which can only be done apprehensively or with pain in those with unstable tears, particularly involving the posterior horn. As part of the physical examination, specific joint line tenderness should also be assessed. Active or passive motion may be restricted because of displaced meniscal fragments. No one test is pathognomonic for the presence of a meniscal tear. However, a composite historical and clinical picture generally yields a presumptive diagnosis.[88] A comprehensive ligamentous exam should also be performed to establish the presence or absence of associated instability. An unstable knee may be causal in the development of a meniscal tear, and the presence of instability may alter treatment of the meniscal lesion. Plain radiographs should be obtained in all suspected cases of a meniscal tear, as mechanical symptoms can also be produced by other joint abnormalities such as loose bodies, osteochondritis dissecans, occult fracture, and tumors. As noted previously, MRI has supplanted arthrography as a diagnostic tool in the detection of meniscal lesions. It is noninvasive, details meniscal pathoanatomy, and is both highly sensitive and specific. Clear-cut indications for the use of MRI in evaluating meniscal lesions are developing.[83] However, when the diagnosis is in question, when establishing a differential diagnosis, and, on occasion, when planning a meniscal repair or partial excision, MRI can give needed information. In acute knee injuries, particularly isolated injuries to the anterior cruciate ligament, clinical examination often fails to elucidate the presence of meniscal injury. MRI is helpful in this situation if the physician plans to treat the ligament injury nonoperatively. The presence of an associated meniscal tear may warrant arthroscopic evaluation and treatment apart from the planned management of the ligament injury.

There is no accepted classification of meniscal tears. Causal mechanisms are categorized broadly as traumatic or degenerative. Tears are generally classified in descriptive terms as to location and configuration. Location in terms of circumference can be in the posterior, middle, or anterior one third of the meniscus (Fig. 49–17A). With regard to the cross-section of the meniscus, tears can be located in the inner, middle, or peripheral third or cross more than one zone (Fig. 49–17B). This has implications for healing, which is possible in the more vascular peripheral third but is unlikely in the inner two thirds. Peripheral detachments can also occur at the meniscocapsular junction. By configuration, meniscal tears are categorized as vertical or horizontal in their cleavage planes (Fig. 49–18). Vertical

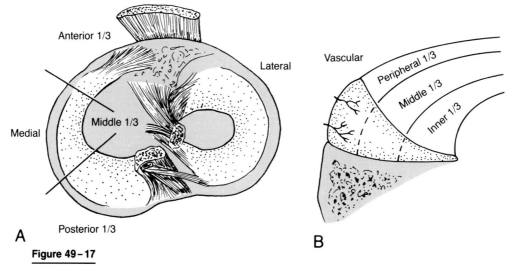

Figure 49–17

A, Meniscal tear sites in relation to circumference. B, Meniscal tear sites in relation to radial diameter.

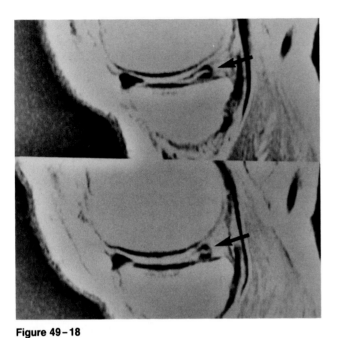

Figure 49-18

MRI scan showing horizontal cleavage tear of the posterior horn of the medial meniscus.

tears may be longitudinal (i.e., bucket-handle), radial, or oblique (flap or parrot-beaked) (Fig. 49–19). Complex tears denote primary and secondary tears and multiple cleavage planes. The most common vertical longitudinal tear involves the posterior third of the medial meniscus (Fig. 49–20). An isolated radial tear is most common to the middle third of the lateral meniscus. An accurate attempt should be made to classify meniscal tears as to location and configuration in operative reports.

Symptomatic meniscal injury warrants arthroscopic treatment, and meniscal preservation should be the goal. The vascular supply to the menisci is from a genicular artery derived from the perimeniscal capillary plexus that penetrates the peripheral 10% to 30% of the medial meniscus and the peripheral 10% to 25% of the lateral meniscus.[81] Tears located within this vascular meniscal zone have excellent healing potential. Asymptomatic, stable, vertical longitudinal tears in the vascularized portion of the meniscus may be treated by skillful neglect with good results.[88] Contributing factors in the decision-making process in terms of meniscal repair vs. excision include associated ligamentous injury and the age, occupation, and sports and activity level of the patient. Meniscal repair in the presence of ligamentous instability in a patient older than 40 yields unsatisfactory results. Arthroscopic or arthroscopically assisted meniscal repair is also a technically demanding procedure, and complications such as peripheral nerve and vascular injury, infection, and arthrofibrosis are more common than in simple arthroscopic partial meniscectomy.[86] Generally, for tears located in the avascular inner two thirds of the meniscus and for flap tears, radial tears, and complex tears, partial arthroscopic excision with balancing of the meniscal rim is recommended. Reparable meniscal tears ideally are those located in the vascular outer third of the body or at the meniscocapsular junction, greater than 1 cm in length, and vertical in their cleavage pattern (Fig. 49–21).[80,85] The chronicity of tear does not adversely affect healing potential. The benefits of partial meniscectomy compared with meniscal repair are less morbidity and a quicker return to activity. Meniscal preservation truly restores optimal knee function and should prevent degenerative changes.

The general principles of meniscal repair include excision of loose or frayed fibrocartilage, preparation of the meniscal surfaces with debridement and abrasion to promote vascular proliferation, and meniscal suture of absorbable nature. Healing potential also has been

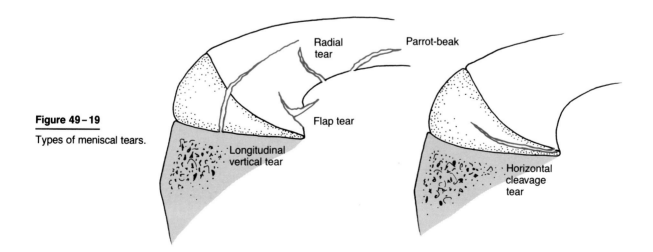

Figure 49-19

Types of meniscal tears.

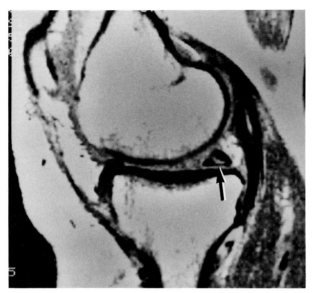

Figure 49-20

MRI scan showing a nondisplaced vertical tear (bucket-handle injury) of the posterior horn of the medial meniscus.

shown to be enhanced by the addition of fibrin clot to the repaired surface.[82] Specific techniques of meniscal repair include arthroscopic, arthroscopically assisted, and open procedures.[85,91,92] The arthroscopically assisted procedure is probably the most commonly used and safest procedure, as it retracts and protects the vital posterolateral or posteromedial structures. Inside-out and outside-in techniques for suture placement are

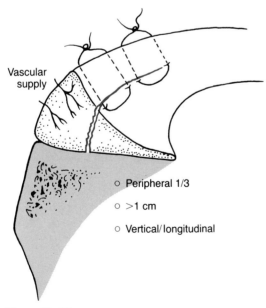

Vascular supply

o Peripheral 1/3

o >1 cm

o Vertical/longitudinal

Figure 49-21

Meniscal repair illustrated for ideal injury type and location.

based on the surgeon's preference. The longevity of meniscal repair is increased by concomitant reconstruction of associated ligamentous instability, usually involving the anterior cruciate ligament.

Rehabilitation following isolated meniscal repair generally includes controlled-motion bracing with avoidance of full flexion and limited weight bearing for four to eight weeks, followed by progression to full weight bearing and an exercise program. No cutting, squatting, or jumping activity is allowed for up to six months following repair. In meniscal repairs associated with ligamentous reconstruction, rehabilitation is dictated by the reconstruction procedure. Excellent results can be anticipated with partial meniscectomy of isolated vertical, longitudinal, or flap tears. Poorer results can be expected with associated chondromalacia, degenerative or complex tears, and ligamentous instability and in knees previously operated on.[87] In properly selected cases for meniscal repair with ligamentous reconstruction, results are comparable with partial excision. The goal of meniscal preservation has prompted research to improve vascular access to the meniscus and early investigation into allograft replacement.

Surgical Approaches to the Acutely Injured Knee

The surgical approach utilized in the acutely injured knee employs the principles of utility and extensibility of incisions. In general, incisions should be straight or gently curved, avoiding transverse placement. Secondary incisions exposing deep capsuloligamentous structures should be parallel to those structures (i.e., avoiding transverse, capsular, or ligamentous incisions that may result in operative injury in addition to primary ligamentous disruption). An exception to this is a gross third-degree rupture in a transverse or oblique fashion that allows direct visualization and repair. Four basic incisions allow treatment of most acute soft tissue knee injuries: medial, lateral, midline, and posterior.[97,98]

MEDIAL INCISION

The medial incision is used to approach the medial collateral ligament, associated capsular structures, and the cruciate ligaments. The incision is generally curved or straight, centering over the adductor tubercle of the medial femoral condyle and carried distally in a parapatellar fashion to the medial border of the tibial tuberosity. With full-thickness anterior and posterior skin flaps, a medial parapatellar arthrotomy incision can be made, and the posteromedial corner can be exposed.

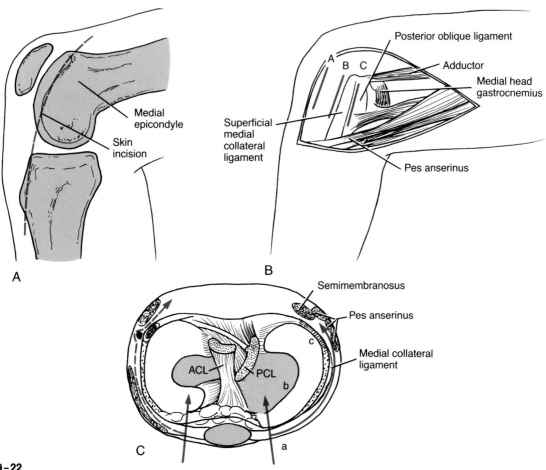

Figure 49–22

A, Skin incision centered or slightly anterior to the adductor tubercle, with the distal extension bordering patellar tendon and tibial tuberosity. The proximal extension can be curved posteriorly if access to the posteromedial corner is desired. *B*, Anterior and posterior flaps mobilized, and the pes anserine group retracted posteriorly. Line A shows the anteromedial parapatellar arthrotomy for approach to the anterior cruciate ligament, the articular surfaces of the medial compartment, and the medial meniscus. Line B shows the midmedial capsular incision for access to the medial collateral ligament complex. Line C shows the posteromedial capsulotomy for the approach to the medial meniscus (open meniscal repair), the posterior capsule, and the posterior cruciate ligament. *C*, Transverse section of the knee with capsular incisions. ACL = Anterior cruciate ligament; PCL = posterior cruciate ligament.

Exposure of the medial collateral ligament can be facilitated by raising a proximally based retinacular flap. Posteromedial exposure for meniscal, capsular, or posterior cruciate repair is through a vertically oriented incision posterior to the medial collateral ligament, superior to the semimembranosus, and anterior to the medial head of the gastrocnemius (Fig. 49–22).

LATERAL INCISION

The lateral incision is used to approach the fibular collateral ligament and associated capsular structures, including the arcuate complex. The lateral incision is centered over the midportion of the lateral femoral condyle and carried in a curved or straight fashion to Gerdy's tubercle. A lateral parapatellar arthrotomy and access to the posterolateral corner are possible with development of full-thickness skin and subcutaneous flaps. The approach to the posterolateral corner is made through a vertical incision posterior and parallel to the fibular collateral ligament. If greater exposure is necessary, detachment of Gerdy's tubercle with bone and proximal retraction exposes the lateral capsular ligamentous structures. The iliotibial band can likewise be split and retracted without distal detachment (Fig. 49–23). Care must be taken to identify and preserve the common peroneal nerve just beneath the biceps femoris.

MIDLINE INCISION

The utility midline incision in acute knee injury is most often used for treatment of extensor mechanism disruption. It can be used in approaching acute anterior

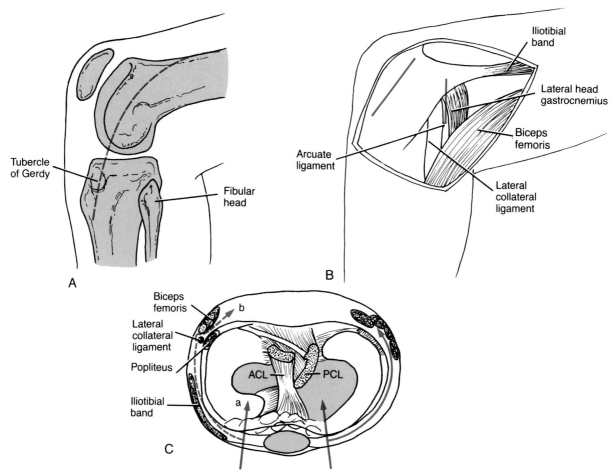

Figure 49-23

A, Skin incision centered over or slightly anterior to the lateral femoral condyle extended distally toward the tubercle of Gerdy and extended proximally in line with the iliotibial band. *B*, Capsular incisions. The iliotibial band can be incised in line with its fibers or reflected proximally with a wafer of bone. Line A shows the anterolateral parapatellar arthrotomy for access to the lateral compartment articular surfaces and the lateral meniscus. Line B shows the posterolateral capsulotomy through the arcuate ligament, for open meniscal repair, and the posterolateral capsule. *C*, Transverse section of the knee with capsular incisions. ACL = Anterior cruciate ligament; PCL = posterior cruciate ligament.

cruciate ligament injury but, unless done through a transpatellar tendon approach, requires patellar dislocation with its subsequent morbidity. For acute primary anterior cruciate ligament reconstruction utilizing the middle third of the patellar tendon, the defect after graft harvest can be opened through division of the fat pad for visualization of the intercondylar notch; however, with expanding arthroscopically assisted techniques, this additional trauma can be avoided.

POSTERIOR INCISION

In acute knee injuries the posterior incision is rarely utilized except in penetrating trauma to the posterior aspect of the knee and in isolated posterior cruciate ligament avulsion fractures in which a direct approach for bone-to-bone surgical stabilization is necessary.

Best done with the patient prone, this involves identification of the sural nerve and short saphenous vein in the midline of the fascial of the proximal calf. These are followed to the popliteal neurovascular structures, and the gastrocnemius muscle heads are separated, medial from lateral. The vessels can be retracted medially or laterally after dividing the tethering geniculate branches. Either gastrocnemius head can be detached proximally to gain access to the posteromedial or posterolateral corner of the knee.[97,98]

REFERENCES

Diagnostic Approach to the Injured Knee

1. Butler, J.C.; Andrews, J.R. The role of arthroscopic surgery in evaluation of acute traumatic hemarthrosis of the knee. Clin Orthop 228:150-152, 1988.

2. DeHaven, K.E. Diagnosis of acute knee injuries with hemarthrosis. Am J Sports Med 8:9–14, 1980.

3. Hughston, J.C.; Andrews, J.R.; Cross, M.J.; Moschi, A. Classification of knee ligament instabilities. Part I. The medial compartment and cruciate ligaments. J Bone Joint Surg 58A:159–172, 1976.

4. Hughston, J.C.; Andrews, J.R.; Cross, M.J.; Moschi, A. Classification of knee ligament instabilities. Part II. The lateral compartment. J Bone Joint Surg 58A:173–179, 1976.

5. Jackson, D.W.; Jennings, L.D.; Maywood, R.M.; Berger, P.E. Magnetic resonance imaging of the knee. Am J Sports Med 16(1):29–38, 1988.

6. Losee, R.E.; Johnson, T.R.; Southwick, W.O. Anterior subluxation of the lateral tibial plateau. A diagnostic test and operative repair. J Bone Joint Surg 50A:211–242, 1968.

7. Munk, P.L.; Helms, C.A.; Genant, N.K.; Holt, R.G. Magnetic resonance imaging of the knee: Current status, new directions. Skeletal Radiol 18:569–577, 1989.

8. Nagel, D.A.; Burton, D.S.; Manning, J. The dashboard knee injury. Clin Orthop 126:203–208, 1977.

9. Noyes, F.R.; Bassett, R.W.; Grood, E.S.; Butler, D.L. Arthroscopy in acute traumatic hemarthrosis of the knee. Incidence of anterior cruciate tears and other injuries. J Bone Joint Surg 62A:687–695, 1980.

10. Polly, D.W.; Callaghan, J.J.; Sikes, R.A.; et al. The accuracy of selective magnetic resonance imaging compared with the findings of arthroscopy of the knee. J Bone Joint Surg 70A:192–198, 1988.

11. Slocum, D.B.; Larson, R.L. Rotatory instability of the knee. Its pathogenesis and a clinical test to demonstrate its presence. J Bone Joint Surg 50A:211–242, 1968.

12. Torg, J.S.; Conrad, W.; Kalen, V. Clinical diagnosis of anterior cruciate instability in the athlete. Am J Sports Med 4(2):84–93, 1976.

Knee Injury in Polytrauma Patients

13. Gillespie, W.J. The incidence and pattern of knee injury associated with dislocation of the hip. J Bone Joint Surg 57B:376–387, 1975.

14. Moore, J.M.; Patzakis, M.J.; Harvey, J.P. Ipsilateral diaphyseal femur fractures and knee ligament injuries. Clin Orthop 232:182–189, 1988.

15. Templeman, D.C.; Marder, R.A. Injuries of the knee associated with fractures of the tibial shaft. Detection by examination under anesthesia: A prospective study. J Bone Joint Surg 71A:1392–1395, 1989.

16. Veith, R.G.; Winquist, R.A.; Hansen, S.T. Ipsilateral fractures of the femur and tibia. A report of fifty-seven consecutive cases. J Bone Joint Surg 66A:991–1002, 1984.

17. Walker, D.M.; Kennedy, J.C. Occult knee ligament injuries associated with femoral shaft fractures. Am J Sports Med 8:172–174, 1980.

18. Walling, A.K.; Seradge, H.; Spiegel, P.G. Injuries to the knee ligaments with fractures of the femur. J Bone Joint Surg 64A:1324–1327, 1982.

Open Knee Injuries

19. Collins, D.N.; Temple, S.D. Open joint injuries. Classification and treatment. Clin Orthop 243:48–56, 1988.

20. Patzakis, M.J.; Dorr, L.D.; Ivler, D.; et al. The early management of open joint injuries. A prospective study of one-hundred and forty patients. J Bone Joint Surg 57A:1065–1071, 1975.

Traumatic Dislocation of the Knee

21. Green, N.E.; Allen, B.L. Vascular injuries associated with dislocation of the knee. J Bone Joint Surg 59A:236–239, 1977.

22. Kennedy, J.C. Complete dislocation of the knee joint. J Bone Joint Surg 45A:889–904, 1963.

23. Meyers, M.H.; Harvey, J.P. Traumatic dislocation of the knee joint. J Bone Joint Surg 53A:16–29, 1971.

24. Meyers, M.H.; Moore, T.M.; Harvey, J.P. Traumatic dislocation of the knee joint. Follow-up notes on articles previously published in the journal. J Bone Joint Surg 57A:430–433, 1975.

25. Quinlan, A.G.; Sharrard, W.J.W. Postero-lateral dislocation of the knee with capsular interposition. J Bone Joint Surg 40B:660–663, 1958.

26. Reckling, F.W.; Peltier, L.F. Acute knee dislocations and their complications. J Trauma 9:181–191, 1969.

27. Roman, P.D.; Hopson, C.N.; Zenni, E.J. Traumatic dislocation of the knee: A report of 30 cases and literature review. Orthop Rev 16(12):33–40, 1987.

28. Sisto, J.D.; Warren, R.F. Complete knee dislocation. A follow-up study of operative treatment. Clin Orthop 198:94–101, 1985.

29. Steadman, J.R.; Montgomery, J.B. Dislocation of the knee in the competitive athlete. In: Spiegel, P.G., ed. Topics in Orthopedic Trauma. Baltimore, University Park Press, 1984, pp. 125–134.

30. Taylor, A.R.; Arden, G.P.; Rainey, H.A. Traumatic dislocation of the knee. A report of forty-three cases with special reference to conservative treatment. J Bone Joint Surg 54B:96–102, 1972.

Anterior Cruciate Ligament Injury

31. Arnold, J.A.; Coker, T.P.; Heaton, L.M.; et al. Natural history of anterior cruciate tears. Am J Sports Med 7(6):305–313, 1979.

32. Carbaud, H.E.; Feagin, J.A. Experimental studies of acute anterior cruciate ligament injury and repair. Am J Sports Med 7:18–22, 1979.

33. Chick, R.R.; Jackson, D.W. Tears of the anterior cruciate ligament in young athletes. J Bone Joint Surg 60A:970–973, 1978.

34. Fetto, J.F.; Marshall, J.L. The natural history and diagnosis of anterior cruciate insufficiency. Clin Orthop 147:29–37, 1980.

35. Fowler, P.J.; Reagan, W.D. The patient with symptomatic chronic anterior cruciate ligament insufficiency. Results of minimal arthroscopic surgery and rehabilitation. Am J Sports Med 15(4):321–325, 1987.

36. Giove, T.P.; Miller, S.J.; Kent, B.E.; et al. Non-operative treatment of the torn anterior cruciate ligament. J Bone Joint Surg 65A:184–192, 1983.

37. Girgis, F.G.; Marshall, J.L.; Monajem, A.R.S. The cruciate ligaments of the knee joint. Anatomical, functional and experimental analysis. Clin Orthop 106:216–231, 1975.

38. Hawkins, R.J.; Misamore, G.W.; Merritt, T.R. Follow-up of the acute nonoperated isolated anterior cruciate ligament tear. Am J Sports Med 14(3):205–210, 1986.

39. Higgins, R.W.; Steadman, J.R. Anterior cruciate ligament repairs in world class skiers. Am J Sports Med 15(5):439–447, 1987.

40. Holden, D.L.; Jackson, D.W. Treatment selection in acute anterior cruciate ligament tears. Orthop Clin North Am 16(1):99–108, 1985.

41. Johnson, R.J. The anterior cruciate: A dilemma in sports medicine. Int J Sports Med 3:71–79, 1982.

42. Kannus, P.; Jarvinen, M. Long-term prognosis of nonoperatively treated acute knee distortions having primary hemarthrosis without clinical instability. Am J Sports Med 15(2):138–143, 1987.

43. Kennedy, J.C.; Weinberg, H.W.; Wilson, A.S. The anatomy and

function of the anterior cruciate ligament. J Bone Joint Surg 56A:223–235, 1974.

44. Lipscomb, A.B.; Johnston, R.K.; Snyder, R.B.; Brothers, R.C. Secondary reconstruction of anterior cruciate ligament in athletes using the semitendinosus tendon. Am J Sports Med 7:81–84, 1979.

45. Marshall, J.L.; Warren, R.F.; Wickiewicz, T.L. Primary surgical treatment of anterior cruciate lesions. Am J Sports Med 10(2):103–107, 1982.

46. Marshall, J.L.; Warren, R.F.; Wickiewicz, T.L.; Reider, B. The anterior cruciate ligament: A technique of repair and reconstruction. Clin Orthop 143:97–106, 1979.

47. McCarroll, J.R.; Rettig, R.C.; Shelbourne, K.D. Anterior cruciate ligament injuries in the young athlete with open physes. Am J Sports Med 16(1):44–47, 1988.

48. McDaniel, W.J.; Dameron, T.B. Untreated ruptures of the anterior cruciate ligament. J Bone Joint Surg 62A:696–704, 1980.

49. Noyes, F.R.; Barber, S.D.; Mooar, L.A. A rationale for assessing sports activity levels and limitations in knee disorders. Clin Orthop 246:238–249, 1989.

50. Noyes, F.R.; Matthews, D.S.; Mooar, P.A.; Grood, E.S. The symptomatic anterior cruciate-deficient knee. Part II: The results of rehabilitation, activity modification, and counseling on functional disability. J Bone Joint Surg 65A:163–174, 1983.

51. Noyes, F.R.; Mooar, P.A.; Matthews, D.S.; Butler, D.L. The symptomatic anterior cruciate-deficient knee. Part I: The long-term functional disability in athletically active individuals. J Bone Joint Surg 65A:154–162, 1983.

52. Odensten, M.; Hamberg, P.; Nordin, M.; et al. Surgical or conservative treatment of the acutely torn anterior cruciate ligament. A randomized study with short-term follow-up observations. Clin Orthop 198:87–93, 1985.

Posterior Cruciate Injury

53. Clancy, W.G.; Shelbourne, K.D.; Zoellan, G.B.; et al. Treatment of knee joint instability secondary to rupture of the posterior cruciate ligament. J Bone Joint Surg 65A:310–322, 1983.

54. Cross, M.J.; Powell, J.F. Long-term followup of posterior cruciate ligament rupture: A study of 116 cases. Am J Sports Med 12(4):292–300, 1984.

55. Dandy, D.J.; Pusey, R.J. The long-term results of unrepaired tears of the posterior cruciate ligament. J Bone Joint Surg 64B:92–98, 1982.

56. Gollehon, D.L.; Torzilli, P.A.; Warren, R.F. The role of the posterolateral and cruciate ligaments in the stability of the human knee. J Bone Joint Surg 69A:233–242, 1987.

57. Hughston, J.C.; Bowden, J.A.; Andrews, J.R.; Norwood, A.A. Acute tears of the posterior cruciate ligament. J Bone Joint Surg 62A:438–450, 1980.

58. Jakob, R.P. The reversed pivot shift sign—a new diagnostic aid for posterolateral rotatory instability of the knee. Acta Orthop Scand 52:18–32, 1981.

59. Loos, W.C.; Fox, J.M.; Blazina, M.E.; et al. Acute posterior cruciate ligament injuries. Am J Sports Med 9:86–92, 1981.

60. Parolie, J.M.; Bergfeld, J.A. Long-term results of nonoperative treatment of isolated posterior cruciate ligament injuries in the athlete. Am J Sports Med 14(1):35–38, 1986.

Medial Collateral Ligament Injury

61. Fetto, J.F.; Marshall, J.L. Medial collateral ligament injuries of the knee: A rationale for treatment. Clin Orthop 132:206–218, 1978.

62. Holden, D.L.; Ebbert, A.W.; Butler, J.E. Non-operative treatment of grade I and grade II medial collateral ligament injuries to the knee. Am J Sports Med 11:340–344, 1983.

63. Indelicato, P.A. Non-operative treatment of complete tears of the medial collateral ligament of the knee. J Bone Joint Surg 65A:323–329, 1983.

64. Sitler, M.; Ryan, J.; Hopkinson, W.; et al. The efficacy of a prophylactic knee brace to reduce knee injuries in football. A prospective, randomized study at West Point. Am J Sports Med 18(3):310–315, 1990.

65. Warren, L.F.; Marshall, J.L. The supporting structures and layers of the medial side of the knee. An anatomical analysis. J Bone Joint Surg 61A:56–62, 1979.

Lateral Collateral Ligament Injury

66. DeLee, J.C.; Riley, M.B.; Rockwood, C.A. Acute posterolateral rotatory instability of the knee. Am J Sports Med 11(4):199–207, 1983.

67. DeLee, J.C.; Riley, M.B.; Rockwood, C.A. Acute straight lateral instability of the knee. Am J Sports Med 11(6):404–411, 1983.

68. Grana, W.A.; Janssen, T. Lateral ligament injury of the knee. Orthopedics 10(7):1039–1044, 1987.

69. Hughston, J.C.; Andrews, J.R.; Cross, M.D.; Moschi, A. Classification of knee ligament instabilities. Part II. The lateral compartment. J Bone Joint Surg 58A:173–179, 1976.

70. Hughston, J.C.; Norwood, L.R. The posterolateral drawer test and external rotational recurvatum test for posterolateral rotatory instability of the knee. Clin Orthop 147:82–87, 1980.

71. Johnson, L.L. Lateral capsular ligament complex. Anatomical and surgical considerations. Am J Sports Med 7:156–160, 1979.

72. Woods, W.G.; Stanley, R.F.; Tullos, H.S. Lateral capsular sign: X-ray clue to a significant knee instability. Am J Sports Med 7:27–33, 1979.

Principles of Ligament Surgery

73. Daniel, D.M. Principles of knee ligament surgery. In: Daniel, D.M.; et al., eds. Knee Ligaments: Structure, Function, Injury, and Repair. New York, Raven Press, 1990.

74. Moller, W. The Knee. Form, Function, and Ligament Reconstruction. New York, Springer-Verlag, 1983.

75. O'Donoghue, D.H. An analysis of end results of surgical treatment of major injuries to the ligaments of the knee. J Bone Joint Surg 37A:1–12, 1955.

76. Woo, S.L.-Y.; Inove, M.; McGurk-Burleson, E. Treatment of the medial collateral ligament injury; structure and function of canine knees in response to differing treatment regimens. Am J Sports Med 15(1):22–29, 1987.

77. Krackow, J.A.; Thomas, S.C.; Jones, C.C. A new stitch for ligament-tendon fixation. J Bone Joint Surg 68A:764–765, 1986.

78. Robertson, D.B.; Daniel, D.M.; Biden, E. Soft tissue fixation to bone. Am J Sports Med 14(5):398–403, 1986.

79. Noyes, F.R. Functional properties of knee ligaments and alterations induced by immobilization. A correlative biomechanical and histologic study in primates. Clin Orthop 123:210–242, 1977.

Meniscal Injury

80. Arnoczky, S.P. Arthroscopic surgery: Meniscus healing. Cont Orthop 10(2):31–39, 1985.

81. Arnoczky, S.P.; Warren, R.F. Microvasculature of the human meniscus. Am J Sports Med 10(2):90–95, 1982.

82. Arnoczky, S.P.; Warren, R.F.; Spivak, J.M. Meniscal repair using an exogenous fibrin clot. J Bone Joint Surg 68A:847–861, 1986.

83. Barronian, A.D.; Zoltan, J.D.; Bucon, K.A. Magnetic resonance imaging of the knee: Correlation with arthroscopy. J Arthros 5(3):187–191, 1989.

84. Day, B.; Mackenzie, W.G.; Shim, S.S.; Leung, G. The vascular and nerve supply of the human meniscus. Arthroscopy 1(1):58–62, 1985.

85. Dehaven, K.E.; Black, K.P.; Griffiths, H.J. Open meniscus repair. Technique and two to nine year results. Am J Sports Med 17(6):788–795, 1989.

86. Fairbank, T.J. Knee joint changes after meniscectomy. J Bone Joint Surg 30B:664–670, 1948.

87. Ferkel, R.D.; Davis, J.R.; Friedman, M.J.; et al. Arthroscopic partial medial meniscectomy: An analysis of unsatisfactory results. Arthroscopy 1(1):44–52, 1985.

88. Fowler, P.J.; Lubliner, J.A. The predictive value of five clinical signs in the evaluation of meniscal pathology. J Arthros 5(3):184–186, 1989.

89. Krause, M.S.; Pope, M.H. Mechanical changes in the knee after meniscectomy. J Bone Joint Surg 58A:599–604, 1976.

90. Levy, I.M.; Torzilli, P.A.; Warren, R.F. The effect of medial meniscectomy on anterior-posterior motion of the knee. J Bone Joint Surg 64A:883–888, 1982.

91. Rosenberg, T.; Scott, S.; Paulos, L. Arthroscopic surgery: Repair of peripheral detachment of the meniscus. Cont Orthop 10(3):43–50, 1985.

92. Scott, G.A.; Jolly, B.L.; Henning, C.E. Combined posterior incision and arthroscopic intra-articular repair of the meniscus. An examination of factors affecting healing. J Bone Joint Surg 68A:847–861, 1986.

93. Small, N.C. Complications in meniscal repair. Comp Orthop 2:109–112, 1987.

94. Walker, P.S.; Erkman, M.J. The role of the menisci in force transmission across the knee. Clin Orthop 109:184–192, 1975.

95. Weiss, C.B.; Lundberg, M.; Hamberg, P.; et al. Non-operative treatment of meniscal tears. J Bone Joint Surg 71A:811–822, 1989.

96. Yocum, L.A.; Kerlan, R.K.; Jobe, F.W.; et al. Isolated lateral meniscectomy. A study of twenty-six patients with isolated tears. J Bone Joint Surg 61A:338–342, 1979.

Surgical Approaches

97. Henry, A.K., Extensile Exposure, Ed. 2. Baltimore, Williams & Wilkins, 1970.

98. Hoppenfeld, S.; deBoer, P.; Surgical Exposures in Orthopaedics. Philadelphia, J.B. Lippincott, 1984.

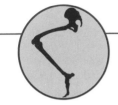

Joseph Schatzker, M.D.

50

Tibial Plateau Fractures

Relevant Anatomy

The medial and lateral tibial plateaux are the articular surfaces of the medial and lateral tibial condyles and articulate with the medial and lateral femoral condyles, respectively. The medial plateau is the larger of the two and is concave from front to back as well as from side to side. The lateral plateau is smaller and higher than the medial and is *convex* from front to back as well as from side to side. The fact that the lateral plateau is higher than the medial must be remembered during internal fixation so that a screw inserted from lateral to medial does not enter the medial articulation. The convexity of the lateral plateau helps the surgeon to identify it on a lateral radiograph of the proximal tibia. The two plateaux are separated from one another by the intercondylar eminence, which is nonarticular and serves as the tibial attachment of the anterior cruciate ligament. The outer portion of each plateau is covered by a cartilaginous meniscus. The lateral meniscus covers a much larger portion of the articular surface than does the medial. The medial articular surface and its supporting medial condyle are stronger than their lateral counterparts. As a result, fractures of the lateral plateau are more common. When fractures of the medial plateau occur, they are invariably associated with more violent injuries and more commonly have associated soft tissue injuries, such as disruptions of the lateral collateral ligament complex, lesions of the lateral peroneal nerve, or damage to the popliteal vessels.

Mechanism of Injury

Injuries to the plateaux occur as a result of (1) a force directed either medially (valgus deformity — the classic "bumper fracture") or laterally (varus deformity), (2) an axial compressive force, or (3) both an axial force and a force from the side. The respective femoral condyle in this mechanism of injury exerts both shearing and compressive forces to the underlying tibial plateau. The resulting fracture is therefore most commonly a split fracture, a depression fracture, or both. Pure split fractures are more common in younger patients in whom the strong bone of the tibial condyle is able to withstand the compressive force of the femoral condyle. With age the dense cancellous bone of the young tibial condyle gives way to much sparser cancellous bone, which changes the physical properties of the condyle; it is no longer able to withstand compressive forces as well. As a result, split depression fractures are common in patients in their fifth decade of life or older.[1,2]

However, fracture patterns are also a reflection of the forces involved. In high-velocity injuries the forces may be so great that the plateaux explode into numerous fracture fragments. The displacement of the various fragments often varies, but the principal shear and compressive forces that have given rise to the injury pattern can still be recognized. In lower velocity injuries the injury pattern and the mechanism of injury are more discernible. Thus the classic "bumper fracture" is a fracture of the lateral plateau, the result of a lateral blow to the leg that creates a valgus deforming force and a loading of the lateral plateau by the overlying femoral condyle. The magnitude of the force determines not only the degree of fragmentation but also the degree of displacement. Thus in addition to the fracture, there may be associated soft tissue lesions such as a tear of the medial collateral ligament or a tear of the anterior cruciate ligament in association with a lateral plateau fracture; or a tear of the lateral collateral ligament complex, the cruciates, and the peroneal nerve; or a lesion of the popliteal vessels associated with a fracture of the medial plateau fracture. The surgeon must also differentiate split fractures that are the result of a shearing force from rim avulsion fractures that are associated with knee dislocations and point to a much more unstable injury.[3]

If an axial force of sufficient severity is exerted on the fully extended knee (e.g., as in a fall from a height), a bicondylar split fracture results. This has been referred to as the "inverted Y" fracture and corresponds to the type V fracture described later. This fracture may be extraarticular if the fracture lines begin in the intercondylar eminence and spare the articular surfaces, or it may be articular.

Consequence of Injury

Tibial plateau fractures pose major threats to the structures and function of the knee joint. Immobilization alone in a plaster cast, if prolonged for more than two to three weeks, may result in an unacceptable degree of stiffness that will not respond to physiotherapy. Traction with early motion will preserve movement but will not ensure reduction, as impacted articular fragments, which are driven into the underlying cancellous bone of the metaphysis and do not have any soft tissue attachment, will not reduce. Unless reduction is achieved, the displacement of the articular fragments may result in joint instability and deformity coupled with a restricted range of motion. The joint depression together with metaphyseal fragmentation may also result in an angular deformity, leading to a major degree of joint overload. Thus unless the joint is reduced anatomically, the alignment of the limb preserved, and motion instituted early (which can only be achieved with an early open reduction and internal fixation), major complications can be anticipated. Delayed mobilization will result in permanent stiffness. Failure to correct instability will result in permanent instability, which alone or when coupled with joint incongruity will lead to posttraumatic arthritis. Even with the most successful form of treatment, depending on the degree of initial joint fragmentation and damage to the articular cartilage, posttraumatic arthritis can develop.

Tibial plateau fractures can be associated with serious soft tissue damage. Tears of the menisci, particularly peripheral detachments, occur, as do tears of the collateral ligaments and of the cruciate ligaments. Avulsion of the infrapatellar tendon together with the tibial tubercle occurs but is rare. Fractures of the lateral plateau are rarely associated with arterial or nerve lesions. However, fractures of the medial plateau, because they invariably are associated with much greater violence and often represent a knee dislocation that has been realigned, are often associated with lesions of the peroneal nerve or the popliteal vessels. The arterial lesions rarely present as hemorrhage. Their common mode of presentation is either as an acute obstruction (because of a complete tear in the vessel or an acute thrombosis) or as a delayed thrombosis or a thrombosis seemingly initiated by the reparative surgery. This occurs because of an injury to the arterial intima sustained at the time of the initial trauma.

Tibial plateau fractures, particularly when associated with extension of the fracture into the diaphysis, may be associated with acute compartment syndromes because of hemorrhage and edema of the involved compartments. Another important mechanism of compartment syndrome development is reperfusion swelling after successful correction of ischemia.

The proximal tibia is subcutaneous except posteriorly. Anteriorly it is covered only by the skin and subcutaneous tissue that cover the few tendons and ligaments that cross the joint. The bone, together with the tendons and ligaments, is very susceptible to injury if skin coverage is lost. Severe contusions of this skin envelope occur particularly with high-energy injuries to the area. Therefore even in the absence of open fractures, the contused soft tissue envelope may be in jeopardy because of instability of the underlying fractures; severe swelling associated with the injury; or any injudicious, traumatizing, poorly timed surgical procedure. Thus fractures of the proximal tibia may become complicated by wound sloughs, infections, and osteomyelitis.

Classification

Most tibial plateau fractures result from a lateral bending force with a simultaneous axial force. However, our experience with tibial plateau fractures has led me to the conclusion that these fractures cannot be viewed collectively, because they differ not only in their pattern of fracture and required treatment but also in their prognosis. We have developed a classification that groups these fractures into six types.[6] Each type represents a group of fractures that are similar in their mechanism of injury and fracture pattern, require a similar approach in their treatment, and have a similar prognosis.

TYPE I

Type I is a wedge fracture or a split fracture of the lateral plateau (Fig. 50–1), the result of bending and axial forces.[4] It occurs in young people in whom the strong

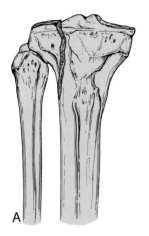
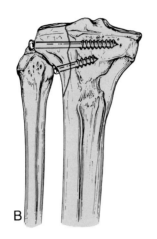

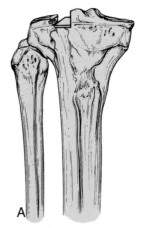
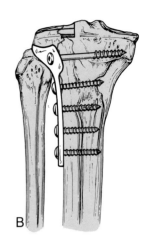

Figure 50-1

A, Type I fracture: a split wedge fracture of the lateral plateau without any joint depression. More or less displacement may be present. Even if displacement is slight, there may be an associated peripheral tear of the lateral meniscus, which can be incarcerated in the fracture. Arthroscopy may be required to exclude a meniscus injury. *B*, Type I wedge fractures can be fixed with lag screws (often with washers) if the bone is of good quality. In older, osteoporotic patients, a buttress plate may be advisable. (Redrawn from Schatzker, J. In: Chapman, M.W. Operative Orthopaedics. Philadelphia, J.B. Lippincott, 1988, Fig. 35-1, p. 422.)

Figure 50-2

A, Type II fracture: a split depression fracture. The depressed fragment may undergo severe fragmentation. These injuries generally occur in patients with decreased bone density. *B*, With a type II fracture, the lateral plateau is exposed beneath the meniscus, and depressed articular surface fragments are carefully elevated en masse by opening the peripheral fracture defect. Sufficient bone graft is inserted into the remaining metaphyseal void. Then the split fragment is reduced and fixed with a buttress plate and lag screws. Allograft may be used in elderly patients. (Redrawn from Schatzker, J. In: Chapman, M.W. Operative Orthopaedics. Philadelphia, J.B. Lippincott, 1988, Fig. 35-3*A*, p. 423.)

cancellous bone of the plateau resists depression. If displaced, this fracture is frequently associated with a peripheral tear of the lateral meniscus, with the meniscus caught in the fracture. It is a partial articular fracture and corresponds to the 41–B1 fracture group of the AO classification.[5]

TYPE II

Type II is a split depression fracture of the lateral plateau (Fig. 50–2). The mechanism of injury is the same as in type I, but the cancellous bone is usually weaker because of some osteoporosis and does not resist depression as it does in the younger population. Therefore in addition to the split or wedge, there is also a depression of the articular surface. The patients are usually somewhat older than those who experience type I fractures; the majority are in their fourth or fifth decade. This is also a partial articular fracture and corresponds to the 41–B3.1 group of the AO classification.[5]

TYPE III

Type III is a pure depression of the lateral plateau (Fig. 50–3). Like type II, this is a very common fracture pattern in patients in their fourth or fifth decade. The depression is usually lateral and central but may involve any part of the articular surface. If the depression

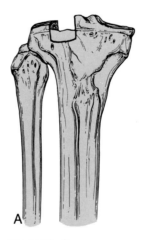
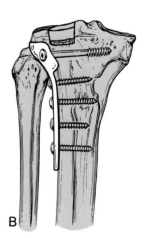

Figure 50-3

A, Type III fracture: a pure depression fracture. The depressions vary in size and degree and may be central or, less commonly, peripheral. Instability may not be present when the depressed area is small or centrally located. An examination under anesthesia may be required to assess stability of a knee with a type III fracture. *B*, If instability is present in a type III fracture, the depressed portion of the tibial plateau is elevated via an appropriately placed window in the metaphysis. Bone graft is packed into the resulting defect. If a large window is required, the cortex must be buttressed with a plate to prevent a split fracture. (Redrawn from Schatzker, J. In: Chapman, M.W. Operative Orthopaedics. Philadelphia, J.B. Lippincott, 1988, Fig. 35-3*A*, p. 423.)

is central, the joint is usually stable, because the depression is usually covered by the large lateral meniscus. If, however, enough of the joint surface is depressed centrally, instability can result. The depression of the articular surface may also be peripheral. Lateral and posterior peripheral depressions are usually associated with a greater incidence of joint instability than are the central depressions. This type corresponds to 41–B2.1 and 41–B2.2 of the AO classification.[5]

TYPE IV

Type IV is a fracture of the medial tibial plateau (Fig. 50–4) and may be a split or a split depression fracture. The medial plateau resists fracture more than the lateral; thus its fractures are usually the result of a much greater force. Medial plateau injuries are most frequently associated with an avulsion of the intercondylar eminence, which may signify rupture of one or both cruciate ligaments. In addition the varus force frequently also results in a rupture of the lateral collateral ligamentous complex. If the displacement at the time of the trauma is sufficient, the fracture may also be associated with a traction lesion of the peroneal nerve or with a lesion of the popliteal artery. Many actually represent a medial dislocation of the knee that has usually been reduced by the time the radiograph is exposed. It is not the fracture of the medial plateau that gives this fracture its bad prognosis, but the associated injuries such as the peroneal nerve lesion, the popliteal

artery lesion, and the rupture of the cruciates and the lateral collateral ligamentous complex. Because of the frequently associated popliteal artery lesion, which may be only an intimal tear, whenever this lesion is recognized the patient should be considered for an arteriogram to evaluate the artery and prevent an intraoperative or postoperative thrombosis. Some of these fractures are also associated with a posterior split of the medial plateau, which causes the femoral condyle to subluxate posteriorly and greatly increases the instability of the joint. These fractures correspond to the 41–B1, 41–B2, and 41–B3 of the AO classification.[5]

TYPE V

Type V is a split fracture of the lateral and medial plateau (Fig. 50–5) and is usually the result of a pure axial load applied to the extended knee. The prognosis depends on whether the fracture line involves the articular surfaces or begins in the intercondylar area and skirts the articular surfaces as it exits in the metaphysis medially and laterally. If the articular surfaces are not involved, the patient's prognosis is correspondingly better. These fractures correspond to the 41–C1 fracture group of the AO classification.

TYPE VI

The hallmark of the type VI fracture is the metaphyseal fracture that separates the articular components from

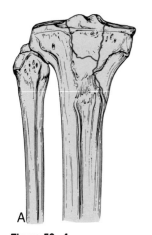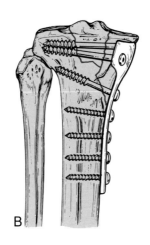

Figure 50–4

A, Type IV fracture: a fracture of the medial plateau, which is frequently associated with a fracture of the intercondylar eminence. This high-energy injury may be associated with neurovascular or other significant soft tissue injury. *B,* Definitive fixation of Type IV (medial plateau) fractures usually requires a medial buttress plate to supplement the lag screws. Lag screws or a wire suture may be needed to anchor an intercondylar eminence fragment. (Redrawn from Schatzker, J. In: Chapman, M.W. Operative Orthopaedics. Philadelphia, J.B. Lippincott, 1988, Fig. 35-4A, p. 424.)

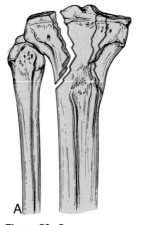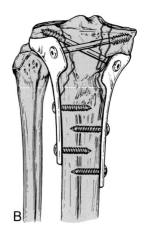

Figure 50–5

A, The type V fracture is a bicondylar fracture that may involve the articular surface. Occasionally, the fracture lines are so close to the intercondylar eminence that the weight-bearing surfaces of the plateaux are not affected. The fracture lines may resemble an inverted Y. *B,* Lag screws with medial and lateral buttress plating provide optimal fixation for Type V plateau fractures. Buttress plates are important to prevent axial collapse. (Redrawn from Schatzker, J. In: Chapman, M.W. Operative Orthopaedics. Philadelphia, J.B. Lippincott, 1988, Fig. 35-5A, p. 424.)

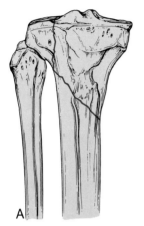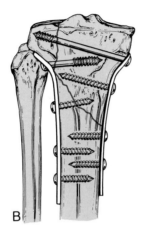

Figure 50-6

A, The hallmark of a type VI fracture is separation of the metaphysis from the diaphysis. Usually, the lateral condyle has a depressed and/or comminuted area, whereas the medial condyle tends to be more intact. Such impaction may involve both condyles. *B*, Two plates are required for optimal fixation of a type VI fracture. Both act as buttresses, but one (a DCP-type plate) must reconnect the metaphysis to the diaphysis, supplementing lag screw fixation if possible. Thus this plate is used for either compression or neutralization. (Redrawn from Schatzker, J. In: Chapman, M.W. Operative Orthopaedics. Philadelphia, J.B. Lippincott, 1988, Fig. 35-6*A*, p. 435.)

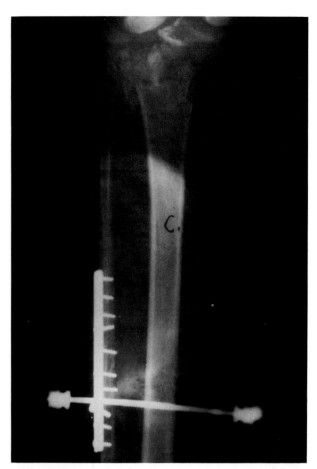

Figure 50-7

Traction fails to reduce the impacted articular fragments, which lack capsular or ligamentous attachments. (From Schatzker, J. In: Chapman, M.W., ed. Operative Orthopaedics. Philadelphia, J.B. Lippincott, 1988, p. 425.)

the diaphysis (Fig. 50-6). Many of these fractures are associated with a depression and impaction of one or both articular surfaces. Traction most frequently fails to reduce the impacted articular fragments and results in distraction of the metaphyseal fracture line (Fig. 50-7). These fractures correspond to the 41–C2 and 41–C3 groups of the AO classification.

FRACTURES OF THE INTERCONDYLAR EMINENCE

Fractures of the intercondylar eminence, when present as isolated injuries, represent avulsion of the anterior cruciate ligament and are not to be included under fractures of the tibial plateau. Occasionally when the fragment is large, it may encroach on the articular surface of the medial tibial plateau. These correspond to the A1 fracture type of the AO classification.

AO CLASSIFICATION OF FRACTURES OF LONG BONES

The Comprehensive Classification of Fractures of Long Bones[5] is a unique classification system because it applies to all long bones rather than being a regionally based classification. Furthermore, it classifies fractures in such a way that they are organized in an ascending order of severity. Thus a type A fracture is generally easier to treat than a type B, and a type C has a worse

prognosis and will be more difficult to manage than a type A or B. In the AO classification, metaphyseal and epiphyseal fractures belong to the fractures of the end segments. They are further divided into partial and complete articular fractures. In the partial articular fracture (the B type), a part of the articular surface retains its continuity with the diaphysis, whereas in the complete articular fracture (the C type), the articular surface has lost all connection to the diaphysis. It is important to recognize that a fracture may be intracapsular and yet extraarticular. In an articular fracture the fracture must involve the articular cartilage.

The AO classification divides the fractures not only into types but also into groups and subgroups. Thus if one considers only the partial and complete articular fractures and excludes the type A metaphyseal fractures, then there are 18 fracture types to consider. If one considers only the groups and omits the subgroups, then there are six types, just as there are in the

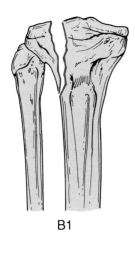

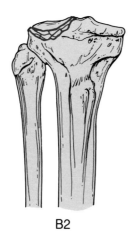

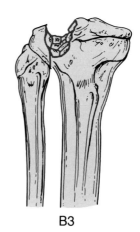

B1   B2   B3

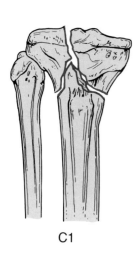

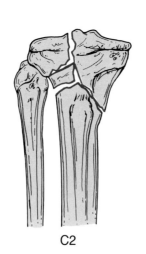

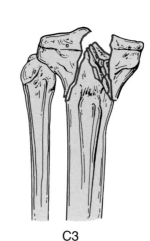

C1   C2   C3

Figure 50–8

The AO classification of fractures of long bones, tibia/fibula, proximal segment. B1, Partial articular fracture, pure split. B2, Partial articular fracture, pure depression. B3, Partial articular fracture, split depression. C1, Complete articular fracture, articular simple, metaphyseal simple. C2, Complete articular fracture, articular simple, metaphyseal multifragmentary. C3, Complete articular fracture, multifragmentary. (Redrawn from Mueller, M.E., et al. The Comprehensive Classification of Fractures of Long Bones. Berlin, Springer-Verlag, 1990, p. 151.)

Schatzker classification (Fig. 50–8). The B group, the partial articular fractures, corresponds to the Schatzker types I, II, III, and IV. The C group corresponds to the Schatzker types V and VI, the complete articular fractures. The AO group C1 corresponds to the Schatzker type V. Group C1 fractures (Fig. 50–9), including subgroups C1.1, C1.2, and C1.3, are all extraarticular as long as they do not involve articular cartilage, and therefore these have a better prognosis than some of the type B fractures. Note also that the medial plateau fracture, type IV in the Schatzker classification, is evident in the AO classification only as subgroups B1.2, B1.3, B2.3, B3.2, and B3.3 (Fig. 50–10). As already mentioned, fracture of the medial tibial plateau is a very serious lesion that deserves more prominent recognition as a separate group rather than as subgroups. A regionally based classification can address with greater precision the regional idiosyncrasies of an injury. The advantage of the AO classification system is clearly its unified approach and consistency in dealing with all fractures.

Diagnosis

HISTORY

The patient is rarely able to relate the exact mechanism of injury, but the history is nevertheless very useful, as it may permit the physician to determine the direction of the force, the deformity produced, and whether the injury was caused by a high- or a low-velocity force. This has an important bearing on the associated soft tissue injuries.

PHYSICAL EXAMINATION

The physical examination is an extremely important aspect of patient evaluation, because it gives invaluable information not available from most laboratory investigations. Physical examination is the most accurate method of evaluation of the soft tissue envelope and its injuries, whether they are closed or open. It is also the most accurate means of evaluation of the neurologic

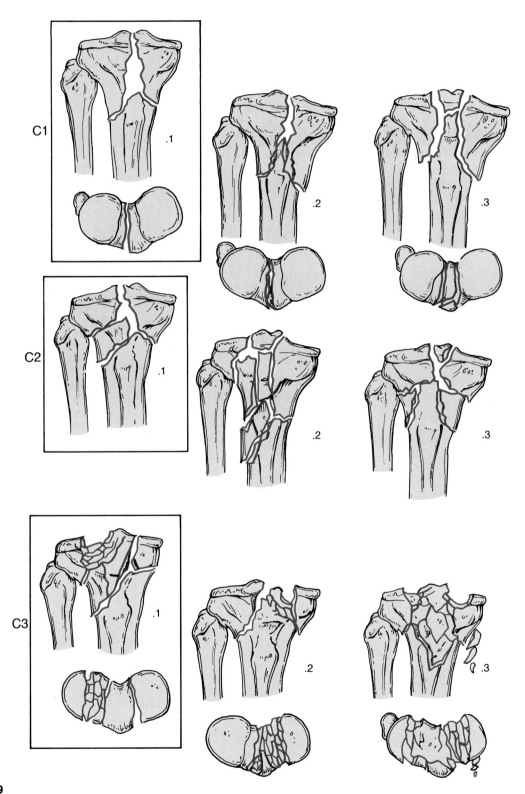

Figure 50–9

Group C fractures. *C1: complete articular fracture, articular simple, metaphyseal simple.* This includes fractures with an intact anterior tibial tubercle and intercondylar eminence, fractures involving the anterior tibial tubercle, and fractures involving the intercondylar eminence. The subgroups are .1, slight displacement; .2, one condyle displaced; and .3, both condyles displaced. *C2: complete articular fracture, articular simple, metaphyseal multifragmentary.* The subgroups are .1, intact wedge (lateral and medial); .2, fragmented wedge (lateral and medial); and .3, complex. *C3: complete articular fracture, multifragmentary.* This includes metaphyseal simple, metaphyseal lateral wedge, metaphyseal medial wedge, metaphyseal complex, and metaphyseal-diaphyseal complex fractures. The subgroups are .1, lateral; .2, medial; and .3, lateral and medial. (Redrawn from Mueller, M.E., et al. The Comprehensive Classification of Fractures of Long Bones. Berlin, Springer-Verlag, 1990, p. 157.)

1751

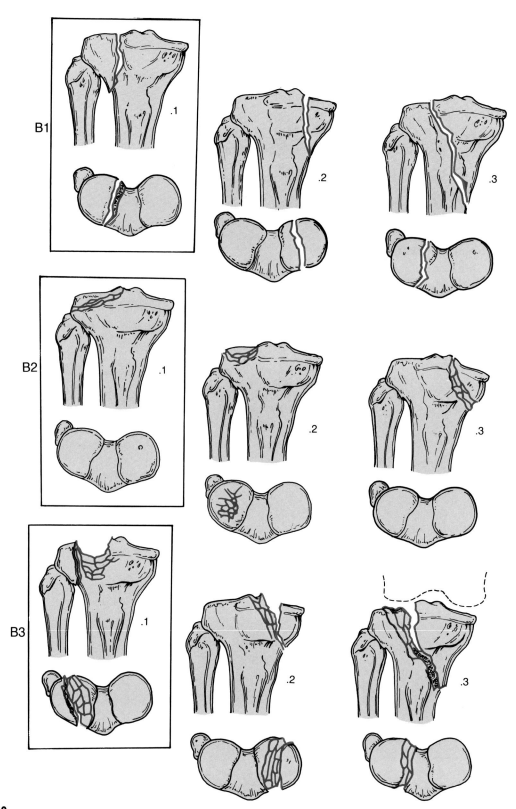

Figure 50-10

Group B fractures. *B1: Partial articular fracture, pure split.* The subgroups are .1, lateral plateau (marginal, sagittal, frontal anterior, or frontal posterior); .2, medial plateau (marginal, sagittal, frontal anterior, or frontal posterior); and .3, oblique, involving the tibial spines and one of the surfaces (lateral or medial). *B2: Partial articular fracture, pure depression.* The subgroups are .1, lateral total (one-piece depression or mosaiclike depression); .2, lateral limited (peripheral, central, anterior, or posterior); and .3, medial (peripheral, central, anterior, posterior, or total). *B3: Partial articular fracture, split depression.* These include anterior lateral depression, posterior lateral depression, anterior medial depression, and posterior medial depression fractures. The subgroups are .1, lateral; .2, medial; and .3, oblique, involving the tibial spines and one of the surfaces (lateral or medial). (Redrawn from Mueller, M.E., et al. The Comprehensive Classification of Fractures of Long Bones. Berlin, Springer-Verlag, 1990, p. 75.)

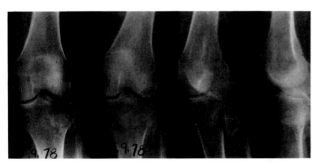

Figure 50-11

Oblique projections provide additional fracture information.

status of the extremity and the most rapid means of evaluation of the vascular status and of the presence or absence of a major tear of a collateral ligament. It is also a fairly accurate guide to compartment pressure and may indicate a compartment syndrome.

IMAGING

Standard Radiographic Views

A radiograph is the only way to assess accurately the fracture pattern and its severity. The standard anteroposterior and lateral views are inadequate and must be supplemented with two oblique projections taken with the leg in internal and external rotation (Fig. 50-11). The internal oblique projects to advantage the lateral plateau, and the external oblique, the medial. The oblique views frequently give information that is completely missed on a standard anteroposterior projection.

Tomography

Whenever there is any uncertainty about the degree of fragmentation or depression of the articular surface, the physician should order anteroposterior and lateral tomographs. These frequently reveal the extent and position of important fracture lines, the number and size of fragments, and the degree of depression (Fig. 50-12).

Computed Tomography Scanning

The computed tomography (CT) scan provides the surgeon with the cross-sectional anatomy of the fracture and with a sagittal reconstruction at any desired depth (Fig. 50-13). We find it an extremely helpful, almost essential, form of imaging for complex fractures. It allows the surgeon to formulate a three-dimensional concept of the fracture and judge its operability. If still in doubt, the surgeon can request a three-dimensional reconstruction to solve any continuing difficulty with the anatomy of the injury. Such complex imaging techniques are usually unnecessary in the simpler fracture patterns.

Arteriography

An arteriogram should be considered whenever there is serious concern about the possibility of an arterial lesion. An intimal tear may be present without a clinically detectable deficit. At surgery, however, such a lesion may lead to an occlusive thrombosis and jeopardize the extremity. The fracture pattern most commonly associated with an arterial injury is the Schatzker type IV, the fracture of the medial plateau

Figure 50-12

Type III fractures are characterized by central depression of the lateral tibial plateau. Note the added detail. *A*, An AP drawing of a tibial plateau fracture. *B*, An AP tomogram of the type of fracture shown in *A*. (*A* Redrawn from Schatzker, J. In: Chapman, M.W. Operative Orthopaedics. Philadephia, J.B. Lippincott, 1988, Fig. 35-2, p. 423.)

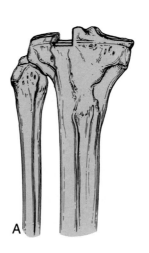

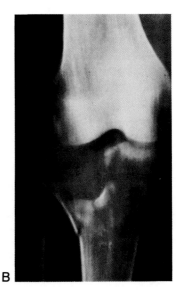

A   B

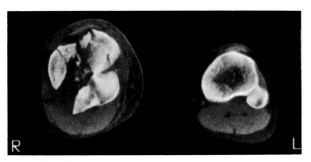

Figure 50–13

CT scan of a type VI fracture of the tibial plateau. Note the cross-sectional anatomy of the fracture. (From Schatzker, J. Fractures of the tibial plateau. In: Chapman, M.W., ed. Operative Orthopaedics. Philadelphia, J.B. Lippincott, 1988, p. 426.)

that frequently presents as a very unstable knee and may have been dislocated at the time of injury. Therefore whenever the surgeon is confronted with a type IV lesion, an arteriogram should be seriously considered as part of the preoperative evaluation.

Management

Until relatively recently major intraarticular fractures remained an unsolved problem, and disability in varying degrees following a major intraarticular fracture was considered unavoidable. Charnley recognized in 1961 that anatomic reduction and early motion were desirable in the treatment of intraarticular injuries,[7] but the techniques of surgery and internal fixation available at the time made these objectives of treatment unattainable. Attempts at early motion following internal fixation frequently resulted in pain because of instability, with resultant loss of fixation and varying degrees of malunion or nonunion. Surgery combined with plaster immobilization resulted in even greater stiffness than plaster immobilization alone. The pathophysiology of joint stiffness was poorly understood, and stiffness following surgery was blamed on the added trauma of surgery[8,9] and on the periarticular location of the fixation device.[8] Therefore surgery was considered the last resort, and nonoperative techniques of treatment of articular injuries were generally favored. The phases of treatment were evaluation, reduction, immobilization, and rehabilitation; thus rehabilitation followed fracture union. This resulted invariably in joint stiffness and led Neer et al.[9] to argue that 70° of knee motion was an acceptable result. Perkins[10] was a great pioneer of early joint rehabilitation and developed successful methods of traction that permitted early motion of joints while providing sufficient immobilization for the fracture to unite. Apley[11,12] applied

these techniques to the treatment of tibial plateau fractures and reported, as did Roberts,[13] what he considered to be satisfactory results, compared with the results of surgery. The difficulty in evaluating these studies is that the authors reported the results of treatment collectively without analyzing the type of tibial plateau fracture that had a satisfactory outcome. The classification employed of "undisplaced, slightly displaced, and severely displaced" amplified by such terms as "vertical or oblique fracture line or split or comminuted"[12] is unable to separate fracture types with intrinsically different prognoses. Furthermore, these authors were comparing the results of the best nonoperative treatment with methods of surgical treatment that are unacceptable by present standards of surgical care. The development by the AO group of atraumatic techniques of open reduction and stable fixation, of new techniques and principles of internal fixation that permitted absolute stability of fixation with early motion without the fear of displacement and malunion or nonunion, and of new implants and instruments that facilitated the attainment of the new goals of open reduction and internal fixation brought about a revolution in fracture surgery.[17]

The following sections analyze the important factors that contribute to proper decision making in fracture treatment and to determination of the "personality" of the injury and indicate the preferred techniques and the results achieved when these techniques were employed.

INDICATIONS FOR TREATMENT: CLOSED VERSUS OPEN

The goals of treatment of any intraarticular fracture are to preserve joint mobility, joint stability, articular surface congruence, and axial alignment; to provide freedom from pain; and to prevent posttraumatic osteoarthritis.

Fractures of the tibial plateau may be either partial or complete articular fractures.[5] They may result in joint incongruity because of displacement of the articular fragments and in joint instability because of depression and displacement of articular fragments or rupture of collateral or cruciate ligaments. They may also result in axial malalignment and deformity as a result of joint depression and associated metaphyseal fracture.

Pauwels[14] demonstrated that if the degree of stress (force/unit area), which results from weight bearing, exceeds the ability of articular cartilage to regenerate or repair itself, then articular cartilage degeneration ensues, leading to posttraumatic osteoarthritis.

Displacement of articular fragments results in a decrease of the available surface area of contact, which results (even in the presence of normal load and normal direction of load application) in a rise in stress. If this rise in stress is coupled with an axial malalignment (the result of joint depression or a metaphyseal fracture), the rise in stress is more significant (Fig. 50–14). These two factors—a decrease in joint surface area and a rise in stress resulting from deformity and an increase in axial loading—may result in posttraumatic osteoarthritis. The likelihood of osteoarthritis is greatly increased if these factors are coupled with instability, which can be the result of either joint depression and incongruity or an associated ligament rupture.

From this we can conclude that in treating intraarticular fractures we must strive to achieve joint congruity and the maximum possible amount of surface area of contact. This can be achieved only by an anatomic reduction of the joint surface. We must also strive to prevent compartment overload by correcting any coexistent axial malalignment.

Mitchell and Shepard,[15] in their studies on the effects

of articular malreduction and unstable fixation on the outcome of articular fractures, have shown that an accurate reduction and stable fixation of intraarticular fragments are necessary for articular cartilage regeneration and that malreduction and instability resulted in rapid articular cartilage degeneration. This not only further supports the need for an anatomic reduction of the joint but also emphasizes the need for stable fixation to enhance articular cartilage regeneration and facilitate early motion by relieving pain, which is often the result of instability and motion at the fracture site.

Schatzker et al.'s review of tibial plateau fractures[6] has allowed the formulation of additional principles of treatment. Tibial plateau fractures treated nonoperatively in plaster casting for a month or longer resulted in marked stiffness of the knee. Patients with similar fractures treated with open reduction and internal fixation combined subsequently with plaster immobilization experienced much greater stiffness of the involved

Figure 50–14

A, In a normal knee the articular surfaces are congruous, and when bearing weight, the medial and lateral compartments share the load almost equally, with the medial taking slightly more than the lateral. *B,* When fractured and partially depressed, the articular surface becomes incongruous, and a smaller portion of the joint carries the full load. The load can be further increased by axial malalignment.

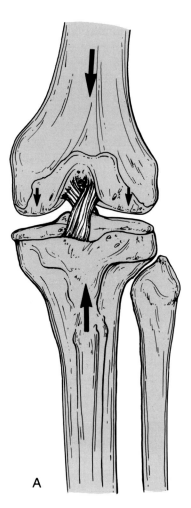

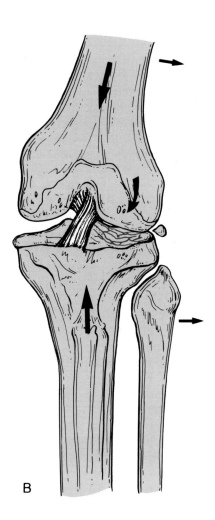

A

B

knee. From this we have concluded that intraarticular fractures, regardless of treatment, must be mobilized early. However, only open reduction and stable fixation permit early motion without loss of articular fragment reduction and consequent malunion or nonunion. Therefore if surgery is inadvisable or not possible, then the joint with an intraarticular fracture should be treated in skeletal traction and early motion in order to preserve motion, even if such treatment may result in joint incongruity or instability. As long as joint mobility is preserved, secondary reconstructive joint salvage procedures, such as intraarticular osteotomies, are possible. These are usually much less successful in the presence of joint stiffness.

Fractures that were initially treated nonoperatively (i.e., by manipulation and traction) often showed persistent displacement of some articular fragments (see Fig. 50–7). If these fractures were then operated on early, the unreduced fragments were always found to be impacted in the metaphysis and required considerable force to be disimpacted and reduced. Thus any displaced articular fragments which do not reduce after suitable closed manipulation and traction can be considered impacted. Their reduction can succeed only by open means. Furthermore, joint depression and articular defects resulting from impacted articular fragments have been found to remain as permanent joint defects. These defects, when examined at the time of late articular reconstructions, have never been found to be filled with fibrocartilage, which would have restored stability. Thus any joint that is unstable as a result of joint depression or displacement will remain unstable unless the depression or displacement is corrected surgically.

From these observations we have formulated the following principles of treatment of tibial plateau fractures:

1. Any tibial plateau fracture that results in joint instability requires an open reduction and internal fixation.

2. Maximum joint congruity can be restored only by open reduction.

3. Stable fixation of articular fragments and anatomic reduction are necessary for articular cartilage regeneration.

4. If an open reduction is indicated but is inadvisable either because of patient or injury factors or because the complexity of the injury exceeds the ability of the treating team, then the fracture must be treated in skeletal traction and early motion.

These principles of treatment are general. When treating a particular patient the surgeon must be governed not only by joint congruity, joint stability, and axial alignment, but also by what we call the "personal-

ity" of the fracture, which is a synthesis of patient factors, injury factors, ability of the treating team, and suitability of the hospital environment.

The following are absolute indications for surgery:
1. An open tibial plateau fracture
2. A tibial plateau fracture combined with
   a. an acute compartment syndrome; or
   b. an acute vascular lesion.

The relative indications and contraindications for surgery must be determined for each patient individually by a careful definition of the personality of the injury.

PERSONALITY OF THE INJURY

If the fracture is displaced and unstable, then joint congruity, axial alignment, and stability most likely will be restorable only by open reduction and internal fixation. However, whether such a course is to be pursued has to be worked out very carefully. This is best done by defining the "personality" of the injury. The concept of the personality of the injury first includes the patient factors: age, history of past health, concurrent health problems, occupation and leisure activities, and expectations of treatment results. For example, the goals of treatment will be very different in an osteoporotic octogenarian than in a healthy young athlete.

Second are the injury factors. Here the surgeon must define very carefully the injury to the soft tissue envelope. Is the fracture open or closed? Associated injuries such as a concomitant neurologic or vascular deficit or an acute compartment syndrome must be determined. Next the morphologic characteristics of the fracture must be defined with great care in order to be able to classify the fracture. From these the surgeon will gain insight into some of the expected difficulties of treatment and will acquire information on the patient's prognosis. This must be combined with an evaluation of the degree of displacement of the fragments and of the mechanism of injury in order to determine the vascularity of the bone and its healing potential. Lastly, the degree of osteoporosis must be determined, because the quality of bone is of paramount importance in judging the operability of a fracture.

Third, in defining the personality of the injury the surgeon must define the treatment team and the treatment environment. This area may be the most difficult, for it forces the surgeon to evaluate objectively his or her own skill and that of his or her assistants and the adequacy of the treatment environment. Without proper fracture classification and proper data bases in which the treatment and its result are carefully documented, the surgeon will continue to treat patients on the basis of anecdotal evidence and frequently fallacious clinical impressions. It is hoped that the emergence of a widely accepted fracture classification[5] and the recently developed trauma data bases, such as those developed by the AO Foundation and the North American AO group and made available to the North American trauma surgeon through the Orthopaedic Trauma Association, will greatly assist surgeons in defining indications for surgery. Until then surgeons must remember that a poorly performed open reduction and internal fixation offers the patient the worst of both worlds. It exposes the patient to all the complications and dangers of surgery without offering any of the described advantages.

NONOPERATIVE TREATMENT

Undisplaced fractures and partial articular fractures, if stable, do not require operative treatment. However, they do require early motion and prevention of displacement. How displacement is prevented will depend on the fracture and on patient compliance. If there is any fear that displacement might occur, the limb should be immobilized in a fracture brace and weight bearing prohibited. We define stability of a partial articular fracture as follows. A fracture is considered stable if, when examined under adequate sedation or, if necessary, general anesthesia, it does not exhibit on varus/valgus stressing more than 10° of instability at any point in the arc of motion from full extension to 90° of flexion. The degree of instability that one is prepared to accept within this range must also be viewed in terms of the personality of the injury. In evaluating a partial articular fracture for stability, one must remember that a peripheral wedge fragment, if it involves the posterior part of the plateau, will not contribute to instability in the frontal plane, and the joint may appear to be perfectly stable on varus/valgus stressing. However, it creates instability in the sagittal plane and is an absolute indication for surgical reduction and stabilization.

If the fracture is unstable but, because of excessive comminution or advanced osteoporosis, is not suited for open reduction and internal fixation, or if it is decided that the fracture should be treated openly but the treatment must be delayed, then the patient must be treated in skeletal traction and early motion. The pin for traction should be inserted at least 4 to 5 in below the lowest discernible fracture line so as to be completely out of the operative field if surgery is to be undertaken. The connection of the traction pin to the traction should have roller bearings.[16] This completely overcomes torquing of the pin with its consequent loosening and possible pin track sepsis.

OPERATIVE TREATMENT

Timing of Surgery

If the decision is made to proceed to surgery, the timing is important. An open fracture should be operated on immediately, as should a fracture associated with an acute compartment syndrome or an arterial lesion. All other tibial plateau fractures must be evaluated individually. If there are no contraindications, it is best to proceed to surgery as soon as possible. However, this should never be at the expense of a careful definition of the injury. The complex tibial plateau fracture must be carefully defined, which will require additional views and special imaging procedures such as tomography or CT scanning. These are not life-threatening injuries, and adequate time should be taken to evaluate the injury. This consideration applies also in polytrauma situations that are discussed later.

If the condition of the patient allows and the fracture is well defined, it is best to deal with it immediately, but the decision to proceed must be made with the realization that a complex fracture may take 3 to 4 hours of surgery, and a delay of 24 to 48 hours will not compromise the treatment of the fracture. Another consideration is the patient in whom the swelling may be so severe or the contusion of the soft tissues such that a delay is indicated. If a delay of more than one to two days is necessary, then the leg should not be immobilized in plaster or another type of splint. This does not prevent shortening and collapse of the fracture, which will make subsequent reduction much more difficult. It is best to place the leg in skeletal traction as already described until such time as an open reduction and internal fixation can be safely carried out.

Planning of the Surgical Procedure

The surgical procedure must be planned carefully. This involves consideration of the surgical approach, which must be atraumatic and extensile and must expose all the component parts of the injury without sacrificing any important structures. It also involves a careful drawing of the fracture pattern with a detailed plan of all the steps in the open reduction and internal fixation. This plan must include an indication of the exact position of all the screws and their function and of the position and the length of the buttress plate.

Positioning of the Patient and Aids to Reduction

The patient should be positioned supine on the operating table in such a way that the footpiece of the table can be adjusted to permit flexion of the knee to 90°. Knee flexion allows the iliotibial band to slip posteriorly off the lateral condyle of the femur, which permits the surgeon to make an incision in the capsule at its attachment to the upper tibia without having to cut through the iliotibial band. However, the surgeon should have no fear of cutting through the iliotibial band at the level of the joint to facilitate exposure, should this prove necessary. At the end of the procedure the iliotibial band should be resutured with a nonabsorbable suture. We have done this many times and have not encountered a single instance of varus instability as a result. The insertion of the iliotibial band should not be osteotomized for the same reason that the tibial tubercle should not be osteotomized in tibial plateau fractures, as reattachment may prove difficult or impossible in an already fractured proximal tibia.

The flexed knee not only facilitates exposure but also greatly aids visualization of the joint. If the table is tilted slightly into the Trendelenburg position, the patient will not slide forward. The dependent position of the leg applies traction, frees an assistant from holding the leg, and allows the surgeon to apply a varus or valgus force by simply pushing on the foot in the desired direction.

Surgical Approaches

We recommend either a straight midline incision or a medial or lateral parapatellar incision, depending on the side involved (Fig. 50–15). We are very much opposed to the lazy S- and the L-shaped incisions and the triradiate "Mercedes star" incision recommended at one time by the AO.[17] Straight longitudinal incisions are best, because they interfere least with the blood supply to the skin flaps and do not interfere with any future reconstructive procedures that might become necessary if the surgical reconstruction should fail or posttraumatic arthritis develop later. The skin incisions must be planned in such a way that they are not positioned directly over an implant. The flaps that are raised must be full thickness, consisting of the subcutaneous fat down to the fascia. This is important to prevent wound edge necrosis.

The meniscus must be preserved and should never be excised to facilitate exposure. The meniscus shares in weight transmission and distributes the weight over a broad surface area.[18,19] This cushioning effect protects the repaired and damaged articular cartilage, prevents the redisplacement of the elevated articular fragments, and enhances cartilage healing. The capsule should be incised horizontally below the meniscus, whether approaching the lateral or the medial side of the joint (Fig.

50–16). This allows the surgeon to pull up on the meniscus and the attached capsule with a sharp small rake retractor, and gain an unobstructed view of the articular surface. If the arthrotomy is made above the meniscus, the meniscus obscures most of the articular surface and interferes with the execution of an anatomic reduction. If a peripheral tear is encountered, or even if there is a tear into the body of the meniscus, this should be repaired at the end of the procedure. Every effort should be made to preserve the meniscus.[20,21]

In order to gain exposure of the depressed articular fragments, the surgeon should make use of the fracture.

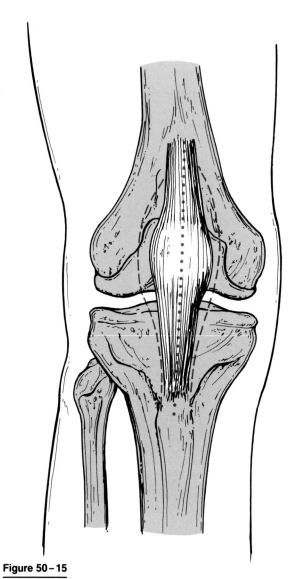

Figure 50–15

The incisions should be straight. An increase in exposure is gained by extension of the incision proximally and distally.

Thus if there is a peripheral wedge fragment, regardless of its size, it should be hinged back on its soft tissue attachment, like opening the cover of a book. This allows perfect visualization of the joint depression. The soft tissue attachment preserves the blood supply to the wedge fragments. Some surgeons advise that whenever there is a wedge fracture, the capsule and the meniscus should not be detached from their tibial attachment, but instead the anterior horn of the meniscus should be detached to the point where the wedge begins, and in this way exposure of the joint depression can be gained. We feel that this has decided disadvantages. One can always repair a peripheral detachment with considerable ease or suture the incision in the capsule, which constitutes a repair of the coronary ligament. It is much more difficult to achieve a secure repair of the detachment of the anterior horn of the meniscus. If there is no wedge or split fragment, the depressed area can be approached from below through a window made in the cortex of the respective tibial condyle.

The surgeon should also be wary of the posterior split or wedge fracture, which may be medial or lateral and associated with any fracture pattern, although it is most commonly associated with a Schatzker type IV fracture

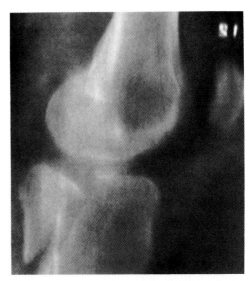

Figure 50-17

Posterior wedge fracture, which is frequently seen best on a lateral tomogram, as shown here. Note the posterior subluxation of the femoral condyles. Frequently plain radiographs fail to reveal important fracture lines, the number of fragments, and their depression. (From Schatzker, J.; Tile, M. Rationale of Fracture Management Care. New York, Springer-Verlag, 1987, p. 287.)

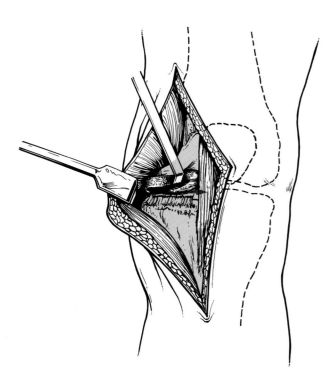

Figure 50-16

The arthrotomy should be made by incising the capsule transversely below the meniscus.

of the medial tibial plateau (Fig. 50-17). Such a posterior wedge cannot be adequately exposed or reduced and fixed from in front. It must be exposed directly either posteromedially or posterolaterally. The surgeon has the option of either reflecting the anterior flaps further back or making a second posteromedial or posterolateral incision. We prefer to make a second incision, because it is less traumatic and affords better access to the fracture.[21]

Occasionally in very severe fractures that involve both tibial plateaux, it is necessary to gain simultaneous exposure of both tibial plateaux. This can be accomplished only when the entire quadriceps mechanism is reflected upward so that as the knee is flexed, both sides of the joint are simultaneously exposed. This type of exposure should not be combined with an osteotomy of the tibial tubercle. In the severe fracture the tibial tubercle and adjacent bone may be the only intact anterior cortex. If this cortex is destroyed, reduction may be made correspondingly more difficult, and it may prove impossible to reattach the tubercle, particularly if the posterior cortex is also comminuted. Furthermore, if the wound should break down over the osteotomy, the osteotomized tubercle could easily become an infected sequestrum, as its only blood supply would be through the tendon. We have found it best to cut the infrapatellar tendon in a Z fashion (Fig. 50–18). At the end of the procedure the cut tendon is resutured together with the incised capsule and quadriceps retinacula. The repair is then protected with a tension band wire passed through the quadriceps tendon at its insertion into the patella, crossed over the front to form a figure of 8, and then tied around a transverse screw inserted through the anterior cortex just below the tibial tubercle. The surgeon must make sure when the wire is tightened that the patella is not pulled down. The wire need not be under great tension; its only function is to protect the tendon repair. The patient should also be warned that this wire usually breaks around the third month following surgery. By that time the tendon is solidly healed, and the wire breakage does not matter. We have had no complications with this approach and have had no secondary ruptures of the tendon or any extensor lags.

Displaced bicondylar (types V and VI) tibial plateau fractures are usually due to high-energy injuries. Damage to the surrounding soft tissue envelope is often severe, even in closed fractures. Extensive surgical exposures required for application of bilateral buttress plates to such a displaced bicondylar plateau fracture may provoke a wound slough and secondary infection.

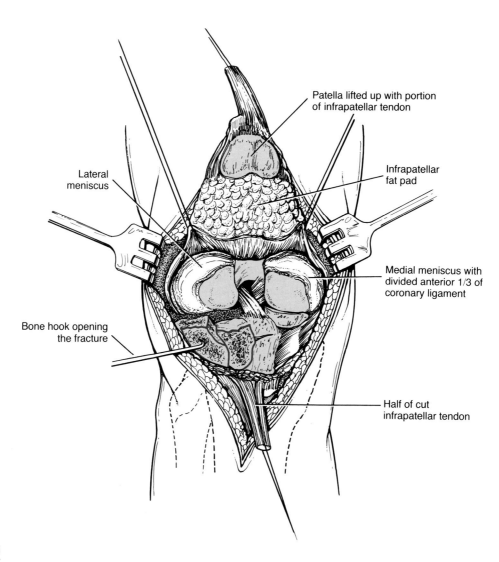

Lateral meniscus

Patella lifted up with portion of infrapatellar tendon

Infrapatellar fat pad

Medial meniscus with divided anterior 1/3 of coronary ligament

Bone hook opening the fracture

Half of cut infrapatellar tendon

Figure 50–18

The best exposure of the depressed fragments is gained by opening the fracture. The lateral wedge is pulled to the side, much like opening the cover of a book. To achieve exposure of bilateral tibial plateau fracture lines, it is best to divide the infrapatellar tendon in a Z fashion and divide across the medial and lateral capsule below the menisci. The capsule, the attached menisci, and the patella are then lifted up to give unlimited exposure of the entire proximal tibia. Osteotomy of the tibial tubercle could enter the main fracture lines and make subsequent fixation very difficult. (Redrawn from Schatzker, J.; Tile, M. Rationale of Fracture Management Care. New York, Springer-Verlag, 1987, p. 289.)

For this reason, some surgeons make an effort to avoid complete exposure of both condyles by using percutaneous lag screws and/or an external fixator opposite a plate to buttress the less unstable plateau (usually medial) if the fracture pattern is suitable.

GENERAL OBSERVATIONS ON OPEN REDUCTION AND INTERNAL FIXATION TECHNIQUES

The Tourniquet and Bone Graft

We prefer to carry out the articular reconstruction with the limb exsanguinated with an inflated pneumatic tourniquet. This controls bleeding and improves visualization. In order to shorten the tourniquet time and the time that the tibial wound is left open, we prefer to obtain the bone graft from the donor site and close this incision before the tibial reconstruction is done.

Order of Fixation

The medial plateau is usually much less comminuted than the lateral; thus when dealing with a severe fracture involving both plateaux, better purchase can be gained with screws in the medial one. However, reconstruction should always begin with the simpler fracture.

In the more complex fracture patterns it is at times very advantageous to rely on indirect reduction techniques to realign the leg and bring about partial reduction of the fracture. This is best done by bridging the flexed knee with one or two AO distractors applied on each side of the knee (Fig. 50-19). As the distractors are opened up, traction is applied, and through ligamentotaxis a considerable portion of the fracture can be realigned. Final adjustments to the reduction can then be done with minimum devitalization of the fragments. This indirect technique aids not only in achieving reduction in difficult situations but also in achieving rapid union because it facilitates preservation of the blood supply to the bony fragments.

METHODS OF ARTICULAR REDUCTION

In a depressed articular fracture, the articular fragments are driven into the supporting cancellous bone of the metaphysis, where they become impacted. The

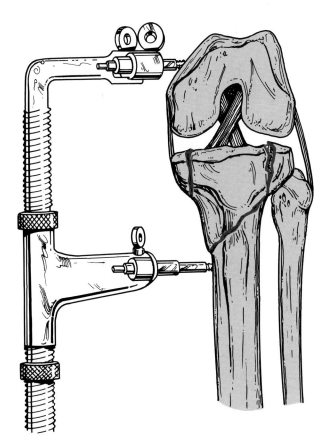

Figure 50-19

One limb of the AO distractor is inserted into the medial condyle while the other is inserted into the subcutaneous anteromedial surface of the tibia. Five-millimeter Schantz screws should be used to anchor the distractor to bone. The AO tubular external fixator can also be substituted for the distractor. (Redrawn from Schatzker, J. In: Chapman, M.W., ed. Operative Orthopaedics. Philadelphia, J.B. Lippincott, 1988, Fig. 35-8, p. 427.)

cancellous bone compacts and holds the fragments together. The reduction of such a fracture should never begin by an attempt to elevate the fragments through the joint, but instead should be accomplished by elevating the fragments en masse from below. Lifting the fragments up through the joint usually results in a number of devitalized loose articular fragments that cannot be put back and fitted together. To reduce a joint depression properly, begin by inserting a periosteal elevator deep into the compacted metaphysis. The reduction is initiated with upward pressure and is then completed by inserting a bone punch deep to the depression and gently tapping the fragments into place until they are slightly overreduced (Fig. 50–20). When elevated in this manner together with the compacted cancellous bone, the fragments do not fall apart but behave as if they were held together.

THE FUNCTION OF THE BONE GRAFT

Once elevated, the fragments tend to fall back into the hole left behind in the metaphysis. Two maneuvers help to prevent this complication. The first is to insert a massive bone graft below the fragments into the hole in the metaphysis that is created when the fragments are elevated. The second is to compress them circumferentially with lag screws through the remaining intact portions of the plateau. When tightened, the lag screws tend to squeeze and narrow the proximal tibia and to provide potential transverse supports. Some surgeons prefer to use cortical slabs to hold up the elevated fragments. We prefer pure cancellous bone autografts obtained from either the iliac crest or the greater trochanter. The cancellous bone adapts better to the shape of the hole and, when firmly compacted with a bone

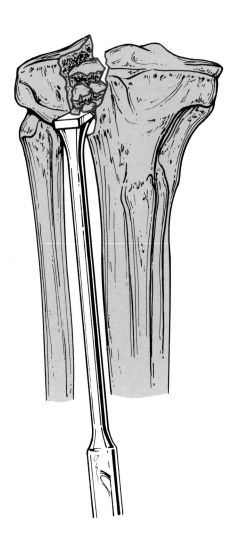

Figure 50–20

An en masse elevation of fragments consists of insertion of a bone punch deep to the depressed fragments. Upward blows on the punch effect the reduction. (Redrawn from Schatzker, J. In: Chapman, M.W., ed. Operative Orthopaedics. Philadelphia, J.B. Lippincott, 1988, Fig. 35-9, p. 428.)

punch, provides excellent support for the articular fragments. Kirschner wires or screws should not immediately be inserted deep to the subchondral bone plate to maintain elevation of the articular fragments. This stiffens the subchondral bone plate and leads to rapid articular cartilage degeneration, which the inexperienced surgeon may interpret as a "late redisplacement" of the elevated fragments or their collapse as a result of avascular necrosis.

THE RATIONALE FOR BUTTRESS PLATING

The plates that are used to support the cortex of a metaphysis and keep it from displacing under axial load are called buttress plates. They must be carefully contoured to the cortex they are supposed to buttress, for if they are accidentally placed under tension, they can cause the very displacement they are supposed to prevent. Therefore whenever a buttress plate is fixed to a bone, the first screw inserted should be through the end toward the diaphysis. The remaining screws should then be inserted one by one in an orderly fashion proceeding toward the joint. The plate need not be fixed to the fragment it is supporting in order to function as a buttress plate. However, the plate must be fixed to the shaft fragment so as to be able to hold up the weight and prevent displacement. Any plate, if carefully contoured, can function as a buttress plate. Because metaphyses in different areas of the body have specific contours, designers (e.g., AO/ASIF) have made available several precontoured and preshaped plates in order to save time in contouring and to make the plate more useful for its specific function. For the proximal tibia there are the regular T plates, which best fit the medial side. For the lateral side there are precontoured T and L plates (Fig. 50–21). It must be remembered that the plates made to buttress the metaphysis are not sufficiently strong to be used as neutralization plates for the diaphysis. Therefore the long T plates should never be used to reattach a complete separation of the metaphysis from the diaphysis (type VI fracture). When dealing with a metaphyseal and a diaphyseal fracture, one must use either a heavier and stronger plate or two plates to do the two jobs. If two plates are chosen, for example, with a fracture of the lateral plateau and a diaphyseal fracture, then the buttress plate would go on the lateral surface and the neutralization plate on the medial surface of the tibia.

THE PLACE OF ARTHROSCOPY

We have used arthroscopy particularly in type I fractures to evaluate the degree of displacement of the articular surfaces and the state of the meniscus. We have not

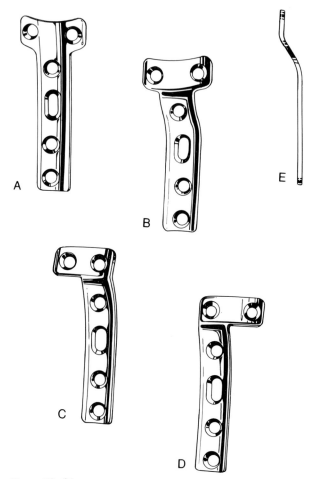

Figure 50–21

Plates available for internal fixation of the proximal tibia. *A* is a flat T-plate that best fits the medial plateau. *B* (seen in profile in E) is more suited for the lateral plateau, as are the 2 L-plates *C* and *D*, for right and left lateral plateaux.

used it as an intraoperative aid to joint reduction and feel that its usefulness in complicated injuries is very limited.

RUPTURED COLLATERAL AND ANTERIOR CRUCIATE LIGAMENTS

A ruptured collateral ligament combined with a plateau fracture requires surgical repair at the time of the open reduction and internal fixation of the fracture. To treat a plateau fracture nonoperatively when it is associated with a disruption of a collateral ligament is to guarantee the patient a poor result. An avulsed anterior cruciate ligament, if it is attached to a sufficiently large fragment of bone to permit a secure fixation of the ligament to the tibia, should also be securely fixed at the time of the open reduction and fixation of the fracture.

If the ligament is disrupted in its substance or lacks a bony fragment, then its repair should be delayed and carried out if or when it is clinically indicated. An acute ligament substitution or repair requiring immobilization and protection, if carried out at the time of fracture repair, can lead to unacceptable stiffness of the joint.

SPECIFIC FRACTURE TYPES

Type I

The wedge or split fracture of the lateral plateau, if displaced, represents an unstable joint and is an absolute indication for open reduction and internal fixation. If there is minimal displacement, however, there may be doubt about the advisability of surgery. We have frequently found the lateral meniscus trapped in the fracture line, even in the presence of relatively minor displacement. Therefore we feel that if there is *any* displacement, the knee should undergo arthroscopy to rule out any meniscal lesion. If there is a peripheral detachment of the meniscus or if this is combined with the meniscus being trapped in the fracture line, then the surgeon must proceed to an open reduction and internal fixation. If the meniscus is sound, the displaced fragments may be manipulated into place under arthroscopic control and then provisionally fixed with K wires. Definitive fixation can then be carried out percutaneously with lag screws without opening the fracture. When an open reduction is necessary in young patients, the fracture requires only lag screws (see Fig. 50-1B). Washers may be used under the heads of the screws to prevent the heads from penetrating the relatively thin cortex. If there is any doubt about the strength of the fixation, the fracture should be buttressed with a plate.

Type II

In the split depression partial articular fracture, the displacement consists of a widening of the joint with spreading apart of the wedge and depression of the articular surface. Depressions of the joint greater than 4 mm are significant if left unreduced and have resulted in joint incongruity, valgus deformity, and a sense of instability,[6] all proportional to the degree of joint widening and depression. Poor results following open or closed treatment may be related to residual joint depression, incongruity, and joint instability.

Closed manipulative reduction combined with traction, or traction alone, has been associated with varying degrees of success. The displaced lateral wedge reduces surprisingly well with traction, but the impacted joint depression cannot be dislodged by traction or manipulation. If left unreduced, these do not fill with fibrocartilage and therefore remain as a permanent defect. Similarly, if treated initially in traction and then in a cast brace (which maintains axial alignment until union), these fractures fail to fill with fibrocartilage. If initially unstable, they remain unstable, and once the fracture brace is discontinued, the deformity recurs. We feel, therefore, that a fracture associated with any degree of instability should have an open reduction and internal fixation. Of particular note is the posterior wedge occasionally associated with this fracture pattern. The posterior wedge signifies posterior instability. Closed methods always fail to bring about its reduction, and if left unreduced, the posterior wedge causes the femoral condyle to subluxate posteriorly in flexion (see Fig. 50–17). Therefore an associated posterior wedge constitutes an absolute indication for open reduction and internal fixation. An associated disruption of a collateral ligament, occurring in up to 10% of these fractures, should be repaired at the time of surgical reconstruction. However, repair of in-substance tears of either cruciate ligament should generally be deferred, as simple suture repairs are of limited value, and substitution or augmentation procedures require patient cooperation, and, often, restriction of motion, with a high risk of permanent stiffness. A repaired collateral ligament is protected in a fracture brace once the knee is fully mobilized.

If there are definite contraindications to surgery or if the patient is very elderly and the bone severely osteoporotic, then the patient should be treated by closed manipulative reduction, skeletal traction, and early motion and should be transferred into a cast brace as soon as the fracture is no longer displaceable, even though it may be still deformable. At no time should the fracture be immobilized in plaster, as such treatment frequently results in a significant degree of joint stiffness.

The elderly patient with severe osteoporosis is a special problem. In these patients the joint depression is frequently very severe, and at the time of open reduction it is extremely difficult, perhaps impossible, to restore the lateral plateau, even with extensive cancellous allografts. In young patients we prefer autogenous bone grafts. However, in the elderly the cancellous bone available from the iliac crest is very sparse, and it is necessary to resort to allografting if a copious amount of cancellous bone is required. In elderly patients cancellous allografts have been shown to incorporate without difficulty. If the lateral plateau in these patients appears to have almost vanished and is almost impossible to reconstruct, then we prefer to initially treat these patients nonoperatively. If the knee remains significantly unstable and deformed once the fracture has united and the knee is mobilized, then we carry out a late arthroplasty with allografting of the defect.

When operatively treated, the type II fracture is stabilized with lag screws and a buttress plate; screws alone are not enough. Without the use of the buttress plate, a recurrence of the deformity is likely, because lag screws alone cannot prevent redisplacement of the split wedge fragment, particularly if the bone is osteoporotic (see Fig. 50-2B).

Type III

The type III fracture is the pure depression fracture of the lateral plateau. The depression may be central or peripheral. If the depression is small, the joint remains stable, and excellent function without joint instability is the usual outcome. It is important when evaluating this fracture to examine the joint, under anesthesia if necessary, testing it from full extension to 90° of flexion. If no valgus instability greater than 5° to 8° is found, it is safe to treat such a joint with early motion without weight bearing. If valgus instability is found and there are no contraindications to surgery, then the depression should be elevated, the metaphysis bone grafted, and the fracture stabilized.

Because there is no split wedge fracture, in order to elevate the joint depression it is necessary to make a small window in the cortex on the undersurface of the lateral tibial condyle, introduce a punch through this hole, and in this way elevate the joint depression. The cortex is usually very thin and may be further weakened by the window. To prevent its fracture under axial load and a consequent deformity, we have buttressed the lateral condyle with a plate in addition to the lag screw fixation (see Fig. 50-3B).

Type IV

Type IV fractures are fractures of the medial plateau. The medial plateau splits usually as a relatively simple wedge, similar to the split wedge fracture of the lateral plateau. However, because of the higher forces involved, there is usually a fracture of the intercondylar eminence and the adjacent bone with its attached cruciate ligaments. Furthermore, there is frequently a disruption of the lateral collateral ligament complex (which may be either a tear through the substance of the ligament or an avulsion of the fibular head) and a traction lesion of the lateral peroneal nerve. In some cases there may also be damage to the popliteal vessels. This injury usually represents a dislocation of the knee that has been realigned before the patient is brought to hospital. The poor prognosis with this injury is the result not of the fracture but of the associated soft tissue inju-

ries. These are unstable injuries that, if displaced, require surgery.

The fracture requires a buttress plate, as do fractures of the lateral plateau (see Fig. 50-4B). This applies also to the occasionally associated posterior split wedge fracture of the medial plateau. The anterior buttress plate is applied to the anteromedial face of the proximal tibial metaphysis deep to the pes anserinus and the anterior fibers of the superficial medial collateral ligament. The posterior buttress plate is applied to the posteromedial edge of the tibia. The posterior wedge fragment is buttressed posteromedially, but it is best to lag it from in front, as it is very difficult to insert a lag screw from back to front on the medial or, for that matter, the lateral side of the knee. In order to reach this posterior wedge fragment, it is best to make a second incision posteromedially or posterolaterally. The frequently avulsed intercondylar eminence with the attached cruciate ligaments should be either fixed back in place with a lag screw or held reduced with a loop of wire tied under tension over the intact anterior cortex. After surgery the knee must be moved through a full range of motion as soon as possible. If the lateral collateral ligaments required repair, then the knee, once mobilized on a continuous passive motion machine, is protected with a fracture brace permitting full range of motion of the knee. Motion takes precedence over cruciate reconstruction. For this reason, even if the cruciate is reattached, a full range of motion is commenced early.

Type V

Type V bicondylar fractures may be either extra- or intraarticular, depending on whether the fracture lines involve the articular surfaces. In shape the fracture resembles an inverted Y. The extraarticular fracture may be successfully managed initially in skeletal traction and subsequently in a fracture brace. Some axial collapse is inevitable, despite traction. This at times results in slight varus/valgus instability that could be symptomatic in athletically active individuals. Therefore in young active individuals, as well as in all patients with fractures involving the articular surfaces, we carry out an open reduction and internal fixation. This bicondylar fracture requires buttressing on both sides; lag screws are never enough to prevent displacement (see Fig. 50-5B).

Type VI

In the difficult type VI fracture pattern, the reconstruction should always begin on the simpler side. For exposure this fracture frequently requires a Z division of the infrapatellar tendon to facilitate visualization of the joint. As in fractures of the distal tibia, it is necessary first to reestablish normal length. This is best and easiest to accomplish if the surgeon uses methods of indirect reduction and applies traction on the flexed knee with two AO distractors (one on each side from femoral condyles to tibial shaft) and then secures fixation first on the side of least comminution. Because this injury involves a fracture that dissociates the metaphysis from the diaphysis, fixation must be carried out with two buttress plates. One of these buttress plates must be strong enough to bridge to the diaphysis and act either as a compression or a neutralization plate. A narrow 4.5 DC plate, rather than a long T plate (which some surgeons have used in error) should be employed. The T plate is too flexible for this purpose, and its use has resulted in fixation failure and nonunion (see Fig. 50-6B). Another alternative is a new, heavier tibial condyle plate.

Fractures of the Intercondylar Eminence

Fractures of the intercondylar eminence not only represent avulsion of the anterior cruciate ligament but also, if large, may at times encroach on and involve the articular surface of the medial tibial plateau. They have been discussed previously in association with tibial plateau fractures. As isolated injuries, if displaced and left unreduced, they not only may give rise to articular surface incongruity but, more importantly, may also represent definite loss of anterior cruciate function. Thus, if displaced, they constitute a clear indication for open reduction and internal fixation. Indeed, such displacement is the only opportunity ever afforded the surgeon to carry out a physiologic repair of the torn anterior cruciate, because the attached fragment of bone facilitates anatomic reattachment of the ligament. Depending on the size of the fragment, it can be secured with one or two small-fragment lag screws inserted from the tibia into the fragment, or, if small or comminuted, it can be secured with a tension band wire passed through holes drilled into the tibia in appropriate locations in relation to the fragment (see chapter 49).

Open Tibial Plateau Fracture

The open fracture of the tibial plateau is a surgical emergency presenting special problems in management. It must be thoroughly debrided and stabilized to prevent infection. The decision as to how best to provide the desired stability presents the most difficult problem in decision making. It is our feeling that in even the most severe open wound, the intraarticular portion of the fracture should be reduced and stabilized (if the fracture configuration allows it) with the minimum possible additional dissection and tissue trauma. The minimum internal fixation used should be in the form of lag screws and K wires. Whether to carry out bone grafting and reconstruction and internal fixation of the metaphyseal component of the fracture must be decided on the basis of the degree of soft tissue injury, the degree of contamination, and the time lapsed from injury to treatment. In the very severe open fracture, once the joint is reduced and stabilized, we attempt to close the joint and stabilize the metaphysis with an external fixator. In fractures of the tibial plateau this usually means bridging the joint with the fixator and immobilizing it until the soft tissue wound is closed. This requires, as a rule, a minimum of two to three weeks and frequently the use of local rotation flaps or even free vascularized tissue flaps to achieve coverage and closure. Once infection has been prevented and the wound closed, the surgeon can review the situation and carry out the necessary metaphyseal reconstruction. Severe open fractures requiring the knee to be bridged with an external fixator for three to four weeks have achieved a surprising range of motion, which would have been completely lost if a too-extensive reconstruction had been done initially and the wound had become infected.

The configuration of the external fixator frame depends on the soft tissue defects one is trying to bridge. A simple anterior half frame consisting of two to three Schanz screws anteriorly in the femur and distally in the tibia joined together on each side with a long tube, with the tubes then joined to each other with a double-tube clamp, is often enough. At times one has to construct a quadrilateral frame with two Steinmann pins through the distal femur and the distal tibia that are then joined together with appropriate tubes and clamps.

In the less severe open fracture, we buttress the metaphysis and leave the wound open. The decision whether to graft an open fracture at the time of the initial reconstruction must be made on the basis of the particular fracture. If bone grafting under an articular elevation is necessary, we tend to do it at the time of the initial reconstruction of the metaphysis.

Tibial Plateau Fractures and the Polytrauma Patient

Tibial plateau fractures are not emergencies unless they are open or associated with a compartment syndrome or a vascular lesion. Therefore if there are indications in the polytrauma patient to defer the treatment of some fractures, the tibial plateau fracture can be included in this list. If the delay in treatment will not exceed 48 hours, the fracture can be safely immobilized in a well-padded plaster cast. A longer delay will lead to shortening, particularly in the more complex type VI (C type) injuries, and to major difficulties in subsequent surgical care. Traction would normally be an ideal alternative but is an unacceptable form of treatment for the polytrauma patient, because the enforced recumbent position is detrimental to the patient's well-being. Under these circumstances we feel it is best to bridge the knee with an external fixator. This will provide immobilization and maintain length until a more suitable form of treatment can be carried out. The type of fixator used is the same as that used for delay of treatment of the open fracture with severe soft tissue lesions.

Postoperative Care

Postoperative care of fractures of the tibial plateau is governed by the findings at surgery and the degree of stability achieved by the internal fixation. If the reduction is satisfactory and the fixation is stable, then we apply a light dressing at the end of the surgery and set the extremity up on a continuous passive motion machine. The machine is set to permit full extension and flexion to 40° to 60°. This is increased to 90° within the first two days. It is important to regain 90° of flexion as quickly as possible. Although the rapid mobilization of the knee may be initially painful, its benefits are definite. At the end of one week it is usually possible to cease continuous passive motion, and patients are able to carry on with their rehabilitation without reliance on aids. If a continuous passive motion machine is not available, then the knee should be immobilized in 60° to 90° of flexion on a very well-padded plaster splint for the first 48 to 76 hours. The splint is then removed, and active motion is encouraged if the wound healing is progressing satisfactorily. Immobilization in flexion greatly accelerates and facilitates postoperative mobilization of the knee. We have not had a single instance of a patient developing a flexion contracture or extensor lag as a result of brief immobilization in flexion. Usually by the end of the first week the patient should have regained 90° of active flexion.

The patients are mobilized with the aid of crutches and non–weight bearing is instituted. In type I injuries and type V extraarticular fractures, partial weight bearing can be started usually after eight weeks and then gradually progressed to full weight bearing. In the more complex intraarticular fractures, weight bearing is withheld for at least 10 to 12 weeks. The duration will depend on the degree of articular surface disruption as well as on the degree of metaphyseal and diaphyseal fragmentation and subsequent union.

We believe in early active motion, as it not only ensures a return of motion to the knee and good function of the soft tissue envelope but also has a very beneficial effect on the healing of articular cartilage.[15,22,23] Early motion, however, does not mean early weight bearing. Premature loading may not only result in loss of reduction, joint incongruity, and malalignment, but can also interfere with healing of articular cartilage.

Disrupted collateral ligaments must be repaired at the time of surgery. Continuous passive motion has a beneficial effect on ligamentous healing.[24,25] At the end of the first week, a ligament repair should be protected with a cast brace set to permit a full range of motion. We are opposed to repairs of in-substance tears of the cruciates at the time of a plateau fracture repair, because an in-substance repair, with or without an augmentation, requires immobilization of the joint. This leads to permanent stiffness, which is unacceptable. The cruciates are left unrepaired. If there is functional cruciate insufficiency after the joint is fully rehabilitated, then a late reconstruction is done. We carry out a meticulous repair of cruciates avulsed with bone, as these can be firmly reattached to permit an unrestricted range of motion. If, at the end of surgery, the surgeon feels the fixation is less than stable, then it must be protected from overload. If only one plateau is involved, a cast brace with the knee stressed in the direction of the normal side is sufficient to prevent overload. If both plateaux are involved, it is necessary to protect the extremity in traction if there is insufficient longitudinal stability to prevent axial collapse. Otherwise a fracture brace can be used, but without stressing it in one direction or other. We prefer a cast brace that also incorporates the foot. This provides more control over the leg and better protects the tibial plateau fracture.

Complications

Recognition of complications and their appropriate treatment are as important as the most important step in the preoperative evaluation of the patient or the operative intervention. General complications such as infection, wound slough, and compartment syndrome will not be discussed here, but some complications of particular importance will be singled out.

FIXATION FAILURE

Occasionally an internal fixation may fail. It is important to recognize such failures early and reoperate as soon as possible. If open reduction and internal fixation were originally indicated, then the recurrent joint malalignment and incongruity should be corrected, unless, of course, specific contraindications to surgery have developed.

LOSS OF ARTICULAR REDUCTION

If a loss of articular reduction occurs because of redisplacement of a major articular fragment, then a revision should be considered as early as possible, particularly if the displacement has resulted in joint instability. As already indicated previously, these joint defects have never been observed to fill with fibrocartilage to provide stability. Whenever we have had occasion to open such a knee, either early or late, we have found the defects filled with fibrous tissue, which fails to provide the joint with any degree of stability.

MALUNION

If a malunion has occurred either because of redisplacement or because of a failure to secure reduction, then an intraarticular osteotomy to realign the joint should be considered. This is possible, however, only with major wedge fragments and not with a central depression of the articular surface. For this reason it is important to follow a patient closely. If a major articular depression has recurred early, then it should be revised immediately, because once the fragments unite in the displaced position, it is impossible to free them and carry out a reduction. Under these circumstances a partial joint replacement, either with a prosthesis or with an allograft, has to be considered.

NONUNION

Nonunion of a tibial plateau fracture is rare. In repairing it, however, attention must be directed to articular surface reduction to secure congruity and correction of the metaphyseal deformity to prevent any axial malalignment and consequent overload of the joint.

Summary and Conclusions

Fractures of the tibial plateau involve a major weight-bearing joint. To preserve normal function, the surgeon must strive to restore joint congruity, normal axial alignment, stability, and a full range of motion. If the fracture is undisplaced or the joint stable, then closed treatment will yield satisfactory results if the joint is moved early; plaster immobilization of even undisplaced fractures has resulted in stiffness. Joint instability and significant incongruity are clear indications for surgical treatment. Moderate osteoporosis is not an argument against open treatment. More than 50% of the patients on whom we have operated have

shown some osteoporosis.[6] The properly executed internal fixation has held, and the results have been very good.

Treatment based on the principles we have emphasized has yielded an 89% acceptable result rate, which is significantly better than that for other methods of treatment.[6] We have achieved these results in patients in whom the tibial plateau fracture was the only major injury. The results in the polytrauma patients with severe associated neurologic complications or severe soft tissue problems have not been as favorable, but even in these patients these principles apply. In the polytrauma population, if there were no other injuries in the involved extremity and their associated injuries did not interfere with their rehabilitation, then the correctly performed surgery led to the same result as in patients with isolated extremity injuries.

REFERENCES

1. Foltin, E. Bone loss and forms of tibial condylar fracture. Arch Orthop Trauma Surg 106(6):341–348, 1987.
2. Foltin, E. Osteoporosis and fracture patterns. A study of split-compression fractures of the lateral tibial condyle. Int Orthop 12(4):299–303, 1988.
3. Moore, T.M. Fracture-dislocation of the knee. Clin Orthop 156:128, 1981.
4. Kennedy, J.C.; Bailey, W.H. Experimental tibial plateau fractures. J Bone Joint Surg 50A:1522–1534, 1968.
5. Mueller, M.E.; Koch, P.; Nazarian, S.; Schatzker, J. The Comprehensive Classification of Fractures of Long Bones. Berlin, Springer-Verlag, 1990.
6. Schatzker, J.; McBroom, R.; Bruce, D. The tibial plateau fracture. The Toronto experience. Clin Orthop 138:94–104, 1979.
7. Charnley, J. The Closed Treatment of Common Fractures. London, Churchill Livingstone, 1961.
8. Stewart, M.J.; Sisk, T.D.; Wallace, S.H. Fractures of the distal third of the femur. A comparison of methods of treatment. J Bone Joint Surg 48A:784–807, 1966.
9. Neer, C.S.; Grantham, S.; Shelton, L. Supracondylar fracture of the adult femur. J Bone Joint Surg 49A:591–613, 1967.
10. Perkins, G. Fractures and Dislocations. London, The Athlone Press, 1958.
11. Apley, A.G. Fractures of the lateral tibial condyle treated by skeletal traction and early mobilization. J Bone Joint Surg 38B:699, 1956.
12. Apley, A.G. Fractures of the tibial plateau. Orthop Clin North Am 10:61–74, 1979.
13. Roberts, J.M. Fractures of the condyles of the tibia. J Bone Joint Surg 50A:1505, 1968.
14. Pauwels, F. Neue Richtlinien fuer die operative Behandlung der Coxarthrose. Verh Dtsch Orthop Ges 48:332–336.
15. Mitchell, N.; Shepard, N. Healing of articular cartilage in intra-articular fractures in rabbits. J Bone Joint Surg 62A:628–634, 1980.
16. Apley, A.G. Personal communication.
17. Mueller, M.E.; Allgoewer, M.; Schneider, R.; Willenegger, H. Manual of Internal Fixation, Ed. 3. New York, Springer, 1991.
18. Schrive, N. The weight bearing role of the menisci of the knee. (Abstract) J Bone Joint Surg 56B:381, 1974.

19. Walker, S.; Erkman, M.J. The role of the menisci in force transmission across the knee. Clin Orthop 109:184–192, 1975.
20. Wirth, C.R. Meniscus repair. Clin Orthop 157:153–160, 1981.
21. Hohl, M.; Moore, T.M. Articular fractures of the proximal tibia. In: McCollister, E.C., ed. Surgery of the Musculoskeletal System, Vol. 7. New York, Churchill Livingstone, 1983, pp. 11–135.
22. Salter, R.; Simmonds, D.F.; Malcolm, B.W.; et al. The biological effects of continuous passive motion on the healing of full thickness defects in articular cartilage: An experimental investigation in the rabbit. J Bone Joint Surg 62A:1232–1251, 1980.
23. Salter, R.B.; Hamilton, H.W.; Wedge, J.H.; et al. Clinical application of basic research on continuous passive motion for disorders and injuries of synovial joints: preliminary report of feasibility study. Tech Orthop 1(1):74–91, 1986.
24. Salter, R. Personal communication.
25. Olerud, S. Personal communication.

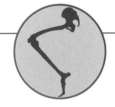

Peter G. Trafton, M.D.

51

Tibial Shaft Fractures

*F*ractures of the tibia are among the most common of serious skeletal injuries. Those who sustain them face a slow recovery, with possible permanent deformity and disability. Those who treat them must deal with complications related to both injury and treatment. Problems are clearly more frequent after more severe injuries. Some claim that more invasive treatments also increase risks, but this is not always true. In treating tibial fractures, the physician does not so much avoid the risk of complications as exchange one risk for another. For example, external fixators reduce the chance of infection for open tibia fractures but carry risks of late loss of alignment, delayed union, and problems with percutaneous pins.[9]

Tibial fractures vary so widely in severity that general prescriptions for treatment are not applicable to each patient. The spectrum of injury extends from trivial enough to be ignored to so severe that amputation is the best treatment. Tibial fractures tax a surgeon's judgment and skill. He or she, after carefully evaluating all aspects of the patient, the injury, and the available options, must select and manage an effective treatment regimen.

Judgment is developed through clinical experience. Therefore it is often helpful to seek the advice of a consultant who has treated many such injuries. Externally proposed "clinical policies" or "standards of care" may offer a reasonable course of treatment, but there are so many variables affecting a given patient's situation that individualized treatment is advisable.

Both operative and nonoperative treatments of tibial shaft fractures have strong advocates. Although at first glance they appear contradictory, each approach is appropriate for a different type of injury. Less severe fractures (the more common ones) generally do well without surgery; the more severe often benefit from it. The question is not whether tibial fractures should be treated operatively, but rather which tibial fractures should be so treated and by what method.

This chapter reviews the spectrum of injuries and the available treatments for tibial shaft fractures. It offers aids to problem solving and clinical decision making in accord with the current experience of orthopedic traumatologists. Each recommendation must be considered in the light of a clinical situation. Much of the controversy associated with treatment of tibial fractures is the result of proponents of a given therapy failing to specify clearly enough the characteristics of the patients for whom they use it. Indeed, some surgeons may not recognize the selection biases affecting the populations they treat. They may thus conclude that a treatment that is successful in their hands will be similarly well suited to all patients with tibial fractures. The physician who wishes to avoid such errors is warned to pay as much attention to the injury and its evaluation as is paid to the treatment.

Following the discussion of tibial shaft fractures, with and without fibular injuries, this chapter includes brief sections on isolated fractures of the fibular shaft, injuries of the proximal tibiofibular joint, and fatigue fractures of both bones.

Pathology

RELEVANT ANATOMY

The lower leg, extending from the knee to the ankle, participates in the structure and function of these important joints. It serves as a weight-bearing support for the body and is also a conduit for the neurovascular supply of the foot and the location of its extrinsic myotendinous units.

The tibia, with its asymmetric surrounding soft tissues, determines the shape of the lower leg. Its roughly triangular external cross section has an anteriorly directed apex. Its anteromedial subcutaneous surface has no muscular or ligamentous attachments from the pes anserinus tendons and tibial collateral ligament of the knee to the deltoid ligament of the ankle. This readily palpable surface is concave medially as it approaches the medial malleolus. Its anterolateral surface forms the medial wall of the anterior muscular compartment of the leg, with the tibialis anterior and, more distally, the neurovascular bundle and extensor hallucis longus muscles adjacent. The tibia's posterior surface, buried under superficial and deep muscle compartments, has attachments from proximal to distal of semimembranosus, popliteus, soleus, tibialis posterior, and flexor digitorum longus muscles. The posterior tibial vessels, tibial nerve, and the flexor hallucis longus muscle approach it distally, curving around the medial malleolus behind the tibialis posterior and flexor digitorum longus.

The adult tibia ranges from less than 30 cm to more than 47 cm in length. The genetic diversity of today's world means that the entire spectrum of tibial sizes may be encountered by any trauma surgeon. The tibia varies not only in length but also in its minimum intramedullary diameter, which may be less than 8 mm to more than 15 mm. Length and internal diameter have significant implications for the sizes of implants required for intramedullary fixation, which is emerging as a valuable treatment for many patients with tibial fractures.

Most of the tibia is comprised of a tubular, cortical diaphysis. Its enlarged proximal and distal ends are formed of cancellous bone, which varies in density according to both location and the individual's metabolic bone status. The cortex surrounding the metaphyseal spongiosa becomes quite thin as distance increases from the diaphysis (Fig. 51–1). Screw purchase in the tibial metaphysis is thus provided by the threads engaging cancellous rather than cortical bone. The transition zone, readily apparent on radiographs, is important to consider. It may be thick enough to require drilling to the outside diameter of the thick shank of a cancellous lag screw, but it might also be so thin that neither drilling nor tapping of threads is necessary.

The proximal tibial metaphysis, with its tibial plateaux, is larger in diameter than the shaft but is similarly triangular in cross section. Laterally it overhangs the interosseous membrane and articulates posterolaterally with the head of the fibula. On its anterior surface is the tibial tubercle with the attached patellar ligament. This may be located sufficiently laterally that an intramedullary nail entry site made through a split

in the patellar ligament is too lateral for insertion of a large-diameter nail. It is important to project the long axis of the diaphysis proximally to determine the entry site for a nail. Also apparent is apex-anterior angulation of the proximal tibia, averaging 15°, which requires a bend in the upper portion of intramedullary nails designed to be inserted by way of an anterior portal. The backward-sloping anterior surface of the tibial metaphysis offers a more or less obvious spot for entry of such an intramedullary nail, above the tibial tubercule and posterior to the patellar ligament. The cancellous bone of the proximal metaphysis can be perforated fairly easily to gain access to the medullary canal. However, the shape of the proximal tibia; its posterior overhang; and its thin, flat posterior wall make it possible to err and perforate the posterior wall with the drill, awl, or intramedullary nail. In addition to directing such devices anteriorly toward the axis of the diaphysis, careful fluoroscopic control of intramedullary surgery helps avoid complications related to this region's anatomy.

Five or ten centimeters distal to the tibial tubercle, the diaphysis becomes distinctly tubular, with thick walls, especially anteriorly, where the prominent crest of the tibia occupies nearly a third of the diameter of the entire bone. This dense cortical bone is difficult to pierce with anything but the sharpest drill and is dense enough to generate significant heat during penetration. It is essential when placing screws or pins across the tibial diaphysis to remember the thickness of the anterior crest and to aim posteriorly enough to bisect the internal rather than the external diameter and thus obtain a true bicortical purchase (Fig. 51–2).

Distally the shaft flares and becomes more rounded as it undergoes a transition from diaphysis to metaphysis. The cortex thins, and the fatty medullary contents are replaced with cancellous bone that is surprisingly dense, especially in the young and active, in the 5 cm or so above the subchondral bone of the transverse tibial plafond, the "ceiling" of the ankle joint. This cancellous bone provides secure purchase for screws and is often compact enough to resist penetration by an intramedullary nail.

The contour of the distal tibia is notable for a somewhat pronounced concavity of its anteromedial surface—enough so as to suggest a varus deformity if one looks at the subcutaneous outline rather than the central axis of the bone. Restoring this distal medial concavity is an essential part of closed reduction of distal tibial shaft fractures. If a cast applied to such an injury is straight along its medial side rather than concave over the distal third, a valgus malalignment is produced. Mast et al. point out that the shape of the tibia's medial surface is fairly constant from patient to

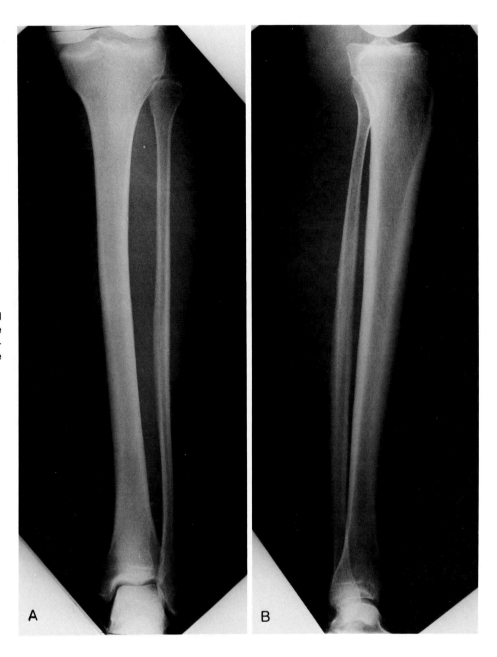

Figure 51-1

A, Anteroposterior and B, lateral radiographs of normal adult male tibia and fibula. Note variable thickness of cortex and typical surface curvatures.

A

B

patient.[173] The radius of the supramalleolar curvature is approximately 20 cm. Because the triangular diaphyseal cross section rounds gently into the pilon, or distal tibial metaphysis, the medial surface turns medially approximately 25°. According to Mast et al., the relative constancy of this surface shape permits precontouring of a plate that can be used to reduce a fracture without complete exposure of all its fragments.[173]

The tibia's medullary canal, extending from the cancellous bone of the proximal metaphysis to that of the distal metaphysis, is significantly more round in cross section than the external appearance of the bone would suggest. Unlike the femur, it is more hourglass than

tubular in shape, with a variably pronounced isthmus that may limit the endosteal contact of an intramedullary nail, even after significant reaming. In the young, the medullary canal tends to be narrow. With aging and the development of osteoporosis, the cortex becomes thinner, the metaphyseal cancellous bone becomes less dense, and the internal diameter of the medullary canal increases. Occasionally the canal becomes large enough to compromise intramedullary fixation.

The diaphyseal blood supply typically reaches the tibia by way of a single nutrient artery, a proximal branch of the posterior tibial.[227] After passing through the most proximal portion of the tibialis posterior, it

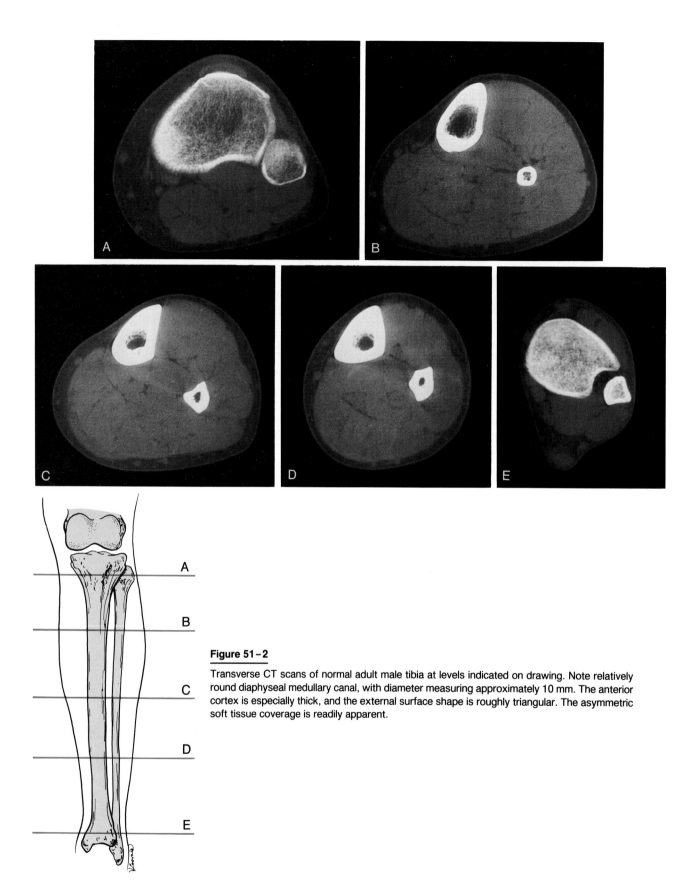

Figure 51-2

Transverse CT scans of normal adult male tibia at levels indicated on drawing. Note relatively round diaphyseal medullary canal, with diameter measuring approximately 10 mm. The anterior cortex is especially thick, and the external surface shape is roughly triangular. The asymmetric soft tissue coverage is readily apparent.

obliquely enters the tibial shaft on its posterior surface in the proximal portion of the middle third of the bone. It is easily injured by displacement of a fracture through its long cortical foramen.[225] Within the medullary canal, it courses proximally and distally, anastomosing with metaphyseal endosteal vessels (Fig. 51–3). A displaced fracture of the diaphysis is thus likely to devascularize the shaft downstream from the nutrient artery. If peripheral soft tissues are significantly stripped, the entire vascular supply can be lost over a distance of several centimeters. This interferes with fracture healing and risks posttraumatic osteomyelitis involving the necrotic, devascularized bone.

Through its intraosseous distribution, the medullary arterial system of the tibia provides nourishment to the majority of the normal diaphysis. The peripheral one fourth to one third is supplied by anastomosing periosteal vessels.[229] This fact is of special significance after reaming for an intramedullary nail, as the combined devascularization caused by both fracture and reaming produces a layer of necrotic bone through much of the diaphysis.[228] The medullary arterial circulation regenerates in a few weeks, if space exists around a medullary nail. This permits revascularization of the inner cortical bone, which also is supported by recruitment of periosteal collateral circulation if the surrounding soft tissues are healthy enough. However, until revascularization has occurred, the dead cortical bone is not able to participate in the healing process and is a large potential sequestrum for infection, as evidenced by the significant risk of medullary osteomyelitis after reaming and intramedullary nailing in open or previously contaminated fractures.

After a fracture, the pattern of blood supply changes with recruitment of peripheral vessels, which take over much of the arterial supply of the cortex and revascularize necrotic areas as well as provide nourishment for the metabolically active peripheral callus.[227,229,269] This process requires healthy surrounding tissues and is most effective in areas with muscles closely applied to the tibia. Those surfaces covered only with periosteum, subcutaneous tissue, and skin are less able to benefit from this temporary extraosseous blood supply. Viable attached muscular pedicles are thus most important to segments of a fractured tibia and should be preserved during surgical exposure for debridement or fixation.

A most important feature of lower extremity anatomy is the relationship between the tibia and the obviously smaller fibula, which is situated posterolaterally and is more surrounded by muscles than its larger neighbor. The fibula is further from the tibia in the proximal half of the leg and approaches it quite closely in the distal half until it lies within a shallow articular facet on the posterolateral surface of the distal tibial

Figure 51–3

A, The arterial blood supply of the intact human tibia arrives primarily by way of a single nutrient artery, a branch of the posterior tibial artery. It enters through an oblique, fairly long foramen angled distally that is usually located in the upper part of the middle third of the tibia. Where the external surface of the tibia is covered only by periosteum, the nutrient artery supplies nearly the full cortical thickness. Where muscles and ligaments are firmly attached, periosteal arterioles supply as much as the outer third of the cortex. A comparatively rich system of metaphyseal arteries is present proximally and distally. These anastomose with the medullary branches of the nutrient artery and provide collateral flow and regenerative potential after injury to this system. *B,* After a fracture, peripheral callus is nourished primarily by a rich vascular plexus derived from the surrounding musculature. The greater the soft tissue injury, the less potential there is for recruiting this blood supply.

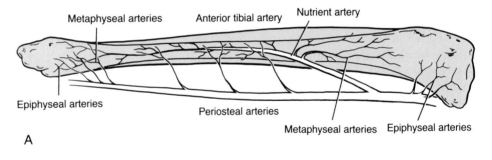

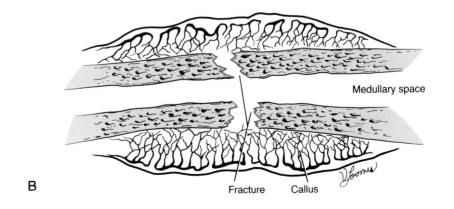

metaphysis. Securely attached to each other, these parallel bones articulate proximally at the superior tibiofibular joint and distally at the inferior one.

The subcutaneous fibular head anchors the lateral collateral ligament of the knee and the biceps femoris tendon. The common peroneal nerve wraps superficially around its neck from an initially posterior location and divides into superficial and deep portions. As it rounds the fibula, the peroneal nerve is at risk of injury from direct blows; from the stretching that occurs with widely displaced fractures or dislocations; and, importantly, from the pressure of casts, splints, and even firm mattresses.

The fibula is described as bearing 6% to 17% of body weight.[160,274] However, function is only slightly affected by absence of its diaphysis or proximal extent.[167] The fibular shaft is a significant muscle origin. Closely accompanied by the peroneal artery, it can be surgically transferred with this as a free or pedicled graft to treat distant or local bone defects.

The distal end of the fibula, or lateral malleolus, has a major role in the structural integrity of the ankle joint. It is securely attached to the distal tibia through the ligaments of the ankle syndesmosis—the anterior and posterior distal tibiofibular ligaments, the inferior transverse ligament, and the interosseous ligament—as well as through the distal interosseous membrane. Disruption of these ligaments, with resultant loss of fibular support for the talus, may occur in association with tibial shaft fractures; therefore the integrity of the ankle joint should always be assessed in patients with tibia fractures.

A thick interosseous membrane connects the lateral crest of the tibia to the anteromedial border of the fibula. Its major fibers run downward and laterally. This membrane is often largely intact after indirect torsional fractures of the tibia, and according to Sarmiento and Latta[247] and others, it is the major limit to shortening of such injuries.[236,261]

Over the top of the interosseous membrane, beneath the proximal tibiofibular joint, the anterior tibial artery and its accompanying veins enter the anterior compartment of the leg. Injury to these structures may be associated with proximal tibial fractures and tibiofibular joint dislocations. Under the distal edge of the interosseous membrane the terminal peroneal artery passes anteriorly to join the vascular anastomoses about the ankle.

The tibia and fibula are surrounded by soft tissues that are most important in any consideration of injuries to this region.[42,43,280,285] In fact, the surgeon who pays more attention to the bones than to these soft tissues may commit irretrievable errors in evaluating and treating fractures of the tibia and fibula. The soft tissue envelope of the leg is injured to a greater or lesser extent whenever a fracture occurs. Open wounds are usually obvious, though they may be small and may underrepresent the extent of damage within. Subcutaneous degloving may result in extensive skin necrosis. Initially, however, such a wound can appear quite benign. Swelling within the fascial compartments of the leg may gradually result in tissue pressures high enough to occlude capillary blood flow, thus producing a compartment syndrome with loss of nerve and muscle tissue. Direct or indirect injuries may occur to the nerves and blood vessels of the leg. Clearly each anatomic element of the leg must be considered together with injuries to its bones and joints.

The skin receives significant blood supply from the underlying fascia by way of small perforating arteries.[283] These are disrupted by subcutaneous dissection or degloving injuries, which separate the subcutaneous fat from the underlying fascia. Therefore dissection should proceed beneath, rather than superficial to, the deep fascia so as to decrease the risk of skin necrosis and take advantage of the subfascial arterial plexus, which is raised off the underlying muscle with the fascia. The dermal plexus is the terminal vascular bed of the skin. Its patency and perfusion are demonstrated clearly by punctate bleeding after tangential excision of a split-thickness layer of skin. This has been used by Ziv et al. to assess viability of degloved skin.[313]

Superficial veins in the subcutaneous tissue of the leg include the saphenous on the medial side and the short saphenous on the lateral. The small saphenous nerve branches that run with the former, as well as the sural nerve near the latter, may be entrapped in a scar or suture, resulting in a painful neuroma. Because the deep venous system may be damaged at the time of injury or may subsequently be occluded by venous thrombosis, it is important to preserve the major superficial veins when operating on a tibia fracture.

The deep fascia of the leg envelops it circumferentially and is adherent to the tibia along its anteromedial surface, as well as proximally and distally, except for small windows for tendons and neurovascular structures. The cylinder thus formed is subdivided into four well-defined longitudinal compartments by septae that attach along the fibula. An anterolateral septum divides the lateral compartment from the anterior. A posterolateral septum lies between the lateral and superficial posterior compartments. Finally, a posterior septum intervenes between the deep and superficial posterior compartments. More proximally, this attaches to the medial tibia. Beyond the midshaft, it attaches to the medial surface of the deep investing fascia so that only a small part of the medial surface of the deep posterior compartment, behind the posteromedial border of the distal half of the tibia, is subcutaneous.

Familiarity with the cross-sectional anatomy of the leg is essential for the fracture surgeon. It guides assessment of the function of structures within each of the four compartments, facilitates surgical approaches, and helps avoid injury to neurovascular and tendinous structures during insertion of percutaneous pins and wires (Fig. 51–4).[77,92,168]

Compartments

The *anterior compartment* contains the dorsiflexors of the ankle and toes: the tibialis anterior, extensor hallucis longus (in its distal half), and extensor digitorum communis (with accompanying peroneus tertius). Its neurovascular (NV) bundle consists of the anterior tibial artery and veins, joined in the proximal part of the compartment by the deep peroneal nerve. The artery is assessed distally by the dorsalis pedis pulse. However, this may fill from the deep plantar arch. The nerve supplies an autonomous sensory zone dorsally on the foot between the bases of first and second toes. It provides motor control for the anterior compartment muscles as well as the short toe extensors. During most of its course through the anterior compartment, the NV bundle lies deep on the interosseous membrane lateral to the tibialis anterior. However, as this muscle becomes tendinous and thinner in the proximal third of the distal quarter, the neurovascular bundle advances anteriorly across the lateral surface of the tibia, where it may be harmed by pins inserted through the bone. A little more distally, it lies anteriorly on the tibia between the tendons of the tibialis anterior and extensor hallucis muscles.

The *lateral compartment,* superficial to the fibula, contains the peroneus brevis and longus muscles, the evertors of the foot. The peroneus longus begins proximally on the lateral aspect of the fibular head. The common peroneal nerve passes under this muscle where it covers the neck of the fibula. The peroneus brevis is beneath the longus, until, at a more distal point, the brevis moves anterior. Thus behind the lateral malleolus, the brevis is the anterior of the two tendons. The superficial peroneal nerve, sensory to the remainder of the dorsum of the foot and motor to the peronei, lies within the lateral compartment, but no major vascular structures are present.

The *superficial posterior compartment* contains the triceps surae, or primary ankle flexors, gastrocnemius, soleus, and plantaris muscles. The sural nerve lies between layers of the posterior fascia of this compartment and provides sensation to the lateral heel. No major artery lies within this compartment, which is the most distensible and least likely to develop elevated pressures after injury.

The *deep posterior compartment* lies underneath (anterior to) the superficial compartment and distal to the popliteal line, with its muscles applied to the posterior surfaces of the tibia, interosseous membrane, and fibula. Within it lie the posterior tibial vessels and tibial nerve, motor to the compartmental muscles and the plantar intrinsic muscles, sensory to the sole of the foot. Also present are the peroneal vessels. The deep posterior compartment muscles are the flexor digitorum longus medially, the flexor hallucis longus laterally, and deep to these, the tibialis posterior. The tibial neurovascular bundle first lies posterior to the popliteus and then posterior to the medial border of the tibialis posterior. The tibial nutrient artery leaves the posterior tibial shortly after it is formed and reaches the bone through the proximal part of the tibialis posterior. The tendon of tibialis posterior passes across the tibia and under the flexor digitorum longus to lie anterior to it and establish the well-known relationship of the deep posterior compartment structures behind the medial malleolus: tibialis posterior, flexor digitorum longus, posterior tibial artery and tibial nerve, and flexor hallucis longus ("Tom, Dick, and Harry") (Table 51–1).

INCIDENCE

Fractures of the tibial shaft have been reported to occur approximately twice a year per 1000 population in Malmö, Sweden.[20b] The rate may be somewhat lower in the United States. Nonetheless, the tibia is the most common diaphyseal fracture.[42,91,165]

MECHANISMS OF INJURY

Tibial fractures have many causes, ranging from simple falls with twisting forces to severe injuries (e.g., being crushed between two automobile bumpers).[220] Severity may be graded in several ways. It is essential to distinguish between high- and low-energy transfer. Indirect fractures, produced by a torsional force acting at a distance, have a typical spiral pattern and usually cause little soft tissue injury. The history of the injury, the physical examination, and the radiograph all corroborate the relatively less forceful nature of this fracture, which was typical of skiers' injuries before safety bindings became common. Even with indirect injuries, however, there is a spectrum of severity. Much more kinetic energy ($\frac{1}{2}MV^2$) is produced by a skiing injury

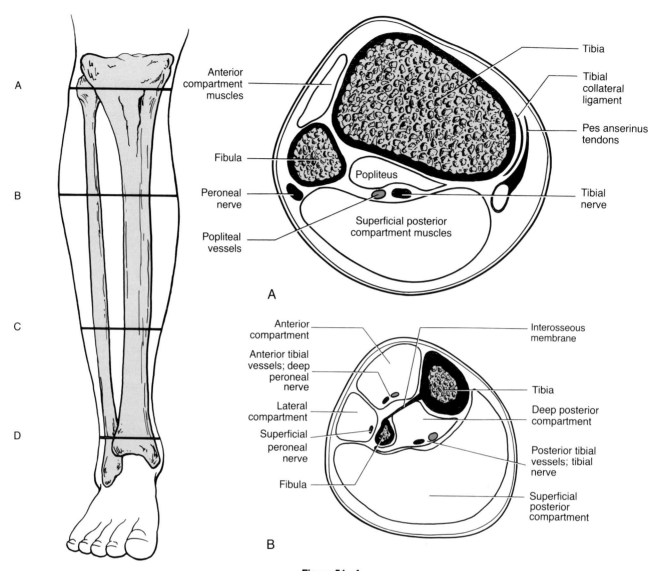

Figure 51-4

than by a simple slip and fall. The amount of comminution of a spiral fracture is proportionate to the amount of energy consumed by its production. The comminuted fragments act as missiles and may cause significant injury to the soft tissues surrounding the fracture. It is thus important to recognize that some indirect tibia fractures are high-energy injuries.[133]

Direct injury mechanisms include bending, as in a skier's "boot-top" fracture, with the top of the boot acting as a fulcrum over which the tibia is broken.[80] Naturally such direct application of force results in a greater or lesser amount (depending on the amount of force) of direct local soft tissue injury. When a great amount of force is involved, as may occur when a pedestrian is struck by an automobile, the extent of injury is correspondingly more severe. Not surprisingly, the prognosis for such injuries is worse.[36] Direct force ap-

plication is often evident by history or appearance of the limb and is also suggested by a fracture pattern that is transverse or has a transverse component on the tension side, with a wedge-shaped butterfly fragment on the side that is compressed during injury.[14,67]

The most severe tibia fractures are those caused by crushing injuries. These have complex highly comminuted or segmental patterns with extensive damage to the surrounding soft tissues. Often the skin is minimally burst, suggesting a so-called "type I" open fracture.[99] However, by definition, type I injuries consist of laceration of the skin envelope by a spike of bone produced in an indirect, torsional injury. The term should not be used for injuries with different mechanisms or radiographic appearances. It is important not to underestimate the severity and consequences of tibial fractures caused by a crushing mechanism.

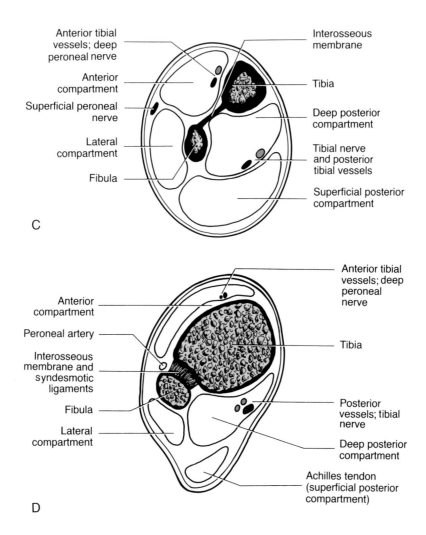

Anterior tibial
vessels; deep
peroneal nerve

Interosseous
membrane

Anterior
compartment

Tibia

Superficial peroneal
nerve

Deep posterior
compartment

Lateral
compartment

Tibial nerve
and posterior
tibial vessels

Fibula

Superficial posterior
compartment

C

Anterior tibial
vessels; deep
peroneal
nerve

Anterior
compartment

Peroneal artery

Tibia

Interosseous
membrane and
syndesmotic
ligaments

Fibula

Posterior
vessels; tibial
nerve

Lateral
compartment

Deep posterior
compartment

Achilles tendon
(superficial posterior
compartment)

D

Figure 51–4

Cross-sectional drawings at indicated levels demonstrate the location of the major nerves and arteries of the leg. Note that the anteromedial surface of the entire tibia, though through a variable arc, is accessible immediately below the skin and subcutaneous tissue. The distal popliteal artery and tibial nerve are in the midline posterior to the proximal tibia. The close proximity of both the anterior tibial artery and the accompanying deep peroneal nerve is an important aspect of the anterolateral tibial surface near the junction of the third and fourth quarters. The posterior tibial artery and tibial nerve are close behind the posteromedial surface of the distal quarter of the tibia.

Table 51–1.

Tests for Assessment of Peripheral Nerves and Compartments of the Leg*

Nerve	Compartment	Motor Function	Sensory Function
Deep peroneal	Anterior	Toe dorsiflexion	Dorsal I–II web space
Superficial peroneal	Lateral	Foot eversion	Lateral dorsum of foot
Tibial	Deep posterior	Toe plantarflexion	Sole of foot
Sural	Superficial posterior	Gastrocsoleus	Lateral heel

* By testing each nerve and associated muscle group, it is possible to assess the status of myoneural tissue within each compartment.

Patients with spinal cord injuries may have high-energy tibial fractures associated with their original injury. These behave as typical high-energy injuries, but management must involve consideration of the patient's neurologic status. Patients with chronic spinal cord injuries and marked osteopenia from disuse can also sustain tibial fractures from either low- or high-energy mechanisms.[82,126]

Some tibia fractures are caused by repeated loading with ultimate failure in a fatigue mode. These fractures, known as fatigue or "stress" fractures, are discussed later. Low levels of force can cause a pathologic fracture (see chapter 17) of the tibia when it is weakened by any of a variety of processes. Conditions that weaken the tibia sufficiently for a fracture to occur under normally applied loads include secondary and primary malignancies, benign neoplasias, dysplasias, infection, and injuries, including surgery.

An additional injury that is all too common in the United States is a fracture caused by a gunshot wound. These injuries are reviewed in chapter 16.

CONSEQUENCES OF INJURY

Fractures of the tibial shaft prevent weight bearing and ambulation, at least initially, and cause pain and instability. If the fracture is open, serious infection may threaten life and limb. These fractures may be associated with immediate or delayed neurovascular deficits that also threaten survival and function of the limb. Although the average tibial fracture heals in approximately 17 weeks, with more time required for complete rehabilitation, some patients are disabled for a year or more.[71] Healing may not occur without additional treatment for nonunion. Deformity may result, either from fracture malalignment or contractures of joints and soft tissues of the ankle and foot.[296] Tibial fractures themselves are rarely lethal injuries now, but their prolonged recovery period and their potential for permanent disability are of great significance.[25,121]

There exists considerable concern that malalignment of a healed tibial shaft fracture may result in posttraumatic arthritis of the ankle or knee. However, this possibility has not been irrefutably established.[157,189,225,281,297] Assuming axial deformity does result in joint damage over time, it is not clear what degree of deformity is significant. The location of the malunion is probably important, with distal deformities more likely to be symptomatic. It may also be that the amount of acceptable deformity varies from patient to patient as well as with the demands placed on the healed limb.[206] Separating the consequences of deformity from those of associated injuries proves difficult,

so that the surgeon must often make judgments about whether to accept a given reduction in the absence of data allowing a reliable prediction of results.

COMMONLY ASSOCIATED INJURIES

As many as 30% of tibial fractures occur in patients with multiple injuries. Potentially, therefore, any injury could be associated, and thus a complete assessment of the patient is mandatory. This should be repeated during the 24 to 48 hours following injury, when the tibial fracture becomes less painful and the patient is better able to identify other sites of discomfort. Injuries to other parts are possible even with low-energy slips and falls; they are not restricted to more typical polytrauma patients. Particular attention must be paid to injuries of the upper extremities, which might interfere with weight bearing for transfers and crutches, and to those involving the opposite leg.[171] Treatment modifications may be required for some or all of the injuries if the patient is to resume ambulation as rapidly as possible.

The most frequent injury associated with a fractured tibia is a fracture of the ipsilateral fibula. This smaller and weaker bone is often disrupted by indirect and direct forces sufficient to fracture the tibia, and injury may occur at the same or at a distant level and may occasionally be segmental. The commonly associated fibular injury is often ignored, because rarely is any specific treatment directed toward the fibula. Some believe that the presence of an intact fibula makes the isolated tibia fracture more prone to complications, such as delayed union and nonunion or varus deformity resulting from maintenance of length on the lateral side.[276] Additionally, it is important not to ignore an associated fibula fracture, as it may provide some helpful opportunities for reconstructing a severely injured leg. Once fixed or healed, it may contribute to stability. It may be used as the basis for bypassing a segmental defect in the tibia and also guides restoration of tibial alignment. In addition to a complete fibular fracture, this bone can be plastically deformed or angulated by a "greenstick" fracture and thus interfere with reduction of a tibial deformity.[87]

Usually the fibula itself fails when forces are sufficient to fracture the tibia. However, as in the Monteggia and Galeazzi fractures of the forearm, there may occasionally be disruption of proximal or distal tibiofibular joints so that the tibial fragments override and shorten in spite of an apparently intact fibula. If such injuries are not recognized, deformity or ankle joint dysfunction may result. Proximal dislocation of the proximal tibiofibular joint may be associated with serious neuro-vascular injury.

Tibial shaft fractures may themselves be segmental, with one or more additional diaphyseal disruptions. Occasionally the second level of injury may be meta-physeal, with intra- or extraarticular fractures that threaten the knee or ankle.[28,288] These vary in the de-gree of displacement and instability. Sometimes such combined injuries make it advisable to modify treat-ment for the diaphyseal injury; therefore it is important that they be identified initially. Generally their treat-ment follows that described in chapters 50 and 52, with alterations as required in the management of the tibial shaft fracture. (For example, an injury that would ordi-narily be treated nonoperatively might be fixed inter-nally to permit early motion of an associated tibial plateau fracture.) More common than fractures at mul-tiple levels, a single transitional fracture may extend from the diaphysis through the metaphysis and into the articular surface.[280] Identification and appropriate management of the articular involvement is crucial to obtaining an optimal result.

Injuries to the supporting ligaments of the knee joint are fairly commonly associated with tibial shaft frac-tures, especially those caused by higher levels of en-ergy.[107,277] In addition to purely ligamentous injuries, fracture-dislocations of the knee may occur, often with associated vascular or neural trauma (Fig. 51–5). Be-cause knee stability is difficult to assess when the tibial shaft is fractured, and because arterial occlusion may be delayed, it is vital not to underestimate the signifi-cance of marginal avulsion and displaced wedge frac-tures of the tibial plateau. They may be the only sign of gross knee instability. Arteriography should be consid-ered for such limbs, in spite of apparently adequate perfusion, to permit identification and repair of an in-timal injury before it thromboses.

Especially in patients with high-energy injuries, tib-ial fractures may be associated with fractures of the ipsilateral femur—the so-called "floating knee in-jury," which has already been discussed (chapter 46). These injuries often involve the knee ligament as well. Fractures and dislocations distal to the tibial injury are also not unusual, so that careful assessment of the foot and ankle are required (Fig. 51–6). Because these areas are covered and splinted in the course of treating the tibial fracture, adequate initial physical exam and ra-diographs are essential if the surgeon is to avoid failing to identify and treat such injuries, which typically in-volve the tarsometatarsal joints, the metatarsals, or the toes.

Involvement of adjacent arteries, veins, and nerves is common with tibial fractures. These structures may

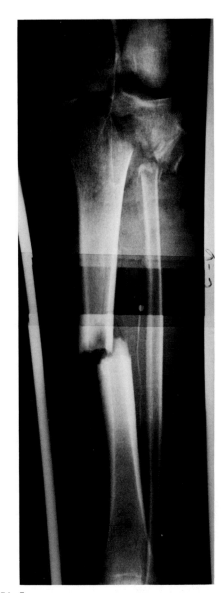

Figure 51–5

Popliteal artery occlusion is demonstrated by this arteriogram, which was done to identify the site of arterial compromise in an ischemic leg with two levels of severe skeletal injury.

have an immediate injury or may develop delayed evi-dence of injury. Because of their profound significance for preservation of limb and function, the neurovascu-lar structures of the leg require repeated assessment during care of a patient with a tibial fracture. Arterial injuries may be occult because of the three arterial con-duits distal to the popliteal "trifurcation." The limb may survive with flow in only a single artery. Another reason that an arterial injury may be inapparent ini-tially is the previously mentioned phenomenon of an intimal tear that may thrombose several hours or days

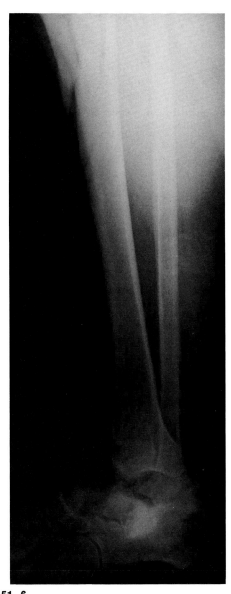

Figure 51–6

Severe fracture-dislocation of the talus associated with a proximal tibial shaft fracture. Less severe injuries to the ankle or foot might be more readily overlooked.

after fracture. Arterial flow may also be compromised by kinking of the vessels in the zone of injury. This may be corrected by reduction of the fracture, but an arteriogram is still advisable to ensure that this temporary mechanism is the only cause of ischemia. Venous injury is often occult, unless a laceration produces copious bleeding from an open fracture wound. Multiple pathways for venous return exist in both deep and superficial systems. Venous injuries may accompany injuries to the arterial side of the circulation. They may also be manifest by deep vein thrombosis, which occurs

in as many as two thirds of tibial fractures, according to Nylander and Semb.[204] Although deep venous thrombosis may be a common phenomenon, only rarely does it seem to progress proximal to the calf veins or lead to clinically evident pulmonary embolism. Late venous insufficiency remains a hazard.[2,223,308]

Development of Classification

Since ancient Egyptian times, many have emphasized that tibial fractures are not all alike, and prognosis varies with the severity of injury. The importance of an open wound extending to the fracture site was recorded in the Edwin Smith Papyrus. Hamilton emphasized the prognostic significance of comminution.[103a] Not until the end of the nineteenth century, when radiography was applied to the diagnosis and treatment of fractures, could fracture configuration and displacement be used for classifying fracture severity.[217] Ellis, in 1958, used displacement, comminution, and wound severity to assign tibial shaft fractures to one of three grades: minor, moderate, and major.[70,71] His "minor" tibial fractures were undisplaced or had only angular deformity; a wound, if present, was only minor; and comminution was either absent or minimal. He defined "moderate" fractures as those with complete displacement but with no more than a minor wound or minor comminution. His "major" tibial fractures included all those with significant comminution or a major open wound. He reviewed 343 conservatively treated tibial fractures and found that average healing times were ten weeks for minor injuries, 15 for moderate, and 23 for major. Delayed union (>20 weeks) occurred in 2% of minor, 11% of moderate, and 60% of major fractures. The importance of injury severity was made clear by Ellis's work, yet many subsequent authors have failed to classify tibial fractures by severity. Instead they group all such injuries together for analysis, reporting "average healing time" for a given treatment without any specification of severity. A few have classified severity differently, most notably Nicoll, who similarly demonstrated the significance of displacement, comminution, and wound severity.[203] He also identified segmental bone loss of a centimeter or more and infection as other factors that delayed healing. Burwell, in 1971, used Ellis's classification system in his report of plate fixation for tibial shaft fractures, the only author to do so prior to Austin's metaanalysis published in 1977.[7,39] Bauer et al. and Edwards et al. noted that the type of trauma (direct or high-energy versus indirect or low-energy) had a significant effect on outcome and related this to the extent of soft tissue damage.[14,67] They suggested that "the prognosis in fractures of the shaft of the tibia was related more to the severity of soft tissue damage than to the bone injury."[67]

Attempts to define the severity of open wounds established an unquestioned relationship between wound severity and complications such as infection, problems with union, and rate of amputation. Most open wound classification systems, as initially proposed, focused on the measurable size of the opening in the skin. However it has become clear that the extent of muscle necrosis, micro- and macrovascular damage, and periosteal stripping are usually of greater significance. Gustilo and colleagues have developed the classification system that is currently used by most North American orthopaedic surgeons.[99] Initially it had three categories, but these have been expanded to five and their specifications refined to emphasize the importance of the entire wound. The type I open fracture has a wound smaller than 1 cm, "usually a moderately clean puncture through which a spike of bone has pierced the skin." There is no crushing and little soft tissue injury. The type II open fracture has a larger wound but no extensive avulsions or crushing of soft tissue and only slight or moderate crushing. All open fractures with severe soft tissue injury and serious contamination are grouped into type III. Because type III represents a considerable spectrum of severity, it was necessary to divide these injuries into three subtypes. In type IIIA injuries, after adequate debridement, there remains sufficient soft tissue coverage of the fractured bone, and delayed closure is possible without local or free muscle flaps. Type IIIB open fractures, with more extensive soft tissue injury, leave the bone exposed and require muscle flap coverage. Type IIIC injuries include all those open fractures associated with an arterial injury that must be repaired. This system is highly predictive of wound infection risk, which, with adequate management, ranges up to 2% for type I, up to 7% for types II and IIIA, from 10% to 50% for type IIIB, and from 25% to 50% for type IIIC.

Gustilo and colleagues specify that open fractures resulting from high-energy or high-velocity trauma, with segmental fractures or severe comminution, should be classified as type III injuries, "regardless of the size of the wound."[99] However, this system permits categorization of open tibia fractures with transverse patterns and some comminution into type I. Edwards has shown that the transverse fracture pattern, caused by a direct rather than indirect mechanism, carries a higher risk of problems.[67] It may thus be appropriate to limit the type I open fracture category to spiral tibial fractures produced by indirect injuries.

Tscherne's grading system similarly uses wound size, contamination, and fracture pattern to grade open fractures.[205] In this system, grade I open fractures have a small puncture wound without skin contusion, negligible bacterial contamination, and a low-energy fracture pattern. Grade II open injuries have small skin and soft tissue contusions, moderate contamination, and variable fracture patterns. Grade III open fractures have heavy contamination, extensive soft tissue damage, and, often, associated arterial or neural injuries. Grade IV open fractures are incomplete or complete amputations. Obviously the location and character of such injuries are also important. A cleanly amputated finger has a much better prognosis for replantation than a crushed or avulsed amputation through the midportion of the tibia.

A most important contribution is Tscherne's emphasis on grading the severity of soft tissue damage in closed as well as open injuries. He has proposed a system for doing this, with four grades of severity for soft tissue injury in closed fractures.[205] Grade 0 injuries result from indirect forces and have negligible soft tissue damage. Grade I closed fractures, which are caused by low- or moderate-energy mechanisms, have superficial abrasions or contusions of the soft tissues overlying the fracture. Grade II closed fractures have significant muscle contusion and may have deep contaminated skin abrasions. Fractures caused by direct violence, such as a "bumper" fracture, and moderate to severe bone injury patterns qualify for this category. There is significant risk of a compartment syndrome. Grade III closed fractures have extensive crushing, subcutaneous "degloving" or avulsion, and perhaps an arterial disruption or established compartment syndrome. It is most important to recognize the wide spectrum of injuries represented by Tscherne's classification. Proper assessment of the degree of soft tissue injury is crucial for determining prognosis and choosing treatment for tibial shaft fractures.

The bony pattern of tibial fractures is evident radiographically. In addition to the fracture's location and displacement, its pattern and comminution should be noted. The pattern may be spiral, oblique, transverse, or segmental. Comminution ranges from none to total circumferential involvement. The extent of comminution has been graded, initially for femoral fractures, by Winquist and Hansen.[115] Their emphasis on the amount of contact between the two major fracture fragments is meaningful with regard to the stability of traditional intramedullary nailing, but with a locked nail, a plate, or an external fixator, these distinctions may be less important.

Johner and Wruhs used fracture morphology to clas-

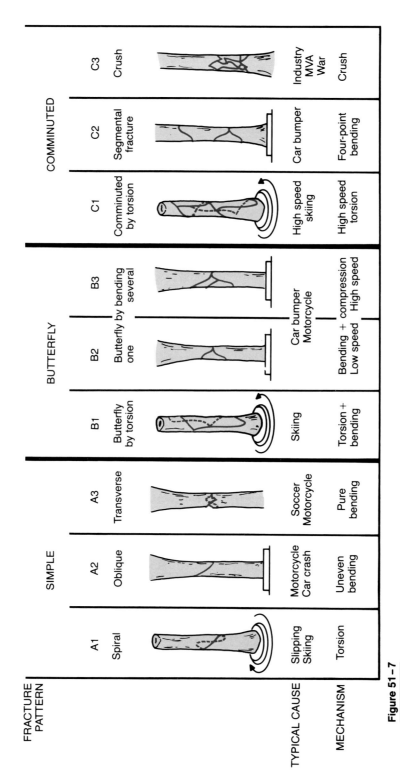

Figure 51–7

Johner and Wruhs' classification system for tibial shaft fractures. Note that neither displacement nor soft tissue wound severity are considered in this system.[133] (Redrawn from Johner, R.; Wruhs, O. Clin Orthop 178:7–25 (Fig. 2), 1983.)

sify tibial shaft fractures treated with AO/ASIF techniques.[133] This classification has been adopted by Müller et al. and the AO/ASIF group in their comprehensive classification of long bone fractures.[201,201a] They recognized the relationship between fracture pattern and injury mechanism: a spiral pattern caused by torsion; an oblique or transverse pattern caused by various modes of bending, often with direct injury; and a segmental or transverse highly comminuted pattern caused by crushing. They also used the extent of comminution, which correlates with absorbed energy, as an indicator of severity. Their resulting classification has three major categories: A, simple, noncomminuted patterns; B, patterns with butterfly or "wedge" fragments; and C, comminuted, including segmental fractures (Fig. 51–7). Although somewhat cumbersome to use with its nine separate categories, this classification is demonstrably well suited to the assessment of results after internal fixation of closed tibial shaft fractures. It is not a comprehensive tibial fracture classification, because it does not include the severity of soft tissue injury, although the authors clearly emphasize the important influence this has on results. Fracture displacement is also not considered, because it has little effect on the outcome of fractures treated by internal fixation. However, it may be quite significant if nonoperative treatment is chosen. Also excluded from Johner and Wruhs' classification is the location of the fracture. Proximal and distal fractures, which can encroach on the knee or ankle and can preclude use of intramedullary nailing, may deserve recognition as separate categories of injury. From Johner and Wruhs' reported results, it is evident that spiral and oblique fractures have the best prognosis after internal fixation. Their A1, A2, B1, and C1 fractures had 91% to 100% good or excellent outcomes. Transverse fractures had intermediate results, with A3 and B2 gaining 80% to 92% good or excellent outcomes. Comminuted or crushing injuries had significantly worse results, with good or excellent outcomes in 75% of B3, 68% of C2, and 50% of C3 tibial fractures.[133]

A fracture classification system should predict results and guide treatment. Because injuries respond differently to different treatments, the choice of treatment may affect the validity of a grading system. For example, Johner and Wruhs found faster recovery of transverse, higher energy fractures treated with intramedullary nails and reported higher infection (17%) and implant failure (5%) rates after plate fixation of type B3 injuries that might have had lower rates of complications if treated with closed locked intramedullary nailing.

Another important limitation of the proposed classification systems for tibial fractures is that they have been validated with end points such as average time to union, risk of nonunion, or risk of infection, rather than ultimate function, risk of deformity, and response to a given treatment.

Current Classification

Although many parameters affect the outcome and choice of treatment for tibial shaft fractures, a matrix of all or even a moderate number of selected factors produces a system that is too complex for clinical use. Thus a classification like Ellis's becomes attractive, although criteria for the categories may require further specification, and certain additional factors may significantly affect both prognosis and choice of treatment within a classification.[7,70,71] Until a better system is validated, Ellis's may be used, as it was by Austin in a prospective study of patellar tendon weight-bearing (PTB) cast treatment.[8] This three-category classification is not the same as the AO/ASIF classification of Johner and Wruhs described previously, for Ellis's emphasizes the benign nature of minimally displaced, low-energy fractures and their suitability for nonoperative treatment. Ellis originally put undisplaced fractures in the minor category and totally displaced ones in the moderate, leaving some question about how to classify partial displacement. Leach's suggestion that up to 50% displacement be accepted in the minor category seems reasonable.[165] Furthermore, Bostman has shown that more than 50% displacement of spiral fractures implies significantly greater soft tissue disruption and greater difficulty maintaining alignment.[30]

In assigning fractures to the appropriate severity group, it is necessary to recognize the preeminence of soft tissue damage, whether or not an open wound is present. Using Tscherne's classification, minor tibial fractures have grade 0 closed or grade I open wounds. Moderate fractures have grade I closed or grade II open injuries. Major severity injuries have grade II or grade III closed injuries or grade II (with a more severe fracture pattern) or grades III or IV open wounds. Using Gustilo's open fracture grading system, type I injuries are minor, type II are moderate, and type III (A, B, or C) are major. When wound severity cannot be judged, as in closed treatment or prior to adequate surgical exploration, the mechanism of injury provides the best guide. This may be indicated by history and also by fracture pattern, as shown by Edwards.[67] Indirect, low-energy (spiral) fractures are minor. Transverse fractures with no comminution or a single butterfly fragment are moderate. High-energy, multiply comminuted or segmental, and crushed fractures are major,

Table 51–2.

Tibial Fracture Classification*

Fracture Characteristic	Minor	Moderate	Major
Displacement	0%–50% diameter	>50%	Tibio-fibular diastasis
Comminution	0–minimal	0 or 1 butterfly fragments	≥ two free fragments or segmental
Wound	Open grade I; closed grade 0	Open grade II; closed grade I	Open grades III–V; closed grades II–III
Available energy (history)	Low	Moderate	High; crushing
Mechanism (fracture pattern)	Spiral	Oblique/transverse	Transverse/fragmented

* After Ellis[71] and Edwards,[67] with Leach's[165] modification. This system incorporates soft tissue wound grading, after Gustilo[99] and Tscherne,[205] and is proposed as a general means for clinical grading of tibial shaft fractures. Use the factor of greatest severity to grade the fracture.

Figure 51–8

Radiographic examples of the three grades of tibial fracture severity. *A*, Minor severity: fracture caused by a simple slip and fall. *B*, Moderate severity: fracture in a pedestrian struck by a slowly moving vehicle. *C*, Major severity: fracture caused by a high-velocity motorcycle crash.

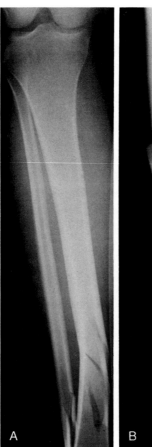
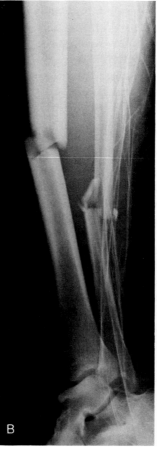
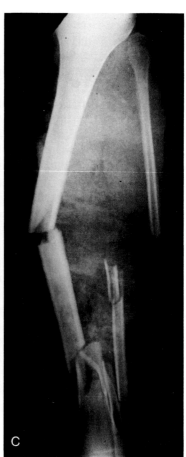

despite a small external wound (Table 51–2 and Fig. 51–8).

Diagnosis

An acute tibial shaft fracture is usually obvious because of the patient's localized pain after injury and the typical physical findings of deformity, tenderness, instability, swelling, and possible open wound. The surgeon's diagnostic efforts primarily involve acquiring the necessary data to plan treatment and excluding injuries elsewhere. Occasionally, undisplaced or incomplete acute injuries or more chronic processes such as fatigue and pathologic fractures can be difficult to identify, and special studies may be required.

HISTORY

The conscious patient can localize injuries by describing where he or she feels pain and by describing its character. Severe, unremitting pain may indicate muscle ischemia. Occasionally a nerve will be caught in fracture fragments so that a particular lancinating pain may be produced by movement of the limb. Absence of sensation can be caused by nerve injury, progressive ischemia, or both.

The time, the place, and the events of the injury should be determined as precisely as possible. Elapsed time is especially important for vascular injuries, compartment syndromes, and open wounds. Certain locales (e.g., barnyards and swamps) are notorious for the presence of virulent microorganisms. Did the patient trip on a curb, or was he or she struck by a car, or run over and crushed by its wheel? The amount of energy involved in causing the injury is perhaps the major determinant of its severity. The mechanism of injury, if known, is a most helpful indicator of this. Reports of bystanders may be helpful. The emergency medical personnel who often bring an injured patient to hospital can provide important information regarding the patient's status and treatment rendered at the scene. They may have detailed knowledge of the injury mechanism, initial deformity, presence of wounds and exposed bone, and neurovascular status of the limb.

Baseline medical information should not be neglected. Previous injuries to the part and any persisting disability should be documented. Exercise tolerance helps identify preexisting peripheral vascular disease. Activity level, both recreational and occupational, may help set functional goals or suggest an injury resulting from overuse. General medical status must include identification of any allergies to medications, the current or recent use of any medications, known medical problems and previous operations, personal or family history of bleeding disorders, and problems with anesthesia or with frequent or poorly healing fractures. Smoking, drinking, and drug use should be determined. Fracture and wound healing problems are more frequent in smokers. A thorough systems review is a helpful screening device. If the patient is unable to provide some or all of this information initially, family and friends can be questioned, and once the patient has recovered sufficiently, the history should be updated as needed.

PHYSICAL EXAMINATION

The strong possibility of multiple injuries, often occult, makes thorough systematic evaluation of the whole patient essential. The principles and practice of initial evaluation and treatment of the trauma patient are taught in the Advanced Trauma Life Support (ATLS) course of the American College of Surgeons and are reviewed in chapter 5.[52]

The injured limb itself must be thoroughly assessed and adequately splinted. If a splint is in place, it should remain in place during the patient's primary survey and in some circumstances may be appropriately left in place during the secondary survey as well, if a reliably described wound will need surgical care and if the distal neurovascular exam is not obscured. Distal perfusion is assessed primarily by pulses, but also by skin color, warmth, and capillary filling. Motor and sensory function are checked in the foot. If an open fracture has been identified in the field and satisfactorily dressed and splinted by a reliable emergency medical team, there is little to be gained by reexposing the wound in the emergency department. Tscherne and Gotzen have shown that this increases the risk of infection and is better deferred until the patient is in the operating room.[285]

Examination of the injured limb includes inspection, palpation, and manipulation and should be goal directed. The surgeon must identify and assess the fracture, establish the presence and severity of soft tissue wounds, and determine the neurologic and vascular status of the injured limb. Furthermore, he or she must also search for associated injuries of the limb above and below the tibia.

A fractured tibia may be more or less deformed, with angulation, shortening, malrotation, or other asymmetry relative to the opposite limb (which may itself be injured). Swelling may be localized or diffuse. An open wound exposing bone fragments leaves no doubt about the presence of a tibial fracture. Palpation allows localization of tenderness, if the patient can cooperate. It may also demonstrate bony irregularity or crepitus.

Palpation may reveal soft boggy swelling typical of a subcutaneous hematoma or degloved area. Alternatively, swelling may be quite tense, suggestive of increased compartmental pressure. Passive manipulation may produce pain and demonstrate instability.

Soft tissue injuries are either open or closed, depending on the integrity of the skin. It is essential to distinguish promptly between the two, because of the well-accepted principle that all open fractures require formal surgical debridement and irrigation, as well as tetanus toxoid and appropriate antibiotics, as soon as possible. A complete circumferential inspection of the limb is essential to avoid missing a small wound. If even a small opening extends through the dermis, it should be presumed to communicate with a nearby fracture. Persistent bloody drainage, perhaps with small fat droplets, is further evidence. In addition to the character and amount of drainage, the wound should be inspected for foreign material as well as obvious anatomic structures. The physician should resist the temptation to probe or explore potential open fracture wounds in the emergency department. Instead, assume that the fracture is open, and proceed to the operating room for formal exploration under optimal conditions. The true severity of soft tissue injury associated with an open fracture is easily underestimated before adequate surgical exploration. Extensively crushed muscle may be present under a small skin laceration. The injury mechanism is a more reliable indicator of soft tissue damage.

In addition to potential open fracture wounds, it is important to note any lacerations or abrasions in areas that might be required for surgical approaches to a closed tibial fracture. Such surgery may best be done immediately or delayed until a contaminated wound has healed.

Impaired perfusion of the injured limb is revealed by skin pallor, coolness, absence of venous and capillary filling, and above all by the absence or significant diminution of palpable pulses. After a tibial fracture, both the dorsalis pedis and posterior tibial pulses should be assessed promptly, marked, and followed closely. Paralysis and loss of sensation may be due to ischemia, which must always be excluded specifically whenever neurologic abnormalities are found in association with a tibial fracture. Swelling may indicate soft tissue edema or venous obstruction or, if rapidly developing, may be the result of arterial hemorrhage. A thrill or bruit suggests an arteriovenous fistula.

Compartmental syndromes are initially characterized by pain, swelling, and loss of neuromuscular function, with pulse and skin perfusion not affected until late in their course. In the patient who is unconscious or insensate, the physician must recognize the special sig-nificance of swelling and induration and promptly assess the tissue pressure in the compartments at risk. When a conscious patient is developing a compartment syndrome, pain can be produced by passively stretching the muscles in the involved compartments (e.g., anterior compartment pain is produced by passively plantarflexing the patient's toes.)

Neurologic function is assessed by specific tests for motor and sensation served by the nerves of the lower leg. Because these nerves lie within different deep fascial compartments, the tests are valuable for identifying compartment syndromes. Sensation is assessed with light touch or pain (e.g., a pinprick). Motor function should be tested with formal manual motor tests requiring the patient to demonstrate maximal power against the examiner's hand. Strength is then graded from 0 to 5 (see Table 51–1). The deep peroneal nerve lies in the anterior compartment. Its sensory area is the dorsal web space between the first and second toes, and its motor test is toe dorsiflexion. The superficial peroneal nerve, located in the lateral compartment, is sensory to the rest of the dorsum of the foot and motor to the foot evertors. The tibial nerve is sensory to the sole of the foot and motor to the toe plantarflexors; it travels through the deep posterior compartment. The sural nerve lies within the superficial posterior compartment and provides sensation to the lateral heel, but no motor activity. An adequate neurologic exam in a limb with a tibial fracture involves testing and recording response in each of the aforementioned nerves. If the exam is initially normal, then a splint or cast that interferes with assessment of pedal pulses, as well as motor and sensory reevaluation of all but the patient's toes, may be applied. However, if there is any question as to neurologic status, then access to the foot must be preserved so that a complete exam can be repeated periodically. This can be achieved by removing the cast or splint from the dorsum of the foot and trimming or windowing over the posteromedial aspect to palpate the posterior tibial pulse as well.

Finally, examination must exclude, as well as possible, any coexisting injuries above or below the tibial fracture. Although pain and instability of the tibia make it difficult to perform a complete exam of the pelvis, thigh, knee, ankle and foot, it is essential not to ignore these regions. The alert patient should be specifically questioned about pain and tenderness. Deformity, wound, and swelling may be present. The iliac crests must be internally and externally stressed to exclude tenderness and instability. The femur, patella, and knee are palpated for tenderness, deformity, crepitus, and effusion. The patellar ligament is checked similarly. Assessment of knee joint stability must usually wait until the patient is under anesthesia and the tibia has been fixed securely. Ankle swelling, tenderness, and crepitus may alert the surgeon to an injury of this joint. The foot must also be assessed carefully, as external deformity may be subtle when there is an injury to the hindfoot or midfoot.

IMAGING

Radiographs

Adequate plain radiographs are an essential diagnostic supplement to the history and physical exam and usually provide definitive diagnosis of a tibial shaft fracture. They offer detailed documentation of fracture configuration, but because they are not similarly informative about radiolucent structures, radiographs tend to divert the surgeon's attention from the all-important soft tissues. It is thus crucial that examination of the patient take precedence over the radiographs and that radiographs be correlated with information from history and physical exam.

Radiographs of the tibia must be obtained whenever significant localized tenderness, pain, or deformity involves the bone. An obvious unstable fracture should be aligned and splinted prior to obtaining radiographs. However, many splinting materials compromise the detail available with current radiographic techniques. Most tibias can be displayed from top to bottom diagonally on a standard 14-in × 17-in film, but the knee and ankle regions receive an oblique beam and deserve their own centered views if there is any question of injury to these regions. It is essential to obtain two perpendicular views, conventionally in the frontal (anteroposterior, or AP) and sagittal (lateral) planes (see Fig. 51–1). It may be difficult to position the injured limb precisely. Certainly it should be rotated as a unit and not twisted through the fracture site. Occasionally an undisplaced spiral fracture may not be apparent on standard films. In this situation, and when one wishes to assess healing, complex deformity, or the placement of hardware or bone grafts, both 45° oblique radiographs are valuable supplements (Fig. 51–9).[5] In any questionable situation, directing the central x-ray beam at the area of interest, rather than at the midtibia, may give more informative results. Fluoroscopically guided spot films can be most helpful in searching for a nonunion cleft or occult injury, as they permit precise rotational alignment. Such positioning is also essential if one wishes to demonstrate the true angle of deformity, as angulation appears less if its plane is not parallel with the film. True length measurements must be obtained with scanographic techniques but can be estimated with a special ruler placed at the level of the tibia (Fig. 51–10). Comparison views of the opposite tibia, if intact, can be invaluable for determining correct length when severe comminution or bone loss is present and for defining the shape of metaphyseal and articular regions of the tibia for preoperative planning. A C-arm fluoroscope can be used to calculate torsional alignment of the tibia, which is poorly demonstrated by routine radiographs.[48,49] In fact, it is essential to remember this limitation of conventional radiography and make an independent assessment of rotational alignment by physical exam for all tibial fractures.

Descriptive Terminology

Conventional techniques and terminology must be used to describe the radiographic appearance of a tibial shaft fracture. Its location, pattern, degree of comminution, extent and direction of displacement, and alignment are all important. The physician should also look for soft tissue abnormalities such as swelling, loss of fat shadows, and the presence of gas or other foreign material.

Other Imaging Techniques

In addition to standard radiographs, other imaging techniques can provide helpful information. Occult problems such as fatigue fractures and pathologic lesions may be localized with technetium phosphate bone scanning. Detailed views of both tibias should be requested. Abnormal early uptake of technetium methylene diphosphonate may be related to delayed fracture union; however, the usefulness of nuclear medicine studies for predicting fracture healing has not been confirmed.[95,265] Indium-labeled white cell scans are probably the best current technique for finding an occult infection but may still yield false-negative or false-positive results.[172,187,250]

Computed tomography (CT) is most helpful for demonstrating transverse images of metaphyseal fractures. This information can be invaluable in preoperative planning. Computer reprocessing can also provide AP and lateral reconstructions that rival standard tomographic techniques, but very thin or overlapping cuts are required. CT imaging offers a precise assessment of rotational alignment and reduction of spiral fractures, should this be needed.[84] The preliminary digital radiograph (scout view) can be used for measuring tibial length. Magnetic resonance imaging (MRI) may be used to demonstrate bone contusions, occult infractions, and fatigue fractures when other studies are negative.[21,166] The MRI findings in tibial fracture healing have recently been reported.[159]

Angiography, using various techniques, demonstrates the status of the leg's arterial tree and may be essential for identifying an intimal injury before it oc-

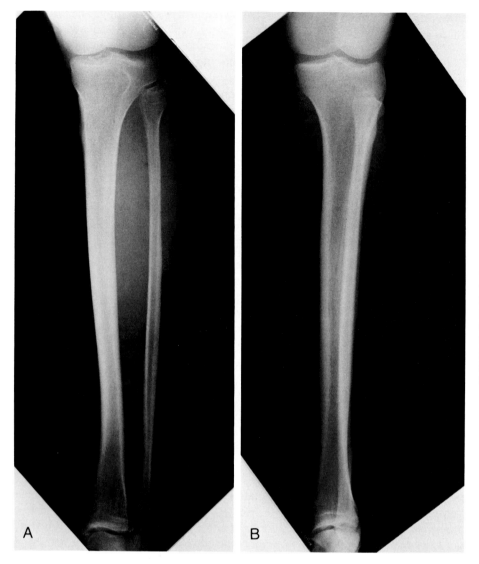

Figure 51–9

Oblique views of the tibia and fibula show spiral fracture lines, comminution, and displacement in the axis perpendicular to the central ray; they may be especially helpful for evaluating metaphyseal fractures proximally and distally. *A,* The internally rotated 45° oblique radiograph provides the best demonstration of bone graft placed along the posterolateral surface of the tibia and interosseous membrane. *B,* Externally rotated 45° oblique radiograph.

cludes completely. Arteriography may be of value in patients whose physical exams show obvious arterial occlusion, but unless it is required to investigate a situation in which several levels of arterial injury may exist, it should be requested cautiously. Direct exploration, perhaps guided by a single-shot intraoperative arteriogram, avoids time-consuming arteriograms in the radiology suite and may permit revascularizing an ischemic leg before irreversible tissue necrosis occurs (see chapter 12).

Venography is the gold standard for assessment of venous circulation. Ultrasound, using the criteria of venous compressibility and flow augmentation, has been shown to be highly effective, as well as safer and much easier, for identification of venous thrombosis in the leg.[81a] However, a cast or splint interferes with the performance of venous ultrasonography.

OTHER STUDIES

Gram stain studies and microbial culture and sensitivity studies are of value whenever an infection is suspected. Routine culture and sensitivity studies have been recommended for open tibial fractures at presentation, prior to debridement, and after debridement and irrigation have been completed. Many infections in such wounds are the result of organisms present when the patient arrives in the hospital.[99,215] However, particularly in more severe wounds, hospital-acquired organisms assume a prominent role in wound colonization and infection. The true value of routine cultures of open fracture wounds has not been established. An urgent Gram stain test may be diagnostic of clostridial myonecrosis and should be promptly obtained whenever this dreaded complication is a possibility.

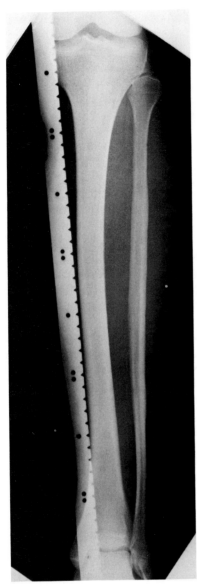

Figure 51–10

A radiodense ruler, as demonstrated, permits reliable estimation of tibial length for choosing an appropriate intramedullary nail. Length can be measured more precisely if a scanogram technique is used with a radioopaque ruler, and separate exposures are made over the proximal and distal ends of the bone, with the central ray perpendicular to the bone at the point of measurement. The leg and ruler must not be moved between exposures.

Ancillary vascular studies may be helpful in assessing the patient with a tibial fracture. Doppler devices may indicate pulsatile arterial flow but can be dangerously deceiving if relied on as indicators of adequate perfusion. Use of the Doppler with a sphygmomanometer cuff about the calf will permit measurement of arterial pressures in the dorsal foot and posterior tibial arteries. This is much more meaningful information but still may fail to rule out an incompletely occlusive intimal

flap tear, which requires arteriography. The increasing availability of equipment for instantaneous measurement of oxygen saturation in skin capillary beds permits assessment and monitoring of skin perfusion.[158] Laser Doppler flowmetry has been proposed as another means of assessing perfusion and can be used intraoperatively to assess blood flow in muscle and bone.[271] In practice, the presence of punctate capillary bleeding from cut tissues, including bone, and capillary flush after release of an arterial tourniquet are both valuable tools for assessment of tissue microperfusion. Temporary split-thickness skin excision is a rapid way of assessing the viability of a degloved flap.[313] Bleeding of the dermal surface after graft harvesting indicates perfusion; the graft is then replaced on such surfaces. Nonbleeding portions of dermal flaps are excised, with application of the split-thickness graft to the underlying muscle and fascia instead.

Reconstitution of the intramedullary blood flow occurs with normal fracture healing. Osteomedullography can be used to investigate this and to diagnose nonunion. Clinically, however, this technique has not proven very useful.

Physical examination is the best early test of peripheral nerve function, but electrodiagnostic studies—particularly nerve conduction velocities, which are immediately affected by neural pathology and do not require a period of delay until classic electromyographic (EMG) changes of denervation have occurred—may be helpful.

Tissue pressure measurement techniques are discussed in chapter 13. Instant-reading, hand-held digital devices are particularly valuable because of their ease of use and ability to obtain multiple measurements quickly. After tibia fractures, pressures are most elevated in the region of the bony injury and are not as high in more remote regions of the same compartment.[114] One or more of the four leg compartments can be involved, with or without open wounds, and the dynamic nature of compartment pressure elevations is such that interpretation of a single pressure measurement must be correlated with the clinical situation.[83] Pressure measurements are helpful to (1) avoid fasciotomy in a swollen limb with normal pressures, (2) assess compartment pressures in unconscious patients or insensate limbs, (3) differentiate among involved and uninvolved compartments, and (4) confirm adequacy of fasciotomy.

The extent of soft tissue injury associated with tibial fractures correlates with serum creatinine phosphokinase activity.[208]

Fracture healing has been assessed investigationally by several types of mechanical tests, although these have not yet found clinical acceptance. Fracture stiffness can be assessed with transducers attached to an external fixator or by measuring radiographic displacement in response to a known force.[58,59,65,106] Ultrasound wave propagation across the fracture site correlates with stiffness and appears to change with fracture healing.

ESSENTIAL STUDIES TO EXCLUDE OTHER INJURIES

A careful history and physical exam, with appropriate radiographic views, should be adequate to exclude other injuries associated with an acute tibial fracture. A high index of suspicion is required. Follow-up assessment with repeated examinations and radiographs is the key to early discovery and treatment of any injuries missed initially and any complications that ensue.

DIFFERENTIAL DIAGNOSIS

A purely soft tissue injury may be present in a patient who appears to have a tibial fracture. Isolated fibular fractures or injuries proximal or distal to the tibial shaft may also become apparent with adequate radiographs. There is usually little confusion about the diagnosis of an acute injury. However, patients without a traumatic episode may have a fatigue fracture, osteomyelitis, a tumor, or pain of neurogenic or vascular origin.

Management of Tibial Fractures

EVOLUTION OF TREATMENT

Fractures have been treated since antiquity by bonesetters in the folk medicine tradition and by surgeons who have recorded their results in learned treatises, such as that reconstructed from an Egyptian papyrus by Edwin Smith. The history of management of severe wounds has in large part been the history of open tibia fracture care.[213] Peltier has reviewed the history of fracture treatment, and the interested reader is referred to his text, as well as to Colton's review in chapter 1, for details.[217]

Watson-Jones, the British surgeon and teacher, had an overwhelming influence on fracture treatment throughout the English-speaking world during the latter half of the twentieth century. He believed that "nonunion is never inevitable and that every fracture will unite if it is immobilized long enough."[298] He recommended immediate anatomic reduction and absolute immobilization in a long-leg, non–weight-bearing plaster cast until union was secure. He further believed that open reduction and internal fixation, if properly

performed and protected postoperatively with plaster, led to healing as rapid as with any other treatment. He thus emphasized reduction and rest until bone union, followed by rehabilitation.

Since the 1960s, fracture treatment can be briefly characterized as a reaction to the principles and practices that Watson-Jones espoused. During this period, both nonoperative and operative tibial fracture treatment have emphasized, and demonstrated the value of, functional regimens that encourage weight bearing, joint motion, or both, depending on fracture characteristics and the chosen treatment. Appreciation of the benefits of both varieties of functional fracture treatment was solidified by Sarmiento's 1974 symposium in *Clinical Orthopaedics and Related Research.*[244] Modern approaches for treating tibial shaft fractures borrow freely from earlier work and emphasize (1) categorization according to severity, (2) nonoperative management of less severe injuries, (3) adequate debridement of necrotic and contaminated tissue in open fractures, (4) external fixation and early soft tissue repair for severe open injuries, (5) minimally traumatic but mechanically sound internal fixation when necessary to preserve alignment, and (6) early bone grafting of severe injuries with a high risk of healing problems.[35,42,43,68,145,231,237,246,280,284,311]

CURRENT TREATMENT ALGORITHM

Faced with a tibial shaft fracture, the surgeon must evaluate the injury, anticipate any problems that might develop, and choose from among several alternatives an appropriate plan of management that will be simultaneously safe and effective. The goal is a healed functional limb with minimal pain and deformity and without an unduly long period of disability. Surprisingly favorable results are often obtained after tibia fractures; they are perhaps too routinely expected. Therefore it is important to establish reasonable goals for a given patient and injury at the outset. Included in these goals should be an acknowledgment of the risks of complications. Definition of goals is a great help for planning treatment. Their clear documentation is of unquestioned value when complications occur or when treatment decisions are reviewed.

The initial evaluation of a tibial fracture must identify the need for urgent limb-saving treatment. Inadequate arterial inflow requires identification and speedy correction; otherwise myoneural necrosis, and often amputation, will result. Compartmental pressure elevation can produce similar problems and similarly requires urgent treatment. These two conditions typically have different presentations. Acute arterial insufficiency is usually present when the patient is first encountered, though its onset may be delayed. Compartment syndromes, on the other hand, generally develop after some hours, although they may occasionally occur early in the patient's course. Each condition requires emergency treatment, and therefore both must be remembered during the early care of a tibia fracture.

Arterial insufficiency requires that the fractured tibia immediately be provisionally reduced and splinted and then reassessed for palpable pulses. With alignment maintained by manual traction, it may be possible to measure arterial pressures at the ankle using Doppler ultrasound. If perfusion is restored by such a reduction, caution is still warranted, for an arterial injury with potential for delayed occlusion may still exist. An arteriogram should be considered. If reduction and splinting do not immediately restore adequate blood flow, then vascular surgery is required if the leg is to be saved.[52,123] The fracture surgeon must obtain immediate consultation and decide whether there are enough time and a need for an arteriogram. Alternatively, the patient is taken directly to the operating room for exploration and repair. Some tibial fractures with arterial injuries, particularly open fractures and those involving long treatment delays or in compromised patients, are best managed with primary amputation.[109,113] The treatment of vascular injuries with tibial fractures is discussed later in this chapter and in chapter 12.

If the injured limb is severely painful or swollen or demonstrates impaired neuromuscular function, an acute compartment syndrome may be present. If persuasive clinical findings are present, the patient must be taken to the operating room immediately for fasciotomies and fracture stabilization. Tissue pressure measurements can aid in making this decision. Compartment syndromes are discussed in chapter 13, and their management with tibia fractures is detailed further later in this chapter.

Severe peripheral nerve deficits should also be identified as early as possible. Although they rarely require primary treatment, their effect on the prognosis and management of the entire injury complex may be considerable, and their prompt identification establishes an important baseline.

In addition to limb or compartmental ischemia, any open fracture wound must be promptly identified, for it requires emergency surgical treatment.[99] Skin wounds in the field of a potential surgical incision indicate relatively immediate surgery, as may exceptionally severe closed soft tissue injuries. If an open fracture is present, a sterile dressing is placed on the wound, with pressure if needed to control bleeding. An appropriately padded splint is applied. Tetanus prophylaxis and parenteral antibiotics are administered, and the patient

is taken to the operating room as soon as practical.[215] Treatment of open tibial shaft fractures is discussed later and also in chapters 14 and 15.

Unless acute arterial insufficiency, compartmental ischemia, or an open wound are present, there is little urgency for definitive reduction and stabilization of a closed tibial shaft fracture. What is important is the application of a well-padded splint, followed by elevation and rest for the injured limb. Repeated manipulations, cast changes or wedging, and the use of prolonged anesthetics while striving for an optimal reduction should not be a part of the early care of the patient with a tibial fracture, for they may add soft tissue injury, are painful, interfere with discovery of developing ischemia, are often followed by the need to loosen or remove a laboriously adjusted cast, and usually must be done at an inconvenient time with insufficient assistance. A much better policy is prompt and gentle realignment of the injured limb, followed by application of a well-padded cast. The quality of the reduction achieved by a single attempt is then a guide for subsequent therapy. Unless an indication for immediate surgery develops, the next phase of treatment is usually best deferred until the patient's swelling is resolving and necessary assistance and equipment are available. In contrast to fractures of the femur or pelvis, tibial fractures are sufficiently supported by such a cast for early mobilization to a sitting position. A long leg cast interferes only minimally with the care of a multiply injured patient. This is not to say that very early open reduction and internal fixation of a tibial fracture cannot be carried out safely.[186,280] However, it is not yet established that the patient will benefit from this approach. On the other hand, should an anesthetic be required for treating other injuries, the fracture surgeon must decide, with due consideration of all aspects of the situation, whether to proceed or to defer definitive fixation of a closed tibial shaft fracture. Studies have shown that traction to regain length of an acute tibial shaft fracture elevates compartmental pressure.[256] Compartment syndromes have occurred after closed intramedullary nailing of such injuries as well, though they may be rare.[186,282] They have also followed repeated attempts at closed reduction and have been missed because the patient was anesthetized during the initial period of painful ischemia.

SPECIAL CONSIDERATIONS FOR POLYTRAUMA PATIENTS

Patients with multiple injuries are more likely to have more severe tibial fractures and thus are more likely to require operative treatment. These fractures may be open, ischemic, or associated with ipsilateral femur fractures (floating knees) or contralateral lower extremity injuries. Regardless of whether the tibia fracture itself requires surgery, the patient usually does for other reasons. Therefore primary management of the tibial fracture takes place in the operating room. If the tibial injury requires surgical care for the indications listed previously, then the major issue becomes one of where its treatment falls in the sequence of procedures that must be carried out. Lifesaving, limb-saving, wound management, and fracture stabilization procedures are generally carried out in that order, with some variations possible if multiple teams make simultaneous procedures possible or if transfers from one operating table to another can be eliminated safely. Although a fracture table may be desirable for intramedullary fixation of the femur, it provides a poor surface for exposure of a tibial fracture, especially if extensive debridement or vascular repair becomes necessary. Therefore with an ipsilateral femur fracture, it may be best to splint the tibia, nail the femur, and then move the patient to a regular or radiolucent operating table for treatment of the tibial injury, unless arterial or compartmental pressure problems are present and require treatment first. Severe, limb-threatening tibial fractures in the polytrauma patient deserve serious consideration of amputation. This expedient debridement of crushed tissue may be in the patient's overall best interests, even if the leg is potentially salvageable. If the polytrauma patient's tibial fracture is a less serious one and its nonoperative management does not compromise overall care of the patient or the injured limb, then primary immobilization as described later is appropriate. If closed nailing is the optimal treatment for the tibial fracture, then delaying this may prove safer, as mentioned previously. Deferring tibial fixation must, however, be weighed against the possibility of unexpectedly prolonged delays. Immediate, extensive external skeletal fixation can provide rapid stabilization of badly injured limbs in severely injured patients.[235] Early fixation of an associated tibial fracture, particularly in the case of an ipsilateral femur fracture, may expedite diagnosis and treatment of an associated knee injury.

THE DECISION FOR OPERATIVE TREATMENT

Limb-threatening tibial fractures require urgent surgery. These include fractures with associated arterial injuries, those with compartment syndromes, and open fractures. Some form of operative fracture fixation is usually advisable, as is correction of the primary problem by vascular repair, fasciotomy, or irrigation and debridement of the open wound. True type I open tibial fractures are an exception. After surgical debridement, cast and brace immobilization are usually sufficient.

With the exception of these limb-threatening conditions, the indications for surgical stabilization of a tibial fracture are relative and require good judgment by the surgeon. This has been adequately discussed by Tile and by Chapman.[42,43,280] Because most low-energy tibial fractures respond well to functional fracture bracing techniques, specific indications must be present for fracture fixation to be recommended. These indications are usually found in more severe injuries and are outlined in Figure 51–11, the recommended algorithm for tibial fracture management.

Unless urgent surgery is required, the tibial fracture is reduced provisionally by gravity manipulation and immobilized in a long-leg cast. If alignment is satisfactory and other indications for surgery are and remain absent, then functional bracing becomes the definitive treatment. Severe (major) injuries, those with unsatisfactory reductions, those with specific indications, and some moderately severe injuries need elective surgical fixation at an appropriate time, usually within the next few days. Specific indications include displaced fractures involving the knee or ankle; segmental fractures; those with ipsilateral femur fractures (floating knees); those with contralateral lower extremity injuries; and perhaps multiply injured patients, if tibial fracture fixation will significantly aid their management.[171,179,290] The rationale for operating on closed tibial fractures of major, and sometimes moderate, severity is the prolonged disability and frequent morbidity associated with these injuries; these are often decreased by appropriate fracture fixation. For some fractures, and some surgeons, surgical fixation of a tibial fracture remains controversial.[61,101,165,209,221] More than one form of management may be appropriate for a given fracture. Figure 51–12 shows examples of fixation options for each of the three grades of tibial fracture severity.

TIBIAL FRACTURES REQUIRING IMMEDIATE SURGERY

Tibial Fractures With Vascular Injuries

The dire prognosis of open tibial fractures with associated arterial injuries has been emphasized by a number of authors.[41,53,109,113,161] If tissue ischemia is present, only prompt successful vascular repair will permit limb salvage. The extent of associated injuries may be such that the salvaged limb is less functional than a prosthesis, in spite of lengthy, elaborate, and potentially dangerous reconstructive procedures. Therefore it is essential to balance carefully the risks and likely functional outcome of salvage attempts against the expectations

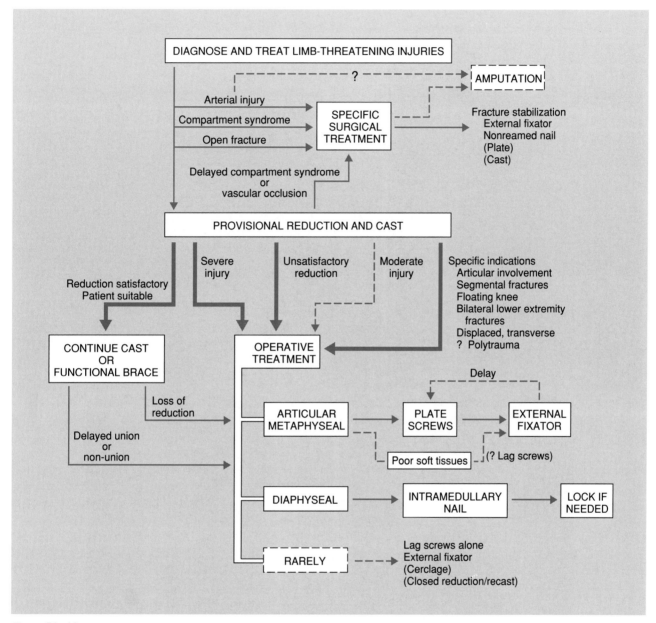

Figure 51–11

Algorithm for management of tibial shaft fractures. The first step is to identify and treat limb-threatening conditions. Next a provisional gravity reduction is usually performed in the emergency treatment area. Depending on the surgeon's assessment, injury characteristics, and the patient's preferences, one of the several listed treatments may be chosen. Response to treatment must be monitored, with changes in therapy instituted as needed.

after primary amputation. Early amputation is often a safer, surer, swifter, and less costly means to restore function than attempts at limb salvage. It must be considered carefully for patients with severe tibial fractures, especially if arterial compromise exists.[25,222] However, when the situation permits, vascular repair can be followed by wound and fracture healing and restoration of normal function (Fig. 51–13). Thus respect for the travails and frequently poor functional

results of attempted limb salvage must be tempered by an awareness that such salvage attempts may be appropriate. Current efforts to establish a rational protocol for making this difficult decision are discussed later in the section on primary amputation.

A patient with a tibial fracture and an arterial injury that causes limb-threatening ischemia is a candidate for arterial reconstruction if flow can be restored within 6 to 8 hours after injury; if there is no anatomic loss of the

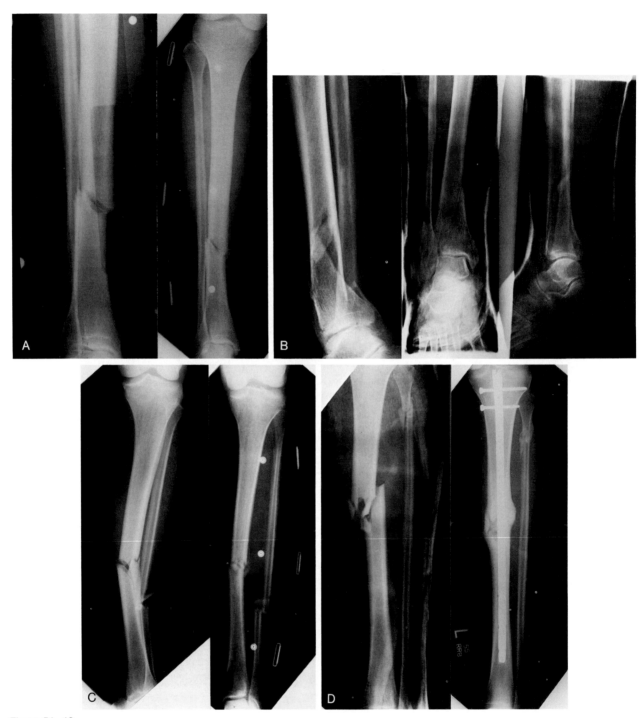

Figure 51–12

Radiographic examples of fracture fixation techniques for each of the three grades of tibial fracture. *A*, Minor-grade fracture of tibial midshaft healing satisfactorily in functional brace. *B*, Minor-grade distal tibiofibular shaft fracture with minimal ankle joint involvement as demonstrated by CT. A functional cast is used for better maintenance of alignment in a distal injury, and weight bearing is initially restricted to 15 to 20 lb. *C*, Moderate severity injury, with stable reduction in provisional cast, healing satisfactorily in functional brace. *D*, Moderate severity tibial fracture. A nonreamed, proximally locked intramedullary nail provides alignment and stability.

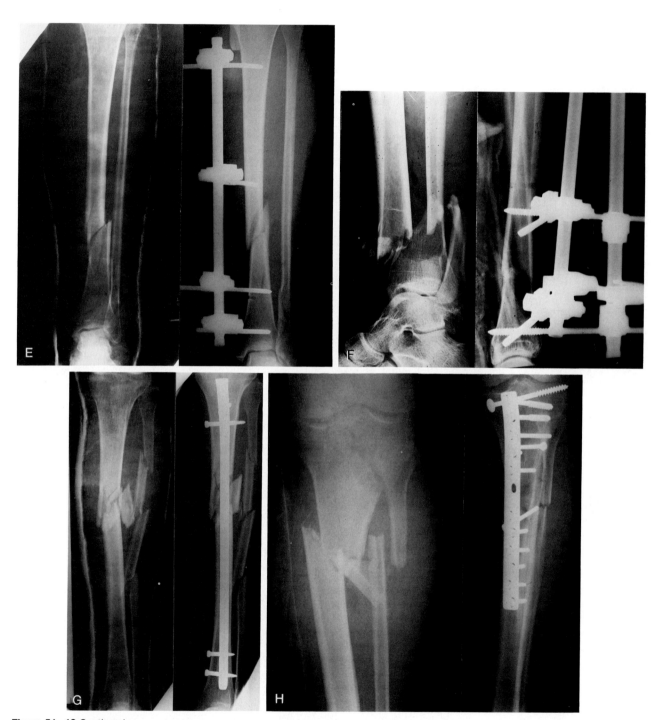

Figure 51–12 *Continued*

E, Moderate severity, spiral, slightly comminuted fracture that developed compartment syndrome after gravity reduction and provisional casting. External fixation was maintained with progressive weight bearing until the fracture became stable, after which a functional brace was used for another six weeks. *F*, Major severity, open, distal tibiofibular fracture treated with a two-plane external fixator. *G*, Major severity, closed, crushing fracture of the tibia and fibula with circumferential fracture comminution. Length and rotational stability secured with a statically-locked reamed intramedullary nail. *H*, Major severity, open intraarticular fracture reduced and stabilized with plate and lag screw fixation. The nonstandard broad plate was used because of extensive comminution and osteopenia. Satisfactory fracture healing resulted and knee function was restored, although scant wound drainage persisted until the fracture had healed and the plate was removed.

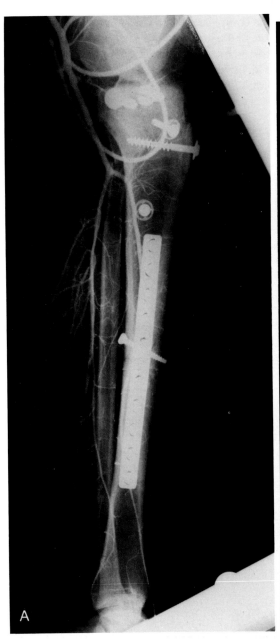

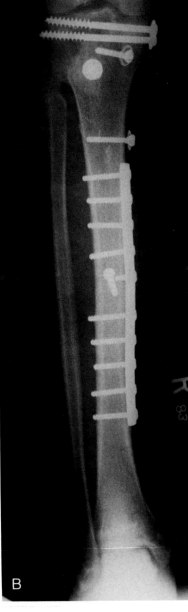

Figure 51–13

A, This "completion arteriogram" demonstrates satisfactory perfusion after arterial repair and fracture fixation in a patient with a grade IIIC open fracture of the proximal tibia with associated fracture-dislocation of the knee (see Figure 51–5 for preoperative appearance). *B*, Fracture healing with essentially normal function six months later. Although many of these injuries have a poor prognosis, limb salvage may occasionally be rewarding. It remains difficult to distinguish between patients who are best treated with amputation and those for whom reconstruction of a severely injured limb should be attempted.

tibial nerve, which provides sensation to the sole of the foot; and if salvage of a useful limb is possible without compromising the patient's overall condition.[162] Prompt diagnosis is established as described previously. Immediate surgery is indicated, with participation and collaboration of both vascular and orthopedic surgeons. Experience, prearranged protocols, and flexibility of both teams are the essentials for optimal results. A vascular injury that does not immediately threaten death of tissue is a less urgent situation than one with established muscle ischemia. In the former situation, skeletal stabilization may be done first, followed by vascular repair. In the latter, perfusion must be reestablished as rapidly as possible, followed by wound and fracture care. In such situations, the use of a temporary arterial shunt permits rapid reperfusion, followed by fracture stabilization and then definitive vascular repair. This is no time for elaborate early fracture repair. An external fixator can be applied as a splint across the tibial fracture site, if there is sufficient bone stock, or across the knee or ankle. Lag screw fixation of an open articular surface fracture is of high priority but should not delay urgent arterial repair. Musculoskeletal structures should be respected during exposure of the injured vessels.

An effective collaborative approach is for both legs to

be prepared and draped. The vascular team then harvests a contralateral saphenous vein graft while the orthopedic team exposes the injured vessels or rapidly applies an external fixator to stabilize the fracture and provide an optimal field for vascular repair. In the case of a type IIIC open fracture, wound debridement and subsequent management must also be considered. Although essential wound toilette must not delay revascularization, the high risk of infection must be acknowledged.[41,99,161] Thorough debridement is required, even though its completion may need to await vascular repair. Pulsatile wound lavage can usually be started without delaying the vascular anastomosis. This, plus antibiotic irrigation, may reduce the risk of bacterial contamination spreading throughout the wound. At the completion of arterial and any necessary venous repair, attention is once again turned to the adequacy of wound debridement. Four compartment fasciotomies are routine after arterial repair because of capillary leakage after blood flow is restored to ischemic tissue.[78] All necrotic tissue, as well as foreign contamination, must be removed. Fracture fixation must be adequate without adding to soft tissue injury. External fixation, possibly with inclusion of the foot, or a locked nonreamed intramedullary nail may be considered. An intraoperative arteriogram is advisable to confirm adequate blood flow after arterial repair and fracture stabilization. A number of recent reports discuss the management of arterial injuries associated with tibial fractures.[53,98,102,123–125,180,210,243,254,266,295]

Wounds should be managed open, as described for open fractures, but exposed blood vessels, especially where repaired, should be covered to prevent a delayed anastomotic rupture. An early return to the operating room for wound assessment and care should be routine.

Tibial Fractures With Compartment Syndromes

Whenever it develops, whether initially or during the subsequent course of a patient with a tibial fracture, a compartment syndrome requires emergency management.[70,83] The diagnosis of compartment syndromes has been discussed previously, and the reader is also referred to chapter 13. A compartment syndrome may develop in any tibia fracture. Low-energy injuries with minimal displacement are still at risk, as are open fractures with large soft tissue wounds.[23] Vigilance is necessary during the first several days after injury.[310]

At the first suggestion of increasing severe pain or neurovascular compromise, it is essential to loosen any cast or splint, cutting or spreading it to leave a wide, troughlike support for the injured limb. If this fails to provide complete relief, a decision must be made as to whether the patient has an established or developing compartment syndrome, whether arterial inflow is obstructed, or whether there is a nerve injury that mimics the motor and sensory changes of a compartment syndrome and also may prevent awareness of ischemic pain.

If increasing pain, swelling, and progressive motor and sensory deficits are present, emergency fasciotomies are indicated. Absence of peripheral pulses raises serious concern about arterial occlusion, though this can also be seen in well-established compartment syndromes. The best course is to perform immediate fasciotomies, followed by an intraoperative arteriogram if pulses do not return when normal compartmental pressures are restored. If the diagnosis is not clear, rapid measurement of pressures in all four compartments, concentrating on the region of the tibial fracture, may be used to identify those patients with some of the signs and symptoms of compartment syndrome but without elevated tissue pressures. They will not benefit from fasciotomy. Such patients should be checked carefully for external pressure over a superficial nerve, especially the peroneal nerve at the proximal fibula. Although low compartmental pressures (under 30 to 35 mm Hg) might dissuade the surgeon from fasciotomy, it is important to remember that the pressure may still be rising. Rather than an absolute tissue pressure measurement, it is important to consider the difference (ΔP) between tissue pressure and mean arterial pressure, as this is a better indicator of the risk of tissue ischemia. A ΔP less than 40 mm Hg appears critical for moderately traumatized muscle.[118] This emphasizes the increased risk of compartment syndrome in hypotensive patients. Continued vigilance and repeated measurements are needed if the patient's neurologic status prevents using the usual clinical symptoms and signs for discovery of compartment syndrome.

Adequate fasciotomy allows unfettered swelling of injured muscles without elevation of interstitial fluid pressure. Local capillary blood flow is preserved. This permits survival of nerve and muscle tissues that are sensitive to ischemia. A wide, truly decompressive fasciotomy is needed if intracompartmental pressure is or may become dangerously elevated. Unlike fasciotomies for exercise-related compartment syndromes, those required after tibia fractures are extensive. It is safest and most appropriate to treat any such leg as though all four compartments are involved. Therefore all four compartments are released to ensure decompression. Two incisions, medial and lateral, are required, and these should be placed well around to the sides of the limb and over muscle so that split-thickness skin coverage will be possible if necessary. The fascia must be divided for the entire length of each compartment (Fig. 51–14) (see chapter 13). Although fibulectomy may theoretically decompress all four compartments, it is never appropriate in the setting of a tibial fracture, as loss of the fibula may compromise reconstruction of the injured leg. A four-compartment fasciotomy using a single lateral incision that is directed both anterior and posterior to the fibula has also been proposed. This approach has two drawbacks: it is less likely to provide adequate decompression than the two-incision technique, and it adds significant soft tissue damage by requiring circumferential fibular dissection.

After fasciotomy, adequate skeletal stabilization is required for wound management and to maintain fracture alignment. External fixation, as advocated by Tscherne and Gotzen, is a safe choice, unless another technique has already been applied.[285] A nonreamed intramedullary nail may also be appropriate. Gershuni and co-workers advise stable internal fixation.[83] Plaster, which is constricting and does not provide as much stability as other techniques, is least desirable. To splint soft tissues well and to control the position of foot and ankle, the external fixator should extend to the forefoot (see later discussion under Application of External Fix-

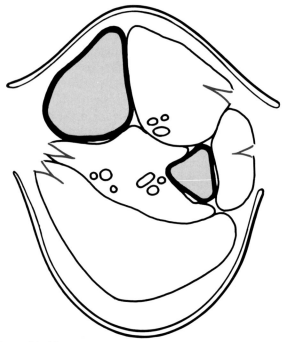

Figure 51–14

The double-incision fasciotomy permits reliable decompression of the fascial compartments of the leg. To ensure that an adequate bridge of anterior skin is left, it is important to place the incisions on midmedial and midlateral sides of the leg. Sufficient length of fasciotomy incisions and release of internal fascial envelopes, such as that around the tibialis posterior, are also important.

ator). Alternatively, a foot plate or plaster splint may be used, but caution and ample padding are required if there is any sensory impairment.

Continuing management of the tibial fracture with compartment syndrome includes delayed wound closure, often with meshed split-thickness skin graft. Depending on fracture severity, delayed bone grafting may be advisable, especially if external fixation is used.

Open Tibial Fractures

Because the tibial shaft is the most common site of significant open fractures (reviewed in detail in chapter 14), the important features of its management are discussed here. Like closed tibial fractures, the spectrum of severity is wide, with several factors affecting outcome. Therefore a single treatment is not best for all open tibial fractures. Although general principles hold true, allowances are appropriately made for the specific features of an individual patient's injury.

The initial evaluation is carried out as described previously. The wound is covered with a sterile dressing, a splint is applied to the leg, and periodic neurovascular monitoring is instituted. Appropriate tetanus prophylaxis is provided: tetanus toxoid (0.5 ml), if immunization status is unknown or more than five years have elapsed since the last dose. If prior immunization is unknown or incomplete, tetanus immunoglobulin (250 U) should be administered, with separate completion of active immunization.[52] Intravenous antibiotics are begun. Unless allergies indicate an alternative choice, a first- or second-generation cephalosporin is routinely administered, with an aminoglycoside for more severe wounds and high-dose penicillin if clostridial contamination is likely.[99,214,215] An alternative to the first-generation cephalosporin and aminoglycoside is the use of a third-generation cephalosporin alone (e.g., cefotaxime).[140]

Any open tibial fracture must be taken promptly to an operating room for thorough debridement and irrigation. Priority for open fracture debridement is immediately after life- and limb-saving care. Formal operative debridement also permits adequate grading of wound severity. The actual severity of a wound becomes apparent during its exposure and debridement. Experience improves the ability to grade and treat an open fracture[214]; good results are less likely when initial operative care is relegated to junior staff.

The wound should be graded, as discussed previously and in chapter 14, and documented in the patient's operative report. Severity is related to the size of the opening in the skin, but even more to other characteristics of the entire wound, including its degree of contamination; the amount of soft tissue necrosis, ischemia, and crushing; the extent that periosteum is stripped from bone; evidence of comminution and of bone loss; injury to neurovascular structures; and the amount of energy absorbed. A significant delay between wounding and debridement may also increase the likelihood of wound problems. A careful determination of wound severity guides both wound care and fracture fixation and establishes the patient's prognosis. By the end of debridement, there should be no doubt about the severity of an open tibial fracture, and it can readily be graded as minor, moderate, or severe (see Table 51–2).

It is easiest to carry out the initial surgical treatment of an open tibial fracture with the patient supine on a radiolucent operating table so that C-arm fluoroscopy can be used if needed to aid with fixation. A tourniquet is placed around the upper thigh to use if necessary to control excessive bleeding, to improve visualization, or to produce a postischemic capillary flush that can be used to help determine tissue viability. Waterproof sterile drapes, instruments and supplies for debridement and irrigation, and sufficient assistance are essential. It may be possible to hold the leg manually or with a support during skin preparation, but this can be difficult if the limb is unstable. An alternative is to carry out the preparation with the leg on waterproof sterile drapes, which are sequentially replaced as the prep progresses. With dressings covering the wounds, gross dirt is removed from the skin. This is often best done with a surgical scrub brush. Hair immediately adjacent to a wound is trimmed or shaved. Degreasing solvents may be required. These solvents, soaps, and alcohols, should be kept out of open wounds. Very contaminated wounds often benefit from pulsating lavage at this stage, but this is usually reserved until after the sterile field has been established. After all soap has been rinsed away and the limb dried, the skin is prepared with a povidone-iodine solution, which need not be excluded from the wound surfaces. The prepped area extends from the toes to the tourniquet. Sterile drapes are applied, allowing circumferential access to the entire limb. A sterile glove or small adhesive drape can cover the toes.

Careful planning is required before incising the skin for debridement. Unless the initial wound is unquestionably adequate, the surgeon must choose between enlarging it or bypassing it with a standard incision. The goal is to obtain adequate access for wound debridement while preserving thick viable tissue flaps that will at least cover bone, tendons, and neurovascular structures. All these are harmed by desiccation and are poorly covered by split-thickness skin grafts. Incisions over muscle can readily be managed with such skin grafts, if delayed suture closure proves impossible.

Because a significant component of skin blood flow is carried at the level of the deep fascia, all surgically created flaps should be fasciocutaneous (i.e., they should include skin, subcutaneous fat, and underlying deep fascia, which is dissected as required from the underlying muscle). This preserves local blood flow and improves flap survival. During exposure of open tibial fractures, the physician should look for degloved flaps of skin and subcutaneous tissue separated from underlying fascia by shearing forces produced by crushing and rollover mechanisms. If there is any question of viability, the technique of split-thickness skin excision can be used to identify the viable portion of the flap, which is preserved while the avascular part is excised down to healthy muscle.[313] It is essential to explore the wound thoroughly, as the fractured end of the tibia can protrude temporarily through a small surface wound and then retract inside, carrying with it a surprising amount of dirt and debris. In addition to foreign material, all necrotic muscle, unattached bone fragments, tags of subcutaneous fat, and exposed fascia should be excised. Necrotic muscle is identified primarily by its lack of bleeding, contractility, and normal elastic consistency. Nerves, superficial and deep veins, arteries, and tendons of functional muscles should be retained, as should the periosteum with blood supply and the paratenon, which protects its tendon from desiccation and necrosis. The physician must remember the possibility of a compartment syndrome developing in an open fracture, for the wound does not reliably decompress even a single compartment.[23] For severe injuries, fasciotomies should be a routine part of the debridement procedure. Copious irrigation, conventionally with warmed Ringer's lactate or normal saline solution, is best delivered with a pulsatile lavage system. This is aided by supporting the leg on an irrigating pan that collects the fluid after it has run through the wound. New gowns, gloves, sterile waterproof drapes, and new sterile instruments are used for the fracture fixation phase of the initial operation for open tibial fractures.

A definitive management plan is developed, based upon the wound, the fracture configuration, the patient's overall status, and the resources available. Any incisions should be planned to accommodate the likely choice of fixation. However, the needs of the wound, rather than the surgeon's choice of stabilization, should ultimately determine all choices made during debridement of an open fracture.

Occasionally a very severe open tibia fracture, especially in a multiply injured patient or one with preexisting medical problems, is better treated with amputation than with salvage. (Amputation is discussed further later in this chapter.) Fractures that have an appropriate bone configuration may be stabilized with a nonreamed nail, though this is still controversial for type III injuries.[44,63,115,120,266a,293,302,306] With the development of nonreamed, lockable intramedullary nails for the tibia, there is little need to consider reamed intramedullary nailing for open fractures. The most severe open tibia fractures are usually managed with external fixation. If the fracture extends into the articular surface of the knee or ankle, then anatomic reduction and lag screw fixation should generally be done primarily, especially if the wound is severe and coverage problems are anticipated.

The next decision, after reconstructing the joint surface is more difficult. The entire tibial injury may be stabilized by external fixation, either from the metaphyseal fragment to the diaphysis or by ligamentotaxis, with the fixator anchored beyond the tibia to the femur proximally or the calcaneus distally.[35] Alternatively, a buttress plate can be used. These options are discussed further later, but it must be emphasized here that the risk of wound complications is higher with plating techniques and is reduced with the external fixator.[9] The plate gives more secure, long-lasting fixation, with the possibility of moving the injured joint as soon as the wound permits, and often gains a good result in spite of problems with infection.[50] However, its application usually requires dissection beyond that produced by the original trauma and debridement. This "adds insult to injury," and is ill advised in most acute open tibial fractures. Occasionally, with low-energy wounds and stable fracture configurations, nonoperative fracture management (also discussed later) is a way to maintain alignment of an open tibial fracture, but it does not provide enough stability of bone and soft tissue to produce the optimal environment for early wound healing and resistance to infection. Ultimately, the choice of fixation for an open tibial fracture is a compromise between that required for the fracture and that required for the soft tissue, with the latter taking precedence.

Whatever fixation is chosen, the open fracture wound should not be closed primarily, but should instead be left open to avoid tension on the soft tissue and resulting microvascular embarrassment. An additional benefit is the opportunity to reassess adequacy of debridement and soft tissue viability early in the postinjury course. The time-honored practice of delayed wound closure has been supported by the experimental studies of Edlich and co-workers and the recent clinical study of Russell et al.[66,238]

Several technical aspects of open wound care are important. Desiccation of exposed tissue must be prevented. Continuous wet dressings can be used, but these may dry or fail to prevent wound contamination. An immediate split-thickness skin graft; allograft or xenograft skin; or artificial skin substitutes (e.g., Epigard, Biobrane, or Op-Site), perhaps using the bead pouch technique described by Henry and co-workers,[74,115a] should be applied. Especially for more distal fractures, the ankle should be splinted to minimize soft tissue motion in the wound area.

Continuing management of the open fracture wound depends on its severity. Type I and many type II wounds can be left covered with sterile dressings and then closed five to seven days after injury either with sutures or by application of a meshed split-thickness skin graft, if the wound edges are not easily brought together. All patients with type III wounds or any questionable type II wound should be returned to the operating room in 24 to 72 hours for thorough reassessment with adequate anesthesia.[35,300] This procedure involves irrigating out all clot, carefully looking for and removing any necrotic tissue, reassessing fracture reduction and stability, and then resuming open wound management in a way that prevents desiccation, as just described. At this time it is too early to proceed with delayed primary closure, although if the wound is clean and viable, then application of a meshed split-thickness skin graft can be considered.

During this return to the operating room, which should be repeated as many times and as frequently as needed, plans for definitive wound closure are formulated and carried out as soon as appropriate.[312] During dressing change and debridement, consulting physicians can inspect the wound together and collaborate on decision making. Type IIIA wounds can usually be closed by suture or by meshed split-thickness skin graft. Type IIIB and IIIC wounds, on the other hand, will usually require muscle flap coverage with either a healthy local muscle or a microvascular free flap. The timing of such a closure should be individualized,[40] but it must be postponed until adequate debridement is ensured. Although there is support in the literature for very early closure of such wounds, application of a muscle flap makes subsequent wound evaluation more difficult.[47,85] When there is a significant possibility of retained nonviable tissue, less hasty coverage is advisable. However, there is no reason to delay once it is clear that the wound is free of necrotic tissue. Failure to achieve adequate debridement and gain wound coverage within the first week or two after injury suggests a higher risk of problems after flap coverage. The greatest difficulty comes with severe wounds in which it is difficult to determine tissue viability until after several debridements.

Attempts to gain coverage with local tissues by using "relaxing incisions" or local rotational flaps are unwise, especially when the amount of soft tissue damage is more severe. These will often result in loss of additional soft tissue. Preservation of injured local skin is best achieved by avoiding incisions that create superficial, narrow, or distally based flaps, by taking pains to place incisions over muscle, and by using tension-free closure with split-thickness skin over viable muscle, or, if this is not possible, by transposing healthy muscle into the wound as a pedicle or free flap, depending on location and available tissue.[182]

Fracture healing of severe open tibial fractures often benefits from a cancellous bone graft, which is especially valuable when external fixation is used. It may be essential if there is a bone defect. Bone grafts should be placed under healthy, well-vascularized tissue, such as the muscles of the deep posterior compartment or perhaps a muscle pedicle flap. In general, it is best to delay such grafts until secure wound healing is present, and to use pure cancellous graft for its greater resistance to infection. In situations in which a graft will be required under a muscle flap, one should consider putting antibiotic-laden acrylic cement beads under the flap and replacing the beads with cancellous bone graft several weeks later.[45]

PRIMARY FRACTURE IMMOBILIZATION

Unless an indication for immediate surgery is identified, the following approach is recommended. Most closed tibia fractures can be aligned quite well with a closed reduction in a dependent position and application of a long-leg cast.[42,43,165,247,280]

Radiographs of the fracture are then obtained, rotational alignment is reconfirmed by visual comparison, and unless a *major* problem with malalignment is noted, the reduction is accepted, at least temporarily. The patient is hospitalized with the leg elevated slightly above heart level and is observed for comfort and neurovascular status. If the cast becomes too tight or the surgeon has serious concern about impending circulatory compromise, then the plaster is loosened and the cast padding divided. If these measures do not maintain or restore satisfactory neurovascular status, then arterial perfusion and compartmental pressures are checked, with further immediate surgical treatment as indicated. With a satisfactory reduction and no evidence of neurovascular compromise, it is expeditious to leave the provisional cast intact. If reduction is not satisfactory or closed treatment is, for some other reason, less desirable, then definitive fixation may be carried out electively after the initial swelling has begun to resolve but without excessive delay.

An alternative to gravity reduction and cast application is the use of skeletal traction applied by way of either the distal tibia or the calcaneus. Either a centrally threaded external fixator pin or a smooth K wire with

ample padding between the skin and tractor bow arms may be used. The leg is supported on a Böhler-Braun or equivalent frame, and traction is limited to the least force needed to maintain length and stability. This can be continued for several weeks until early consolidation makes an initially unstable reduction manageable in a cast.[148]

Procedure

Advance preparation is a great aid to reduction and cast application. Before beginning, it is necessary to have close at hand ample cast padding, usually as 4-in rolls; plaster rolls, 4- to 6-in; plaster splints or fiberglass cast material if desired; a bucket of cool water; and a cast saw. The patient's radiographs should be visible on a viewbox. A seat is helpful for the person applying the cast. The task requires at least two people: one to hold the leg and the other to apply the cast. The patient must be as comfortable as possible, and his or her cooperation and understanding should be encouraged. An intravenous line should be in place. Analgesia is often best provided with intravenous narcotics (e.g., morphine sulfate, 3 to 8 mg, titrated as needed). Naloxone and other similar medications and resuscitation equipment should be readily available. A hematoma block with 1% lidocaine may be considered, but only with scrupulous attention to sterile technique, and awareness of the risk of systemic effects (myocardial depression, seizures).

The patient is positioned recumbent on an examining or operating table. Both legs are checked to ensure that rotational alignment and contours of the normal limb are used to guide the reduction. This can be facilitated by hanging both legs over the end of the table, or the injured leg can be abducted at the hip and hung over the table's side. There must be enough room to allow padding and plaster to be rolled around the upper calf. The assistant holds the forefoot, steadying the leg and maintaining its alignment, especially regarding rotation and foot position. Rotational alignment is not fixed with the knee flexed but can be gauged fairly well using the relationship of second toe to tibial tubercle, as demonstrated by the opposite limb. The assistant's fingers are placed under the plantar surface, with the thumb over the dorsum of the foot. Thus plantarflexion and inversion (supination) are controlled, both of which tend to occur and subsequently interfere with weight bearing in this cast. Although ankle equinus is occasionally the alternative to apex posterior angulation of a distal tibial fracture site, it may often be avoided if, as Sarmiento suggests, the initial cast is applied with the foot in neutral.[245-247]

The assistant maintains foot position as chosen while

ample cast padding is rolled (over the thumb and fingers) onto the foot and up as high on the leg as the flexed knee will allow (Fig. 51–15). Developing soft tissue edema and the leg's characteristic bony prominences argue for thick padding, as does the likelihood that the cast will need to be cut in the near future, while the leg is still swollen. Because the patient will be supine, extra padding is required posterior to the heel, where much of the weight will be borne. The malleoli, the fibular head and neck with the surrounding peroneal nerve, and the subcutaneous tibial border also require extra padding. The padding is palpated to ensure its adequacy, supplemented if necessary, and then a thin plaster (ten layers at most) is rolled on from the toe metatarsophalangeal joints to an inch or two below the top of the padding at the knee. The plantar surface may be extended to support the toes, but the dorsum is trimmed proximal to all five metatarsophalangeal joints.

Plaster is still easier to apply and mold than fiberglass. However, it should be left thin to simplify alterations and avoid unnecessary weight. Overlying fiberglass reinforcement can be applied in a day or two, once it is clear that the cast will be left in place. As the plaster sets, molding is carried out to make the shape of the medial border of the cast similar to that of the patient's opposite leg; a straight cast usually results in valgus malalignment. Ensure that the foot position has been maintained.

Once the lower leg portion is firm, it is used to hold the leg horizontal, with the knee flexed 10° to 15° and the thigh sufficiently clear of the table surface to allow padding to be extended proximally an inch beyond the intended top of the cast, approximately two thirds of the way up the thigh. Plaster is then rolled on, overlapping by 4 to 6 inches the top of the previously applied lower portion. It is essential that there be adequate padding at the junction of the two

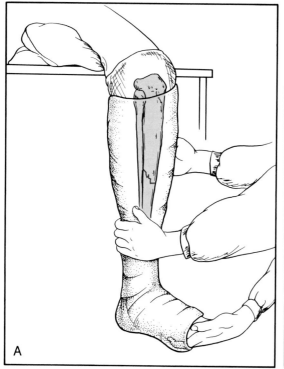

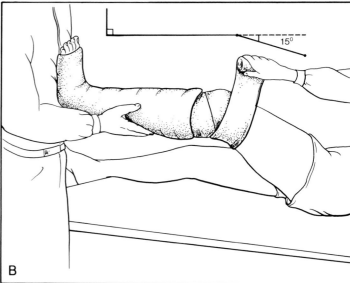

Figure 51–15

Most acute tibial shaft fractures will reduce fairly satisfactorily if they are hung over the side of an examining table with the foot correctly rotated and supported in neutral. *A*, The leg must hang far enough away from the table to allow circumferential access. A pad under the proximal thigh may help. It is imperative to have an assistant hold the foot and steady the leg. The surgeon ensures that alignment is correct and applies ample cast padding, especially over the posterior heel, malleoli, and proximal fibula; the fracture site; and where the cast will be cut. Plaster is rolled on over the padding, leaving a segment of padding exposed just below the knee to be overlapped later by the above-knee part of the plaster. Gentle molding by the surgeon often improves alignment, especially by making the medial surface slightly concave to match that of the normal leg. Six to eight layers of plaster are usually sufficient, perhaps with extra reinforcement at the knee and ankle. *B*, Once the lower portion of the cast is firm, it is used to support the limb in correct rotation and with the knee flexed approximately 15°. Cast padding is then rolled over the thigh, and an upper cuff of stockinette is applied if desired. Padding of the patella and hamstring tendons is important. Plaster is then applied approximately two thirds of the way up the thigh, overlapping the lower-leg part of the cast by 4 to 6 in. The padding is turned down over the top of the cast to avoid a sharp edge. The leg must be supported until the plaster is hard; then rotational alignment is checked by comparison with the opposite leg, and AP and lateral radiographs of the full tibia are obtained.

segments, but no padding should lie between the layers of plaster.

As soon as is practical, AP and lateral radiographs are obtained of the entire tibia within the cast, and a decision is made as to the provisional adequacy of reduction and plaster. Only if there is marked deformity or risk of skin compromise should the appearance of these radiographs lead to changing the cast. Adjustments such as wedging, applying a new cast, or changing to another mode of treatment are better deferred until swelling has resolved.

The long-leg cast just applied may need to be loosened to accommodate potential or actual swelling of the injured limb. Although it is wise to always provide for such swelling, many low-energy tibia fractures can remain, without loosening, in an intact cast; routine splitting of all such casts results in unnecessary manipulation and may compromise the security of the cast during weight bearing.

A cast may be loosened in several ways. If swelling is severe and likely to progress, the cast should be converted to a posterior trough splint. This is done by removing the anterior third of the cast and bending both sides outward wide enough to permit removal of the leg and avoid any pressure on the sides of the limb. The padding is cut anteriorly and folded outward to allow examination of the limb and to ensure that the padding itself is not a source of constriction. Removal of part of the medial wall at the ankle can allow assessment of the posterior tibial pulse (Fig. 51–16). A practical concern about removing strips and windows from casts is that the stability of the cast may be compromised. The result can be a plaster cast that fails to immobilize the injured limb and does not prevent pain and additional tissue trauma. To avoid such problems, use fiberglass reinforcement or judicious alterations in the plaster (delayed until it has hardened and is more

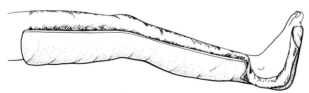

Figure 51–16

A cast can be loosened somewhat by cutting its anterior surface from top to bottom, using a cast spreader to open the cut, and then bending the sides out and stretching the cast padding to loosen it as well. To accommodate significant swelling or to permit adequate observation of a severely injured limb while maintaining an adequate splint, the long-leg cast can be converted into a trough splint, after it has hardened adequately, by removing an anterior strip approximately one third the cast circumference in width. The cast padding is cut and turned back, and the sides of the cast are bent outward to eliminate pressure on the leg. The trim line is placed posteriorly, if needed, in the area of the posterior tibial pulse to permit its palpation in cases of potential vascular injury.

able to retain its shape and strength); and reassess the adequacy of the plaster frequently.

Removal of an anterior strip prevents ongoing use of the cast. An alternative is to split the cast anteriorly after it has hardened for an hour or two and to widen this cut sufficiently with cast spreaders so that the padding is stretched and subsequent loosening of the cast will be easy. This "univalve" cast may be salvaged after swelling recedes by squeezing it together and encircling it with adhesive tape just tightly enough to provide adequate support. Once a final adjustment has been made, fiberglass reinforcement is added to make the cast strong enough to begin ambulation. It is important to realize that this technique of cast spreading does not provide adequate decompression in the presence of serious swelling. In addition to longitudinal cuts in the cast, windows may be removed to check questionable areas of skin, to relieve pressure over a bony prominence, or to assess pulses. The removed plaster window should be retained and taped securely in place when the opening is not in use. Doing this adds to the strength of the cast and maintains enough overlying pressure to avoid "window edema"—swelling of the soft tissues into the window defect.

If the cast is left intact, then there must be fail-safe arrangements for it to be released if the patient develops significant pain or neurovascular compromise. Although this generally requires hospitalization, occasionally a patient may be sent home if he or she has a low-energy injury, is able to use crutches and to transfer, and has adequate assistance and prompt transportation back to the hospital. Whether as an outpatient or in the hospital, the patient should keep the injured leg elevated and should be followed closely for increasing pain, decreasing sensation, and loss of palpable toe muscle strength. Pain after a tibial fracture is largely relieved by adequate splinting. Narcotic analgesics are usually required, but standard doses of morphine or meperidine should be effective and should be required progressively less frequently. After a day or two, oral narcotics should be sufficient during the daytime, with injectable narcotics needed only at night. Lack of response to analgesia suggests neurovascular problems.

DEFINITIVE TREATMENT MODALITIES

Nonoperative Treatment (Functional Cast or Brace)

Sarmiento, perhaps the most eloquent advocate and teacher of nonoperative functional treatment of tibial fractures, originally conveyed the impression that most such injuries could be managed according to his guidelines.[244] However, in a recent report of tibial shaft fractures treated with functional braces, he emphasized that the technique was applied to selected patients and that many other tibial fractures were treated operatively.[245,246] He stated that high-energy tibial fractures and fractures in patients with multiple injuries or ipsilateral femur fractures were usually treated with surgical fixation, which was also indicated for fractures with excessive initial shortening, segmental bone loss, and neurovascular damage and for those whose alignment was not maintained satisfactorily in the initial cast or subsequent brace.

Functional treatment of tibial fractures has yielded low rates of nonunion, infection, and significant malunion. However, it is important to recognize that properly managed closed functional treatment has been effective only for selected low-energy tibial fractures.[8,62,101,219] Functional bracing is unsuitable, at least in the early stages, for tibial fractures with significant associated soft tissue injury. Using the classification system described previously, functional bracing, as a primary treatment, should be restricted to tibial fractures of minor severity. Occasional moderate severity injuries can also be managed in this way.

Functional bracing begins with a closed gravity realignment and application of an initial cast. Rarely, it may be considered if manipulation under anesthesia can provide an assuredly stable closed reduction. In addition to injury severity, the adequacy of reduction in this cast and the patient's subsequent clinical course are the most important determinants of whether closed functional treatment is appropriate. The amount of soft tissue damage determines the shortening that may occur. Ultimate shortening is usually predictable from the amount of shortening apparent on the initial radiographs. Brace treatment is generally not appropriate if there is more than 1 cm shortening, as measured by fragment overlap or by scanogram in plaster. Poor control of angulation in a plaster long-leg cast is also a contraindication to functional bracing, unless it can be expected that a properly applied brace or functional patellar tendon weight-bearing (PTB) cast will improve angular alignment. Angulation on either the AP or lateral radiograph should not exceed 5°.

Significant comminution and displacement of more than a third of the shaft diameter are relative contraindications to closed functional treatment because of their association with delayed healing when this treatment is used. Closed functional treatment is not optimal for patients with intraarticular fractures that would prevent weight bearing, for patients with bilateral lower extremity injuries who could walk on a tibial fracture if it were fixed with an intramedullary nail, for patients with high-energy injuries with extensive closed or open soft tissue injuries, and for patients with ipsilateral

femur fractures.[171,280,290] Elderly and infirm patients may be better able to care for themselves after fracture fixation if fixation permits weight bearing sooner with greater comfort and less encumbrance.[239] Unreliable patients, who may not return faithfully for follow-up visits during the four to seven months typically required for fracture healing, may have lower risks if internal fixation can be done in a way that permits unrestricted weight bearing. If this is not possible, then internal fixation is not as safe as closed treatment.[144]

Fracture braces and functional casts rely on soft tissues, primarily the interosseous membrane, to prevent shortening while the surrounding cast controls angulation and rotation.[236,247] When soft tissue disruption is considerable, a simple closed reduction cannot stabilize a displaced oblique or spiral fracture or one with significant comminution. A transverse fracture, however, may have its length and stability restored with a closed reduction and cast application under anesthesia, if end-on-end apposition can be maintained. This has been advocated for such injuries. These injuries are so readily and safely treated with closed intramedullary nailing (described later), that it seems inappropriate to subject a patient to anesthesia for a closed reduction without offering the benefit of stable fixation as well.

Functional cast or brace treatment is advisable after removal of an external fixator. Its use for this purpose is discussed in the section on external fixation.

The following protocol for closed functional treatment of tibial shaft fractures is similar to that which Sarmiento and his co-workers have developed.[245–247] The first stage involves application of a gravity reduction cast, as previously described. An acceptable reduction must be confirmed. After an initial day or two of elevation, usually in the hospital, ambulation is encouraged, with weight bearing as tolerated using a removable cast boot. Crutches or a walker are recommended for as long as needed. The patient is asked to elevate the limb when not walking and to do isometric exercises with the immobilized muscles and active and passive exercises for the toes. He or she should be reassured about the inevitable motion of fracture fragments felt inside the cast. In addition to the exercise program, physical therapy is helpful for gait training on a level surface, and on stairs and for transfers. Once patients are comfortable and mobile enough to manage at home and any necessary assistance has been arranged, they are discharged to outpatient follow-up. They are instructed to promptly report any cast problems, increasing pain, or excessive swelling that is not promptly relieved by rest, elevation, and mild analgesics. An office or clinic visit a week or two following discharge permits assessment of comfort, gait, swelling, neuromotor function, cast integrity, and clinical as well as radiographic alignment.

Although some patients may benefit from a PTB walking cast, as originally advocated by Sarmiento, a prefabricated functional PTB brace from knee to foot, with a hinged ankle, has largely replaced this, unless a satisfactorily fitting brace is not available or offers inadequate control, as may happen with a very distal fracture (Fig. 51–17). The PTB cast or brace is applied when the patient can comfortably bear partial weight in the long-leg cast and early fracture consolidation is likely. This usually occurs between three and five weeks after injury. It is advisable to delay applying the PTB brace for a longer period, but preferably not more than six weeks, after more severe injuries. Proximal tibial fractures may be better controlled in a long-leg cast. If knee motion is desired for such patients, hinges and a thigh cuff can be added to the below-knee portion of the cast. An effective method for doing this is to use a fiberglass below-knee cast, to which are attached the hinges and adjustable thigh cuff of a commercially available modular fracture brace. This allows adjustment of the thigh cuff for comfort and maximal support.

A prefabricated fracture brace that follows Sarmiento's principles usually provides excellent fracture control while permitting satisfactory function for the majority of patients with low-energy tibial shaft fractures.[246,258] When such a brace must be worn for many months and the commercially available devices do not provide an adequate fit, a custom-molded bivalve total contact brace can be fabricated by an orthotist. This may have either a fixed or a hinged ankle, depending on the degree of immobilization desired. Lippert and Hirsch demonstrated that ankle immobilization decreases displacement of fracture fragments with activity.[170]

Radiographs through the cast or brace are initially

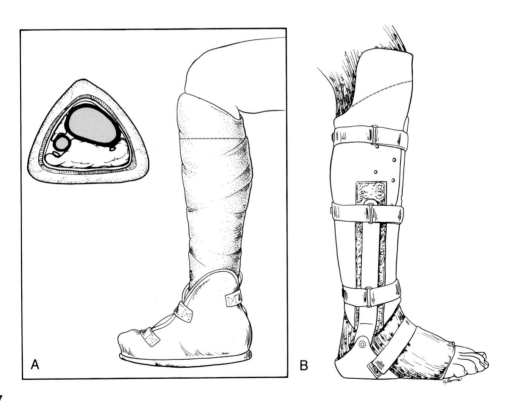

Figure 51–17

A, A patellar tendon–bearing (PTB) functional cast is applied after soft tissue swelling has resolved and the fracture has become somewhat "sticky" and less tender. If a neutral position was obtained initially, then the ankle can be maintained in a PTB cast. Such a cast is pointless unless the foot is plantigrade, for the patient will not otherwise be able to bear weight. The top of the cast is trimmed a little lower anteriorly than was originally proposed by Sarmiento[247] and low enough posteriorly to permit 90° knee flexion. The upper part of the PTB cast is molded into a triangular cross section, flaring upward and outward over the anterior surfaces of the tibial plateaux (see inset). This produces a bulge over the proximal fibula and peroneal nerve while providing a molded fit for the anterior surfaces of the proximal tibia, thus supporting it, and gaining rotational control. The PTB cast is used chiefly for distal fractures in which a brace with ankle motion might not provide adequate control and for patients whom commercially available prefabricated braces do not fit. *B*, A prefabricated fracture brace is often applied to tibia fractures instead of a PTB cast. It may not fit well or provide adequate support for a distal fracture, and it often requires some proximal trimming or padding for comfort and fracture support. The brace is applied over a thick Spandex stocking. A sneaker or walking shoe goes on over the heel cup and helps maintain alignment of the brace on the leg.

checked every two to three weeks to ensure maintenance of satisfactory alignment. Minor degrees of angulation can be corrected with cast changes or wedging. However, the latter may render the cast less suitable for weight bearing, so that once the fracture is "sticky" enough to permit only bending rather than translation of fragments, it is better to change the cast or move on to the brace rather than adjust alignment with wedging.

When sufficient function and comfort are possible in a long-leg weight-bearing plaster cast and satisfactory fracture alignment has been maintained, the patient may progress to the prefabricated fracture brace. The cast is removed in the clinic, and the nearly pain-free limb is supported as needed while a thick elastic fracture-brace sock is applied and the fracture brace secured snugly over it. Trimming and occasionally padding of this brace may be needed for comfort and optimal fracture control. The heel cup and ankle hinge must be sized and adjusted correctly. A lace-up training or walking shoe helps hold the brace in place. Tightness is adjusted to provide support with comfort, and the patient is once again encouraged to bear as much

weight as tolerated, gradually discarding crutches or cane as these become unnecessary. Many feel that beginning weight bearing before six weeks after injury is significantly beneficial for tibial fracture healing.[117,247]

Roentgenograms are obtained in the brace initially and again in a week or two, at which time it is also essential to confirm that the brace fits well, without skin or nerve irritation, and that the patient is maintaining and adjusting it properly. Thereafter (usually from six to eight or more weeks after a low-energy tibial shaft fracture) it is usually possible to monitor the patient with monthly visits and radiographs. The brace is continued until the patient is fully weight bearing without discomfort, tenderness and warmth are absent at the stable fracture site, and radiographs in the AP, lateral, and both oblique projections confirm union with mature bridging callus (see later discussion of assessment of fracture healing).

At this point, some residual muscle weakness and atrophy persist, the patient's endurance is not yet normal, and the skeleton is weaker than normal as a result of disuse atrophy. Therefore a continuing rehabilita-

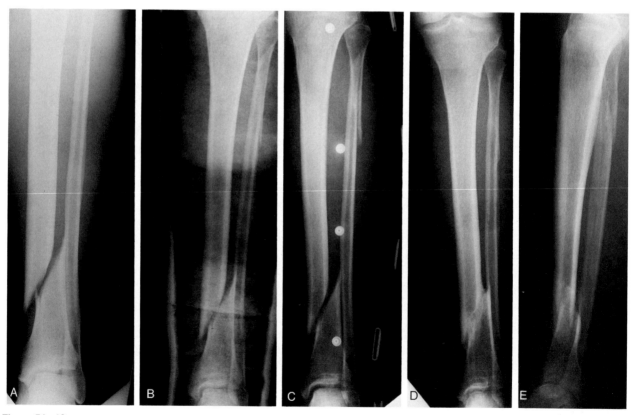

Figure 51–18

Successful functional brace treatment of a minor severity, distal tibiofibular shaft fracture. *A,* Initial injury, caused by a slip and fall. *B,* Appearance after gravity reduction and medially based opening wedge. *C,* Twelve weeks after injury. The patient was fully weight bearing in a fracture brace, since its application at six weeks. *D,E,* Healed fracture, 1 cm short, nine months after injury. The patient was fully functional, and without complaint.

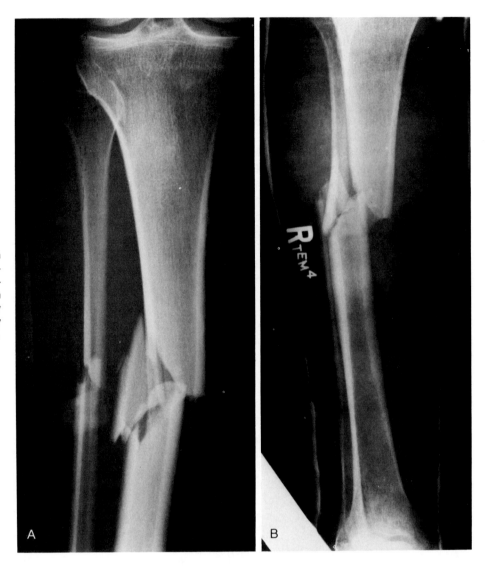

Figure 51–19

A,B, Unsatisfactory reduction three weeks after injury in a well-molded long-leg cast. The 79-year-old patient was unable to walk in the cast but became ambulatory readily and healed uneventfully after closed intramedullary nailing.

tion program with avoidance of risk and contact sports is advised, while encouraging repetitive loading to increasing tolerance. These graded, progressively increasing exercises should continue until the patient's activity level and tolerance reach an appropriate goal. This often requires 6 to 12 months from the time of injury.

An open wound may be difficult to manage in a prefabricated plastic brace. If it is more than a minimal wound, then a cast may be better. Skin problems associated with braces are rare but should be watched for. If they develop, padding or other brace adjustments may be required. All patients need at least two socks, one to wash and the other to wear. If loss of alignment occurs, remanipulation may be done in the clinic, followed by reapplication of a long-leg cast.

Results of functional cast and brace treatment of tibia fractures are excellent with appropriate patient selection and management. Using the criterion of 5° as the maximum acceptable angulation during brace treatment, Sarmiento et al.'s recent series reported only a 4% incidence of angulation more than 10° after fracture union.[246] Shortening should be no more than that present initially. Most fractures in properly selected patients should heal within four or five months. Complications are rare. Functional recovery will be adequate, within a year or so, for approximately 80% of patients, though many will have at least some residual symptoms.[8,61,62,121,209,219,270] Examples of closed functional treatment of tibial fractures are shown in Figures 51–18 and 51–19.

Intramedullary Nailing

Intramedullary nailing has only recently been acknowledged as a valuable treatment for tibial shaft fractures. This contrasts with its overwhelming acceptance for femoral fractures. However, now that biologic and mechanical principles are understood, implants have improved, and techniques are better known, intramedullary nailing of tibial fractures offers substantial benefits when applied correctly and with appropriate indications. It is important to recognize differences between the femur and tibia with regard to intramedullary fixation. For example, reaming has a well-established place in femoral nailing to enlarge the medullary canal for insertion of a larger diameter implant with tighter fixation over longer segments of the proximal and distal shaft fragments. The medullary canal of the tibia, however, has a typically short isthmic segment with a small internal diameter, in spite of thick cortical walls. Therefore reaming does not provide the same improvement of fracture control. With smaller medullary canals, extensive reaming may be required for insertion of larger implants. Reaming causes necrosis of the adjacent diaphyseal bone. This is of little clinical relevance with most closed fractures but results in unacceptable risks of infection and osteomyelitis in open injuries.[7,20,26,115,175,224]

Several varieties of intramedullary nail are available for fixation of the tibia. Nails are often categorized as "reamed" and "nonreamed," depending on whether enlargement of the medullary canal with power reamers is an intended part of nail insertion. This is not so much a property of the nail as of the technique employed. Nails for which reaming is generally required have outside diameters of 11 mm or more. Such nails are now routinely available with holes for proximal and distal locking screws. They may be used without screws, or appropriate locking screws may be placed proximally, distally, or both, to improve fixation.[69,141,207] Depending on the tibia's intramedullary diameter, reaming may or may not be required for any nail. Other things being equal, small-diameter nails have less bending strength, which is proportional to the cube of the nail's radius.

Single intramedullary nails intended for use without reaming have diameters of 8 to 10 mm. Ender nails, with diameters of 3.5, 4, and 5 mm, are usually inserted two or more at a time through two separate insertion sites. These smaller diameter nails can be inserted without reaming, but they may not control fracture alignment well, particularly length and rotation, especially if a fracture is comminuted. Therefore vigorous efforts are currently underway to develop and test tibial intramedullary nails that can be inserted without reaming and also permit interlocking.[33,63,115] The tibia's small medullary canal makes it difficult to design an implant system in which both nail and locking screws will have adequate strength. One 10-mm nail system has an internal device that can be deployed distally for locking. In large enough tibias, this can be inserted with little or no reaming. Clinical experience with nonreamed locking intramedullary nails is insufficient to determine risks of mechanical failure. In theory, however, they offer a relatively atraumatic means of stabilizing serious tibia fractures.

The text that follows discusses intramedullary nailing in general, reviews indications for different varieties of nails, and describes techniques for intramedullary nailing of tibial fractures, indicating individual variations where appropriate. Examples of intramedullary nail fixation for the tibia are shown in Figure 51–20.

Intramedullary nails control diaphyseal fractures with an interference fit against the internal surface of the medullary canal. The nail is generally effective at controlling bending and lateral displacement. Its longitudinal shape and its diameter affect stability and fracture alignment. Because the medullary canal of the tibia is relatively straight in the A-P plane, a straight medullary nail usually restores axis alignment, but a curved nail or nails must be properly positioned to avoid producing deformity. If two Ender nails are inserted with the concavity of both curves facing anteriorly, a characteristic anterior "dishing" of the bone is common. An elastic or loosely fitting nail permits greater motion at the fracture site. More rigid tubular nails, especially if inserted with a tight fit into a reamed canal, allow less motion, but all intramedullary nails act as splints, limiting motion rather than providing rigid fixation.[218] Thus fracture healing occurs mostly through proliferation of peripheral callus. This may be delayed if the surrounding soft tissues or tibial blood supply are badly injured. With axial loading, the fracture ends telescope together until weight is borne by the bone. If there is significant comminution or obliquity with a canal diameter greater than the nail's, then excessive shortening may occur. To prevent shortening and control rotation, proximal and distal locking devices can attach the nail to the bone above and below the fracture. However, such a statically locked nail must endure the full axial stresses of any weight borne before the bone heals.

The several components of a statically locked nail are thus at risk of fatigue failure, which is most likely at the distal interlocking screw holes or in the screws themselves. Clinically, distal tibial fractures close to the nail's distal locking screws are most at risk of causing nail failure. Implant material and design, especially outside diameter, determine the strength and endurance of intramedullary nails. Tibial nails in particular have a small margin of safety.[218] Thus it is much more important to protect them from excessive loading and extremes of bending using crutches or functional braces until fracture consolidation has developed. Another way to deal with problems of fatigue and weak-

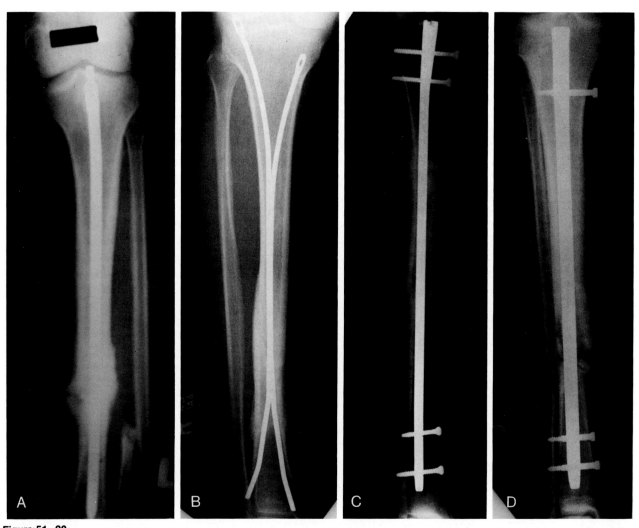

Figure 51-20

Examples of intramedullary fixation for tibial shaft fractures. *A*, Lottes nail. *B*, Ender nails in patient with major severity, open, comminuted injury. Wound and fracture healed benignly. The prominent lateral nail was associated with some knee pain until removal. *C*, Nonreamed, static-locked intramedullary nail in patient with a healing comminuted major severity injury. *D*, Reamed, locked nail in patient with closed major severity injury.

ness of a small tibial nail is to exchange it for one of larger size, if the fracture has not healed after several months have elapsed. Exchanging the nail is not technically difficult. However, the necessary reaming may risk infection, if bacterial contamination remains from the original injury.

As with the femur, stiffer nails must be carefully inserted through an entry portal that lies on the long axis of the tibial shaft. This is necessary to avoid difficulties during insertion that result in implant deformation, fracture displacement, or damage to the bone. This entry site usually lies slightly medial to the tibial tuberosity, and encroaches upon the anterior surface of the tibial plateau.

Intramedullary nailing, with or without reaming, affects endosteal blood circulation. There is immediate loss of medullary arterial flow with a variable thickness of bone necrosis around the nail. To compensate, the periosteal blood supply assumes a larger role in perfusing the cortex. If immobilization is sufficient and there is sufficient space between the nail and the internal surface of the cortex, then the medullary arterial system regenerates within a few weeks. There is significantly less cortical necrosis with a loosely fitting intramedullary nail than with a snug nail after reaming.[228] For this reason, nonreamed nails are thought to have a lower risk of infection and are thus preferable for open tibial fractures.

Indications

Intramedullary nails are especially suitable for closed, displaced, transverse middiaphyseal tibial fractures with little comminution.[26,207,262] If reaming is avoided in open injuries and locking nails are used when necessary, then nailing may provide excellent stability for tibial fractures of minor, moderate, and major severity.[31,156] Closed nailing after reaming offers fracture control for weight bearing with a low risk of infection or other treatment complications. It is only necessary that good technique be used and that the fracture be far enough from each end of the bone that good control can be achieved (Fig. 51–21). Generally this means that the fracture must not significantly involve either metaphysis. The stability of fractures with shorter proximal or distal fragments, comminution, or a more oblique pattern is significantly improved by locking either or both ends of the nail.

Nailing is of special benefit to patients with floating knees, contralateral injuries that will delay weight bearing on the opposite side, or upper extremity injuries

that interfere with crutch use, and in less compliant patients. Segmental tibial fractures, which have a very high risk of nonunion, are especially amenable to nailing, but technical details are important.[191,212] Intramedullary nailing can simplify the management of those tibial fractures with intact fibulas that angulate in a cast (approximately 25%).[169] A major advantage of a reamed nail for a closed tibial fracture is that it permits secure interlocking if this is necessary. It may also offer improved stability, greater strength, and earlier unsupported weight bearing. For uncontaminated and uninfected delayed unions and nonunions, reamed nailing usually provides an excellent and reliable functional treatment, if the fracture is appropriately located and the nail can be inserted with a closed technique or with minimal soft tissue stripping (Fig. 51–22).[263] For some

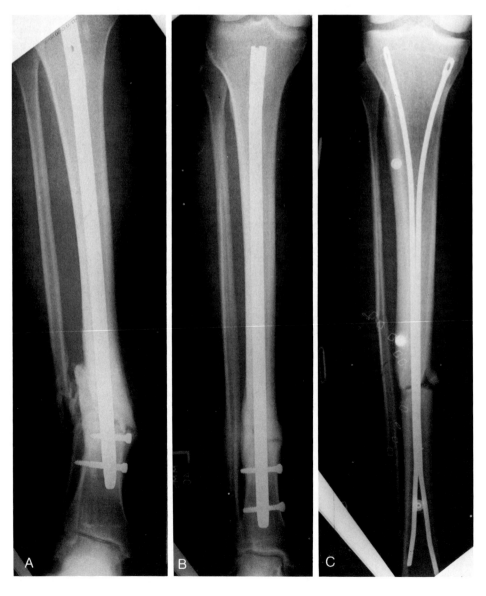

Figure 51–21

An intramedullary nail must be long enough and adequately fixed in the distal fragment. Degree of comminution, level, and pattern of fracture each affect stability and suggest the need for improved distal fixation. *A*, A 6'6", 270-pound patient with a nail too short to control his comminuted fracture. Not surprisingly, posterolateral bone grafting did not help either. Better external support and avoidance of unprotected weight bearing might have maintained his initially satisfactory reduction, but the use of distal locking screws was not sufficient. See Figure 51–48 for salvage results. *B*, Distal, moderate severity fracture healing uneventfully following fixation with a distally locked, nonreamed nail. *C*, Another large patient with tibia too long for the available locking nonreamed nails. Ender nails offer a better selection of lengths and provide satisfactory stabilization for this moderate severity, open fracture. A functional brace was used for the first six weeks.

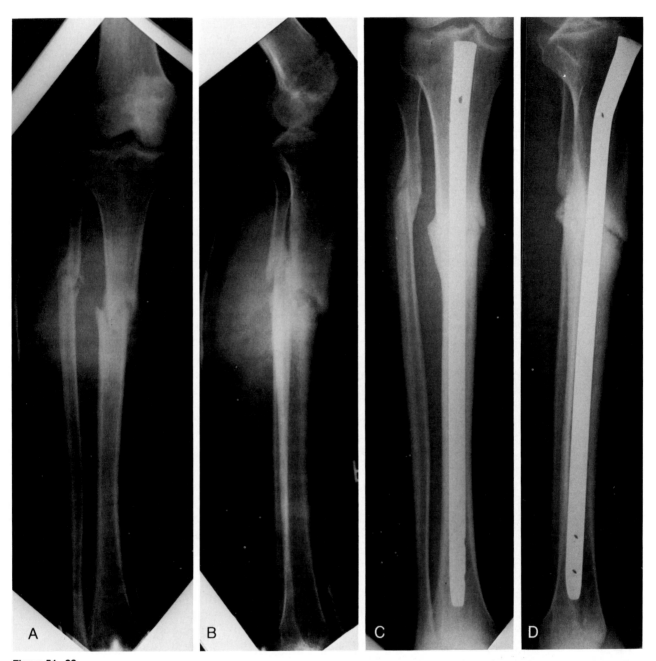

Figure 51-22

A,B, Six months after closed fracture and weight bearing in a PTB cast, this patient still has pain at his somewhat mobile fracture site. *C,D,* The fracture was clinically united 3 months after nailing. He is shown here 12 months after injury and 3 months after he returned to work.

high-risk patients, even those with infected nonunions, intramedullary nailing may be the best of several problematic alternatives.[194]

Nonreamed intramedullary nails are often effective for closed tibial fractures, although they do not provide as much stability.[120,178,190,198,252,253,306,307] Most importantly, they permit safe intramedullary fixation of suitable open tibial fractures. Recent prospective controlled studies have demonstrated that such nails have

fewer problems than does external fixation for treatment of type I and type II open tibial fractures.[120,266a,302] Sufficient data are not yet available to convincingly demonstrate their performance in type III injuries. It is probably safer to limit the use of nonreamed nails to those type III open tibial injuries with optimal fracture patterns and without high-grade bacterial contamination. Ender and Lottes nails may fail to control length and rotation in comminuted tibial fractures. Locked nonreamed nails offer this control but are more at risk of mechanical failure if significant weight bearing precedes fracture healing.

The use of any intramedullary nail after an external fixator appears to have an increased risk of intramedullary infection, although the effect of reaming in such a situation is not completely clear.[175,181] If infection occurs during external fixation, even if it is treated successfully, its recurrence after subsequent intramedullary nailing must be a real concern. Although delays of several weeks or more between fixator removal and nailing may somewhat decrease the risk of infection, the risk remains elevated when compared with that in a fracture in which infection has not occurred. Therefore it seems wise to make an early choice between external fixation and a nonreamed intramedullary nail for stabilization of an open tibial fracture. Good clinical studies show that the nail is superior to the fixator for patients with "axially stable" fracture patterns. With significantly comminuted injuries, however, the relative merits of locked nonreamed nailing and of external fixation remain to be clarified. In spite of the increased risk of infection, it may still be appropriate to treat a nonunion after external fixation with an intramedullary nail, if it is the most satisfactory alternative and if steps are taken to minimize risks.[137,155,194]

Timing

Fractures that need immediate surgery for soft tissue considerations may be treated immediately with intramedullary nails. Although reamed nails have been used, nonreamed nails may be safer, given their lower risk of infection.[22,44,141] It is important to be aware that restoration of length decreases muscular compartment volume, raising the possibility of compartment syndrome, especially if fascial compartments remain intact (as they may with closed nailing).[282] Therefore careful monitoring is advisable, unless fasciotomies are done with debridement.

Closed fractures that would benefit from reamed nailing rarely need immediate fixation and can be provisionally stabilized with a cast. Therefore reamed nailing can generally be delayed until soft tissue swelling is resolving and the patient's neurovascular status is secure. Too long a delay can be a problem if there is significant shortening. Temporary skeletal traction on a Böhler-Braun frame with a calcaneal pin can be used, after the acute swelling resolves, to maintain or restore length before surgery. This may avoid a difficult intraoperative reduction with resultant risk of compartment and peripheral nerve problems.[26,226]

Preoperative Preparation

Adequate radiographs of the injured limb are needed to ensure that the injury is suitable for intramedullary nailing and to identify knee or ankle involvement. Occasionally an undisplaced metaphyseal fracture can be fixed with cancellous lag screws prior to intramedullary nailing. Measurement of the opposite intact tibia (tibial tubercle to medial malleolus) is a good guide to nail length. If there is extreme comminution of the tibia and fibula so that radiographic interpretation is difficult, then measuring the uninjured limb is essential. This can be confirmed radiographically with a radiopaque ruler, or a provisionally selected implant, fluoroscoped if necessary through its sterile packaging. Because many tibial intramedullary nails are not yet available in adequate lengths for very tall patients, it is essential to know what size nail is likely to be required. For safety, larger and smaller nails should be available as well. It is valuable to have a full complement of both nonreamed and locking nails so that intraoperative problems do not preclude some form of satisfactory intramedullary fixation. All instruments required for nail insertion must be on hand and in working order. The surgeon should review and know the technical details of the selected implant system. Image intensification fluoroscopy and an appropriate operating table as discussed later, are also essential.

Anesthesia and Positioning

A general or a spinal anesthetic is appropriate. Perioperative antibiotics are routine. A tourniquet may aid exposure but must never be used during reaming, as absence of blood flow increases the extent of thermal necrosis. The patient is positioned supine on a conventional operating table with a radiolucent extension or on a fracture table adapted for intramedullary nailing of the tibia. Patients with open fractures should not have their leg placed in traction until after adequate debridement has been accomplished with the leg free. This requires another operating surface for debridement (e.g., table extension or Mayo stand). Skin preparation and sterile draping are repeated after traction is applied to the leg. If a fracture table is used, then a calcaneal pin and an appropriate table attachment that controls rotation and angulation will be required if distal interlocking is likely. The proximal leg support must be well padded. It is positioned posterior to the distal femoral shaft, not in the popliteal fossa, to avoid excessive pressure on neurovascular structures.

The leg is positioned with the knee flexed more than 90° to permit free access to the entry site. There must be adequate fluoroscopic visualization in the AP and lateral planes from the tibial plateaux to the ankle. Usually the opposite leg is extended close to and below the injured one. If hip motion is adequate, the uninjured leg may be alternatively flexed, abducted, and externally rotated to allow bilateral access. The surgeon stands on the medial side of the injured leg, with the fluoroscope on the lateral, as this simplifies insertion of locking screws (Fig. 51–23). Adequate imaging and provisional closed fracture reduction are confirmed before draping; then double-check rotational alignment and secure it.

Instead of a fracture table, a radiolucent operating table or extension may be used. The injured leg is draped free; the fluoroscope, with sterile cover, is on the lateral side; and the surgeon is on the medial side. Ender nails, using medial and lateral proximal portals, can be inserted with the knee extended on such a table. However, the midanterior portal used by other nonreamed and reamed nails requires that the knee be flexed to 90° or more. This is especially important with some of the newer nonreamed locking nails, although it is not so crucial with the distally curved Lottes nail. Closed nailing is very difficult without stabilizing the fracture site so that reduction can be maintained while the knee is flexed. The new AO/ASIF bone distractor,

with a longer shaft, has enough span to distract and stabilize the fracture.[173] Use of the distractor is described later. After it is applied, the hip and knee are flexed and the foot placed on the operating table surface during reduction, reaming, and nail insertion. An external fixator frame can be similarly used (Fig. 51–24).[299]

Surgical Techniques

If the fracture is open, irrigation and debridement are done first, as previously described; the leg is reprepped and redraped; and generally only a nonreamed nailing technique is chosen. DiPasquale et al. have used "minimal reaming" of only the proximal tibia down to, but not across, the site of the nutrient artery to allow use in smaller canals of a 10-mm nail designed for insertion without reaming.[63]

Anterior Entry Site. If a fracture table is used and provisional reduction has already been confirmed,

Figure 51–23

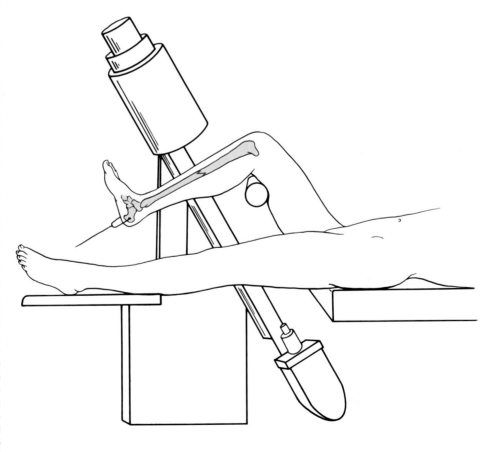

Position of patient on fracture table for closed intramedullary nailing of tibia. This illustrates one type of table. It is important to be familiar with the available equipment to ensure easy, safe positioning and surgery. It is essential that the patient's knee be flexed to at least 90°, and that the thigh rest on a well-padded support that is proximal to the popliteal fossa. The foot of the injured limb may be secured in a boot, but if distal interlocking is done, a calcaneal pin is necessary for support with adequate access to the distal tibia. A good table provides a pin holder with positive control of alignment in all planes. Rotational alignment of the fractured tibia must be assessed and corrected as needed. However, the position of the thigh may affect tibial rotation. The opposite limb must be placed so it does not interfere with either the surgeon or the fluoroscope. A satisfactory method is to extend the uninjured limb beside and below the flexed, injured leg. The surgeon stands on the side opposite the fractured tibia, with the C-arm fluoroscope on the same side as the fracture. After positioning the patient and the injured leg, it is important to check that fluoroscopy is satisfactory in both AP and lateral planes throughout the length of the tibia. Repositioning of the legs and the table may be necessary.

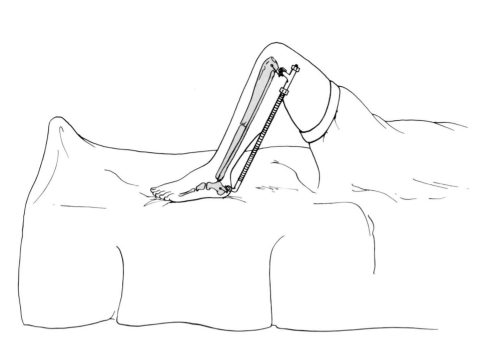

Figure 51-24

An alternative to a fracture table for intramedullary nailing of a tibial fracture is a radiolucent operating table or extension, with a bone distractor used, if necessary, to obtain and maintain provisional reduction of the tibial fracture. This permits the knee and hip to be flexed and the foot placed on the table during reaming and nail insertion. Some manual support of the fracture is usually needed to control angulation. The surgeon stands on the medial side of the injured leg, with the C arm placed on the lateral side. Folded sterile linen placed under the injured tibia permits elevation above the opposite leg for the fluoroscopic lateral view. The distractor can be placed on either the medial or lateral side of the limb, with care to avoid injury to vital structures and to position the distractor so that it does not interfere with nail insertion (including insertion instruments). The distractor's distal pin can be placed in the tibia, just above the plafond for better control of the fracture.

then the next step is preparation of the insertion site. The incision is centered over the long axis of the tibia just medial to the patellar ligament and extends proximally from the level of the tibial tubercle to the midportion of the patella. Distally the incision is carried to bone, but proximally only to the deep fascia, so that skin flaps retract out of the way of reamers and nail, and the knee joint is not entered. The infrapatellar fat pad is pushed proximally and posteriorly into the knee joint with an elevator, thus baring the anterior surface of the proximal tibia, from which the periosteum is reflected over a 1-cm diameter area after incising it with an electrocautery. The patellar ligament is retracted laterally as needed to gain access to this site, which must lie on the long axis of the tibia slightly medial and proximal to the tibial tubercle and close to, if not on, the anterior edge of the tibial plateau. The cortical bone is thin here and is easily perforated with a Küntscher pistol-grip awl. This should be large enough to prepare for the proximal end of the nail, if a nonreamed system is used, or it will be necessary to enlarge the first few centimeters of the canal according to the nail manufacturer's directions. It is important to stay central in the proximal tibia, with awareness of its apex anterior angulation. Initially the awl is directed posteriorly. While rotating the awl through enough of an arc to enlarge the round hole, it should be advanced gradually, changing

its angulation from posterior to anterior in order to end up within and parallel to the medullary canal of the shaft. Fluoroscopy in the AP and, especially, lateral planes should confirm this to help avoid posterior cortical perforation and too superficial an entry (Fig. 51-25).

Reaming and Nailing. If the canal will be reamed, then an appropriate guide wire with a beaded tip is passed across the fracture site and down into the dense bone of the distal tibial metaphysis. This is confirmed on AP and lateral views. Closed manipulation, guided by the subcutaneous anterior tibial crest, makes this a usually easy procedure in relatively fresh fractures. By subtracting the length of the exposed guide wire from that of another of the same length, the intramedullary length can be determined. Reaming is then done over the guide wire with cannulated power reamers. Fracture alignment is maintained manually as each reamer is passed across it. Depending on the reamers used and the size and shape of the nail, it is usual to ream 0.5 to 1 mm larger than the nail's nominal diameter. Generally no more than 2 to 4 mm of reaming is carried out after the first reamer makes contact with the cortex, but it is desirable to ream enough to use a nail diameter that provides adequate strength and fit. Next the reaming guide wire is exchanged for the driving guide wire, if necessary. The canal is irrigated with antibiotic solu-

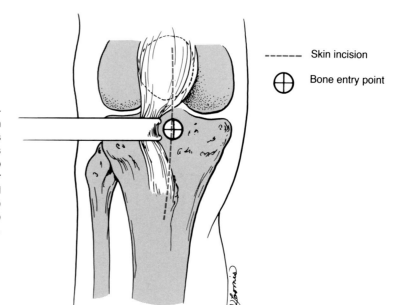

------- Skin incision

⊕ Bone entry point

Figure 51-25

The entry portal for an intramedullary tibial nail is approached through a midline longitudinal incision from midpatella to the level of the tibial tubercle. The fascia is incised medial to the patellar ligament; its paratenon is left intact if possible. The ligament is retracted laterally to permit access to the entry site just distal to the anterior margin of the knee joint and on the long axis of the tibial shaft. The bone here is easy to perforate with a sharp Küntscher awl, which must be turned as it passes into the metaphysis to lie on the central axis of the tibial shaft.

tion, and the chosen nail, which is as long as possible without distracting the fracture by impinging on dense distal metaphyseal bone or protruding above the cortex at the insertion site, is inserted with the appropriate instruments. Liberal biplanar fluoroscopy helps ensure that reduction is maintained and that the nail is passed across the fracture zone without producing comminution. The nail must advance with each hammer blow, or else it should be removed in favor of a smaller size nail or to allow additional reaming. It is occasionally necessary to release all traction and provide firm manual support for the foot to avoid distracting the fracture during the last stage of nail insertion because of the density of distal tibial metaphyseal bone.

Interlocking. Proximal locking screws are easily placed with the insertion guide, if the guide is true to the holes in the nail. This should routinely be checked during assembly of the device. Its bolt may loosen during driving and should be tightened again before drilling for locking screws. If the nail system has an AP locking screw proximally, then great caution, with frequent fluoroscopy, must be used to ensure that the drill bit does not break as it obliquely encounters the posterior cortex and that it does not penetrate beyond this cortex to jeopardize the popliteal neurovascular structures.[305] Proximal locking helps to keep the nail from backing out into the knee if it loosens or the fracture telescopes and it also provides angular and rotational control of a shorter proximal fragment.

Distal interlocking can be achieved with deployment of the internal fins of the Brooker tibial nail, which has an external diameter of 1 cm, thus somewhat restricting its unreamed use.[33] Otherwise, if more control is needed than is achieved by impaling the tip of the nail

into the dense distal metaphyseal bone, then distal locking screws must be inserted with fluoroscopic guidance.[150,156] An alternative is to fix the fibula with a plate or to use a temporary bent-knee long-leg cast to control rotation and loading until fracture consolidation is sufficient. Distal locking screws are best inserted from the medial side in a manner similar to that used for the femur.

Use of the AO Distractor. If, instead of a fracture table, the longer AO/ASIF distractor is used with a radiolucent table or extension, then the first step after prepping and draping is insertion of the distractor. A proximal Schanz screw is placed horizontally, just below and parallel to the articular surface, parallel with the knee joint axis, and sufficiently posterior to the nail entry site that it will not interfere with reaming and nailing. Fluoroscopy aids in positioning this screw. The distal Schanz screw can be placed at the distalmost point of the tibia for better control of reduction or in the calcaneal tuberosity, where it will not need to be removed during nailing. With the fracture reduced, both screws should be approximately parallel to the coronal plane of the leg. Once the two Schanz screws are in place, the distractor is attached securely, and its threaded length adjustment is used to apply traction across the fracture site. This stabilizes the leg.

After the entry site is prepared, the knee and hip are flexed with the foot resting on the table surface. Typically mild apex anterior angulation of the fracture is controlled with manual pressure during reduction, reaming (if it is carried out), and nail insertion.

Proximal locking screws are placed with the knee flexed, as required by the insertion device, which impinges on the knee in extension. Distal locking is easier

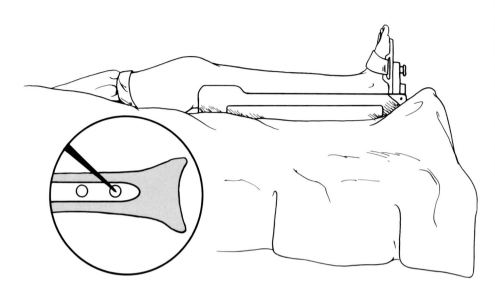

Figure 51–26

Insertion of distal locking screws is usually straightforward when the patient is on a fracture table. The essential first step is orienting the C-arm fluoroscope so that its central ray is perpendicular to the nail and centered over the hole for the locking screw. The distal holes must appear to be perfectly round. This is difficult when the leg is lying free on the operating table but can be simplified by positioning the leg in extension on enough padding so that it is above the uninjured limb, with the foot pointing straight up. (Rotational alignment of the fracture must be maintained.) The leg is more stable if a radiolucent positioning aid is used, as illustrated (see text). With the leg thus supported, the chosen technique for insertion of distal locking screws can be followed most readily.

if the foot is positioned neutrally in a radiolucent holder (e.g., A.L.A.R.M.)* so that the central ray of the fluoroscope can be easily aligned concentrically with the nail's distal locking holes (Fig. 51–26). The distal screws are then inserted using the surgeon's preferred technique. (For example, an incision is made to expose the bone surface; a sharp awl is placed with the aid of the fluoroscope in the center of the round image of the locking hole and then turned so that it is coaxial with the central x-ray beam. This is used to make a pilot hole for drilling the bone; this also follows the central beam. Finally the length is measured and the locking screw is inserted.)

If Ender nails are used with medial and lateral proximal portals, the AO/ASIF distractor can be applied in the midline anteriorly from the tibial tubercle to the anterior distal tibial shaft. Caution should be used to avoid overpenetration of the proximal Schanz screw.

Ender Nails. Ender's C-shaped, flexible stainless steel nails are available in 4.5-mm, 4.0-mm, and 3.5-mm diameters and in various lengths. The smaller diameter nails are not long enough for tall patients with slender medullary canals. Originally intended for intertrochanteric femur fractures, Ender nails are also well suited for tibial shaft fractures.[120,178,190,212,253,306,307] Usually two nails are inserted from medial and lateral portals in the proximal tibia and passed distally across the fracture, using a closed or open technique (used for an open fracture), and into the distal metaphysis. Better

stability can be achieved if the medullary canal is filled by using larger diameter nails or more nails. Ender nails, like other nonlocked devices, may not provide adequate control of length in comminuted fractures, but their control of rotation, albeit elastic, is good enough that proper rotational alignment must be achieved prior to passing the nails across the fracture, as subsequent correction is unreliable. Angular alignment is affected by the orientation of the curvature of the Ender nails, which can be turned so that the convexity of the nail resists undesirable angulation. Satisfactory alignment can usually be achieved with two nails if the one inserted from the medial portal lies in the coronal plane with its convexity laterally directed and the one inserted from the lateral portal has its convexity oriented anteriorly. Some adjustment of rotational alignment of the nails aids passing them across the fracture site and helps to achieve the desired reduction.

The proper length for Ender nails can be estimated by the distance from the tibial tubercle to the medial malleolus. The patient is positioned and prepared in either manner described previously. Insertion sites are developed in the proximal tibia, the lateral one in Gerdy's tubercle and the medial one approximately halfway between the anterior and posterior borders of the medial metaphyseal flare and just proximal to the tibial tubercle. Five-centimeter incisions are started at the selected insertion sites and carried proximally in line with the tibial shaft (Fig. 51–27). Except for the entry portal itself, the incision need go no deeper than to the deep fascia, so that it permits the nail to lie obliquely in the wound without injuring the skin dur-

---

*Manufactured by M. C. Johnson Co., Inc., Leominster, MA 01453.

Figure 51-27

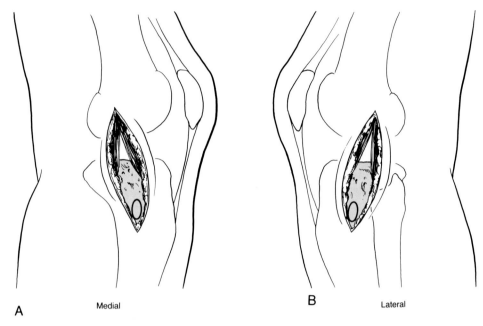

A Medial   B Lateral

Ender nails are usually inserted from medial *(A)* and lateral *(B)* portals in the proximal tibia. The incisions are approximately 8 cm long, in line with the tibial shaft, and extend proximally from the bony insertion portals. These are mid-medial and midlateral at approximately the level of the tibial tubercle. The lateral site is the palpable bone of Gerdy's tubercle. The incisions extend proximally, (only as deep as the fascia) to avoid trauma to the skin during insertion of the nail, which would otherwise press against it. The entry portal is prepared by elevating the periosteum over a small area and then perforating the tibia with a drill or Küntscher awl, which is rotated to parallel the shaft and stay within the medullary canal, into which the Ender nail is then inserted.

ing insertion. A drill bit or Küntscher awl is used to begin the portal. This is then enlarged and connected with the medullary canal of the shaft with the awl, turning it to avoid penetration through the opposite cortex. Taking advantage of its curvature, as described by Rush[237a] (whose rods can be used similarly), the first Ender nail is inserted just across the fracture site, following which reduction, including rotational alignment, is adjusted; the next Ender nail is also passed across the fracture site. Next the fracture is compressed by manual pressure on the foot to avoid distraction as the rods are driven into the distal tibial metaphyseal bone under fluoroscopic guidance. With the nails thus anchored, rotational alignment is usually reliable, but shortening and, occasionally, angulation can occur if there is significant comminution. Additional stability can be achieved, if it is needed and the opportunity exists, by plating the fibula or by using external support with a prefabricated fracture brace or long- or short-leg cast until early stability is present. Most patients with Ender nail fixation of tibial shaft fractures can bear full weight, often without external support, by six weeks or less after injury. This technique usually controls alignment and permits relatively prompt return to function. For many patients, Lottes, Ender, or other nonreamed nailing permits control of tibial fracture alignment, with low risks, except for limited stability in comminuted fractures.

Complications

Technical problems can usually be anticipated and prevented. These include malreduction, fracture com-

minution, incarceration of a nail, impaired fixation, and neurovascular injury.[226,262,305] Familiarity with technique and attention to detail minimizes their occurrence. Deliberate, step-by-step technique ensures that the fracture is satisfactorily aligned while a nail of appropriate size is placed across it. Fluoroscopy in two planes aids smooth passage of the nail into the medullary canal and across the fracture. Spot images should be checked often. The nail should advance with each hammer blow. If it fails to, or if its audible pitch rises, then the nail may be about to jam. It should be withdrawn and exchanged for a smaller one, or the canal should be reamed larger. Proper positioning and padding and the avoidance of overly forceful traction with a fracture table will reduce the risks of neurovascular injury.

Nailing done too soon after injury probably increases the risk of compartment syndrome, as does an attempt to forcibly regain length in a short period of time under anesthesia.[186,256,282] Because compartment syndromes are theoretically possible after any tibial nailing procedure, the patient must be closely monitored during the early postoperative period, with pressure measurement or fasciotomy as indicated.

Infection, a worrisome problem if it extends through the medullary canal, is rare if reamed nailing is not used for open fractures and if closed or minimally invasive reductions are used.[26,216] Some experience and good technique are important for avoiding an increased incidence of infection.[22] Alertness should permit early discovery of infection using intramedullary aspiration and culture. Low-virulence intramedullary infections may be managed with appropriate antibiotics, retention of a secure nail, or reaming a small amount and inserting a larger nail. Rarely an especially aggressive and unresponsive intramedullary infection occurs that requires nail removal, external fixation, antibiotics, canal irrigation, and often bone grafting to obtain union.[216]

Late insertion site pain is not unusual, especially if hardware is prominent. It usually resolves after implant removal. Efforts should be made to minimize the nail's prominence by choosing its length carefully, monitoring insertion with radiographs, and locking proximally when advisable.

Postoperative Care

Nail insertion wounds are routinely closed, with liberal use of closed suction drainage, although brisk intramedullary bleeding should be allowed to clot by delaying application of suction to a drain placed in continuity with the medullary canal. Open fracture or fasciotomy wounds are managed as previously described. Elevation and observation for neurovascular problems are necessary for the first day or two, after which the patient is encouraged to ambulate, if other problems permit. External support may be advisable. Most patients are more comfortable for the first few days if a posterior splint is used to stabilize the ankle, though this is needed less with proximal fractures. Continued external support may range from none at all, with a strong nail and good bone contact, to a prefabricated fracture brace or even a long-leg bent-knee cast if comminution, weaker locking screws, a less strong nail, or impaired patient cooperation are considerations. Intramedullary nails vary significantly with regard to strength and stiffness. Their fatigue life is unknown. Tibial anatomy also varies from person to person and from one spot to another in a given tibia. These facts, plus the wide spectrum of tibial fracture configurations, make it essential to individualize postoperative care for patients with nailed tibial fractures.

The surgeon must decide the stability and strength of the fracture montage, which, like a chain, is limited by its weakest link. Although more than a PTB fracture brace is rarely necessary, the surgeon must make this decision and ensure that proper protection is provided. Rarely is it necessary to continue external support for more than six weeks. From removal of any initial splint until rehabilitation is advanced, a short-leg elastic stocking may be valuable to control edema and perhaps reduce the risk of deep vein thrombosis. The amount of weight bearing that can be allowed is similarly an important and individualized decision. When the nail acts primarily as a gliding splint and bone contact allows the tibia to bear compressive loads, full weight bearing can

be allowed as soon as the patient can tolerate it. If comminution or poor contact are present, then significant weight bearing must be deferred to prevent fracture telescoping or failure of locked intramedullary fixation.[51] With early and progressive healing, as revealed by periodic radiographs, weight bearing can be increased progressively, generally after about six weeks. At a minimum, isometric and toe mobility exercises are begun for all patients as soon as possible in the postoperative period. The patient should not sit with the leg dependent for the first few weeks. Instead it should be elevated on a couch or footstool when the patient is not walking.

Once they are comfortable, ambulatory, and without evidence of complications, patients with intramedullary tibial fixation are ready for outpatient management. Instructions are provided for bracing and weight bearing as detailed previously. Follow-up visits are needed at regular intervals until the fracture is healed and the limb rehabilitated. If there are no apparent problems, radiographs need be obtained only every four to six weeks and should be monitored for bridging callus, which signifies the appropriateness of full weight bearing. Oblique views, as well as AP and lateral, may be valuable to assess fracture healing. When some bridging callus is evident, and after the fibula has healed, there is usually little reason to be concerned about persistent, slowly healing fracture lines. If no bridging callus at all is present at five or six months, it may be wise to change to a larger reamed nail or to add bone graft. The timing of such a rarely needed procedure is adjusted according to the estimated durability of the patient's nail.

Removal of locking screws is rarely necessary to gain union. If done before healing of at least the fibula, it may result in loss of alignment. However, once length and rotation are stable, it may be wise to remove at least the distal locking screws from the nonreamed tibial nails to reduce the risk of late failure, which can occur even after fracture healing. The intramedullary nail itself should be left in place until the fracture is well healed, with mature, remodeled callus on four-view radiographs. This is usually a year or more after injury. Symptoms at the insertion site are common if the nail is prominent but usually resolve after the nail is removed. Many patients will request this when so informed. At present, removal of asymptomatic nails may be considered optional, but there may be severe difficulty removing a slotted nail that has been in place for many years. Therefore routine removal after fracture healing should be considered for younger patients and those with prominent hardware.

When planning removal of an intramedullary nail, it is important to ensure that healing is complete. This usually requires 12 to 18 months and is signified by obliteration of fracture lines and complete cortical remodeling. The surgeon must correctly identify the type of implant and obtain the necessary instruments for nail extraction. The manufacturer's instructions should be reviewed preoperatively, as instrumentation might be used differently during removal than during insertion.

Results

When patients are selected appropriately and the procedure is technically done well, satisfactory results are usual for the vast majority of tibial fractures treated with intramedullary nailing.[26,44,69,115,120,141,156,169,178,190,191,207,252,262,295,303,306,307] Techniques must be mastered and attention devoted to detail.[22,226] Infections occur no more frequently than with other treatments, provided reaming is not done for open fractures and nailing is done closed.[26] Nonunions, malunions, and fixation failures are exceptional, with an incidence generally well under 5% each. More rapid return to unsupported weight bearing and to work are typical when compared with other methods.[224]

External Fixation

Only since the mid 1970s has external fixation gained a significant role in the treatment of tibial fractures, primarily open fractures with severe soft tissue injuries. This is especially evident when reviewing Sarmiento's 1974 symposium on tibial fractures.[244] No article was devoted solely to external fixation, though the technique was mentioned almost in passing by Karlstrom and Olerud, who did show illustrations of three cases treated with Hoffmann devices using the Videl-Adrey method with transfixion pins.[145] They reported their early impression that this technique aided in reducing the infection rate for open tibia fractures and described it in more detail the next year.[146] The advantages of external skeletal fixation compared with casts or traction were soon confirmed by many others.[35,56,60,68,163,188,248,249,268] Figure 51–28 illustrates the Videl-Adrey technique for application of the Hoffmann external fixator.

Because of these advantages and a general dissatisfaction with available alternatives for treating severe open tibia fractures, many clinicians adopted external fixation using transfixion pins inserted in the coronal

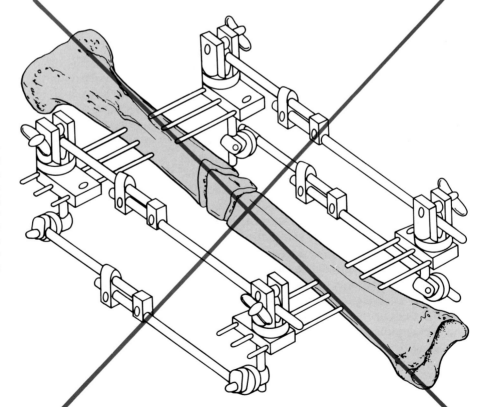

Figure 51–28

This drawing illustrates, for historical purposes, the so-called quadrilateral external fixator frame constructed with Hoffmann components as advocated by Videl and Adrey. It offers no more stability than anterior unilateral frames. Its transfixion pins are more prone to complications than are half pins inserted through thinner anterior soft tissues.

plane, as proposed by Videl and Adrey and soon widely taught.[76,92,94,146,291] This was in fact similar to the traditional pins and plaster technique, with improved wound access and easier adjustability but poorer control of the foot and ankle.[4] The benefits of this method of external fixation were soon found to be mixed and accompanied by their own complications.[232] Pin site infections ranged from local cellulitis to osteomyelitis with ring sequestra. The fixators were awkward and so heavy that without overhead suspension, heel pressure sores were seen. Transfixed and tethered soft tissues were associated with foot and ankle joint stiffness and contractures in nonfunctional positions, especially if provisions were not made for supporting the foot and ankle in neutral.[275] Though more open than a cast, the bulky frames often interfered with soft tissue transfer procedures. Pins sometimes limited potential muscle flaps. Pin trauma occasionally resulted in immediate or delayed neurovascular compromise. Partly because they were used for more severe fractures, external fixators were associated with delay or failure of fracture healing.[1,105,202] A proposed solution was to retain the external fixator only as long as needed for soft tissue healing. After restoration of an intact soft tissue envelope, the fixator would be replaced by a cast or fracture brace, with weight bearing encouraged. The hope was that functional weight-bearing treatment in a cast or brace would effectively stimulate fracture healing, as it seemed to for less severe fractures. However, results were not always as desired. Even though many fractures seemed quite solid immediately after fixator removal, they had rarely developed significant callus, and within a few days the fracture was obviously mobile. Loss of alignment often followed, and such fractures healed slowly if at all.

Recognition of these and other shortcomings led to a series of major improvements in the use of external fixators, which are reviewed in chapters 10 and 14. Predrilled holes for external fixation pins reduce the risks of thermal necrosis, infection, and pin loosening. Three-piece insertion guides, with two nested sleeves and an inner trocar, also limit soft tissue injury. The guide is inserted through a cutaneous stab incision, and the pilot hole is drilled through the inner sleeve, which is removed while the outer one is held securely against the bone. Its inner diameter accommodates the chosen pin size and aids in finding the hole as well as protecting tissue. Power instruments are used for predrilling, whereas hand braces are used for pins. Attention to cross-sectional anatomy reduces the risk of injury to vital structures.[77,92,168]

Mechanical investigations demonstrated that "rigid" quadrilateral frames with transfixion pins in the coronal plane actually were quite flexible in the sagittal plane. Behrens, Hierholzer, and colleagues returned to the concept of unilateral frame types, using stiffer components than those developed by Hoffmann.[15,17,18,119] Such unilateral frames could be applied in one or two planes. Clinical trials soon showed that satisfactory fracture control could be provided by a single-plane unilateral frame constructed with 5-mm threaded pins inserted into the tibia through its subcutaneous anterior border. By avoiding transfixion pins and using half pins that penetrate only the anterior skin and subcutaneous tissue, many pin site problems can be avoided. Contractures are less likely, and functional weight bearing may be allowed, if the fracture configuration and healing permit.

Behrens's three basic principles of external fixation are a helpful guide.[17,18] First, the fixator should pose a low risk to vital structures. Second, it should allow easy access to the wounded area. Third, it should be mechanically adequate for the needs of the patient and the injured limb. For the tibia, these principles are met by using anterior half pins; single- or, occasionally, double-plane anterior frames that allow free access to the rest of the leg; and system components with adequate strength, stiffness, and adaptability to (1) provide initial rigid support for maximal stability during wound coverage, (2) permit progressive weight bearing as fracture configuration and healing permit, and (3) allow progressive frame adjustments that diminish rigidity and permit progressive cyclic loading of the healing fracture.

Because the major bending moments on the tibia during gait are in the sagittal plane, placement of the fixator pins and frame near this plane improves stability.[16] Additional considerations are the use of an external fixator that is sufficiently radiolucent to permit informative radiography and light enough to decrease the risk of pressure sores and maximize the patient's mobility. Carbon-fiber reinforced radiolucent connecting rods help meet these goals (Fig. 51-29).

Fracture immobilization is increased by using two connecting rods, by increasing the number of pins above the minimum of four, by increasing the distance between the two pins in each fragment, by decreasing the distance between the connecting rod and the tibia, and by adding another anteromedial unilateral single-plane montage with separate pins in a different plane and connecting it to the first. Although the optimal stiffness for a tibial external fixator is not known, the following ideas have been tentatively accepted:

1. Fracture immobilization is a result of the combination of the frame and the reduced fracture fragments.

2. Bone contact that supports loading may be stabilized by interfragmentary compression with the frame.

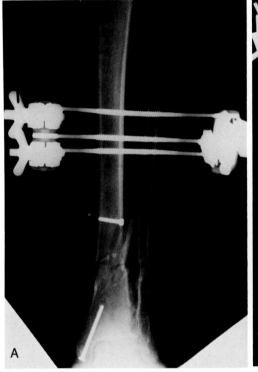
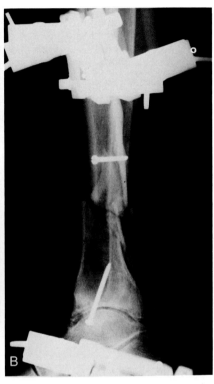

Figure 51–29

Radiolucent carbon-fiber external fixator rods are lightweight and make radiographic follow-up easy. The patient, who also had an open proximal femur fracture, sustained this open tibial shaft fracture around one of several screws placed many years previously. His ankle arthritis was minimally symptomatic. The proximal transfixion pins are above the point where the anterior tibial artery crosses the tibial shaft, but they should still be avoided, as half pins have fewer soft tissue complications and work at least as well.

3. Loading, when the bone configuration or healing permits, may facilitate fracture healing. This may be intermittent, partial, and for only brief periods of time each day.[151-153]

4. More rigid fixators are better early after injury.

5. More rigid fixators have fewer pin problems.

6. Rigid fixators can and probably should be made less so as fracture healing progresses.[19,164,278,294]

7. More rigid fixators are preferable when there is segmental bone loss or comminution and when there are wound healing problems or infection.

8. Bone grafting through healthy soft tissues may accelerate fracture healing or reduce nonunion rate.[20,24]

Applying these principles, Behrens and co-workers reported union of 75 fractures and nonunions of the tibia in a median time of slightly more than six months, with a low rate of pin complications and good preservation of knee and ankle motion. Median time to partial weight bearing was slightly more than one month, and to full weight bearing, slightly more than two.[15] Bone grafts were used frequently. Behrens and colleagues pointed out that the type of fixator did not seem as important as the principles, though stiffness and strength did need to be considered in choosing fixator configuration. Others have reported similarly good results with external fixation of tibial fractures using different external fixator systems in a similar man-

ner.[35,56,60,68,188,248,249,268] External fixation is discussed in more detail in chapter 10.

The high risk of delayed union or nonunion in severe tibial fractures is evident. Early, preemptive bone grafting is coming into favor for reducing this risk.[20,24,43,99,280] Such an approach is especially valuable for patients in external fixators, where alignment may be lost if the frame is removed before the fracture is healed. Timing of such bone grafts is important and depends at least in part on the severity of the original wound and the type of soft tissue coverage, if any, that has been required. Too early a graft may increase the rate of wound complications.[20,99] This is discussed further in the section on bone grafting.

Control of the position and motion of the foot and ankle is especially important in severe injuries of the lower half of the tibia. Early experience with the Videl-Adrey frame soon revealed that foot and ankle stiffness remained a frequent problem after the tibial fracture healed. Equinus and equinovarus deformities were common and posed worse functional problems than did limited motion alone. With a tibial external fixator, often hung from an overhead frame for elevation and to avoid heel pressure, the patient's foot falls into an equinus deformity. Soft tissue scarring related to wound, fracture, and fixator pins, especially if transverse and through the muscles, contributes to ankle and foot stiffness. To avoid stiffness in a dysfunctional position, some form of foot splint is required during the early stages of external fixation for a tibial fracture.[275] Elaborate foot plates and orthoses, often with elastic supports, have been tried. For more proximal and less severe injuries, a well-padded foot splint attached with a webbing strap to the fixator pins is adequate. For more distal and more severe injuries in which absolute control of soft tissue motion may be important for wound healing, the most reliable technique is to extend the fixator frame into the metatarsals.[35,68] This prevents contractures of the ankle and provides excellent soft tissue immobilization. This portion of the fixator can be removed after early wound healing has occurred, generally within two to four weeks, after which active and passive exercises, splinting, or both, are used as needed.

Current advocates of external fixator treatment for severe tibial fractures stress that the fixator is but one element of a comprehensive plan, which includes aggressive wound debridement; prompt coverage of any significant defect with healthy, vascular muscle tissue; and early bone grafting. To reduce the risk of fracture deformation and nonunion after fixator removal, such a plan often includes continuing fixation until the fracture is healed and sequential frame modifications to permit progressive weight bearing by the bone.[19,35,278] Alternative approaches stress early weight bearing or external mechanical loading in a "dynamized" fixator that controls angulation and rotation while allowing axial compression.[60,152,164,188]

So-called "minimal internal fixation," with lag screws used to coapt fracture fragments, may be chosen to augment the stability provided by external fixators.[27,195,267,268] However, a potential problem is posed by the fact that the external fixator may need to be removed before sufficient fracture healing has occurred to provide the stability required for unprotected loading of the minimally fixed fracture site. Early bone grafting, dynamization of the fixator, or external bracing may thus be required. Results have been mixed.

An emerging application of external fixation is its use for traction osteogenesis or bone transport techniques developed by Ilizarov (see chapter 21).[211] Others have demonstrated that such applications do not require the use of Ilizarov's ring fixator with crossed transfixing K wires under tension. However, the techniques for correction of complex deformities are better established with such frames. Currently there appear to be few accepted indications for primary use of the Ilizarov fixator for acute tibial fractures.

Although there is a secure place for external fixation in our armamentarium of treatments for tibial fractures, it is not always the best form of immobilization for these injuries. Speigel and co-workers and Hol-

brook et al. have recently presented prospective, randomized comparative studies showing that nonreamed intramedullary nails (e.g., Lottes, Ender) are at least as effective and better tolerated than external fixators for certain open tibial fractures, provided the fracture is not excessively comminuted.[120,266a] Others have had similar experience.[302] It remains to be seen what role will be assumed by nonreamed interlocking nails for more comminuted open tibial fractures. Furthermore, it must be stated that some minor open tibia fractures can be managed so well with functional weight-bearing casts and braces that there are no benefits to be gained from the risks of external fixation.

Choice of External Fixator

A number of different external fixator systems have been developed to address different needs. There is no firm evidence that one fixator is better than another, in spite of striking differences in design and cost. Single-unit fixators are available with adjustments that permit progressive fracture loading.[60,164,188] Modular frames also can be applied or altered sequentially to allow similar loading of the healing fracture.[19,35,248,268,278,294]

Because single-unit fixators are more limited in their applications, the physician may prefer a modular fixator system that allows construction of frames for all long bones and crossing of knee and ankle joints to support them without additional immobilization. This capability is especially helpful for proximal and distal tibial fractures and those with associated periarticular soft tissue injuries. Although universal connecting joints permit adjustment of the initial reduction, they may compromise the strength and stiffness of the frame. Pin clamps designed for closely spaced pin clusters limit fixator stiffness, because maximal pin separation is prevented. Thus, for example, modified Hoffmann apparatus pin clamps with longer spans have been developed to increase the rigidity attainable with this system.[294]

Pin diameter is necessarily a compromise between maximal stiffness and reasonable size for the bone in question. For the tibia, 4.5-mm or 5.0-mm diameter threaded, self-tapping stainless steel half pins are appropriate; some fixators use 6-mm pins. Pins should be inserted with predrilling and a guide-sleeve system. Connecting rods of carbon-fiber–plastic composites are light and radiolucent. These are beneficial for both of these reasons, but if presterilized, they make it more difficult to choose and assemble an external fixator frame from stock components. It is helpful to assemble a complex frame from unsterile components and then sterilize them prior to applying the fixator. For more standard frames, a kit of essential sterile modular components is effective and simple. With care and monitoring, many external fixator components can be reused for a number of patients at significant cost savings, although this practice is often discouraged for nonclinical reasons.

Application of the External Fixator

As previously mentioned, a number of different systems are available for externally fixing the tibia. Figure 51–30 illustrates one such alternative, the AO tubular system assembled and applied according to Behrens's principles. Modifications of this frame accommodate proximal and distal lesions as well as the need for more rigid immobilization. It can be used, when needed, to bridge and support the knee, ankle, and foot. It can readily be "dynamized" to permit axial loading with weight bearing while maintaining control of angulation and rotation. Although the pins used in this example are the newer AO/ASIF 4.5-mm external fixator pins with short threaded tips, this type of frame can also be applied with 5-mm Schanz screws. Design improvements continue to be made in external fixator pins.

The most important constraint posed by this technique is that the fracture must be satisfactorily reduced before the frame assembly is completed, as subsequent adjustments require either interposition of a less rigid universal joint or replacement of some of the pins.

All required instruments and equipment are assembled before fixation is begun. A power drill, sharp 3.5- and 4.5-mm bits, and an appropriate table surface are required. An image intensifier can help confirm reduction, pin placement, and length. Prior to applying the external fixator, any open wound is thoroughly debrided, and a new, sterile prep and drape are carried out.

For a typical mid-diaphyseal tibial fracture, a connecting tube of appropriate length is fitted with four pin-holding clamps and capped to keep them on the tube. If the fracture is comminuted over more than half its circumference or is so oblique that it cannot bear some load during gait, then a stacked frame is prepared using two such connecting tubes. Making this decision and assembling the frame with both tubes at the beginning is much easier than trying to keep the pins aligned so that a second tube can be applied after all four pins have been placed and secured to the first tube.

The plane of the fixator is determined, either straight anterior to posterior through the crest of the tibia, which may be difficult to drill through, or anteromedial to posterolateral, with the pins directed through the thinner subcutaneous tibial cortex. The proximal pin is inserted, preferably at the junction of the diaphysis and metaphysis, to gain purchase in thick cortical bone. If,

because of fracture proximity or to increase the span between pins, a more proximal position is selected, then a 5.0-mm Schanz screw with longer thread than the 4.5-mm AO external fixator pin should be used.

A 10-mm skin incision is made at the chosen site and carried bluntly down to the bone. Using the triple drill guide consisting of a trocar and two nesting sleeves, a 3.5-mm hole is drilled through both cortices, with as large a chord as possible across the medullary canal. Guard against sliding subperiosteally if the drill meets the cortex obliquely. Removing the inner sleeve with the 3.5-mm drill, overdrill the near cortex with the 4.5-mm drill, and insert the 4.5-mm external fixator pin so that its blunt tip protrudes approximately 2 mm through the opposite cortex. Provisionally align the fracture, and use the external fixator tube assembly to confirm the position of the distal pin. Placing this in cortical bone may provide more secure purchase, but sometimes the dense cancellous bone of the tibial pilon must be used. If a cancellous insertion site is chosen, the hole is drilled only with the 3.5-mm drill, and a 5.0-mm Schanz screw is used. Otherwise, the previously described procedure is repeated, with insertion of a 4.5-mm external fixator pin.

The fixator tube assembly is then attached to the two pins with its outer clamps. The fracture is reduced and held either manually or with a clamp through the open wound. Then the pin clamps are tightened securely to hold a provisional reduction, which can be checked radiographically if desired. However, the fixation is quite tenuous at this point. Ensure that the connecting tube is as close as possible to the pretibial skin without interfering with dressing application and wound care. Confirm also that the ends of the tube do not impede positioning or movement of the knee or ankle. If a stacked frame with two connecting tubes will be used, the second tube with four attached clamps is then applied over the first.

With the triple drill guide placed through the inner clamps, the remaining two 4.5-mm cortical half pins are inserted at least 1 cm proximal or distal to the fracture site, ensuring that any undisplaced comminution is given a sufficiently wide berth. The clamp is tightened around the first such pin. The reduction is confirmed, and the second pin is similarly inserted. Then all clamps are tightened to the tubes and pins, and the reduction is once again confirmed, preferably with full-length AP and lateral radiographs (Fig. 51–31).

The fixator should be extended to the foot when there is an associated unstable foot or ankle injury, when a nerve injury renders the foot insensate and at risk of pressure sores, and whenever there is a severe soft tissue injury of the lower half of the leg (Fig.

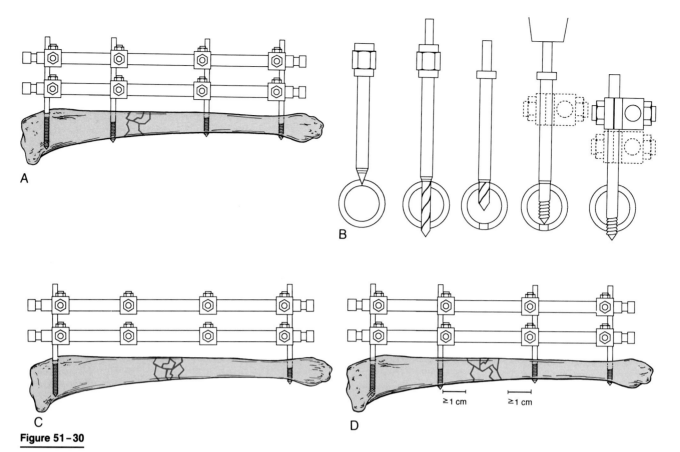

Figure 51–30

A, Double-bar, unilateral, single-plane external fixator. This provides adequate support for most tibial diaphyseal fractures. As healing progresses, it can be "dynamized" by loosening the bar clamps connecting the closer bar to both pins on one side of the fracture and the bar clamps connecting the farther bar to the pins on the opposite side of the fracture. This permits the bars to slide through the clamps and telescope slightly with loading of the fracture site. Control of rotation and angulation is maintained.

B, Pins are inserted into the bone perpendicular to its long axis so as to form a major chord on cross section. Insertion sites are located on the subcutaneous surface of the tibia, avoiding muscle-tendon units and neurovascular structures, especially when penetrating the far side of the bone. The following technique is for 4.5 mm external fixator pins with short, threaded tips designed to screw only into the far cortex. A 1-cm skin incision is deepened bluntly to the bone. A "triple drill guide" consisting of a trocar, inner 3.5-mm internal diameter (ID) sleeve, and outer 4.5-mm ID sleeve is held against the tibial cortex, and a 3.5-mm hole is drilled with a power drill through both near and far cortices. This drill is removed with the inner 3.5-mm sleeve, and a 4.5-mm drill is used to further enlarge the near cortex through the remaining 4.5-mm sleeve. The short threaded (self-tapping) 4.5 mm pin is inserted by hand through this same sleeve for guidance and protection of the soft tissues and advanced until its tip just protrudes through the far cortex. Alternatively, longer threaded Schanz screws can be used without the extra drill step. However, with their thinner root diameter, such pins are more flexible and do not provide as rigid fixation. The triple drill guide fits through the adjustable pin clamps of the fixator system and can be used to align pins and clamps after the initial pins are placed.

C, Construction of the double-bar fixator is begun by provisionally aligning the fracture and inserting the proximal and distal pins. These should lie in the plane chosen for the fixator—generally on the anteromedial aspect of the tibia. Two bars of appropriate length are chosen, and each is fitted with four adjustable clamps. The end clamps on each bar are placed over the proximal and distal pins, and the fracture is reduced before they are tightened. This type of fixator is not adjustable after it is attached to the bone, so reduction must be accomplished first and maintained during application of the fixator.

D, While the fracture is held reduced, the inner two pins are inserted in turn using the triple drill guide placed through each pair of inner clamps as shown. The pins should be at least 1 cm away from the fracture site. The adjustable clamps can be tightened onto the bars to stabilize the drill sleeves and ease insertion. Each pin must be positioned so as to gain secure purchase in the bone. If this is not achieved, modifications must be made, which usually involve reinsertion of one or more pins. Before inserting an inner pin, confirm that the fracture remains reduced.

E, A single-bar, single-plane, unilateral fixator with four 4.5- or 5-mm pins is sufficient for most middiaphyseal tibial fractures without extensive bone loss or comminution.

F, If comminution or bone loss is extensive, the double-bar or "stacked" frame is advisable. An alternative is to use a two-plane unilateral fixator with separate or interconnected anterior and anteromedial frames.

G, Variations provide adequate external fixation for proximal and distal fractures. This diagram shows a two-plane unilateral frame stabilizing a proximal tibial fracture. This can also be done with a cluster of transfixion pins parallel to the joint surface (see Figure 51–33).

H, A similar two-plane unilateral external fixation montage is used for a distal tibial fracture. Note the interconnecting rods between the two planes of the fixator.

I, Pin placement into short juxtaarticular segments can be avoided by spanning the adjacent joint and stabilizing, though less rigidly, the proximal or distal tibia by means of "ligamentotaxis." This distal fracture is stabilized with a frame connected to a transfixion pin in the calcaneus, as well as to the first and fifth metatarsal bases, to hold the foot in neutral.

Illustration continued on following page

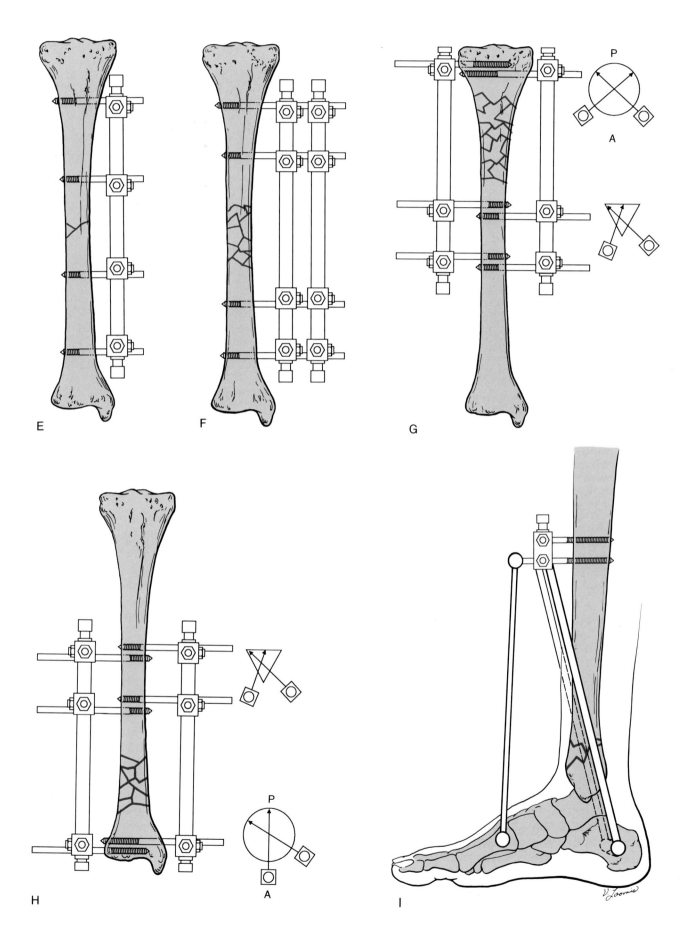

E

F

G

P

A

H

P

A

I

V. Loomis

1827

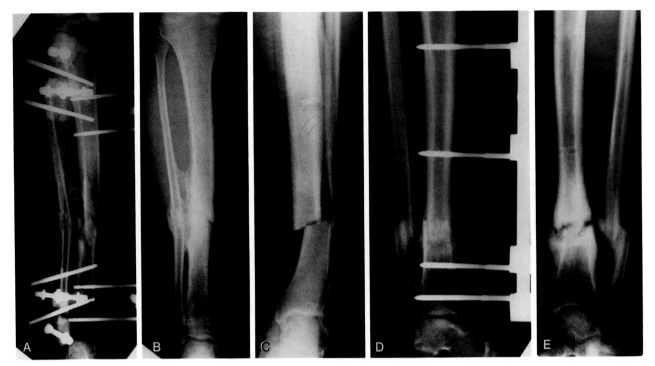

Figure 51-31

A,B. Major severity, open tibial fracture treated with external fixation and delayed posterolateral bone grafting, followed by gradually progressive weight bearing in sequentially disassembled fixator. Healing was uneventful, with satisfactory alignment maintained. Note radiolucent fixator rods. *C,D.* Moderate severity, open fracture treated with external fixation without bone graft but progressive weight bearing with dynamization of fixator frame. In spite of significant callus proliferation, union was delayed. *E,* Appearance one year after injury. Bone grafting after wounds have healed is wise for externally fixed tibia fractures of more than minor severity.

51–32). This may be done in several ways. One or two small half pins can be inserted into the subcutaneous border of the first metatarsal shaft. The fifth metatarsal can be used similarly. Alternatively, a single transfixion pin can be placed transversely through the midfoot between dorsal and plantar neurovascular and musculotendinous structures. If there is a significant ankle injury, it is wise to also stabilize the heel with one to three transfixion pins through the posterior calcaneal tuberosity. When the indication for stabilizing the foot and ankle is a soft tissue injury, a simple metatarsal extension is sufficient, if it holds the foot in neutral. Medial and lateral pins may be necessary to avoid inversion or eversion of the forefoot. The fixator segment that extends to the foot and ankle should be removed as soon as it is no longer needed.

External fixation of the knee is especially valuable for proximal tibial injuries (including those with associated articular damage, knee dislocations and fracture-dislocations, severe soft tissue injuries, and small proximal tibial fragments) and for fractures or dislocations with vascular injuries that require repair (Fig. 51–33). The simplest such frame consists of a stacked fixator with two tubes connecting two long Schanz screws in the anterior distal femoral shaft with two

similar screws in the anterior tibial shaft. Using long screws permits some flexion of the knee, in spite of the straight tubes. More flexion can be provided, at the expense of stability, if adjustable couplings are used at the knee. The technique of application is essentially as described previously for the tibial shaft fixator. Pins through the quadriceps may have a greater risk of soft tissue problems, but the absence of knee motion while the pins are in place seems to reduce such difficulties. Fixation across the knee should be considered a temporary solution; other stabilization must be found for the tibia fracture within six or eight weeks. This might involve internal fixation or a proximal tibial external fixator anchorage once soft tissues permit. Occasionally, a fracture brace may be appropriate. Manipulation of the knee under anesthesia when the femoral pins are removed helps restore motion promptly.

A small proximal tibial fragment can be stabilized with an external fixator using a cluster of two or three transfixion pins inserted from lateral to medial, with fluoroscopic guidance, close to and parallel with the articular surface. This cluster can be attached to anterior half pins distally. One alternative is to use half pins in the proximal piece inserted from either side of the patellar ligament, also with fluoroscopic guidance, to

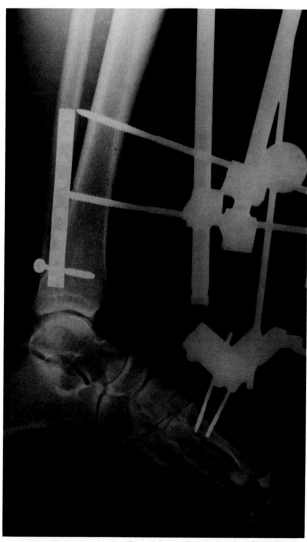

Figure 51–32

Extension of external fixation across the ankle and into the foot provides effective, atraumatic immobilization for optimal soft tissue healing and avoids contractures and pressure sores. In this case, "forearm" Hoffmann frame parts have linked the distal 5-mm tibial fixator pin to 3-mm pins in the first metatarsal.

ensure optimal anchorage without violating the knee joint or neurovascular corridors. Another, using different fixator equipment, involves use of crossed, tensioned Kirschner wires and a partial ring fixator, connected to diaphyseal half-pins.

Small distal supramalleolar fragments can usually be controlled similarly. If there is articular involvement, extension of the frame distally with transfixion pins in the calcaneus may be helpful for control of alignment and stability.

Dynamization of a tibial external fixator is possible in several ways. Using the stacked, double-tube unilateral half frame assembly described previously, loosen the pin clamps from one tube proximal to the fracture and from the other distally. This permits telescoping of the frame without rotation or angulation. This allows significant weight to be borne by the fracture without loss of alignment when the fracture configuration is sufficiently stable or when adequate healing has occurred. A single-plane, single-rod fixator frame can be dynamized by loosening the two central pin clamps and by increasing the distance of the frame from the tibia.[19]

Results

Reported results of external fixation are inconsistent, perhaps even more than might be expected of a treatment that is generally reserved for more severe tibial fractures. Strong proponents acknowledge the long treatment course associated with external fixation, but some control this successfully with aggressive soft tissue coverage, early bone grafting, and progressive dynamization with weight bearing. Many investigators have been most enthusiastic, reporting a high union rate and acceptable morbidity.[20a,35,60,68,164,188] Others have reported nonunion rates approaching 40%, malunion rates of more than 20%, prolonged times before healing, and frequent pin and other complications. Compared with nonreamed nails, external fixators have been less effective.[120,266a,302]

Loss of fracture alignment after fixator removal remains a significant challenge to the surgeon, as do pin tract problems, difficulties gaining union, and loss of joint motion. Experience, commitment, planning, and attention to detail may be important keys to the successful use of an external fixator for severe tibial fractures when soft tissue injury is severe and nonreamed nailing is not applicable. See chapter 10 for more information on external skeletal fixation.

Pins and Plaster

For many years, the use of casts incorporating transfixation pins proximal and distal to the fracture was a standard treatment for unstable tibial fractures. This eliminated the need for continuous traction and permitted ambulatory management. This approach has been reviewed by Anderson et al.[4] For those patients with severe fractures who did not develop nonunions, they reported an average time to unsupported full weight bearing of 7.5 months. When modern external fixation techniques are not available, pins and plaster provide a satisfactory alternative, but this method is cumbersome, obstructs modern wound management, is associated with a prolonged treatment course, and should be considered archaic when the surgeon has access to newer alternatives that permit joint motion or

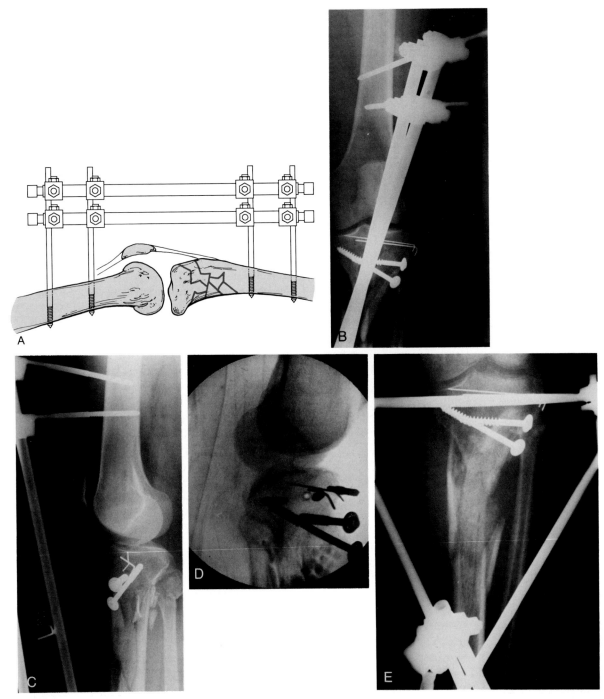

Figure 51-33

A, Schematic drawing of double-bar anterior half pin external fixator placed across knee for proximal tibial fracture. Initial AP *(B)* and lateral *(C)* radiographs after irrigation and debridement and internal fixation of articular surface component of injury. *D,* Fluoroscopy was performed for precise placement of proximal tibial transfixion pins seven weeks after injury after successful gastrocnemius flap coverage with antibiotic cement beads in fracture defect. *E,* AP radiograph after conversion to below-knee fixation and exchange of autogenous bone graft for antibiotic cement beads.

weight bearing. In some situations, however, it remains valuable.[13]

Cerclage Wiring

Few authors recommend cerclage wiring for tibial shaft fractures.[34,100] Those injuries for which it may seem most suited (i.e., spiral fractures without comminution) rarely need internal fixation, as previously discussed. Unless placed percutaneously with great care to avoid neurovascular injury, cerclage wiring is likely to be more invasive than intramedullary nailing, which is therefore a better choice. Pure lag screw fixation (see later discussion) may also be a better choice for long spiral fractures in good quality bone.

Screw and Plate Fixation

Postoperative infection, wound slough, and problems with fracture union were commonly seen after plate fixation of tibial shaft fractures when this treatment first became popular during the 1950s.[39,110,183,264] Such frequent complications encouraged a strong shift toward nonoperative treatment of closed tibial fractures in the 1960s and 1970s. Plating of tibial shaft fractures was not universally rejected, however. The Swiss AO group developed implants and technical expertise and reported plating results as good as those of any other treatment.[237] However, it soon became apparent that good results were not guaranteed by using Swiss implants. Considerable experience and expertise are necessary if complications are to be minimized. Proper patient selection is also important. Crushed soft tissues, tenuous skin flaps, severe open wounds, and other signs of high-energy trauma suggest a high risk of problems after plate fixation of tibial fractures.

In fresh tibial fractures, plates are best suited for displaced fractures that involve the articular surface. Plates should also be considered when fixation is required for fractures of the proximal or distal metaphysis that are not suitable for intramedullary nailing (Figs. 51–34 and 51–35).

Very rarely, a plate may be the best alternative for an open tibial fracture, but only when its mechanical stability is essential, the overlying soft tissues are adequate, and additional damage will not result from the required exposure.[50] Exceptional surgical experience and skill, as well as careful judgment, are required. Bach and Hansen have shown that the use of a plate rather than external fixation for open fractures carries an increased rate of infection, wound problems, and fixation failure.[9] Apparently the additional soft tissue trauma required for plating and the presence of a large foreign body negate any beneficial effect conferred by improved fracture stability. If the mechanical benefits of plating are essential for long-term management of a tibial fracture with a significant soft tissue injury, then consideration should be given to provisional external fixation, with plating done some weeks later when uncomplicated wound healing is more likely.

Plate fixation of closed tibial fractures may be used after arterial repair, particularly if the needed exposure has been created during the approach to the injured vessels (see Fig. 51–13). Plates should be used with great caution, however, in open fractures that require vascular repair, as the infection rate is especially high in this setting, and external fixation is generally preferred.

Exceptionally, when a long comminuted span of diaphysis is exposed by an open fracture, neither an ex-

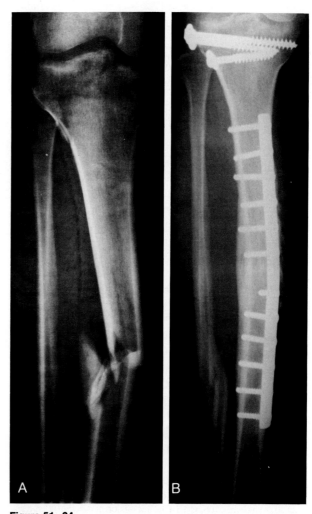

Figure 51–34

Plate fixation of closed tibial shaft fracture with associated intraarticular proximal tibia fracture that compromised intramedullary nail entry site. *A*, Preoperative AP radiograph. *B*, 18 months later. Patient is asymptomatic.

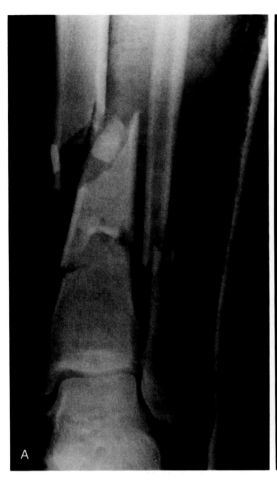

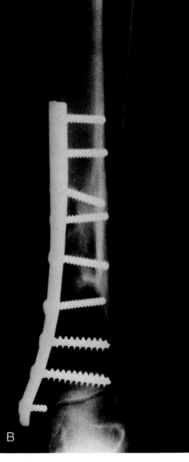

Figure 51–35

Open comminuted distal tibial metaphyseal fracture. External fixation carries less risk of wound infection but does not stabilize the fracture as well as a plate. The soft tissue wound was judged to be suitable for plating with minimal additional dissection. *A*, Preoperative AP radiograph. *B*, Seven months later. Wound and fracture healing were benign, and the patient is asymptomatic and fully active. A longer plate with 4 screws in the proximal Tibia would have been safer.

ternal fixator nor statically locked nonreamed intramedullary nailing satisfactorily stabilizes the multiple fragments. If the open fracture wound offers sufficient access for plating without additional soft tissue dissection, and if the fracture fragments are viable and not badly contaminated, then plate and screw fixation may be appropriate. Such an injury must be treated with great care to avoid additional soft tissue stripping and bone devascularization. If healthy soft tissue flaps do not permit early tension-free wound closure, then prompt muscle pedicle or free-flap closure will generally be required. Bone grafting after soft tissue healing may also be advisable for such injuries.

Plate fixation of tibial shaft fractures is most important for proximal and distal injuries adjacent to or involving knee or ankle joints. Treatment and outcome are dictated by articular involvement, with the diaphyseal injury being of secondary importance. Technical aspects of plate fixation are covered in the preceding and following chapters on tibial plateau and ankle fractures. If significant articular involvement is present, the reader should consult the appropriate section. With regard to the tibial shaft, several issues, including surgical approach, reduction techniques, and type of implant, will be reviewed.

Surgical Approach

With its triangular external cross section, the tibial shaft offers three potential surfaces for plate application. The medial and lateral are readily available from an anterior approach. The less accessible posterior surface may also be mechanically less satisfactory for plate fixation (Fig. 51–36).

It is vital to assess carefully the condition of the skin and soft tissues before choosing plate fixation and before exposing the tibia. The subcutaneous anteromedial surface of the tibia is often injured, and it may not be suitable for plate application, especially after direct local trauma. There is a high risk of wound slough if an incision is made near contusions, lacerations, or abrasions. For this reason, many believe that the anteromedial surface should rarely, if ever, be used for acute tibial fractures. A safer alternative may be the anterolateral surface, which is covered by the anterior compartment muscles. However, each injured leg should be evaluated on the basis of its own characteristics and

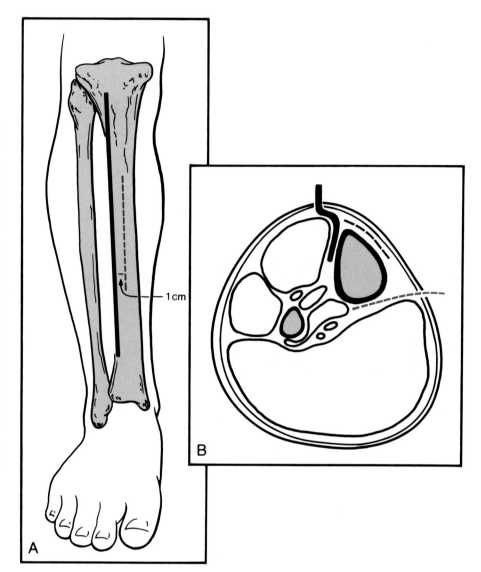

Figure 51-36

A, The standard anterior skin incision 1 cm lateral to the anterior tibial crest is used to approach either anterolateral or anteromedial surfaces. Distally the incision follows the medial border of the tibialis anterior as it crosses the tibia. The posteromedial approach is used for a double-incision fasciotomy and should never be employed together with the anterior incision, as the intervening skin bridge is too narrow and will slough. However, it can be used to plate the tibia on the anteromedial or, rarely, the posterior surface. *B*, The approach to the tibia should be carried directly through and then beneath the fascia. A fasciocutaneous flap is elevated, rather than dissecting in the subcutaneous plane. Once the bone is reached, dissection is subperiosteal. It is important to avoid stripping soft tissues from both anteromedial and anterolateral surfaces of the tibia; the soft tissue on one side or the other should be left undisturbed.

those of the injury. The presence of a posteromedial incision for vascular repair or fasciotomy provides easy access to the medial surface of the tibia, which might also be the best site for a plate if extensive soft tissue wounds mandate from the outset the use of a muscle pedicle flap for medial coverage. In such a situation, there seems to be little merit to detaching any remaining anterior compartment muscles from the bone fragments. An anterolateral incision risks slough of the intervening skin flap, if it is combined with one on the posteromedial leg.

The tibia is approached with the patient supine and a pneumatic tourniquet in place about the upper thigh. The tourniquet is usually inflated, but may not be for severely injured limbs. The leg is prepared sterilely and draped free on the standard or radiolucent operating table. Additional padding under the ipsilateral buttock may help obtain easy access to the lateral calf.

The same skin incision is used to access both the anteromedial and anterolateral tibial surfaces. The incision should be made over the muscles of the anterior compartment at least 1 cm lateral to the anterior tibial crest (see Fig. 51–36). If there is significant soft tissue contusion, a more lateral incision ensures that bone and hardware will remain covered by soft tissue, even if skin closure is not possible. The incision is carried down directly through the deep fascia without creating subcutaneous flaps. Preservation of a fasciocutaneous flap comprised of skin, subcutaneous tissue, and underlying deep fascia is important, because the dermal blood supply depends on vascular connections with the fascia.[283] The resulting anterior flap is elevated from the underlying muscles and reflected medially as needed for exposure. A longer incision is safer than overvigorous retraction. Self-retaining retractors should be used briefly and gently or not at all.

Depending on the surgeon's choice, the tibial shaft is next exposed on *either* its anterolateral or anteromedial aspect. To preserve blood supply, only minimal soft tissue should be reflected from the other surface. The tibia can be exposed either subperiosteally or extraperiosteally. Fracture healing after plate fixation appears to be equivalent with either exposure, but injured muscles do better with a subperiosteal dissection.[3,303]

Reduction Techniques

Mast and others have led a shift in emphasis from interfragmentary reduction and fixation, which generally require more bone exposure, to "indirect reduction" techniques in which soft tissue attachments are spared and the fracture is reduced by distraction or application of appropriately precontoured plates.[173,174] The "classic" AO technique for plate fixation involves provisional reduction, initial fixation with interfragmentary lag screws, and, finally, application of a neutralizing plate, which is contoured to match the surface of the reassembled tibia.[201] As mentioned, this requires significant exposure to gain reduction and to apply bone-holding clamps. The use of alternative soft tissue sparing techniques may decrease the complications of both wound and fracture healing.

The AO distractor is a helpful instrument for gaining indirect reduction (Fig. 51–37). A plate attached appropriately to one major fragment can be used to manipulate it relative to the other, often with the aid of the articulated tension device or a bone spreader and screw (Fig. 51–38).

Type of Implant

The currently optimal plate for almost all tibial fractures extending into the diaphysis is the so-called narrow AO dynamic compression plate from the large fragment set. The plate holes are shaped so that a properly placed screw causes the plate to slide along the bone, thus increasing compression forces between fracture fragments. Each end hole is slightly larger, so that a 6.5-mm diameter cancellous screw can be directed at a greater angle than it can through the other holes. This helps when the plate is used either proximally or distally but does not readily allow use of multiple metaphyseal cancellous screws. It is therefore less suited for buttress applications than the thinner and much more flexible metaphyseal plates. Recently introduced plates for the proximal tibial condyles combine the features of the narrow dynamic compression plate for the shaft and a thinner, broader proximal segment with multiple holes for cancellous screws to fix and support fractures involving the tibial plateaux (Fig. 51–39).

The broad plate with staggered holes for 4.5-mm screws is stiffer and more bulky than is appropriate for

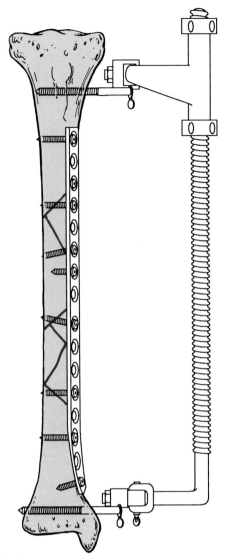

Figure 51–37

The AO bone distractor permits indirect, less traumatic reduction of a tibial shaft fracture. Traction reduction minimally disturbs soft tissue attachments of bone fragments and allows less traumatic application of an appropriately contoured plate.

the tibia. However, on occasion it may be chosen to span a significant comminuted zone or an area of segmental bone loss. Rarely, the 95° condylar blade plate is helpful for proximal tibial fractures involving the transitional zone between metaphysis and diaphysis. It provides better control of angulation for comminuted fractures when cortical contact cannot be restored on the side opposite the plate.

A tibial plate should be sufficiently long that four secure screws attach each end to the proximal and distal fragments. (Some advocate seven cortices in each fragment, accepting one screw with poor purchase on either the near or far cortex.) Be cautious about undis-

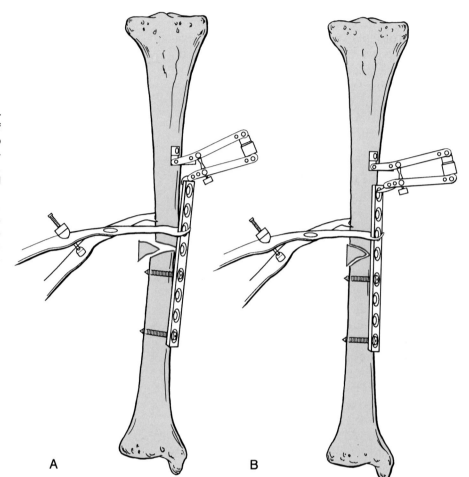

Figure 51-38

A plate can also be used as a reduction aid. It is first contoured, if necessary, and then attached to one end fragment and used to manipulate it relative to the other, often with the aid of the articulated tension device, as shown here. *A,* Tension device used as distractor. *B,* Tension device used to compress fracture fragments. It may be possible to tease comminuted fragments into place and gain interfragmentary compression through them for additional stability, but this may be less important than preserving soft tissue attachments. (Redrawn with modifications from Figure 3.10 Mast J, Jakob R, Ganz R. Planning and Reduction Technique in Fracture Surgery. New York, Springer-Verlag, 1989.)

A   B

placed comminution. Poor quality radiographs and fracture planes visible only on oblique views may significantly compromise a screw's holding power, as may osteopenic bone. In such situations, a slightly longer plate is safer. Where a plate lies over cancellous bone, it is generally preferable to use 6.5-mm cancellous screws. Unlike the cortex, cancellous bone should not be tapped prior to screw insertion. The metaphyseal cortex is usually thin and provides neither additional purchase nor an impediment to insertion of a cancellous screw. Furthermore, screw purchase in cancellous bone is improved by allowing it to cut its own threads.

Pure Lag Screw Fixation. Although plating is the basic extramedullary technique for internal fixation of tibial shaft fractures, there are situations in which screws alone may be chosen. Long spiral fractures (at least three times the shaft diameter) without comminution are most suited to lag screw fixation. The technique of lag screw insertion is important and has been well defined. In long spiral fractures with good bone quality, three lag screws are inserted both perpendicular to the long axis of the tibia and also perpendicular to the fracture line on the transverse plane in which the

screw lies. The screws should be spaced evenly, spiral with the fracture, bisect the surface of each fragment, and be well back from the thin, fragile fracture ends.[132,197,201] The shorter the obliquity or the greater the presence or likelihood of comminution, the more lag screw fixation must be protected with a neutralization plate. However, the soft tissue consequences of applying a plate must be balanced against its benefits.

Bone Grafting of Plated Fractures

It is now well recognized that a fracture that does not heal soon enough will result in failure of internal fixation. Therefore bone grafting should be considered for fractures with more than minimal bone loss or with increased risk for delayed or nonunion because of a high-energy mechanism of injury. If the soft tissue condition permits, graft may be added during plate fixation of a tibial fracture. However, if the fracture is open or there is significant soft tissue injury, then it is safer to delay grafting. For minor wounds, this might be done by way of the wound at the time of delayed primary closure, but after significant injury, it should be delayed for several weeks to minimize risk of wound prob-

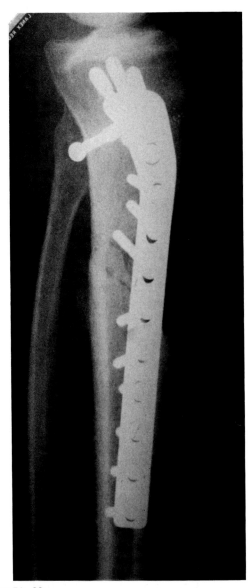

Figure 51-39

Lateral condylar plate for proximal tibial fractures. The distal portion is a narrow 4.5-mm screw dynamic compression plate. The proximal part is thinner and flared for multiple cancellous thread screws.

lems.[20] Occasionally a young patient will demonstrate radiographically evident periosteal callus formation by that time, thus obviating the need for grafting. If not, it is generally best to graft early rather than wait until fixation failure indicates the need.

Wound Management

After plate fixation of a closed tibial fracture, the wound can usually be closed primarily over suction drains. The fascia is left open to decrease the risk of compartment syndrome, and sutures are placed as gently as possible in the skin, which should never be grasped directly with forceps. After application of a sterile dressing and adequate padding, the foot and ankle are splinted in neutral, and the leg is moderately elevated during the initial postoperative period. There is no evidence to support more than brief use of prophylactic antibiotics, although their perioperative administration is valuable. Patients are much more comfortable in a splint than with the foot and ankle free following fixation of all but the most proximal tibial fractures. Early motion, if desired, may begin within a few days. A splint may still be helpful between exercise sessions for comfort and to avoid contractures. In some very badly injured limbs in which the knee or ankle require stabilization, an external fixator might be used provisionally for this purpose after an associated tibial fracture has been plated.

If a plate is applied to an open fracture, the wound should not be closed primarily. In some such situations in which the plate is inserted through a completely separate wound, the surgical wound might be closed while the original injury is left open for delayed closure by suture or skin graft. However, with severe injuries it is unwise to close any wound until the limb has been reevaluated again in the operating room.

Rehabilitation After Plating

One of the advantages of plate fixation for tibial fractures is that it usually provides sufficient stability for motion of adjacent joints and myotendinous units. This helps prevent stiffness and speeds early recovery. However, it is essential to delay significant weight bearing on the plated tibial fracture until healing is advanced enough to protect the fixation from cyclic loading and resulting failure. Optimally this can be done with limited weight bearing on crutches, using only an elastic stocking as needed to control edema. However, when patient cooperation is questionable or fixation is tenuous, additional external support must be used. In the most unreliable patient, this might be a long-leg cast with the knee flexed and the dorsum of the foot removed to permit ankle dorsiflexion above neutral. A functional cast or fracture brace could also be employed, but there are no definitive data to indicate how much protection braces offer to plated tibial fractures.

Periodic outpatient follow-up is required until the fracture is healed and the patient rehabilitated. The patient is instructed to report promptly any pain or wound problems. Unless problems are noted, radiographs are needed only every four to six weeks until union has occurred. Very limited weight bearing (15 to 20 lb) during the first six weeks after internal fixation of a tibial fracture may be gradually increased during the second six weeks, if radiographs demonstrate maintenance of fixation and progressive obliteration of any fracture lines. Weight bearing should increase more slowly after more severe injuries. Hardware removal should be delayed at least 18 months, or more for severe injuries.[201]

External callus is rarely seen with rigid internal fixation, unless bone graft has been used to obtain it. When it is observed unexpectedly but does not bridge the fracture site, such wispy "irritation callus" may indicate excessive loading and relative instability. This is an indication to reduce loading until the callus becomes radiographically mature. If healing of a plated tibial fracture does not progress, serious consideration should be given to early revision of fixation, rather than delaying necessary surgery while the tibia becomes more osteoporotic.[81,234]

Ankle and subtalar range-of-motion exercises should be carried out early after plating of a tibial fracture to minimize late disability resulting from contractures of the ankle joints. Low-resistance strength and endurance exercises are progressively increased as the fracture heals, and functional rehabilitation is completed once bone healing and soft tissues permit. By four or five months, most plated tibial fractures are healed enough for unsupported weight bearing. Rarely is it wise for the patient to return to contact sports and risk activities in fewer than nine months. Time estimates for tibial fracture healing must be adjusted upward for more severe injuries, with the clinical and radiographic progress of healing critically reassessed to ensure that union is complete before excessive loading is begun. Local pain, warmth, swelling, and tenderness may indicate mechanical instability or occult infection. Adequate radiographs, wound aspiration, sedimentation rate, and perhaps indium-labeled leukocyte scans may be helpful in questionable cases.

Results

When plate fixation is done with great skill for appropriate patients, the results are gratifying, and the few complications are usually manageable. Few series are as impressive as that of Rüedi and co-workers, who reported good or very good outcomes in 98% of closed and 88% of open fractures.[237] Complications occurred in 6% of closed and 32% of open fractures. However, after successful management, they had little effect on the end result. Nonunion occurred in less than 1% of closed and 7% of open fractures. Infections followed plate fixation after 12% of open fractures. Other authors have been enthusiastic about plate fixation,[50,90,231,289] but complication rates have been high (19% to 30%), especially after open fractures.[61,110,183,231] Two randomized trials have compared plate fixation with other treatments. Bach and Hansen found external fixation more satisfactory than plating for type II and type III open fractures.[9] Van der Linden and Lars-

son had better results with plates than with non–weight-bearing cast treatment of closed fractures from predominantly low-energy injuries, but there were more complications with plates used to treat open injuries.[289]

Primary Amputation

Indications

Every appropriate effort should be made to salvage a severely injured leg and restore its function. Modern fracture care makes this possible for the vast majority of tibial fractures. However, if limb salvage poses excessive risks to the individual, if the functional end result will be worse than with a prosthesis, or if the time required will cause intolerable psychosocial problems, then amputation may be the best course.[109,113,124a] The dismal results for salvage of type IIIC open tibial fractures reported by Caudle and Stern raise serious questions about salvage for such injuries.[41] It is especially important to avoid delaying an amputation that is inevitable from the outset of treatment. Bondurant and co-workers and Pozo et al. have emphasized the mortality, morbidity, extensive treatment, and costs associated with delayed amputation after severe tibial fractures.[25,222] Early amputation of unsalvageable limbs will reduce futile suffering and expense and expedite rehabilitation. Pozo et al.'s 15 patients with infected nonunions and delayed amputations averaged 12 operations, eight months total hospitalization, and more than 50 months before amputation. In contrast, they reported that only six months rehabilitation time was required before employment after a below-knee amputation, although patients could not always return to their previous job.

Lange et al. have proposed two absolute indications for amputation in open tibial fractures associated with arterial injuries: crush injury with warm ischemia time >6 hours and anatomic division of the tibial nerve in adults. They also offer these relative indications: serious associated polytrauma, severe ipsilateral foot injuries, and an anticipated protracted course to salvage.[161,162] Howe and colleagues have proposed a salvage index based on the arterial injury level, the severity of bone and muscle injury, and the elapsed time from injury to surgery.[124] Others have also proposed guidelines for which severely injured limbs are best amputated.[96,98,131,161,185,222,225] Age, physiologic condition, wound contamination, and necrosis of a substantial intercalary segment of calf musculature are additional potentially significant factors; as yet there is no prospectively validated and universally accepted system for determining the appropriateness of amputation. In the absence of secure indications for amputation, good judgment is required. Therefore it is appropriate to seek knowledgeable consultation or to refer such patients to treatment centers with the necessary experience.

Technique

Amputation for trauma is both a debriding and a function-restoring procedure. After a tibial fracture, modifications of standard amputations can often improve the residual limb. At the outset, it is important that all necrotic and contaminated tissue be removed. It is also important to preserve a functional knee, if possible, with sufficient tibial length below it for prosthesis use.[10,32,72,73,200] The benefits of a functioning knee are so significant that a stump that includes no more than the tibial tubercle is worth saving. A length of bone 12 to 18 cm below the medial knee joint line generally is adequate. There is little benefit to going much below the midtibia, as such levels pose cosmetic challenges to the prosthetist. Healthy, full-thickness skin cover is desirable, but split-thickness skin over muscle is also satisfactory. It is essential to debride thoroughly and not attempt to preserve unsalvageable tissue. It is also important not to discard valuable tissue below the level of amputation. Uneven skin flaps may take advantage of an asymmetric level of injury. One compartment may contain viable muscle, which can be turned proximally over the end of the bone. Weight-bearing skin or a composite tissue graft may be transferred from the foot as a neurovascular pedicle flap or, exceptionally, as a free flap.[104,241] The amputated part is a valuable tissue bank for reconstructive use. Cancellous bone, tendon, and split-thickness skin can be harvested and used, depending on the patient's injuries; a pure "guillotine" amputation may sacrifice tissue excessively. The wounds should never be closed, but should be managed instead like any severe open fracture, with early return to the operating room for redebridement as needed and, ultimately, delayed closure. If this is done within five to seven days, there is rarely a problem with contraction of the flaps, which could interfere with closure after longer delays. It is usually better to begin with bone and tissue flap lengths that permit delayed closure, rather than to insist on a transverse amputation that subsequently requires more proximal reamputation. Whenever possible, myofascial flaps, anchored to bone under adequate tension and cushioning the end of the stump, will provide an optimal limb. A rigid postoperative dressing protects the residual limb and helps avoid knee flexion contracture during the early stages of recovery.

If the soft tissue injury requires it, the longest possible higher amputation is the only alternative. Maximal length can often be obtained with a knee disarticulation, which is manageable with modern prosthetic techniques.[10,128] Heroic attempts to salvage a below-knee level may be rewarded by significantly improved function if they succeed, but they should not be considered if they risk the patient's life or threaten salvage of a long above-knee stump.

Bone Grafting

Bone grafting has several roles to play in the care of tibial fractures. Traditionally it has been reserved for those fractures that fail to unite. Acutely its need is obvious if a segment of the tibia is missing. Over the past several years, a number of authors have reported favorably on their experience with early bone grafting after severe tibia fractures to reduce the time to healing, prevent nonunion, and improve the chances of restoring normal strength to the bone.[20,24,43,99,280]

Timing

Recognizing the value of bone grafting, one might advocate the procedure as soon as possible after injury for patients who are likely to need it. This would result in some grafts being applied to tibias that would have healed anyway, while at the same time reducing the number of nonunions. However, its major drawback is that wound infection may occur, with loss of the grafted bone and development of the very complications that the operation was done to avoid. Optimal timing is not yet clear. Some recommend grafting less severe injuries at the time of delayed wound closure.[42,43,99] Behrens and co-workers found a high failure rate, usually because of infection, if such bone grafting was done during the first week. They pointed out that delayed healing was not unusual for benign-appearing tibial fractures treated with fixators.[20] Blick and colleagues recommend early grafting, based on the history of high-energy trauma. They suggest waiting two weeks after closure by suture, skin graft, or local muscle flap, but six weeks after a free muscle graft.[24] For this reason, Behrens and others have advised delaying until the wounds are well healed and sufficient time has elapsed for soft tissue revascularization (e.g., six weeks or more). On the other hand, if the soft tissue condition does permit, there is little to be gained by waiting, except perhaps in very young patients, whose periosteum may produce enough bridging bone to make grafting unnecessary. Unless the patient is infected or the nutritional status has not yet been optimized, bone grafting should be carried out for most severely comminuted tibial shaft fractures that have been treated with external fixators or plates and perhaps with nonreamed intramedullary nails as well. Haines et al. reported a series of 91 displaced tibia fractures in which bone grafting was done in 22 cases (24%) to obtain union within 35 weeks of injury.[101] Well-defined indications for early bone grafting of tibial fractures do not yet exist, but the procedure is becoming accepted in many centers that treat severe injuries.[35,285] Possible alternatives, such as injections of autologous bone marrow, remain experimental.[55]

Technique

The optimal graft is autogenous cancellous bone. This may be obtained in considerable quantities from the iliac crest, especially the posterior portion. Optimal graft placement is under a healthy layer of muscle, either preexisting normal tissue or a muscle pedicle flap, if required for coverage. It remains unclear whether posterolateral grafting is better than the use of a pocket under a muscle flap. As Christian et al. have shown, space can be reserved for such a bone graft by placing antibiotic-laden polymethylmethacrylate (PMMA) beads under the muscle flap.[45] Then, once the soft tissues are healed, bone graft is exchanged for the beads. Collaboration with the surgeon who transferred the flap is essential to avoid damage to its vascular pedicle. While protecting the adjacent muscle, the tibial surface is cleared of all soft tissue. Any necrotic cortex is removed while using a sharp osteotome to turn up superficial osseous flaps to expose bleeding bone.

Phemister's technique of raising periosteal flaps from the anterior surfaces of the tibia and placing graft within the pockets thus formed is not well suited to recent injuries. Rarely is the anterior soft tissue in condition for this procedure until months have elapsed after injury.[112,130] However, the posterior soft tissues are often healthy, and early grafting can be done using the posterolateral approach described by Harmon (Fig. 51 – 40).[111,259,260] This is far easier if the patient is prone because of the posterior location of the fibula. An external fixator, if present, is left in place unless its pins are loose. Sterile, folded linen bolsters may help position an externally fixed tibia. The interval between the lateral and the posterior compartments is identified distally, where the peronei are tendinous. Dissection is carried medially around the fibula to the interosseous membrane distal and proximal to the zone of injury, which is then exposed, progressing from normal to injured tissue. The large veins of the deep and superficial calf muscle compartments are avoided by retracting rather than entering these spaces. After subperiosteally exposing the posterior tibial surface for 4 to 5 cm proximal and distal to the fracture, the cortex is "petalled" with a sharp osteotome. The fracture site is not taken down or excised, although a small tissue sample is ob-

tained for culture. Then previously harvested cancellous graft is laid against the bleeding tibial cortex, as described previously. Graft should extend along the interosseous membrane to the fibula, if fibular reinforcement is desired. Because incorporation of the fibula to form a synostosis may interfere with ankle function, this is not chosen unless it is necessary to reinforce a tibial defect. An oblique radiograph is best for assessing placement of the graft and should be obtained intraoperatively.[5] Only the skin is closed over a suction drain, and the ankle is splinted in neutral. Rehabilitation resumes when the wound is healed, with weight bearing as soon as appropriate.

ASSESSMENT OF HEALING

Union of a tibial fracture is often more a matter of judgment than an obvious end point. Because progressive remodeling and increasing strength follow successful union, union should be seen as an important threshold rather than termination of the healing process. However, an operational definition is essential, for union implies that external support and restrictions on activity can be discontinued. Conventionally, union is diagnosed when fracture motion is not evident, the patient can walk without pain or support, and radiographs demonstrate bone continuity.

Diagnosis of healing is based on history, physical examination, and radiographs. The patient is asked about pain at the fracture, especially with activities, and can usually be fairly precise about when it ceased. He or she should report the ability to bear full weight without use of crutches or cane. The elapsed time since injury must also be considered in reference to the severity of the original injury. In Ellis's series, for example, 80% of minor (undisplaced) tibial fractures had healed by approximately 12 weeks.[71] Eighty percent of moderate (displaced, noncomminuted) fractures healed by 15 weeks, but 27 weeks were required to achieve union in 80% of tibial fractures with major severity (complete displacement with significant comminution or significant open wound).

On physical examination, a healed fracture exhibits no motion or pain with bending stress in any direction. Some local tenderness to direct pressure may be noted. Increased warmth, typical of healing fractures, is less apparent.

Anteroposterior and lateral radiographs are standard for monitoring alignment of tibial fractures, but the addition of both 45° oblique views aids in the evaluation of healing. New bone formation (radiographic callus) should bridge the fracture defect on each radiograph. A nonunion, if present, will usually be evident

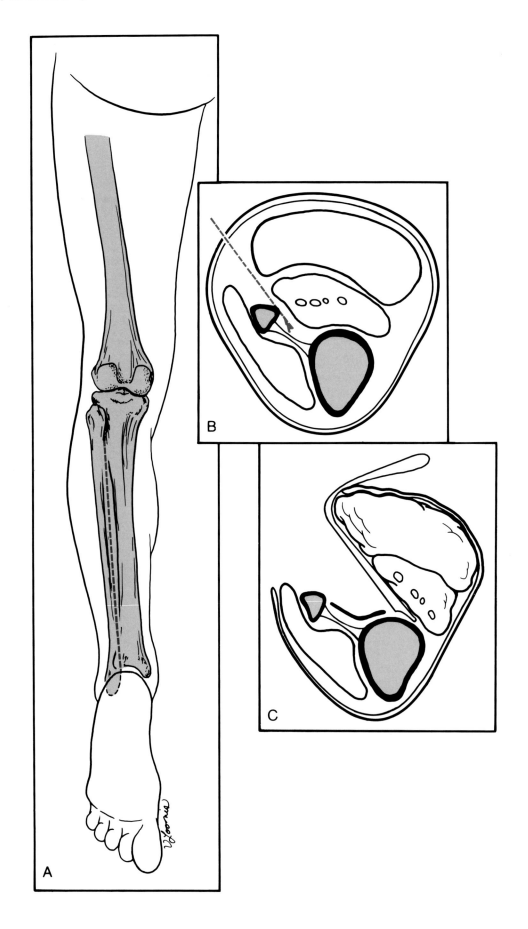

on at least one of the four views. Tomograms may be helpful but are often no more conclusive than well-exposed standard films. Unless movement is obvious on physical exam, stress films are rarely helpful. Carefully standardized stress radiographs have been used to calculate fracture site stiffness. Followed over time, failure of stiffness to increase in the typical fashion indicates nonunion.[65] Panjabi and colleagues have demonstrated that clinicians are not reliably able to assess bone strength from a single set of radiographs.[211a] Hammer and co-workers showed this clearly for tibial fractures.[108] The patient's *serial* films should be reviewed carefully for signs of problems: progressive deformity, hardware failure, lack of maturing callus, and an increasingly evident fracture cleft.

It is important to be aware of differences in apparent healing related to different techniques of fracture management. Immediately after removal of a rigid external fixator, a fracture site can feel very stiff, even though minimal radiographic callus is present. When reexamined a day or two later, obvious motion is often present. Fracture mobility and tenderness are abolished by internal fixation, unless it fails. Therefore these important signs of incomplete healing are usually absent after internal fixation, and radiographic evaluation becomes much more important.

Anatomic reduction and interfragmentary compression are hallmarks of rigid internal fixation. If achieved, the fracture line may not be evident on the initial postfixation radiographs. Fractures thus fixed exhibit essentially no external callus formation, if rigid immobilization is maintained. In this situation, healing is diagnosed primarily by absence of pain and absence of radiographic signs of instability (e.g., external callus, loss of fixation, or bone resorption around implants) as the patient progresses from non–weight bearing to full weight bearing over an appropriate time period, according to the surgeon's judgment and experience.

ASSESSMENT OF RESULTS

Outcome after a tibial fracture is most affected by the severity of injury but also depends on treatment and the occurrence of certain complications, particularly infection. There are no uniformly accepted criteria for rating results. Only rarely has severity of injury been used to stratify patients in reports of a given treatment,[7,149] and therefore it is difficult to use published results to compare treatments. There are few prospective, randomized comparisons of treatment for tibial shaft fractures. Until more such data are available, conclusions about therapeutic choices must be tentative.

A number of factors are important for assessing results of tibia shaft fractures. Most reports omit one or more of them. For example, Anderson et al. used only shortening and angulation to classify results of pins and plaster treatment into categories of excellent, good, fair, and poor. They rejected joint motion as a criterion because of confounding variables such as "associated fractures involving the knee or ankle, associated injuries of other long bones, and the age and motivation of the patient."[4] However, Horne and colleagues and Hutchins found that ankle motion was a major determinant of symptoms and function after tibial fractures.[121,124a]

It is clear that nonunion, osteomyelitis, gross deformity, amputation, and severe pain are undesirable outcomes. They are often used as criteria for a poor result. However, nonunion or infection, after corrective treatment, may ultimately yield a very satisfactory limb, whereas a united fracture, albeit with deformity, contractures of foot and ankle, and poor function, might in some series be reported as a satisfactory result. Obviously the factors considered have a large bearing on the authors' conclusions about efficacy of treatment, as do the definitions employed for fracture union and for significant deformity.

Figure 51–40

Posterolateral bone grafting is done using the approach described by Harmon.[111] *A*, The patient is positioned prone, with the posterior ilium and entire leg prepared. The leg is exsanguinated with elevation or an Esmarch tourniquet. The skin incision is shown. The peroneal tendons are identified distally and retracted laterally to gain access to the posterior aspect of the fibula. *B*, The deep posterior compartment muscles are elevated from the fibula and retracted medially, taking care to avoid injuring the large veins of the posterior calf as well as other neurovascular structures. This is easiest if a long incision is used and the fracture site is approached from normal tissue planes, with the interosseous membrane identified proximally and distally first to aid dissection in abnormal tissue. *C*, After exposing the fracture or nonunion, tissue is taken for routine culture, and the tibia is bared approximately 5 cm proximally and distally and its surface "feathered" with a sharp osteotome. At this time the tourniquet is deflated to check for significant bleeding and for bone perfusion. Separately harvested cancellous or corticocancellous autogenous iliac crest graft is packed in against the tibia, and across the interosseous membrane to the fibula, if this is desired. An oblique radiograph taken perpendicular to the interosseous membrane (internally rotated) is advisable to ensure adequate placement of the graft. A large suction drain is placed under the muscles, and only the skin is closed. Even if the fracture is stable, the foot is initially splinted in neutral position to protect against soft tissue motion.

Time for healing is an understandable focus of studies on tibial fracture treatment. A figure such as the number of months until union seems concrete and objective, but in reality, judgments are made about healing at outpatient visits occurring at intervals of at least several weeks. Furthermore, they are arbitrary, based on symptoms, function, and radiographic appearance. The precision and significance of several-week differences in healing time must therefore be questioned.

Factors that give a fair picture of results include final deformity (rotation, length, and angulation), actual times to both union and completion of rehabilitation, ultimate function, and mobility of the joints of foot and ankle. Also important, but rarely included, are length of hospitalization, associated costs and complications, number of operations, and requirements for outpatient rehabilitation. Patients are concerned not only about function, but also about the appearance of the leg.

The relative importance of these various factors is not clear, nor is the way they are best stratified. How much angulation and how much shortening are acceptable? Merchant and Dietz's and Kristensen et al.'s long-term follow-up studies failed to show a threshold beyond which angular deformity compromises late results.[157,189] Others, however, support the well-accepted concept that excessive angulation is a problem.[18,122,225]

When results are assessed is also important, particularly if the factors studied are slow to recover. An example is mobility of the hindfoot, which may be limited a year after injury but improve by two years. It is unclear how long it takes for results to become final, especially with regard to function. Digby and co-workers studied function after cast brace treatment of a group of predominantly low-energy tibial fractures. With a mean follow-up of 47 weeks (range, 26 to 98), she reported that 27% of patients had not recovered the ability to run.[62]

In addition to *what* and *when*, *how* results are presented is also a consideration. Especially in a mixed series, average time to fracture union may be misleading, in spite of its often being all that is provided. Austin showed the value of a cumulative healing curve, with percentage healed on the ordinate and weeks since injury on the abscissa.[7] Figure 51–41 illustrates this format. Rightward displacement of the healing curve, its more gradual slope, and its failure to arrive at 100% healing are typical of sets of more severe injuries and less successful treatment. If injury severity is stratified, effects of treatment become clear when groups of patients are presented this way. Figure 51–42 demonstrates the importance of both fracture severity and treatment by presenting the nonoperative results of Ellis's[71] and Burwell's[39] similarly stratified series of plated tibial fractures.[7] This format displays the rela-

tively poorer results of this plated series, especially for more severe injuries. Also apparent is the relatively smaller difference between minor and moderate injuries, classified by Ellis, compared with that between his moderate and major ones. The distinction between minor and moderate, which seems irrelevant with cast treatment, does become apparent in Burwell's plated series.

Another important concept revealed by cumulative healing curves is that there is often quite substantial overlap among groups (i.e., some severe injuries do heal within the same length of time as minor ones).

Austin used cumulative percentage curves to report his prospective study of Sarmiento's PTB cast for tibial fractures (Fig. 51–43).[8] Of particular note was the marked difference between minor and moderate severity groups, although the latter was rather small. Ninety percent of minor fractures had healed by 20 weeks, but it took 47 weeks for 90% of the moderate ones (completely displaced, minor comminution, minor wound) to heal with this treatment.

Cumulative percentage curves can be used to report end points other than fracture healing, as in Figure 51–44, which shows time until return to work after transverse tibial fracture.[3a]

Bauer and colleagues classified final results of tibial fractures into three grades: good (minimal or no complaints, full or slightly limited function), fair (minor

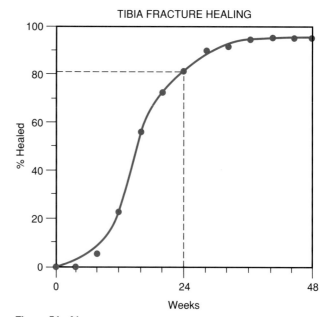

TIBIA FRACTURE HEALING

Figure 51–41

The time required for union of tibial fractures is best understood when plotted as percentage healed against elapsed time. Note that 80% of this pooled series of tibia fractures have healed at 24 weeks. (Redrawn from Austin, R.T. Injury 9:3–101, 1977.)

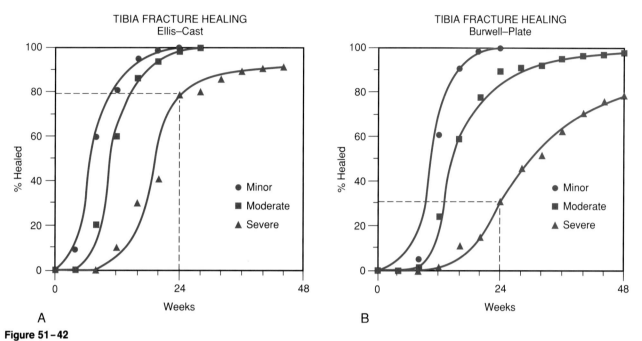

Figure 51–42

Austin[7] plotted Ellis's[71] data for cast treatment *(A)* and Burwell's[39] data for plating of minor, moderate, and major severity tibial shaft fractures *(B)*, as shown here, with separate curves for cumulative percentage healed versus elapsed time for each of the three Ellis severity grades. This clarifies differences in outcome and their potential meaning for an individual patient's fracture healing. (Redrawn from Austin, R.T. Injury 9:3–101, 1977.)

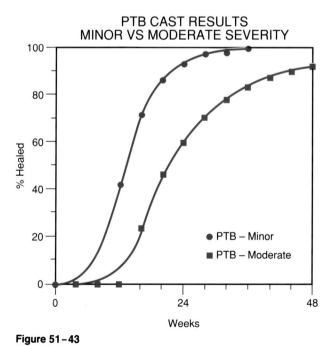

Figure 51–43

Differences in healing time between minor and moderate severity fractures treated by Austin in PTB casts with early weight bearing.[8] (Plotted from data of Austin, R.T. Injury 9:3–101, 1977.)

complaints or limitation of function), and poor (major complaints; nonunion, draining wound, amputation, or poor function of knee or ankle).[14] Edwards expanded on this scheme and used eight different parameters, plus nonunion, osteomyelitis, and amputation to classify results.[67] His system, shown in Table 51–3, considers pain; ability to work; gait; sports activity; motion of knee, ankle, and foot; and leg swelling. Notably absent is any reference to deformity. Edwards reported the following overall results: for 149 spiral fractures: good, 83%; fair, 17%; and poor 0%; for 149 closed transverse fractures: good, 75%; fair, 20%; and poor 5%; and for 106 open transverse fractures: good, 59%; fair, 26%; and poor, 14%.[67]

Johner and Wruhs used a four-level scale for classifying results of tibial fractures (Table 51–4).[133] They included deformity, which has often been omitted, but otherwise assessed factors similar to Edwards'. Although some overlap exists between categories, their "excellent" and "good" categories correspond fairly well to Edwards' "good," and "poor" has essentially the same criteria in both studies. Using this rating system, they reported results at four to eight years for 283 patients with mostly closed injuries (84%) classified by fracture morphology (see Fig. 51–7). All were treated with skeletal fixation using a plate (67%), nail (30%), or external fixator (3%). Eighty-six percent of the group had good or excellent results, 9% had fair results, and

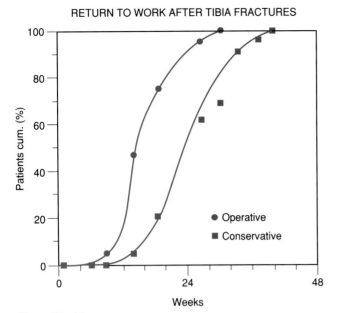

RETURN TO WORK AFTER TIBIA FRACTURES

Figure 51–44

Cumulative percentage of patients returned to work versus time since injury in a retrospectively matched series of transverse tibia fractures from the files of the Swiss National Insurance Company.[3a] In this series 50% of patients treated operatively had returned to work by 14 weeks, compared with 22 weeks for 50% of the nonoperatively managed patients. Note that all patients in both groups did return to work in fewer than 40 weeks after injury. (Drawn from data presented by Allgöwer, M. AO/ASIF Dialogue 1:1, 1985.)

5% had poor results. When reviewed separately for different categories, however, the percentage with good or excellent results ranged from 50% to 100%. Consistent with many other observers, these investigators found that spiral or oblique fractures (A1, A2, B1, C1), with mostly indirect mechanisms, had the best results (93% to 100% good or excellent). Transverse fractures resulting from direct force application (A3, B2) had slightly poorer outcomes (80% to 92% good or excellent). Comminuted transverse fractures (B3, C2, C3) with direct application of greater forces, had the poorest results, ranging from 50% to 75% good or excellent. It must be emphasized that the cases reported by Johner and Wruhs, from the University Orthopaedic Clinic in Bern, Switzerland, were treated by experts in internal fixation and included a higher proportion of closed and low- to moderate-energy injuries than might be seen in a center that deals exclusively with serious polytrauma.

Many reports of tibial fracture treatment provide data of limited and uncertain applicability to a given surgeon's patient and treatment options. These have been summarized extensively and are not reviewed in detail here.[42,43,145,149,165,284] Although they may be used to establish global rates of various complications and time required for healing, they are rarely stratified according to injury severity. A substantial amount of recently published data has been reviewed by Keller.[149] He found average times to union ranging from three to

Table 51–3.

Edwards' Classification System for Results Following Tibial Fracture Treatment

	Good	Fair	Poor
1. Pain	Little or none	Slight	Severe
2. Work capacity	Normal	Difficulty or inability to do heavy work	Markedly decreased; light seated work only
3. Limp	None	Slight with or after severe exercise	Constant
4. Sports activity	Normal	Decreased ability	Short walks only
5. Knee motion	Stable; full extension; loss of flexion less than 20°	Stable; full extension; flexion to at least 90°	Lack of full extension; flexion to less than 90°
6. Ankle motion	Less than 10° loss of dorsiflexion; less than 20° loss of plantarflexion	Dorsiflexion over 90°; less than 30° loss of plantarflexion	Dorsiflexion less than 90°; more than 30° loss of plantarflexion
7. Foot motion	Less than 25% decrease of pro- and supination	Moderately decreased	Severely decreased
8. Swelling of lower leg	Slight, only after exercise	Slight	Constant

Poor results also include:
1. Amputation
2. Osteomyelitis with recurrent drainage
3. Pseudarthrosis

Source: Edwards, P. Acta Orthop Scand (Suppl) 76:33, 1965.

Table 51–4.

Johner and Wruhs's Criteria for Evaluation of Final Results After Tibial Shaft Fracture

	Excellent (Left = Right)	Good	Fair	Poor
Nonunion, osteitis, amputation	None	None	None	Yes
Neurovascular disturbances	None	Minimal	Moderate	Severe
Deformity				
Varus/valgus	None	2°–5°	6°–10°	>10°
Anteversion/recurvation	0°–5°	6°–10°	11°–20°	>20°
Rotation	0°–5°	6°–10°	11°–20°	>20°
Shortening	0–5 mm	6–10 mm	11–20 mm	>20 mm
Mobility				
Knee	Normal	>80%	>75%	<75%
Ankle	Normal	>75%	>50%	<50%
Subtalar joint	>75%	>50%	<50%	
Pain	None	Occasional	Moderate	Severe
Gait	Normal	Normal	Insignificant limp	Significant limp
Strenuous activities	Possible	Limited	Severely limited	Impossible

Source: Johner, R.; Wruhs, O. Clin Orthop 178:12, 1983.

more than eight months, with delayed union rates of 0% to 83%. Reported nonunion rates were from 0% to 35%. Malunions, if mentioned, were reported in 0% to 60% of fractures. Loss of motion was also rarely reported but ranged from 0% to 20%. Early deep wound infections ranged from 0% to 6.6% after operations on closed fractures and from 0% to 24% after open fractures. Osteomyelitis occurred in 0% to 5.5% of closed fractures and in 0% to 23% of open ones. It is essential to remember, as pointed out by Watson-Jones, that "it means nothing to find that 1074 fractures of the tibia had an average time of union of 17 weeks. The figure depends wholly upon the proportion of simple uncomplicated fractures uniting in about ten weeks, difficult fractures uniting in 10 to 20 weeks, infected fractures uniting in 6 to 12 months, and avascular fractures uniting in one to three years."[298]

The best comparison between treatments is made by a prospective, randomized study; few of these have been presented for tibial fractures. This may be partly because of the need for stratification, so that appropriate groups for comparison become quite small, if only a single institution is involved. Hopefully the future will see well-conceived, carefully executed multicenter prospective studies of tibial fracture treatment, so that clinical impressions can be replaced by reliable data.

To date, prospective clinical trials have shown the superiority of Lottes nailing to cast treatment for unselected fractures,[210a] of plating to non–weight-bearing casts for closed displaced tibial shaft fractures,[289] of external fixation to plating for grade II and III open fractures,[9] of Lottes nailing to external fixation,[266a] and

of Ender nailing to external fixation for axially stable open fractures.[120]

Complications

Because the essence of treating tibia fractures is the avoidance of complications, most complications have already been mentioned. This section reviews the recognized complications of tibial fractures and summarizes briefly the essentials of diagnosis and treatment (see also chapter 18). Complications of tibial fractures are listed in Table 51–5.

FRACTURE SITE PROBLEMS

Deep Infection

The presence of a deep infection is usually heralded by increasing pain, drainage from the wound, or development of a sinus. Wound exploration with deep tissue cultures or, occasionally, aspiration permits early diagnosis. It is not very meaningful to distinguish between acute deep fracture site infections and so-called chronic osteomyelitis. Both processes involve necrotic, devascularized bone. Effective treatment requires surgical removal of such sequestra. Antibiotics may be helpful, but they are only an adjunct. Stability is crucial and is best provided surgically, if the fracture is not united. Usually external fixation provides the best combination of rigidity and less invasive surgery without introduction of a foreign body into the infected area. Var-

Table 51–5.

Complications of Fractures of the Tibia and Fibula

Bone and fracture site
 Deep infection
  Acute
  Chronic osteitis, drainage, or osteomyelitis
 Bone loss
 Delayed union
 Nonunion
 Malunion
 Loss of alignment in cast or brace
 Fixation problems
  Failure of hardware
  Failure of bone
 Refracture

Skin and subcutaneous tissue
 Wound slough
 Wound infection (superficial)
 Pressure sore

Nerve
 Direct injury
 Pressure from cast or brace
 Ischemic damage (compartment syndrome)
 Reflex sympathetic dystrophy

Vascular
 Arterial occlusion
 Venous insufficiency
 Deep venous thrombosis
 Compartment syndrome

Joint motion
 Associated joint surface fracture
 Contracture
  Knee
  Ankle
  Subtalar
  Foot and toe
 Late arthritis (secondary to deformity)
 Fatigue fracture distally

Functional
 Pain
 Disability (temporary vs. permanent)
  Objective
   Muscle strength
   Endurance
  Subjective
  Activities of daily living
  Work
  Sport

Cosmesis

ious host factors, especially local vascularity and systemic nutrition also play significant roles.[46] The sequence for treatment is usually (1) debridement, (2) stabilization with external fixation, (3) provision of healthy soft tissue cover with muscle pedicle or free muscle flap grafts, and (4) bone graft of any resulting defect.[6,37,75,86,177,272,286,300,309] Adequate debridement may require creation of a defect in the tibia, the management of which is discussed later (Fig. 51–45).

If an infected tibial fracture is satisfactorily stabilized by an intramedullary nail, it may be best to continue with intramedullary stabilization until the fracture is healed.[138,139] Adequate drainage and debridement are of course indicated, as may be bone grafting. Suppressive antibiotics are chosen according to sensitivity studies on cultures from deep tissue specimens. If the nail is loose, its removal and exchange for a larger one may provide both increased stability and a measure of debridement by gently reaming the canal to a larger diameter. The reamings are cultured to confirm appropriate antibiotic choices. Rarely, a flagrant infection after intramedullary nailing will not respond to such treatment and requires nail removal, extensive intramedullary debridement, and external fixation.[216]

The treatment of infected nonunions is discussed further in chapters 20 and 21.

Bone Loss

Loss of bone may occur with an open fracture or be the result of subsequent infection and necessary debridement. Loss of either an intercalary segment or a substantial paraxial portion requires restoration of bone substance to obtain fracture union or to prevent pathologic fracture through a seriously weakened area. Soft tissue defects are frequently present and usually need repair before bone grafting.[6,12,45,86,176,182,255,300,309,312]

There are occasional reports of replacing extruded fragments of the tibia after sterilization.[103] Although this may work, the risks of infection and delayed reincorporation of the bone increase the attractiveness of other alternatives, primarily autogenous cancellous bone graft. Allografts (if no infection is present), free vascularized autografts, and Ilizarov traction osteogenesis are other possibilities (see chapters 15, 20, and 21).[127,211,240,273]

Delayed Union

The term "delayed union" describes an ununited fracture that continues to show progress toward healing or has not been present long enough to satisfy an arbitrary time criterion for nonunion. The lack of precision in its definition decreases its value in reports of results. Retarded progress of union is especially evident after more serious fractures, as in Edwards' series, in which only 23% of grade III open fractures had healed by six months.[68] It is essential for the surgeon to recognize

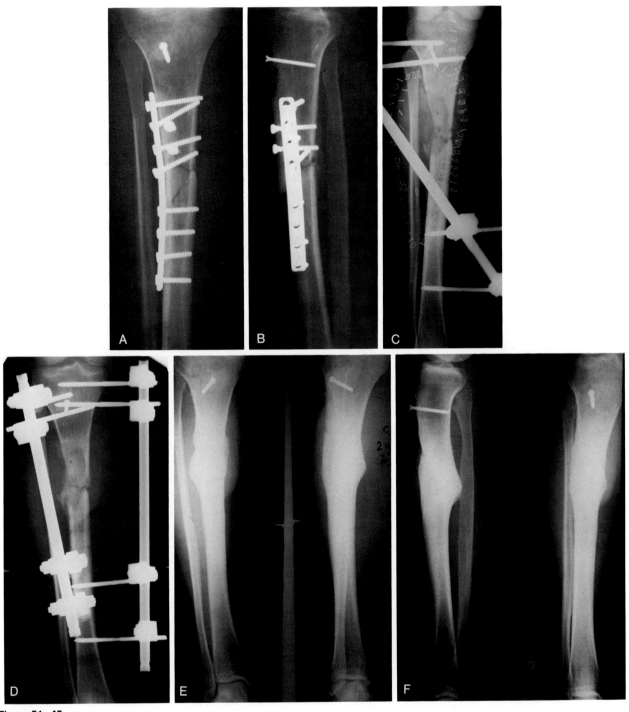

Figure 51–45

Infected draining tibial shaft fracture with exposed hardware after plate fixation. *A,B,* The hardware became loose prior to fracture healing. *C,* The plate and screws were removed and an external fixator was applied, using an oblique frame for stability and easy access for serial wound debridement. This was followed by medial gastrocnemius muscle pedicle flap and cancellous bone grafting once the wound was clean and the bone entirely covered by healthy granulation tissue. *D,* Once the wounds were healed, the fixator was modified for additional fracture stability to gain purchase of additional pins in the osteoporotic proximal metaphysis. *E,F,* Healed fracture. The wound healed as well, and the patient is minimally symptomatic.

delayed healing, search for causes, and make appropriate decisions about treatment.

It is usually difficult to identify a definite cause for retarded healing of a given fracture, but occult infection is a possibility that must always be considered.[172] Poor local blood supply, bone loss, excessive mechanical instability, and, for some fractures, insufficient functional use are some of the potential contributors to delayed healing that can be addressed in the treatment of delayed union of the tibia (Fig. 51–46). Fracture malalignment may need correction to prevent potential adverse effects on the mechanical environment, as well as to promote union. The factor most commonly associated with delayed union of tibia fractures is the severity of the original injury. Many other possible local and systemic contributing factors are discussed in chapter 20.

Continued weight bearing in an appropriate brace or cast will often lead to union of a fracture that is being treated closed.[209,247] The same treatment may be appropriate for fractures that have been fixed with an intramedullary nail, but if union does not occur, the nail will fail and become more difficult to extract. The best treatment for a nailed tibial fracture that is not uniting is usually a reamed nail of larger diameter. This is advisable if union is not evident by six to nine months. Because the durability of an intramedullary nail depends on several factors, some judgment is necessary, especially for smaller diameter locked nails. The risk of activating an infection by substituting a reamed nail for a nonreamed nail originally placed for an open fracture is as yet unknown. In such a patient, an onlay bone graft may be a safer alternative.

If a delayed union is noted after plate fixation and there is no infection, then intramedullary fixation may also be appropriate.[81,234] If flagrant infection is present, then debridement, often followed by change of fixation from plate to external fixation, and subsequent bone

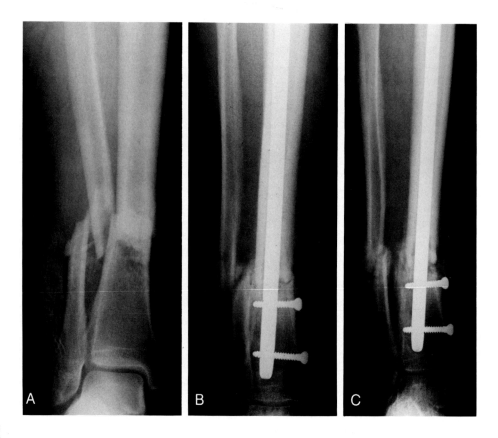

Figure 51–46

A, Open, moderate severity distal tibiofibular fracture treated with irrigation and debridement, a distally locked nonreamed intramedullary nail, and delayed split-thickness skin grafting. *B,* Five months after injury, the patient had mild pain on weight bearing, fluffy callus without union, some resorption about his hardware distally, and questionable motion at the fracture site, with slight tenderness. Fatigue failure of the 9-mm intramedullary nail was a concern, especially because the fracture site was so close to the upper of the two distal locking screws. An orthosis was prescribed. *C,* Six weeks later he was bearing full weight in his ankle-foot orthosis without any pain and had a stable, nontender fracture. Sclerosis of the proximal fracture end probably represents avascular necrosis caused by the fracture or by interference with medullary diaphyseal blood flow by the snugly fitting, nonreamed nail. The fracture subsequently healed, after which fracture of the nail was noted at the upper distal locking hole.

grafting will be required. However, with a suppressed or quiescent infection, a secure plate will often permit fracture union, especially if bone graft is added. Control of infection then follows fracture healing.[37]

Delayed union is especially common after external fixation, which is generally used for more severe fractures. If the fixator must be removed before the fracture has consolidated, loss of alignment may follow. Therefore, as discussed previously, the physician should routinely consider early bone grafting and progressive weight bearing after appropriate fixator modifications or, alternatively, plan on conversion from external fixation to a plate as soon as soft tissue healing permits.[233]

Fibular osteotomy has been recommended as a stimulus for tibial fracture union. Although it might counteract a tendency to varus deformity produced by an intact fibula and might produce more loading of a tibial fracture, osteotomy of the fibula is not a very successful means of achieving union.[94] It may also increase instability and deformity.

Various types of electrical stimulation have been advocated for problems of fracture healing.[11,116,193] A recent study indicates that at least one variety of magnetic stimulation is more effective than a placebo, though less so than most reports of surgical techniques.[257]

As long as a tibial fracture is satisfactorily aligned, progressing toward union, and not causing more pain or disability than the patient can tolerate, then the physician should continue the treatment course or increase functional weight bearing with appropriate external support, unless risk of fixation failure prevents this.[54,57] However, if unacceptable deformity, an excessively prolonged course, or a high likelihood of nonunion become evident, it is appropriate to reexamine the alternatives and perhaps choose another treatment option. The choice must meet the patient's needs, especially correction of any deformity, but should also have a high likelihood of achieving union within a reasonable length of time. It should interfere as little as possible with the patient's activities and have a low risk of complications compared with the other alternatives.

Loss of Reduction in a Cast or Brace

Acceptable alignment may be gained and lost during treatment of a fracture. This occasionally occurs with failure of internal fixation but is more common with a cast or brace. Alignment loss is a significant risk after removal of an external fixator, as stability is hard to assess, and less control is provided by a cast.

During nonoperative treatment of a tibial fracture, periodic radiographs are required to identify loss of satisfactory alignment. Reduction goals are usually set more strictly than guidelines for acceptable deformity after healing. This is reasonable, because osteotomy of a healed fracture usually has a higher risk-to-benefit ratio than does correction of deformity in an ununited one. Most references give guidelines of 5° to 10° maximal varus-valgus angulation, 10° to 20° sagittal plane angulation, up to 1.5 or even 2 cm shortening, and up to 15° internal or 20° external rotation.[42,43,165,225,280,287] Appearance of the limb and unwillingness to accept any deformity have become issues for some patients. It is important to acknowledge that some, usually slight, deformity is an expected outcome of closed treatment for tibial shaft fractures and that this is rarely, if ever, of any consequence to long-term outcome.

If alignment of a tibial fracture becomes unacceptable during closed treatment, correction may be possible by manipulation and revision of the cast or brace. This may require return to a long-leg cast, perhaps with temporary restriction of weight bearing. If adequate correction cannot be obtained and maintained, then an alternative treatment should be selected and carried out before the fracture heals unsatisfactorily. Depending on the deformity, its mobility, and the fracture configuration, this may require a carefully planned open reduction.[174] If so, bone grafting should be considered. Closed reduction and fixation with an intramedullary nail is a better option, if possible. Rarely, an external fixator may be used to realign a healing fracture.[93]

Fixation Failure

Fracture fixation depends on a composite of bone and hardware. Either, or both, may fail and result in loss of fixation. Bone may be deficient, most often because of osteoporosis or unrecognized comminution. Internal fixation may prove inadequate because of insufficient length, too few screws, too weak an implant, poor technique, or too much loading, or because the fracture does not heal within a reasonable period of time. Clues to failing fixation are provided by development of deformity, by loosening or plastic deformation of implants, and by the appearance of peripheral callus in a fracture that is thought to be rigidly fixed. The possibility of fixation failure must be anticipated whenever progressive fracture healing is not radiologically evident.

Treatment generally requires at least decreased loading and, if failure has occurred, revision of the fixation. Unless infection is present, failed diaphyseal plate fixation without infection is often best revised with an intramedullary nail.[81] If the problem is metaphyseal, new lag screws and a plate are usually needed.[234] External fixators may require new pins or possibly removal and replacement with a plate, unless healing is sufficient for removal of the fixator without later loss of alignment.[233] Reaming and insertion of a larger nail is usually the best choice when healing does not progress after intramedullary fixation. Various methods have been devised to help remove retained fragments of a broken intramedullary nail.[64,79]

Whenever a fracture is not healing as expected, the possibility of a deep infection must be excluded by appropriate tissue cultures.[172] These should be obtained prior to revision of fixation if there is any indication of sepsis.

When fixation is not adequate and fracture fragment mobility is noted, some mechanical change is warranted; this usually means revision of fixation. If failure has not yet occurred, onlay bone grafting may provide the necessary stimulus to healing. Revision strategies to be avoided are plating after intramedullary nailing, flexible intramedullary nailing after rigid fixation, and external fixation without bone grafting. Intramedullary nailing after external fixation is risky because of the likelihood of bacterial contamination from pin sites or the initial injury.[175,181] Adequate debridement, prolonged delay, and preoperative or intraoperative medullary cultures with appropriate antibiotic coverage, are all ways to decrease the risk of intramedullary sepsis.[137,155,194]

Nonunion

Like the diagnosis of delayed union, calling an ununited fracture a nonunion is also an arbitrary decision, until radiographic criteria are met. Time limits that have been used range from five months to more than a year.[57,94,112,117] A good working definition for nonunion is that of Heppenstall: a fracture that has shown no radiologic progress toward union during a three-month period.[117] If extending the definition of nonunion leads to long delays before treating a disabling condition, even if it may eventually heal, there is little benefit to the patient. However, if that patient is functional, comfortable, and not losing alignment or fixation, then weight-bearing treatment may reasonably be continued for prolonged periods. Noninvasive electrical stimulation may also be considered. However, disability, pain, malalignment (especially if progressive), and actual or impending hardware failure should lead to a prompt change in treatment. Electrical stimulation is not appropriate in the presence of unacceptable deformity.

Treatment of nonunion is discussed further in chapters 20 and 21.

Malunion

The significance of residual deformity after union of a tibial fracture remains uncertain. It is generally addressed in terms of single parameters: angulation in coronal or sagittal planes, shortening, or rotational deformity. No information is available regarding combinations of these elements. Puno and others have pointed out that the location of the deformity is important. Angulation is more significant, in terms of its effect on ankle loading, with more distal fracture sites.[225,297] Kettlekamp et al., looking at knee joint arthritis, demonstrated abnormal joint loading as a result of tibial deformity.[154] This seemed more of a problem with varus than with valgus deformities. They pointed out that very long-term studies are needed to demonstrate the relationship between deformity and arthritis, as more than 30 years had elapsed between fracture and arthrosis in their small series of patients. Merchant and Dietz reported long-term follow-up (average, 29 years) for 37 patients with closed or type I open tibial fractures.[189] Seventy-eight percent of the ipsilateral ankles had a good or excellent result, and 92% of the knees had an excellent result. They found no significant difference among groups of patients with 5° or less angulation, 5° to 10° angulation, and more than 10° angulation. Pain and radiographic appearance did not correlate with deformity. Outcomes were not demonstrably worse in more distal fractures with deformity. They concluded that there remains no established limit for acceptable angulation of a healed tibial fracture. Kristensen et al., in a similar long-term follow-up study, concluded that deformity of up to 15° did not produce ankle complications.[157] Nonetheless, some patients with deformity after tibial shaft fractures are symptomatic. Perhaps, as Olerud has pointed out, there are individual variations in the ability to compensate.[206]

Because it is not possible to predict which patients with deformity will be symptomatic, it remains appropriate to strive for restoration of normal alignment during treatment of tibial fractures. There is no strong clinical evidence, however, for aggressive treatment to correct asymptomatic malalignment simply to ward off the possibility of late posttraumatic arthrosis.

For symptomatic patients with significant deformity, an osteotomy is the appropriate treatment. A complete preoperative evaluation and careful planning are essential for best results.[122,134,139,173,174,201] Graehl and colleagues have advocated a supramalleolar osteotomy through rapidly healing cancellous bone to correct frontal plane deformity.[89] Their patients had a number of complications, in contrast to results reported by Janssen and Dietschi for supramalleolar wedge osteotomies.[129] Mast, Sangeorzan and colleagues, and Horster have described various techniques for wedge osteotomies.[122,174,242] Complex deformities can be corrected by osteotomy through the site of malunion with plate and screw fixation or intramedullary nailing.[134,139] If the bone configuration permits, osteotomy and intramedullary nailing may provide durable fixation in satisfactory alignment, but extensive soft tissue stripping from the diaphyseal osteotomy site may make

it wise to add bone graft. Interlocking nails offer more secure control of alignment than do simple nails and might be preferable after tibial osteotomy (Figs. 51–47 through 51–49).

Shortening of up to 2 cm can be tolerated by most patients, although a shoe lift or innersole may be appreciated.[97] Many patients are unhappy about this possibility, however. Minor rotational deformities are not a problem, but Van Der Werken and Marti advise osteotomy if external rotation is greater than 20° or if internal rotation is greater than 15°.[287]

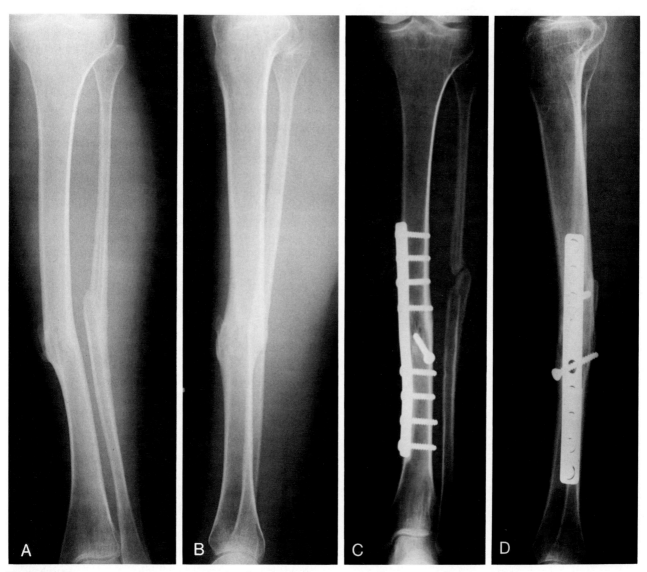

Figure 51–47

Midtibial osteotomy for malunion of previous left tibiofibular fracture. In addition to the evident 10° valgus deformity, the patient had 35° internal rotation, ¾-in shortening, knee pain, and an unsightly gait. *A,B,* Preoperative AP and lateral radiographs, respectively. *C,D,* Healed osteotomy of tibia and fibular nonunion, with fixation still in place. The patient had relief of deformity and knee pain, ½-in residual shortening, and mild hardware tenderness after derotational wedge osteotomy with distal sliding that gained approximately ¼-in length.

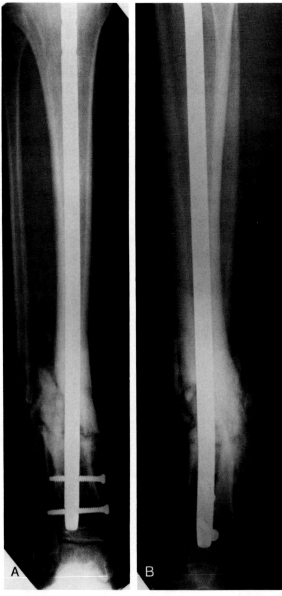

Figure 51-48

Intramedullary nailing can be used to salvage a nonunion after aseptic failure of plate or nail fixation. Caution should be used, however, regarding intramedullary nailing after external fixation. A,B, AP and lateral radiographs, respectively, after osteotomy of tibia and fibula and revision of intramedullary nailing. (Preoperative radiograph is shown in Figure 51–21A.) Posterolateral bone graft had been done before the fracture healed in a valgus position, which was intolerable to this active man with a prior subtalar arthrodesis.

Refracture

Excessive loading prior to fracture healing may result in deformation of an incompletely healed fracture. White and co-workers defined four stages of fracture healing, demonstrating flexible and then more rigid failure, followed by high-energy failure through the fracture site, and finally, failure adjacent to the healed fracture.[301] The greater polar moment of inertia of the larger diameter healed callus and adjacent disuse osteopenia presumably play roles in this. The clinical relevance of such refracture from torsional loading of healed spiral tibial fractures has been demonstrated by Böstman.[29]

Refracture can also occur when hardware is removed too early. This is more likely with plate fixation, as a satisfactory reduction obliterates the fracture line, and visible callus does not form. Although waiting at least 18 months is generally sufficient, higher energy fractures or those with greater devascularization may heal slower. Removal of screws and external fixator pins transiently weakens bone, so that significant cast or PTB functional brace protection, with gradually progressive weight bearing to allow remodeling and restoration of strength, is mandatory if fracture through screw holes in the tibia is to be avoided.[38] The length of time for the human tibial diaphysis to regain its strength after screw removal is not known for certain, but a waiting period of at least six weeks before unsupported weight bearing and 12 weeks before contact or risk activities are conventional restrictions. It has been asserted that plates cause progressive disuse osteopenia as a result of stress protection. However, recent studies indicate that the osteopenia, which is well localized under the plate, is probably a result of interference with local vascularity[218] and is not progressive.[279] Therefore leaving an appropriately chosen plate in place long enough to obtain complete healing should cause no concern. This reduces, rather than increases, the risk of refracture.

Wound Slough

Wound healing difficulties often result from damage sustained at the time of injury, especially if degloving occurs, with loss of the radially oriented blood supply to the skin. Not unusually, the problem becomes evident after a surgical incision is placed through the injured area. Deep abrasions, crushing, significant swelling, and fracture blisters are some of the indicators of an area of risk. Problems can often be avoided by resisting the temptation to operate through such an area until it has recovered.

The combination of contused and poorly perfused tissue, an open wound, and bacterial contamination predisposes to infection, which may remain superficial or, because of proximity to the fracture site, may involve it as well. In the absence of significant infection, a superficial wound will heal, unless there is inadequate local blood supply, fracture instability, edema, or external pressure. It is important to recognize early a skin

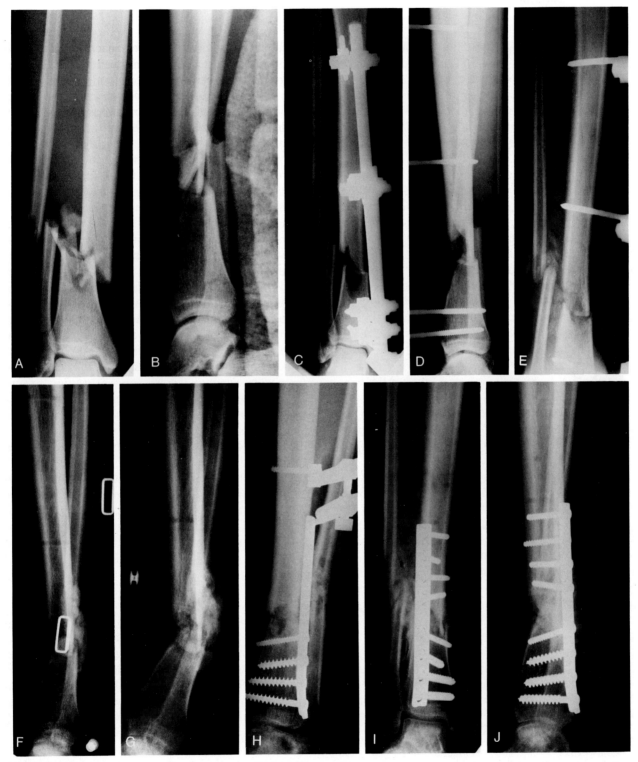

Figure 51–49

A,B, AP and lateral radiographs, respectively, of major severity, open, crushed distal tibiofibular shaft fracture. Note disruption of interosseous membrane proximally, indicated by diastasis on radiograph. *C,D,* Radiographs after irrigation, debridement (including removal of avascular bone fragments), and external fixation, which extended to the foot. *E,* Six weeks after injury, when the wound was healed, a posterolateral bone graft was done. *F,* Progressive weight bearing was begun six weeks later, and the fixator was removed when the patient was fully weight bearing, four months after injury. *G,* Although the fracture appeared united clinically and was protected with crutches, a brace, and, subsequently, a cast, significant apex posterior angulation (25°) developed. *H,* Correction was accomplished with a posterior tension band plate. The fracture site was still mobile through a small cleft. No additional bone graft was applied. *I,J,* Three months later the fracture was united with satisfactory alignment, and the patient had a normal pain-free gait.

flap that is in jeopardy. Correction of some or all of these factors might salvage it. If full-thickness necrosis does occur and the fracture site is exposed before the formation of well-organized callus, the risk of a deep wound infection is high. Immediate debridement of such a flap and replacement with viable soft tissue coverage may prevent a deep infection and promote fracture healing.

A small wound, especially if it does not communicate with a fresh fracture hematoma, will often heal satisfactorily with minimal treatment. Bone with intact periosteum will rapidly be covered by granulation tissue. If it is bare and necrotic, this process takes much longer, though it may still occur, especially in smaller wounds. Even exposed hardware may be covered by secondary wound healing, though the process is slow and often punctuated by episodes of infection with pain, swelling, erythema, and drainage. Such problems often occur after a draining wound heals completely and may be less frequent if a small opening remains. Although a chronic infection persists around such an exposed plate, bone healing often continues slowly if the fixation is secure. Once the fracture is united, removal of the plate and superficial debridement of its bed is often followed by secondary wound healing and resolution of active or recurrent flares of infection, unless sequestra remain.[37]

It is important to recognize that many fractures with exposed bone or hardware can unite without hardware removal or surgical soft tissue coverage. There are no well-supported guidelines for treating established soft tissue sloughs. In many situations, slowly progressive healing may be more acceptable than aggressive debridement and soft tissue coverage. If fixation is secure, healing is progressing, and infection does not remain active, simple wound care may be all that is required until the fracture is healed. Then it is often quite simple to proceed with hardware removal, debridement, and delayed coverage. If progress is not satisfactory, and especially if fixation becomes unstable, then a change in treatment is required. This usually entails hardware removal and radical debridement of necrotic bone and soft tissue. External fixation, muscle flap coverage, and delayed bone grafting offer an effective salvage.[45,86,88,101,176,300,311] Alternatively, the Ilizarov techniques of bone transport and nonunion treatment may be considered.[202]

Superficial Wound Infection

Superficial wound infections occasionally develop during open treatment of closed fractures, as well as after open tibial injuries. Definition and diagnosis are im-

portant, because trivial treatment of a deep infection is usually ineffective. Even worse, failure to identify and treat a deep infection promptly and appropriately may compromise its definitive care. Therefore any pain, tenderness, redness, swelling, and (presumably) superficial drainage should be seen first as a possible indication of a deep infection, if they persist beyond the normal first few days of wound inflammation.[37] Adequate deep cultures are essential, if there is any indication of infection extending below the subcutaneous tissue. These can usually be obtained by needle aspiration with sterile technique. The fracture hematoma and the area around any hardware should be sampled and studied with Gram stain as well as culture and sensitivity tests. If no fluid can be aspirated, introduction of a small volume of nonbacteriostatic saline may permit a culture. A more certain test is operative exploration of the wound, with tissue samples obtained under direct vision for bacteriologic studies. Because it leads to prompt definitive diagnosis and care, formal surgical exploration of a possibly infected wound is safer than merely opening it on the ward and instituting dressing changes. Early aggressive management of a significant infection minimizes recovery time and improves results. However, there are patients with superficial erythema, possibly a bacterial cellulitis, who have no signs of deep infection and who respond in a few days to rest, elevation, and antibiotic treatment appropriate for gram-positive cocci. Some infections are undoubtedly superficial, though the burden of proof is on the treating surgeon. In time, a significant deep infection may become manifest.

PRESSURE SORES

The use of casts and splints always risks development of a pressure sore, typically occurring over a bony prominence. It is crucial to be aware of this, especially if the patient's level of consciousness or peripheral sensation is impaired or his or her nutrition is poor, and to pad appropriately all areas at risk, including the fibular head and neck, posterior heel and Achilles tendon, malleoli, anterior tibial crest, and the fracture site. Early inspection of such areas through a cast window may permit correction of a problem before major tissue loss occurs. It is important to manage such a window with care. It should be well placed and be large enough to see the area in question. After windowing a cast, the removed piece of plaster should be replaced over adequate padding. Adhesive-backed foam padding can be applied directly to the removed piece of plaster. Failure to close a window can lead to localized swelling (window edema) and more pressure problems around the edge of the window. Replaced or not, a window weakens a cast, perhaps too much for weight bearing or even for it to remain a satisfactory splint. Reinforcement, preferably with fiberglass cast tape, or replacement of the cast may be needed.

Although pressure sores are usually associated with casts and splints, they may also occur during treatment with external fixation. Occasionally this is from pressure of a malpositioned frame component, but more often it is because the entire weight of the leg is borne by the patient's heel on an inadequately padded bed surface. Because of obtundation, pain, or other impediment to moving the leg, a pressure sore develops on the posterior heel. This may be prevented by suspending the leg from the fixator frame or by using padding that distributes the weight over the entire posterior surface of the leg. Should a pressure sore develop, immediate relief of pressure and appropriate wound care techniques must be employed.

NERVE INJURIES

Direct injuries to the peripheral nerves of the leg may result from laceration, contusion, traction, or a combination of these mechanisms at the same time as the tibial fracture.[196] It is thus vital to perform and document a detailed neurologic examination as soon as possible during the patient's care. If a complete exam is impossible, the possibility of an occult nerve injury must be kept in mind and precautions taken, including a complete documented examination as soon as it is feasible. Nerve injuries can occur during treatment as well as from the initial trauma. Obviously care must be taken during surgical approaches and application of fixation, including percutaneous pins or wires for external fixators. Pressure injury from a cast, particularly over the peroneal nerve as it rounds the proximal fibula, is a well-known complication. The same may occur from pressure of a splint, traction frame, fracture table, and even the hospital bed. If loss of peroneal nerve function occurs, the subcutaneous course of this nerve must be inspected. It is important never to blame a nerve injury, including "tourniquet palsy," for loss of motor or sensory function in a patient who is developing a compartment syndrome. Although pain is usually present with compartment syndromes, if a sensory deficit is already present, or if the painful period is missed for some reason, then this initially treatable cause of impaired neural function may be ignored.[310] Impaired motion or sensation can also be a sign of arterial injury.

Reflex sympathetic dystrophy may follow any injury to the lower extremity.[251] This subject is reviewed in chapter 19.

VASCULAR PROBLEMS

The diagnosis and treatment of arterial injuries associated with tibial fractures is discussed previously, as well as in chapter 12. It is important to remember that onset of vascular occlusion can be delayed. Adequate patient monitoring must include continued assessment of vascular status. Later, false aneurysms and arteriovenous fistulas may be found.

Venous insufficiency may be the result of an associated acute injury, as well as of deep venous thrombosis, which is common and can occur at any point during recovery from a tibial fracture.[204] This is most often limited to the deep veins of the calf and is rarely recognized. It usually has no evident sequelae, but occasionally thrombosis may progress proximally, or pulmonary embolism may occur. Risk factors for pulmonary embolism should be assessed and anticoagulation considered for high-risk patients after the early stages of injury. Certainly, symptoms and signs that suggest a pulmonary embolism after a tibial fracture must be evaluated seriously with a ventilation-perfusion (V/Q) scan and pulmonary angiogram, if indicated. For tibia fracture patients without elevated risk factors, it is probable, though not proven, that the risks of routine prophylactic anticoagulation exceed the benefit (see chapter 18). Chronic venous stasis is a potentially challenging problem after tibia shaft fractures complicated by venous thrombosis.[2,223] The relative rarity of chronic swelling is fortunate, given the prevalence of venous occlusion, but it is usual for a patient to have some degree of foot and calf edema during the months after a tibial fracture. Elastic support stockings are thus frequently beneficial until the tendency for swelling abates.

COMPARTMENT SYNDROMES

Compartment syndromes, listed here for completeness, have been discussed previously in this chapter and more thoroughly in chapter 13.

ASSOCIATED FATIGUE FRACTURE

During rehabilitation after a period of prolonged nonweight bearing, some patients will develop pain and well-localized tenderness in a metatarsal, the calcaneal tuberosity, or the distal fibula. Radiographs are usually normal initially. Results of other studies may become positive, confirming a fatigue fracture. Usual treatment is temporary reduction of weight bearing, rather than external immobilization.

LIMITED JOINT MOTION

Injuries to the articular surfaces of the knee, ankle, subtalar joint, or foot are obvious causes of impaired motion, posttraumatic arthritis, and pain. They are discussed in chapters 50 and 52 and are mentioned here only to remind the reader that early recognition is necessary for effective treatment of these injuries (Fig. 51–50).[28,288] Bowing of an intact fibula associated with a shortened tibial fracture may cause ankle symptoms.[142]

Contractures also involve these same joints after tibia fractures, even without direct articular injury. Such problems are rare at the knee; most are probably the result of unrecognized knee injuries.[107,179,277,290] Some loss of knee motion may result from prolonged immobilization. Contractures are more significant problems in the ankle and foot, as demonstrated and discussed by McMaster after closed treatment and Merriam and Porter after open treatment and confirmed by Horne et al.[121,184,192] Most common is subtalar stiffness, without bony damage, present in 72% of patients in McMaster's series and in 50% of Merriam and Porter's. Motion was

better preserved after internal fixation and in both groups was only occasionally severe enough to be a functional problem (12% after closed treatment and 16% after open treatment). Operative fracture fixation, followed by early motion, does appear to decrease foot and ankle stiffness.[262,289] Some, but not all, studies suggest that contractures are related importantly to the amount of soft tissue damage, especially in the lower half of the leg. Unrecognized deep posterior compartment syndrome can also cause contractures, especially of the forefoot and toes.[143] Rupture or loss of the posterior tibial tendon may cause a pes planus deformity.

Failure to immobilize the foot and ankle in a functional position results in far more disability than mere loss of motion. A fixed equinovarus deformity is to be avoided at all costs. This can usually be done with a cast or splint. More severe open injuries are especially well managed by extending the external fixator out to the foot. Edwards' patients with severe open tibial fractures had only a 5% incidence of major problems with foot and ankle contractures.[68] Toe flexion contractures can generally be prevented by repeated passive manipula-

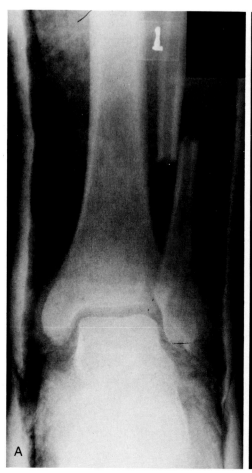
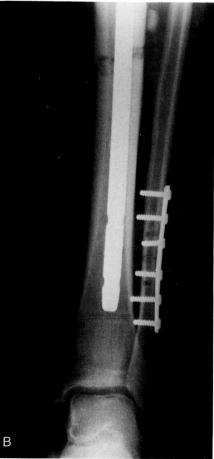

Figure 51–50

Ankle joint injury is occasionally associated with a tibial shaft fracture. Anatomic reduction and fixation provide the best opportunity for normal function of the ankle and may be required to gain satisfactory reduction of both fractures. *A*, Radiograph obtained when patient was first seen, three weeks after injury. *B*, After open reduction and internal fixation of both fractures. The transverse lucency distal to the tibial nail was left by a bone distractor screw.

tion but occasionally persist or recur and, if symptomatic, benefit from surgical correction.

Recovery of ankle and, especially, foot mobility is slow after tibial fractures but often occurs if a patient can initiate weight bearing with the foot in a functional position.[262] If weight bearing must be delayed, then maintenance of a neutral position is important, as are early vigorous, active range-of-motion exercises.

LATE ARTHRITIS

Direct joint damage is a well-accepted cause of posttraumatic arthritis. Less securely documented is the role that posttraumatic skeletal deformity plays in development of such arthritis. Still less certain are thresholds beyond which deformity carries a significant risk of arthritis. This issue is discussed further in the previous section on malunion. Long-term follow-up studies of tibia fractures are rare.[154,157,189] If significant deformity is present with radiologically mild arthritis, an osteotomy, as discussed previously, may relieve symptoms.

Once severe arthritis develops, correction of deformity may still be advisable, but arthrodesis of the symptomatic distal joints is the best method to manage disabling symptoms that do not respond to conservative therapy, which consists of well-cushioned footgear, bracing of the foot and ankle, oral antiinflammatory agents, and reduced activity.

FUNCTIONAL DISABILITIES

Few reports detail the functional results after tibial fractures. It is not clear how long complete recovery takes. Depending on severity of injury, the frequency of good or excellent results ranges from 50% to 100%.[14,67,133] At five years, Peter and colleagues found minimal problems after low-energy fractures treated with functional braces, but only half had returned to skiing by one year after injury.[219] Digby, at 47 weeks follow-up, noted that 82% had returned to employment, and 79% had recovered the ability to run.[62] Horne et al., with a 68-month follow-up, reported that only 21% were asymptomatic, and only 40% could participate in all activities without difficulties. Nineteen percent had severe, constant pain; 60% had visible deformity; 24% had modified their work; and 52% had reduced walking tolerance. Symptoms correlated best with reduced ankle, rather than subtalar, motion, and this was more common in more distal fractures.[121] Hutchins and Moore et al. reviewed the long-term results of severe, complicated injuries.[124a,199] Although fractures usually healed without draining wounds, the final function and appearance rarely approached the status before injury.

Further work is necessary to adequately document the relationships among functional results, fracture severity, and treatment, including rehabilitation.

POOR COSMETIC RESULT

Deformity of bone and soft tissues can produce an unsightly leg that may be more or less objectionable to the patient. Injury severity and problems during treatment are major determinants of the leg's appearance. Some improvement may be possible with delayed plastic and reconstructive surgery.

Fibular Fractures

The anatomy and function of the fibula have been discussed previously in the section on anatomy. Weight bearing is not a major function for the fibula under normal conditions.[323] It has been claimed to carry approximately 17% of body weight, but it may be closer to 6%.[318,323] Proximally, it anchors the lateral supports of the knee. Distally, it is the crucial lateral buttress for the talus and ankle joint. Although structural continuity of the fibula is not important if the tibia is intact, patients with tibial fractures are often aided by fibular union, and occasionally its fixation is indicated as a means of restoring stability and alignment. If used to substitute for the tibia in one of the so-called fibula pro tibia operations, it can hypertrophy significantly, albeit gradually. As helpful as an intact fibula can be, it will occasionally disturb the healing of a tibia shaft fracture, producing a varus deformity or possibly delaying union.[324] This possibility must be considered whenever the fibula heals, as it usually does, before the tibia, or whenever the tibia alone is fractured. Ender nail fixation of an isolated tibial fracture may counteract the detrimental effects of the intact fibula.[320]

Isolated acute fractures of the fibula are perhaps best considered as diagnostic challenges. If indeed it is an isolated fracture, the consequences are almost always minor, and only symptomatic treatment is required. However, the situation may not be as it seems. Common associated injuries involve nerves and vessels, ligaments of the knee or ankle, and compartment syndromes, in addition to tibial shaft fractures.[314,316,321] Indirectly produced fibular fractures are caused by external rotation of the foot. This often produces a distal fibular fracture at or slightly above the ankle syndesmosis, but occasionally it is much higher. This so-called Maisonneuve fracture is discussed further in the next chapter. If the medial ankle disruption is purely ligamentous, and if the talus is not displaced very far laterally, then this injury complex may not be suspected. A spiral fracture pattern, ankle pain, tenderness, and instability are clues to the diagnosis of the Maisonneuve fracture. Clearly the ankle must be examined carefully whenever there is a fracture that involves the fibula.

Proximal fibular fractures may be caused by avulsions of the attachments of the fibular collateral ligament and biceps femoris tendon.

If the injury involves a blow to the lateral aspect of the calf during weight bearing, the resulting valgus force on the knee may tear the medial collateral ligament. Superficial, deep, or common peroneal nerves may be injured initially or may become involved because of progressive elevation of compartmental pressure in the anterior and lateral compartments. Because the fibula is contiguous with all four compartments, the deep and superficial posterior spaces are potentially involved as well. Even if the knee is stable, the possibility of a vascular injury, especially to the anterior tibial artery, must be considered.[314] Therefore assessment of the patient with a fibula fracture must include a detailed neurovascular examination, repeated if symptoms increase, or if the patient's consciousness is compromised. Knee and ankle stability must be confirmed as well. Rarely, especially in the young, the fibula may be bowed rather than fractured, and this may interfere with reduction of an angulated tibia fracture.[315,317]

Treatment of truly isolated fibular shaft fractures need only be symptomatic. A well-padded splint or cast may be useful briefly for comfort, but this is not required, and if the patient is comfortable, a lightly wrapped elastic bandage support is applied over adequate padding. Elevation, ice, crutches (with weight bearing as tolerated), and analgesics as needed are all helpful. Once pain and swelling have largely resolved (usually one to two weeks), progressive weight bearing is encouraged, and activities are allowed as the patient's capacity permits. Functional recovery is usually nearly complete by six to eight weeks, if the foregoing scheme is followed.

Rare indications do exist for fixation of fractures of the fibular shaft; generally it is needed to augment other fixation for a severe tibial fracture. If required, fixation is best done with a 3.5-mm, small-fragment dynamic compression plate with a minimum of three secure screws on each side of the fracture. If comminution or significant devascularization are present, bone grafting may be valuable as well. Be cautious not to injure the common peroneal nerve with an operation on the proximal fibula.

Complications after fibular shaft fracture include the neurovascular problems and associated injuries mentioned previously. Prompt recognition and treatment of arterial injuries and compartment are essential. Mino and Hughes have reported late entrapment and palsy of the superficial peroneal nerve by fracture callus.[321] Nonunion occurs occasionally but is rarely symptomatic. If treatment is indicated, a fibular nonunion should respond to compression plate fixation, with or without bone graft, based on pattern and vascularity of the fracture.

Injuries of the Proximal Tibiofibular Joint

The proximal tibiofibular joint is not a frequent site of recognized injuries but is at risk from both indirect and direct trauma.[325,327,333,338] Ogden's and Resnick's comprehensive reviews have established our understanding of these injuries, which may occur with, or independent of, tibial shaft fractures.[334,336] Awareness is necessary so that early appropriate treatment can be carried out. Recurrent dislocations are rare.[331,339] Reports and reviews of proximal tibiofibular joint injuries tend to focus on isolated injuries. It is important to look for disruption of this joint whenever a displaced tibial fracture is associated with an intact fibula.

Anatomically, the proximal tibiofibular joint has two major patterns: horizontal and oblique. Ogden used 20° as the dividing point between the two, although acknowledging a continuum from horizontal to 76°. The more vertical joints had a smaller contact area. He felt that an important role of the proximal tibiofibular joint is to permit slight rotation and relieve rotational stress at the ankle, a function that is lost after tibiofibular synostosis, below or at the level of the joint. The more vertical joints, perhaps because of less ability to accommodate rotation, seemed more frequent among those with dislocations. It is not clear how much weight is borne by the proximal joint, but it may be that the variation in joint anatomy signifies a similar variability in its loading.[329]

There are four types of proximal tibiofibular joint injuries: subluxation, anterolateral dislocation, posteromedial dislocation, and superior (or proximal) dislocation. Their mechanisms, consequences, and treatments are different. Common to all are complaints of local pain, tenderness, and frequent distally radiating paresthesias, with or without objective peroneal nerve involvement. Local deformity may be masked by soft tissue swelling initially. Subtle findings may render early diagnosis difficult (Fig. 51–51).

Subluxation of the proximal tibiofibular joint is associated with generalized ligamentous laxity. Hypermobility of the joint is associated with local tenderness. If symptoms do not resolve with observation or a brief

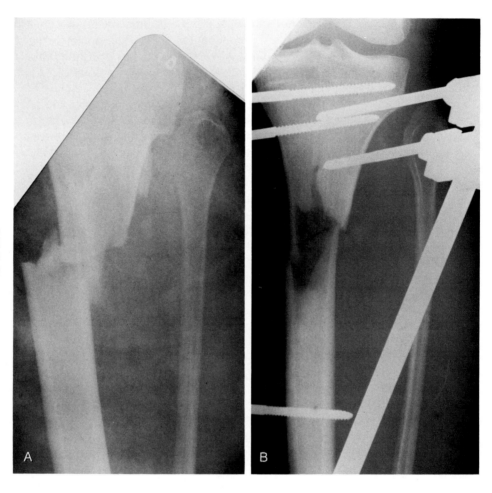

Figure 51–51

Proximal dislocation of the fibula associated with a severe proximal tibial fracture. *A,* After provisional casting. *B,* After debridement and external fixation.

period of splint or cast immobilization, and especially if peroneal nerve palsy does not recover promptly, then fibular head resection is indicated.[334]

Anterolateral dislocation of the proximal tibiofibular joint is usually caused by an acute indirect injury produced by a relative internal rotation of the proximal shank on the inverted talus, with the knee flexed and the anterior and lateral compartment muscles contracting.[337] The fibular collateral ligament and biceps tendon are relaxed, and the rotational stress, combined with tension in the anterolateral muscle groups, tends to spring the proximal fibula laterally and forward. Examination reveals prominence of the fibular head and an abnormal anteriorly curving course of the biceps tendon.[330] Associated injuries may interfere with its recognition.

Treatment is by closed reduction, unless diagnosis is excessively delayed.[328,333–335] The knee is flexed to at least 70°, and the foot is dorsiflexed, pronated, and externally rotated. Direct pressure on the fibular head (but not over the peroneal nerve) then displaces it abruptly posteriorly over the lateral tibial ridge and back into its sulcus on the proximal tibia. The reduc-

tion is usually quite stable. Ogden recommends active rehabilitation after two to three weeks of immobilization. However, 8 of his 14 patients had recurrent pain and subjective instability. For this, he advises fibular head resection, which was successful in the four patients so treated. Proximal arthrodesis is not recommended, as it is associated with development of subsequent ankle joint symptoms, presumably because of loss of rotation of the lateral malleolus. Difficulty obtaining fusion was also noted, along with hardware failure and symptomatic nonunion. Should ankle symptoms occur after proximal tibiofibular synostosis, a segmental fibulectomy, distal to the synostosis, or a fibular head resection is Ogden's recommendation. However, if this is delayed too long, ankle arthrosis may progress to the point that symptoms are not relieved.[332]

Posteromedial proximal tibiofibular joint dislocation is a rare injury and is usually caused by direct, high-energy trauma. It is likely to be associated with damage to the lateral supporting structures of the knee joint. Nonoperative treatment has poor results. Surgical repair of the injured structures, including open reduction and temporary screw fixation of the proximal fibula, is likely to offer the best results. It is essential to identify and protect the peroneal nerve during any such procedure.

Superior proximal tibiofibular joint dislocations are the result of a severe leg injury with a displaced tibial shaft fracture and an intact fibula.[326] Although most isolated tibial shaft fractures are caused by lower energy injuries and thus have an overall improved prognosis, it is important to look for these rare injuries that have failed through the proximal tibiofibular joint rather than the fibular shaft. This dislocation, because of the force required to produce it, is associated with neurovascular injuries and compartment syndromes. Anatomic reduction and secure stabilization of the tibial fracture usually reduce the proximal tibiofibular joint. If this is unsuccessful, then closed or open reduction, perhaps with provisional stabilization, is probably warranted. Retention of the proximal fibula at this time seems wise, as it may be needed to reconstruct the leg. Persistent local symptoms may require later fibular head resection.

Fatigue Fractures

Fatigue fractures occur when repetitive loading exceeds a bone's capacity to remodel in response to cyclic stress application.[340] They have often been called "stress fractures," but "fatigue" is a more correct mechanical term for their etiology. They are most commonly seen in individuals, such as soldiers, dancers, and runners, who place significant demands on their lower extremities.[342,344-346,348,350,351,353-355] A careful history usually reveals recently increased impact loading, such as an intensified or altered training schedule or a change in footgear or exercise surface. Occasionally, aggressive resumption of weight bearing after a period of disability provokes a fatigue fracture in a patient recovering from a previous injury.[358] There may be a relationship to decreased bone mass.[352]

The location of fatigue fractures is typical and is perhaps related to specific activities.[354] The bones of the foot, particularly the metatarsals, are often reported as the most frequent site of fatigue fractures, but the tibia and fibula are also significantly involved.[355] The posterior surface of the tibial diaphysis, ranging from the proximal third to the junction of the middle and distal thirds, is the usual location. The fibula also may be affected, particularly its distal third.[356]

The osseous failure of a fatigue fracture may be only microscopic, with pain, swelling, tenderness, and increased warmth as its clinical manifestations. Usually, no radiologic abnormality is noted until periosteal or intraosseous new bone formation is evident. A very fine radiolucent defect may be present. A technetium 99m methylene diphosphonate (MDP) bone scan usually shows well-localized uptake of radionuclide in the area of a fatigue fracture.[351,354,355] Increased temperature by thermography and pain induction by ultrasound are noninvasive, economical tests, one or both of which will have positive results in most patients with fatigue fractures and normal radiographs.[342] This combination can be used instead of the frequently requested bone scan, if objective confirmation is desired.

Differential diagnosis of fatigue fractures is important to ensure timely, appropriate treatment. Tumor, infection, exertional compartment syndrome, and so-called "medial tibial stress syndrome" must be considered. History, exam, and radiographs should allow each of these to be distinguished. In medial tibial stress syndrome, there is more diffuse area of hyperactive bone resorption and remodeling without microfractures. This is demonstrated by a more diffusely increased uptake of technetium 99m MDP. Chronic recurrent exertional compartment syndromes show typical activity-related changes in physical findings and compartmental pressure measurements. Infections and tumors may have only localized morphologic findings evident on high-quality radiographs or CT scans. Magnetic resonance imaging shows abnormalities, but the specificity of this very sensitive examination is still being refined.[341,357] A typical clinical and radiologic course is often the best confirmation for a diagnosis of fatigue fracture. Only very exceptionally will a biopsy for tissue diagnosis be necessary.

Because fatigue fractures have mechanically weakened bone, catastrophic failure may occur with an obvious displaced fracture and may perhaps be preceded by local pain and associated with radiolucencies or new bone formation that might generate concern about other types of pathologic fractures. Early recognition and appropriate treatment with reduced activity and external support, if needed, should prevent catastrophic failures of fatigue fractures.

Treatment of fatigue fractures of the tibia and fibula is conservative. Even if catastrophic failure occurs, the fracture usually is a result of low-energy trauma and is generally amenable to nonoperative treatment with a cast or brace and early weight bearing.[343,348,355] If failure has not occurred but is thought to be a risk because of an obvious radiolucent defect, then external support may be advisable, just as it is if activity restriction does not control symptoms. Otherwise, weight bearing is restricted with crutches, and less demanding activities are gradually resumed, avoiding those that produce pain. Once the patient's symptoms have resolved and radiographs show progressive healing of any defect, a carefully monitored, gradually increased rehabilitation program will help the patient return to his or her desired level of performance. Good coaching regarding technique and proper footgear are important aspects of such a rehabilitation program.[347] Two to three months may be required for resolution of the problem, which can recur if resumption of activity is too vigorous.

REFERENCES

Tibial Shaft Fractures

1. Aho, A.J.; Nieminen, S.J.; Nylamo, E.I. External fixation by Hoffmann-Vidal-Adrey osteotaxis for severe tibial fractures. Treatment scheme and technical criticism. Clin Orthop 181:154–164, 1983.
2. Aitken, R.J.; Mills, C.; Immelman, E.J. The postphlebitic syndrome following shaft fractures of the leg. A significant late complication. J Bone Joint Surg 69B:775–778, 1987.
3. Alexander, A.H.; Cabaud, H.E.; Johnston, J.O.; Lichtman, D.M. Compression plate position. Extraperiosteal or subperiosteal. Clin Orthop 175:280–285, 1983.
3a. Allgöwer, M. Modern concepts of fracture treatment. AO/ASIF Dialogue 1:1, 1985.
4. Anderson, L.D.; Hutchins, W.C.; Wright, P.E.; Disney, J.D. Fractures of the tibia and fibula treated by casts and transfixing pins. Clin Orthop 105:179–191, 1974.
5. An, H.S.; Ebraheim, N.B.; Savolaine, E.R.; et al. The value of internal oblique radiographs for posterolateral bone grafting of the tibia. Clin Orthop 238:209–210, 1989.
6. Asko-Seljavaara, S.; Slatis, P.; Kannisto, M.; Sundell, B. Management of infected fractures of the tibia with associated soft tissue loss: Experience with external fixation, bone grafting and soft tissue reconstruction using pedicle muscle flaps or microvascular composite tissue grafts. Br J Plast Surg 38:546–555, 1985.
7. Austin, R.T. Fractures of the tibial shaft: Is medical audit possible? Injury 9:3–101, 1977.
8. Austin, R.T. The Sarmiento tibial plaster: A prospective study of 145 fractures. Injury 13:10–22, 1981.
9. Bach, A.W.; Hansen, S.T. Jr. Plates versus external fixation in severe open tibial shaft fractures. A randomized trial. Clin Orthop 241:89–94, 1989.
10. Banerjee, S.N., ed. Rehabilitation Management of Amputees. Baltimore, Williams and Wilkins, 1982.
11. Barker, A.T.; Dixon, R.A.; Sharrard, W.J.; Sutcliffe, M.L. Pulsed magnetic field therapy for tibial non-union. Interim results of a double-blind trial. Lancet 1:994–996, 1984.
12. Barquet, A.; Masliah, R. Large segmental necrosis of the tibia with deep infection after open fracture. Acta Orthop Scand 59:443–446, 1988.
13. Bassey, L.O. The use of P.O.P. integrated transfixation pins as an improvisation on the Hoffmann's apparatus: Contribution to open fracture management in the tropics. J Trauma 29:59–64, 1989.
14. Bauer, G.C.H.; Edwards, P.; Widmark, P.H. Shaft fractures of the tibia: Etiology of poor results in a consecutive series of 173 fractures. Acta Chir Scand 124:386–395, 1962.
15. Behrens, F.; Comfort, T.H.; Searls, K.; et al. Unilateral external fixation for severe open tibial fractures. Preliminary report of a prospective study. Clin Orthop 178:111–120, 1983.
16. Behrens, F.; Johnson, W.D.; Koch, T.W.; Kovacevic, N. Bending stiffness of unilateral and bilateral fixator frames. Clin Orthop 178:103–110, 1983.
17. Behrens, F. General theory and principles of external fixation. Clin Orthop 241:15–23, 1989.
18. Behrens, F. A primer of fixator devices and configurations. Clin Orthop 241:5–14, 1989.
19. Behrens, F.; Johnson, W. Unilateral external fixation. Methods to increase and reduce frame stiffness. Clin Orthop 241:48–56, 1989.
20. Behrens, F.; Johnson, J.; Guntzburger, T.; et al. Early bone grafting for tibial fractures. J Orthop Trauma 3:156, 1989.
20a. Behrens, F.; Seals, K. External fixation of the tibia. Basic concepts and prospective evaluation. J Bone Joint Surg 68B:246–254, 1986.
20b. Bengner, V.; Ekbom, T.; Johnell, O.; et al. Incidence of femoral and tibial shaft fractures. Acta Orthop Scand 61:251–254, 1990.
21. Berger, P.E.; Ofstein, R.A.; Jackson, D.W.; et al. MRI demonstration of radiographically occult fractures: What have we been missing? Radiographics 9:407–436, 1989.
22. Bintcliffe, I.W.; Scott, W.A.; Vickers, R.H. The case for an open approach to tibial nailing. Injury 15:407–410, 1984.
23. Blick, S.S.; Brumback, R.J.; Poka, A.; et al. Compartment syndrome in open tibial fractures. J Bone Joint Surg 68A:1348–1353, 1986.
24. Blick, S.S.; Brumback, R.J.; Lakatos, R.; et al. Early prophylactic bone grafting of high-energy tibial fractures. Clin Orthop 240:21–41, 1989.
25. Bondurant, F.J.; Cotler, H.B.; Buckle, R.; et al. The medical and economic impact of severely injured lower extremities. J Trauma 28:1270–1273, 1988.
26. Bone, L.B.; Johnson, K.D. Treatment of tibial fractures by reaming and intramedullary nailing. J Bone Joint Surg 68A:877–887, 1986.
27. Bosse, M.J.; Staeheli, J.W.; Reinert, C.M. Treatment of unstable tibial diaphyseal fractures with minimal internal and external fixation. J Orthop Trauma 3:223–231, 1989.
28. Böstman, O.M. Displaced malleolar fractures associated with spiral fractures of the tibial shaft. Clin Orthop 228:202–207, 1988.
29. Böstman, O.M. Rotational refracture of the shaft of the adult tibia. Injury 15:93–98, 1983.
30. Böstman, O.M. Spiral fractures of the shaft of the tibia. Initial displacement and stability of reduction. J Bone Joint Surg 68B:462–466, 1986.
31. Böstman, O.M.; Vainionpaa, S.; Saikku, K. Infra-isthmal longitudinal fractures of the tibial diaphysis: Results of treatment using closed intramedullary compression nailing. J Trauma 24:964–969, 1984.
32. Bowker, J.H. Surgical techniques for conserving tissue and function in lower-limb amputation for trauma, infection, and vascular disease. Instruct Course Lect 39:355–360, 1990.
33. Brooker, A.F. Jr; Epps, H.; Constable, D. New tibial interlocking nail system. J Orthop Trauma 1:257–259, 1987.
34. Buhler, J. Percutaneous circlage of tibial fractures. Clin Orthop 105:276–282, 1974.
35. Burgess, A.R.; Poka, A.; Brumback, R.J.; Bosse, M.J. Management of open grade III tibial fractures. Orthop Clin North Am 18:85–93, 1987.
36. Burgess, A.R.; Poka, A.; Brumback, R.J.; et al. Pedestrian tibial injuries. J Trauma 27:596–601, 1987.
37. Burri, C. Post-traumatic Osteomyelitis. Bern, Hans Huber, 1975.
38. Burstein, A.H.; Currey, J.; Frankel, V.H.; et al. Bone strength.

The effect of screw holes. J Bone Joint Surg 54A:1143–1156, 1972.

39. Burwell, H.N. Plate fixation of tibial shaft fractures. J Bone Joint Surg 53B:258–271, 1971.

40. Byrd, H.S.; Spicer, T.E.; Cierney, G. III. Management of open tibial fractures. Plast Reconstr Surg 76:719–730, 1985.

41. Caudle, R.J.; Stern, P.J. Severe open fractures of the tibia. J Bone Joint Surg 69:801–807, 1987.

42. Chapman, M.W. Fractures of the tibia and fibula. In: Chapman, M.W., ed. Operative Orthopaedics. Philadelphia, J.B. Lippincott, 1988.

43. Chapman, M.W. Fractures of the tibial and fibular shafts. In: Evarts, C.M., ed. Surgery of the Musculoskeletal System, Vol. 4. New York, Churchill Livingstone, 1990, pp. 3741–3799.

44. Chiron, H.S. Open fractures of the shaft of the tibia treated by intramedullary nailing. Bull Hosp Jt Dis Orthop Inst 42:92–102, 1982.

45. Christian, E.P.; Bosse, M.J.; Robb, G. Reconstruction of large diaphyseal defects in grade-IIIB tibial fractures without free fibular transfer. J Bone Joint Surg 71A:994–1004, 1989.

46. Cierny, G. III. Chronic osteomyelitis: Results of treatment. Instr Course Lect 39:495–507, 1990.

47. Cierny, G. III; Byrd, H.S.; Jones, R.E. Primary versus delayed soft tissue coverage for severe open tibial fractures. A comparison of results. Clin Orthop 178:54–63, 1983.

48. Clementz, B.G.; Magnusson, A. Assessment of tibial torsion employing fluoroscopy, computed tomography and the cryosectioning technique. Acta Radiol 30:75–80, 1989.

49. Clementz, B.G. Assessment of tibial torsion and rotational deformity with a new fluoroscopic technique. Clin Orthop 245:199–209, 1989.

50. Clifford, R.P.; Beauchamp, C.G.; Kellam, J.F.; et al. Plate fixation of open fractures of the tibia. J Bone Joint Surg 70B:644–648, 1988.

51. Cohn, B.T.; Bilfield, L. Fatigue fracture of a tibial interlocking nail. Orthopedics 9:1215–1218, 1986.

52. Committee on Trauma, American College of Surgeons. Advanced Trauma Life Support Program. Chicago, American College of Surgeons, 1989.

53. Cone, J.B. Vascular injury associated with fracture-dislocations of the lower extremity. Clin Orthop 243:30–35, 1989.

54. Connolly, J.F. Common avoidable problems in nonunions. Clin Orthop 194:226–235, 1985.

55. Connolly, J.F.; Guse, R.; Tiedeman, J.; Dehne, R. Autologous marrow injection for delayed unions of the tibia: A preliminary report. J Orthop Trauma 3:276–282, 1989.

56. Court-Brown, C.M.; Hughes, S.P. Hughes external fixator in treatment of tibial fractures. J R Soc Med 78:830–837, 1985.

57. Csongradi, J.J.; Maloney, W.J. Ununited lower limb fractures. West J Med 150:675–680, 1989.

58. Cunningham, J.L.; Evans, M.; Harris, J.D.; Kenwright, J. The measurement of stiffness of fractures treated with external fixation. Eng Med 16:229–232, 1987.

59. Cunningham, J.L.; Evans, M.; Kenwright, J. Measurement of fracture movement in patients treated with unilateral external skeletal fixation. J Biomed Eng 11:118–122, 1989.

60. De Bastiani, G.; Aldegheri, R.; Renzi Brivio, L. Dynamic axial fixation. A rational alternative for the external fixation of fractures. Int Orthop 10:95–99, 1986.

61. Den Outer, A.J.; Meeuwis, J.D.; Hermans, J.; Zwaveling, A. Conservative versus operative treatment of displaced noncomminuted tibial shaft fractures. A retrospective comparative study. Clin Orthop 252:231–237, 1990.

62. Digby, J.M.; Holloway, G.M.; Webb, J.K. A study of function after tibial cast bracing. Injury 14:432–439, 1983.

63. DiPasquale, T.; Helfet, D.; Sanders, R.; et al. The treatment of open and/or unstable tibial fractures with an unreamed double-locked tibial nail. Abstract. J Orthop Trauma 4:223, 1990.

64. Dugdale, T.W.; Degnan, G.G.; Bosse, M.J.; Reinert, C.M. A technique for removing a fractured interlocking tibial nail. J Orthop Trauma 2:39–42, 1988.

65. Edholm, P.; Hammer, R.; Hammerby, S.; Lindholm, B. The stability of union in tibial shaft fractures: Its measurement by a non-invasive method. Arch Orthop Trauma Surg 102:242–247, 1984.

66. Edlich, R.F.; Rodeheaver, G.; Thacker, J.G.; Edgerton, M. Technical factors in wound management. In: Hunt, T.K.; Dunphy, J.E., eds. Fundamentals of Wound Management. New York, Appleton-Century-Crofts, 1979, pp. 424–426.

67. Edwards, P. Fracture of the shaft of the tibia: 492 consecutive cases in adults: Importance of soft tissue injury. Acta Orthop Scand (Suppl) 76:1–83, 1965.

68. Edwards, C.C.; Simmons, S.C.; Browner, B.D.; Weigel, M.C. Severe open tibial fractures. Results treating 202 injuries with external fixation. Clin Orthop 230:98–115, 1988.

69. Ekeland, A.; Thoresen, B.O.; Alho, A.; et al. Interlocking intramedullary nailing in the treatment of tibial fractures. A report of 45 cases. Clin Orthop 231:205–215, 1988.

70. Ellis, H. Disabilities after tibial shaft fractures: With special references to Volkmann's ischaemic contracture. J Bone Joint Surg 40B:190–197, 1958.

71. Ellis, H. The speed of healing after fracture of the tibial shaft. J Bone Joint Surg 40B:42–46, 1958.

72. Epps, C.H. Jr. Amputation of the lower limb. In: Evarts, C.M., ed. Surgery of the Musculoskeletal System. New York, Churchill Livingstone, 1990, p. 5075.

73. Epps, C.H. Jr. Principles of amputation surgery in trauma. In: Evarts, C.M., ed. Surgery of the Musculoskeletal System. New York, Churchill Livingstone, 1990, p. 5075.

74. Esterhai, J.L. Jr. Management of soft-tissue wounds associated with open fractures. Instr Course Lect 39:483–486, 1990.

75. Esterhai, J.L.; Sennett, B.; Gelb, H.; et al. Treatment of chronic osteomyelitis complicating nonunion and segmental defects of the tibia with open cancellous bone graft, posterolateral bone graft, and soft-tissue transfer. J Trauma 30:49–54, 1990.

76. Etter, C.; Burri, C.; Claes, L.; et al. Treatment by external fixation of open fractures associated with severe soft tissue damage of the leg. Biomechanical principles and clinical experience. Clin Orthop 178:80–88, 1983.

77. Faure, C.; Merloz, P. Transfixation. An Atlas of Anatomical Sections for the External Fixation of Limbs. New York, Springer-Verlag, 1987.

78. Feliciano, D.V.; Cruse, P.A.; Spjut-Patrinely, V.; et al. Fasciotomy after trauma to the extremities. Am J Surg 156:533–536, 1988.

79. Franklin, J.L.; Winquist, R.A.; Benirschke, S.K.; Hansen, S.T. Jr. Broken intramedullary nails. J Bone Joint Surg 70A:1463–1471, 1988.

80. Freeman, J.R.; Weaver, J.K.; Oden, R.R.; Kirk, R.E. Changing patterns in tibial fractures resulting from skiing. Clin Orthop 216:19–23, 1987.

81. Galpin, R.D.; Veith, R.G.; Hansen, S.T. Treatment of failures after plating of tibial fractures. J Bone Joint Surg 68A:1231–1236, 1986.

81a. Froehlich, J.; Dorfman, G.S.; Cronan, J.J.; et al. Compression ultrasonography for the detection of deep venous thrombosis in patients who have a fracture of the hip. A prospective study. J Bone Joint Surg 71A:249–256, 1989.

82. Garland, D.E.; Saucedo, T.; Reiser, T.V. The management of

tibial fractures in acute spinal cord injury patients. Clin Orthop 213:237–240, 1986.

83. Gershuni, D.H.; Mubarak, S.J.; Yaru, N.C.; Lee, Y.F. Fracture of the tibia complicated by acute compartment syndrome. Clin Orthop 217:221–227, 1987.

84. Gershuni, D.H.; Skyhar, M.J.; Thompson, B.; et al. A comparison of conventional radiography and computed tomography in the evaluation of spiral fractures of the tibia. J Bone Joint Surg 67A:1388–1395, 1985.

85. Godina, M. Early microsurgical reconstruction of complex trauma of the extremities. Plast Reconstr Surg 78:285–292, 1986.

86. Goldstrohm, G.L.; Mears, D.C.; Swartz, W.M. The results of 39 fractures complicated by major segmental bone loss and/or leg length discrepancy. J Trauma 24:50–58, 1984.

87. Golimbu, C.; Firooznia, H.; Rafii, M.; Waugh, T. Acute traumatic fibular bowing associated with tibial fractures. Clin Orthop 182:211–214, 1984.

88. Gordon, L.; Chiu, E.J. Treatment of infected non-unions and segmental defects of the tibia with staged microvascular muscle transplantation and bone-grafting. J Bone Joint Surg 70A:377–386, 1988.

89. Graehl, P.M.; Hersh, M.R.; Heckman, J.D. Supramalleolar osteotomy for the treatment of symptomatic tibial malunion. J Orthop Trauma 1:281–292, 1987.

90. Grassi, G.; Nigrisoli, P.; Brandigi, S.; Petrini, A. A survey of 240 cases of fractures of the tibia treated by AO compression plating. Ital J Orthop Traumatol 10:131–142, 1984.

91. Grazier, K.L.; Holbrook, T.L.; Kelsey, J.L.; Stauffer, R.N. The Frequency of Occurrence, Impact, and Cost of Musculoskeletal Conditions in the United States. Chicago, American Academy of Orthopaedic Surgeons, 1984.

92. Green, S.A. Complications of External Fixation. Springfield, IL, Charles C Thomas, 1981.

93. Green, S.A.; Garland, D.E.; Moore, T.J.; Barad, S.J. External fixation for the uninfected angulated nonunion of the tibia. Clin Orthop 190:204–211, 1984.

94. Green, S.A.; Moore, T.A.; Spohn, P.J. Nonunion of the tibial shaft. Orthopedics 11:1149–1157, 1988.

95. Gregg, P.J.; Clayton, C.B.; Fenwick, J.D.; et al. Static and sequential dynamic scintigraphy of the tibia following fracture. Injury 17:95–103, 1986.

96. Gregory, R.T.; Gould, R.J.; Peclet, M.; et al. The mangled extremity syndrome (M.E.S.): A severity grading system for multisystem injury of the extremity. J Trauma 25:1147–1150, 1985.

97. Gross, R.H. Leg length discrepancy: How much is too much? Orthopedics 1:307–310, 1978.

98. Guercio, N.; Orsini, G. Fractures of the limbs complicated by ischaemia due to lesions of the major vessels. Ital J Orthop Traumatol 10:163–165, 1984.

99. Gustilo, R.B.; Merkow, R.L.; Templeman, D. Current concepts review. The management of open fractures. J Bone Joint Surg 72A:299–303, 1990.

100. Habernek, H.; Walch, G.; Dengg, C. Cerclage for torsional fractures of the tibia. J Bone Joint Surg 71B:311–313, 1989.

101. Haines, J.F.; Williams, E.A.; Hargadon, E.J.; Davies, D.R. Is conservative treatment of displaced tibial shaft fractures justified? J Bone Joint Surg 66B:84–88, 1984.

102. Hall, R.F. Jr; Gonzales, M. Fracture of the proximal part of the tibia and fibula associated with an entrapped popliteal artery. A case report. J Bone Joint Surg 68A:941–944, 1986.

103. Hallock, G.G.; Sussman, D.; Rhodes, M. Lower limb salvage with autoclaved autogenous tibial diaphysis: Case report. J Trauma 29:528–530, 1989.

103a. Hamilton, FH. A Practical Treatise on Fractures and Dislocations. Philadelphia, Blanchard and Lea, 1860.

104. Hamm, J.C.; Stevenson, T.R.; Mathes, S.J. Knee joint salvage utilising a plantar musculocutaneous island pedicle flap. Br J Plast Surg 39:249–254, 1986.

105. Hammer, R.R. External fixation of tibial shaft fractures. A review of 42 fractures by the Hoffman-Vidal-Adrey external fixation system. Arch Orthop Trauma Surg 104:271–274, 1985.

106. Hammer, R.R. Strength of union in human tibial shaft fracture. A prospective study of 104 cases. Clin Orthop 199:226–232, 1985.

107. Hammer, R.R. Tibial shaft fracture associated with silent isolated partial rupture of the anterior cruciate ligament. Arthroscopy 1:128–130, 1985.

108. Hammer, R.R.; Hammerby, S.; Lindholm, B. Accuracy of radiologic assessment of tibial shaft fracture union in humans. Clin Orthop 199:233–238, 1985.

109. Hansen, S.T. Jr. The type-IIIC tibial fracture. Salvage or amputation. Editorial. J Bone Joint Surg 69A:799–800, 1987.

110. Harley, J.M.; Campbell, M.J.; Jackson, R.K. A comparison of plating and traction in the treatment of tibial shaft fractures. Injury 17:91–94, 1986.

111. Harmon, P.H. A simplified posterior approach to the tibia for bone-grafting and fibular transference. J Bone Joint Surg 27A:496, 1945.

112. Harrington, I.J.; Barrington, T.W.W.; Evans, D.C.; et al. Delayed union and nonunion of the tibia: Experience in a community teaching hospital. Can J Surg 30:204–206, 1987.

113. Heatley, F.W. Severe open fractures of the tibia: The courage to amputate. Editorial. Br Med J 296:229, 1988.

114. Heckman, M.M.; Whitesides, T.E.; Grewe, S.R. Spatial relationships of compartment syndromes in lower extremity trauma. Orthop Trans 11:537, 1987.

115. Henley, M.B. Intramedullary devices for tibial fracture stabilization. Clin Orthop 249:87–96, 1989.

115a. Henry, S.L.; Osterman, P.; Seligson, D. Prophylactic management of open fractures with the antibiotic bead pouch technique. Orthop Trans 13:748, 1989.

116. Heppenstall, R.B. Constant direct-current treatment for established nonunion of the tibia. Clin Orthop 178:179–184, 1983.

117. Heppenstall, R.B.; Brighton, C.T.; Esterhai, J.L. Jr; Muller, G. Prognostic factors in nonunion of the tibia: An evaluation of 185 cases treated with constant direct current. J Trauma 24:790–795, 1984.

118. Heppenstall, R.B.; Sapega, A.A.; Scott, R.; et al. The compartment syndrome. An experimental and clinical study of muscular energy metabolism using phosphorus nuclear magnetic resonance spectroscopy. Clin Orthop 226:138–155, 1988.

119. Hierholzer, G.; Rüedi, T.; Allgöwer, M.; Schatzker, J. Manual on the AO/ASIF Tubular External Fixator. New York, Springer, 1985.

120. Holbrook, J.L.; Swiontkowski, M.F.; Sanders, R. Treatment of open fractures of the tibial shaft: Ender nailing versus external fixation. A randomized prospective comparison. J Bone Joint Surg 71A:1231–1238, 1989.

121. Horne, G.; Iceton, J.; Twist, J.; Malony, R. Disability following fractures of the tibial shaft. Orthopedics 13:423–426, 1990.

122. Horster, G. Corrective osteotomies of the tibial shaft. In: Hierholzer, G.; Muller, K.H., eds. Corrective Osteotomies of the Lower Extremity after Trauma. New York, Springer-Verlag, 1985, pp. 127–139.

123. Howard, P.W.; Makin, G.S. Lower limb fractures with associated vascular injuries. J Bone Joint Surg 72B:116–120, 1990.

124. Howe, H.R. Jr; Poole, G.V. Jr; Hansen, K.J.; et al. Salvage of

lower extremities following combined orthopedic and vascular trauma. A predictive salvage index. Am Surg 53:205–208, 1987.

124a. Hutchins, P.M. The outcome of severe tibial injury. Injury 13:216–219, 1982.

125. Ichtertz, D.R.; Slabaugh, P. Thrombosis of the tibial artery associated with simultaneous fractures of the femur, tibia, and fibula. Report of a case. J Bone Joint Surg 69A:775–777, 1987.

126. Ingram, R.R.; Suman, R.K.; Freeman, P.A. Lower limb fractures in the chronic spinal cord injured patient. Paraplegia 27:133–139, 1989.

127. Ito, T.; Kohno, T.; Kojima, T. Free vascularized fibular graft. J Trauma 24:756–760, 1984.

128. Jansen, K.; Jensen, J.S. Operative technique in knee disarticulation. Prosthet Orthot Int 7:72–74, 1983.

129. Janssen, G.; Dietschi, C. Supramalleolar corrective osteotomy after fractures of the leg. Orthopedics 112:444–449, 1974.

130. Jayaswal, A.; Bhan, S.; Dave, P.K.; Chandra, P. Modified Phemister grafting in potentially infected nonunion of tibial shaft fractures. Int Surg 70:67–70, 1985.

131. Johansen, K.; Helfet, D.H.; Howey, T.; et al. Objective criteria accurately predict amputation following lower extremity trauma. J Orthop Trauma 3:166, 1989.

132. Johner, R.; Joerger, K.; Cordey, J.; Perren, S.M. Rigidity of pure lag-screw fixation as a function of screw inclination in an in vitro spiral osteotomy. Clin Orthop 178:74–79, 1983.

133. Johner, R.; Wruhs, O. Classification of tibial shaft fractures and correlation with results after rigid internal fixation. Clin Orthop 178:7–25, 1983.

134. Johnson, E.E. Multiplane correctional osteotomy of the tibia for diaphyseal malunion. Clin Orthop 215:223–232, 1987.

135. Johnson, E.E.; Marder, R.A. Open intramedullary nailing and bone-grafting for non-union of tibial diaphyseal fracture. J Bone Joint Surg 69A:375–380, 1987.

136. Johnson, E.E.; Urist, M.R.; Finerman, G.A. Distal metaphyseal tibial nonunion. Deformity and bone loss treated by open reduction, internal fixation, and human bone morphogenetic protein (HBMP). Clin Orthop 250:234–240, 1990.

137. Johnson, E.E.; Simpson, L.A.; Helfet, D.L. Delayed intramedullary fixation after failed external fixation of the tibia. Clin Orthop 253:251–257, 1990.

138. Johnson, K.D. Indications, instrumentation, and experience with locked tibial nails. Orthopedics 8:1377–1383, 1985.

139. Johnson, K.D. Management of malunion and nonunion of the tibia. Orthop Clin North Am 18:157–171, 1987.

140. Johnson, K.D.; Bone, L.B.; Scheinberg, R. Severe open tibial fractures: A study protocol. J Orthop Trauma 2:175–180, 1988.

141. Kaltenecker, G.; Wruhs, O.; Quaicoe, S. Lower infection rate after interlocking nailing in open fractures of femur and tibia. J Trauma 30:474–479, 1990.

142. Karkabi, S.; Reis, N.D. Fibular bowing due to tibial shortening in isolated fracture of the tibia: Failure of late segmental fibulectomy to relieve ankle pain. Arch Orthop Trauma Surg 106:61–63, 1986.

143. Karlstrom, G.; Lonnerholm, T.; Olerud, S. Cavus deformity of the foot after fracture of the tibial shaft. J Bone Joint Surg 57A:893–900, 1975.

144. Karlstrom, G.; Olerud, S. The management of tibial fractures in alcoholics and mentally disturbed patients. J Bone Joint Surg 56B:730–734, 1974.

145. Karlstrom, G.; Olerud, S. Fractures of the tibial shaft. A critical evaluation of treatment alternatives. Clin Orthop 105:82–115, 1974.

146. Karlstrom, G.; Olerud, S. Percutaneous pin fixation of open

147. Karlstrom, G.; Olerud, S. External fixation of severe open tibial fractures with the Hoffmann frame. Clin Orthop 180:68–77, 1983.

148. Kay, L.; Hansen, B.A.; Raaschou, H.O. Fractures of the tibial shaft conservatively treated. Injury 17:5–11, 1986.

149. Keller, C.D. The principles of the treatment of tibial shaft fractures. A review of 10,146 cases from the literature. Orthopedics 6:993–1106, 1983.

150. Kempf, I.; Grosse, A.; Rigaut, P. The treatment of noninfected pseudarthrosis of the femur and tibia with locked intramedullary nailing. Clin Orthop 212:142–154, 1986.

151. Kenwright, J.; Richardson, J.B.; Goodship, A.E.; et al. Effect of controlled axial micromovement on healing of tibial fractures. Lancet 2:1185–1187, 1986.

152. Kenwright, J.; Goodship, A.E. Controlled mechanical stimulation in the treatment of tibial fractures. Clin Orthop 241:36–47, 1989.

153. Kenwright, J. The influence of cyclical loading upon fracture healing. J R Coll Surg 34:160, 1989.

154. Kettelkamp, D.B.; Hillberry, B.M.; Murrish, D.E.; Heck, D.A. Degenerative arthritis of the knee secondary to fracture malunion. Clin Orthop 234:159, 1988.

155. Klemm, K.W. Treatment of infected pseudarthrosis of the femur and tibia with an interlocking nail. Clin Orthop 212:174–181, 1986.

156. Klemm, K.W.; Borner, M. Interlocking nailing of complex fractures of the femur and tibia. Clin Orthop 212:89–100, 1986.

157. Kristensen, K.D.; Kiaer, T.; Blicher, J. No arthrosis of the ankle 20 years after malaligned tibial-shaft fracture. Acta Orthop Scand 60:208–209, 1989.

158. Kwong, L.M.; Johanson, P.H.; Klein, S.R. Postocclusive transcutaneous oximetry in followup assessment of tibial nonunion and healed tibia fractures. J Trauma 28:947–954, 1988.

159. Laasonen, E.M.; Kyro, A.; Korhola, O.; Bostman, O. Magnetic resonance imaging of tibial shaft fracture repair. Arch Orthop Trauma Surg 108:40–43, 1989.

160. Lambert, K.L. Weight-bearing function of the fibula. J Bone Joint Surg 54A:507–513, 1971.

161. Lange, R.H. Limb reconstruction vs. amputation. Decision making in massive lower extremity trauma. Clin Orthop 243:92–99, 1989.

162. Lange, R.H.; Bach, A.W.; Hansen, S.T. Jr; Johansen, K.H. Open tibial fractures with associated vascular injuries: Prognosis for limb salvage. J Trauma 25:203–208, 1985.

163. Larsson, K.; Van Der Linden, W. Open tibial shaft fractures. Clin Orthop 180:63–67, 1983.

164. Lazo-Zbikowski, J.; Aguilar, F.; Mozo, F.; et al. Biocompression external fixation. Sliding external osteosynthesis. Clin Orthop 206:169–184, 1986.

165. Leach, R.E. Fractures of the tibia and fibula. In: Rockwood, C.A. Jr.; Green, D.P., eds. Fractures In Adults, Vol. 2. Philadelphia, J.B. Lippincott, 1984, pp. 1593–1663.

166. Lee, J.K.; Yao, L. Occult intraosseous fracture: Magnetic resonance appearance versus age of injury. Am J Sports Med 17:620–623, 1989.

167. Lee, E.H.; Goh, J.C.H.; Helm, R.; Pho, R.W.H. Donor site morbidity following resection of the fibula. J Bone Joint Surg 72B:129–131, 1990.

168. Lehman, W.B.; Paley, D.; Atar, D. Operating Room Guide to Cross Sectional Anatomy of the Extremities and Pelvis. New York, Raven Press, 1989.

169. Levy, A.S.; Levitt, L.E.; Gunther, S.F.; Wetzler, M.J. The role

of Ender rodding in tibial fractures with an intact fibula. J Orthop Trauma 4:75–80, 1990.

170. Lippert, F.G. III; Hirsch, C. The three dimensional measurement of tibial fracture motion by photogrammetry. Clin Orthop 105:130–143, 1974.

171. Marcus, R.E.; Hansen, S.T. Jr. Bilateral fractures of the tibia: A severe injury associated with multiple trauma. J Trauma 27:415–419, 1987.

172. Marsh, J.; Nepola, J.; Seabold, J. Subclinical infection in delayed union of fractures. J Orthop Trauma 3:169, 1988.

173. Mast, J.; Jakob, R.; Ganz, R. Planning and Reduction Technique in Fracture Surgery. New York, Springer-Verlag, 1989.

174. Mast, J.W. Preoperative planning in the surgical correction of tibial nonunions and malunions. Clin Orthop 178:26–30, 1983.

175. Maurer, R.C.; Dillin, L. Multistaged surgical management of posttraumatic segmental tibial bone loss. Clin Orthop 216:162–170, 1987.

176. Maurer, D.J.; Merkow, R.L.; Gustilo, R.B. Infections after intramedullary nailing of severe open tibial fractures initially treated with external fixation. J Bone Joint Surg 71A:835–838, 1989.

177. May, J.W. Jr.; Jupiter, J.B.; Weiland, A.J.; Byrd, H.S. Current concepts review. Clinical classification of post-traumatic tibial osteomyelitis. J Bone Joint Surg 71A:1422–1428, 1989.

178. Mayer, L.; Werbie, T.; Schwab, J.P.; Johnson, R.P. The use of Ender nails in fractures of the tibial shaft. J Bone Joint Surg 67A:446–455, 1985.

179. McAndrew, M.P.; Pontarelli, W. The long-term follow-up of ipsilateral tibial and femoral diaphyseal fractures. Clin Orthop 232:190–196, 1988.

180. McCabe, C.J.; Ferguson, C.M.; Ottinger, L.W. Improved limb salvage in popliteal artery injuries. J Trauma 23:982–985, 1983.

181. McGraw, J.M.; Lim, E.V. Treatment of open tibial-shaft fractures. External fixation and secondary intramedullary nailing. J Bone Joint Surg 70A:900–911, 1988.

182. McGregor, J.C. Current thoughts on soft tissue repair of compound injuries of the lower limb (excluding the foot). J R Coll Surg Edinb 33:294–298, 1988.

183. McMahon, A.J.; Wilson, N.I.; Hamblen, D.L. Compression-fixation of long bone fractures: Problems and pitfalls revisited. Injury 20:84–86, 1989.

184. McMaster, M. Disability of the hindfoot after fracture of the tibial shaft. J Bone Joint Surg 58B:90–93, 1976.

185. McNutt, R.; Seabrook, G.R.; Schmitt, D.D.; et al. Blunt tibial artery trauma: Predicting the irretrievable extremity. J Trauma 29:1624–1627, 1989.

186. McQueen, M.M.; Christie, J.; Court-Brown, C.M. Compartment pressures after intramedullary nailing of the tibia. J Bone Joint Surg 72B:395–397, 1990.

187. Mead, L.P.; Scott, A.C.; Bondurant, F.J.; Browner, B.D. Indium-111 leukocyte scanning and fracture healing. J Orthop Trauma 4:81–84, 1990.

188. Melendez, E.M.; Colon, C. Treatment of open tibial fractures with the Orthofix fixator. Clin Orthop 241:224–230, 1989.

189. Merchant, T.C.; Dietz, F.R. Long-term follow-up after fractures of the tibial and fibular shafts. J Bone Joint Surg 71A:599–606, 1989.

190. Merianos, P.; Cambouridis, P.; Smyrnis, P. The treatment of 143 tibial shaft fractures by Ender's nailing and early weight-bearing. J Bone Joint Surg 67B:576–580, 1985.

191. Merianos, P.; Papagiannakos, K.; Scretas, E.; Smyrnis, P. Ender nails for segmental tibial fracture. Early weight bearing in 22 cases. Acta Orthop Scand 59:297–301, 1988.

192. Merriam, W.F.; Porter, K.M. Hindfoot disability after a tibial shaft fracture treated by internal fixation. J Bone Joint Surg 65B:326–328, 1983.

193. Meskens, M.W.; Stuyck, J.A.; Mulier, J.C. Treatment of delayed union and nonunion of the tibia by pulsed electromagnetic fields. A retrospective follow-up. Bull Hosp Jt Dis Orthop Inst 48:170–175, 1988.

194. Miller, M.E.; Ada, J.R.; Webb, L.X. Treatment of infected nonunion and delayed union of tibia fractures with locking intramedullary nails. Clin Orthop 245:233–238, 1989.

195. Mills, R.M. Minimal internal and external fixation in oblique lower extremity fractures: A report of five cases and description of technique. J Orthop Trauma 3:250–256, 1988.

196. Mino, D.E.; Hughes, E.C. Jr. Bony entrapment of the superficial peroneal nerve. Clin Orthop 185:203–206, 1984.

197. Moed, B.R.; Morawa, L.G.; Pedersen, H.E. Screw fixation of closed oblique and spiral fractures of the tibial shaft. Clin Orthop 177:196–202, 1983.

198. Mollica, Q.; Gangitano, R.; Russo, T.C.; Longo, G. The measurement of relative interfragmentary deformation in diaphyseal fractures of the lower extremity stabilised by flexible endomedullary nailing. A radiographic analysis. Ital J Orthop Traumatol 13:353–364, 1987.

199. Moore, T.J.; Green, S.A.; Garland, D.E. Severe trauma to the lower extremity: Long-term sequelae. South Med J 82:843–844, 1989.

200. Moore, T.J. Amputations of the lower extremities. In: Chapman, M.W., ed. Operative Orthopaedics. Philadelphia, J.B. Lippincott, 1988, pp. 603–615.

201. Müller, M.E.; Allgöwer, M.; Schneider, R.; Willenegger, H. Manual of Internal Fixation. Techniques Recommended by the AO-ASIF Group, Ed. 3. New York, Springer-Verlag, 1990.

201a. Müller, M.E., Nazarian, S., Koch, P.; et al. The Comprehensive Classification of Fractures of Long Bones. New York, Springer-Verlag, 1990.

202. Nesbakken, A.; Alho A.; Bjersand, A.J.; et al. Open tibial fractures treated with Hoffmann external fixation. Arch Orthop Trauma Surg 107:248–252, 1988.

203. Nicoll, E.A. Fractures of the tibial shaft: A survey of 705 cases. J Bone Joint Surg 46B:373–387, 1964.

204. Nylander, G.; Semb, H. Veins of the lower part of the leg after tibial fractures. Surg Gynecol Obstet 134:974–976, 1972.

205. Oestern, H.J.; Tscherne, H. Pathophysiology and classification of soft tissue injuries associated with fractures. In: Tscherne, H.; Gotzen, L., eds. Fractures With Soft Tissue Injuries. New York, Springer-Verlag, 1984, pp. 1–9.

206. Olerud, C. The pronation capacity of the foot—its consequences for axial deformity after tibial shaft fractures. Arch Orthop Trauma Surg 104:303–306, 1985.

207. Olerud, S.; Karlstrom, G. The spectrum of intramedullary nailing of the tibia. Clin Orthop 212:101–112, 1986.

208. Oni, O.A.O.; Fenton, A.; Iqbal, S.J.; Gregg, P.J. Prognostic indicators in tibial shaft fractures: Serum creatinine kinase activity. J Orthop Trauma 3:345–347, 1989.

209. Oni, O.O.; Hui, A.; Gregg, P.J. The healing of closed tibial shaft fractures. The natural history of union with closed treatment. J Bone Joint Surg 70A:787–790, 1988.

210. Op Den Winkel, R.; Wernet, E.; Glaser, F. Repair of vascular injuries associated with tibial shaft fractures—early and late results. Vasa 16:354–357, 1987.

210a. Owen, C.A.; Covin, J.J.; Kang, L.W. Fractures of the shaft of the tibia and fibula. J Bone Joint Surg 49A:194, 1967.

211. Paley, D.; Catagni, M.A.; Argnani, F.; et al. Ilizarov treatment of tibial nonunions with bone loss. Clin Orthop 241:146–165, 1989.

211a. Panjabi, M.M.; Lindsey, R.W.; Walter, S.D.; White, A.A. III. The clinicians ability to evaluate the strength of healing fractures from plain radiographs. J Orthop Trauma 3:29–32, 1989.

212. Pankovich, A.M.; Shantharam, S.S.; Stein, J.I. The Ring butterfly fragment in diaphyseal fractures: Its importance in flexible intramedullary nailing. J Orthop Trauma 2:18–21, 1988.

213. Paré, A. The classic: Compound fracture of leg, Paré's personal care. Clin Orthop 178:3–6, 1983.

214. Patzakis, M.J.; Wilkins, J.; Tillman, M.M. Considerations in reducing the infection rate in open tibial fractures. Clin Orthop 178:36–41, 1983.

215. Patzakis, M.J.; Wilkins, J.; Moore, T.M. Use of antibiotics in open tibial fractures. Clin Orthop 178:31–35, 1983.

216. Patzakis, M.J.; Wilkins, J.; Wiss, D.A. Infection following intramedullary nailing of long bones: Diagnosis and management. Clin Orthop 212:182–191, 1986.

217. Peltier, L.F. Fractures. A History and Iconography of their Treatment. San Francisco, Norman Publishing, 1990.

218. Perren, S.M. The biomechanics and biology of internal fixation using plates and nails. Orthopedics 12:21–34, 1989.

219. Peter, R.E.; Bachelin, P.; Fritschy, D. Skiers' lower leg shaft fracture. Outcome in 91 cases treated conservatively with Sarmiento's brace. Am J Sports Med 16:486–491, 1988.

220. Pope, M.H. The biomechanics of tibial shaft and knee injuries. Clin Sports Med 1:229–239, 1982.

221. Pospisil, M.; Wierer, I.; Franz, J. Treatment of fractures of the leg in elderly patients. (Analysis of 240 cases treated in 1968–1979). Acta Univ Carol [Med] (Praha) 31:153–163, 1985.

222. Pozo, J.L.; Powell, B.; Andrews, B.G.; et al. The timing of amputation for lower limb trauma. J Bone Joint Surg 72B:288–292, 1990.

223. Pun, W.K.; Chow, S.P.; Fang, D.; et al. Posttraumatic oedema of the foot after tibial fracture. Injury 20:232–235, 1989.

224. Puno, R.M.; Teynor, J.T.; Nagano, J.; Gustilo, R.B. Critical analysis of results of treatment of 201 tibial shaft fractures. Clin Orthop 212:113–121, 1986.

225. Puno, R.M.; Vaughan, J.J.; Von Fraunhofer, J.A.; et al. A method of determining the angular malalignments of the knee and ankle joints resulting from a tibial malunion. Clin Orthop 223:213–219, 1987.

226. Reinders, J.; Mockwitz, J. Technical faults and complications in interlocking nailing of femoral and tibial fractures. Acta Orthop Belg 50:577–590, 1984.

227. Rhinelander, F.W. Tibial blood supply in relation to fracture healing. Clin Orthop 105:34–81, 1974.

228. Rhinelander, F.W. The vascular response of bone to internal fixation. In: Browner, B.D.; Edwards, C.C., eds. The Science and Practice of Intramedullary Nailing. Philadelphia, Lea & Febiger, 1987, pp. 25–59.

229. Rhinelander, F.W.; Wilson, J.W. Blood supply to developing, mature, and healing bone. In: Sumner-Smith, G., ed. Bone in Clinical Orthopaedics. Philadelphia, W.B. Saunders, 1982, pp. 81–158.

230. Rommens, P.; Broos, P.; Gruwez, J.A. External fixation of tibial shaft fractures with severe soft tissue injuries with Hoffmann-Vidal-Adrey osteotaxis. Arch Orthop Trauma Surg 105:170–174, 1986.

231. Rommens, P.; Schmit-Neuerburg, K.P. Ten years of experience with the operative management of tibial shaft fractures. J Trauma 27:917–927, 1987.

232. Rommens, P.; Gielen, J.; Broos, P.; Gruwez, J. Intrinsic problems with the external fixation device of Hoffmann-Vidal-Adrey: A critical evaluation of 117 patients with complex tibial shaft fractures. J Trauma 29:630–638, 1989.

233. Rommens, P.M.; Van, Raemdonck, D.E.; Broos, P.L. Reos-

teosynthesis of the tibial shaft. Part I. Change of procedure after external fixation. Acta Chir Belg 189:281–286, 1989.

234. Rommens, P.M.; Van Raemdonck, D.E.; Broos, P.L. Reosteosynthesis of the tibial shaft. Part II. Changement of procedure after plate osteosynthesis. Acta Chir Belg 89:287–292, 1989.

235. Rooser, B.; Hansson, P. External fixation of ipsilateral fractures of the femur and tibia. Injury 16:371–373, 1985.

236. Rosati, E.; Medina, M.A. The role of the tibiofibular interosseous membrane in the repair of fractures of the tibia and fibula. Ital J Orthop Traumatol 13:521–525, 1987.

237. Rüedi, T.H.; Webb, J.K.; Allgöwer, M. Experience with a dynamic compression plate (DCP) in 418 recent fractures of the tibial shaft. Injury 7:252–257, 1976.

237a. Rush, L.V. Manual of Rush Pin Technics. A System of Fracture Treatment. Meridian, MS, Rush-Berivon, 1988.

238. Russell, G.G.; Henderson, R.; Arnett, G. Primary or delayed closure for open tibial fractures. J Bone Joint Surg 72B:125–131, 1990.

239. Salai, M.; Israeli, A.; Amit, Y.; et al. Closed intramedullary nailing of tibial fractures in elderly patients. J Am Geriatr Soc 32:939–941, 1984.

240. Salibian, A.H.; Anzel, S.H.; Salyer, W.A. Transfer of vascularized grafts of iliac bone to the extremities. J Bone Joint Surg 69A:1319–1327, 1987.

241. Sanders, W.E. Amputation after tibial fracture: Preservation of length by use of a neurovascular island (fillet) flap of the foot. A brief note. J Bone Joint Surg 71A:435–437, 1989.

242. Sangeorzan, B.J.; Sangeorzan, B.P.; Hansen, S.T. Jr.; Judd, R.P. Mathematically directed single-cut osteotomy for correction of tibial malunion. J Orthop Trauma 3:267–275, 1989.

243. Sangiuolo, P.; Minieri, F.; Calise, F.; et al. Arterial injuries of the lower limb with associated fractures. Mt Sinai J Med 53:554–557, 1986.

244. Sarmiento, A., ed. Tibial fractures. Clin Orthop Vol. 105, pp. 2–282, 1974.

245. Sarmiento, A.; Sobol, P.A.; Sew Hoy, A.L.; et al. Prefabricated functional braces for the treatment of fractures of the tibial diaphysis. J Bone Joint Surg 66A:1328–1339, 1984.

246. Sarmiento, A.; Gersten, L.M.; Sobol, P.A.; et al. Tibial shaft fractures treated with functional braces. Experience with 780 fractures. J Bone Joint Surg 71B:602–609, 1989.

247. Sarmiento, A.; Latta, L.L. Closed Functional Treatment of Fractures. New York, Springer-Verlag, 1981.

248. Schmidt, A.; Rorabeck, C.H. Fractures of the tibia treated by flexible external fixation. Clin Orthop 178:162–172, 1983.

249. Schroder, H.A.; Christoffersen, H.; Sorensen, T.S.; Lindequist, S. Fractures of the shaft of the tibia treated with Hoffmann external fixation. Arch Orthop Trauma Surg 105:28–30, 1986.

250. Seabold, J.E.; Nepola, J.V.; Conrad, G.R.; et al. Detection of osteomyelitis at fracture nonunion sites: Comparison of two scintigraphic methods. AJR 152:1021–1027, 1989.

251. Seale, K.S. Reflex sympathetic dystrophy of the lower extremity. Clin Orthop 243:80–85, 1989.

252. Sedlin, E.D.; Zitner, D.T. The Lottes nail in the closed treatment of tibia fractures. Clin Orthop 192:185–192, 1985.

253. Segal, D. Flexible intramedullary nailing of tibial shaft fractures. Instr Course Lect 36:338–349, 1987.

254. Segal, D.; Brenner, M.; Gorczyca, J. Tibial fractures with infrapopliteal arterial injuries. J Orthop Trauma 1:160–169, 1987.

255. Seyfer, A.E.; Lower, R. Late results of free-muscle flaps and delayed bone grafting in the secondary treatment of open distal tibial fractures. Plast Reconstr Surg 83:77–84, 1989.

256. Shakespeare, D.T.; Henderson, N.J. Compartmental pressure changes during calcaneal traction in tibial fractures. J Bone Joint Surg 64B:498–499, 1982.

257. Sharrard, W.J.W. A double-blind trial of pulsed electromagnetic fields for delayed union of tibial fractures. J Bone Joint Surg 72B:347–355, 1990.

258. Sherman, K.P.; Shakespeare, D.T.; Nelson, L.; Fyfe, C. A simple adjustable functional brace for tibial fractures. Injury 17:15–18, 1986.

259. Simon, J.P.; Hoogmartens, M. The value of posterolateral bone-grafting for non-union of the tibia. Acta Orthop Belg 50:557–564, 1984.

260. Simpson, J.M.; Ebraheim, N.A.; An, H.S.; Jackson, W.T. Posterolateral bone graft of the tibia. Clin Orthop 251:200–206, 1990.

261. Skraba, J.S.; Greenwald, A.S. The role of the interosseous membrane on tibiofibular weightbearing. Foot Ankle 4:301–304, 1984.

262. Slatis, P.; Rokkanen, P. Closed intramedullary nailing of tibial shaft fractures. A comparison with conservatively treated cases. Acta Orthop Scand 38:88–100, 1967.

263. Sledge, S.L.; Johnson, K.D.; Henley, M.B.; Watson, J.T. Intramedullary nailing with reaming to treat non-union of the tibia. J Bone Joint Surg 71A:1004–1019, 1989.

264. Smith, J.E.M. Results of early and delayed internal fixation for tibial shaft fractures. A review of 470 fractures. J Bone Joint Surg 56B:469–477, 1974.

265. Smith, M.A.; Jones, E.A.; Strachan, R.K.; et al. Prediction of fracture healing in the tibia by quantitative radionuclide imaging. J Bone Joint Surg 69B:441–447, 1987.

266. Snyder, W.H. III. Popliteal and shank arterial injury. Surg Clin North Am 68:787–807, 1988.

266a. Speigel, J.; Bray, T.; Chapman, M.; Swanson, T. The Lottes nail versus AO external fixation in open tibia fractures. Orthop Trans 12:656, 1988.

267. Spiegel, P.G.; Vanderschilden, J.L. Minimal internal and external fixation in the treatment of open tibial fractures. Clin Orthop 178:96–102, 1983.

268. Steinfield, P.H.; Cobelli, N.J.; Sadler, A.H.; Szporn, M.N. Open tibial fractures treated by anterior half-pin frame fixation. Clin Orthop 228:208–214, 1988.

269. Strachan, R.K.; McCarthy, I.; Fleming, R.; Hughes, S.P.F. The role of the tibial nutrient artery. Microsphere estimation of blood flow in the osteotomized canine tibia. J Bone Joint Surg 72B:391–397, 1990.

270. Suman, R.K. Functional bracing in lower limb fractures. Ital J Orthop Traumatol 9:201–209, 1983.

271. Swiontkowski, M.F. Criteria for bone debridement in massive lower limb trauma. Clin Orthop 243:41–47, 1989.

272. Taine, W.H.; Gillespie, W.J. Post-traumatic osteomyelitis (fifteen months to rehabilitate from tibial fracture). Orthopedics 8:565;568–569;688, 1985.

273. Takami, H.; Doi, T.; Takahashi, S.; Ninomiya, S. Reconstruction of a large tibial defect with a free vascularized fibular graft. Arch Orthop Trauma Surg 102:203–205, 1984.

274. Takebe, K.; Nakagawa, A.; Minami, H.; et al. Role of the fibula in weightbearing. Clin Orthop 184:289–292, 1984.

275. Taylor, G.J.; Allum, R.L. Ankle motion after external fixation of tibial fractures. J R Soc Med 81:19–21, 1988.

276. Teitz, C.C.; Carter, D.R.; Frankel, V.H. Problems associated with tibial fractures with intact fibulae. J Bone Joint Surg 62A:770–776, 1980.

277. Templeman, D.C.; Marder, R.A. Injuries of the knee associated with fractures of the tibial shaft. Detection by examination under anesthesia. J Bone Joint Surg 71A:1392–1395, 1989.

278. Tencer, A.F.; Claudi, B.; Pearce, S.; et al. Development of a variable stiffness external fixation system for stabilization of segmental defects of the tibia. J Orthop Res 1:395–404, 1984.

279. Terjesen, T.; Nordby, A.; Arnulf, V. The extent of stress-protection after plate osteosynthesis in the human tibia. Clin Orthop 207:108–112, 1986.

280. Tile, M. Fractures of the tibia. In: Schatzker, J.; Tile, M., eds. The Rationale of Operative Fracture Care. New York, Springer-Verlag, 1987, pp. 297–341.

281. Ting, A.J.; Tarr, R.R.; Sarmiento, A.; et al. The role of subtalar motion and ankle contact pressure changes from angular deformities of the tibia. Foot Ankle 7:290–299, 1987.

282. Tischenko, G.J.; Goodman, S.B. Compartment syndrome after intramedullary nailing of the tibia. J Bone Joint Surg 72A:41–44, 1990.

283. Tolhurst, D.E.; Haeseker, B.; Zeeman, R.J. The development of the fasciocutaneous flap and its clinical applications. Plast Reconstr Surg 71:597–605, 1983.

284. Trafton, P.G. Closed unstable fractures of the tibia. Clin Orthop 230:58–67, 1988.

285. Tscherne, H.; Gotzen, L. Fractures with Soft Tissue Injuries. New York, Springer-Verlag, 1984.

286. Valenti, J.R.; Arenas, A.; Barredo, R.; et al. Treatment of infected tibial pseudarthrosis by external fixation with the Wagner device. Arch Orthop Trauma Surg 102:256–259, 1984.

287. Van Der Werken, C.; Marti, R.K. Post-traumatic rotational deformity of the lower leg. Injury 15:38–40, 1983.

288. Van Der Werken, C.; Zeegers, E.V. Fracture of the lower leg with involvement of the posterior malleolus; a neglected combination? Injury 19:241–243, 1988.

289. Van Der Linden, W.; Larsson, K. Plate fixation versus conservative treatment of tibial shaft fractures. A randomized trial. J Bone Joint Surg 61A:873–878, 1979.

290. Veith, R.G.; Winquist, R.A.; Hansen, S.T. Jr. Ipsilateral fractures of the femur and tibia. A report of fifty-seven consecutive cases. J Bone Joint Surg 66A:991–1002, 1984.

291. Velazco, A.; Fleming, L.L. Open fractures of the tibia treated by the Hoffmann external fixator. Clin Orthop 180:125–132, 1983.

292. Velazco, A.; Fleming, L.L.; Nahai, F. Soft-tissue reconstruction of the leg associated with the use of the Hoffmann external fixator. J Trauma 23:1052–1057, 1983.

293. Velazco, A.; Whitesides, T.E. Jr.; Fleming, L.L. Open fractures of the tibia treated with the Lottes nail. J Bone Joint Surg 65A:879–885, 1983.

294. Vossoughi, J.; Youm, Y.; Bosse, M.; et al. Structural stiffness of the Hoffmann simple anterior tibial external fixation frame. Ann Biomed Eng 17:127–141, 1989.

295. Voto, S.J.; Pigott, J.; Riley, P.; Donovan, D. Arterial injuries associated with lower extremity fractures. Orthopedics 11:357–360, 1988.

296. Waddell, J.P.; Reardon, G.P. Complications of tibial shaft fractures. Clin Orthop 178:173–178, 1983.

297. Wagner, K.S.; Tarr, R.R.; Resnick, C.; et al. The effect of simulated tibial deformities on the ankle joint during the gait cycle. Foot Ankle 5:131–141, 1984.

298. Watson-Jones, R.; Coltart, W.D. Slow union of fractures, with a study of 804 fractures of the shafts of the tibia and femur. Clin Orthop 168:2–16, 1982.

299. Webb, L.X.; Bosse, M.J.; Staeheli, J.W.; Naylor, P.T. Closed intramedullary nailing of the tibia without a fracture table—a simple technique. Exhibit At the Annual Meeting of AAOS, New Orleans, February 1990.

300. Weiland, A.J.; Moore, J.R.; Hotchkiss, R.N. Soft tissue procedures for reconstruction of tibial shaft fractures. Clin Orthop 178:42–53, 1983.

301. White, A.A. III; Panjabi, M.M.; Southwick, W.O. The four

biomechanical stages of fracture repair. J Bone Joint Surg 59:188–192, 1977.

302. Whitelaw, G.P.; Wetzler, M.; Nelson, A.; et al. Ender rods versus external fixation in the treatment of open tibial fractures. Clin Orthop 253:258–269, 1990.

303. Whiteside, L.A.; Lesker, P.A. The effects of extraperiosteal and subperiosteal dissection. II. On fracture healing. J Bone Joint Surg 60A:26–30, 1978.

304. Wihlborg, O. The effect of a change in management of displaced tibial shaft fractures. Rigid fixation versus conservative treatment. Helv Chir Acta 53:191–199, 1986.

305. Williamson, D.M.; Kershaw, C.J. Serious vascular complication of locked tibial nailing. Injury 20:310–312, 1989.

306. Wiss, D.A. Flexible medullary nailing of acute tibial shaft fractures. Clin Orthop 212:122–132, 1986.

307. Wiss, D.A.; Segal, D.; Gumbs, V.L.; Salter, D. Flexible medullary nailing of tibial shaft fractures. J Trauma 26:1106–1112, 1986.

308. Wolfe, J.H. Postphlebitic syndrome after fractures of the leg. Br Med J [Clin Res] 295:1364–1365, 1987.

309. Wood, M.B.; Cooney, W.P.; Irons, G.B. Lower extremity salvage and reconstruction by free-tissue transfer. Analysis of results. Clin Orthop 201:151–161, 1985.

310. Wright, J.G.; Bogoch, E.R.; Hastings, D.E. The "occult" compartment syndrome. J Trauma 29:133–134, 1989.

311. Yaremchuk, M.J.; Brumback, R.J.; Manson, P.N.; et al. Acute and definitive management of traumatic osteocutaneous defects of the lower extremity. Plast Reconstr Surg 80:1–14, 1987.

312. Yaremchuk, M.J. Acute management of severe soft-tissue damage accompanying open fractures of the lower extremity. Clin Plast Surg 13:621–632, 1986.

313. Ziv, I.; Zeligowski, A.; Mosheiff, R.; et al. Split-thickness skin excision in severe open fractures. J Bone Joint Surg 70B:23–26, 1988.

Fibular Fractures

314. al-Awami, S.M.; Sadat-Ali, M.; Sankaran-Kutty, M. Arterial injury complicating fracture of the fibula: A case report. Injury 18:214–215, 1987.

315. Golimbu, C.; Firooznia, H.; Rafii, M.; Waugh, T. Acute traumatic fibular bowing associated with tibial fractures. Clin Orthop 182:211–214, 1984.

316. Hall, R.F. Jr.; Gonzales, M. Fracture of the proximal part of the tibia and fibula associated with an entrapped popliteal artery. A case report. J Bone Joint Surg 68A:941–944, 1986.

317. Karkabi, S.; Reis, N.D. Fibular bowing due to tibial shortening in isolated fracture of the tibia: Failure of late segmental fibulectomy to relieve ankle pain. Arch Orthop Trauma Surg 106:61–63, 1986.

318. Lambert, K.L. Weight-bearing function of the fibula. J Bone Joint Surg 54A:507–513, 1971.

319. Lee, E.H.; Goh, J.C.H.; Helm, R.; Pho, R.W.H. Donor site morbidity following resection of the fibula. J Bone Joint Surg 72B:129–131, 1990.

320. Levy, A.S.; Levitt, L.E.; Gunther, S.F.; Wetzler, M.J. The role of Ender rodding in tibial fractures with an intact fibula. J Orthop Trauma 4:75–80, 1990.

321. Mino, D.E.; Hughes, E.C. Jr. Bony entrapment of the superficial peroneal nerve. Clin Orthop 185:203–206, 1984.

322. Skraba, J.S.; Greenwald, A.S. The role of the interosseous membrane on tibiofibular weightbearing. Foot Ankle 4:301–304, 1984.

323. Takebe, K.; Nakagawa, A.; Minami, H.; et al. Role of the fibula in weightbearing. Clin Orthop 184:289–292, 1984.

324. Teitz, C.C.; Carter, D.R.; Frankel, V.H. Problems associated with tibial fractures with intact fibulae. J Bone Joint Surg 62A:770–776, 1980.

Proximal Tibiofibular Joint Injuries

325. Andersen, K. Dislocation of the superior tibiofibular joint. Injury 16:494–498, 1985.

326. Brana, V.A.; Mieres, B.P.; Montes, M.S. Traumatic luxation of the proximal tibiofibular joint, superior variety. A case report. Acta Orthop Belg 49:479–482, 1983.

327. Clews, A.G. Dislocation of the upper end of the fibula. Can Med Assoc J 98:169–170, 1968.

328. Crothers, O.D.; Johnson, J.T.H. Isolated acute dislocation of the proximal tibiofibular joint. J Bone Joint Surg 55A:181–183, 1973.

329. Eichenblat, M.; et al. The proximal tibio-fibular joint. Anatomic study with clinico-pathologic correlation. Int Orthop 7:31, 1983.

330. Falkenberg, P.; Nygaard, H. Isolated anterior dislocation of the proximal tibiofibular joint. J Bone Joint Surg 65B:310–311, 1983.

331. Giachino, A.A. Recurrent dislocations of the proximal tibiofibular joint. Report of two cases. J Bone Joint Surg 68A:1104–1106, 1986.

332. Karkabi, S.; Reis, N.D. Fibular bowing due to tibial shortening in isolated fracture of the tibia: Failure of late segmental fibulectomy to relieve ankle pain. Arch Orthop Trauma Surg 106:61–63, 1986.

333. Kiester, P.D.; Connolly, J.F. Fibular head dislocation—another differential in the diagnosis of knee injury. Nebr Med J 70:26–27, 1985.

334. Ogden, J.A. Subluxation and dislocation of the proximal tibiofibular joint. J Bone Joint Surg 56A:145–154, 1974.

335. Parkes, J.C.; Zelko, R.R. Isolated acute dislocation of the proximal tibiofibular joint. J Bone Joint Surg 55A:177–180, 1973.

336. Resnick, D.; et al. Proximal tibiofibular joint: Anatomic, pathologic, and radiologic correlation. Am J Radiol 131:133, 1978.

337. Sharma, P.; Daffner, R.H. Case report 389: Idiopathic, anterolateral dislocation of the fibula at the proximal tibiofibular joint. Skeletal Radiol 15:505–506, 1986.

338. Thomason, P.A.; Linson, M.A. Isolated dislocation of the proximal tibiofibular joint. J Trauma 26:192–195, 1986.

339. Weinert, C.R. Jr.; Raczka, R. Recurrent dislocation of the superior tibiofibular joint. Surgical stabilization by ligament reconstruction. J Bone Joint Surg 68A:126–128, 1986.

Fatigue Fractures

340. Burr, D.B.; Milgram, C.; Boyd, R.D.; et al. Experimental stress fractures of the tibia. Biological and mechanical aetiology in rabbits. J Bone Joint Surg 72B:370–375, 1990.

341. Castillo, M.; Tehranzadeh, J.; Morillo, G. Atypical healed stress fracture of the fibula masquerading as chronic osteomyelitis. A case report of magnetic resonance distinction. Am J Sports Med 16:185–188, 1988.

342. Devereaux, M.D.; Parr, G.R.; Lachmann, S.M.; et al. The diagnosis of stress fractures in athletes. JAMA 252:531–533, 1984.

343. Dickson, T.B. Jr; Kichline, P.D. Functional management of stress fractures in female athletes using a pneumatic leg brace. Am J Sports Med 15:86–89, 1987.

344. Dowey, K.E.; Moore, G.W. Stress fractures in athletes. Ulster Med J 53:121–124, 1984.
345. Dugan, R.C.; D'Ambrosia, R. Fibular stress fractures in runners. J Fam Pract 17:415–418, 1983.
346. McBride, A.M. Stress fractures in runners. Clin Sports Med 4:737–752, 1985.
347. Miller, H.G. Stress fracture of the fibula: Secondary to pronation? J Am Podiatr Med Assoc 75:211–212, 1985.
348. Morris, J.M.; Blickenstaff, L.D. Fatigue Fractures—A Clinical Study. Springfield, IL, Charles C Thomas, 1967.
349. Mubarak, S.J.; et al. Medial tibial stress syndrome (a cause of shin splints). Am J Sports Med 10:201–205, 1982.
350. Nix, R.A. Stress fractures in the lower extremity. J Arkansas Med Soc 80:10–13, 1983.
351. Nussbaum, A.R.; Treves, S.T.; Micheli, L. Bone stress lesions in ballet dancers: Scintigraphic assessment. AJR 150:851–855, 1988.
352. Pouilles, J.M.; Bernard, J.; Tremollieres, F.; et al. Femoral bone density in young male adults with stress fractures. Bone 10:105–108, 1989.
353. Read, M.T. Runner's stress fracture produced by an aerobic dance routine. Br J Sports Med 18:40–41, 1984.
354. Rupani, H.D.; Holder, L.E.; Espinola, D.A.; Engin, S.I. Three-phase radionuclide bone imaging in sports medicine. Radiology 156:187–196, 1985.
355. Sullivan, D.; Warren, R.F.; Pavlov, H.; Kelman, G. Stress fractures in 51 runners. Clin Orthop 187:188–192, 1984.
356. Synnott, J.L.; Barry, O.C. Bilateral stress fractures of the fused lower fibular epiphysis. Ir J Med Sci 153:252–254, 1984.
357. Yao, L.; et al. Occult intraosseous fracture: Detection with MR imaging. Radiology 167:749–751, 1988.
358. Zlatkin, M.B.; Bjorkengren, A.; Sartoris, D.J.; Resnick, D. Stress fractures of the distal tibia and calcaneus subsequent to acute fractures of the tibia and fibula. AJR 149:329–332, 1987.

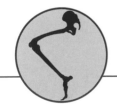

Peter G. Trafton, M.D.
Timothy J. Bray, M.D.
Lex A. Simpson, M.D.

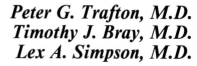

Fractures and Soft Tissue Injuries of the Ankle

*T*here is no unequivocal boundary marking the proximal or distal limits of the ankle region. Structure, function, and injuries have no borders here and often require that the leg and foot be included in any regional assessment or treatment. This chapter considers injuries of the tibiotalar joint from the supramalleolar region of the tibia and fibula distally to the talus. Trauma to the talus itself is reviewed in chapter 53. In addition to ankle joint injuries, this chapter also deals with local injuries of the structures crossing the joint.

The ankle is a complex hinge in which both bone and ligaments play important and inseparable parts.[105] Its satisfactory function depends significantly on its precise structural integrity. As a weight-bearing joint, the ankle is exposed to forces that transiently exceed 1.25 × body weight with normal gait and that may exceed 5.5 × body weight with vigorous activities. Normal gait requires adequate dorsiflexion and plantarflexion. Inversion and eversion, as well as accommodation to rotational stresses, are provided by the subtalar joint, whose function is linked closely with that of the ankle.[92a,132] The ankle is not intrinsically stable in any position and requires support from the muscles that cross it.

The overlying skin is thin, with a tenuous blood supply.[213] Tendons rather than muscle bellies cross the joint and provide no coverage for it. After severe injuries, ankle wounds, both traumatic and surgical, may have problems healing. An injury of the ankle region can involve, in addition to bone, articular surface, and ligament, any of the tendons, nerves, or blood vessels that cross it.

Management of ankle injuries depends first on a thorough evaluation identifying both the anatomic structures involved and the severity of the damage.[79,210] Once the injuries are defined, optimal treatment generally entails as anatomic a repair as possible while avoiding any additional compromise to the region.

Anatomy and Biomechanics

ANATOMY

Ankle anatomy has been thoroughly reviewed by several authors.[79,202] Distally the tibial shaft flares, and the bone changes from tubular cortical to metaphyseal and cancellous (Fig. 52–1). In the young active adult, the distal tibia may be exceptionally dense. This supramalleolar portion of the ankle is referred to as the "pilon tibiale," using the French word for "pestle," the shape of which it resembles. Fractures involving this region are thus "pilon" fractures, a term that is generally reserved for those injuries with significant supramalleolar involvement as well as extension into the weight-bearing, horizontal articular surface of the distal tibia. This part of the proximal articular surface of the ankle joint is called the "plafond," which means the "ceiling." The AO/ASIF has contributed to our awareness of the distinction between *malleolar fractures,* which may have associated involvement of the plafond, and

Figure 52–1

Normal anteroposterior (A), lateral (B) and mortise (C) views of the ankle. The tibiotalar joint demonstrates congruent articular surfaces, normal subchondral bone outline, and uniform width of cartilage space. The overlap of tibia and fibula at the incisural notch is evident. D, Computed tomogram through another patient's ankle shows that medial and lateral joint spaces are not necessarily parallel. Note again the congruent fit of talus in mortise.

pilon fractures, where the focus of the injury is primarily supramalleolar.[200]

The anteromedial aspect of the distal tibia is notable for the prominent medial malleolus, which carries the medial articular surface of the ankle mortise. It is smaller than the lateral malleolus and can be divided into an anterior colliculus, covered laterally with articular cartilage, and a posterior colliculus. The superficial deltoid (medial collateral ligament) is attached at the anterior colliculus and distally goes to the talus, calcaneus, and navicular, but provides little stability to the ankle joint itself. The primary medial stabilizer is the deep portion of the deltoid ligament, which is attached to the posterior colliculus, the somewhat shorter posterior part of the malleolus. This nearly transverse, synovial-covered, essentially intraarticular ligament is not accessible from outside the joint, unless the talus is displaced laterally or the medial malleolus can be

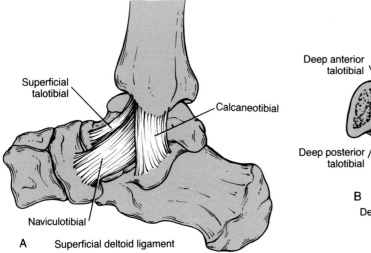

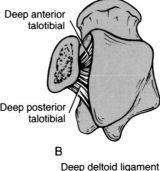

Figure 52–2

The medial collateral ligament of the ankle. A, The superficial fibers connecting the medial malleolus to the talus, calcaneus, and navicular have a roughly triangular appearance and suggest the name "deltoid." B, The much more important deep fibers run nearly transversely from the posterior colliculus to the talus posterior to its medial articular facet.

turned distally through a fracture or osteotomy (Fig. 52–2). Any repair of the deltoid ligament that does not include this structure does not restore ligamentous stability.

The shape of the articular surface of the distal tibia is concave, with the anterior and, especially, posterior lips projecting more distally. The posterior lip of the plafond is the anchorage for the posterior part of the inferior tibiofibular syndesmotic ligaments. It does not limit movement of the talus the way the medial and lateral malleoli do. However, it is not uncommonly injured along with the lateral and medial malleoli, becoming the "third malleolus." This is the basis for the term "trimalleolar" fracture to describe injuries involving both the medial and lateral malleoli along with the posterior lip.[79]

The ankle joint surface has a slight central prominence oriented anteroposteriorly. The articular surface contour of the talar dome matches the curved plafond very closely. Slight lateral displacement of the talus results in a considerable reduction of the contact area between the two bones. According to Ramsey and Hamilton, a 1-mm lateral shift produces a 42% decrease in joint contact area.[183a] It is presumed that increased joint pressure, caused by the same amount of force being borne by a smaller area, results in degenerative changes of the articular cartilage, a common problem after severe injuries in which loss of the congruent relationship between talus and tibia occurs. However, more recent studies of ankle joint contact stresses suggest that neither lateral talar shift nor displacement of posterior malleolar fragments increases peak stress.[245] It is possible that high joint contact stress is not the primary cause of posttraumatic arthrosis.

Laterally, the distal tibia is indented by a shallow groove or incisura for the fibula (Fig. 52–3). This is formed by a larger anterior tubercle (Chaput's, or Tillaux-Chaput's) and a significantly smaller posterior tubercule.

The most significant ligamentous complex of the ankle is that which unites the distal tibia and fibula. This so-called syndesmosis is comprised of five distinct portions (Fig. 52–4). Anteriorly the *anteroinferior tibiofibular ligament* (AITFL) runs obliquely slightly distally from the anterior lateral tubercle of the tibia (Chaput's) to the anterior portion of the lateral malleolus, where its attachment is occasionally referred to as Wagstaffe's tubercle. The *posteroinferior tibiofibular ligament* (PITFL) runs obliquely distally from the posterior tubercle (Volkmann's, or third or posterior malleolus). It is distinguished from a fibrocartilaginous but otherwise similar connection between the tibia and fibula that lies just distally and is called the *inferior transverse tibiofibular ligament*. A short and variable dis-

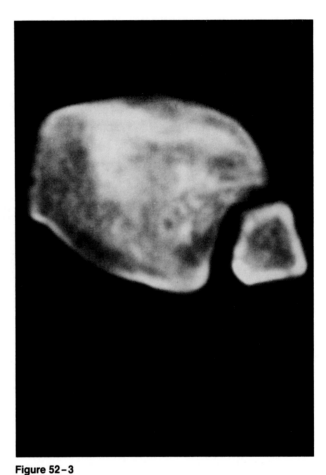

Figure 52–3

Computed tomogram just above the ankle shows the prominent anterior tubercle, which overlaps the more posterior fibula and helps form the incisural notch.

tance above the ankle, the *tibiofibular interosseous membrane* thickens and becomes the *interosseous ligament*. These five structures comprise collectively the "syndesmosis" and are largely responsible for the structural integrity of the ankle mortise. If they fail and the fibular malleolus displaces laterally, then the talus follows it and loses its normal relationship with the weight-bearing surface of the tibial plafond.[120,183a,256] This lateral talar shift is not reliably prevented by an apparently intact deltoid ligament and forms the basis for the now well-appreciated need to reestablish the anatomic relationship of the lateral malleolus to the distal tibia when it has been disrupted in a malleolar injury.

The lateral collateral ligament complex is made up of three portions (Fig. 52–5). The *anterior talofibular ligament* is directed anteromedially to the lateral neck of the talus. The bulky and stout *posterior talofibular ligament* is posteromedially attached to the posterior process of the talus. Both of these are essentially thicken-

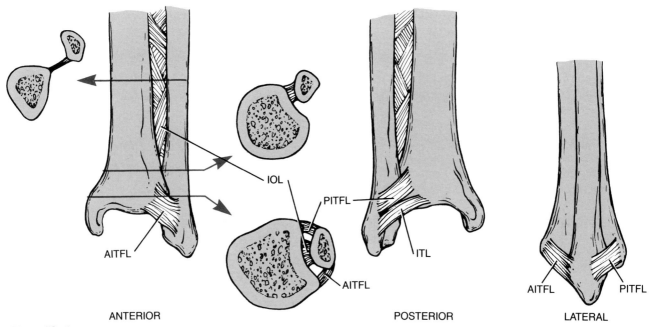

Figure 52-4

The ligaments of the distal tibiofibular syndesmosis. The lower part of the interosseous membrane thickens to form the interosseous ligament (IOL). Just above the plafond lie the anterior inferior tibiofibular ligament (AITFL) and the posterior inferior tibiofibular ligament (PITFL), with more distal fibers called the "inferior transverse ligament." (Redrawn from Hamilton, W.C. Traumatic Disorders of the Ankle [Fig. 1–7]. New York, Springer-Verlag, 1984.)

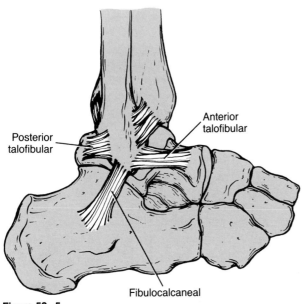

Figure 52-5

The three components of the lateral collateral ligament are the anterior and posterior talofibular and, between them, the calcaneofibular, which crosses the talus. The orientation of anterior talofibular and fibulocalcaneal ligaments is demonstrated in Figure 52–13.

ings, along with the superficial deltoid ligament medially, in an otherwise structurally unimpressive and redundant ankle joint capsule. The middle part of the ankle's lateral collateral ligament complex is the *fibulocalcaneal ligament.* This runs obliquely posteriorly and distally deep to the peroneal tendons, more or less perpendicularly across the posterior facet of the subtalar joint, and attaches to the calcaneous just posterior to the proximal extent of its peroneal tubercle. An additional, inconstant posterolateral extracapsular ligamentous structure is the so-called fibulotalocalcaneal ligament, a local thickening of the deep aponeurosis of the leg that resists extreme foot dorsiflexion.[202]

A number of important structures cross the ankle joint and must be considered with any approach to diagnosis and treatment of ankle injuries.

Superficially and posteriorly, the powerful plantarflexor of the ankle, the tendo calcaneus or Achilles tendon, is prominent, with a thin tendon sheath and little subcutaneous tissue between it and the overlying skin. Just lateral to the Achilles tendon lies the sural nerve. The sural nerve supplies the skin of the lateral heel and midfoot and is at risk of painful entrapment in a surgical scar. The plantaris tendon runs along the medial border of the Achilles tendon and attaches to the calcaneus just medial to it. This small-diameter tendon may be used for tendon or ligament repairs in the ankle region and elsewhere.

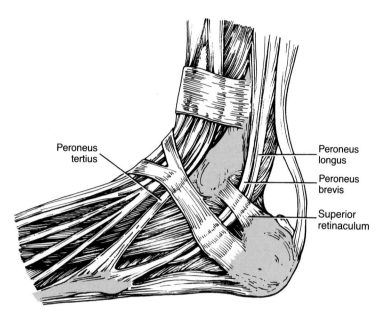

Figure 52-6

The lateral ankle is crossed posteriorly by the peroneus brevis and peroneus longus tendons, restrained primarily by their superior retinaculum posterior to the distal part of the lateral malleolus. The Achilles tendon is most posterior. The peroneus tertius and toe extensors are anterior.

On the lateral side of the ankle, the peroneus brevis and peroneus longus tendons, the latter more posteriorly, course around the posterior surface of the lateral malleolus (Fig. 52-6). They are tethered there by the superior peroneal retinaculum, which, with its fibrocartilaginous attachment may be avulsed from the fibula and permit anterior dislocation of the tendons. Such a dislocation is not prevented by the more anteriorly located inferior peroneal retinaculum, a prolongation of the inferior extensor retinaculum. The peroneal tendons are superficial to the fibulocalcaneal ligament. As they reach the lateral border of the foot, the peroneus longus crosses plantarward under the peroneus brevis and traverses the foot under the long plantar ligament to insert on the proximal first metatarsal and

first cuneiform. The peroneus brevis inserts on the base of the fifth metatarsal, from which, with an inversion injury, it may be avulsed with a small bone fragment.

On the medial side of the ankle, several important structures lie posterior to the medial malleolus, anchored there by the flexor retinaculum, which runs from the posteroinferior surface of the malleolus to the medial surface of the tuberosity of the calcaneus. Its malleolar attachment is a fibrocartilaginous pulley for the most anterior of the flexor tendons, the tibialis posterior, behind which lie, in order, the flexor digitorum longus; the posterior tibial artery and associated veins with the tibial nerve; and, most posteriorly, crossing the posterior surface of the ankle joint, the flexor hallucis longus (Fig. 52-7). Each tendon lies in a well-devel-

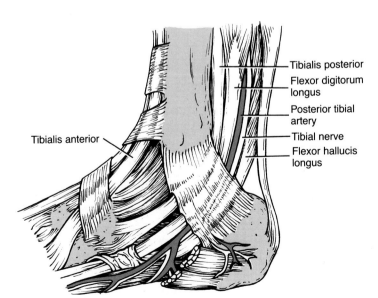

Figure 52-7

The structures crossing the medial ankle anteriorly include the tibialis anterior tendon, saphenous vein, and saphenous nerve. Behind the medial malleolus lie the important tibialis posterior, flexor digitorum longus, the posterior tibial artery and veins, the tibial nerve, and the posteriorly located flexor hallucis longus.

oped tunnel. Should a flexor tendon rupture or be lacerated, it may retract beyond the surgeon's view, with the result that the injury is not recognized. Posterior tibial tendon laceration occurs frequently enough with medial malleolus fractures that the surgeon should identify this tendon when the fracture exposes its tunnel.

A centimeter or two anterior to the medial malleolus lies the saphenous vein with its accompanying saphenous nerve (usually two or more small branches). The vein is valuable for fluid administration, as it is rapidly available by cutdown regardless of whether a patient is in shock. It is also important for venous

drainage of an injured foot and should be spared in such situations whenever possible. The saphenous nerve is at risk of entrapment in a local surgical or traumatic scar, with resultant formation of painful neuromas. It should be identified and preserved or resected in a manner that allows the proximal end to retract well away from any wound.

On the anterior aspect of the ankle, the extensor retinacula restrain the extensor tendons, anterior tibial vessels, and deep peroneal nerve as they leave the anterior compartment of the leg and cross onto the dorsum of the foot (Fig. 52–8). Proximal to the ankle, the transverse fibers of the superior extensor retinaculum run from the anteromedial subcutaneous surface of the tibia to the anterolateral surface of the distal fibula. The inferior extensor retinaculum is Y shaped. Its base attaches to the calcaneus laterally. The proximal medial limb attaches to the medial malleolus and the distal to the deep fascia medial to the navicular. The inferior extensor retinaculum thus lies over the anterior ankle joint capsule. Under it, from lateral to medial, are the peroneus tertius, the extensor digitorum longus tendon, the deep peroneal nerve, the anterior tibial artery (becoming the dorsalis pedis), the extensor hallucis longus tendon, and the tibialis anterior tendon. The last runs somewhat obliquely to insert on the medial surface of the first cuneiform and the base of the first metatarsal.

Significant individual variation in ankle joint anatomy and mechanics should be recognized and considered in attempts to define normality and to treat injuries. The use of the opposite ankle as a control is helpful, but it is important to recognize the normal range of asymmetry that may account for some differences. For example, 3% of normal individuals will have a 10° difference between ankles in talar tilt measured on inversion stress radiographs.[79]

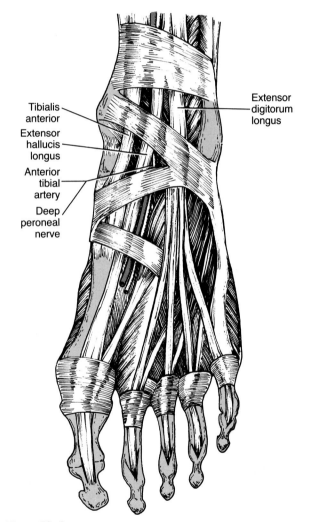

Tibialis anterior

Extensor hallucis longus

Anterior tibial artery

Deep peroneal nerve

Extensor digitorum longus

Figure 52–8

The anterior ankle is crossed by the dorsiflexors: tibialis anterior, extensor hallucis longus, extensor digitorum longus, and the occasionally absent peroneus tertius tendons. The anterior tibial vessels and deep peroneal nerve are just lateral to the extensor hallucis longus. The superior (transverse) and inferior (cruciate) retinacula provide pulleys for the dorsiflexors. The origin of the short extensors is from the anterolateral calcaneus beneath the long toe extensor tendons.

ANKLE BIOMECHANICS

Ankle Joint Mechanics

The "empiric ankle axis" can be estimated by palpating the tips of the medial and lateral malleoli.[92a,132] It passes just below these, directed medially to laterally both posteriorly and inferiorly (Fig. 52–9). In 80% of ankles, normal motion is simple rotation around this axis.

The obliquity of the empiric ankle joint axis varies from person to person. Its angle with the midline of the tibia in the coronal plane averages 82° (i.e., 8° varus angulation). This varies from 74° to 94°, with a standard deviation of 3.6°. External tibial torsion in the transverse plane increases during childhood. In the adult it measures approximately 22° relative to the midpoints of the proximal tibial condyles, ranging

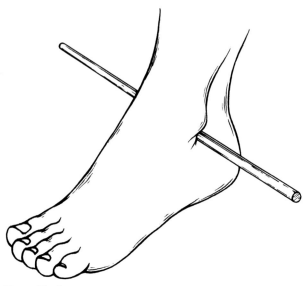

Figure 52-9

A line joining the tips of the medial and lateral malleoli is a close approximation of the axis of the ankle joint. Inman[92a] has called this the "empirical axis of the ankle."

from $-4°$ to $+56°$, with a standard deviation of $10°$.[92a]

The actual axis of the ankle joint is more oblique than the joint surface. The joint surface of the tibial plafond is also angled in the coronal plane relative to the midline of the tibia but in the *opposite* direction to the ankle joint axis. Its average is 3° of valgus angulation, ranging from $-2°$ to $+10°$. The angle between the two, the talocrural angle, is an indicator of normal lateral malleolar alignment. It normally ranges from $83°$ to $+4°$ and is normally within 2° of the opposite ankle (Fig. 52-10).[92,177]

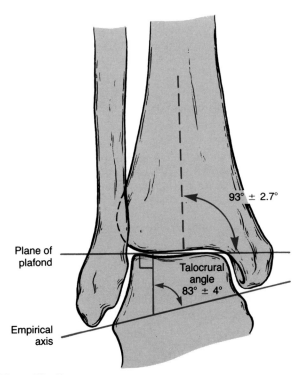

Figure 52-10

The tibiotalar articular surface (plafond) usually has a slight lateral tilt, averaging 3°. The empirical axis is in a relatively varus position, as indicated by the talocrural angle, formed by the intersection of a line perpendicular to the plafond with the empirical axis. This averages $83° \pm 4°$ and is a reliable radiographic indicator of the relationship among malleoli and plafond. It should be very similar to that of the opposite ankle.

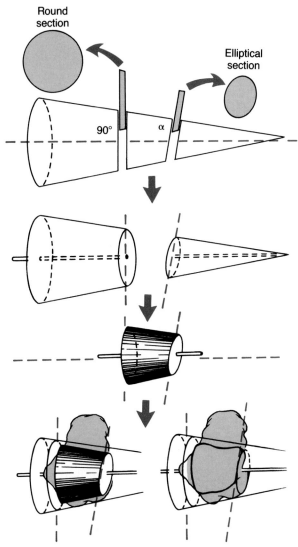

Figure 52-11

The puzzling shape of the talus and mortise, which maintain a congruent fit throughout the range of ankle motion, is explained by Inman's demonstration that the joint surface is a segment (frustum) of a cone, the axis of which lies on the ankle's empirical axis. The smaller fibular facet is elliptical because of its obliquity. The larger medial articular facet is round, since it is perpendicular to the axis of the cone. (Redrawn from Inman, V.T. The Joints of the Ankle. © Williams & Wilkins, Baltimore, 1976.)

The fit of talus in mortise is precise, making it the most congruent of the weight-bearing joints.[92a] Both mortise and talar trochlea are narrower posteriorly, with the amount, as well as the degree of parallelism of the malleolar articular surfaces, varying among individuals. The fit of talus in mortise remains congruent throughout the ankle's range of motion, as Inman[92a] demonstrated, because the joint surface is a portion of a frustum of a cone, the axis of which is the ankle's axis of rotation (Fig. 52–11). Therefore there is little if any change in mortise width during ankle motion (0 to 2 mm, according to Inman).[92a] The effect of the ankle's oblique axis is an obligatory internal and external rotation of the foot with plantar- and dorsiflexion, respectively (Fig. 52–12).

Lindsjö et al. measured motion of the loaded ankle, noting, with hip and knee flexed and the foot on a 30-cm high stool, a mean of 32° dorsiflexion and 45° plantar flexion.[124a] They stated that although normal gait required at least 10° dorsiflexion, athletic activities were limited if loaded dorsiflexion was less than 20° to 30°.

Because the medial and lateral facets of the ankle mortise vary in their relationship to each other and to the ankle joint axis, a mortise view radiograph will not necessarily show symmetric width of the ankle joint's "cartilage space."

Average in vivo subtalar motion is approximately 40°, ranging from 20° to 62°.[92] The orientation of the subtalar joint is 23° ± 11° (range, 4° to 47°), internally rotated relative to the long axis of the foot in the transverse plane and elevated anteriorly from the horizontal by 42° ± 9° (range, 20.5° to 68.5°) relative to the horizontal in the sagittal plane.[92a] During walking on level ground, average subtalar motion for a normal foot is 6°.[132]

Ankle Ligament Mechanics

Medial Collateral Ligament

The deltoid ligament lies near the apex of the cone on which the surface of the ankle joint lies. It is thus able to accommodate to the relatively smaller distance the talus travels on this side of the joint.[92a,132,187]

Lateral Collateral Ligament

Because the lateral side of the joint has a greater radius of curvature, a larger distance is traveled on this side during the same arc of rotation. The lateral collateral ligament is thus more complex, being comprised of three portions.[185] The anterior part, the anterior talofibular ligament, lines up with the fibula during plantarflexion and in this position functions as a true collateral ligament, resisting inversion of the talus in the mortise. With dorsiflexion, the fibulocalcaneal ligament is brought into alignment with the fibula and becomes the functional collateral ligament. Inman[92a] demonstrated considerable variation (70° to 140°) in the relationship between these two portions of the lateral collateral complex (Fig. 52–13). He hypothesized that ankle inversion laxity may be present in those individuals with a relatively greater arc between the anterior talofibular and fibulocalcaneal ligaments, as a significant part of their ankle range of motion would be without an appropriately positioned lateral collateral ligament.

An important corollary of the relative positions of the components of the ankle's lateral collateral ligament complex is that assessment of stability must be done with regard to the position of the ankle joint. The anterior talofibular ligament resists inversion in plantarflexion. It also resists anterior subluxation of the talus when the ankle is in neutral, as demonstrated by

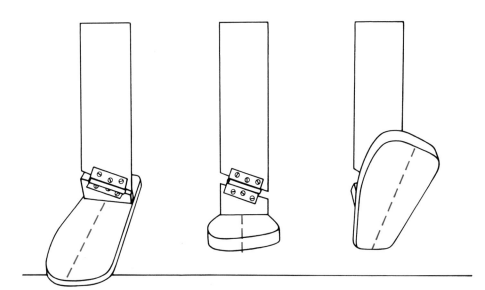

Figure 52–12

The obliquity of the ankle axis produces relative medial deviation (internal rotation) with plantarflexion, and relative lateral deviation of the foot (external rotation) with dorsiflexion. (Redrawn from Mann, R., ed. Surgery of the Foot, 5th ed. [Fig. 1–12]. St. Louis, 1986, The C.V. Mosby Co.)

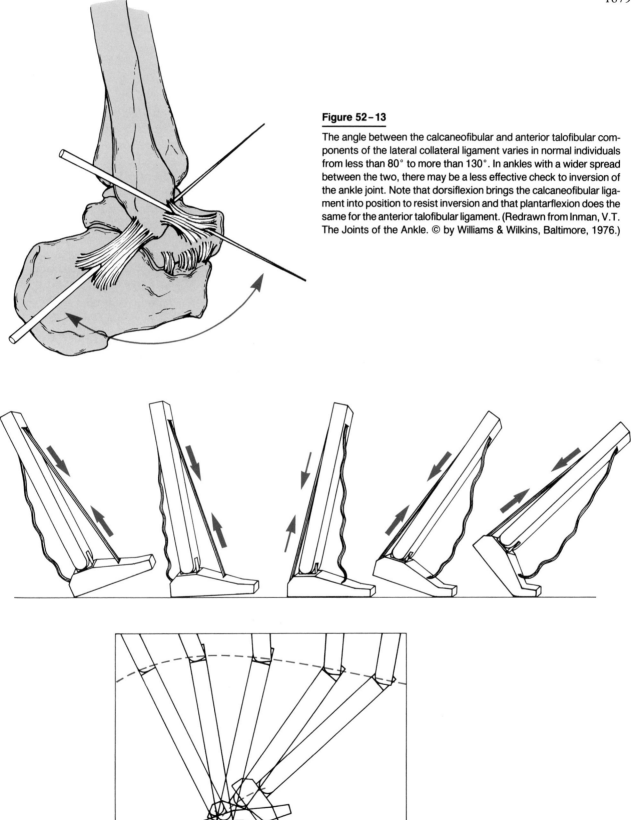

Figure 52–13

The angle between the calcaneofibular and anterior talofibular components of the lateral collateral ligament varies in normal individuals from less than 80° to more than 130°. In ankles with a wider spread between the two, there may be a less effective check to inversion of the ankle joint. Note that dorsiflexion brings the calcaneofibular ligament into position to resist inversion and that plantarflexion does the same for the anterior talofibular ligament. (Redrawn from Inman, V.T. The Joints of the Ankle. © by Williams & Wilkins, Baltimore, 1976.)

Figure 52–14

Ankle mechanics during gait. At heel strike, the dorsiflexors slow plantarflexion produced by the moment arm of the heel. Forward momentum of the body next produces ankle dorsiflexion. This is restrained by the plantarflexors, which stabilize the foot during terminal stance. (Redrawn from Inman, V.T., Ralston, H.J.,Todd, F. Human Walking Vol. 1, [Fig. 1–9]. © Williams & Wilkins, Baltimore, 1981.)

the so-called anterior drawer test. The fibulocalcaneal ligament resists inversion when the ankle is dorsiflexed. Because either or both components may be incompetent, an adequate examination requires testing inversion instability in both dorsiflexion and plantarflexion.

The relationship of the fibulocalcaneal ligament to the subtalar joint is important. Normally it lies on the conical plane of motion of this joint and thus does not interfere with it.[92a] If it is to be reconstructed surgically, deviation from its normal location may compromise subtalar joint movement.

Biomechanics of Gait

The ankle helps to smooth the vertical movement of the body's center of gravity and decrease the transient ground reaction force during forward progression.[132] This minimizes the energy cost of walking and the impact on the lower extremity. At heel strike, the ankle begins to plantarflex against the force of the anterior compartment muscles contracting eccentrically. As the leg accepts weight, foot pronation and knee flexion decelerate the body's fall. The plantarflexed ankle begins to dorsiflex. With further plantarflexion, the heel elevates and the foot supinates, thus becoming rigid and propelling the body upward and forward (Fig. 52–14). During this process the tibia rotates — internally during swing and externally during stance — about its long axis. Inman points out that because of the obliquity of the subtalar joint axis, internal and external rotation of the tibia are linked respectively to pronation and supination of the foot.[92a] It is important to remember that during stance phase the foot is fixed on the ground and becomes the fixed point of reference for movements of the leg and body.

Mann describes three intervals of stance phase.[132] In the first portion, from heel strike to foot flat, the initially slightly dorsiflexed ankle plantar flexes to approximately 18° and then begins to dorsiflex, reaching neutral by the end of this phase. The anterior tibial muscles contract throughout this phase, the foot progressively pronates through the subtalar joint, and internal rotation of the tibia continues.

In the second part, or foot flat period of stance, the ankle moves from neutral to approximately 18° of dorsiflexion, with heel rise beginning just before plantarflexion starts to end this phase. During the second phase, the plantarflexors of the superficial and deep posterior calf compartments are active, controlling the forward motion of the tibia on the talus (i.e., contracting eccentrically while the ankle dorsiflexes). Early in this phase, the internally rotated tibia begins to externally rotate, and the foot supinates, becoming more rigid, supported also by the intrinsic muscles of the foot.

In the third and final portion of stance phase, the ankle plantarflexes from its extreme of dorsiflexion to a little more than 10° plantarflexion, with continuing contraction of the posterior calf muscles. The tibia remains externally rotated and the foot supinated; the latter is made even more rigid by the windlass action of the dorsiflexed toes, tightening the plantar fascia and elevating the longitudinal arch of the foot.

Mann emphasizes that the ankle joint's oblique axis determines relative motion of the leg.[132] Heel strike and plantarflexion produce apparent in-toeing. In midstance, the ankle dorsiflexes as the tibia moves forward. This results in internal rotation of the leg. When the heel begins to rise and plantarflexion occurs, the tibia externally rotates. The amount of observed rotation of the leg is greater than that accounted for by ankle joint obliquity and is in fact accomplished through motion of the subtalar joint, which is also oblique.

Evaluation of the Injured Ankle

HISTORY

The major points to be gained from the history of a patient with an injured ankle are (1) how, when, and where the injury happened, (2) preexisting status of the injured part, and (3) overall medical condition of the individual.

The mechanism of injury is only occasionally presented in a way that provides definitive understanding of the direction and magnitude of applied force and a good clue to the diagnosis. ("I stepped on a pebble and my foot turned inward until I felt a pop on the outside of my ankle.") More often the actual details are more vague, but still helpful ("motorcycle crash"; "tripped and fell down the stairs"; "jumped off a deck and landed flat-footed"). The location is important in assessing the likely extent of contamination of an open wound. Elapsed time, correlated with the extent of swelling, helps assess the patient's suitability for certain types of surgery.

The status of the leg prior to the present injury is also important. This includes, for example, whether the part was normal, incompletely recovered from a prior injury, subject to recurrent instability or pain, or untrustworthy since a stroke. Symptoms to be sought are those suggestive of neurologic difficulty, especially peripheral neuropathy, most often caused by diabetes mellitus. Similarly critical is evidence of vascular disease, venous stasis ulcers, claudication, or chronic infection. Other factors include pain, deformity, or altered function affecting the ankle or any other part of the leg. Choice of treatment may be profoundly altered by these factors.

Systemic illness clearly has an impact on overall patient management and often on local treatment choice as well. An inveterate smoker may have a higher risk of wound and fracture healing problems. An alcoholic may not be able to cooperate with limited weight-bearing without external immobilization. A patient with limited cardiorespiratory disease may not be able to handle the energy cost of walking in a long-leg cast. A patient with injuries of the opposite leg that prevent weight-bearing will require different rehabilitation plans than a patient with an isolated pilon fracture. Information on medications, drug allergies, and familial problems must be obtained from the patient or from family members or friends.

PHYSICAL EXAMINATION

Physical examination of the injured ankle is conducted differently depending on the injury. A brief inspection may reveal severe deformity or an open wound. The challenge then is to identify all elements of the injury and to proceed rapidly with the treatment required to reduce a dislocation, relieve tension on overlying soft tissues, or decontaminate and appropriately treat an open wound. Some parts of the exam may not be possible to perform or may even be inappropriate until later in the patient's course. (For instance, an adequate distal motor exam may be unobtainable while a fracture-dislocation is markedly displaced. Any significant wound exploration should be deferred until the patient is in the operating room.)

On the other hand, if the patient complains of an ankle injury, but the problem is not obvious, it is necessary to carry out a systematic assessment of each structure in the region before an injury can be excluded or identified. Because injuries often occur in constellations but may coexist seemingly at random, it is especially important not to terminate the evaluation after the first positive finding on either physical examination or radiography.

The ankle should be inspected circumferentially for open or impending wounds; crushed, abraded or swollen areas; and bony deformity. Pallor may suggest ischemia. Any open wound, even a small one, may communicate with underlying crushed tissues, a fracture, or the ankle joint itself. It is vital to correlate the appearance of the wound with the patient's history. For example, a small opening in the skin of a patient whose ankle was run over by a car does *not* indicate a grade I open fracture. Is there apparent rotational deformity? A transverse, seemingly shallow, laceration along the lat-

eral surface of the ankle, just distal to the lateral malleolus, may be the result of rupture of the overlying skin with a severe inversion injury and complete failure of the lateral collateral ligaments. Such a laceration extends into the ankle joint.

The vascular exam must include palpation of the posterior tibial and dorsalis pedis pulses. Swelling or deformity may interfere with this. A Doppler device may help identify the pulses, but it reliably indicates good flow only if local arterial pressure is measured with a pneumatic cuff on the calf. Skin temperature, capillary filling after blanching pressure, venous engorgement, and edema should each be noted. A decision must be made about the adequacy of perfusion, both before and after any treatment, with measures taken to rapidly identify and correct the cause of ischemia.

The nerves that cross the ankle are assessed by testing light touch and pain sensation in each of their sensory areas. The sural nerve supplies the lateral heel and lateral border of the foot. The sole of the foot is innervated by the medial and lateral plantar nerves, branches of the tibial nerve, which also gives medial calcaneal branches. The plantar intrinsic muscles of the foot are supplied by this system but are hard to test because of the long motors of the toes. Pain produced in the sole of the foot by forced passive dorsiflexion of the toes may indicate ischemia of these muscles.

The medial border of the foot is innervated by the saphenous nerve. The dorsal web space between the great and second toes is the territory of the deep peroneal nerve. This nerve gives motor branches to the extensores breves on the dorsum of the foot. Their contraction can be palpated locally, if swelling is not excessive. The superficial peroneal nerve provides sensation for the majority of the dorsum of the foot.

Function of the tendons crossing the ankle may be difficult to assess but must be checked initially and then reviewed as a more thorough examination becomes possible. It is necessary to assess the strength generated, not just the apparent motion of the part.

The Achilles tendon is checked by palpation for tenderness or a defect and by means of Thompson's test, strong active plantarflexion of the ankle. In Thompson's test, plantarflexion is produced in response to the examiner's squeezing the calf of a relaxed (usually kneeling) individual (Fig. 52–15).

The peroneus longus and brevis lie behind the lateral malleolus and may be locally tender or palpably displaced if they have been dislocated from their superior retinaculum. The peroneals evert the foot and should be checked, if possible, before a cast is applied that prevents this maneuver.

The anterior compartment muscles dorsiflex the ankle and toes. Extension of both the hallux and the

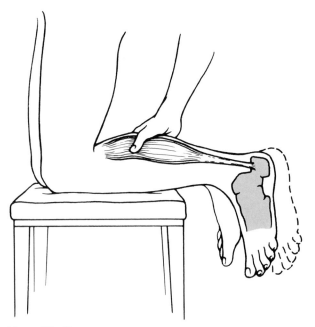

Figure 52-15

Compression of the calf muscles normally produces plantarflexion of the ankle. If the Achilles tendon is ruptured, this response is greatly diminished or absent.

lesser toes should be confirmed. A palpable contraction of the tibialis anterior is often present. This tendon rarely ruptures because of attrition, but may be tender and nonpalpable if this has occurred.

The deep posterior compartment muscles are the long flexors of the hallux and digitorum, as well as the tibialis posterior. This important support for the longitudinal arch of the foot may be injured along with other ankle structures and may also rupture on an attritional basis or in association with inflammatory arthritis. It inverts and plantarflexes the foot and should be palpable when performing these tasks. The toe flexors are tested by checking the strength of that activity. These tendons should be palpated for tenderness behind the medial malleolus, where dislocation from beneath the flexor retinaculum occurs occasionally.

It is essential to realize that ankle pain may be the complaint of a patient with a developing calf compartment syndrome.[8] Impaired distal motor and sensory function may be the early manifestation of such a problem, which should suggest a careful search for calf tenderness, induration, and stretch-induced pain within involved muscle groups. When in doubt, measurement of calf compartment pressures may be diagnostic.

Systematic palpation to localize tenderness is an important part of examining the less severely injured ankle. The cooperative patient with normal sensation

and no overbearing pain can often define the injured area quite precisely because of the superficial location of most of the ankle's structures.

Each of the traversing structures reviewed previously must be checked for tenderness. Each bony prominence should be assessed as well. Is a malleolus diffusely tender, or only where a ligament attaches to it? Is tenderness localized over one or more parts of the lateral collateral ligament, the nearby anterior syndesmosis, or the superficial deltoid ligament? The deep deltoid ligament is intraarticular, nonpalpable, and may be ruptured without much medial tenderness, a vital point to remember in assessing its integrity. The posterior syndesmotic ligaments are also buried more deeply and may be ruptured without well-localized tenderness. The entire fibula must be palpated, because routine radiographic exposures often will not demonstrate the occasional fracture of the upper fibula associated with disruption of the ankle joint (Maisonneuve fracture).

Examinations for range of motion and stability should be deferred if an obvious injury is present, based either on physical examination or on radiographs, which are often obtained prior to the orthopedist being asked to see a patient with an ankle injury. Otherwise, joint motion should be checked. Active and passive dorsiflexion and plantarflexion must be compared with those of the contralateral side, because of the wide range of normal values. The average is about 30° dorsiflexion and about 30° to 45° plantarflexion.[124a,210] In assessing the ankle's range of motion, it is important to recognize that a surprising amount of dorsiflexion and plantarflexion occurs in the tarsal and tarsometatarsal joints. A better estimate of true ankle motion is obtained, as Segal suggested, by measuring the angle between the tibia and the weight-bearing surface of the foot while the patient dorsiflexes maximally. The angle between the plantar surface of the heel (only) and the tibia is the measure of plantarflexion.[210]

Inversion and eversion are intimately associated with ankle motion and should be assessed as well. They normally occur at the subtalar joint, although an ankle with lateral collateral ligament insufficiency may invert at the tibiotalar joint as well. Inversion stress radiographs are necessary to distinguish this and are thus required if excessive inversion is noted on exam or a history of recurrent inversion injuries is obtained. Anterior displacement of the foot relative to the tibia can be produced by performing an "anterior drawer" test (Fig. 52-16). This implies laxity of the anterior fibulotalar component of the lateral collateral complex. It may be easier to perform with the patient prone.[78]

Instability of the mortise, with laxity or rupture of the syndesmotic ligaments, is suggested by sideways move-

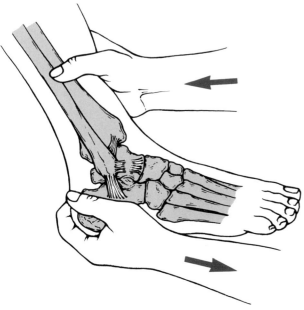

Figure 52-16

Anterior displacement of the foot relative to the tibia by the so-called "anterior drawer test" indicates insufficiency of the anterior talofibular ligament. This should be compared with the opposite side and may be quantified radiographically.

ment of the talus within the mortise. This may produce pain and may also be associated with a sensation of the talus moving laterally or clicking back against the medial malleolus after having been subtly displaced away from it. A stress view mortise radiograph may be helpful in confirming this finding. The tibia is rotated internally to bring the malleoli into a plane parallel with the film. The talus is then pulled laterally or externally rotated and is held in this position while the radiograph is exposed. A control view of the other side may be helpful. Remember that even a 1-mm lateral shift of the talus significantly decreases ankle joint contact area.[183a]

It is important to check other regional structures that might be injured in association with the ankle or that might lead the patient to complain of ankle symptoms, in spite of that region not being directly involved. In particular, fractures of the anterior process of the calcaneus, the lateral process of the talus, or the base of the fifth metatarsal may be missed, as might a fracture elsewhere in the calcaneus or talus, a fracture of the navicular, or osteoligamentous injuries of the midfoot, (e.g., a tarsometatarsal dislocation) (see chapter 53).[103] Any findings suggesting foot abnormalities should lead to a request for additional radiographic projections of the foot, as routine ankle radiographs poorly demonstrate foot abnormalities.

RADIOGRAPHIC IMAGING

Routine studies for the ankle include anteroposterior (AP), lateral, and internally rotated mortise views.[47,68,153,154] If proximal tenderness has been noted, full-length views of the fibula are essential, as are all other radiographs necessary to evaluate symptoms and signs of other potential injuries proximal to the ankle. The same holds true, as just noted, for radiographs of the foot.

Additional radiographic studies of the ankle may include one or more of several views. Forty-five-degree oblique radiographs can help identify and assess articular involvement and anatomic details of fractures affecting the distal tibial metaphysis. Weight-bearing views of the ankle demonstrate the thickness of articular cartilage as well as joint congruity during loading. They are a valuable part of follow-up evaluations after ankle fractures (Fig. 52-17). Stress views are the basis for confirming ligamentous instability. Comparison with the opposite ankle is helpful, but symmetric laxity is not reliably present in normal individuals. Furthermore, in normal ankles the range of inversion laxity varies considerably.[192,199a] Therefore judgment must be used in interpreting stress radiographs. In general they are not indicated for assessment of an acute ligamentous injury, but can be helpful in planning the appropriate management of a chronically unstable ankle.

For assessment of the lateral collateral ligament complex, an anterior drawer lateral view is obtained with the foot supported by a pad under the heel and a posteriorly directed force applied to the distal tibia. Brostrom claims that as little as 3-mm anterior talar displacement indicates rupture of the anterior fibulotalar ligament.[31]

Inversion instability of the tibiotalar joint is demonstrated by inversion stress radiographs.[47,89,192,242] These are perhaps most consistently obtained with specific positioning and loading jigs, but the clinical value of such devices has not been established. As noted in the section on biomechanics, an inversion stress radiograph in plantarflexion demonstrates the competence of the anterior fibulotalar ligament, and one in dorsiflexion demonstrates the fibulocalcaneal ligament. Gross instability (more than 25° talar inversion) in neutral strongly suggests incompetence of both the anterior and middle portions of the lateral collateral complex. Inversion instability may also be caused by excessive laxity of the subtalar joint. This may be demonstrable with appropriate stress radiographs.[28,259]

Ankle arthrograms and peroneal tenograms have been advocated for assessment of collateral ligament integrity.[242] Leakage of dye will occur when there is a complete tear of the joint capsule, such as produced by

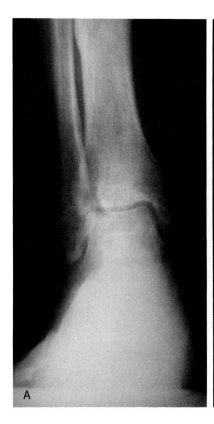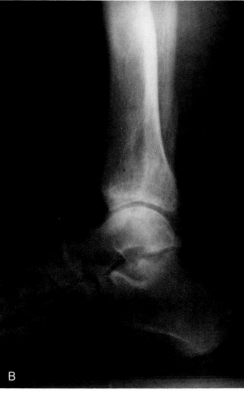

Figure 52–17

Weight-bearing radiographs demonstrate the true thickness of the articular cartilage and the congruence of the loaded ankle joint, AP *(A)* and lateral *(B)* views.

a lateral collateral ligament rupture.[23] This can also produce an abnormal communication between the ankle joint and the peroneal tendon sheath, which lies immediately superficial to the fibulocalcaneal ligament. With the present trend toward functional management of lateral collateral ligament injuries, clinical justification for confirming a complete lateral collateral ligament rupture is lacking, and these studies are rarely indicated unless some special indication exists for surgical repair.[54]

Standard tomography (laminagrams) in AP and lateral projections may be helpful in documenting articular surface deformity, fracture comminution, and osteochondral lesions of the talus (Fig. 52–18).[34]

Computed tomography (CT), especially if carefully done with thin sections and maintenance of patient positioning, can be even more informative, as it provides a cross section of the joint that clarifies the relationship of the fibula to the tibia, as well as the fit of the talus within the mortise and the status of soft tissue structures.[196–198] Precise measurements are readily obtainable. The extent and location of articular surface involvement are obvious, and planning of surgical approaches is facilitated. Computer reconstructions in sagittal and coronal planes currently provide essentially as much information as standard tomography, which does not offer the cross-sectional view (Fig. 52–

19). Although CT scans are rarely needed for evaluation and treatment of routine malleolar injuries, they are very helpful when there is significant plafond involvement.[129,153,154] If a CT scan is desired after an ankle has been externally fixed, replacement of the metal connecting rods with radiolucent carbon-fiber composite rods makes it possible to obtain high-quality CT studies. CT cuts through the ankle region can be made transversely, parallel to the tibiotalar articular surface, or coronally, nearly perpendicular to the injury, by flexing the knee and tilting the CT gantry. The first are best for assessment of the mortise and pilon region. The last are now standard for calcaneal fractures and subtalar joint visualization. CT studies may also aid the evaluation of patients with chronic pain after inversion injuries.[150]

Magnetic resonance imaging (MRI) can be valuable for assessing some ankle region injuries, especially occult tendon ruptures and articular surface disruptions (Fig. 52–18F).[48,195,201,258]

Bone scanning with technetium 99m diphosphonate or an equivalent agent can be helpful in localizing stress or other occult fractures, infections, and neoplastic lesions.[34,139,143,175]

Ankle arthroscopy via anteromedial, anterolateral, or posterolateral portals may be helpful for diagnosing and occasionally treating osteophytes, loose bodies, os-

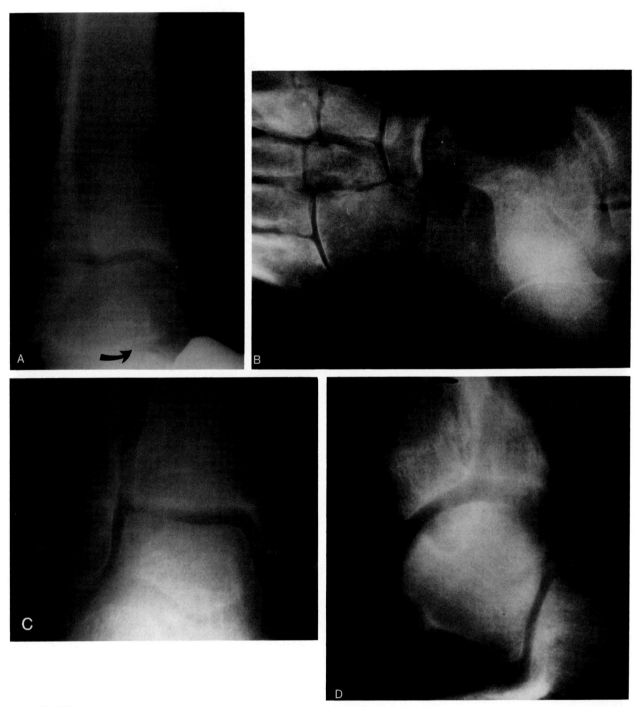

Figure 52–18

Painful episodes of giving way developed nine months after ankle and tibia fractures sustained in a fall from a scaffold. Weight-bearing radiographs are shown in Figure 52–17. *A*, No instability is evident on an inversion stress radiograph. *B*, An oblique radiograph of the foot shows no abnormality of the anterior process of the calcaneus. *C*, A repeated plain film taken 2½ months later suggests a defect in the lateral talar dome. *D*, Lateral tomogram reveals a cystic lesion of the talar dome.

Illustration and legend continued on following page

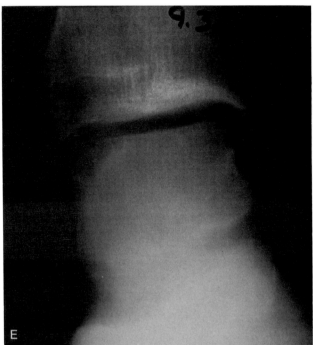

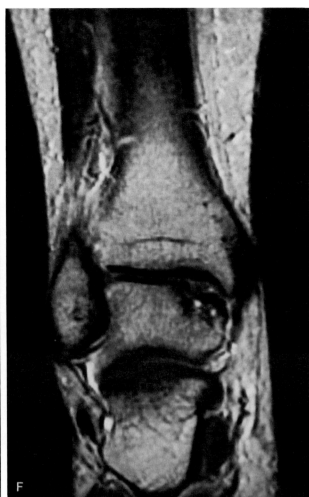

Figure 52–18 *Continued*

E, AP tomogram further localizes the lesion. This underlay a typical small osteochondral fracture, which responded to excision and drilling of the defect. *F*, MRI coronal view of *another patient* clearly shows an osteochondral lesion of the talar dome.

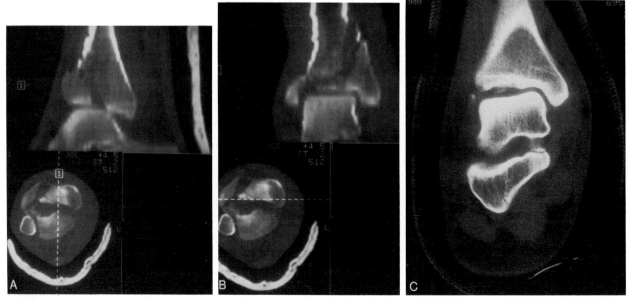

Figure 52–19

Computed tomography of the ankle provides helpful detailed views of the pathologic anatomy of ankle injuries. *A* and *B* show a transverse CT scan with sagittal and coronal plane reconstructions. *C*, Coronal plane computed tomogram of *another patient* showing impaction of the anterior lateral margin of the distal tibia.

teochondral fractures, ligamentous laxity, and synovitis.[126,127,173,182] Smaller arthroscopes are helpful; the technology continues to develop. Some means of ankle distraction aids entry and visualization.[239] Arthroscopy is presently of greatest value for assessing ankles that remain painful after injury, often because of anterolateral soft tissue impingement or osteochondritis dissecans.[59,83,137,174]

Table 52–1.
Injuries of the Ankle Region

Bone injuries (fractures)
  Malleolar
  Metaphyseal — split
  Metaphyseal — impacted
  Ligamentous avulsion
  Joint capsule avulsion
  Other nearby fractures
    Base of fifth metatarsal
    Lateral process of talus
    Anterior process of calcaneus
    Tarsometatarsal complex
    Many other possibilities

Articular surface injuries
  Fractures, as above, with articular involvement
  Osteochondral fractures (predominantly talus)

Ligament injuries
  Lateral collateral complex injuries
  Syndesmosis injuries
  Medial collateral injuries
  Injuries to other nearby ligaments
    Subtalar
    Tarsometatarsal
    Midtarsal

Soft tissue envelope injuries
  Laceration
  Contusion extending to crush injury
  Avulsion/degloving
  Foreign body retention
  Edema
  Preexisting compromise

Tendon injuries
  Intrinsic injury
    Rupture
    Laceration
  Retinacular injury
    Rupture; tendon dislocation

Nerve injuries
  Laceration
  Contusion
  Entrapment

Vascular injuries
  Arterial
  Venous

OTHER STUDIES

Arteriography, noninvasive vascular studies, and pulse oximetry can be helpful for assessing and monitoring perfusion distal to an injured ankle. Compartment pressures may need to be measured in the leg or foot. Nerve conduction velocities and electromyography (EMG) may be helpful for assessing lesions of the tibial nerve, such as tarsal tunnel syndrome.

ESSENTIAL STUDIES TO EXCLUDE OTHER INJURIES

A careful history and physical examination are the basis for identifying all of a trauma patient's injuries. Assessment (and documentation) of peripheral pulses is essential to avoid missing limb-threatening ischemia. If the patient is not conscious or is not able to cooperate, then routine radiographs of the pelvis and spine are essential. An ankle fracture may be the only outward sign of a fall from a height or a high-velocity motor vehicle crash. Inspection, palpation, and assessment of range of motion and stability of the lower extremity proximal to the ankle are essential. Radiographs up to and including the pelvis should be obtained, unless the physical exam is completely normal.

DIFFERENTIAL DIAGNOSIS

It is wise to modify the traditional concept of differential diagnosis when dealing with trauma, especially in the ankle region. Rather than thinking in terms of a list of potential diagnoses to be excluded one by one, the surgeon must remain constantly aware of the likelihood of more than one lesion.[70,114,158,163,249] Remember that ankle pain may be the complaint of a patient with a leg compartment syndrome, proximal neurovascular compromise, or a foot injury. Table 52–1 is a list of various injuries that can affect the structures of the ankle.

Management of Ankle Fractures

GENERAL PRINCIPLES

Adequate assessment and treatment of the entire patient and the entire injured limb generally have a higher priority than assessment and treatment of the ankle (see chapter 5). However, significant permanent disability, including amputation, can be prevented by adequate care of an ankle injury. After life- and limb-saving measures are under way, the ankle injury must not be neglected. Priorities for the ankle itself include both diagnosis and treatment, in the following order: (1)

assurance of adequate blood flow; (2) provisional reduction of marked deformity or dislocation; (3) care of any open wound or other injury to the skin and soft tissue envelope; (4) precise reduction of skeletal deformity, which must be maintained through healing; (5) repair of tendons and nerves; (6) rehabilitation; and (7) identification and treatment of any complications that develop.

Without adequate perfusion, the foot will not survive. Therefore it is crucial to recognize ischemia. Except in the case of a mangled foot and ankle, it is unusual for an ankle-level arterial injury to be limb-threatening, probably because three arteries cross the region. Thus if the foot is ischemic, one must look for a more proximal arterial lesion. Some injuries are unsalvageable, or an attempt at salvage may pose too much of a threat to the patient. For such patients an early amputation is the best treatment. This topic is discussed in further detail in chapter 51. An exceptional patient with an injury that is more of a laceration than a crush may be a candidate for local microvascular reconstruction or even replantation of a traumatic incomplete or complete amputation.

Marked deformity, usually resulting from a dislocation, fracture-dislocation, or severely displaced fracture, poses a threat to the local perfusion of skin stretched over bony prominences. It promotes local swelling and may also interfere with distal blood circulation. In addition it is often quite painful and may produce repeated injury to articular cartilage rubbing against a sharp bony edge. Therefore provisional reduction to improve local perfusion and prevent further injury is urgent. Application of a very well padded splint should follow. Although not always successful, an attempted manipulation in the emergency department often yields at least some improvement and is an appropriate part of applying a splint. It is better to return exposed and contaminated bone to the wound than to splint it in a position of excessive deformity. Because urgent operative wound care must soon follow, the benefits of correcting deformity outweigh the theoretical risks of introducing additional contamination into an already dirty wound.

Care of the soft tissues, including any open wound, is a vital element in the management of an injured ankle. There is a surprising spectrum of both open and closed soft tissue injuries.[241] Some low-energy ankle injuries have so little soft tissue damage that it may be ignored. There is little swelling, and surgery, if indicated, can be carried out safely any time after the injury. These injuries may lull the surgeon into thinking that all ankle injuries can be similarly treated. A high-energy injury with extensive displacement of comminuted, impacted, and transverse fractures may not exhibit much

swelling during the first few hours, especially if the patient is in shock. However, such fractures are accompanied by a high degree of soft tissue trauma, even if there is no open wound, and have a very low tolerance for extensive surgical approaches. Although all operations on ankle fractures must be done as atraumatically as possible, such severe crushing injuries should be approached with trepidation, if at all.[27,53,234,236] Certainly if there is evidence of soft tissue compromise — marked swelling, blistering, abrasions, or early eschar formation — whatever the fracture pattern, the surgeon must consider external fixation and should be willing to delay open reduction for several weeks if necessary until the soft tissues recover.

Open wounds involving fractures and dislocations of the ankle must be recognized as *additional* soft tissue damage, and not, by themselves, as the entire extent of injury.[43,241] Each such open wound should be treated as any open fracture, with sterile dressing, splint, tetanus prophylaxis, and urgent intravenous antibiotics (generally a first-generation cephalosporin for less severe wounds, with an aminoglycoside or substitution of a third-generation cephalosporin for those that are more severe). In addition to these adjuncts, prompt surgical debridement and irrigation in an operating room is the key step in minimizing the risk of serious infection. If a fracture is present, immediate fixation with appropriate techniques offers better results.[20,30,65,74,231,252] With less severe injuries, fixation techniques are essentially the same as for closed injuries. For more severe injuries, it may be appropriate to minimize the extent of surgical exposure and to employ external fixation to immobilize both the foot and ankle. In either case, the original open wound is left open for delayed closure.

Articular fractures of the ankle have the best prognosis when they heal in an alignment as close as possible to their original anatomy. It is generally accepted that the quality of the reduction is more important than whether it was achieved with an open or closed technique. With this recognition and with the development of internal fixation methods that reliably maintain the tibiotalar relationship, open treatment of malleolar fractures has become more popular. When AO principles and techniques are properly applied to malleolar fractures, good results can be obtained in up to 90% of external rotation-abduction malleolar fractures.[51a,91,124] Other fixation techniques have their proponents, but they are now less widely favored, at least in North America.[1,2,26,36,86,145,169] As Olerud and Molander have shown, less rigid fixation with wires, pins, or staples works well for more stable unilateral injuries, but when there is involvement of both sides of the ankle, reduction is more likely to be lost.[169]

Anatomic reduction and stable fixation may also

benefit the patient with a fracture involving the tibial pilon, but complications can be significant, especially in those injuries with extensive crushing of bone and soft tissue.[27,53,213,234] For these very severe injuries, an acceptable overall realignment of ankle and foot can often be achieved with external fixation. Through a minimal exposure, articular surface congruity may be restored acutely, especially during treatment of an open wound. Alternatively, with external fixation of a severe closed ankle injury, open reduction and internal fixation, often with bone grafting, can be deferred until the soft tissues have optimally recovered.

Fractures of the ankle vary widely in severity. Their effect on ankle stability and on the articular surface may range from minimal to profound. Treatment of the fracture itself will depend on its location, size, displacement, and effects on joint stability. Opinions and recommendations for management of ankle fractures range equally widely, from nonoperative management to anatomic repair of every fragment. Clearly the treating surgeon must make a decision based on the reported results of injuries and treatment, the patient's injury and other characteristics, and his or her own personal experience and expertise. Stable restoration of normal anatomy in the safest and most reliable way ought to be the basic guideline for treatment of articular fractures about the ankle.[36,37,79,236]

If any tendon injury accompanies or is the major component of ankle trauma, its surgical repair must be considered.[62] In some patients, closed nonoperative treatment of a ruptured Achilles tendon may be appropriate. Unless repaired early, failure of the posterior tibial tendon usually results in a symptomatic flat foot deformity.[132] Lacerations or ruptures of other tendons may also prove less disabling if they are repaired. Therefore such tendon injuries will often require surgical treatment, but only if there is an open wound will such treatment be urgent.

The most disabling nerve injury of the ankle region is loss of the tibial nerve, which provides sensation for the sole of the foot. Some have advocated amputation when adults sustain this injury along with an otherwise treatable arterial injury, because of the high risk of neurotrophic ulcers and their complications.[114a] Such problems are more common when the foot and ankle are stiff and deformed and do not necessarily accompany absence of plantar sensation. If nerve continuity is present, functional recovery may occur, even after many months. A temporary but prolonged period of dysesthesia may accompany recovery of tibial nerve function, either spontaneously or after repair. It may also persist after an injury to the nerve and may respond to nerve repair. Experience with treatment of lower extremity nerve injuries is rare. Sedel recom-

mends that microsurgical repair be considered for complete lesions of the major lower extremity nerves.[209] Seddon, reviewing a large number of patients, few of whom were treated surgically, recommended against nerve repair but emphasized the good functional result that can be obtained, even with a complete tibial nerve palsy.[40,209a]

Injuries of the other nerves crossing the ankle can become painful because of neuromas that are caught in the scar. This problem may be prevented by transecting the injured nerve and burying it deeply in soft tissue away from scar and moving structures.

The ankle's ligaments are frequently damaged. The syndesmosis (distal tibiofibular ligaments) may be disrupted in association with a fibular fracture. If it is unstable after the associated fracture has been repaired, surgical fixation of the syndesmosis is the safest way of ensuring healing with stability in the correct position. This may not be required, especially if the AITFL or PITFL has caused an avulsion fracture that permits stable repair of the ligament's attachment. Assessment of the stability of the tibiofibular relationship (as discussed later) is an essential part of the operative treatment of any malleolar injury with a fibular fracture above the level of the plafond.

Acute surgical repair of the completely ruptured lateral collateral ligament complex has been advocated by a number of authors.[31,57] Although this may improve apparent stability, it does not seem to provide a better result than functional treatment, which has now become the more favored approach, even for vigorous athletes.[56,224] Should late instability occur, delayed repair is as successful as primary suture, but it is not frequently required after adequate functional management and rehabilitation.[35,117]

The medial collateral ligament is rarely injured without a malleolar fracture. In such cases, deltoid ligament failure is often the equivalent of a medial malleolar fracture, and unless the talus is visibly displaced when radiographs are taken, the injury may be overlooked. Its repair has been advocated for unstable malleolar injuries, but this does not effectively stabilize the talus and is unnecessary if the lateral malleolus has been restored securely to its anatomic location.[2,11,51a,81,254] Isolated late insufficiency of the deltoid ligament is practically unheard of in spite of nonoperative treatment, so skepticism about the need for primary repair of ruptured deltoid ligaments seems warranted.

Rehabilitation of ankle injuries emphasizes maintenance of a neutral functional position, protection of the injured area from excessive forces, restoration of motion, and progressive resumption of weight bearing as soon as possible. Many different approaches and recommendations exist. Whether one is better than another remains questionable.[1,211] The surgeon who has managed the entire treatment of a patient with an ankle fracture and knows the quality of bone and fixation is best equipped to manage the rehabilitation phase, as this information is not as readily available to therapists and other personnel. Finally, restoration of strength, endurance, and agility are necessary before a patient completes his or her recovery.

Complications that may develop during care of ankle injuries are discussed later. Especially important to avoid or recognize are infection, skin slough, malalignment, loss of fixation, nonunion, and reflex sympathetic dystrophy with its variants.[37,213,236a,252a] Infection after open injury or surgical treatment may be occult and may involve the ankle joint itself. Diagnosis relies on a high index of suspicion and aspiration of the joint for Gram's stain, cell count, culture, and sensitivity procedures. Wound exploration in the operating room may also be required. Skin sloughs, unless very small, will often require plastic surgical repair, usually with a free flap in this region, which has limited local soft tissue. Malalignment can be identified with adequate intraoperative radiographs. Patients being treated with cast immobilization require regular follow-up radiographs with strict assessment according to standard criteria for reduction. Fixation loss can be prevented by good technique and appropriate postoperative management. If it should occur, reoperation is usually indicated. Nonunions, if symptomatic, generally need open reduction and bone grafting, especially if malaligned. The evaluation and treatment of reflex sympathetic dystrophy is considered in chapter 19. Even after apparently satisfactory fracture healing with an anatomic reduction, minor degrees of arthrosis are common, and 25% to 30% of patients have at least some degree of subjective complaints.[17]

SPECIAL CONSIDERATIONS FOR POLYTRAUMA PATIENTS

As noted previously, most other injuries take precedence over definitive treatment of the ankle. Evaluation with as much history as possible, a brief physical exam, and application of a well-padded splint with provisional reduction of dislocation or gross deformity may be all that can be done for some time. Adequate radiographs are necessary for definitive diagnosis and treatment. If life- or limb-threatening injuries require urgent attention, radiographs of the ankle should be deferred until the earliest appropriate time and can certainly be obtained in the operating room. Although operative treatment of an open wound should be accomplished as soon as possible, fracture fixation may need to be deferred for some time. If soft tissue injury is

severe or if a distraction force is needed to maintain reduction, an external fixator including the tibia, calcaneus, and metatarsals is advisable and can be applied rapidly. This maintains a neutral foot position, provides access to soft tissue wounds, and permits suspension and continuous elevation of the injured limb. For less severe injuries, a plaster cast or splint will maintain a provisional reduction and allow the patient to be mobilized in bed and chair while maintaining as much elevation as possible of the injured leg. It is important to use a lot of padding, especially posterior to the heel. If the injury is rotationally unstable, a short extension onto the thigh with the knee moderately flexed improves the effectiveness of such a cast or splint. It is important to gain the best possible provisional reduction and immobilization, for the multiply injured patient may not be able to return to the operating room as soon as initially planned for definitive care of the ankle. Marked displacement may cause further damage to the soft tissues. Ankle injuries for which operative treatment is optimal can often have this deferred for up to a week or two without significantly compromising the ultimate result, if the patient's overall condition makes this advisable and if adequate interim management is provided for the ankle.

DEFINITIVE TREATMENT

Malleolar Fractures

Malleolar injuries are the most common significant lower extremity fracture.[50] Thus most orthopedic surgeons are frequently called on to treat them. Understanding and philosophy of management of these injuries have changed significantly since the 1970s. Current approaches appear to produce better results with fewer problems and more rapid rehabilitation. However, some controversies remain, and complications still occur.

Malleolar fractures primarily involve the lateral or medial malleolus and often other parts of the ankle as well. They are produced indirectly by shearing and tensile forces applied through the talus. Most malleolar fractures occur when the foot, including the talus, is fixed on the ground by the body's weight. A relative bending moment is produced with rotation either in the coronal plane, so that the talus either adducts or abducts relative to the tibia, or in the transverse plane, so that there is relative internal rotation of the tibia on the talus. Conventionally a skeletal deformity is usually described in terms of displacement of the distal part. Therefore, these injuries are referred to as "external rotation" injuries.[123] These mechanisms of injury produce characteristic fracture patterns that can be classified in terms of severity and stability based on the sequence of failure observed in cadaver experiments. It is important to recognize that exceptions do occur and that a given injury pattern may have an atypical mechanism or more than one possible cause. It is also likely that more than a single force vector was acting during the injury. This may result in variable impaction of the weight-bearing plafond, if the joint was loaded when the injury occurred. This in fact seems to be a major element in the production of large posterior lip fractures, anterior lip fractures, and those transitional malleolar injuries that have significant associated metaphyseal components.

Classification

Hamilton has thoroughly and lucidly discussed malleolar fractures in his text *Traumatic Disorders of the Ankle*.[79] A number of other helpful summaries are also available.[49,79,236,247,251,251a,251b,252a] This section reviews the pathophysiologic findings of Lauge-Hansen and others to provide an understanding of injury patterns as related to mechanism. It then offers the Danis-Weber (AO) classification as a practical clinical scheme and uses it as the basis for discussing treatment of malleolar fractures.[123] As will become evident, the details of treatment depend more on the actual anatomy of a

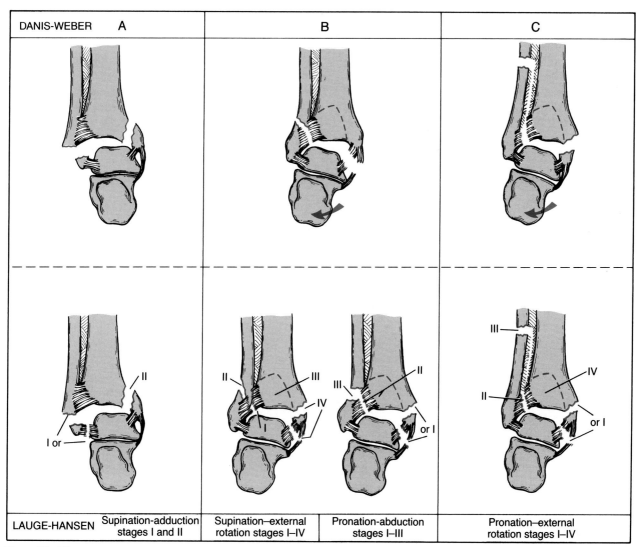

Figure 52-20

Correlation of the Danis-Weber (AO/ASIF) and Lauge-Hansen classification systems for malleolar fractures. The Danis-Weber system is based on the level of the fibular fracture, and the Lauge-Hansen system is based on experimentally verified injury mechanisms. Type B injuries can be produced by two mechanisms; suppination–external rotation or pronation-abduction. See text.

bone and ligament injury than on its classification according to any system. The more thoroughly the surgeon understands the fracture anatomy, the better he or she can plan and carry out effective treatment.

It is important to clarify Lauge-Hansen's terminology before considering his experiments and classification. His names for fracture types refer to how he caused them in experiments with cadaver legs that were secured proximally while he manipulated the foot. The first part of the name is the position of the foot — either supination or pronation. The second part of the name indicates the force that was applied to cause the observed injury — external rotation, abduction, or adduction. Unfortunately, Lauge-Hansen used the word "eversion" to mean external rotation and thus magnified the complexity of his terminology.[118,119] Figure 52–20 illustrates the Lauge-Hansen malleolar fracture classification and the corresponding Danis-Weber categories.

Supination-Adduction. Adducting the supinated (inverted) foot, usually from unanticipated weight bearing on the lateral border, is the most common mechanism

of injury to the ankle. Failure occurs first on the lateral side, which is under tension, and is usually limited to the lateral collateral ligament, which may be avulsed with a portion of the distal fibula. This mechanism thus produces the typical inversion sprain. Avulsion fractures are recognizable as characteristically transverse, perpendicular to the applied force. Such fractures of the lateral malleolus are distal to the plafond and are the hallmark of the type A injury of Danis and Weber. The second stage of this injury, produced by continued adduction of the supinated foot, is a shearing, medially displaced fracture of the medial malleolus, which is pushed medially by the talus. This causes a vertical fracture line that is distinct from the horizontal failure produced by tensile loading. This mechanism accounts for 10% to 20% of malleolar fractures (Fig. 52–21).[79]

The characteristic vertical appearance of the medial malleolar fracture reveals the injury mechanism, even if the lateral failure is purely ligamentous. It is important to note that an undisplaced or minimally displaced medial malleolus fracture may be produced by this mechanism without lateral failure if sufficient preexist-

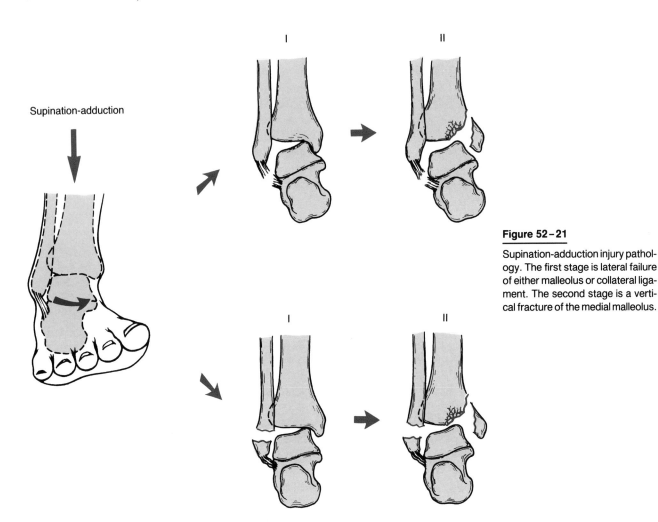

Supination-adduction

I   II   I   II

Figure 52–21

Supination-adduction injury pathology. The first stage is lateral failure of either malleolus or collateral ligament. The second stage is a vertical fracture of the medial malleolus.

ing lateral laxity is present. Because of the compressive forces applied medially, supination-adduction may produce impaction of the medial plafond in addition to the medial malleolus fracture (Fig. 52–22).

Oblique fractures of the medial malleolus are not often differentiated from vertical ones. Giachino and Hammond point out that they should be, because of their mechanism involving dorsiflexion as well as abduction and external rotation, which also produces a frequently occult, impacted anterolateral tibial plafond fracture.[67a] These oblique medial malleolus fractures are avulsion injuries rather than impacted ones and therefore are unstable in tension and better suited to internal fixation.

Supination–External Rotation. External rotation of the supinated foot produces a very common fracture pattern and is the cause of 40% to 75% of malleolar fractures.[79] The pattern is a spiral oblique fracture of the lateral malleolus, beginning at the level of the tibia plafond and extending a variable distance proximally (Fig. 52–23). The plane of this injury is predominantly

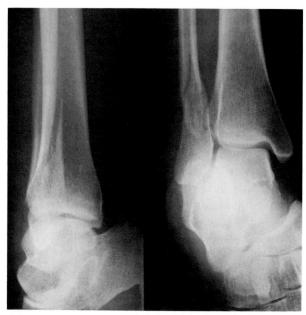

Figure 52–23

A slightly displaced supination–external rotation fracture of the lateral malleolus shows the typical pattern of fibular fractures caused by this mechanism. The overall plane of the fracture is oblique, from low anteriorly to high posteriorly, so that displacement is more evident on the lateral than on the AP view.

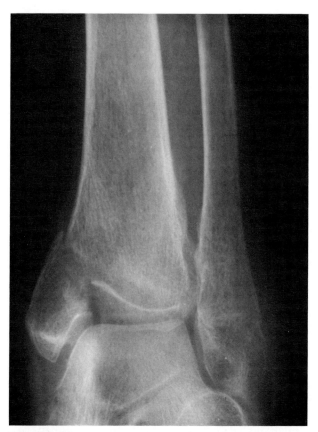

Figure 52–22

A supination-adduction, stage II fracture with significant impaction of the medial tibial plafond. The type A lateral malleolus fracture is undisplaced on this radiograph but was unstable to examination during surgery.

frontal, so it is typically more evident on the lateral than the AP or mortise radiograph, unless there is significant displacement. This characteristic fracture of the fibula is one of the two seen in the Danis-Weber type B injury, into which category it falls by virtue of its origin at the level of the tibial plafond. The mechanism of the fibular fracture is a rotational shearing force produced by pressure on the fibula by the talus while the tibia internally rotates, usually because of the body falling to the opposite side.[134]

Lauge-Hansen demonstrated that during external rotation injuries, failure of structures around the ankle occurs sequentially in a characteristic order. In supination–external rotation injuries, the first to fail is the AITFL, followed by the fibula, then the PITFL, and then the medial side of the ankle mortise, where tensile failure may produce either a rupture of the deltoid ligament or a transverse avulsion fracture of the medial malleolus (Fig. 52–24). Knowledge of the several components and sequence of injury brings some order to an otherwise chaotic collection of bone and ligament injuries. This can help the surgeon identify an occult ligamentous injury or guide treatment.

Note that in supination–external rotation injuries the fibular fracture is at or just above the level of the plafond, so that even with failure of the anteroinferior and posteroinferior tibiofibular ligaments, the more

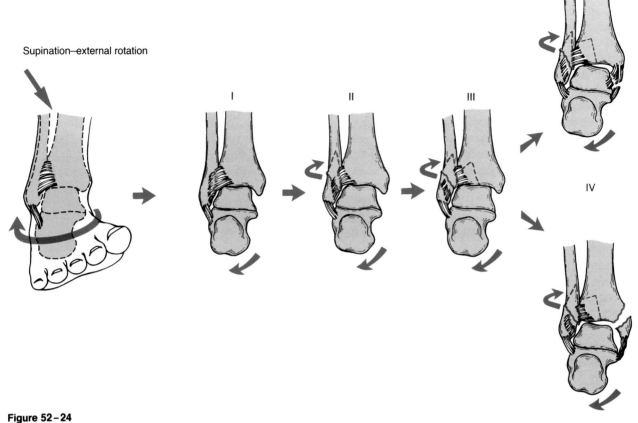

Supination–external rotation

Figure 52–24

Supination–external rotation injury pathology. The first stage is failure of the AITFL. The second stage is a spiral lateral malleolar fracture at the level of the plafond. The third stage is PITFL failure. The fourth stage is medial failure of either malleolus or the deltoid ligament.

proximal syndesmotic components stabilize the fibular shaft. Thus open reduction and internal fixation (ORIF) of the fibular fracture should restore the proper relationship of the lateral malleolus to the distal tibia. Stability is not guaranteed, however, because it depends on the soft tissues. It must be confirmed for each patient at operation.

Although the general pattern of each type of malleolar fracture is usually consistent, a moderate amount of variation is seen. Thus the supination–external rotation injury can be identified by its typical fibular fracture pattern. If explored surgically, the anteroinferior tibiofibular ligament disruption is obvious. The disruption may be through the substance of the ligament, by avulsion of a bone fragment from Chaput's tubercle on the tibia, or by avulsion of its fibular attachment, called Wagstaffe's (Le Fort's) tubercle. This ligament can guide reduction of the normal tibiofibular relationship, and its repair may aid in the secure healing of the syndesmosis. Although most supination–external rotation fibular fractures are at the level of the ankle joint, the same pattern, from the same mechanism, is occasionally seen at a higher level.[171]

The PITFL is next in order of failure. Because of its location, it is not as often exposed during surgical treatment of malleolar fractures. It may fail in substance or by avulsion of its tibial attachment, often as a small, extraarticular "posterior malleolar" fragment, but occasionally as a large, intraarticular one. These posterolateral tibial tubercular avulsion fractures are sometimes referred to as Volkmann's fragments.

The medial and final component of the supination–external rotation injury may be either a fracture of the medial malleolus or a rupture of the deltoid ligament.[98] Rarely, a hybrid lesion is seen, with fracture of the anterior colliculus representing superficial deltoid failure and rupture of the fibers of the deep deltoid, while the posterior colliculus remains intact.[216]

The surgeon must remember that an ankle with a radiologically apparent supination–external rotation fracture of the lateral malleolus may have a completely unstable stage IV injury, with the deltoid ligament ruptured medially, or a stable stage II injury, with an intact posterior syndesmosis and medial complex. Lateral talar shift, a posterior lip fragment, and significant displacement of the fibular fracture are all evidence for more than a stage II injury. Differential diagnosis is important, because true stage II injuries do well with nonoperative weight-bearing treatment, even though some potential lateral mobility of the talus is present.[16,36,89,112] However, if the injury is an unrecognized stage IV, then talar subluxation, malunion, and arthrosis are potential sequelae that are preventable with surgery. Certainly, follow-up radiographs are an important part of the nonoperative management of stage II supination–external rotation injuries for early identification of the lateral malleolus fracture with an unrecognized deltoid ligament disruption.

Pronation-Abduction. Forced abduction of the pronated foot is responsible for this category of ankle injuries, also classified by Danis and Weber as type B because the fibular fracture produced by this mechanism is also adjacent to the tibial plafond. This pattern comprises 5% to 21% of malleolar fractures.[79] Pronation-abduction fibular fractures are distinguished from supination–external rotation injuries by their different pattern, which is transverse and often laterally comminuted, as bending forces applied to the fibula result in medial tension and lateral compression (Fig. 52–25). Some such injuries may be hybrids, with initiation by abduction, followed by rotation externally about the axis of the posteroinferior tibiofibular ligament.[69] The transverse orientation and lateral comminution, which may be extensive, make open reduction and internal

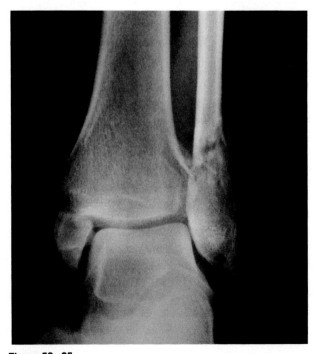

Figure 52–25

Pronation-abduction fracture demonstrating laterally comminuted, fairly transverse fibular fracture just above the plafond.

fixation of pronation-abduction injuries more difficult than it usually is for supination–external rotation injuries.

Lauge-Hansen demonstrated that the initial stage of failure (essentially a mirror image of the supination-adduction pattern) is medial tensile failure, either through the deltoid ligament or with a transverse avulsion fracture of the medial malleolus. The second stage is rupture or avulsion of the anteroinferior and posteroinferior tibiofibular ligaments of the syndesmosis. The third stage is the fibular fracture (Fig. 52–26). Limbird and Aaron have recently emphasized, as initially demonstrated by Coonrad, that these injuries may have an associated impaction fracture of the lateral plafond, also analogous to the supination-adduction pattern.[122a] Although the syndesmotic fibers proximal to the level of a pronation abduction fracture are usually intact, the fracture itself may be proximal enough that these fibers offer little stability to the tibiofibular relationship. Therefore, after repair of a pronation abduction fibular fracture, as with a supination–external rotation fracture, it is important to assess the stability of the syndesmosis.

Pronation–External Rotation. With external rotation of the pronated foot, Lauge-Hansen produced another pattern of malleolar injury (Fig. 52–27). In this case, the initial failure occurs on the medial side with either deltoid ligament rupture or avulsion of the medial malleolus. In the second stage, the anteroinferior tibiofibular ligament fails. The pathognomonic third stage is a spiral or oblique fracture, which typically runs from anterior proximally to posterior distally, rather than the reverse pattern seen in supination–external rotation fractures.[171] The location of the pronation–external rotation fibular fracture is its most important characteristic, for it is above the level of the ankle joint plafond. This level of fibular fracture is the hallmark of the Danis-Weber type C malleolar injury (Fig. 52–28). The fourth stage is disruption of the PITFL osteoligamentous complex. Pronation–external rotation injuries comprise 7% to 19% of malleolar fractures.[79]

Thus disruption occurs in the same direction around the ankle as it does with supination–external rotation injuries, but the starting point is medial instead of anterior. Because supraarticular fibular fractures can also be produced by supination–external rotation, a stage IV injury may be assigned to one category or the other on the basis of the appearance of the fibular fracture.[171,172] Furthermore, a type C fibular fracture with little displacement may be a stable stage II supination–external rotation fracture.

Significance of Classification. An important point about the supraarticular type C fibular fracture is that the entire ligamentous connection between the distal

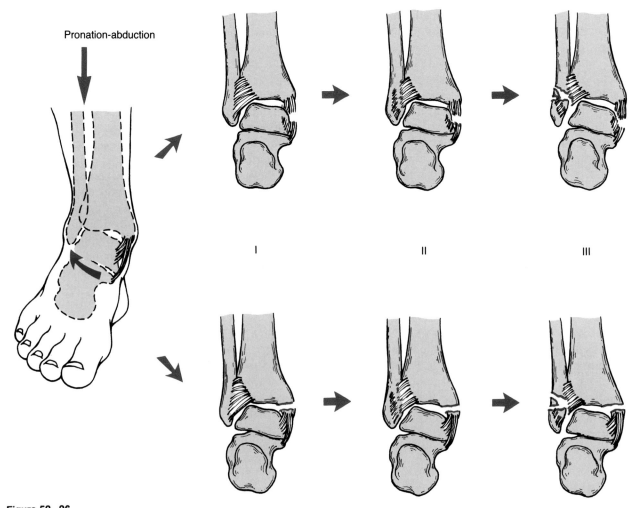

Pronation-abduction

I

II

III

Figure 52–26

Pronation-abduction injury pathology. The first stage is medial failure of either malleolus or the deltoid ligament. The second stage is syndesmosis (AITFL and PITFL) disruption. The third stage is a bending fracture of the lateral malleolus with a transverse, laterally comminuted pattern.

tibia and fibula may have failed, whether through the radiolucent ligaments or by avulsion of a bone fragment. The need for operative stabilization of the syndesmosis is more likely with type C injuries and may be confirmed by a stress test after fixation of the fibular fracture. Occasionally, remaining ligamentous connections are sufficient, and additional syndesmosis fixation is not necessary. If the supraarticular fibular fracture is caused by a stage II supination–external rotation mechanism, as demonstrated by Pankovich, displacement will be less, and the ankle may be quite stable.[171,236a] The *potential* for instability of the syndesmosis is the rationale for the separate category of type C injuries in the Danis-Weber classification system.[189]

Neither Lauge-Hansen's nor the Danis-Weber classification provide with their categories a complete indication of the pathology present and the treatment required.[123] A Lauge-Hansen grade IV supination–

external rotation injury may or may not have an unstable syndesmosis, a posterior articular lip fracture, an unstable fracture-dislocation, or a medial malleolus fracture. It may even have a high fibular fracture. A Danis-Weber type A injury may, or may not have a lateral malleolus fracture, a medial malleolus fracture, or a medial articular plafond impaction. However, with a little more anatomic detail, such classification systems provide an efficient means of categorizing and describing malleolar injuries and developing a treatment plan. The new AO fracture classification system expands that of Danis and Weber by providing this additional detail. It is helpful for research and descriptive purposes but is too complex for daily clinical use.[161]

Atypical Malleolar Fractures. A certain number of malleolar fractures are not classifiable according to the schemes presented. Those caused by direct crushing or angulating forces, as seen often in open injuries, often fall into this category.[65] The so-called Bosworth fracture-dislocation has a fracture just above the plafond with marked external rotation of the foot. The end of the proximal fibular segment is incarcerated behind the tibia and usually requires open reduction.[87] Very rarely, the fibula may be dislocated anteriorly.[207] In cases of atypical malleolar fractures, careful analysis of the pathoanatomy should lead to appropriate anatomic reduction.[166]

Treatment

Using the Danis-Weber classification, this section reviews the general principles of treatment for each injury pattern. Thereafter, details of operative management will be provided. The basis of treatment for malleolar fractures is the secure restoration of a normal tibiotalar relationship. This means anatomic repositioning of the talus under the plafond, with anatomic realignment of the articular surface of the lateral malleolus to the plafond as well. In a malleolar injury, the lateral malleolus not only follows the talus, but also, if it heals anatomically, maintains talar location as well.

Assessing the reduction of the talus requires adequate radiographs and careful scrutiny of the relationships between the plafond and talar dome, between the lateral articular surface of the talus and the lateral malleolus, and between the lateral malleolus and the distal tibial articular surface.[176,229] Reduction of the fibular fracture site is also helpful. If it is displaced, the ankle joint cannot be anatomically reduced. Length, rotation, and obliquity of the distal fibula are all important aspects of a successful reduction. The fibula must be appropriately seated in its incisural notch. Because of its greater distal diameter, proximal displacement of the lateral malleolus interferes with the fit of the malleolus in the notch, displacing the fibula laterally and thus widening the mortise. A comparison radiograph of the opposite ankle, and occasionally a CT scan, are helpful tools for assessing the adequacy of lateral malleolus reduction.

Figure 52–29 demonstrates the radiologic landmarks for assessing the relationship of the lateral malleolus to both the talus and the distal tibia. It is important to remember that a good closed reduction and a well-molded cast often align the talus satisfactorily.

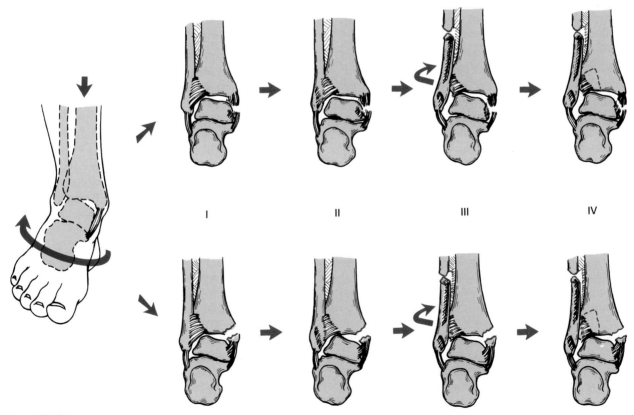

Figure 52–27

Pronation–external rotation injury pathology. The first stage is medial failure of either malleolus or the deltoid ligament. The second stage is AITFL disruption. The third stage is a spiral fracture of the fibula above the level of the plafond. The fourth stage is PITFL failure, demonstrated as a posterior malleolar failure.

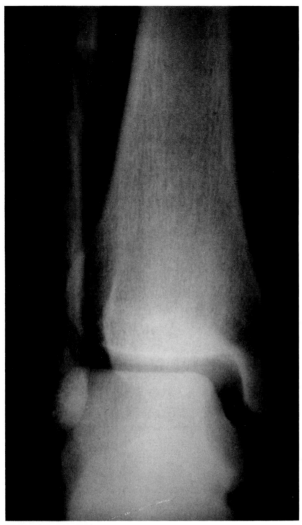

Figure 52-28

Radiograph of pronation–external rotation ankle fracture. This stage IV injury has a ruptured deltoid ligament; a laterally displaced fibula, indicating complete syndesmosis disruption; and a supraarticular short spiral fracture of the fibula, with orientation from low medial to high lateral.

However, unless the lateral malleolus heals anatomically, it will not be able to maintain talar position after the cast is removed. Therefore the surgeon must assess the position not only of the talus, but also of the lateral malleolus. Failure to reduce the fibula anatomically with a closed reduction is a prime justification for opening an unstable malleolar fracture in an effort to minimize the risk of posttraumatic arthrosis. This goal is more relevant in the young, active, healthy individual, for slight deviations from an anatomic alignment are often well-tolerated by an older, more sedentary patient. There are as yet no conclusive and well-accepted criteria, based on long-term clinical outcome studies, for the limits of a satisfactory reduction. Other factors also affect the results.[17] The importance of an accurate reduction has been convincingly demonstrated for more severe injuries[124], but minor degrees of displacement in relatively stable injuries do not have dire consequences, as shown by two long-term follow-up studies.[16,36,112]

Treatment Principles

Type A Injuries. Type A injuries, caused by supination-adduction mechanisms, produce a tensile failure on the lateral side with either lateral collateral ligament disruption or a transverse distal fracture of the lateral malleolus. On the medial side, an oblique medial malleolus fracture may be present, rarely without any lateral lesion. The medial malleolar fracture may be more or less displaced, may extend into the posterior articular surface, and may be associated with an impacted fracture of the medial plafond beginning just lateral to the malleolar fracture line. The syndesmosis is only rarely affected.

Truly undisplaced fractures of either malleolus do not require surgical treatment and can be managed well with a short-leg cast. Some displaced supination-adduction fractures of the medial malleolus with either a fracture or a ligament rupture laterally can be reduced with a maneuver that reverses the mechanism of injury and corrects both angulation and displacement by abducting the hindfoot. Overreduction is not likely, so a significant force can be applied and the position maintained with a well-padded short-leg cast molded medially over the talus and calcaneus to maintain a valgus alignment of the hindfoot. Radiographic monitoring of the reduction is necessary.

If there is significant articular surface impaction, plafond incongruity resulting from a posteromedial fracture line, or an inadequate closed reduction, then ORIF is indicated. Isolated, purely ligamentous lateral injuries can be managed satisfactorily nonoperatively (see Collateral Ligament Injuries). However, repair of the lateral collateral ligament is a small procedure that may protect the medial reconstruction. A type A lateral malleolus fracture should generally be fixed for similar reasons, unless the medial side is very secure and the lateral malleolus is completely undisplaced. Medial malleolar fractures should be fixed, unless an anatomic closed reduction is obtained and preserved. The same is true if there is plafond distortion by either a posteromedial fragment or an impacted area that requires elevation and usually bone grafting of the resulting defect (Fig. 52-30). Depending on bone quality, security of fixation, and extent of plafond involvement, postoperative weight bearing may need to be restricted.

Type B Injuries. Type B injuries may be caused by either a supination–external rotation or a pronation-abduction mechanism. The syndesmosis is occasion-

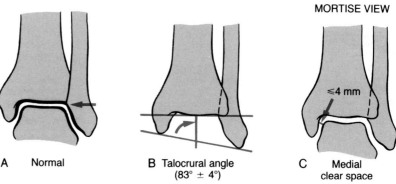

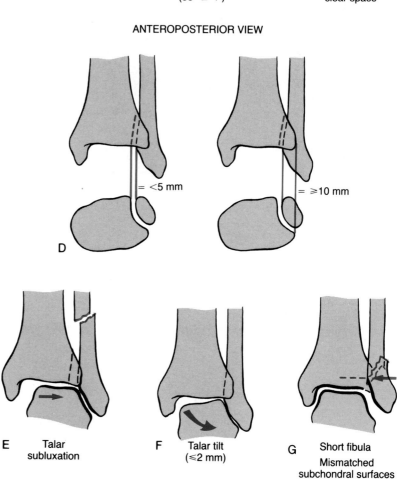

Figure 52–29

Restoration of the ankle mortise requires anatomic reduction of the lateral malleolus so that its articular surface is congruous with the reduced talus. *A*, On a mortise radiograph, the condensed subchondral bone should form a continuous line around the talus, and there should be no proximal displacement, malrotation, or angulation of the lateral malleolus. *B,C*, A proper talocrural angle and normal joint space width also indicate normality. The medial joint space should be less than 4 mm and the superior joint space within 2 mm medially of its width laterally. *D*, Adequate tibiofibular overlap on the AP view indicates a proper syndesmotic relationship. The space between the medial wall of the fibula and the incisural surface of the tibia should be less than 5 mm. The anterior tubercle of the tibia should overlap the fibula by at least 10 mm. *E,F*, Talar malalignment is indicated by its lateral displacement or tilt into valgus. *G*, Although the talus may be reduced by external pressure, its alignment is not maintained by a shortened, malrotated lateral malleolus, as shown.

ally disrupted. The medial injury may be an avulsion fracture of the medial malleolus, a deltoid ligament rupture, or (occasionally) a combined lesion. Anatomic reduction and fixation of the medial malleolus cannot be counted on to reduce and maintain talar alignment (Fig. 52–31).[11,64,81,120,254] Depending on the mechanism and stage, either or both of the inferior tibiofibular ligaments may be ruptured, but above the level of injury, the ligamentous connections between the tibia and fibula are usually maintained. Often, but not always, they adequately stabilize the syndesmosis

after the distal fibular fragment is securely and anatomically reattached to the proximal one.

As discussed previously, the fibular fracture configuration depends significantly on the mechanism of injury. In supination–external rotation fractures, the characteristic spiral oblique fracture usually begins in an almost transverse plane distally on the anterior surface of the fibula. It then spirals lazily externally, extending a variable length up the fibula to exit proximally on its posterior surface. Occasionally the long posterior spike of the distal fragment may be commi-

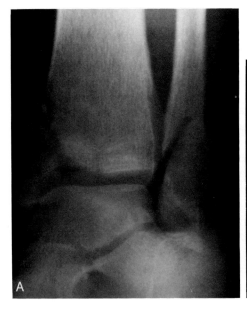

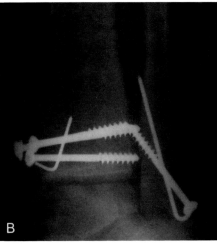

Figure 52-30

This stage II supination-adduction fracture has significant plafond impaction medially. The impacted fragment was reduced through the medial malleolar fracture plane. The defect was filled with local cancellous graft, and the fracture stabilized with cancellous screws and a Kirschner wire.

nuted. The more transverse, often laterally comminuted, pronation–external rotation fibular fracture is usually recognizable as different, even though its primary location is the same. Transitional forms incorporating some external rotation about the intact PITFL are typically spiral but are oriented differently, from low medial to high lateral, and begin above the plafond level.

In addition to the constant pathognomonic fibular fracture and the possibility of some form of medial side disruption, type B injuries may have associated posterior lip fractures of larger or smaller size, with or without articular surface involvement. Also, with prona-

tion-abduction injuries there may occasionally be impaction of the lateral tibial plafond. This may require elevation and bone grafting if a significant portion of the plafond is involved. Fragments and deformation of the tibia may prevent satisfactory reduction of the fibula unless they are corrected. Anteriorly the AITFL may be avulsed with a bony fragment of the anterior tibia or fibula or may be a pure soft tissue injury.

Treatment of type B malleolar fractures is determined by the severity and anatomy of the injury. Undisplaced injuries usually represent lesser degrees of severity and are well suited to nonoperative manage-

Figure 52-31

In spite of anatomic reduction of the medial malleolus, the talus is laterally subluxated, as it is not stabilized by the malreduced lateral malleolus.

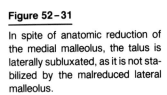

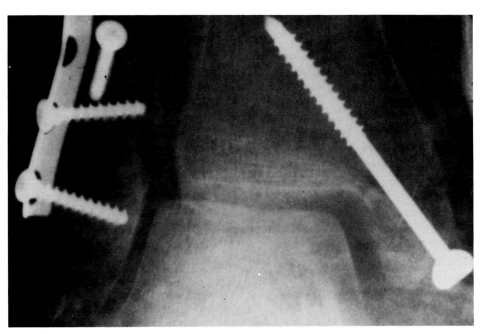

ment. Grade I supination–external rotation injuries, with damage limited to the AITFL are hard to confirm but are recognized injuries. Such "anterior syndesmosis sprains" are slow to heal. A more common example is the undisplaced or minimally displaced (up to 2 or 3 mm) spiral fracture of the lateral malleolus exhibiting the pattern described previously but unassociated with lateral displacement or tilt of the talus or evidence of medial side injury. Because the radiographic appearances are similar, it is essential to differentiate this injury from unstable stage IV injuries with deltoid disruption. A short-leg walking cast or functional brace for six weeks permits functional treatment of stable type B supination–external rotation fractures of the lateral malleolus. Radiographs taken in the cast about 10 to 14 days after injury should be checked for talar shift to aid in identifying a missed supination–external rotation stage IV deltoid injury.

Closed reduction may succeed for displaced supination–external rotation injuries. The knee is flexed, and the foot is distracted, pulled anteriorly, and *internally rotated.* Assessment of reduction should ensure not only reposition of the talus relative to the plafond, but also anatomic reduction of the lateral and (if present) medial malleolar fracture. More than 2 to 3 mm of displacement of a malleolus or of a plafond fragment is a reason to consider ORIF.

Where local and systemic conditions permit, ORIF of displaced external rotation injuries usually provides the best results and the quickest restoration of function. In general, the most secure fixation is with an interfragmentary lag screw and a small plate for added strength. The plate may be applied posterolaterally, as advocated by Weber,[33,206] or directly laterally. Syndesmosis stability must be confirmed, for occasionally such marked tibiofibular instability is present that it is necessary to employ syndesmosis transfixation or repair the inferior tibiofibular ligaments, if this is possible with security.

With anatomic reduction of the lateral malleolus and a stable syndesmosis, talar position will be maintained; there is no benefit from repair of a torn deltoid ligament.[11,51a,81,254,257] To avoid the occasional symptomatic medial malleolus nonunion, most surgeons prefer to fix all but the smallest medial malleolar fractures associated with displaced ankle injuries.

It is helpful to recognize the mechanism of injury of type B injuries, for pronation-abduction fractures require a different technique of closed reduction and may pose different surgical challenges than do fractures associated with supination–external rotation. Stage I pronation-abduction injuries have only isolated medial side lesions. If the injury is ligamentous, repair is not required, and functional treatment is appropriate. The same is true for undisplaced medial malleolar frac-

tures, which may deserve fixation if there is more than 2 to 3 mm displacement. Stage II injuries add complete distal syndesmosis disruption, but unless a large avulsed fragment results in plafond or syndesmosis incongruity, treatment is the same. Stage III injuries may be markedly displaced and usually require fixation of the fibular fracture, although closed reduction by supination and adduction may be successful.

In pronation-abduction fractures, lateral comminution of the fibular fracture is frequently seen. This may be so severe as to defy anatomic reduction by reassembly of the fragments. In such a situation, it is best to realign the talus and reduce the lateral malleolus to it with provisional K wire fixation to the tibia or talus. The reduction is confirmed with a mortise radiograph checked against a control view of the other side. Then one can proceed with buttress plate fixation and possibly bone grafting of a very comminuted fibular fracture. Often, initial reduction and fixation of the much less complex medial malleolus fracture can aid repair of the comminuted lateral side of the ankle. In true pronation-abduction lateral malleolus fractures, it is rarely possible to use a lag screw between the proximal and distal fragments, and as a result, lateral fixation may be less secure.

Type C Injuries. The mechanism of type C malleolar injuries is classically pronation–external rotation. Stage I involves bony or ligamentous failure medially. In stage II the AITFL fails, along with the interosseous ligament and some of the interosseous membrane. Stage III is the supraarticular fibular fracture at a variable height above the plafond. In significantly higher fractures, such as the Maisonneuve, it is probably unlikely that the interosseous membrane tear ascends as high as the fibular fracture. Rather, the intact proximal interosseous membrane does not interfere with torsional failure of the proximal fibula after the more distal soft tissues rupture. Finally, the fourth stage involves PITFL rupture. Anterior and especially posterior tubercular fractures may be a part of inferior syndesmotic ligament failure and may involve the articular plafond.

Rarely, a type C malleolar fracture is stable, undisplaced, and amenable to nonoperative management. Much more frequently, there is displacement and syndesmosis instability. Restoration of stability will require anatomic open reduction and internal fixation of the fibular fracture. Next the syndesmosis is assessed and, if it is unstable or remains displaced, fixed in a position of anatomic alignment. Reduction and fixation of a large or destabilizing plafond fragment and of a medial malleolar fracture complete the reconstruction of displaced type C injuries. When the fibular fracture is very proximal, it is sufficient to regain length and rotation with only a distal exposure. After anatomic reduction of the lateral malleolar articular surface, confirmed by a comparison radiograph, one or two transfixion screws are placed to maintain this position during ligamentous healing of the syndesmosis. Type C malleolar injuries have a greater risk of syndesmosis disruption and instability, even after fixation of the fibular fracture. This category therefore serves to warn the surgeon of the need to assess syndesmosis stability. Particularly deceiving is the high Maisonneuve fracture with only a deltoid ligament tear medially. Only subtle malalignment of the fibular malleolus indicates the existence and nature of the injury.

Nonoperative Treatment of Malleolar Fractures. Undisplaced malleolar fractures can usually be satisfactorily treated with the ankle in neutral in a short-leg walking cast. Rotational control is improved with triangular proximal molding of the cast to fit the proximal tibia without pressure on the peroneal nerve. Medial or lateral distal molding of the cast can resist varus or valgus angulation. It is important to distribute the contact area widely over the hindfoot, rather than just around the malleoli, and to avoid focal pressure on bony prominences with thin overlying soft tissues.

Optimally, a closed reduction is performed with a general or regional anesthetic that provides total relaxation and relief of pain. A satisfactory closed reduction becomes harder to achieve if more than a day or so has elapsed since injury. Closed reduction is usually best achieved by reversing the mechanism of injury that produced the displacement and fracture pattern evident on initial radiographs. Some distraction as well will help to disengage fragments and ease the realignment of the talus with the mortise. Reduction of the talus, rather than direct pressure on the malleoli, brings them back into position and maintains alignment.

Thus a type A *supination-adduction* fracture is reduced by abducting (everting) the hindfoot and molding the medial side of the distalmost part of the cast to retain this position. Three-point fixation is provided by a lateral mold proximal to the ankle and another medial molded area extending along the proximal medial tibial shaft.

Type B *supination-external rotation* fractures are reduced with (1) distraction, (2) anterior traction, (3) internal rotation, and (4) medial displacement of the talus. A long-leg cast with the knee flexed is necessary to maintain the foot's internally rotated position that resists redisplacement. Pronation is not necessary, and the foot should be in a relatively neutral position. Although it may be tempting to supinate the hindfoot in an effort to restore fibular length, this rarely works and may result in difficulties regaining a plantigrade foot. The long-leg, bent-knee, internally rotated cast for a

supination–external rotation ankle fracture is best applied with the patient supine, hip and knee flexed, hip abducted, and the foot held in internal rotation as shown in Fig. 52–32. The entire cast from toes to mid thigh can be applied at one time, after the reduction maneuver, if the foot and leg are held in the proper position by an assistant. The weight of the externally rotated leg counteracts the internal rotation moment applied to the foot and stabilizes the reduction. With adequate padding, molding of the cast is primarily over the lateral foot, around but not directly on top of the lateral malleolus (Fig. 52–33).

Type B *pronation-abduction* fractures are reduced by distraction and adduction. The presence of an intact medial malleolus or at least an overhanging remnant thereof often prevents overcorrection, and provides a template for anatomic reduction. If there is no medial buttress (i.e., the medial malleolar fracture is at or above the plafond), the ankle may be so unstable that a satisfactory closed reduction is not possible. Although rotation does not usually need to be corrected, its control may enhance stability; thus a long-leg, bent-knee cast is better if the reduction is unstable. The weight of

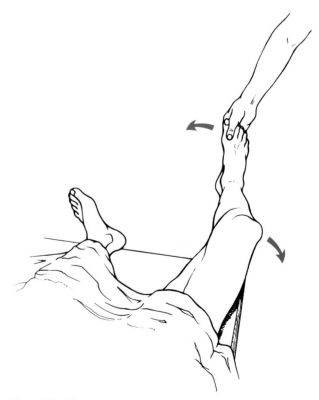

Figure 52–32

External rotation deformity can be reduced by internally rotating the foot relative to the abducted and flexed proximal leg. A well-padded long-leg cast is applied while the leg is held in this position.

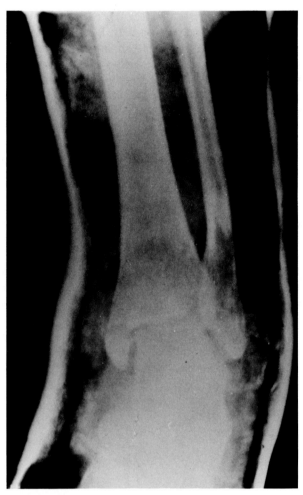

Figure 52-33

Molding of this cast over the lateral hindfoot, combined with moderate internal rotation, holds the talus anatomically reduced. The malleoli reduce with it, as they are attached by the collateral ligaments.

the leg can be positioned to maintain a varus force on the ankle during reduction and cast application.

Type C *pronation–external rotation* fractures are best reduced with (1) distraction, (2) anterior displacement, (3) internal rotation, and (4) medial displacement, similarly to supination–external rotation injuries. A long-leg, bent-knee, internally rotated cast is applied, as shown in Figure 52–32, with the foot held gently internally rotated but otherwise as neutral as possible.

Although a closed manipulation will usually restore the talotibial relationship, it rarely reduces the lateral malleolus anatomically. Because some shortening or malrotation is likely to remain, the lateral malleolus will not be able to maintain the precise alignment of the talus after a cast is removed and normal weight bearing is resumed. Thus ORIF is generally preferred.

If closed reduction is chosen for treatment of a displaced malleolar fracture, it is important to monitor the reduction until healing is secure, for if it is lost, prompt rereduction or open reduction and internal fixation may still provide a satisfactory result. In general, adequate monitoring requires radiographs in the cast at seven to ten days and again at three weeks. If reduction is maintained at three weeks, it is unlikely that it will displace during the next three weeks in a non–weight-bearing cast. Many regimens have been proposed for immobilization after closed reduction of a displaced malleolar fracture. We generally advocate six weeks in a non–weight-bearing cast molded primarily to preserve the reduction. Following this, another two to three weeks in a plantigrade short-leg walking cast or brace provides additional protection and helps with rehabilitation. Variations from this protocol may be advisable based on bone quality, fracture stability, and patient characteristics.

When the cast is removed, the patient may need to resume crutch use for awhile, even if he or she was able to manage without them while in the cast. Stretching, progressive strengthening, endurance, and agility exercises are required for several months if optimal results are to be achieved as rapidly as possible. After cast removal, an elastic stocking may be needed for a month or two to control edema. Elevation of the leg when not actually walking also helps.

Operative Treatment

Initial Care and Timing of Surgery. Displaced malleolar fractures often involve significant subluxation or dislocation of the tibiotalar joint. To minimize pain, swelling, and additional local trauma, such injuries should be treated with a prompt provisional reduction and immobilization in a safe, effective splint. Evaluation of skin and neurovascular status precedes this, with follow-up reassessment periodically thereafter.

If possible, a formal closed reduction maneuver is carried out in the emergency department with appropriate analgesia. Then a very well padded cast is applied. This provides the best possible splint. Extra padding is necessary to accommodate swelling and protect the skin from the cast saw blade. Once hard, the cast can be split and spread or bivalved, if necessary, to accommodate swelling. Radiographs are obtained in the cast to assess reduction, which should be repeated immediately only if there is gross deformity with skin or neurovascular compromise. An *anatomic* reduction obtained without the foot being placed in an extreme position suggests consideration of nonoperative management, unless the fracture is very unstable. Unsuccessful closed reduction in this setting may still be improved with a manipulation under anesthesia, but if an anesthetic is required, many surgeons now feel that only strong local contraindications would dissuade them from ORIF of an unstable malleolar fracture.

If an abrasion of any significance is present about an injured ankle, its contamination and bacterial colonization should delay surgery until the skin has healed. Therefore such ankles may best be treated with urgent surgery to permit ORIF before the wound surface poses an increased risk of infection. A povidone-iodine dressing over such a superficial skin wound may reduce the rate of bacterial colonization. If there is only slight soft tissue injury, indicated by mild initial displacement and little swelling, then ORIF can be done essentially electively during the early postinjury period, although it becomes progressively less easy after a week or so and is often very difficult after three weeks, because of early fracture healing and disuse osteoporosis, which is a potentially severe problem in older women.[19,37] Because it is associated with a reduced likelihood of anatomic reduction, delay in ORIF of malleolar fractures beyond two weeks is associated with poorer results. However, if an anatomic reduction is achieved, the outcome may closely approach that achieved by early surgery.[63] It is wise to remember that unappreciated swelling may increase the risk of such procedures during the first several days after injury. Therefore, during the early postinjury period, the skin should be assessed just prior to inducing anesthesia for ORIF of an ankle fracture. If significant soft tissue injury with marked swelling and blisters are evident, ORIF should be delayed until the local tissues have recovered, which may take seven to ten days or more of strict elevation. The return of cutaneous wrinkles indicates the resolution of edema. If soft tissue trauma is exceptionally severe, it is often best to treat the ankle with closed reduction and external fixation, deferring open reduction, if it is required, until the risk of wound slough has diminished.

It is important not to accept poor ankle alignment and an inadequate splint because early surgery is planned. The opportunity to operate may be lost for a variety of reasons, and the ankle may suffer additional insult without proper early care.

Choice and Planning of Fixation. A satisfactory fixation technique must have a low risk of failure, must resist the forces that are likely to cause redisplacement of the fracture, and must not be likely to increase comminution or cause displacement during its application. Many techniques of malleolar fracture fixation have been advocated.[15] The ones described here are essentially those advocated by the Swiss AO.[85,160,247] They have been generally accepted and work well for the authors.[159] Less rigid techniques have also been advocated, and although they are often successful, especially in more stable injuries, they are not as reliable as those

of the AO in maintaining reduction of bimalleolar or trimalleolar and equivalent fractures.[169]

Adequate preoperative radiographs are required for planning fixation. Comparison views of the uninjured ankle can be very helpful. A precise preoperative plan guides positioning and choice of incision and also provides a shared operative strategy that increases the efficiency of the entire surgical team.[141a]

Lateral Malleolus Fractures. A secure anatomic repair of a displaced lateral malleolus fracture is one of the most important steps in operative management of a malleolar fracture because of the role this structure plays in maintaining tibiotalar alignment.

Because of its posterior location, the fibula is easier to approach if a cushion is placed under the supine patient's ipsilateral buttock to internally rotate the trunk and leg. A safety strap about the pelvis allows the table to be tilted further if needed. A pneumatic tourniquet is a conventional adjunct but may wisely be omitted in patients with impaired perfusion or vascular disease.

A longitudinal lateral incision provides adequate ac-

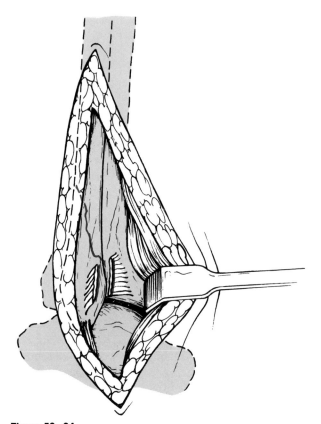

Figure 52–34

The incision to repair a lateral malleolar fracture should provide access to the anterolateral ankle joint, as well as the anterior inferior tibiofibular ligament. This is necessary to search for osteochondral injuries and especially to ensure anatomic repair of the mortise.

cess to the distal fibula. Because the primary purpose of the procedure is to reconstruct the alignment and integrity of the ankle joint, and not to improve the appearance of the fibular fracture, it is important that the lateral incision also permit exposure of the anterior syndesmosis, in particular the AITFL and the superolateral corner of the anterior ankle joint (Fig. 52–34). Inspection of the relationship of the talus, tibial plafond, and lateral malleolus reveals the congruity, or lack thereof, of the articular surfaces. This area is better seen if the distal end of the incision is angled slightly anteriorly and carried sufficiently distally. The distal end of the incision permits an arthrotomy for irrigation and inspection of the ankle joint to identify and remove loose osteochondral fragments and intraarticular clot. The proximal extent of the incision is determined by the requirements for fixation of the fibular fracture.

Flaps should be kept as thick as possible and handled gently. A more extensive fasciotomy may be wise in patients with more soft tissue swelling. If an anteromedial incision is also used, then the lateral incision must be more posterior, as it also should for access to the posterolateral tibia through the interval between the peronei and the Achilles tendon or for posterior plate fixation of a supination–external rotation fibular fracture. The sural and superficial peroneal nerves have branches in the region of this lateral incision and

should be protected or resected and buried away from the scar to avoid a painful neuroma.

Through this lateral incision it is possible to repair the lateral ligaments, as well as to fix fractures of the lateral malleolus. The torn lateral collateral ligament complex is reapproximated with interrupted, medium-weight sutures. A small, very distal fibular avulsion fracture can be reattached with sutures to bone or soft tissue or with a small-fragment or minifragment screw and plastic ligament washer, whose small spikes prevent pressure necrosis of the soft tissue it secures to bone.[92,194] A larger avulsed fragment of the distal lateral malleolus, typical of type A injuries, is best fixed with either a tension band wire or a small oblique screw. Fixation must resist distraction forces produced by inversion of the hindfoot (Fig. 52–35). Reduction is obtained by clearing clot and minimally reflecting the periosteum to see the bony apposition. The distal fragment is grasped with a small forceps, guided into place, and held with a sharp dental probe. For tension band wiring, it is fixed with two 1.25- or 1.6-mm K wires, which may be oblique or intramedullary. Advancing and then withdrawing them will permit their impaction into the bone after the exposed ends are cut and bent into a J shape (Fig. 52–36). The figure-of-eight 1.25-mm tension band wire can be anchored proximally by passage through a transverse drill hole in the fibula or,

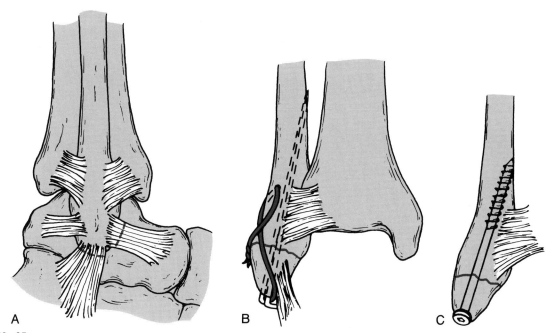

Figure 52–35

Repair of type A lateral ankle injuries. *A*, ligament tears are sutured. Low transverse fibular fractures are reduced anatomically and fixed with K wires and a tension band *(B)* or a small oblique lag screw *(C)* that penetrates and anchors in the medial cortex proximally. (*A*, Redrawn from Müller, M.E., et al. Manual of Internal Fixation, 2nd ed. New York, Springer-Verlag, 1979. *B*, Redrawn from Heim, U.; Pfeiffer, K.M. Small Fragment Set Manual: Technique Recommended by the ASIF Group, 2nd ed. New York, Springer-Verlag, 1982.)

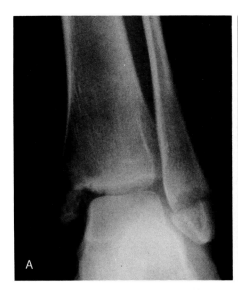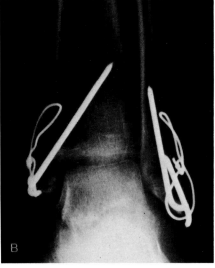

Figure 52–36

A, Type A bimalleolar fracture with significant comminution of a small medial malleolar fragment. *B,* Kirschner wires with tension bands provide fixation.

more easily, around a small cortical screw. If an oblique lag screw is chosen instead, provisional fixation of the fragment with a small K wire aids in holding position during the steps of screw placement.

Supination–external rotation type B injuries, as discussed previously, generally cause a spiral fracture that distally exits the anterior surface of the fibula at or just above the level of the plafond. The malleolar fragment carries the lateral attachment of the AITFL. This structure can often be a guide to reduction. Comminution produced by its avulsion from either the tibia or fibula may add another element of complexity.

The same lateral incision is used, extending sufficiently proximal to provide easy access to the posterior proximal end of the distal fragment. Unless excessively comminuted, this posterior spike can guide restoration of length and rotational alignment. It can often be repositioned first, and held in place while the reduction is completed. After exposure of the fracture and the anterior surface of the fibula proximal to it, the joint is explored, aided by an intraarticular angled retractor anteriorly. Then the distal fibula is grasped with a pointed forceps, such as a towel clip, and teased into place with traction and repositioning of both foot and fracture fragment as needed (Fig. 52–37). Be cautious with strong forces if the bone is osteopenic. Simultaneous control of the proximal fibular fragment with a bone clamp may aid reduction. A small, pointed or lobster-claw reduction forceps is used to oppose the fracture as proximal and distal pieces are realigned.

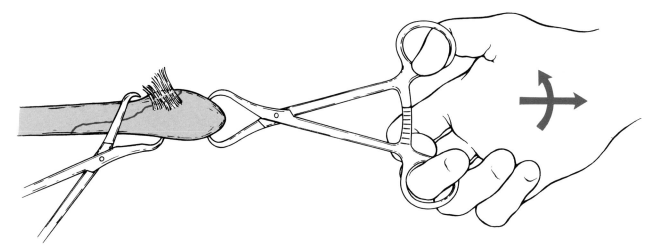

Figure 52–37

Reduction of the common supination–external rotation lateral malleolar fracture requires grasping the distal fragment (cautiously if the patient is osteopenic) and bringing it into precise alignment with the proximal fragment, after which a reduction forceps is tightened, perpendicular to the fracture plane.

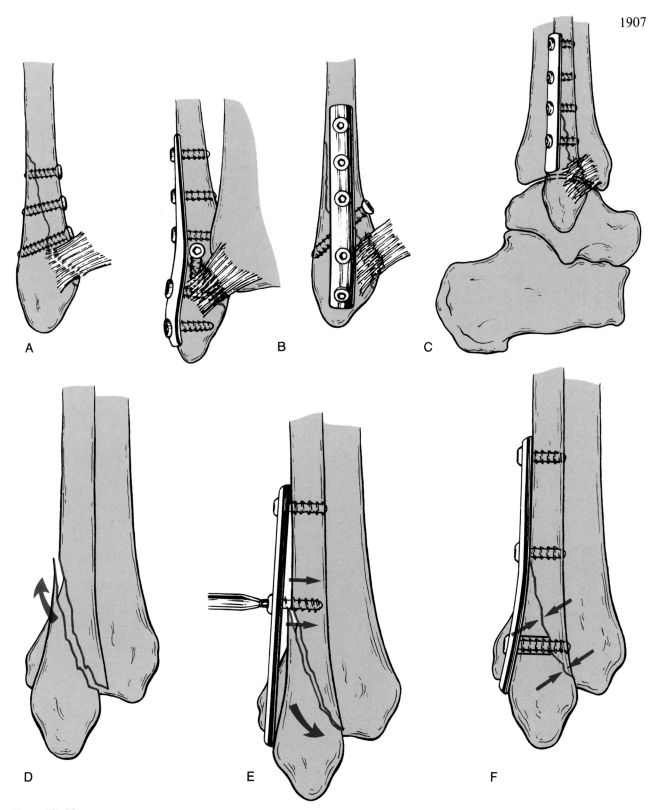

Figure 52–38

Repair of type B lateral malleolar injuries. *A,* A long spiral fracture can be repaired with two or more lag screws. External protection is required. *B,C,* A single lag screw and one-third tubular neutralization plate is more secure. *D,E,* An antiglide plate (one-third tubular) can be applied posteriorly, where it resists proximal displacement of the distal fragment. *F,* A lag screw can be used with a posterior plate, either through the plate, as illustrated, or previously placed from anterior to posterior (see Fig. 52–40). The principle of the posterior antiglide plate is illustrated. (*A,* Redrawn from Müller, M.E., et al. Manual of Internal Fixation, 2nd ed. New York, Springer-Verlag, 1979. *B,* Redrawn from Heim, U.; Pfeiffer, K.M. Small Fragment Set Manual: Technique Recommended by the ASIF Group, 2nd ed. New York, Springer-Verlag, 1982. (*D–F,* Modified from Brunner, C.F., Weber, B.G. Special Techniques in Internal Fixation. New York, Springer-Verlag, 1982.)

The reduction forceps should be applied perpendicular to the fracture plane, or it may cause redisplacement. It should not interfere with placing an anteroposterior lag screw perpendicular to the fracture, and it should not be so close to the end of the proximal piece that it produces comminution. A satisfactory reduction opposes the fracture line on the anterior and lateral surfaces of the fibula, restores the position of the proximal spike, places the AITFL so that its ends lie anatomically, and restores the relationship of the lateral malleolus, lateral plafond, and lateral edge of the talar dome, as seen in the anterolateral corner of the mortise. If reduction is not readily achieved, the possibility of a medial obstruction — fracture fragments or an intraarticular flexor tendon — must be excluded by exploration of the medial side of the joint.

If a truly anatomic reduction has been achieved, a lag screw is applied perpendicular to the fracture using a 3.5-mm cortical screw with the anterior cortex overdrilled. Two or more such lag screws can be used as the entire fixation, if the bone is of excellent quality and a cast will be used for protection. More secure fixation is achieved with a one-third tubular plate contoured to fit the concave, slightly spiral, lateral surface of the fibula. This is usually applied with three or four screws proximal to the fracture's distal obliquity and at least two in the distal fragment, placed carefully and checked with radiographs to ensure that they do not enter the joint space (Figs. 52–38 and 52–39).

Alternatively, as proposed by Brunner and Weber, a similar plate can be applied on the posterolateral surface of the fibula, where it overlies the posterior fracture spike of the distal fragment and prevents its gliding proximally.[33,206] This is less prominent laterally and may be better tolerated, although it requires more posterior exposure (Fig. 52–40). Any technique that is used for fixation of the lateral malleolus must resist proximal migration or rotation of the distal fragment. Therefore most intramedullary techniques are risky, though special devices such as the Inyo nail may be successful.[146,147]

Pronation-abduction type B injuries cause a transverse and often comminuted fracture at or just above the level of the plafond. Depending on the extent of comminution, reduction of the lateral malleolus may be quite difficult. Preoperative radiographs will usually define the pathology and allow a modified operative plan.[122a] Lateral plafond impaction may need to be elevated through or around the fibular fracture; a CT scan may be a considerable aid to planning. The medial side of the ankle is a helpful guide to reduction. If its malleolus is intact, the talus can be pushed back medially against it. If there is a transverse fracture that can readily be fixed, it, too, will provide support. With the talus reduced against the medial side of the mortise, the lateral shoulder of the talus provides a template for reduction of the lateral malleolus. Provisional fixation with K wires to the talus and/or tibia permits radio-

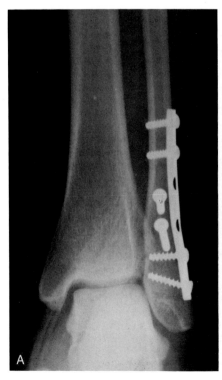 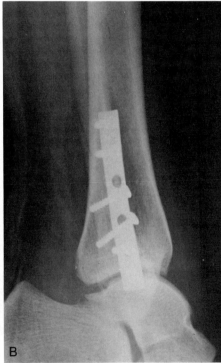

Figure 52–39

This type B lateral malleolar fracture has been fixed anatomically with two lag screws across the fracture line, barely visible at its most proximal extent on the lateral view. A one-third tubular plate adds support to the fracture, with cortical screws proximally and cancellous fully threaded screws distally. Screws probably could have been placed through the empty holes and into the anterior portion of the proximal fibular fragment.

Figure 52-40

This type B fracture was reduced anatomically and fixed with a single anteroposterior lag screw perpendicular to the fracture plane. An antiglide plate was then applied to the posterolateral surface of the malleolus, avoiding prominent lateral hardware. With an undisplaced medial malleolus fracture, the patient is fully weight bearing in a PTB cast. A, AP radiograph. B, lateral radiograph.

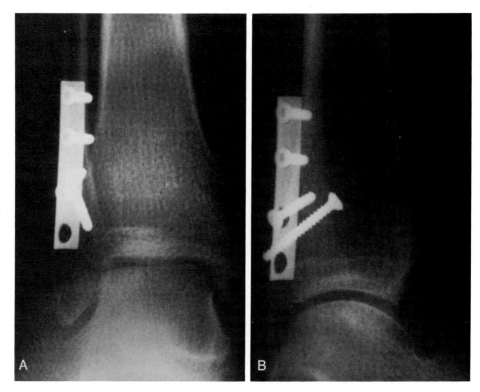

graphic confirmation of reduction (Fig. 52–41). This is compared with a mortise view of the opposite ankle, and if reduction is satisfactory, a plate (either a one-third tubular or, if the fracture is very comminuted and the patient is large, a stouter 3.5-mm dynamic compression plate) is applied as a buttress. Bone graft may aid healing of a comminuted fibular fracture. Indirect reduction techniques can help with these very challenging fracture reductions (see Fig. 52–45).[140,141]

The AITFL disruption should be repaired, at least to confirm appropriate reduction of the syndesmosis. Avulsion of the ligament with or without a fragment of bone from the Wagstaffe (Le Fort) or the Chaput tubercles can often be repaired with a small screw or ligament washer. A mechanically insecure horizontal mattress suture will appose the ends of a rupture in substance and may improve the ultimate quality of the healed ligament (Fig. 52–42).

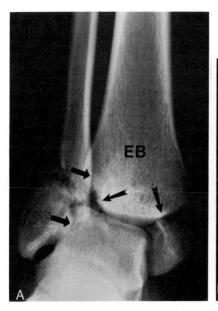
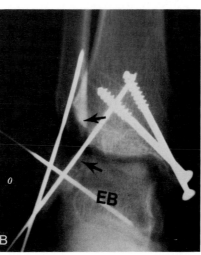

Figure 52-41

A, A pronation-abduction type B fracture with lateral plafond impaction. B, The fracture has been realigned by reduction and fixation of the medial malleolus, followed by provisional K-wire fixation of the lateral malleolus. Radiographic confirmation of this reduction precedes definitive internal fixation and bone grafting of the fibula. (A From Limbird, R.S.; Aaron, R.K. Laterally comminuted fracture dislocation of the ankle. J Bone Joint Surg 69A:881–885, 1987.)

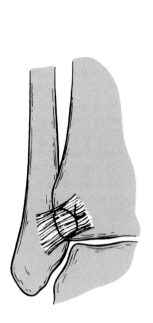
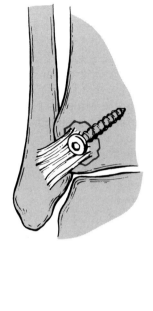
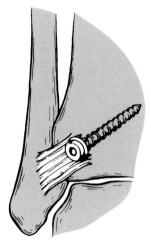

Figure 52–42

The anteroinferior tibiofibular ligament ends should appose perfectly
if reduction is precise. The ligament
can be repaired with a horizontal
mattress suture, with a screw
through an avulsed bone fragment,
or with a small spiked plastic ligament washer.

Repair of the PITFL is not as easy but has been recommended as justification for reduction and fixation of all posterolateral tibial lip (Volkmann's) fragments, even those that are extraarticular, because of the presumed benefit of immediate syndesmosis stabilization (Fig. 52–43).[84] Possibly this may eliminate the need for syndesmosis transfixation. Strong evidence that refixation of the PITFL to the distal tibia makes a difference in outcome has not yet been provided.[82] The value of fixation of a small Volkmann's fragment thus remains controversial.

After fixation of the lateral malleolus, it is important to assess stability of the syndesmosis by externally rotating the foot and pulling the repaired fibula laterally with an encircling clamp. The anterolateral corner of the malleolus is observed, and demonstrable laxity of more than 3 or 4 mm with such maneuvers should be considered as an indication for use of a syndesmosis transfixation screw.[69,79,101,102,162,229]

In higher lateral malleolus fractures (those seen with type C injuries), the fracture is often relatively transverse. Fixation with an interfragmentary lag screw may be impossible, but comminution is not as frequent a problem as it is in typical pronation-abduction injuries (Fig. 52–44). If comminution and shortening of the fibula are significant, then indirect reduction using a small distractor or a plate with a tension device or bone spreader to regain length may be very helpful (Fig. 52–45).[141] Provisional fixation and confirmation of reduction by radiographs and direct visualization of the ankle joint are essential. The surgeon should resist the temptation to reduce the high lateral malleolus fracture

Figure 52–43

The posteroinferior tibiofibular ligament can be repaired by reduction
and fixation of a posterolateral
avulsion fracture (Volkmann's
fragment) of the distal tibia.

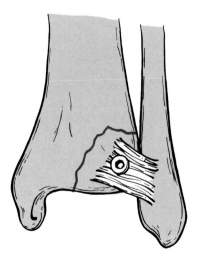

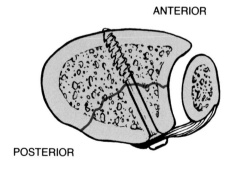

ANTERIOR

POSTERIOR

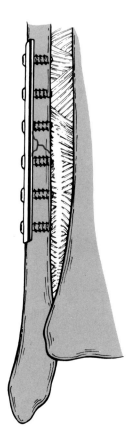

Figure 52-44

Repair of type C lateral malleolar fractures requires precise anatomic reduction of the articular fragment and usually plate and screw fixation of the fracture. Occasionally the fracture will permit use of a lag screw as well, but more often it is transverse or comminuted. A one-third tubular, small-fragment plate or a 3.5-mm DC plate is most often used, with three or four screws above and below the fracture. (Redrawn from Heim, U.; Pfeiffer, K.M. Small Fragment Set Manual: Technique Recommended by the ASIF Group, 2nd ed. New York, Springer-Verlag, 1982.)

without exposing the joint and should not be misled by an apparent reduction of a comminuted fracture site. Ankle joint restoration, not fibular fracture reduction, is the goal (Figs. 52-46 and 52-47). Use of a syndesmosis transfixation screw without precise fibular fracture reduction is unlikely to provide an anatomic reduction because of difficulty assessing and obtaining length and rotational alignment. Therefore this approach should also be avoided.

Only very proximal fibular fractures (upper third) with mortise disruption are reasonably treated without direct reduction and fixation, but mortise reconstruction and transfixation must be done with great care.

Syndesmosis Transfixation. Syndesmosis stability is checked by laterally displacing the distal fibula from the tibia while observing the relationship of the two bones. If more than 3 to 4 mm of lateral shift of the

talus occurs, then instability is present. This has been called the Cotton Test (Fig. 52-48).[229] Gross displacement indicates the need for surgical stabilization of the syndesmosis.

There are many different beliefs regarding indications and technique for stabilizing a disrupted syndesmosis. Little hard data support the advice, so skepticism is warranted. Like other controversial topics, it may be that controversy flourishes because there is little difference in outcome. The problem is that sometimes, after seemingly satisfactory reduction of the medial and lateral malleoli, the space between the tibia and fibula widens, and the talus fits loosely in the mortise. Pain, instability, and posttraumatic arthrosis may follow. It is clear that the fibula bears some weight and that in some individuals, at least, it moves slightly relative to the tibia with normal gait.[92a,162,229] The strength of the forces that displace the fibula laterally are not known. Significantly controversial issues include (1) when syndesmosis fixation is necessary (i.e., internal fixation between the tibia and fibula that prevents diastasis), (2) how such fixation should be carried out, (3) what activities should be permitted when the distal tibia and fibula are fixed together, and (4) how long such fixation should be retained.

Obvious distal tibiofibular diastasis on initial or subsequent radiographs or gross mechanical instability of the syndesmosis signals the possible need for syndesmosis transfixation. The amount of fibular motion that indicates critical instability is not certain.[92,101,102,162] Slight laxity (up to 2 to 3 mm) of a well-reduced fibula, especially if there is a good end point, rarely indicates a significant risk of late diastasis. Adjunctive syndesmosis stabilization through repair of avulsed inferior tibiofibular ligaments may improve such a situation. There is some evidence that stability increases over time.[169] The use of a long-leg, non-weight bearing cast for a few weeks may also prevent loss of alignment in questionable cases. It is vital to remember that if the fibula is not satisfactorily reduced initially, then it is unlikely that transfixation of the syndesmosis will yield an acceptable result.

TECHNIQUES. Inman, who agreed with Grath, quoted Grath's study as evidence that only slight lateral motion (0 to 2 mm) of the lateral malleolus occurred with full ankle dorsiflexion.[75,92a] Olerud demonstrated loss of 0.1° of dorsiflexion for every degree of plantarflexion the ankle was in at the time the syndesmosis was fixed.[167a] For this reason, it seems wise to fix the syndesmosis with the talus held fully dorsiflexed. Fixation is usually obtained by placing one or two screws from posterolaterally in the fibula to anteromedially in the tibia about 1.5 to 3.0 cm above the plafond (Fig. 52-49). Direct observation of the ankle joint provides as-

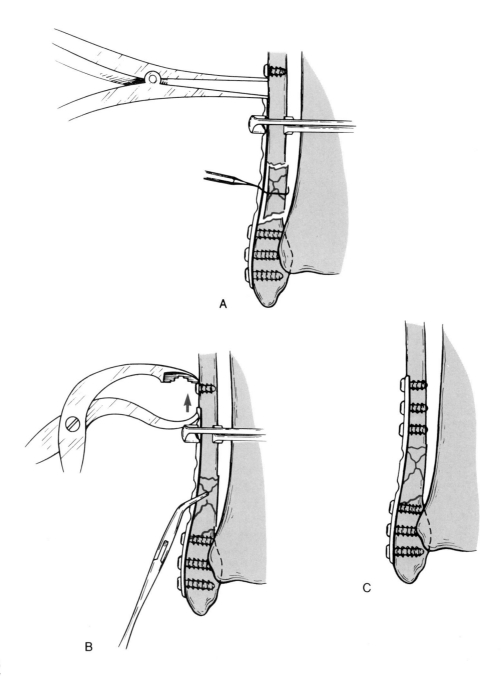

Figure 52 – 45

When a type C fibular fracture is comminuted, a plate can be used for indirect reduction while leaving soft tissue attachments on comminuted fragments. *A*, The plate is contoured and attached distally and controlled proximally with a clamp, and a bone spreader is used against a more proximal, temporary screw to push the distal fragment into a reduced position. Comminuted fragments may be teased gently into place. *B*, If fracture configuration permits, compression across it may be obtained with a small Verbrugge clamp hooked over the proximal screw. Lateral malleolar length *must* be maintained. *C*, The plate is then attached proximally. It is not necessary to place screws into small comminuted fragments. (Redrawn from Mast, J., et al. Planning and Reduction Techniques in Fracture Surgery [Fig. 3–18]. New York, Springer-Verlag, 1989.)

Figure 52-46

A, Type C bimalleolar fracture. B, Typical fixation with a one-third tubular plate and lag screw for a comminuted fragment and two 4.0-mm cancellous lag screws for the medial malleolus.

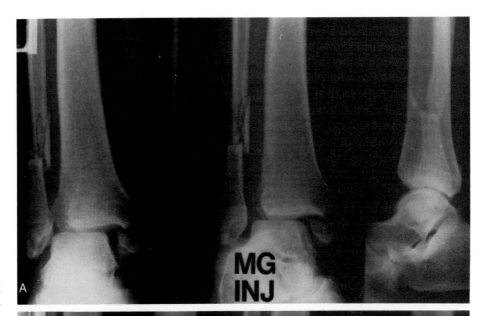

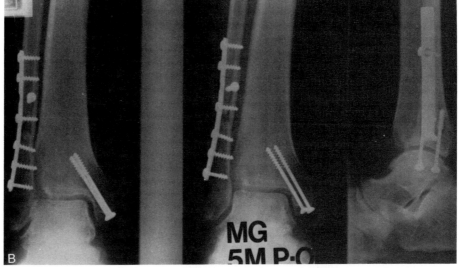

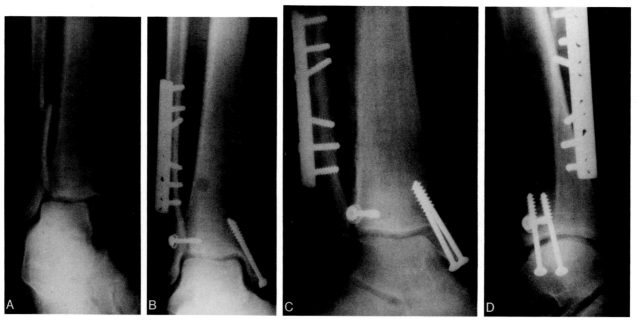

Figure 52–47

A, A Type C, atypically high pronation-abduction fracture, indicated by a transverse, laterally comminuted fracture. Injury was caused by a heavy blow to the lateral leg, just above the ankle. *B,* Intraoperative mortise radiograph showing a 3.5-mm DC plate fixation, additional repair of the syndesmosis with a screw and ligament washer to reattach the AITFL to the tubercle of Chaput, and two 4.0-mm cancellous lag screws for the medial malleolus. *C,D,* Ten weeks later both fractures had healed. Note heterotopic ossification of the torn lower interosseous membrane.

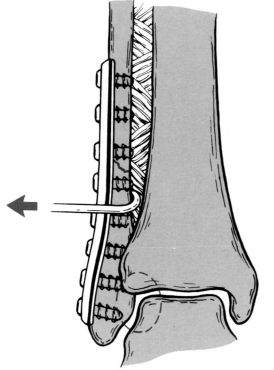

Figure 52–48

After repair of the fibula fracture, syndesmosis stability is confirmed by attempting to displace the malleolus laterally while observing the anterolateral corner of the joint for excessive movement of the fibula and talus. (Redrawn from Müller, M.E., et al. Manual of Internal Fixation, 2nd ed. New York, Springer-Verlag, 1979.)

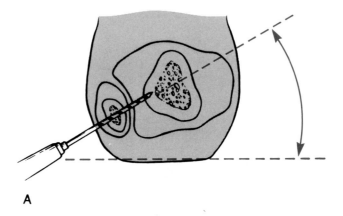

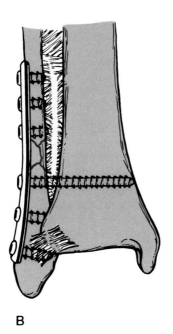

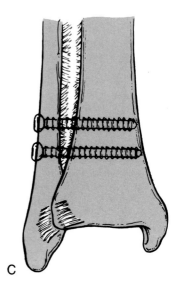

Figure 52–49

A, A syndesmosis transfixation screw must be inserted with care from posterolaterally in the fibula to anteriorly in the tibia. The appropriate angle is approximately 30° from the coronal plane. *B,* The fibula must be held reduced during screw placement, and the ankle should be fully dorsiflexed. In this example, screw is inserted through the fibular plate. *C,* Here, two screws are used for improved control when a proximal fibular fracture is not internally fixed. (Redrawn from Heim, U.; Pfeiffer, K.M. Small Fragment Set Manual: Technique Recommended by the ASIF Group, 2nd ed. New York, Springer-Verlag, 1982.)

surance that the screw is at the desired distance from it. It is essential that the tibiofibular relationship be anatomic when such screws are inserted. Provisional K-wire fixation or an appropriate clamp may help with this (Fig. 52–50). The AO group advocates use of a fully threaded screw, a "position screw," with threads tapped in a pilot hole in both the fibula and tibia. This allows essentially no motion between the two bones unless the screw loosens, as it often does. It avoids the risk of overtightening inherent with a lag screw but permits no adjustment of the relationship between the fibula and tibia from that existing when the screw is placed between the bones. The optimal type of screw is also debated and is as yet unproved. Generally a 4.5- or 3.5-mm cortical screw is chosen. Some advocate its insertion only part way through the tibia, so that the screw soon loosens. There is a small incidence of screw fracture, and a retained fragment in the tibia is

traumatic to remove. Use of a stronger screw, limited weight bearing, early screw removal, provision for some motion around the screw, and use of other devices are various ways to avoid screw failure.[58,90,92a,101,102,162]

Aware of the risks of overtightening a lag screw, others advocate use of the original AO 4.5-mm malleolar screw for syndesmosis fixation (Fig. 52–51). With the fibula reduced, a 3.2-mm drill is used to prepare a hole through the fibula and tibia. The screw length is chosen to penetrate deeply into the tibial metaphysis, approximately 3 cm above the plafond. The fibula and tibia are held reduced with the ankle fully dorsiflexed. Reduction is ascertained by inspection of the superolateral corner of the mortise. This is observed as the screw is inserted. The screw is tightened only enough to prevent lateral displacement of the fibula without compression of the mortise, which can be observed through

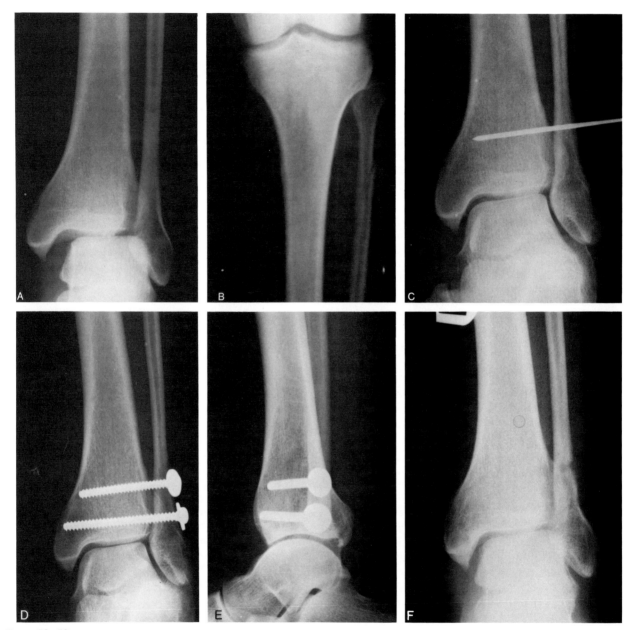

Figure 52–50

Maisonneuve fracture. *A*, Ankle radiograph shows mortise widening and lateral displacement of the talus. *B*, A spiral fracture of the proximal fibula is present. *C*, Intraoperative radiograph confirms satisfactory reduction of a provisionally fixed syndesmosis. *D,E,* Definitive fixation with two 4.5-mm cortical position screws threaded into both fibula and tibia. *F*, One year after injury, fixation has been removed, and the ankle mortise remains congruent.

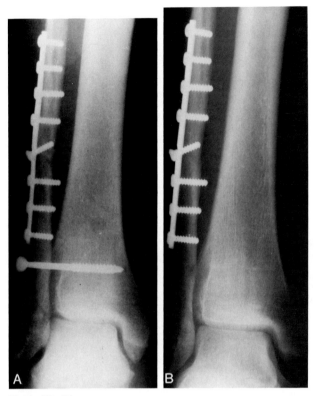

Figure 52–51

The syndesmosis was unstable after reduction and fixation of this type C supraarticular lateral malleolus fracture. *A*, The syndesmosis was stabilized with a 4.5-mm malleolar screw inserted with the syndesmosis held reduced and the ankle fully dorsiflexed. The screw was tightened just enough to retain the position of the fibula in the incisural notch, with direct inspection of the ankle to ensure that it was not compressed. *B*, The patient was allowed to bear weight with the screw in place; it was removed at three months. A year after injury, the patient had a stable syndesmosis and normal, pain-free ankle function.

the arthrotomy. The screw head retains the fibula laterally, preventing displacement. Its nonthreaded shaft is slightly loose within the fibula, permitting a small amount of motion of the bone around the screw, which is anchored securely in the tibia.

The purpose of transfixing the syndesmosis with a screw is to maintain the distal tibiofibular relationship until the syndesmotic ligaments have healed enough to do so on their own. How long it takes for sufficient ligament healing is not certain, but inference from clinical and experimental studies of the healing of other ligaments suggests that at six weeks little strength has returned. Therefore the frequent recommendation of only six weeks transfixation seems risky. A related issue is the weight-bearing regimen prescribed during and after syndesmosis screw fixation, ranging from no weight bearing to full weight bearing.

In attempting to choose the best approach, the surgeon finds an opinionated literature with little supporting data. Two of the authors use 4.5- or 3.5-mm cortical position screws, delay weight bearing for the first six weeks, and do not routinely remove the screws. This approach has an approximately 10% incidence of screw breakage. The other author generally uses a 4.5-mm malleolar screw, encourages full weight bearing in a short-leg cast if the fibula has been fixed securely, and leaves the screw in place for a minimum of three months.

Posterior Tibial Lip Fracture Reduction and Fixation. A posterior lip fracture may be associated with essentially any mechanism of malleolar fracture and may be caused by the interplay between tensile forces applied through the PITFL and compressive weight-bearing forces applied by the talar dome (Fig. 52–52). The posteromedial lip of the mortise may also be fractured by the supination-adduction mechanism.[79] Posterior lip fragments are often difficult to assess in fracture-dislocations until a provisional reduction has been achieved. They are best demonstrated by a transverse CT scan (Fig. 52–53). On the AP or mortise radiograph, the posterior lip fragment can often be observed as a double density superimposed on the tibial metaphysis. These views help in assessing the proximal extent and width of the fragment and in determining whether it is posteromedial or posterolateral in location. Comminution and obliquity of the posterior lip fragment may not be easily appreciated on the lateral ankle radiograph. Because of obliquity, the apparent size of the fragment may differ from reality. A transverse CT scan provides an explicit image of the size, location, comminution, and displacement of posterior lip fractures. The ankle should be inspected carefully for posterior subluxation of the talus relative to the tibia; this is more common with larger posterior lip fragments.

Occasionally loss of the posterior lip produces such instability that the talus redislocates posteriorly and cannot be held reduced in a cast (Fig. 52–54). Dorsiflexion tends to aggravate this situation by increasing the tension on posterior myotendinous units. Small posterior lip fragments may be extraarticular avulsions. Larger ones, however, do involve the joint. Most authors agree that if more than 25% to 35% of the joint surface is involved, the fragment should be reduced and fixed to stabilize the ankle and decrease the risk of posttraumatic arthrosis caused by irregularity of the joint surface.[79,145,251a,251b] Although closed reduction of a displaced posterior lip fragment is rarely successful, such fragments are usually connected to the distal fibular fragment by the PITFL. Therefore precise open reduction of the lateral malleolus often results in a close,

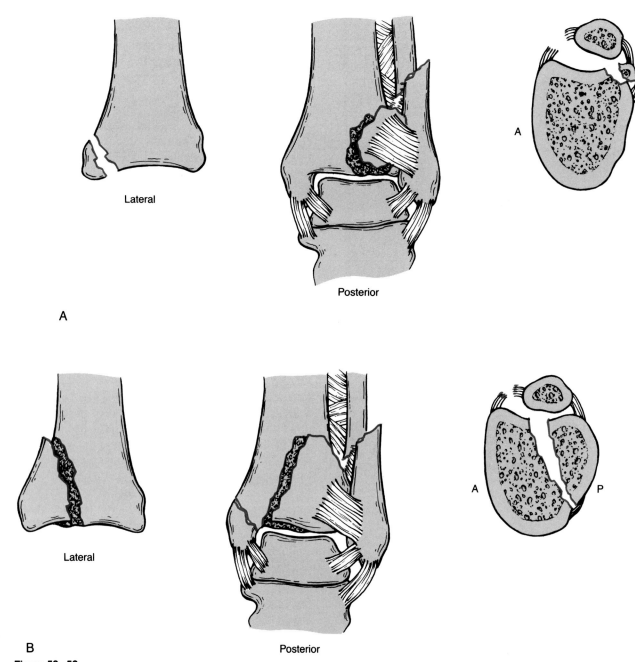

A

Lateral

Posterior

A

P

B

Lateral

Posterior

A

P

Figure 52–52

Posterior malleolar fractures may be small (A), often extraarticular, or they may be large articular fragments that require reduction to prevent posterior dislocation of the talus (B). Careful inspection of AP and mortise radiographs often reveals whether the fragment is more medial or lateral in location. (Redrawn from Heim, U.; Pfeiffer, K.M. Small Fragment Set Manual: Technique Recommended by the ASIF Group, 2nd ed. New York, Springer-Verlag, 1982.)

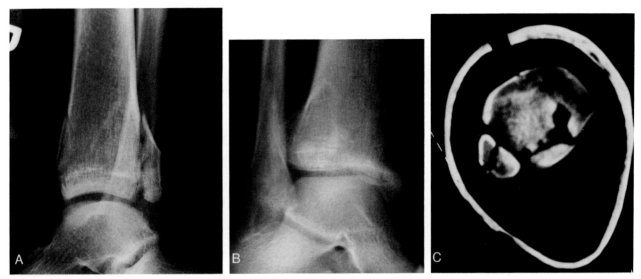

Figure 52–53

Lateral (A) and oblique (B) radiographs demonstrate a small, displaced posterior lip fracture. C, The CT scan shows impaction, interposed fragments, and significant displacement just above the articular surface.

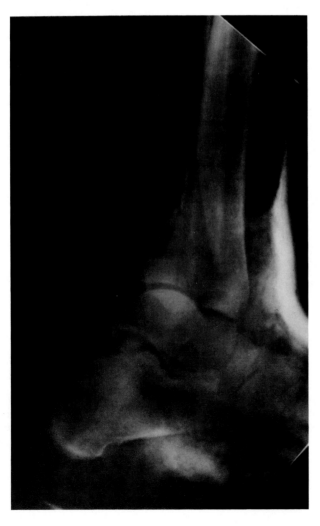

Figure 52–54

After an attempted closed reduction, posterior dislocation persists. Note that the ankle has been dorsiflexed to neutral, probably increasing the tension in posterior soft tissues and adding to the difficulty of regaining tibiotalar alignment.

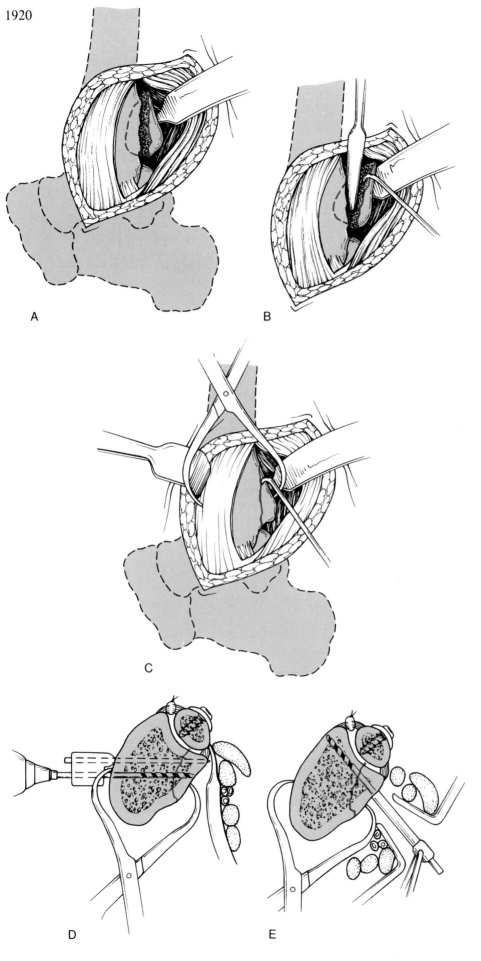

Figure 52–55

Reduction and fixation of a posterior malleolar fragment through a posteromedial approach. The flexor tendons and neurovascular bundle are retracted posteriorly with a Hohmann retractor, the fragment is manipulated into place, and provisional fixation is made, often with a pointed reduction clamp. Occasionally the articular surface reduction can be seen directly through an unreduced medial malleolar fracture. A confirmatory radiograph should be taken. Definitive fixation is obtained with anteroposterior lag screws or occasionally, as also shown, with a screw inserted through the interval between the Achilles tendon and the structures behind the medial malleolus. (Redrawn from Heim, U.; Pfeiffer, K.M. Small Fragment Set Manual: Technique Recommended by the ASIF Group, 2nd ed. New York, Springer-Verlag, 1982.)

A

B

C

D

E

if not anatomic, realignment of the posterior tibial lip fragment. Some suggest that this is all that is necessary, unless the weight-bearing surface of the plafond is distorted or posterior subluxation of the talus persists.[82] Others advise routine fixation of all posterior lip fragments.[84] The optimal approach remains controversial.

Indications for reduction and fixation of posterior lip fragments thus depend significantly on the judgment of the surgeon. Posterior talar subluxation or dislocation, plafond articular incongruity, and possibly stabilization of the syndesmosis are the usual reasons for ORIF of a posterior lip fragment.

The surgical approach should be guided by the location of the fragment, by the incisions required for treatment of associated components of the ankle injury, and by the preoperative plan for fixation.[85] Generally some direct access to the posterior fragment is necessary, although often the articular surface reduction is not fully visualized. When the joint surface is not seen and its reduction is judged by the extraarticular portion of the fracture line, it is wise to obtain an intraoperative lateral radiograph following provisional K wire or clamp fixation of the fragment before definitive screws are inserted. Revision of fixation may not be possible after lag screws have been placed.

Posterior lip fragments can best be reattached with one or two lag screws, occasionally supplemented with K wires, washers, or, rarely, a small buttress plate. It is important to avoid penetrating the ankle joint with such implants, but they must be close to it to obtain good fixation, as the distal base of the wedge-shaped fragment is thickest. The most secure fixation is provided by interfragmentary fixation with lag screws, which must glide through the fragment adjacent to their head and be threaded only into the opposite fragment. Such screws can be placed from posterior to anterior if the fragment is exposed using a posterolateral incision. Otherwise they must be inserted from anterior to posterior using the anteromedial incision or a small anterolateral stab incision. Screws placed from posteriorly can be either 4.0- or, very rarely, 6.5-mm cancellous lag screws or fully threaded screws inserted through a predrilled sliding hole in the posterior fragment. Lag screws inserted from anteriorly pose the problem of gaining maximal purchase in the posterior fragment without having threads on both sides of the fracture line. It is rare, and difficult to ensure, that a partially threaded lag screw is appropriate for this. Sometimes cutting off a portion of the screw's tip will permit 4.0-mm cancellous screws to be used this way. A better technique is to overdrill a gliding hole and place the appropriate insert drill sleeve in the anterior metaphyseal fragment before reduction. Then the posterior lip fragment is reduced and provisionally fixed, its

alignment is confirmed by a lateral radiograph, and the threaded hole is drilled through the sleeve and tapped if necessary. Finally the fragments are lagged together with a fully threaded 3.5- or 4.5-mm cortical screw of appropriate length. In general, anteroposterior screws are better suited for larger posterior fragments. The choice of whether to use a medial or lateral insertion site can be made according to the obliquity of the fragment and the need for other incisions. Unless the piece is small, a second screw or at least a heavy K wire may be advisable to prevent rotation around a single implant. Small posterior fragments are best fixed with screws inserted from posterior to anterior, with care taken to avoid the joint surface, which is convex proximally.

Reduction of posterior lip fragments can be done indirectly through either posteromedial or posterolateral incisions. The choice is often best made by the location of the fragment on the AP radiograph. Posteromedial exposure is by retraction of the flexor tendons and neurovascular bundle from the posteromedial tibial cortex (Fig. 52–55). As illustrated in the figure, it may be possible to insert a posteroanterior screw in such a fragment through a plane between the deep flexors and the Achilles tendon.

Posterolateral exposure of a posterior lip fragment is through the interval between the peroneal tendons and the Achilles tendon (Fig. 52–56). Attention must be taken to protect the sural nerve. This approach is greatly facilitated by having the patient lie prone or on the unaffected side. Unfortunately, both these positions hamper medial exposure and interfere with reduction and fixation of the medial malleolus. For the prone patient, internal rotation of the leg, aided by a cushion anterior to the opposite hip, eases access to the medial malleolus, if it must also be fixed.

Through either a posterolateral or a posteromedial approach, the fragment is retracted and hematoma removed from the fracture cleft with irrigation and suction. The peripheral margin of the fracture is used as a guide to fragment reduction, perhaps aided by a small arthrotomy or occasionally by visualization of the plafond through the bed of an as-yet-unreduced medial or lateral malleolar fracture. A sharp dental pick, K wires, and the three-hole pointed drill guide aid reduction. Provisional fixation from the anterior tibia to the posterior lip fragment is achieved with K wires or occasionally large, pointed reduction forceps. Unless the articular surface is well seen, a lateral radiograph of the provisional reduction should be obtained before definitive fixation. Final intraoperative radiographs are then routinely obtained after all fixation is in place but before the sterile field is broken, in case changes are required (Figs. 52–57, 52–58, and 52–59).

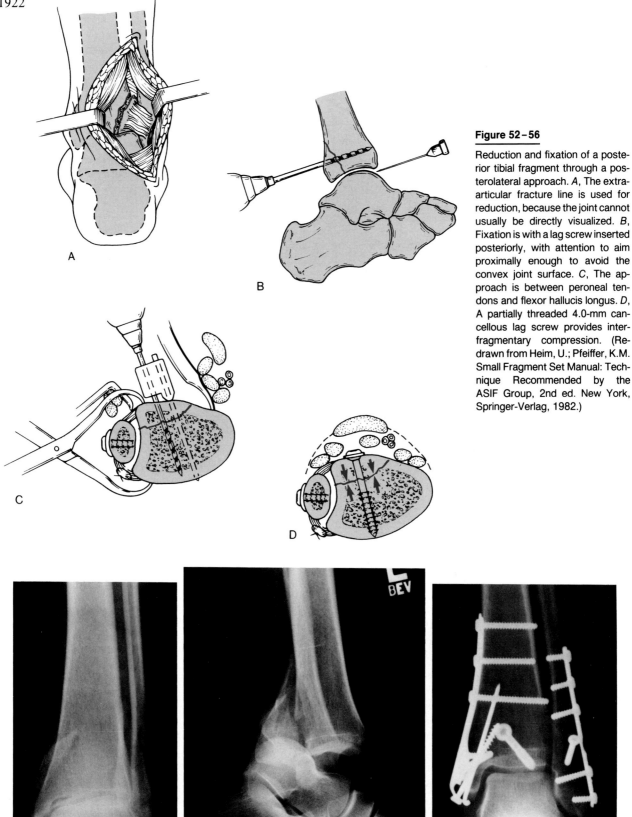

Figure 52–56

Reduction and fixation of a posterior tibial fragment through a posterolateral approach. *A*, The extra-articular fracture line is used for reduction, because the joint cannot usually be directly visualized. *B*, Fixation is with a lag screw inserted posteriorly, with attention to aim proximally enough to avoid the convex joint surface. *C*, The approach is between peroneal tendons and flexor hallucis longus. *D*, A partially threaded 4.0-mm cancellous lag screw provides interfragmentary compression. (Redrawn from Heim, U.; Pfeiffer, K.M. Small Fragment Set Manual: Technique Recommended by the ASIF Group, 2nd ed. New York, Springer-Verlag, 1982.)

Figure 52–57

A, B, Fracture-dislocation of the ankle with a large posterior lip fragment and extensive medial malleolar comminution. *C,* A cannulated posterior malleolar screw placed over a provisional K wire. A medial coverleaf plate and standard lateral malleolar construct complete the fixation.

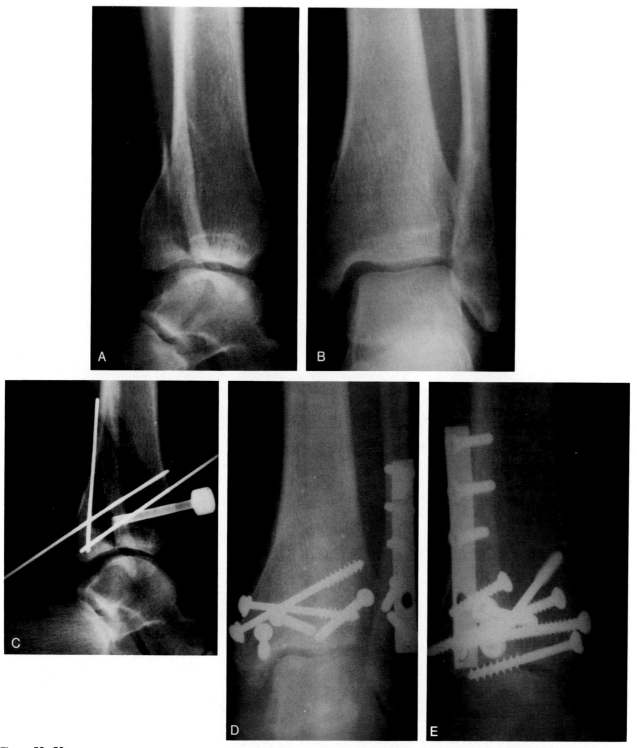

Figure 52–58

A, Articular incongruence is primarily caused by a large, displaced posterior malleolar fragment. *B*, A comminuted medial malleolar fracture is also present. *C*, After predrilling the anterior distal tibia for a 3.5-mm sliding hole, the insert drill sleeve is placed, and a provisional reduction accomplished with K wire fixation. This radiograph confirms anatomic realignment of the joint surface. *D,E* Fixation was completed with multiple lag screws and a fibular plate. The fracture healed uneventfully.

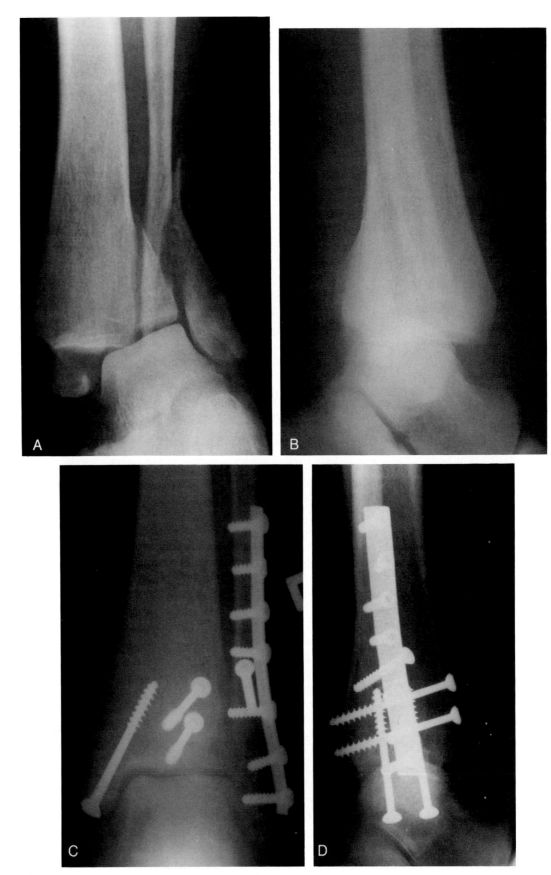

Figure 52–59

A,B, Trimalleolar fracture-dislocation with a significant posterior lip fragment. *C,D,* Fixation with two 4.0-mm cancellous lag screws inserted from front to back. It was fortunate that the threads were the right length for this fixation, which would have been impaired had they crossed the fracture line.

Clearly, in view of the many options and multiple steps involved in fixing a trimalleolar fracture, the surgical team will be aided and the result often improved by careful preoperative assessment and a detailed, explicit preoperative plan for positioning, exposure, reduction, fixation, and radiographic documentation. If many radiographs will be needed or if parts of the reduction and fixation are to be done without direct visualization, the use of image-intensification fluoroscopy may be helpful, and appropriate positioning and use of the table should be planned. Image quality, however, may lack the detail obtained with standard radiographs, which are the best confirmation of final reduction and fixation.

When there is a large posterior lip fracture, extensive visualization of the plafond is possible by delivering the distal tibia through a medial incision, as has been advocated by Shelton and described recently by Grantham.[74] Both advise release of the posterior lip fragment from its attached PITFL and a careful search for any comminuted fragments of articular surface in the joint. The entire distal tibial plafond is delivered through an approximately 7-in medial incision while the talus, lateral and medial malleolar fragments, and foot are dislocated laterally. This requires release and posterior retraction of the posterior tibial tendon sheath. According to the technique's proponents, comminution and bone grafting, if needed, can readily be dealt with through this approach. After reconstruction of the plafond, the talus is relocated, and the lateral and medial malleoli are fixed in the usual fashion.

Anterior Lip Fractures. The location and character of anterior lip injuries will determine the approach and fixation. A CT scan may be helpful for preoperative planning. If extensive comminution of the anterior lip is a relatively isolated injury, an anterolateral arthrotomy lateral to the extensor tendons may be the best access. Extensive comminution may require buttress fixation, with a small plate. An avulsed Tillaux fragment (anterolateral articular surface) should be reduced and fixed with a lag screw. An impacted anterolateral fragment may be excised, if small, or elevated with bone grafting, if it involves a significant part of the articular surface.

Medial Malleolar and Ligamentous Injuries. Operative treatment of medial ankle disruptions in malleolar injuries may not always be necessary. Since recognition of the vital role of the lateral malleolus, many authors have reported satisfactory results with anatomic repair of the lateral malleolus and nonoperative management of complete deltoid ligament disruptions. In general, fractures of the medial malleolus should be reduced and fixed to add stability, maintain joint congruity, and decrease the rather low risk of a symptomatic medial malleolar nonunion.

A straight, slightly oblique, or curving incision is made according to the surgeon's preference and the planned fixation (Fig. 52–60). Anteriorly, the saphenous vein and its accompanying cutaneous nerve branches should be protected. The incision should permit an anteromedial ankle arthrotomy as well as visualization of both the anterior and medial aspects of any malleolar fracture. The joint is inspected and any loose osteochondral shards removed. Retraction of the malleolar fragment demonstrates the flexor tendons, which are occasionally injured. The tibialis posterior is most commonly involved, and it should be checked to exclude injury.[52,205,220] Local comminution may be associated with posterior tibial tendon involvement.[228]

The medial surface of the plafond should be assessed through the fracture site, especially in supination-adduction injuries, to search for an impacted area that may need elevation and bone grafting of any resulting defect. Usually only a small amount of graft is required, and this can be obtained from the more proximal part of the tibial pilon or, through a separate incision, from Gerdy's tubercle (Figs. 52–61 and 52–62).

If repair of the deltoid ligament is desired, its deep portion must be visualized, usually posteriorly after retraction of the tendons, and sutures placed before the lateral side has been fixed. The talus must be displaced laterally to permit this. Depending on the location of

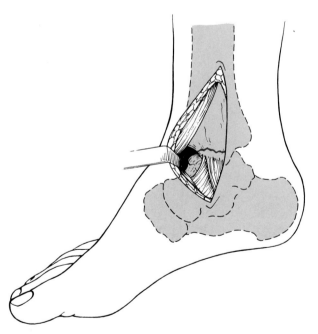

Figure 52–60

The medial malleolus is approached through a longitudinal incision that allows access to the anterolateral corner of the ankle joint and as much of the distal tibia as required. A longer incision is better than too-vigorous retraction. Attention is paid to the saphenous nerve branches, which may cause a painful neuroma if caught in the scar.

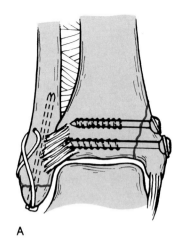

A

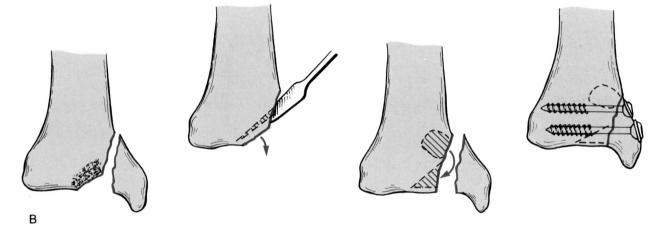

B

Figure 52–61

A, The vertical type A medial malleolar fracture is fixed with two or more lag screws inserted perpendicular to the fracture. The use of washers or, rarely, a buttress plate is wise. *B*, If there is impaction of the medial plafond, the articular cartilage and subchondral bone are carefully pried en masse back into place against the reduced talus, and bone graft is inserted into the defect before the medial malleolus is repaired. (*A*, Redrawn from Heim, U.; Pfeiffer, K.M. Small Fragment Set Manual: Technique Recommended by the ASIF Group, 2nd ed. New York, Springer-Verlag, 1982. *B*, Redrawn from Müller, M.E., et al. Manual of Internal Fixation, 2nd ed. New York, Springer-Verlag, 1979.)

the tear, sutures may be placed through drill holes in the malleolus or talus to provide secure reattachment. A few sutures in the superficial deltoid may improve the appearance of the repair but will probably add little to stability of the ankle.

Avulsion fractures of the medial malleolus are best reduced after exposing both the anterior and medial aspects of the fracture by sharply turning back the periosteum and attached fascia. The fragment is grasped with a small towel clip or pointed reduction forceps and maneuvered into place with this and the aid of a sharp dental pick. It can be held in place with this or with a bone hook while two fixation points are achieved. For smaller fragments, especially if incipient comminution is noted, two small K wires (1.2- or 1.6-mm) may be

chosen. For intermediate fragments, use one wire and a 2.0- or 2.5-mm drill bit to prepare a hole for a 4.0-mm partially threaded cancellous screw. For larger fragments, two such drills are used for provisional fixation and replaced one at a time with the 4.0-mm partially threaded screws. Cancellous screws for fixation of medial malleolar fractures should be inserted so as to avoid comminution of the fragment (i.e., not too close to its edge and not overtightened). They should be oriented perpendicular to the plane of the fracture. To obtain a lag effect, their threads must not cross the fracture. They should be seated in the dense bone of the central distal tibial metaphysis and thus should be approximately 40-mm long. Do not attempt to anchor them in the far cortex, which is too thin to provide than through a transverse drill hole (Figs. 52–63 and 52–64).

If the medial malleolar fracture is vertical or oblique, as in supination-adduction (type A) injuries, the orientation of lag screws to fix the fracture will be different. They must be inserted perpendicular to the fracture and thus are fairly transverse. Washers are more likely to be needed because of the thinner medial cortex, and occasionally even a small medial buttress plate is advisable, if the bone is osteopenic or excessively comminuted. Three or more screws may be used with vertical fractures if the medial fragment is large enough.

Intraoperative Radiographs. Adequate intraoperative radiographs must be obtained to confirm the re-

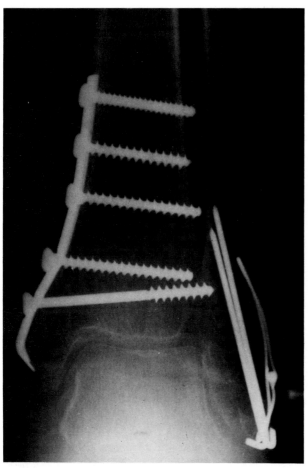

Figure 52–62

Occasionally the supination-adduction medial malleolus fracture requires buttress support, analogous to an impacted tibial plateau fracture. A one-third tubular plate has been flattened, cut through the distal hole to provide prongs for additional fixation, and secured with multiple screws. This weight-bearing radiograph was taken nine months after fixation of the fracture seen in Figure 52–22.

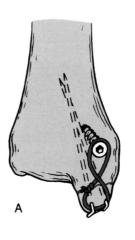
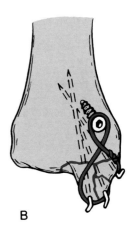
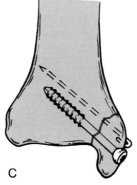
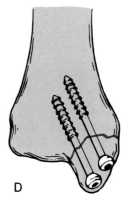

A   B

C   D

Figure 52–63

Fixation of avulsion fractures of the medial malleolus depends on their size and comminution. Small or comminuted fragments are best repaired with K wires and a tension band wire. A larger piece can be fixed with a single K wire and a lag screw, or two lag screws. Usually 4.0-mm partially threaded lag screws are used. They are inserted perpendicular to the fracture line. Provisional fixation of a medial malleolar fragment is often better done with K wires or 2.5-mm drill bits, rather than clamps, which might comminute or displace it.

much purchase. This can cause either the drill or the screw to deviate during the insertion process and thus lead to malreduction or comminution of the malleolar fragment. Although tapping of cancellous bone is not needed and may reduce the pull-out strength of screws, the use of an appropriate tap through the malleolus and just across the fracture may ease screw insertion and reduce risk of comminution. A preliminary small incision of the superficial deltoid fibers before drilling the pilot hole will aid this.

When the medial malleolar fragment is too small for screws or if comminution develops, the use of K wires with a figure-of-8 tension band can provide satisfactory fixation. The ends of the K wires are bent over and gently impacted over the tension band. Proximal anchorage for the wire can be over a screwhead rather

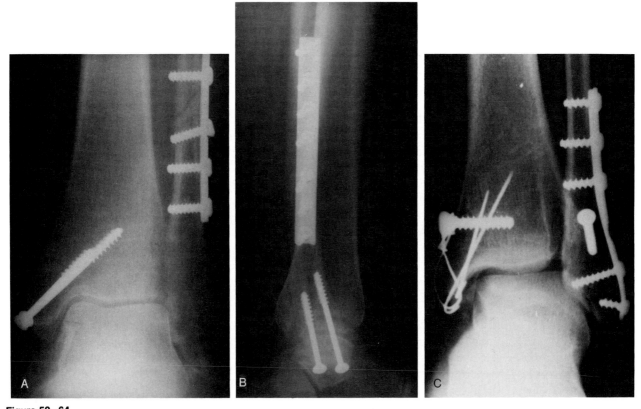

Figure 52-64

Medial malleolus fixation with two 4.0-mm cancellous lag screws. *A*, Mortise, *B*, Lateral, radiographs. Note insertion of the threads only into the densest bone of the central metaphysis and their posterior orientation to accommodate the anteriorly situated medial malleolus. *C*, K-wires and a tension band loop are more appropriate for a small or comminuted medial malleolar avulsion. Note the use of a screw for proximal anchorage of the wire.

duction and fixation of any periarticular fracture, and this holds true for malleolar injuries. In general, AP, lateral, and mortise exposures are made during or just prior to wound closure. More reproducible radiographs can be obtained with a radiolucent positioning jig (e.g., A.L.A.R.M., manufactured by M.C. Johnson Co. Inc., Leominster, Massachusetts 01453). The ankle should be in neutral during AP, mortise, and lateral radiographs, and the radiographs should be carefully checked for adequate positioning and exposure, malleolar fracture reduction (especially the talotibial relationship), the tibiofibular relationship (syndesmosis), the articular surfaces, the length and rotation of the lateral malleolus, and the location of any inserted hardware.

Wound Closure and Postoperative Care. The wounds are irrigated and closed atraumatically, usually with interrupted nonabsorbable skin sutures, although some urge that deeper tissues be approximated as well. Small suction drains may decrease problems from hematomas. Generally, a very well padded, loosely wrapped short-leg splint is applied to hold the ankle fully dorsiflexed. Such a splint can be used until the sutures are removed and the surgeon's choice of subsequent immobilization is applied. It is important to splint the ankle in as much dorsiflexion as possible, for this is hard to regain if an equinus contracture is allowed to develop.

According to Ahl and co-workers,[1] it makes little difference to most patients what postoperative immobilization regimen is followed, though with tenuous fixation, osteopenic bone, or an uncooperative or neuropathic patient, more rather than less protection may be advisable. Accordingly, the ankle may be placed in a long- or short-leg non–weight-bearing cast, a short-leg walking cast, a hinged brace, a removable bivalved cast, or an elastic support with crutches to limit weight bearing.[37,49,51a,60,61,102,113,124,125,159,194,211,225] After the first six weeks (if the fracture is only malleolar) or longer (if there is plafond involvement), progressive unrestricted weight bearing can usually be allowed with safety. Crutches are appropriate until the patient is walking well without a limp and radiographic healing is advanced. Range-of-motion, strengthening, endurance, and agility exercises are also necessary elements of the rehabilitation program, which usually lasts several months before the patient can return to vigorous work and athletics. Some swelling of the soft tissues frequently persists for months.[55]

Results of Treatment

The outcome of an injury is best judged by how much it affects the patient. Pain, impaired function, deformity, and loss of motion are all important factors. A variety of rating systems have been proposed for the subjective and objective components of clinical results of ankle injuries. Results are usually stratified into groups for analysis. Criteria for this are not uniform, so it is unwise to compare published series directly. Rating and scoring systems often give different levels of importance to different variables, and most include several interrelated aspects of ankle function or anatomy. Some systems consider only functional outcome; others include clinical exams and radiographic findings. Some rely heavily on the ability to work or participate in sports, criteria that are irrelevant to certain categories of patients. An example of an ankle scoring system is that of Baird and Jackson, modified from Weber's, that was presented by Hughes et al. (Table 52–2).[11,91,247] Note that fewer than 80 points on their scale is considered a poor result. Another, more functionally oriented, alternative is that of Mazur et al. (Table 52–3).[144] Olerud and Molander offer yet another (Table 52–4).[168]

Radiographic results may be assessed separately or combined with subjective and objective clinical data.[11,99,176] Both the quality of reduction after healing and the presence of degenerative changes are pertinent. Joy et al. presented objective techniques for measurement of malleolar and talar displacement.[99] Goergen et al. emphasized the value of adequately positioned radiographs for such assessments.[68] Pettrone and co-workers demonstrated the predictive validity of radiographic criteria—particularly displacement of either malleolus, syndesmosis widening, and increased clear space between the medial malleolus and the medial surface of the talus.[176] In a prospective study, Phillips et al. noted that the significant indicators of a poor result after severe external rotation ankle fractures were talar subluxation on the lateral radiograph and lateral malleolar shortening, as measured directly or by a different talocrural angle from the normal side (see Fig. 52–10).[177]

Osteoarthritis of the ankle joint, rare except after injury, is manifested by osteophyte formation, narrowing of the radiolucent cartilage space, and subchondral sclerosis and cyst formation. Radiographs made during weight bearing have not always been used to diagnose joint narrowing. The changes of osteoarthritis tend to

---

Table 52–2.

Ankle Scoring System*

	Points
Pain	
A. No pain	15
B. Mild pain with strenuous activity	12
C. Mild pain with activities of daily living	8
D. Pain with weight-bearing	4
E. Pain at rest	0
Stability of ankle	
A. No clinical instability	15
B. Instability with sports activities	5
C. Instability with activities of daily living	0
Ability to walk	
A. Able to walk desired distances without limp or pain	15
B. Able to walk desired distances with mild limp or pain	12
C. Moderately restricted in ability to walk	8
D. Able to walk short distances only	4
E. Unable to walk	0
Ability to run	
A. Able to run desired distances without pain	10
B. Able to run desired distances with slight pain	8
C. Moderate restriction in ability to run, with mild pain	6
D. Able to run short distances only	3
E. Unable to run	0
Ability to work	
A. Able to perform usual occupation	10
B. Able to perform usual occupation with restrictions in some strenuous activities	8
C. Able to perform usual occupation with substantial restrictions	6
D. Partially disabled; selected jobs only	3
E. Unable to work	0
Motion of the ankle	
A. Within 10° of uninjured ankle	10
B. Within 15° of uninjured ankle	7
C. Within 20° of uninjured ankle	4
D. <50% of uninjured ankle, or dorsiflexion < 5°	0
Radiographic result	
A. Anatomic with intact mortise (normal medial clear space, normal superior joint space, no talar tilt)	25
B. Same as A with mild reactive changes at the joint margins	15
C. Measurable narrowing of superior joint space, with superior joint space >2 mm, or talar tilt >2 mm	10
D. Moderate narrowing of the superior joint space, with superior joint space between 2 and 1 mm	5
E. Severe narrowing of the superior joint space, with superior joint space < 1 mm, widening of the medial clear space, severe reactive changes (sclerotic subchondral bone and osteophyte formation)	0
Maximum possible score	100

* Excellent = 96 to 100 points, good = 91 to 95 points, fair = 81 to 90 points, and poor = zero to 80 points.
Source: Baird, R.A.; Jackson, S.T. J Bone Joint Surg 69A(9):1347, 1987.

Table 52-3.

Ankle Evaluation Grading System (Wearing Shoes)

Pain			Support			Ability to rise on toes (stability)	
None, or patient ignores it	50		None	6		Able to rise on toes × 10 repetitions	5
Slight when going up or down stairs or walking long distances (no restriction of activities of daily living)	45		Cane, long walks only	5		Able to rise on toes × 3 repetitions	3
			Cane, full time	3		Able to rise on toes × 1 repetition	1
			Two canes or crutches	1		Unable to rise on toes	0
Moderate when going up or down stairs or walking long distances; none during level gait; occasional non-narcotic medication needed	40		Walker required or unable to walk	0		Total ___	
			Total ___			Running	
						Able to run as much as desired	5
During level gait, with more pain on stairs; none at rest; daily medication used	25		Hills (up)			Able to run but limited	3
			Climbs normally	3		Unable to run	0
			Climbs with foot externally rotated	2		Total ___	
At rest or night plus during walking; narcotic medication required	10		Climbs on toes or by side-stepping	1			
			Unable to climb hills	0		Range of motion	
Continuous, regardless of activity	0		Total ___			Dorsiflexion beyond neutral	
Disabled because of pain	0					40°	5
Total ___			Hills (down)			30°	4
			Descends normally	3		20°	3
			Descends with foot externally rotated	2		10°	2
Function			Descends on toes or by side-stepping	1		5°	1
Limp, antalgic			Unable to descend	0		0°	0
None	6		Total ___			Total ___	
Slight	4						
Moderate	2		Stairs (up)				
Marked	0		Climbs normally	3		Plantarflexion	
Total ___			Needs banister	2		40°	5
			Steps up with normal foot only	1		30°	4
			Unable to climb stairs	0		20°	3
Distance			Total ___			10°	2
Unlimited	6					5°	1
4-6 blocks	4		Stairs (down)			0°	0
1-3 blocks	2		Descends normally	3		Total ___	
Indoors only	1		Needs banister	2			
Bed to chair	0		Steps down with normal foot only	1			
Unable to walk	0		Unable to descend stairs	0			
Total ___			Total ___				

Source: Mazur, J.M. et al. J Bone Joint Surg 61A:966, 1979.

develop early (within two to three years) after injury and may not progress.[124] Although the significance of slight joint narrowing is not clear, poor clinical results are associated with more advanced osteoarthritis.

A number of factors affect the outcome of ankle fractures. A very important one is the severity of the original injury. This is indicated primarily by the amount of damage to the plafond and by the amount of impaction, comminution, or displacement of the posterior lip fracture. Involvement of multiple structures is also pertinent, so that higher grade injuries, using the Lauge-Hansen system, have a poorer prognosis, as do trimalleolar fractures when compared with those involving a single malleolus. Some, but not all, reports suggest that women and older patients experience poorer results, although they may be less troubled because of reduced functional demands. The fracture type (Lauge-Hansen or AO/ASIF) carries variable prognostic weight, depending on the study.[79,124] The

presence of a posterior lip fracture, even when small, adversely affects the prognosis of malleolar fractures.[85,96]

A recent significant finding is the benign nature and good outcome of supination–external rotation grade II lateral malleolar fractures.[16,36,112,244] Prolonged follow-up after nonoperative treatment in a short-leg weight-bearing cast reveals an extremely low incidence of arthrosis and symptoms, in spite of an initial 2- to 3-mm displacement of many of these isolated injuries. It is important to distinguish these from the very similar supination–external rotation type IV injuries with deltoid ligament ruptures medially, as they have a much worse prognosis.

The adequacy of reduction after fracture healing is a very significant determinant of outcome. Lindsjö reported 87% good-to-excellent results in 217 patients with well-reduced, originally displaced malleolar fractures, compared with 68% good-to-excellent results in

Table 52–4.
The Ankle Score

I. Pain (25 points)	None	25 points
	While walking on uneven surface	20
	While walking on even surface outdoors	10
	While walking indoors	5
	Constant and severe	0
II. Stiffness (10 points)	None	10
	Stiffness	0
III. Swelling (10 points)	None	10
	Only evenings	5
	Constant	0
IV. Stair climbing (10 points)	No problems	10
	Impaired	5
	Unable	0
V. Running (5 points)	Possible	5
	Impossible	0
VI. Jumping (5 points)	Possible	5
	Impossible	0
VII. Squatting (5 points)	No problems	5
	Unable	0
VIII. Supports (10 points)	No support	10
	Taping, wrapping	5
	Stick or crutch	0
IX. Work, activities of daily life (20 points)	Same as before injury	20
	Loss of tempo	15
	Change to a simpler job/half time	10
	Disabled, strongly impaired work capacity	0

Source: Olerud, C.; Molander, H. Clin Orthop 206:255, 1986.

89 patients with inadequate reductions.[124] These patients were treated with AO fixation techniques and had a higher incidence of maintained reduction and of good outcomes than those in a series reported by Cedell with less rigid fixation.[35a] Similar good results following anatomic reduction and rigid fixation were reported by others, including Hughes et al., from several Swiss centers.[51a,91,130] Satisfactory outcomes were achieved in 78% to 83% of type A, 76% to 83% of type B, and 62% to 85% of type C malleolar injuries. A comparable group of patients with similar injuries treated nonoperatively had satisfactory results in 71% to 75% of type A, 35% to 43% of type B, and 23% to 37% of type C fractures.

Results with less satisfactory approaches to reduction and internal fixation (i.e., medial fixation alone, approximate reduction, or avoidance of lateral plates) are generally poorer as well, though they are not strictly compared in the literature.[99,145,170,176,177]

Subjective complaints are common after malleolar fractures, even after several years. Many authors report an approximately 30% incidence of such symptoms, although there is evidence that the symptoms gradually improve.[16,17,121] The reported incidence of significant posttraumatic osteoarthritis after malleolar fractures ranges from negligible in supination–external rotation type II injuries to 37% or more in more severely displaced patterns, especially if posterior malleolar involvement is present.[16] It is also clear that the incidence of arthritis is much greater if a malleolar fracture heals with significant displacement.[91,176,260]

Distal Tibial Metaphyseal Fractures (Pilon Fractures)

Fractures significantly involving the weight-bearing articular surface and the overlying metaphysis of the distal tibia have achieved deserved notoriety as a severe and challenging subset of ankle injuries. Although both medial and lateral malleoli are often involved, and although there may be a posterior malleolar fragment as well, the focus of injury is above the malleoli. The extent of involvement and frequent comminution of both the plafond articular surface and the distal tibial metaphysis generally serve to distinguish these injuries from trimalleolar fractures, although there is no absolute boundary between them. Severe pilon fractures are often similar to both-column acetabular fractures in that no portion of the tibial articular surface remains attached to the more proximal skeleton. (The reader is reminded that the term "pilon" describes not the

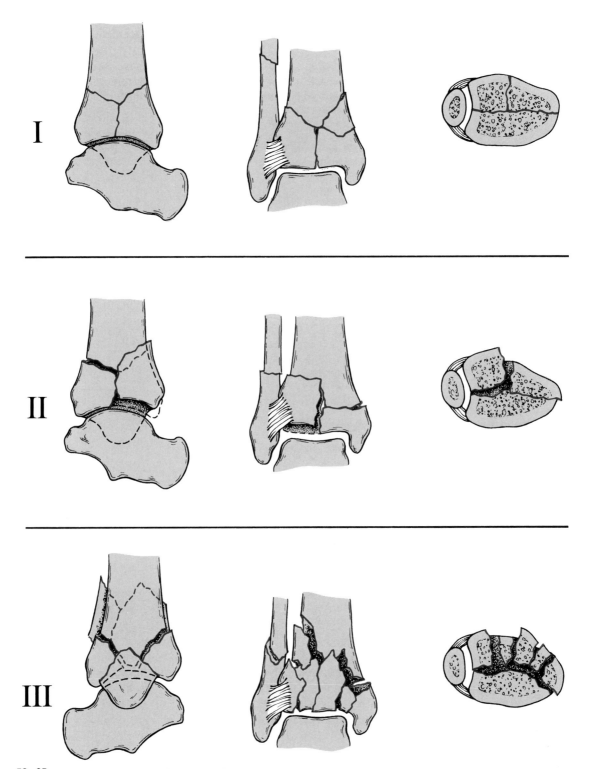

Figure 52–65

The Rüedi and Allgöwer classification for pilon fractures. Type I is undisplaced, with splitting fracture lines. Type II has displacement of the articular surface, with split type fractures. Type III is a crush or impacted injury with comminution and displacement of the articular surface. (Redrawn from Müller, M.E., et al. Manual of Internal Fixation, 2nd ed. New York, Springer-Verlag, 1979.)

mechanism but the region, which resembles the pestle used with a pharmacist's mortar.) A fall from a height or a motor vehicle crash is the typical mechanism. Associated injuries are thus to be expected.

Tibial pilon fractures are produced by either or both of two types of force: *shearing forces* that split apart bone fragments or *compressive forces* (from axial loading) that crush and impact them. Radiographs of the injured area usually provide graphic documentation of the interplay between these two types of force. Severity of injury is greater when there has been more comminution, displacement, and impaction. With either mechanism, significant damage may occur to the thin soft tissue envelope that surrounds the ankle. Although an open wound may or may not be present, forces absorbed by the soft tissues at the moment of injury can be severe enough to cause necrosis or to prevent healing of a surgical incision.

In understanding these challenging fractures, it is important to categorize them according to injury severity. Results are far better and complications much less common in those pilon fractures that have less comminution, crushing, and displacement.[10,27,170,236] To make this distinction, the classification proposed by Rüedi

and Allgöwer[200] is helpful, effective, and well recognized (Fig. 52–65). Grade I injuries are those with no significant articular displacement. These are generally cleavage fractures without separation of bone fragments. Grade II injuries have significant displacement of articular surface cleavage fracture lines, but the joint surface itself is not crushed or grossly comminuted (Fig. 52–66). Grade III injuries have significant comminution and impaction involving both the articular surface and the metaphyseal bone (Fig. 52–67).

The AO classification system has since been altered so that type I injuries may have articular displacement but are not comminuted or impacted. Type 2 injuries have impaction involving only the supraarticular metaphysis, and type 3 injuries, in addition to impaction, have comminution and crushing of the articular surface.[161]

Mast has offered another variation on classifications for metaphyseal fractures of the distal tibia. His type I fractures consist of malleolar fractures with significant posterior lip articular fragments. Type II fractures are spiral fractures of the distal tibia with extension into the plafond, as described by Maale and Seligson.[128] Type III injuries are "central compression injuries" catego-

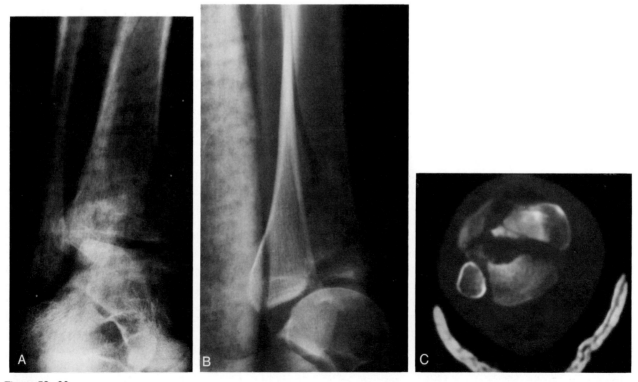

Figure 52-66

A type II (split) pilon fracture caused by a fall. *A,* Anteroposterior, *B,* Lateral, radiographs. The posterior fragment is not displaced far from the shaft, whereas the talus is anteriorly dislocated along with the anterior lip fragment. *C,* The CT scan demonstrates some comminution and a slight amount of impaction anterolaterally.

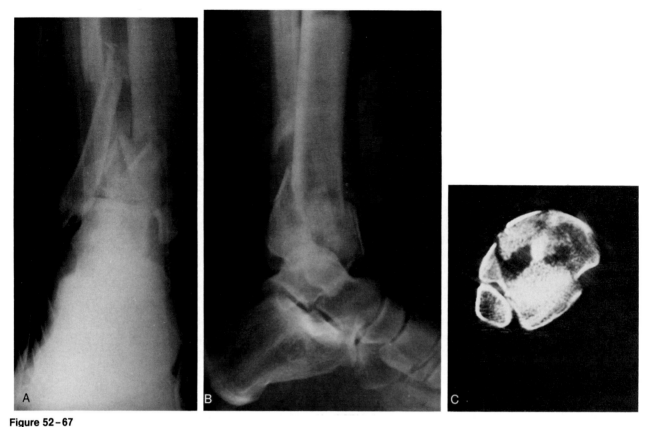

Figure 52-67

A type III (impacted) pilon fracture caused by an automobiile crash. There is extensive comminution and crushing evident on AP and lateral views (*A* and *B*, respectively). The CT scan *(C)* was made after application of an external fixator with radiolucent connecting rods, and it confirms the crushing nature of the injury, as well as the persistence of articular surface displacement.

rized into three subgroups according to Rüedi and Allgöwer.[128,141a,142]

Pronation-Dorsiflexion Injuries

Lauge-Hansen described a pronation-dorsiflexion injury mechanism, although he never duplicated it experimentally.[79] He developed this category and its stages by studying roentgenograms and described (1) an oblique medial malleolar fracture, (2) a large anterior lip fracture, (3) a supraarticular fibular fracture, and (4) a posterior tibial fracture, often connecting with the stage II anterior fracture. The resulting injury has many of the characteristics of pilon fractures, although it does not have their comminution. Most authors pay little attention to this proposed mechanism, which adds little to our understanding or treatment of complex fractures of the distal tibia.

Ovadia and Beals reviewed 145 pilon fractures, separating them into five groups according to severity as indicated by comminution and displacement, with categories similar to Rüedi and Allgöwer's three grades. They clearly demonstrated the validity of such an approach, but using five instead of three grades seemed to add little additional information.[170]

Several other important variables affect outcome and decision making for pilon fractures. These include severity of soft tissue injury; quality of bone stock; associated injuries; and preexisting medical problems, including alcoholism, peripheral vascular disease, and possibly diabetes mellitus. Age alone does not appear to have much of an effect. In addition to these patient-related variables, surgeon-related issues are also important. Results are better for surgeons who have greater experience with these injuries, presumably because of better decision making, as well as more facility with techniques of gentle soft tissue handling and rigid internal fixation.[200]

Treatment

Undisplaced fractures of the tibial pilon do well with either operative or nonoperative treatment.[170] When displacement is present, the general principles of managing articular injuries apply to this region, but with some important caveats.[236] Open anatomic reduction, rigid fixation, and early motion are desirable. However, if soft tissue injury is severe, wound slough and infection may occur, potentially leading to chronic infection or amputation. If fracture comminution and impaction are severe, anatomic reduction may be technically impossible. Furthermore, with a high-energy crushing injury of the articular surface, there may be irreversible damage to the articular cartilage, with inevitable post-traumatic osteoarthritis.

Given a displaced pilon fracture, the surgeon must decide whether the patient's fracture is fixable, how best to minimize the risk of problems with soft tissue healing, and whether the outcome is likely to be improved by open treatment when compared with the alternatives of closed reduction and casting, calcaneal pin traction, or external fixation. If ORIF is chosen, a thorough analysis of the injury and a carefully formulated preoperative plan are likely to improve the result and aid the surgeon's task. Open treatment of properly selected pilon fractures does indeed seem to improve results, although this belief is based on uncontrolled comparisons among published series or retrospectively selected patients.[170,200] Although Ovadia and Beals found that operated patients had better results than nonoperatively treated ones in all severity grades, only 40% of their most severe injuries had a good or excellent result after ORIF.[170] Bourne found so many complications after ORIF of grade III injuries, with only 32% satisfactory functional results, that he expressed little enthusiasm about the benefits of ORIF for this most severe category of pilon fractures.[27] Other authors have also reported poor results from ORIF of severe tibial pilon fractures or have suggested less invasive alternatives.[25,52,214,234] It seems wise to be cautious about operating on such injuries (Fig. 52–68).

Operative Treatment

Timing of Surgery. If ORIF is chosen, it is important to operate when the risk of additional soft tissue damage is least. Certainly marked edema, skin blistering, or deep abrasions indicate an unhealthy soft tissue envelope. An ankle with such an appearance should not be operated on until complete skin healing has occurred, which may take seven to ten days or more. It has been suggested that if a severely injured pilon fracture can be fixed before such changes become evident, they may be avoidable.[213,236] This assertion has not been proved. Furthermore, it is possible that an urgent operation may prevent the surgeon from preoperatively identifying the status of the soft tissues. Certainly urgent ORIF by an inexperienced, poorly prepared surgeon is not likely to improve the outcome. It is probably safer to use an external fixator or calcaneal traction, if deformity must be reduced and stability provided for severe pilon fractures.[25,214] ORIF, if appropriate, can be done

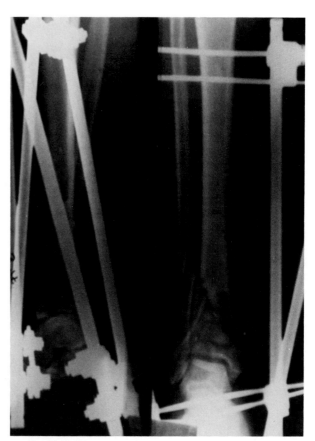

Figure 52–68

This highly comminuted pilon fracture with severe soft tissue involvement has been immobilized in an external fixator from tibia to calcaneus. Ligamentotaxis provides alignment and stability for the fracture and soft tissue envelope.

once the soft tissues have recovered and without struggling to regain length and overall alignment.

Strategy and Preoperative Planning. The classic steps for ORIF of a pilon fracture are (1) reduction and fixation of the fibula, (2) reduction and fixation of the tibial articular surface, (3) bone grafting of any resulting metaphyseal bone defect, and (4) application of a buttress plate (Fig. 52–69).[160,200] An adequate preoperative plan depends on a clear demonstration of the fracture anatomy with AP, lateral, and, usually, mortise and oblique radiographs of the injured limb. Mortise and lateral radiographs of the opposite ankle provide a model for reduction. Because of normal variation, it is especially helpful to use the patient's own anatomy as a control. A CT scan in the transverse plane can be very helpful and may be supplemented with multiplanar or three-dimensional reconstructed images.

Using these data, AP and lateral tracings of the fracture fragments are prepared and are reassembled to fit the outline of the normal ankle, as advocated by Müller

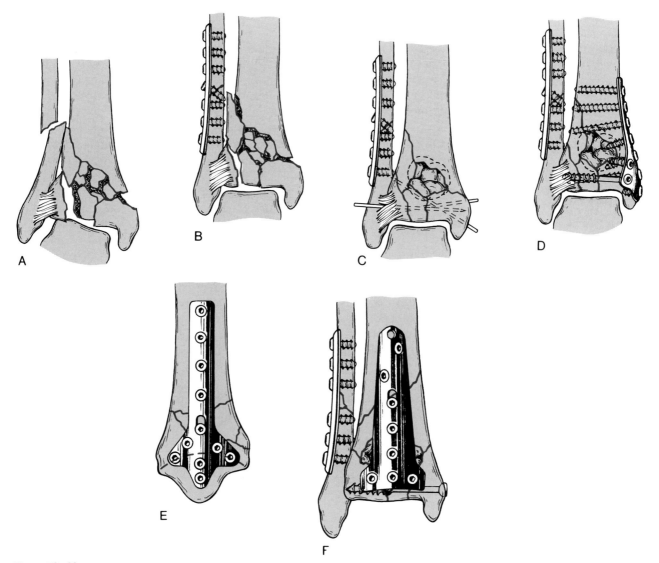

Figure 52–69

The steps for repair of a displaced, impacted pilon fracture, after Rüedi and Allgöwer. First the fibula is reduced and fixed. Then the articular surface is reduced and provisionally fixed. Bone graft is used to fill the resulting metaphyseal defect. Finally, a buttressing plate is applied. This may be a cloverleaf or DC plate medially or the large-fragment spoon plate anteriorly. (Redrawn from Müller, M.E., et al. Manual of Internal Fixation, 2nd ed. New York, Springer-Verlag, 1979.)

and co-workers and illustrated by Mast and colleagues.[141,160] Fixation implants and their location are drawn in, and a sequential list of the operative steps is prepared. Such a plan is invaluable in the care of these severe injuries. As each step is considered, the alternatives can be weighed and the entire procedure visualized as a whole as well as a series of tasks. All necessary instruments and implants can be made available, and all members of the team can be clear about the plan.

Incisions. A pneumatic tourniquet is advisable. The incision for operative treatment of a pilon fracture will depend on the status of the soft tissues and the fracture anatomy. In approximately 85% of such injuries, there will be a fibular fracture. This fracture is best approached through a posterolateral incision to ensure an adequate anterior bridge of tissue between it and the anteromedial incision for the distal tibia (Fig. 52–70). A *minimum* of 7 cm has been advised.[200] Both incisions must be marked with a pen before either is made. The standard anteromedial incision begins proximally just lateral to the anterior tibial crest and spirals distally just medial to the tibialis anterior tendon, the paratenon of which should be preserved if possible. In both incisions, full-thickness flaps should be employed. The skin is handled extremely gently with sharp hooks and retraction sutures instead of forceps. Blunt dissection

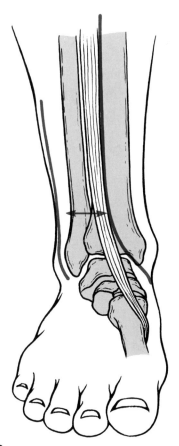

Figure 52-70

The AO/ASIF incisions for repair of a plateau fracture. At least a 7-cm bridge must be maintained between the anteromedial and postero-lateral incisions. Soft tissue injury or fracture configuration may require modifications of these incisions. (Redrawn from Müller, M.E., et al. Manual of Internal Fixation, 2nd ed. New York, Springer-Verlag, 1979.)

should be cautious, spreading tissue just enough to identify structures without disturbing the subcutaneous vascular plexus. Structures are divided sharply, and the underlying fascia is reflected with the skin to preserve fasciocutaneous flaps. Deep retractors are used gently and intermittently. Indirect reduction techniques are employed whenever possible. For example, a bone distractor applied between the tibia and the talus can facilitate reduction and minimize added soft tissue trauma.[140] A plate applied to one side of the fracture may be used with a spreader against a screw to reduce and then fix a suitable fracture.[141]

Reduction and Fixation of the Fracture Elements. Reduction of a fibular fracture, if one is present, is an important aid for reconstruction of the ankle. The fibula provides a reference for length and is usually attached to some of the lateral tibial metaphyseal-articular fragments, as well as to the talus. If anatomically reduced and securely fixed, it can be the basis for resto-

ration of the joint. However, malreduction will interfere with each subsequent stage of the procedure. Usually a plate, often the 3.5-mm dynamic compression (DC) variety, is best for fixing the fibula, with three or four screws in both the proximal and distal fragments. If the fibular fracture is a low one, the one-third tubular plate may be more appropriate.

With the talus realigned relative to the tibial shaft, often aided by the use of a bone distractor, its articular surface can be used as a template for reduction of the tibial plafond and medial malleolus, which are held in place with provisional K wires and any definitive lag screws that are appropriate at this stage. Intraoperative radiography, perhaps with an image-intensifier fluoroscope, but subject to confirmation with high-quality permanent films, may be helpful during this process. Finally, the diaphyseal-metaphyseal junction is reduced, cancellous or corticocancelleous bone graft is used to fill any defects, and an appropriate buttress plate is applied. Depending on fracture configuration, the plate selected may be the cloverleaf small-fragment plate, used with 3.5- and 4.0-mm screws and perhaps modified by removal of one or more of the distal projections, as well as by necessary contouring. Alternatively, if significant coronal plane disruption is present, the large-fragment spoon plate, designed for the anterior distal tibia, may be helpful. If the fracture zone is long, an appropriately contoured 4.5-mm standard DC plate may be valuable for larger patients. Occasionally T plates may be selected and contoured to fit the medial distal tibia. Whenever possible, interfragmentary lag screws are used for stability. Small fragments and comminuted areas may require supplementary K wires for definitive fixation. The goal is to obtain sufficient fracture stability to avoid loss of alignment and permit active range-of-motion exercises as soon as the soft tissue has healed (Figs. 52-71, 52-72, and 52-73).

Aftercare. The wounds are closed atraumatically, often over small suction drains, with interrupted dermal or Allgöwer-Donati sutures.[160] A very well padded, nonconstricting splint is applied to ensure maintenance of a neutral ankle position, and the leg is elevated moderately. Over the next days the wound is observed, and if a slough of any significance occurs, then prompt coverage with a free muscle flap should be seriously considered.[71,215] When wound healing is secure, active range-of-motion exercises are begun, with the ankle otherwise held in a neutral position using a bivalved short-leg cast or splint. Once good ankle control and early healing have been obtained, a cooperative patient may omit the splint, and *minimal* weight bearing can be allowed on crutches. Unless the patient is reliably able to protect the limb, better external immobilization is recommended. Although progression to full weight

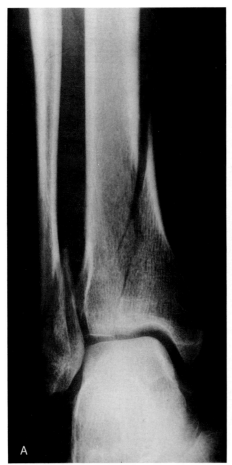
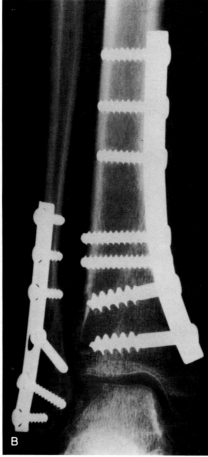

Figure 52–71

A, Type I (split and minimally displaced) pilon fracture. B, One year after anatomic reduction and rigid fixation.

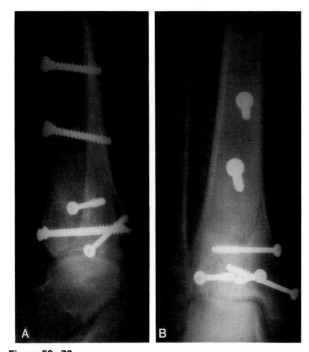

Figure 52–72

Fixation with multiple lag screws of a type II pilon fracture, shown preoperatively in Figure 52–66.

bearing may be possible about three months after fixation of less comminuted fractures, it may be wise to continue partial weight bearing for a longer period if there are areas of defect in the articular cartilage.[236]

Less Invasive Options. When fracture displacement is significant, but soft tissues do not permit ORIF as described previously, other alternatives must be considered. Chief among these is external fixation.[25] Although it may not permit immediate motion of the injured ankle, it provides absolute stability, which may aid healing of injured soft tissue. It also avoids a dysfunctional contracture. Effective external fixation for the ankle and foot can be obtained with two or three 5-mm anterior half pins in the distal tibial shaft, one or more 4-mm transfixion pins through the calcaneus, and 3-mm half pins in the first and fifth metatarsals (Fig. 52–74). Use of ring fixators with tensioned K wires in the reconstructed distal tibia is currently being explored. A hybrid fixator may be constructed with half pins proximally, a partial ring with transfixion wires for the metaphysis, and extensions into the foot as needed.[169a]

Fixation of the forefoot in neutral is important, both to keep it plantigrade and to minimize soft tissue mo-

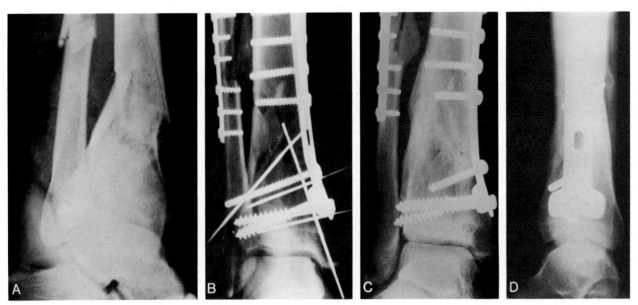

Figure 52–73

A, Type III pilon fracture, severely comminuted with an open wound. *B,* Intraoperative radiograph confirming satisfactory alignment. *C,D,* At one year follow-up with anatomically preserved joint and axial alignment.

Figure 52–74

External fixation for severe ankle fractures. The illustration shows a frame of Hoffmann type components anchored proximally with two or three 5-mm half pins in the distal tibial shaft. Four-millimeter transfixion pins are placed through the calcaneal tuberosity. A double-ball joint clamp on the half pins connects to bars that go to single-ball joint clamps on the calcaneal pins. Control of the forefoot is obtained with 3-mm half-pins inserted into the first and fifth metatarsals and connected as shown. Radiolucent rods can be used to permit radiographs and CT scans of the ankle.

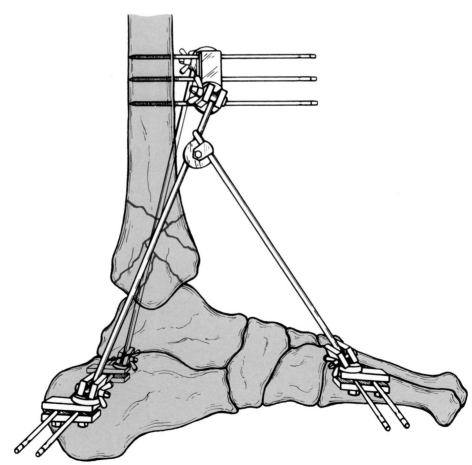

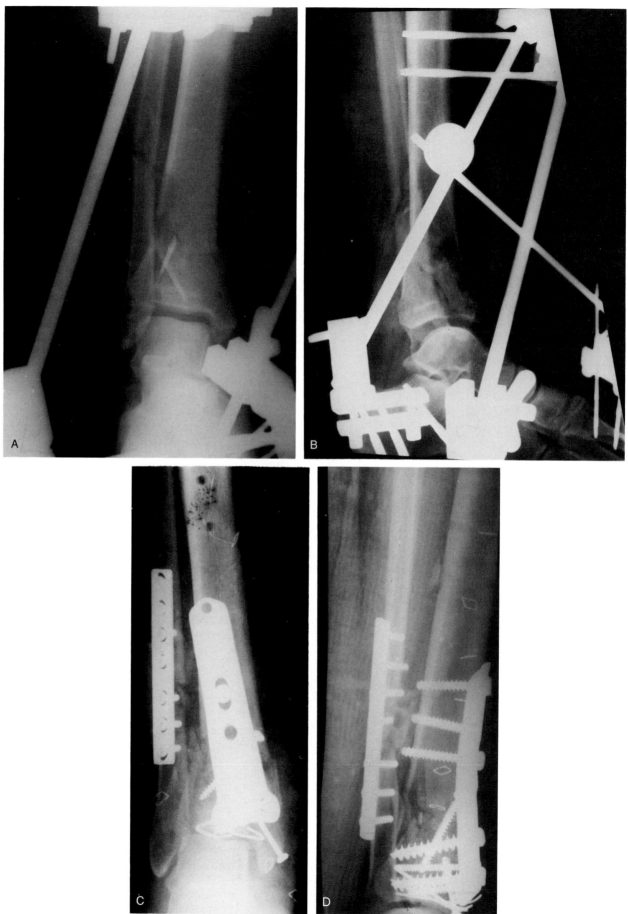

See legend on opposite page

tion in the ankle wound. External fixation, which can be rapidly applied, is very helpful for a seriously injured patient. It provides optimal control for the pilon fracture while permitting a challenging ORIF to be deferred until a more opportune time (Fig. 52–75). Maintenance of length and overall alignment by ligamentotaxis aids the delayed ORIF. If an open wound is present, it can be debrided and closed at an appropriate time. With external fixation instead of a plate, reassembly of the plafond fragments and lag screw fixation may be done with a less extensive exposure. Bone grafting can be deferred as well. It is also possible to use an external fixator in place of a plate to buttress medial comminution without soft tissue exposure.[191] Fixation of a fibular fracture, if one is present, can increase stability of the pilon injury, but rarely by itself is it as effective as external fixation. It should be emphasized that minimal soft tissue stripping and the gentlest possible exposure, together with indirect reduction techniques, are the keys to low complication rates following ORIF of pilon fractures (Figs. 52–76 and 52–77).[141a] Every effort should be made to employ these methods.

Other less invasive options include limited internal fixation, often including at least the fibula. Either a cast or skeletal traction is necessary protection when less than rigid fixation is employed.[45] Soft tissue management and prevention of deformity must be considered. Delayed bone grafting of a residual metaphyseal defect may be needed to prevent late angulation of the fracture.

The Unreconstructible Pilon Fracture. Some tibial pilon fractures have so much comminution, so much articular damage, or such poor bone stock that they are not amenable to internal fixation or will have predictably poor results. In these situations primary ankle arthrodesis has occasionally been advised.[229] Preservation of a plantigrade foot and soft tissue healing are the first priorities. If there is any question about the soft tissue status, these goals should be obtained initially with external fixation. Arthrodesis can be deferred until bone comminution has consolidated and the soft tissue envelope has fully recovered. If appropriate, internal fixation alone can be used for an arthrodesis, or the external fixator can be continued until union is sufficient for a cast to be trusted.[108,229,236]

Results of Treatment

Marked variation in the severity of pilon fractures makes summary evaluation and comparison of different treatment methods difficult. If complications are avoided, articular surface impaction and comminution are not severe, and an anatomic reduction is achieved, followed by early active motion, then most patients seem satisfied. Ovadia and Beals considered an excellent outcome to be a pain-free patient who had returned to all activities without a limp.[170] A good result was a patient who had mild pain after vigorous activity, slightly modified recreational activities, and otherwise resumed preinjury activities without a limp or medication. Their proportion of patients in these categories fell rapidly from 100% in the least severe fractures to 22% in the most severe category, with operatively treated patients having a somewhat better outcome. Bourne's review of the literature found successful outcomes in 29% to 55% in most series, though as many as 70% to 90% of patients treated by AO techniques had acceptable results.[27] Stratifying his patients according to severity, he, too, found that just under a third of patients with type III fractures had satisfactory results. Rüedi and Allgöwer feel that subjective results improve over time, in spite of persistent restriction of motion.[200] Complications after operative treatment of pilon fractures are frequent and often severe.[53,213,234]

Soft Tissue Injuries of the Ankle

LATERAL COLLATERAL LIGAMENT INJURIES

Ankle "sprains" are very frequent injuries and are thus familiar to both patients and physicians.[184,204] They are the most common injury resulting from recreational sports, have a considerable socioeconomic impact, and have generated an abundant literature that has been extensively reviewed.[101a,117,200a,221] According to Brostrom, common ankle sprains have complete ligament ruptures in 75% of cases. Two thirds of these are isolated injuries of the anterior fibulotalar ligament.[31,186]

This section emphasizes (1) the need for appropriate diagnosis, (2) the currently favored nonoperative man-

Figure 52–75

A,B, Type III pilon fracture in external fixation with plantigrade foot ensured by extension of frame to the first metatarsal. Some articular surface displacement persists, as seen on the lateral view and on the CT scan, shown in Figure 52–67. In spite of delayed surgery, open reduction, internal fixation, and bone grafting were followed by soft tissue slough that required free muscle flap coverage. Note excessive valgus reduction in *C.*

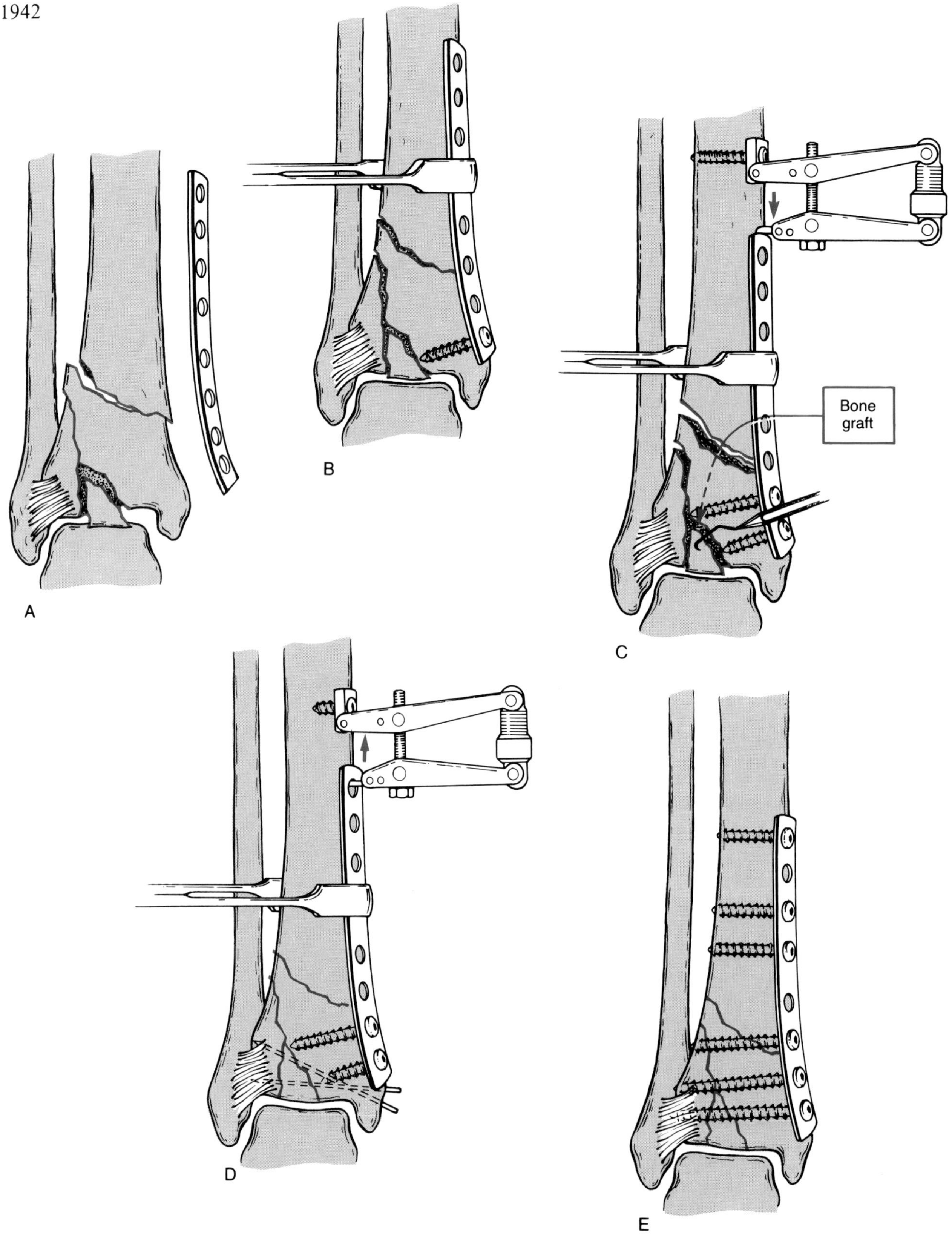

Figure 52–76

Indirect reduction of some pilon fractures can be achieved with a properly contoured 4.5-mm DC plate attached to the distal fragment and used with the tension device reversed to push the fragment into alignment. After this, the articular surface is anatomically reduced, bone graft is added as needed, and screws are inserted through or separate from the plate to gain secure fixation. If the medial cortex will not overcompress, tension can be added to the plate, as shown in D. (Redrawn from Mast, J.; Jakob, R., Ganz, R. Planning and Reduction Technique in Fracture Surgery. New York, Springer-Verlag, 1989.)

Figure 52–77

The AO bone distractor is another vital aid for reduction of pilon fractures. Anchoring 5-mm Schanz screws are placed parallel to the plafond in the tibia proximally and in the talar neck, just anterior to the medial malleolus. Distraction permits atraumatic reduction of impacted, comminuted bone fragments with a minimum of soft tissue stripping. Standard fixation and bone grafting are then applied. (Redrawn from Mast, J.; Jakob, R., Ganz, R. Planning and Reduction Technique in Fracture Surgery. New York, Springer-Verlag, 1989.)

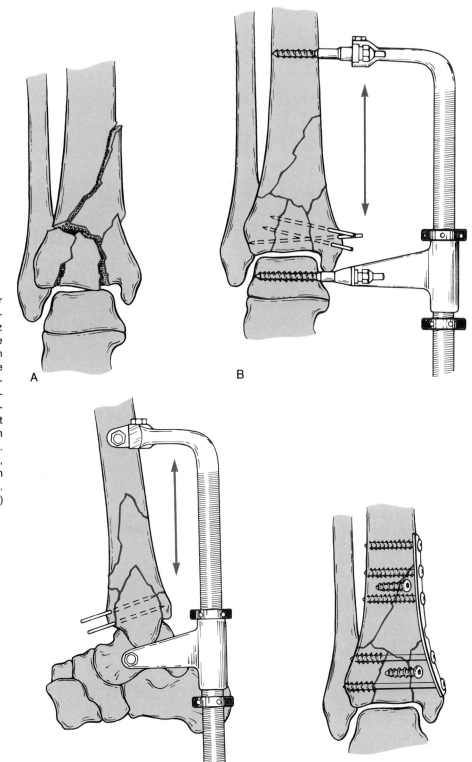

agement of essentially all closed lateral collateral ligament ruptures, and (3) late instability resulting from functional or mechanical causes and its management.

Diagnosis

The complaint of a "sprain" by a patient with a swollen, tender ankle is so common in the urgent care setting that it is often disregarded if ankle radiographs fail to reveal a fracture. Systematic evaluation is necessary to avoid missing a less obvious injury. The patient's description of the injury is important, and it should be determined whether the onset was sudden, with an injury episode, or gradual. An inversion mechanism, with the foot forcibly supinated, as has been previously discussed, produces failure of the lateral collateral ligament (LCL) complex. The anterior fibulotalar ligament is the structure most likely to be partially or completely torn. If the foot was dorsiflexed, the fibulocalcaneal ligament may also be involved. If it was plantarflexed, the anterior capsule is often torn as well. If the applied force *externally* rotated the foot (often in a pronated position), the injury is likely to involve the tibiofibular syndesmosis and possibly the deltoid ligament (see the previous discussion on pronation–external rotation injuries in the section on malleolar fractures). If no fracture is present on the ankle radiographs, this injury may be mistaken for a lateral collateral sprain, in spite of syndesmotic involvement and the risk of a higher fibular fracture or talar instability in the mortise. Tendon ruptures or dislocations have characteristic histories of failure under load, without extreme twisting of the ankle. It is important to ask about prior difficulties with the ankle to identify attritional problems and chronic conditions.

Physical examination is often difficult because of tenderness.[157] Status of the skin and neurovascular function is important. Very forceful inversion injuries may rupture the lateral ankle skin, producing a characteristic transverse wound that looks almost as though it were made with a scalpel. Peroneal nerve palsies and occasionally delayed compartment syndromes accompany inversion sprains.[114,163] Localization of tenderness is essential to identify the injured structures. If the lateral collateral ligament complex is involved, there will be tenderness over the anterior fibulotalar ligament and possibly over the fibulocalcaneal ligament, the anterior capsule, and the medial collateral ligament. LCL injuries should not produce tenderness over the syndesmosis, the malleoli themselves, the proximal fibula, or the Achilles or other tendons, although the nearby peroneal tendons may be rather sensitive. Rarely, an LCL disruption occurs in company with a lateral malleolar fracture.[249]

Assessment of stability is the basis for confirming and grading a ligament injury. This is often difficult in the case of an acute ankle injury and is even harder after a day or two have elapsed. Anterior drawer motion of the plantigrade foot is a sign of anterior fibulotalar laxity. This can be confirmed and quantitated by stress radiography. Inversion laxity may be caused by deficiencies of the fibulocalcaneal ligament (in dorsiflexion) or the anterior fibulotalar ligament (in plantarflexion). This is hard to judge because of patient discomfort and the normal motion of the subtalar joint, which itself may be unstable in as many as 10% of patients with inversion laxity.

Confirmation of ligament rupture is possible with peroneal tenography or ankle arthrography, but neither defines the degree of instability. This can be done with stress films, with or without special apparatus or anesthesia.[4,115] With general anesthesia, stress radiographs are quite accurate (92%), but accuracy with local anesthesia falls to 68% (Fig. 52–78).[89] Although academically interesting, such studies do not convincingly improve patient outcome after acute ankle sprains, so they are rarely indicated.

It is vital to inspect carefully the standard radiographs of a patient with a presumed ankle sprain. Osteochondral fractures of the talus may be present on either the lateral or medial dome; their identification is necessary for proper management (see chapter 53).[79,256] A fracture of the lateral process of the talus may simulate an LCL sprain, as may a fracture of the anterior process of the calcaneus. The latter is hard to see without oblique radiographs of the foot, though its characteristic tenderness is more anterior. Avulsion of the base of the fifth metatarsal may occur with an inversion injury with or without associated ankle LCL rupture.

Small ligamentous avulsion fractures from the lateral malleolus or ankle capsular attachments are occasionally seen with sprains and should not affect treatment or outcome. Brostrom found these in 14% of patients using standard radiographs.[31] Meyer and colleagues reported them in 42% of patients using high-resolution CT.[150]

Treatment

The goals of treatment for LCL injuries are to achieve rapid and complete rehabilitation with minimal morbidity and cost and the lowest possible risk of late instability. Many approaches, with a great number of variations, have been reported.[95] At present there appears to be little justification for primary surgical repair, which has been shown by several randomized prospective studies not to improve the outcome of either isolated ruptures of the anterior fibulotalar ligament or those

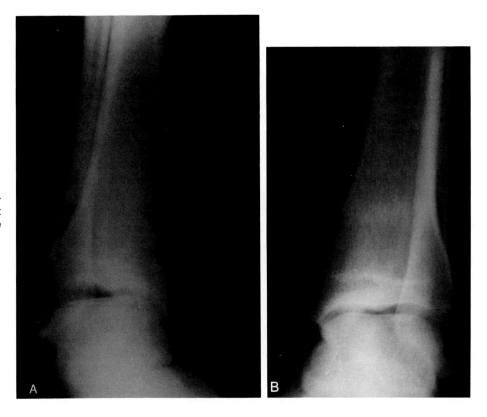

Figure 52-78

Inversion stress radiographs demonstrate (A) 14° varus tilt of right talus versus (B) 2° varus on the left.

with concomitant fibulocalcaneal rupture.[56,111,224] Furthermore, late reconstructions, for those who need them, are no less successful than early repair.[35]

Optimal nonoperative management of ankle LCL sprains has not been definitively established.[20,179,218,221,224] Because late instability may be caused by functional or anatomic causes[7a,117,201] and may respond to appropriate rehabilitation measures, including exercises for muscle strength and agility, such measures may have a role in the management of acute injuries, as may various physical modalities that increase comfort and provide support for the ankle. On the other hand, many patients with these common injuries do so well with independent rehabilitation programs that routine prescription of physical therapy and long-term bracing carries a significant unnecessary economic burden.

The patient with an acute ankle LCL sprain may have a *minor injury* with tenderness, slight swelling, and little difficulty walking. More demanding activities may be symptomatic, and the risk of reinjury is probably significant if he or she returns immediately and without protection to challenging activities. The patient with a *moderate injury* has significant swelling and tenderness, walks with difficulty on the ankle, and is unable to participate in vigorous work or sports. The patient with a *severe LCL injury* has such significant pain and tenderness that he or she is unable to bear

weight without rigid immobilization or crutches and usually has documentable evidence of a complete disruption of both the anterior fibulotalar ligament and the fibulocalcaneal ligament.

Treatment of minor ankle sprains is directed at relief of symptoms and prevention of further injury. This consists of reduced activity, stretching and strengthening exercises, and the use of a training type brace that provides proprioceptive input. Moderate and severe ankle sprains are difficult to differentiate precisely without anesthesia. Therefore similar treatment regimens are advised. Although a more precise diagnosis might expedite rehabilitation for athletes under pressure to return to competition earlier, it is unnecessary and not cost effective in the majority of cases. Progressive return to normal activity can be determined by the patient's clinical course.

The acutely injured ankle with a moderate or severe sprain is best immobilized in a well-padded plaster splint. Ice, elevation, and crutch walking are advised. Within two or three days, as the acute swelling diminishes, the patient is reassessed. Generally, a stirrup splint with pneumatic cushions (e.g., Aircast, or equivalent) is applied over a sock or a light, loose elastic wrap, and the patient is encouraged to bear weight progressively as tolerated and to discard the crutches as soon as comfort and security permit (Fig. 52-79).[20,183] For a noncompliant patient with a severe injury, a cast

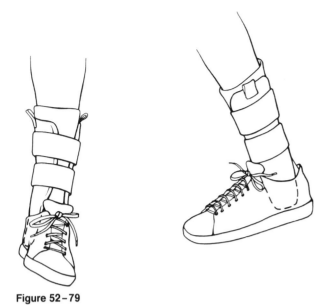

Figure 52-79

A stirrup splint with air-filled cushions and velcro fasteners provides secure, functional support for a lateral collateral ligament injury after the acute pain and swelling have resolved.

may be considered. Generally, however, it is withheld unless the patient is so disabled that rigid external support is necessary for comfort. In such a case, a short-leg walking cast can be applied as soon as swelling permits and used for one to three weeks until full weight bearing is possible in the cast. At this point, the functional brace is substituted.

An important part of the aftercare of an acute LCL ankle sprain is a functional rehabilitation program. This usually consists of progressive resumption of activity, stretching and strengthening exercises, functional bracing or taping, and proprioceptive drills. Many such regimens have been described and are reported in the literature.[5,12,18,40,46,67,117,156]

SYNDESMOSIS SPRAINS

Identified by the history of an external rotation injury and tenderness over the anterior inferior tibiofibular ligament (AITFL), these less frequent ligamentous injuries of the ankle are slower to recover and may benefit from a somewhat more restrictive approach to management, including a period of a few weeks in a non-weight bearing cast.[20,101] It is important to exclude the diagnosis of complete ligamentous disruption with displacement of the fibula from the incisural notch. This is suggested by mortise widening or by a separation of 5 mm or more between the fibula and lateral border of the notch on mortise radiographs. Remember that a high fibula fracture or plastic deformation of the fibula may accompany these injuries. Precise documentation

of the distal tibiofibular anatomy is readily obtained with a CT scan. If displacement is present, closed management is not likely to replace the fibula, and ORIF is indicated. In the absence of displacement of the fibula, protection and progressive rehabilitation are advised.

LATE INVERSION INSTABILITY

Chronic instability has been reported to follow 20% to 40% of acute inversion ankle sprains.[88] The patient reports recurring inversion sprains or the feeling that the ankle will "give way" in this manner. Prospective randomized studies provide little support for the belief that acute surgical treatment reduces this risk.[56,111,117,224] However, more effective early nonoperative management may be beneficial.

Instability may be mechanical, with documentable inversion laxity of the ankle or subtalar joint.[7a,28,117,149,259] It may also have functional causes, such as impaired proprioception and balance or, rarely, peroneal rupture or palsy.[67,77,110,240] History, examination, and stress radiographs usually permit diagnosis of the cause of ankle instability. If a trial of intensive rehabilitation is unsuccessful and mechanical instability is present, then some form of lateral ligamentous reconstruction is appropriate. High success rates have been reported for treatment of recalcitrant mechanical instability by most of these various procedures, which range from repair of the residual ligament to its advancement, or to its augmentation with local or more distant tendon grafts. If subtalar instability is present, the ligament reconstruction must address this, but otherwise there appears to be little basis for choosing one type of reconstruction over another.[3,6,7,22,32,97,100,164,190,201,219,243,250]

ANKLE DISLOCATIONS

Ankle Dislocations Without Fracture

Although most ankle dislocations are part of a complex malleolar injury, the tibiotalar joint rarely dislocates without a fracture.[44,238] Approximately a third are open, with an associated risk of infection that can be diminished with appropriate wound care and delayed closure.[107] Neurovascular injuries are frequently associated with these dislocations. Closed reduction is usually successful, with a generally satisfactory result and little risk of long-term functional instability or arthritis. The results of open dislocations are poorer.

Occasionally there is a complete dislocation of the talus, with dislocation from the subtalar and talonavicular joints as well. These "extruded talus" lesions are usually open and have a high risk of sepsis, avascular necrosis, and ultimate amputation. Talectomy and early tibiotalar arthrodesis may be the best means of salvaging a functional foot.[107]

Occasionally ankle pain, rather than a sensation of instability per se, is a residual problem after an ankle inversion injury. This may be the result of one or more of several factors. An osteochondral fracture of the talus should be considered.[79,254] There may be impingement on the talus by a hypertrophic anteroinferior tibiofibular ligament.[14] Another possibility is a posttraumatic sinus tarsi syndrome, with damage to the restraining ligaments of the subtalar joint, which can be demonstrated by posterior subtalar arthrography.[151] CT or MRI evaluation and ankle arthroscopy may help with the evaluation and management of these often puzzling injuries.

Tibiofibular Diastasis

Widening of the ankle mortise occurs occasionally without obvious fracture.[131,139] This may be occult, with a syndesmosis disruption that requires stress radiographs for confirmation. It may also be frank and visible on routine radiographs (Fig. 52–80). Edwards and DeLee have described four types of this rare injury.[55a] In type I, there is a direct lateral displacement of the otherwise normal fibula. This is best treated with open reduction and syndesmosis transfixation. Type II injuries are similar but have plastic deformation of the fibula and may need an osteotomy as well as open reduction of the distal fibula. Type III injuries have posterolateral rotary subluxation. Type IV have interposition of the superiorly dislocated talus. Types III and IV are usually managed well with closed reduction and cast immobilization, according to Edwards and DeLee.[55a]

MEDIAL COLLATERAL (DELTOID) LIGAMENT RUPTURES

The deltoid ligament usually is injured as a component of a malleolar fracture and has been discussed previously. Rarely, it appears as an isolated injury.[93] Nonoperative management should provide satisfactory stability, unless unrecognized syndesmosis disruption is present.

ACHILLES TENDON RUPTURES

A myriad of pathologic conditions may affect the Achilles tendon, including Achilles tendinitis, partial or incomplete ruptures of the tendon, bursitis, and tenosynovitis. Because of the large mass of the triceps surae and its importance in control of the tibiotalar

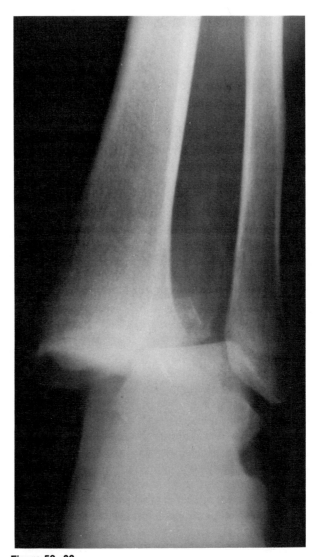

Figure 52–80

Tibiofibular diastasis with a small posterior avulsion fracture of the tibia in a teenaged patient. Plastic deformation of the fibula required osteotomy and fibular fixation.

relationship during walking, running, and jumping, the Achilles tendon is subjected to large loads on a regular, recurrent basis. Achilles tendinitis is an overuse syndrome and must be differentiated from more acute problems such as tears, partial tears, muscle strains, and thrombophlebitis. Radiographic examinations are usually noncontributory except in the case of a large posterosuperior calcaneal spur. Most of the overuse syndromes respond to a shoe lift, contrast baths, and oral antiinflammatory agents. Injections with steroid preparations should be discouraged, as they damage the collagen matrix and may result in iatrogenic tendon ruptures.

Ruptures of the Achilles tendon are usually secondary to forced dorsiflexion of the plantarflexed foot.

Most patients are usually middle-aged "weekend athletes." Not uncommonly, rupture occurs in high-demand sports such as basketball, football, or tennis. A possible contributory factor may be the failure to stretch and appropriately warm up for the sporting event. Rarely, these ruptures accompany fractures of the ankle.[138]

The examination of the patient with an acute Achilles tendon rupture usually demonstrates a defect in the heel cord with exquisite pain and inability to plantarflex the ankle completely. Swelling may obscure the tendon defect. The Thompson test is performed by manually squeezing the calf while the patient is kneeling. This normally produces passive plantarflexion of the ankle. The injured Achilles tendon will demonstrate less plantarflexion than the normal calf while performing the test (see Fig. 52–15).

The treatment for Achilles tendon rupture includes conservative management with the foot held in the plantarflexed position for at least 8 to 12 weeks, open management with primary repair and preservation of the tenosynovium, percutaneous repair through small stab incisions, and open repair with or without augmentation. The literature offers various opinions about the results of treatment.[76] A large, randomized study demonstrated little difference in outcome, and similar complication rates, between nonoperative and operative treatments.[162a] However, it is usually suggested that the elite-level athlete or the serious amateur athlete should be treated with operative repair. This may offer a more functional result than that of conservative management. The reported risk of re-rupture is lower after surgical treatment, unless care is taken with nonoperative treatment.[19a,24,106]

Surgical technique should include a posteromedial skin incision rather than one in the midline, which could be associated with shoe wear problems as well as skin sloughs. The paratenon should be preserved and repaired, if possible, to prevent adhesions between the skin and tendon repair. The tendon ends are reapproximated with appropriate suture techniques in the manner of Bunnell or Kessler.[237] Loose ends of the tendon can be sutured into bundles before being reconnected.[21] The plantaris tendon can be used to augment the primary repair if it does not appear strong enough. Dacron mesh or other fabric can also be used to reinforce an Achilles tendon repair. An alternative technique relies on a suture placed percutaneously through the tendon ends, which are not exposed in an effort to avoid skin complications, which are a reported problem with open repairs. After primary repair or augmentation, short-leg immobilization for six to eight weeks is usually adequate, followed by use of a heel lift to protect the repair for an additional six weeks.

Late repairs of neglected Achilles tendon ruptures can be augmented with a "turn down" of the gastrosoleus fascia, a strip of fascia lata, plantaris tendon, or fabric, as previously mentioned.[13]

LESS COMMON TENDON INJURIES

Other less common tendon injuries around the ankle include ruptures and dislocations of the peroneal or posterior tibial tendons.[122,178,208,231] Any ankle tendon is at risk of laceration in an open wound. Loss of peroneal tendon function may be manifest as inversion instability.[110,235]

Peroneal Tendon Dislocations

Dislocations of the peroneal tendon are fairly rare and usually result from forced dorsiflexion or forced inversion. The injury is easily misdiagnosed as an ankle sprain and treated with early mobilization, with attendant risk of redislocation or chronic dislocation. Radiographic evaluation of a patient with a peroneal tendon dislocation reveals a small fleck of bone off the posterior aspect of the lateral malleolus. This is well seen by CT.[196,197,223] Such an avulsion fragment, in association with the classic physical findings of pain *behind* the lateral malleolus and localized swelling, is the hallmark of the diagnosis.

If reduction of the dislocated tendons is stable, these injuries can be treated with closed reduction of the tendons and a below-knee walking cast for six to eight weeks. In some cases, little intrinsic stability exists after retinacular rupture, and open reduction with retinacular repair or reconstruction is advisable.

Recurrent dislocation (or subluxation), however, poses a more difficult reconstructive problem. Surgical alternatives include transfer of the lateral Achilles tendon sheath, fibular osteotomy to create a deeper pulley for the tendons, or rerouting peroneal tendons under the calcaneal fibular ligament.[39,51,72,116,135,152,180,181,217,227]

Posterior Tibial Tendon Ruptures

Acute posterior tibial tendon ruptures are difficult to diagnose and frequently are unrecognized for long periods of time.[2,32,66,209] Occasionally they accompany malleolar fractures.[104,205,228] They are usually found in patients in their fourth to sixth decades who present with a recently developed, painful flatfoot deformity. Standing radiographic evaluations classically show a flatfoot deformity with asymmetry of the talo-navicular-cuneiform arch. The tendon can be visualized by CT and MRI, which greatly aid diagnosis.[195,198] Complete ruptures that have been diagnosed early can be treated with repair, usually with augmentation from the adjacent toe flexor. However, chronic posterior tendon ruptures may require a subtalar or triple arthrodesis, depending on the severity of symptoms. Rarely, dislocations of the posterior tibial tendon may occur.[155,222,226]

Complications

Shelton and Anderson have provided a thorough and exceptionally detailed analysis of the complications of ankle injuries and their treatment. Based on our review of the literature and extensive personal experience, this definitive work is strongly recommended.[213,236,236a,251b,253] Other reviews also deserve mention.[236,236a,251b,253]

Most complications of ankle injuries relate to one of three basic areas: infection, soft tissue problems, or malunion and arthrosis (osteoarthritis).

INFECTION

The open ankle fracture is at highest risk for developing an infection after internal fixation. However, several large series of open ankle fractures treated with immediate internal fixation have had acceptable rates of infection. The main reason for this success is a combination of appropriate perioperative antibiotics, compulsive surgical technique, and open wound management. The improved outcome of open ankle fractures treated with appropriate wound care and immediate internal fixation justifies this change from traditional orthopedic teaching.[29,30,43,65,74,252]

Infection may be difficult to identify after surgical treatment of an ankle fracture. It may be limited to a surgical wound but often involves the ankle joint. Aspiration of the joint and proper evaluation of its fluid are thus mandatory whenever an infection is possible. Studies should include Gram's stain, cell count, and culture and sensitivity.

If an infection ensues after open reduction and internal fixation of the ankle, then an aggressive approach must be undertaken with immediate surgical debridement, multiple deep wound cultures, open wound management, and appropriate antibiotics. The ankle joint should not be left open but should be closed over a suction tube to prevent any accumulation of pus under pressure. If the ankle joint cannot be closed, then serious consideration must be given to early local soft tissue transfers or free microvascular tissue transfer.

There may be disagreement between infectious dis-

ease consultants and orthopedic surgeons as to the necessity of hardware removal in the event of an infection. If the hardware is providing stability, even in the face of gross infection, it should generally not be removed until the fracture has united. Instability of the infected fracture fragments provides a less desirable biologic environment in which to fight infection. Obtaining a durably functional ankle without chronic infection requires a combination of adequate debridement of necrotic and infected bone and soft tissue, anatomic reduction, rigid stability, appropriate antibiotics, occasional soft tissue coverage (which might entail a free muscle flap), and, ultimately, an aggressive postoperative ankle rehabilitation program.[76] If internal fixation does not provide adequate stability, then external fixation should be used instead, generally with distal purchase in both calcaneus and forefoot.

MALUNION

Malunion of an ankle fracture may be caused by an inadequate closed reduction or by loss of such a reduction. If caused by one of these, then early recognition and correction, usually with ORIF, may resolve the problem, although the difficulties of a late operation must be remembered. Malalignment may follow ORIF if reduction is inadequate and not recognized, or if it is lost because of failure of fixation. This may result from an uncooperative or neuropathic patient or from mechanical problems of fixation or bone quality. The risk of inadequate reduction of an ankle fracture is significantly increased in severe injuries with comminution, impaction, bone loss, and obscured landmarks for reduction.

The operating surgeon must compulsively examine the intraoperative radiographs to be absolutely certain that an anatomic reduction has been achieved. This is a not infrequent source of error. Well-positioned and satisfactorily exposed AP, lateral, and mortise views must be obtained intraoperatively and carefully reviewed, perhaps by comparison with the opposite side, to be sure that the bony relationships are appropriate.

The most common malunion of the ankle has been reported to be shortening and malrotation of the fibula. Weber and Simpson have described a corrective osteotomy to bring the fibula back to length and restore appropriate rotation.[248] This requires preoperative planning, the use of intraoperative distraction, bone grafting, and rigid fixation.[253] If the fibula has been brought to appropriate length and reduced, then aggressive physical therapy should follow. This osteotomy may have limited application, as many malunions of the ankle are associated with pain and severe degenerative changes. If loss of motion, pain, and severe degenerative changes are present, the lengthening-distraction osteotomy may not be enough to provide the patient with a functional ankle. However, such a procedure, along with correction of all other deformities affecting the ankle, should be seriously considered unless end-stage functional impairment is present, as nearly three fourths of such patients can have significant, long-lasting improvement.[136,246,248,255]

POSTTRAUMATIC ARTHRITIS

Posttraumatic arthritis may be manageable with reduced activity, nonsteroidal antiinflammatory medication, a well-cushioned shoe with a heel lift, or a fixed-ankle short-leg brace with a cushioned rocker heel. If these measures are inadequate, then arthrodesis is a reasonable consideration (Fig. 52–81).[144,199] Ankle replacement arthroplasties have not proved as successful

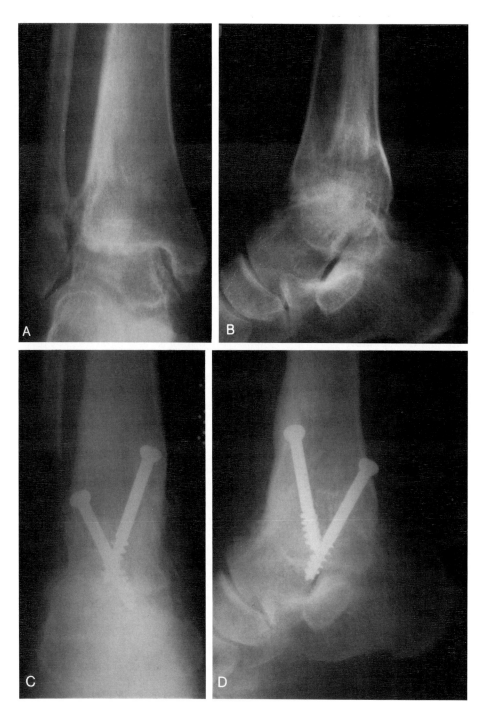

Figure 52–81

A,B, Posttraumatic arthrosis several years after malleolar ankle fracture. *C,D,* Because of progressive, severe symptoms, unresponsive to conservative treatment, an arthrodesis was performed, with good result.

as arthrodesis for most patients with posttraumatic arthritis. Occasionally, however, removal of osteophytes especially from the anterior ankle, with open or arthroscopic techniques can significantly improve symptoms.

TIBIOFIBULAR SYNOSTOSIS

After disruption of the tibiofibular syndesmosis, heterotopic bone occasionally forms in the soft tissues between the tibia and fibula and may unite to both to produce a synostosis. It occurs with and without syndesmosis transfixation screws and is probably dependent primarily on the severity of the original injury. It may be completely asymptomatic or may be associated with pain during push-off. If so, its excision may help relieve symptoms.[73,83,127]

NONUNION

Nonunions of the ankle, albeit rare, are usually treated with small autogenous cancellous bone grafts and stable internal fixation. Medial malleolar nonunions with interposed periosteum have been successfully treated with currettage of the fibrous interface, packing of cancellous bone grafting, and rigid screw fixation. Fibular nonunions result from unreduced significant displacement, comminution, or bone loss. In the case of bone loss or comminution, bone grafting should be considered. When this is anticipated, the iliac crest should be prepared. An alternative is Gerdy's tubercle in the proximal tibia, where a small to moderate amount of cancellous graft is available.

WOUND SLOUGHS

Soft tissue wounds around the ankle usually result from high-energy trauma. Open ankle fractures are usually treated as mentioned previously with aggressive surgical debridement, immediate internal fixation, and delayed wound closure. In the event of a superficial skin loss, the wound can be treated with wet to dry dressing changes for a five- to seven-day period and then followed by split-thickness skin grafting with a one to one-and-a-half mesh. Alternatively, skin substitutes (e.g., Epigard) or Seligson's bead pouch technique can be used, especially if there is exposed bone and tendon, to prevent dessication and infection.

With the sophistication of microvascular transfer techniques, consultation with a microvascular surgeon well versed in orthopedic injuries can provide reconstructive options not previously available.[71,215] Small, well-perfused free tissue transfers may be more cosmetic and more functional than the split-thickness skin graft that was previously placed on granulating periosteum. The free tissue transfer can salvage the ankle after a potentially catastrophic injury, especially in the event of an open joint. If severe cartilage injury has occurred to either the tibial or the talar articular surface, ankle arthrodesis may be required.[38] The free tissue transfers provide a much more appropriate surgical soft tissue environment for arthrodesis.

REFERENCES

1. Ahl, T.; Dalen, N.; Holmberg, S.; Selvik, G. Early weight bearing of displaced ankle fractures. Acta Orthop Scand 58(5):535–538, 1987.
2. Ahl, T.; Dalen, N.; Selvik, G. Ankle fractures. A clinical and roentgenographic stereophotogrammetric study. Clin Orthop 245:246–255, 1989.
3. Ahlgren, O.; Larsson, S. Reconstruction for lateral ligament injuries of the ankle. J Bone Joint Surg 71B(2):300–303, 1989.
4. Ahovuo, J.; Kaartinen, E.; Slatis, P. Diagnostic value of stress radiography in lesions of the lateral ligaments of the ankle. Acta Radiol 29(6):711–714, 1988.
5. Allen, M.J.; McShane, M. Inversion injuries to the lateral ligament of the ankle joint. A pilot study of treatment. Br J Clin Pract 39(7):282–286, 1985.
6. Andersen, E.; Hvass, I. Treatment of lateral instability of the ankle—a new modification of the Evans repair. Arch Orthop Trauma Surg 106(1):15–17, 1986.
7. Anderson, M.E. Reconstruction of the lateral ligaments of the ankle using the plantaris tendon. J Bone Joint Surg 67A(6):930–934, 1985.
7a. Anonymous. Residual disability after ankle joint injury. Editorial. Lancet 1:1056, 1989.
7b. Anonymous. Achilles tendon rupture. Editorial. Lancet 1:1427–1428, 1989.
8. Arciero, R.A.; Shishido, N.S.; Parr, T.J. Acute anterolateral compartment syndrome secondary to rupture of the peroneus longus muscle. Am J Sports Med 12(5):366–367, 1984.
9. Arrowsmith, S.R.; Fleming, L.L.; Allman, F.L. Traumatic dislocations of the peroneal tendons. Am J Sports Med 11(3):142–146, 1983.
10. Ayeni, J.P. Pilon fractures of the tibia: A study based on 19 cases. Injury 19(2):109–114, 1988.
11. Baird, R.A.; Jackson, S.T. Fractures of the distal part of the fibula with associated disruption of the deltoid ligament. Treatment without repair of the deltoid ligament. J Bone Joint Surg 69A(9):1346–1352, 1987.
12. Balduini, F.C.; Vegso, J.J.; Torg, J.S.; Torg, E. Management and rehabilitation of ligamentous injuries to the ankle. Sports Med 4(5):364–380, 1987.
12a. Barber, F.A.; Britt, B.T.; Ratliff, H.W.; Sutker, A.N. Arthroscopic surgery of the ankle. Orthop Rev 17:446–451, 1988.
13. Barnes, M.J.; Hardy, A.E. Delayed reconstruction of the calcaneal tendon. J Bone Joint Surg 68B:121–124, 1986.
14. Bassett, F.H. III; Gates, H.S. III; Billys, J.B.; et al. Talar impingement by the anteroinferior tibiofibular ligament. A cause of chronic pain in the ankle after inversion sprain. J Bone Joint Surg 72A(1):55–59, 1990.
15. Bauer, M.; Johnell, O.; Redlund-Johnell, I.; Johnsson, K. Ankle fractures. Foot Ankle 8(1):23–25, 1987.
16. Bauer, M.; Jonsson K.; Nilsson, B. Thirty-year follow-up of ankle fractures. Acta Orthop Scand 56(2):103–106, 1985.

17. Bauer, M., Bergstrom, B., Hemborg, A., Sandegard, J. Malleolar fractures: Nonoperative versus operative treatment: A controlled study. Clin Orthop 199:17–27, 1985.
18. Baxter, D.E. Ligamentous injuries. In: Mann, R.A. Surgery of the foot, Ed. 5. St. Louis, C.V. Mosby, 1986, pp. 456–472.
19. Beauchamp, C.G.; Clay, N.R.; Thexton, P.W. Displaced ankle fractures in patients over 50 years of age. J Bone Joint Surg 65B:329–332, 1983.
20. Bergfeld J.A.; Cox, J.S.; Drez, D.; et al. Symposium: Management of acute ankle sprains. Contemp Orthop 13:83–116, 1986.
21. Beskin, J.L.; Sanders, R.A.; Hunter, S.C.; et al. Surgical repair of Achilles tendon ruptures. Am J Sports Med 15:1–8, 1987.
22. Bjorkenheim, J.M.; Sandelin, J.; Santavirta, S. Evans' procedure in the treatment of chronic instability of the ankle. Injury 19(2):70–72, 1988.
23. Bleichrodt, R.P.; Kingma, L.M.; Binnendijk, B.; Klein, J.P. Injuries of the lateral ankle ligaments: Classification with tenography and arthrography. Radiology 173(2):347–349, 1989.
24. Bomler, J.; Sturup, J. Achilles tendon rupture. An 8-year follow up. Acta Orthop Belg 55(3):307–310, 1989.
25. Bone, L.; Stegemann, P.; McNamara, K.; Seibel, R. The use of external fixation in severe fractures about the ankle. Orthop Trans 14:265, 1990.
26. Bostman, O.; Hirvensalo, E.; Vainionpaa, S.; et al. Ankle fractures treated using biodegradable internal fixation. Clin Orthop 238:195–203, 1989.
27. Bourne, R.B. Pylon fractures of the distal tibia. Clin Orthop 240:42–46, 1989.
28. Brantigan, J.W.; Pedegana, L.R.; Lippert, F.G. Instability of the subtalar joint. J Bone Joint Surg 59A:321, 1977.
29. Bray, T.J. Soft-tissue techniques in the management of open ankle fractures. Tech Orthop 2:20–28, 1987.
30. Bray, T.J.; Endicott, M.; Capra, S.E. Treatment of open ankle fractures. Immediate internal fixation vs closed immobilization and delayed fixation. Clin Orthop 240:47–52, 1989.
31. Brostrom, L. Sprained ankles. Anatomic lesions in recent sprains. Acta Chir Scand 128:483–495, 1964.
32. Brostrom, L. Sprained ankles VI. Surgical treatment of chronic ligament ruptures. Acta Chir Scand 132:551–565, 1966.
33. Brunner, C.F.; Weber, B.G. Special Techniques in Internal Fixation. Berlin, Springer-Verlag, 1982.
34. Burkus, J.K.; Sella, E.J.; Southwick, W.O. Occult injuries of the talus diagnosed by bone scan and tomography. Foot Ankle 4(6):316–324, 1984.
35. Cass, J.R.; Morrey, B.F.; Katoh, Y.; Chao, E.Y. Ankle instability: Comparison of primary repair and delayed reconstruction after long-term follow-up study. Clin Orthop 198:110–117, 1985.
35a. Cedell, C.A. Supination-outward rotation injuries of the ankle. Acta Orthop Scand (Suppl) 110:1, 1967.
36. Cedell, C.A. Is closed treatment of ankle fractures advisable? Editorial. Acta Orthop Scand 56(2):101–102, 1985.
37. Chapman, M.W. Fractures and fracture-dislocations of the ankle. In: Mann, R.A. Surgery of the Foot, Ed. 5. St. Louis, C.V. Mosby, 1986, pp. 568–591.
38. Cierny, G. III; Cook, W.G.; Mader, J.T. Ankle arthrodesis in the presence of ongoing sepsis. Indications, methods, and results. Orthop Clin North Am 20(4):709–721, 1989.
39. Clancy, W.G. Jr. Specific rehabilitation for the injured recreational runner. Instr Course Lect 38:483–486, 1989.
40. Clawson, D.K.; Seddon, H.J. The late consequences of sciatic nerve injury. J Bone Joint Surg 42B:213, 1960.
41. Clohisy, D.R.; Thompson, R.C. Jr. Fractures associated with neuropathic arthropathy in adults who have juvenile-onset diabetes. J Bone Joint Surg 70A(8):1192–1200, 1988.
42. Cohen, I.; Lane, S.; Koning, W. Peroneal tendon dislocations: A review of the literature. J Foot Surg 22(1):15–20, 1983.
43. Collins, D.N.; Temple, S.D. Open joint injuries: Classification and treatment. Clin Orthop 243:48–65, 1989.
44. Colville, M.R.; Colville, J.M.; Manoli, A. II. Posteromedial dislocation of the ankle without fracture. J Bone Joint Surg 69A(5):706–711, 1987.
45. Connolly, J.F.; Peterson, D.A. Explosion dorsiflexion fracture-dislocation of the ankle—an indication for closed functional traction treatment. Nebr Med J 70(10):374–377, 1985.
46. Cox, J.S. Surgical and nonsurgical treatment of acute ankle sprains. Clin Orthop 198:118–126, 1985.
47. Daffner, R.H. Ankle trauma. Radiol Clin North Am 28(2):395–421, 1990.
48. Daffner, R.H.; Riemer, B.L.; Lupetin, A.R.; Dash, N. Magnetic resonance imaging in acute tendon ruptures. Skeletal Radiol 15(8):619–621, 1986.
49. Dahners, L.E. The pathogenesis and treatment of bimalleolar ankle fractures. Instr Course Lect 39:85–94, 1990.
50. Daly, P.J.; Fitzgerald, R.H. Jr.; Melton, L.J.; Ilstrup, D.M. Epidemiology of ankle fractures in Rochester, Minnesota. Acta Orthop Scand 58(5):539–544, 1987.
51. Das, De S.; Balasubramaniam, P. A repair operation for recurrent dislocation of peroneal tendons. J Bone Joint Surg 67B(4):585–587, 1985.
51a. DeSouza, L.J.; Gustillo, R.B.; Meyer, T.J.; Results of operative treatment of displaced external rotation-abduction fractures of the ankle. J Bone Joint Surg 67A:1066–1074, 1985.
52. DeZwart, D.E.; Davidson, J.S.A. Rupture of the posterior tibial tendon associated with fracture of the ankle. J Bone Joint Surg 65A:260–262, 1983.
53. Dillin, L.; Slabaugh, P. Delayed wound healing, infection, and nonunion following open reduction and internal fixation of tibial plafond fractures. J Trauma 26:1116–1119, 1986.
54. Dory, M.A. Arthrography of the ankle joint in chronic instability. Skeletal Radiol 15(4):291–294, 1986.
55. Drabu, K.J. Soft-tissue swelling following fractures of the ankle. Injury 18(6):401–403, 1987.
55a. Edwards, G.S.; DeLee, J.C. Ankle diastasis without fracture. Foot Ankle 4:305–312, 1984.
56. Evans, G.A.; Hardcastle, P.; Frenyo, A.D. Acute rupture of the lateral ligament of the ankle. To suture or not to suture? J Bone Joint Surg 66B(2):209–212, 1984.
57. Eyring, E.J.; Guthrie, W.D. A surgical approach to the problem of severe lateral instability at the ankle. Clin Orthop 206:185–191, 1986.
58. Farhan, M.J.; Smith, T.W. Fixation of diastasis of the inferior tibiofibular joint using the syndesmosis hook. Injury 16(5):309–311, 1985.
59. Ferkel, R.D.; Fischer, S.P. Progress in ankle arthroscopy. Clin Orthop 240:210–220, 1989.
60. Fernandez, G.N. Internal fixation of the oblique, osteoporotic fracture of the lateral malleolus. Injury 19(4):257–258, 1988.
61. Finsen, V.; et al. Early postoperative weightbearing and muscle activity in patients who have a fracture of the ankle. J Bone Joint Surg 71A:23–27, 1989.
62. Floyd, D.W.; Heckman, J.D.; Rockwood, C.A. Jr. Tendon lacerations in the foot. Foot Ankle 4(1):8–14, 1983.
63. Fogel, G.R.; Morrey, B.F. Delayed open reduction and fixation of ankle fractures. Clin Orthop 215:187–195, 1987.
64. Fowler, P.J.; Regan, W.D. Management of the deltoid ligament disruption in fracture-dislocation of the ankle. J Bone Joint Surg 69B:504, 1987.

65. Franklin, J.L.; Johnson, K.D.; Hansen, S.T. Immediate internal fixation of open ankle fractures. J Bone Joint Surg 66A:1349–1356, 1984.

66. Funk, D.A.; Cass, J.R.; Johnson, K.A. Acquired adult flat foot secondary to posterior tibial-tendon pathology. J Bone Joint Surg 68A(1):95–102, 1986.

67. Gauffin, H.; Tropp, H.; Odenrick, P. Effect of ankle disk training on postural control in patients with functional instability of the ankle joint. Int J Sports Med 9(2):141–144, 1988.

67a. Giachino, A.A.; Hammond, D.I. The relationship between oblique fractures of the medial malleolus and concomitant fractures of the anterolateral aspect of the tibial plafond. J Bone Joint Surg 69A:381–384, 1987.

68. Goergen, T.G.; Danzig, L.A.; Resnick, D.; Owen, C.A. Roentgenographic evaluation of the tibiotalar joint. J Bone Joint Surg 59A:874–877, 1977.

69. Golterman, A.F.L. Diagnosis and treatment of tibiofibular diastasis. Arch Chir Neerl 16:185, 1964.

70. Goris, R.J. Irreducible subluxation of the tibio-talar joint due to a fracture of the calcaneus. Injury 18(5):358–360, 1987.

71. Gould, J.S. Reconstruction of soft tissue injuries of the foot and ankle with microsurgical techniques. Orthopedics 10(1):151–157, 1987.

72. Gould, N. Technique tips: Footings. Repair of dislocating peroneal tendons. Foot Ankle 6(4):208–213, 1986.

73. Gould, N.; Flick, A.B. Post-fracture, late debridement resection arthroplasty of the ankle. Foot Ankle 6(2):70–82, 1985.

74. Grantham, S.A. Trimalleolar ankle fractures and open ankle fractures. Instr Course Lect 39:105–111, 1990.

75. Grath, G.-B. Widening of the ankle mortise: A clinical and experimental study. Acta Chir Scand 263(suppl):1, 1960.

76. Green, S.A.; Roesler, S. Salvage of the infected pilon fracture. Tech Orthop 2:37–41, 1987.

77. Gross, M.T. Effects of recurrent lateral ankle sprains on active and passive judgments of joint position. Phys Ther 67(10):1505–1509, 1987.

78. Gungor, T. A test for ankle instability: Brief report. J Bone Joint Surg 70B(3):487, 1988.

79. Hamilton, W.C. Traumatic Disorders of the Ankle. New York, Springer-Verlag, 1984.

80. Harper, M.C. An anatomic study of the short oblique fracture of the distal fibula and ankle stability. Foot Ankle 4(1):23–29, 1983.

81. Harper, M.C. The deltoid ligament: An evaluation of need for surgical repair. Clin Orthop 226:156–168, 1988.

82. Harper, M.G.; Hardin, G. Posterior malleolar fractures of the ankle associated with external rotation-abduction injuries: Results with and without internal fixation. J Bone Joint Surg 70A:1348–1356, 1988.

83. Hawkins, R.B. Arthroscopic treatment of sports-related anterior osteophytes in the ankle. Foot Ankle 9(2):87–90, 1988.

84. Heim, U.F. Trimalleolar fractures: Late results after fixation of the posterior fragment. Orthopedics 12(8):1053–1059, 1989.

85. Heim, U.; Pfeiffer, K.M. Small Fragment Set Manual. Technique Recommended by the ASIF Group, Ed. 2. New York, Springer-Verlag, 1981.

86. Hirvensalo, E. Fracture fixation with biodegradable rods. Forty-one cases of severe ankle fractures. Acta Orthop Scand 60(5):601–606, 1989.

87. Hoblitzell, R.M.; Ebraheim, N.A.; Merrit, T.; Jackson, W.T. Bosworth fracture-dislocation of the ankle. A case report and review of the literature. Clin Orthop 255:257–262, 1990.

88. Homminga, G.N.; Kluft, O. Long-term inversion stability of the ankle after rupture of the lateral ligaments. Neth J Surg 38(4):103–105, 1986.

89. Hoogenband, C.R.; Moppes, F.I.; Stapert, J.W. Clinical diagnosis, arthrography, stress examination and surgical girding after inversion trauma of the ankle. Arch Orthop Trauma Surg 103:115–119, 1984.

90. Hooper, J. Movement of the ankle joint after driving a screw across the inferior tibiofibular joint. Injury 14(6):493–506, 1983.

91. Hughes, J.L.; Weber, H.; Willenegger, H.; Kuner, E.H. Evaluation of ankle fractures: Non-operative and operative treatment. Clin Orthop 138:111–119, 1979.

92. Hurson, B.J.; Sheehan, J.M. Use of spiked washers in the repair of avulsed ligaments. Acta Orthop Scand 52:23–26, 1981.

92a. Inman, V.T. The Joints of the Ankle. Baltimore, Williams and Wilkins, 1976.

93. Jackson, R.; Wills, R.E.; Jackson, R. Rupture of deltoid ligament without involvement of the lateral ligament. Am J Sports Med 16(5):541–543, 1988.

94. Jahss, M.H. Spontaneous rupture of the tibialis posterior tendon: Clinical findings, tenographic studies, and a new technique of repair. Foot Ankle 3(3):158–166, 1982.

95. Jaskulka, R.; Fischer, G.; Schedl, R. Injuries of the lateral ligaments of the ankle joint. Operative treatment and long-term results. Arch Orthop Trauma Surg 107(4):217–221, 1988.

96. Jaskulka, R.A.; Ittner, G.; Schedl, R. Fractures of the posterior tibial margin: Their role in the prognosis of malleolar fractures. J Trauma 29(11):1565–1570, 1989.

97. Javors, J.R.; Violet, J.T. Correction of chronic lateral ligament instability of the ankle by use of the Brostrom procedure. A report of 15 cases. Clin Orthop 198:201–207, 1985.

98. Johnson, D.P.; Hill, J. Fracture-dislocation of the ankle with rupture of the deltoid ligament. Injury 19(2):59–61, 1988.

99. Joy, G.; Patzakis, M.J.; Harvey, J.P. Precise evaluation of the reduction of severe ankle fractures. J Bone Joint Surg 56A:979–993, 1974.

100. Karlson, J.; Bergsten, T.; Lansinger, O.; Peterson, L. Reconstruction of the lateral ligaments of the ankle for chronic lateral instability. J Bone Joint Surg 70A:581–588, 1988.

101. Katznelson, A.; Lin, E.; Militiano, J. Ruptures of the ligaments about the tibio-fibular syndesmosis. Injury 15(3):170–172, 1983.

101a. Kay, D.B. The sprained ankle: Current therapy. Foot Ankle 6:22–28, 1985.

102. Kaye, R.A. Stabilization of ankle syndesmosis injuries with a syndesmosis screw. Foot Ankle 9(6):290–293, 1989.

103. Keene, J.S.; Lange, R.H. Diagnostic dilemmas in foot and ankle injuries. JAMA 256(2):247–251, 1986.

104. Kelbel, M.; Jardon, O.M. Rupture of tibialis posterior tendon in a closed ankle fracture. J Trauma 22(12):1026–1027, 1982.

105. Kelikian, H.; Kelikian, A.S. Disorders of the Ankle. Philadelphia, W.B. Saunders, 1985.

106. Kellam, J.F.; Hunter, G.A.; McElwain. Review of the operative treatment of Achilles tendon rupture. Clin Orthop 201:80–83, 1985.

107. Kelly, P.J.; Peterson, F.P. Compound dislocations of the ankle without fractures. Am J Surg 103:170, 1986.

108. Kenzora, J.E.; Simmons, S.C.; Burgess, A.R.; Edwards, C.C. External fixation arthrodesis of the ankle joint following trauma. Foot Ankle 7(1):49–61, 1986.

109. Kerr, H.D. Posterior tibial tendon rupture. Ann Emerg Med 17(6):649–650, 1988.

110. Konradsen, L.; Sommer, H. Ankle instability caused by peroneal tendon rupture. A case report. Acta Orthop Scand 60(6):723–724, 1989.

111. Korkala, O.; Rusanen, M.; Jokipii, P.; et al. A prospective study

of the treatment of severe tears of the lateral ligament of the ankle. Int Orthop 11(1):13–17, 1987.

112. Kristensen, K.D.; Hansen, T. Closed treatment of ankle fractures. Stage II supination-eversion fractures followed for 20 years. Acta Orthop Scand 56(2):107–109, 1985.

113. Kristiansen, B. Results of surgical treatment of malleolar fractures in patients with diabetes mellitus. Dan Med Bull 30(4):272–274, 1983.

114. Kym, M.R.; Worsing, R.A. Jr. Compartment syndrome in the foot after an inversion injury to the ankle. A case report. J Bone Joint Surg 72A(1):138–139, 1990.

114a. Lange, R.H.; Back, A.W.; Hansen, S.T. Jr.; Johansen, K.H. Open tibial fracture with associated vascular injuries. Prognosis for limb salvage. J Trauma 25:203, 1985.

115. Larsen, E. Experimental instability of the ankle. A radiographic investigation. Clin Orthop 204:193–200, 1986.

116. Larsen, E.; Flink-Olsen, M.; Seerup, K. Surgery for recurrent dislocation of the peroneal tendons. Acta Orthop Scand 55(5):554–555, 1984.

117. Lassiter, T.E. Jr.; Malone, T.R.; Garrett, W.E. Jr. Injury to the lateral ligaments of the ankle. Orthop Clin North Am 20(4):629–640, 1989.

118. Lauge-Hansen, N. Fractures of the ankle. Analytic historic survey as basis of new experimental roentgenologic and clinical investigations. Arch Surg 56:259–317, 1948.

119. Lauge-Hansen, N. Fractures of the ankle II. Combined experimental-surgical and experimental-roentgenologic investigation. Arch Surg 60:957–985, 1950.

119a. Lea, R.B.; Smith, L. Nonsurgical treatment of tendo-Achilles rupture. J Bone Joint Surg 54A:1398, 1972.

120. Leeds, H.C.; Ehrlich, M.G. Instability of the distal tibiofibular syndesmosis after bimalleolar and trimalleolar ankle fractures. J Bone Joint Surg 66A(4):490–503, 1984.

121. Lehto, M.; Tunturi, T. Improvement 2–9 years after ankle fracture. Acta Orthop Scand 61(1):80, 1990.

122. LeMelle, D.P.; Janis, L.R. Longitudinal rupture of the peroneus brevis tendon: A study of eight cases. J Foot Surg 28(2):132–136, 1989.

122a. Limbird, R.S.; Aaron, R.K. Laterally comminuted fracture dislocation of the ankle. J Bone Joint Surg 69A:881–885, 1987.

123. Lindsjö, U. Classification of ankle fractures: the Lauge-Hansen or AO system? Clin Orthop 199:12–16, 1985.

124. Lindsjö, U. Operative treatment of ankle fracture-dislocations: A follow-up study of 306/321 consecutive cases. Clin Orthop 199:28–38, 1985.

124a. Lindsjö, U.; Danckwardt-Lillieström, G.; Sahlstedt, B. Measurement of the motion range in the loaded ankle. Clin Orthop 199:68–71, 1985.

125. Litchfield, J.C. The treatment of unstable fractures of the ankle in the elderly. Injury 18(2):128–132, 1987.

126. Lundeen, R.O. Arthroscopic evaluation of traumatic injuries to the ankle and foot. Part II: Chronic posttraumatic pain. J Foot Surg 29(1):59–71, 1990.

127. Lundeen, R.O. Medial impingement lesions of the tibial plafond. J Foot Surg 26(1):37–40, 1987.

128. Maale, G.; Seligson, D. Fractures through the weightbearing surface of the distal tibia. Orthopedics 3:517–521, 1980.

129. Magid, D.; Michelson, J.D.; Ney, D.R.; Fishman, E.K. Adult ankle fractures: Comparison of plain films and interactive two- and three-dimensional CT scans. AJR 154(5):1017–1023, 1990.

130. Mak, K.H.; Chan, K.M.; Leung, P.C. Ankle fracture treated with the AO principle—an experience with 116 cases. Injury 16(4):265–272, 1985.

131. Manderson, E.L. The uncommon sprain. Ligamentous diastasis of the ankle without fracture or bony deformity. Orthop Rev 15(10):664–668, 1986.

132. Mann, R.A. Biomechanics of the foot and ankle. In: Mann, R.A. Surgery of the Foot and Ankle, Ed. 5. St. Louis, C.V. Mosby, 1986.

133. Mann, R.A.; Thompson, F.M. Rupture of the posterior tibial tendon causing flat foot. Surgical treatment. J Bone Joint Surg 67A(4):556–561, 1985.

134. Markolf, K.L.; Schmalzried, T.P.; Ferkel, R.D. Torsional strength of the ankle in vitro. The supination-external-rotation injury. Clin Orthop (246):266–272, 1989.

135. Martens, M.A.; Noyez, J.F.; Mulier, J.C. Recurrent dislocation of the peroneal tendons. Results of rerouting the tendons under the calcaneofibular ligament. Am J Sports Med 14(2):148–150, 1986.

136. Marti, R.K.; Raaymakers, E.L.F.B.; Nolte, P.A. Malunited ankle fractures. The late results of reconstruction. J Bone Joint Surg 72B:709–713, 1990.

137. Martin, D.F.; Curl, W.W.; Baker, C.L. Arthroscopic treatment of chronic synovitis of the ankle. Arthroscopy 5(2):110–114, 1989.

138. Martin, J.W.; Thompson, G.H. Achilles tendon rupture. Occurrence with a closed ankle fracture. Clin Orthop 210:216–218, 1986.

139. Marymont, J.V.; Lynch, M.A.; Henning, C.E. Acute ligamentous diastasis of the ankle without fracture. Evaluation by radionuclide imaging. Am J Sports Med 14(5):407–409, 1986.

140. Mast, J. Reduction techniques in fractures of the distal tibial articular surface. Tech Orthop 2:29–36, 1987.

141. Mast, J.; Jakob, R.; Ganz, R. Planning and Reduction Technique in Fracture Surgery. New York, Springer-Verlag, 1989.

141a. Mast, J.W.; Spiege, P.G.; Pappas, J.N. Fractures of the tibial pilon. Clin Orthop 230:68–82, 1988.

142. Mast, J.W.; Spiegel, P.G. Complex ankle fractures. In: Meyers, M.H., Ed. The Multiply Injured Patient with Complex Fractures. Philadelphia, Lea and Febiger; 1984.

143. Maurice, H.; Watt, I. Technetium-99m hydroxymethylene diphosphonate scanning of acute injuries to the lateral ligaments of the ankle. Br J Radiol 62(733):31–34, 1989.

144. Mazur, J.M.; Schwartz, E.; Simon, S.R. Ankle arthrodesis: Long term follow-up with gait analysis. J Bone Joint Surg 61A:964–975, 1979.

145. McDaniel, W.J.; Wilson, F.C. Trimalleolar fractures of the ankle. Clin Orthop 122:37–45, 1977.

146. McLennan, J.G.; Ungersma, J. Evaluation of the treatment of ankle fractures with the Inyo nail. J Orthop Trauma 2(4):272–276, 1988.

147. McLennan, J.G.; Ungersma, J.A. A new approach to the treatment of ankle fractures. The Inyo nail. Clin Orthop 213:125–136, 1986.

148. McMaster, J.H.; Scranton, P.E. Tibiofibular synostosis. A cause of ankle disability. Clin Orthop 111:172–174, 1975.

149. Meyer, J.M.; Garcia, J.; Hoffmeyer, P.; Fritschy, D. The subtalar sprain. A roentgenographic study. Clin Orthop 226:169–173, 1988.

150. Meyer, J.M.; Hoffmeyer, P.; Savoy, X. High resolution computed tomography in the chronically painful ankle sprain. Foot Ankle 8(6):291–296, 1988.

151. Meyer, J.M.; Lagier, R. Post-traumatic sinus tarsi syndrome. Acta Orthop Scand 48:121–128, 1977.

152. Micheli, L.J.; Waters, P.M.; Sanders, D.P. Sliding fibular graft repair for chronic dislocation of the peroneal tendons. Am J Sports Med 17(1):68–71, 1989.

153. Mitchell, M.J.; Ho, C.; Howard, B.A.; et al. Diagnostic imaging

of trauma to the ankle and foot: I. Fractures about the ankle. J Foot Surg 28(2):174–179, 1989.

154. Mitchell, M.J.; Ho, C.; Howard, B.A.; et al. Diagnostic imaging of trauma to the ankle and foot: Part II. J Foot Surg 28(3):266–271, 1989.

155. Mittal, R.L.; Jain, N.C. Traumatic dislocation of the tibialis posterior tendon. Int Orthop 12(3):259–260, 1988.

156. Molnar, M.E. Rehabilitation of the injured ankle. Clin Sports Med 7(1):193–204, 1988.

157. Montague, A.P.; McQuillan, R.F. Clinical assessment of apparently sprained ankle and detection of fracture. Injury 16(8):545–546, 1985.

158. Montane, I.; Zych, G.A. An unusual fracture of the talus associated with a bimalleolar ankle fracture. A case report and review of the literature. Clin Orthop 208:278–281, 1986.

159. Morris, M.; Chandler, R.W. Fractures of the ankle. Tech Orthop 2:10–19, 1987.

160. Müller, M.E.; Allgöwer, M.; Schneider, R.; Willenegger, H. Manual of Internal Fixation. New York, Springer-Verlag, 1979.

161. Müller, M.E.; Nazarian, S.; Koch, P. Classification AO des Fractures. New York, Springer-Verlag, 1987.

162. Needleman, R.L.; Skrade, D.A.; Stiehl, J.B. Effect of the syndesmotic screw on ankle motion. Foot Ankle 10(1):17–24, 1989.

162a. Nistor, L. Surgical and non-surgical treatment of Achilles tendon rupture. J Bone Joint Surg 63A:394–399, 1981.

163. Nitz, A.J.; Dobner, J.J.; Kersey, D. Nerve injury and grades II and III ankle sprains. Am J Sports Med 13(3):177–182, 1985.

164. Noyez, J.F.; Martens, M.A. Secondary reconstruction of the lateral ligaments of the ankle by the Chrisman-Snook technique. Arch Orthop Trauma Surg 106(1):52–56, 1986.

165. Nugent, J.F.; Gale, B.D. Isolated posterior malleolar ankle fractures. J Foot Surg 29(1):80–83, 1990.

166. O'Leary, C.; Ward, F.J. A unique closed abduction-external rotation ankle fracture. J Trauma 29(1):119–121, 1989.

167. Oden, R.R. Tendon injuries about the ankle resulting from skiing. Clin Orthop 216:63–69, 1987.

167a. Olerud, C. The effect of the syndesmotic screw on the extension capacity of the ankle joint. Arch Orthop Trauma Surg 104:299–302, 1985.

168. Olerud, C.; Molander, H. Atypical pronation-eversion ankle joint fractures. Arch Orthop Trauma Surg 102(3):201–202, 1984.

169. Olerud, C.; Molander, H. Bi- and trimalleolar ankle fractures operated with nonrigid internal fixation. Clin Orthop 206:253–260, 1986.

169a. Ordway, C.B.; Weiner, L.; Bergman, M.; et al. Wire tension techniques combined with minimal internal fixation for treatment of juxtaarticular fractures. Exhibit 3608. 58th Annual Meeting of the American Academy of Orthopaedic Surgeons. Anaheim, CA, November 7–12, 1991.

170. Ovadia, D.N.; Beals, R.K. Fractures of the tibial plafond. J Bone Joint Surg 68A:543–551, 1986.

171. Pankovich, A.M. Fractures of the fibula proximal to the distal tibiofibular syndesmosis. J Bone Joint Surg 60A:221–229, 1978.

172. Pankovich, A.M. Maisonneuve fracture of the fibula. J Bone Joint Surg 58A:337–342, 1976.

173. Parisien, J.S. Ankle and subtalar joint arthroscopy. An update. Bull Hosp Jt Dis Orthop Inst 47(2):262–272, 1987.

174. Parisien, J.S.; Vangsness, T. Operative arthroscopy of the ankle. Three years' experience. Clin Orthop 199:46–53, 1985.

175. Paulos, L.E.; Johnson, C.L.; Noyes, F.R. Posterior compartment fractures of the ankle. A commonly missed athletic injury. Am J Sports Med 11(6):439–443, 1983.

176. Pettrone, F.A.; Gail, M.; Pee, D.; et al. Quantitative criteria for prediction of results after displaced fracture of the ankle. J Bone Joint Surg 65A:667–677, 1983.

177. Phillips, W.A.; Schwartz, H.S.; Keller, C.S.; et al. A prospective, randomized study of the management of severe ankle fractures. J Bone Joint Surg 67A(1):67–78, 1985.

178. Plattner, P.F. Tendon problems of the foot and ankle. The spectrum from peritendinitis to rupture. Postgrad Med 86(3):155–162, 167–170, 1989.

179. Pointer, J. Using an Unna's boot in treating ligamentous ankle injuries. West J Med 139(2):257–259, 1983.

180. Poll, R.G.; Duijfjes, F. The treatment of recurrent dislocation of the peroneal tendons. J Bone Joint Surg 66B(1):98–100, 1984.

181. Pozo, J.L.; Jackson, A.M. A rerouting operation for dislocation of peroneal tendons: operative technique and case report. Foot Ankle 5(1):42–44, 1984.

182. Pritsch, M.; Horoshovski, H.; Farine, I. Ankle arthroscopy. Clin Orthop 184:137–140, 1984.

183. Raemy, H.; Jakob, R.P. Functional treatment of fresh fibular ligament injuries using the Aircast ankle brace. Swiss J Sports Med 31:53–57, 1983.

183a. Ramsey, P.; Hamilton, W. Changes in tibiotalar area of contact caused by lateral talar shift. J Bone Joint Surg 58A:356–357, 1976.

184. Rasmussen, O. Stability of the ankle joint. Analysis of the function and traumatology of the ankle ligaments. Acta Orthop Scand (Suppl) 211:1–75, 1985.

185. Rasmussen, O.; Jensen, I.T.; Hedeboe, J. An analysis of the function of the posterior talofibular ligament. Int Orthop 7(1):41–48, 1983.

186. Rasmussen, O.; Kromann-Andersen, C. Experimental ankle injuries. Analysis of the traumatology of the ankle ligaments. Acta Orthop Scand 54(3):356–362, 1983.

187. Rasmussen, O.; Kromann-Andersen, C.; Boe, S. Deltoid ligament. Functional analysis of the medial collateral ligamentous apparatus of the ankle joint. Acta Orthop Scand 54(1):36–44, 1983.

189. Riegels-Nielsen, P.; Christensen, J.; Greiff, J. The stability of the tibio-fibular syndesmosis following rigid internal fixation for type C malleolar fractures: an experimental and clinical study. Injury 14(4):357–360, 1983.

190. Riegler, H.F. Reconstruction for lateral instability of the ankle. J Bone Joint Surg 66A(3):336–339, 1984.

191. Ries, M.D.; Meinhard, B.P. Medial external fixation with lateral plate internal fixation in metaphyseal tibial fractures. Clin Orthop 256:215–223, 1990.

192. Rijke, A.M.; Jones, B.; Vierhout, P.A. Stress examination of traumatized lateral ligaments of the ankle. Clin Orthop 210:143–151, 1986.

193. Roberts, R.S. Surgical treatment of displaced ankle fractures. Clin Orthop 172:164–170, 1983.

194. Robertson, D.B.; Daniel, D.M.; Biden, E. Soft tissue fixation to bone. Am J Sports Med 14:398–403, 1986.

195. Rosenberg, Z.S.; Cheung, Y.; Jahss, M.H.; et al. Rupture of posterior tibial tendon: CT and MR imaging with surgical correlation. Radiology 169(1):229–235, 1988.

196. Rosenberg, Z.S.; Feldman, F.; Singson, R.D. Peroneal tendon injuries: CT analysis. Radiology 161(3):743–748, 1986.

197. Rosenberg, Z.S.; Feldman, F.; Singson, R.D.; Kane, R. Ankle tendons: Evaluation with CT. Radiology 166(1, pt. 1):221–226, 1988.

198. Rosenberg, Z.S.; Jahss, M.H.; Noto, A.M.; et al. Rupture of the posterior tibial tendon: CT and surgical findings. Radiology 167(2):489–493, 1988.

199. Ross, S.D.; Matta, J. Internal compression arthrodesis of the ankle. Clin Orthop 199:54–60, 1985.

199a. Rubin, G.; Witien, M. The talar tilt angle and fibular collateral ligaments. J Bone Joint Surg 42A:311–326, 1960.

200. Rüedi, T.P.; Allgöwer, M. The operative treatment of intraarticular fractures of the lower end of the tibia. Clin Orthop 138:105–110, 1979.

200a. Ryan, J.B.; Hopkinson, W.J.; Wheeler, J.H.; et al. Office management of the acute ankle sprain. Clin Sports Med 8:477–495, 1989.

201. Sammarco, G.J.; DiRaimondo, C.V. Surgical treatment of lateral ankle instability syndrome. Am J Sports Med 16(5):501–511, 1988.

202. Sarrafian, S.K. Anatomy of the Foot and Ankle. Philadelphia, J.B. Lippincott, 1983.

203. Sartoris, D.J.; Resnick, D. Magnetic resonance imaging of tendons in the foot and ankle. J Foot Surg 28(4):370–377, 1989.

204. Schaap, G.R.; de Keizer, G.; Marti, K. Inversion trauma of the ankle. Arch Orthop Trauma Surg 108(5):273–275, 1989.

205. Schaffer, J.J.; Lock, T.R.; Salciccioli, G.G. Posterior tibial tendon rupture in pronation-external rotation ankle fractures. J Trauma 27(7):795–796, 1987.

206. Schaffer, J.J.; Manoli, A. II. The antiglide plate for distal fibular fixation. A biomechanical comparison with a lateral plate. J Bone Joint Surg 69A:596–604, 1987.

207. Schatzker, J.; Johnson, R.G. Fracture-dislocation of the ankle with anterior dislocation of the fibula. J Trauma 23(5):420–423, 1983.

208. Scheller, A.D.; Kasser, J.R.; Quigley, T.B. Tendon injuries about the ankle. Clin Sports Med 2(3):631–641, 1983.

209. Sedel, L. The surgical management of nerve lesions in the lower limbs. Clinical evaluation, surgical technique and results. Int Orthop 9:159–170, 1985.

209a. Seddon, H.J. Surgical Disorders of Peripheral Nerves, Ed. 2. London, Churchill Livingstone, 1975.

210. Segal, D. Introduction. In: Yablon, I.G.; Segal, D.; Leach, R.E. Ankle Injuries. New York, Churchill Livingstone, 1983.

211. Segal, D.; Wiss, D.A.; Whitelaw, G.P. Functional bracing and rehabilitation of ankle fractures. Clin Orthop 199:39–45, 1985.

212. Segal, D.; Yablon, I.G. Bi-malleolar fractures. In: Yablon, I.G.; Segal, D.; Leach, R.E., eds. Ankle Injuries. New York, Churchill Livingstone, 1983, pp. 31–70.

213. Shelton, M.L.; Anderson, R.L. Jr. Complications of fractures and dislocations of the ankle. In: Epps, C.H. Jr., ed. Complications in Orthopaedic Surgery, ed. 2, Vol. 1. Philadelphia, J.B. Lippincott, 1986, pp. 599–648.

214. Shelton, M.; James, R.; Shelton, Y. Pilon fractures—a new classification and treatment. Orthop Trans 13:762, 1989.

215. Sherman, R.; Wellisz, T.; Wiss, D.; et al. Coverage of type III open ankle and foot fractures with the temporoparietal fascial free flap. Orthop Trans 14:265, 1990.

216. Skie, M.; Woldenberg, L.; Ebraheim, N.; Jackson, W.T. Assessment of collicular fractures of the medial malleolus. Foot Ankle 10(3):118–123, 1989.

217. Slatis, P.; Santavirta, S.; Sandelin, J. Surgical treatment of chronic dislocation of the peroneal tendons. Br J Sports Med 22(1):16–18, 1988.

218. Smith, R.W.; Reischl, S, The influence of dorsiflexion in the treatment of severe ankle sprains: An anatomical study. Foot Ankle 9(1):28–33, 1988.

219. Snook, G.A.; Chrisman, O.D.; Wilson, T.C. Long-term results of the Chrisman-Snook operation for reconstruction of the lateral ligaments of the ankle. J Bone Joint Surg 67A(1):1–7, 1985.

220. Soballe, K.; Kjaersgaard-Anderson, P. Ruptured tibialis posterior tendon in a closed ankle fracture. Clin Orthop 231:140–143, 1988.

221. Soboroff, S.H.; Pappius, E.M.; Komaroff, A.L. Benefits, risks, and costs of alternative approaches to the evaluation and treatment of severe ankle sprain. Clin Orthop 183:160–168, 1984.

222. Soler, R.R.; Gallart Castany, F.J.; Riba Ferret, J.; et al. Traumatic dislocation of the tibialis posterior tendon at the ankle level. J. Trauma 26(11):1049–1052, 1986.

223. Solomon, M.A.; Gilula, L.A.; Oloff, L.M.; Oloff, J. CT scanning of the foot and ankle: 2. Clinical applications and review of the literature. AJR 146(6):1204–1214, 1986.

224. Sommer, H.M.; Arza, D. Functional treatment of recent ruptures of the fibular ligament of the ankle. Int Orthop 13(2):157–160, 1989.

225. Sondenaa, K.; Hoogaard, U.; Smith, D.; et al. Immobilization of operated ankle fractures. Acta Orthop Scand 57:59–61, 1986.

226. Stanish, W.D.; Vincent, N. Recurrent dislocation of the tibialis posterior tendon—a case report with a new surgical approach. Can J Appl Sport Sci 9(4):220–222, 1984.

227. Stein, R.E. Reconstruction of the superior peroneal retinaculum using a portion of the peroneus brevis tendon. A case report. J Bone Joint Surg 69A(2):298–299, 1987.

228. Stein, R.E. Rupture of the posterior tibial tendon in closed ankle fractures. Possible prognostic value of a medial bone flake: Report of two cases. J Bone Joint Surg 67A(3):493–494, 1985.

229. Stiehl, J.B. Ankle fractures with diastasis. Instr Course Lect 39:95–103, 1990.

230. Stiehl, J.B. Concomitant rupture of the peroneus brevis tendon and bimalleolar fracture. A case report. J Bone Joint Surg 70A(6):936–937, 1988.

231. Stiehl, J.B. Open fractures of the ankle joint. Instr Course Lect; 39:113–117, 1990.

232. Stiehl, J.B.; Dollinger, B. Primary ankle arthrodesis in trauma: Report of three cases. J Orthop Trauma 2:277–283, 1988.

233. Szczukowski, M. Jr.; St. Pierre, R.K.; Fleming, L.L.; Somogyi, J. Computerized tomography in the evaluation of peroneal tendon dislocation. A report of two cases. Am J Sports Med 11(6):444–447, 1983.

234. Teeny, S.; Wiss, D.A.; Hathaway, R.; Sarmiento A. Tibial plafond fractures: Errors, complications, and pitfalls in operative treatment. Orthop Trans 14:265, 1990.

235. Thompson, F.M.; Patterson, A.H. Rupture of the peroneus longus tendon. Report of three cases. J Bone Joint Surg 71A(2):293–295, 1989.

236. Tile, M. Fractures of the distal tibial metaphysis involving the ankle joint: The Pilon Fracture. In: Schatzker, J.; Tile, M., eds. The Rationale of Operative Fracture Care. New York, Springer-Verlag, 1987, pp. 343–369.

236a. Tile, M. Fractures of the ankle. In: Schatzker, J.; Tile, M., eds. The Rationale of Operative Fracture Care. New York, Springer-Verlag, 1987, pp. 371–405.

237. Tonino, P.; Shields, C.L.; Chandler, R.W. Rupture of the Achilles tendon. Techn Orthop 2:6–9, 1987.

238. Toohey, J.S.; Worsing, R.A. Jr. A long-term follow-up study of tibiotalar dislocations without associated fractures. Clin Orthop 239:207–210, 1989.

239. Trager, S.; Frederick, L.D.; Seligson, D. Ankle arthroscopy: A method of distraction. Orthopedics 12(10):1317–1320, 1989.

240. Tropp, H.; Odenrick, P.; Gillquist, J. Stabilometry recordings in functional and mechanical instability of the ankle joint. Int J Sports Med 6(3):180–182, 1985.

241. Tscherne, H.; Gotzen, L. Fractures with Soft Tissue Injuries. Berlin, Springer-Verlag, 1984.

242. Van den Hoogenband, C.R.; van Moppes, F.I.; Stapert, J.W.; Greep, J.M. Clinical diagnosis, arthrography, stress examination and surgical findings after inversion trauma of the ankle. Arch Orthop Trauma Surg 103(2):115–119, 1984.

243. Van der Rijt, A.J.; Evans, G.A. The long-term results of W son-Jones tenodesis. J Bone Joint Surg 66B(3):371–375, 198.

244. Veldhuizen, J.W.; van Thiel, T.P.; Oostvogel, H.J.; Stapert, J.W. Early functional treatment of supination-eversion stage-II ankle fractures: Preliminary results. Neth J Surg 40(6):155–157, 1988.

245. Vrahas, M.; Veenis, B.; Nudert, S.; et al. Intra-articular contact stress with simulated ankle malunions. Orthop Trans 14:265, 1990.

246. Ward, A.J.; Ackroyd, C.E.; Baker, A.S. Late lengthening of the fibula for malaligned ankle fractures. J Bone Joint Surg 72B:714–717, 1990.

247. Weber, B.G. Die Verletzungen des Oberen Sprunggelenkes. Bern, Hans Huber, 1966.

248. Weber, B.G.; Simpson, L.A. Corrective lengthening osteotomy of the fibula. Clin Orthop 199:61–67, 1985.

249. Whitelaw, G.P.; Sawka, M.W.; Wetzler, M.; et al. Unrecognized injuries of the lateral ligaments associated with lateral malleolar fractures of the ankle. J Bone Joint Surg 71A(9):1396–1399, 1989.

250. Williams, J.G. Plication of the anterolateral capsule of the ankle with extensor digitorum brevis transfer for chronic lateral ligament instability. Injury 19(2):65–69, 1988.

251. Wilson, F.C. The pathogenesis and treatment of ankle fractures: classification. Instr Course Lect 39:79–83, 1990.

251a. Wilson, F.C. The pathogenesis and treatment of ankle fractures, historical studies. Instr Course Lect 39:73–78, 1990.

251b. Wilson, F.C. Fractures and dislocations of the ankle. In: Rockwood, C.A. Jr.; Green, D.P., eds. Fractures in Adults, Ed. 2. Philadelphia, J.B. Lippincott, 1984.

252. Wiss, D.A.; Gilbert, P.; Merritt, P.O.; Sarmiento, A. Immediate internal fixation of open ankle fractures. J Orthop Trauma 2(4):265–271, 1988.

252a. Yablon, I.G. Complications and their management. In: Yablon, G.; Segal, D.; Leach, R.E. Ankle Injuries. New York, Churchill Livingstone, 1983.

253. Yablon, I.G. Treatment of ankle malunion. Instr Course Lect 33:118–123, 1984.

254. Yablon, I.G.; Keller, F.G.; Shouse, L. The key role of the lateral malleolus in displaced fractures of the ankle. J Bone Joint Surg 59A:169–173, 1977.

255. Yablon, I.G.; Leach, R.E. Reconstruction of malunited fractures of the lateral malleolus. J Bone Joint Surg 71A:521–527, 1989.

256. Yablon, I.G.; Segal, D.; Leach, R.E. Ankle Injuries. New York, Churchill Livingstone, 1983.

257. Zeegers, A.V.; van der Werken, C. Rupture of the deltoid ligament in ankle fractures: should it be repaired? Injury 20(1):39–41, 1989.

258. Zeiss, J.; Saddemi, S.R.; Ebraheim, N.A. MR imaging of the peroneal tunnel. J Comput Assist Tomogr 13(5):840–844, 1989.

259. Zell, B.K.; Shereff, M.J.; Greenspan, A.; Liebowitz, S. Combined ankle and subtalar instability. Bull Hosp Jt Dis Orthop Inst 46(1):37–46, 1986.

260. Zenker, H.; Nerlich, M. Prognostic aspects in operated ankle fractures. Arch Orthop Trauma Surg 100(4):237–241, 1982.

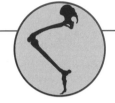

Sigvard T. Hansen, Jr., M.D.

53

Foot Injuries

Compared with the extensive literature published in the past 25 years about fractures in the lower extremity, little has been written about the treatment of fractures in the foot. Advances in fracture treatment using open reduction and internal fixation (ORIF) have demonstrated that function in the lower extremity is markedly improved when normal anatomy is retained and prolonged casting is avoided. The principles of internal fixation also apply to the foot, where excellent functional results have been realized with ORIF. Because the lower extremity cannot function normally without a sound foot, the lack of interest in modern internal fixation for foot fractures is difficult to understand.

Readers seeking information about biomechanics, history, or a review of treatments for foot fractures are referred to previous authors. Inman et al., Mann, and others have outlined the complex biomechanics of the foot, which rely on normal motion, alignment, and stability.[16,20] DeLee has contributed a monumental historical work on the treatments of fractures, dislocations, and other injuries in the foot in Mann's most recent text.[11,20] My goal in this chapter is to describe the role that modern internal fixation techniques play in restoring function and preventing fracture disease in foot injuries.

Adapting internal fixation techniques to fractures in the foot is consistent with the fundamental principles of fracture treatment described by the Arbeitsgemeinschaft für Osteosynthesefragen (AO) group in the *Manual of Internal Fixation.*[22] The *Manual of Internal Fixation* identifies four goals of internal fixation: (1) to achieve anatomic reduction, (2) to preserve the blood supply during surgery, (3) to apply stable internal fixation that meets the biomechanical demands of the affected region, and (4) to mobilize the injured limb as early as possible.

Not all fractures require internal fixation to heal with satisfactory functional results. Diaphyseal fractures in the tibia and the humerus, for example, frequently can be treated nonoperatively in a cast in a satisfactory manner. Intraarticular fractures, on the other hand, require near-perfect anatomic reduction of joint surfaces and repair of any surrounding torn ligaments, tendons, and joint capsules before full functional recovery can be anticipated. Precise anatomic restoration and repair of surrounding tissues cannot be achieved without ORIF.

Whereas full range of motion is essential in some joints in the foot for normal foot function, others function well without mobility. Generally speaking, joint motion may be lost in the flat joints in the midfoot without risking impaired function. Loss of motion in the intertarsal joints and the tarsometatarsal joints, which are predominantly flat joints, affects the overall function of the foot very little. In the forefoot, loss of motion in the interphalangeal (IP) joint of the great toe and the proximal and distal IP joints of the remaining toes has, in marked contrast to the fingers, very few consequences unless the toes are significantly deformed. All these injuries may be treated nonoperatively.

In contrast, many of the 26 bones and numerous joints in the foot are intricately interrelated and require near-full range of motion before the remainder can function normally. Open reduction and internal fixation are indicated in injuries to articular surfaces and to areas that affect articular congruity indirectly. Hindfoot joints, for example, must retain normal motion to cushion heel strike, smoothly exchange weight from hindfoot to forefoot, and provide a strong push-off during gait. Those joints that interact with others and must retain individual motion for normal or near-normal function of the hindfoot are the ankle (tibiotalar and fibulotalar), the subtalar (talocalcaneal), the talonavicular, and the calcaneocuboid. The calcaneocuboid, a flat joint in the midfoot, is an exception to the rule that motion in flat joints may be sacrificed without losing function. Normal motion of the calcaneocuboid must be maintained in order for the talocalcaneal and talonavicular joints to function during inversion and eversion of the hindfoot. Similarly, normal motion in the metatarsophalangeal (MTP) joints is essential for normal motion in the forefoot, especially for dorsiflexion of the toes during toe-off.

Being dependent in position, the foot is prone to inadequate circulation and poor venous and lymphatic return and, subsequently, to fracture disease. These conditions may lead to secondary complications such as joint stiffness, disuse osteoporosis, and muscle wasting, which can develop gradually after injury. Early motion and protected weight bearing during the healing phase mitigate these conditions. Recognizing the benefits of early motion and weight bearing and identifying which joints must move and which need not move are two extremely important factors to be taken into consideration when choosing the appropriate treatment for an injury, particularly for a navicular fracture or a tarsometatarsal fracture-dislocation.

The following sections will outline the causes of injury, the commonly seen complications, and the recommended treatments for various foot fractures. The sections on rehabilitation will emphasize the importance of initiating motion very soon after surgery and maintaining partial weight bearing throughout the healing phase in those joints where normal motion is essential for foot function.

Fractures of the Talus

Of all the bones in the foot, the most important to fix internally as anatomically as possible and to mobilize soon after injury is the talus.

ANATOMY

The articular surfaces of the head, the superior body, and the inferior body of the talus make possible flexion and extension of the ankle, inversion and eversion of the hindfoot, pronation during early stance phase, supination during late stance phase, and normal push-off. More than 60% of the surface of the talus is articular, and unless its various joints have near-full range of motion, normal gait mechanics will be impossible.

Fractures of the body and neck of the talus usually occur from high-energy injuries. Fractures of the head, midbody, and posterior body are less common but may occur from certain kinds of axial load or high-energy injuries. Osteochondral fractures are often seen with ankle sprains, subtalar sprains, and fracture-dislocations. Adequate definition of talar injuries has been aided significantly by use of computed tomography (CT) and magnetic resonance imaging (MRI). CT is especially helpful in preoperative planning for complex fractures, where it supplements plain radiographs, including oblique views of the ankle and foot. MRI provides detailed information about soft tissues and cartilage lesions.

AVASCULAR NECROSIS

Because no tendons or muscles attach into the talus, there is limited blood supply in this area, and the talus is prone to vascular deficiency and avascular necrosis, particularly after the body has been subluxated or dislocated. Evidence suggests that immediate compression-fixation may lessen the amount of avascular necrosis, and we believe that ORIF should be attempted in all talus fractures.

The Hawkins classification grades talar neck fractures according to how much the body fragments are dislocated from the neck, the ankle, or the subtalar joint and predicts the amount of avascular necrosis that may be expected.[15] Depending on the combined degree of injury, the risk of avascular necrosis in the body runs from less than 5% to 90% or more:

Type I: The talar neck fracture is undisplaced; the risk of AVN to the body is less than 10%.
Type II: The body is slightly displaced from one of the two joints; the risk of AVN to the body is less than 40%.
Type III: The body is displaced in both the ankle and the subtalar joints; the risk of AVN to the body is greater than 90%.
Type IV: Added by Canale and Kelly (i.e., not part of Hawkins' original classification), this category includes subluxation of the head, dislocation of the body on both sides, and extrusion of the body; the risk of AVN to the body approaches 100%.[6]

Fortunately, avascular necrosis is usually an incomplete phenomenon, and the presence of partial necrosis does not guarantee a poor result. In fact, compressing the two talar fragments tightly together with lag screws may permit early revascularization of the fracture site and limit the final amount of avascular necrosis in the body.

Kirschner wires were traditionally used to treat talar neck fractures but are no longer advisable, as they do not provide sufficiently stable fixation for revascularization to occur. Optimal conditions for revascularization are provided when the fracture interfaces are absolutely immobilized as early as possible by two screws in compression or by one large compression screw and a Kirschner wire. Fixation with this combination of hardware is significantly stronger than that using Kirschner wires alone. In addition, screw fixation is more beneficial to ultimate joint function because it allows early motion in the foot.

Revascularization is much more likely to occur with compression-fixation than with fusion. If symptomatic avascular necrosis does appear, we replace the avascular portion of the talus with a large tricortical block of posterior iliac crest or other cancellous bone and carry out a panarthrodesis with screw fixation. Although this tibiotalar-talocalcaneal fusion results in a fairly rigid hindfoot and produces some disability in a heavy patient or one in whom accurate alignment was not originally achieved, the pan-talar arthrodesis maintains the normal size and shape of the hindfoot and preserves the midtarsal joints. Much of the symptomatic discomfort that remains may be alleviated with well-cushioned rocker-bottom shoes.

FRACTURES OF THE NECK OF THE TALUS

The type of talar fracture that is most frequently seen in trauma centers is a fracture of the neck and the anterior body caused by a high-energy injury. A foot that is on the pedal of an automobile at the moment of a head-on collision or on the floor of an airplane when it strikes the ground is subject to excessive dorsiflexion and axial loads that may fracture the talus, usually at the neck or anterior body. Whether to reduce a talar neck fracture using a closed or an open technique is determined by the severity of the injury according to Hawkins' classification.

Closed Reduction

A minimally displaced Hawkins type I fracture may be anatomically reduced using a closed technique by plantarflexing the foot with distraction while inverting it and then compressing the fracture while returning the foot to a neutral position. Fixation is provided by two preliminary guiding Kirschner wires inserted almost parallel into the body of the talus from a posterior position and a cannulated 7.0-mm or 6.5-mm screw placed over one of the Kirschner wires.

If this fails, anatomic reduction may be achieved using an alternative technique. A cancellous 6.5-mm lag screw may be inserted with image intensifier guidance in place of one of the Kirschner wires. A fracture fixed firmly with this approach accommodates early motion and has little chance of being displaced. Treat-

ing an undisplaced or a minimally displaced talar neck fracture in a cast precludes early motion and should be considered only a temporary measure that postpones internal fixation, not an acceptable method of treatment that replaces it.

The talus consists of very dense bone and must have a gliding hole drilled into it before a 6.5-mm screw can be inserted. A 4.5-mm gliding hole must be drilled into the posterior body fragment and a 3.5-mm hole into the distal or head fragment, whether or not a tap is used. In very dense young bone, both fragments of the talus should be drilled with a 4.5-mm drill to prevent the

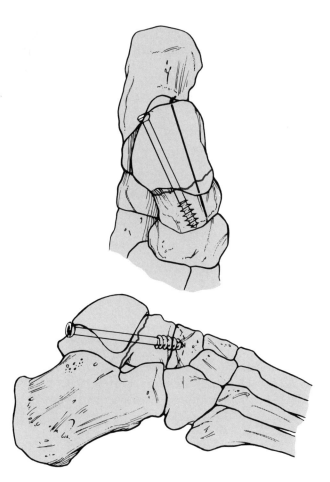

Figure 53 – 1.

In a talar neck fracture that can be reduced closed, the ideal fixation is a 6.5-mm lag screw to compress the fracture and a Kirschner wire placed nearly parallel to control rotation. This combination of fixation is strong enough to allow early motion and limited weight bearing in a fracture that is not significantly comminuted. The drill hole in the body fragment must be 4.5-mm in diameter, and the hole for the threads in the neck and head fragment should be 3.5-mm in diameter. Since the talus is extremely dense, especially in a young patient, excessive force would be needed to glide a large lag screw through 3.2-mm drill holes. A Cincinnati or a vertical lateral incision provides the best access.

screw from binding in or splitting the fragments of bone. If the drilled hole is too small, the head will tend to rotate, but rotation may be prevented by placing a Kirschner wire parallel and close to the periphery of the fracture. If only one screw is used, the Kirschner wire may be left in place during the healing phase to prevent rotation while the lag screw compresses the two fragments together (Fig. 53–1).

Open Reduction

Closed anatomic reduction usually cannot be achieved in a displaced Hawkins type II or a comminuted fracture, and these types of fractures must be exposed through long medial incisions. If lateral visualization is needed, the medial incision may be combined with an Ollier-like lateral incision or an anterolateral longitu-

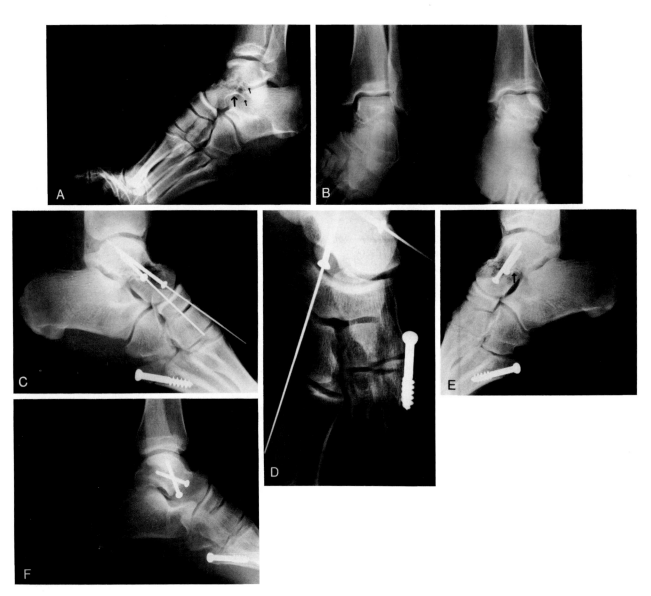

Figure 53–2.

(A), A lateral-view x-ray film reveals a high-energy closed fracture of the neck of the talus and, incidentally, a displaced metaphyseal fracture at the base of the fifth metatarsal. (B), Anteroposterior (AP) and mortice views show a minimally displaced comminuted fracture of the talus.

Radiographic lateral (C) and AP (D) views show guide wires and cannulated screws in place in the neck of the talus. The fracture was reduced and fixation was applied through medial and lateral incisions. Note that the large 6.5-mm screw stabilizes the fifth metatarsal fracture in near-anatomic position. (E), The postoperative x-ray film, lateral view, shows near-anatomic reduction and fixation of the talus with two 3.5-mm screws. (F), Three months postoperation, x-ray films show solid anatomic union of both fractures. Thanks to early motion and partial weight bearing, little demineralization has occurred in the bone.

dinal incision. The medial approach allows visualization of the sustentaculum and the talonavicular joint, whereas the lateral incision exposes the articular surface of the ankle and the posterior facet.

By combining these incisions, a surgeon may open the fracture and visualize it adequately without disturbing the blood supply in the dorsal part of the talar neck. The deltoid ligament, which is attached to the medial body and may be seen through the medial incision, provides a very important blood supply and must be kept intact. Another advantage of combining these incisions is that the fracture may be reduced more accurately without rotational or angular deformities. Comminution on one or both sides of the fracture often makes accurate reduction difficult (Fig. 53–2).

Two lag screws are used for compression-fixation after appropriate gliding holes are drilled. A 3.5-mm gliding hole is drilled into the head and neck of the talus, and a 2.5-mm thread hole is drilled into the body across the fracture site. The first screw is usually placed from a lateral position, but the point of entry varies depending on the fracture line. The lateral screw is ideally inserted from the extraarticular side if the lateral flare of the neck is part of the distal fragment. The screw must be placed as perpendicular as possible to the fracture line to provide strong anatomic compression (Fig. 53–3).

The medial screw provides good purchase when it is either placed through a tubercle in the neck or countersunk into the medial edge of the articular surface of the talonavicular joint. The primary purpose of the second screw is to provide more compression, but it also prevents rotation.

We use two 3.5-mm cortical screws to fix talus fractures because they have strong shanks and good holding power in spite of their seemingly shallow thread configuration. The screws self-tap and actually have more holding power than pretapped screws in dense cancellous bone. Gaps in the cortical bone that are caused by comminution may allow the head to angle in a varus direction and should be filled with cancellous bone graft to prevent this eventuality.

Reducing the body of the talus may be more difficult in displaced Hawkins type III or IV (Canale and Kelly) fractures.[6] In these severe fractures, the long flexor, the flexor hallucis, or the posterior tibial tendon may obstruct the partially extruded body, but in our opinion, attempts to replace the talus and to apply compression-fixation should always be made. The body may still be attached to the deltoid ligament, even if the body is completely extruded and few or no soft tissue attachments can be seen.

A long posteromedial vertical incision allows visualization of the posterior tibial neurovascular bundle and

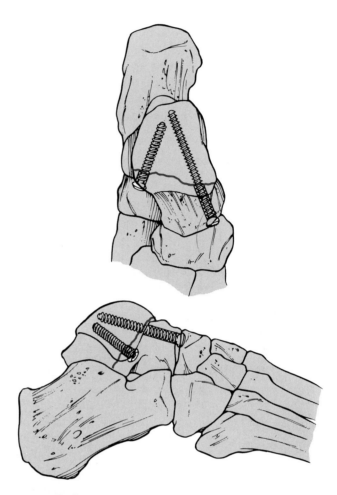

Figure 53–3.

Two 3.5-mm cortical screws are placed across a fracture located at the base of the neck of the talus. The first screw, which is placed medially, is countersunk into the articular surface. The second screw is placed through a 3.5-mm gliding hole in the sinus tarsi into a 2.5-mm thread hole in the body. In this case, both screws are relatively perpendicular to the fracture line.

the toe flexors while protecting them from injury. Reducing the body may be difficult but is made easier when the anatomy can be visualized and when a temporary screw is used as a handle (Fig. 53–4A–F).

The posterior tibial artery, which is also located here, is a major source of blood to the body of the talus, and severing this artery increases the risk of avascular necrosis. Every attempt should be made to keep the posterior tibial tendon intact when the body of the talus has been dislocated at the subtalar joint, because if the deltoid ligament remains attached, the body may retain enough vascularity to survive without requiring a major arthrodesis in the future. If the ankle or the subtalar joint is highly unstable, a Kirschner wire may be passed upward through the os calcis and both joints and extended into the distal tibia to stabilize the joints after

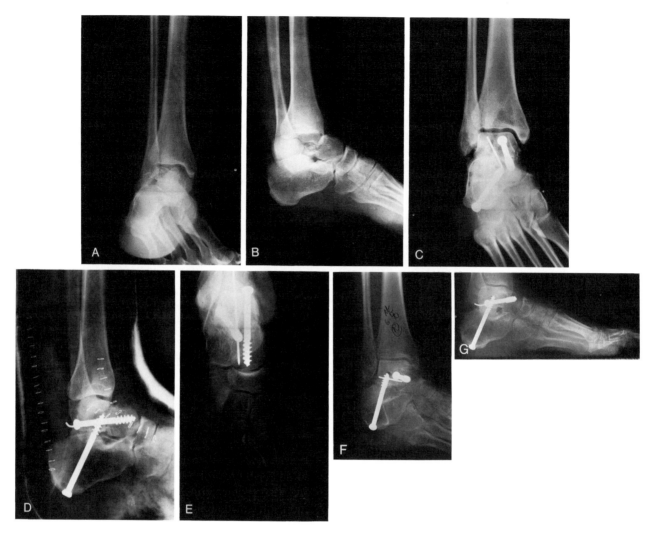

Figure 53–4.

The ankle of a patient who was injured in a high-speed motor vehicle accident is seen in a mortice view x-ray film (*A*). The patient's foot was on the brake pedal as the automobile struck a bridge abutment. The patient experienced immediate deformity and pain in the ankle posterior to the medial malleolus. (*B*), A lateral x-ray film of the same patient shows the body of the talus extruded from the talocalcaneal space. The talus body was rotated 90° in two planes and was located posteromedially, under the neurovascular bundle, where it was tethered only by the deltoid ligament. (*C*), The postoperative mortise view of the ankle shows the talar body restored into the mortise and fixed to the neck and head fragment with a 6.5-mm cancellous screw and a Kirschner wire, which were inserted posterior to anterior. A second screw was added across the traumatically denuded subtalar joint.

(*D*), The lateral view postoperative x-ray film in splint shows the fixation of the talus in place. When the fracture was visualized from the posteromedial approach, the articular cartilage in the subtalar joint was seen to be completely destroyed. A 6.5-mm screw was placed from the calcaneus into the talus to fuse this joint, since it eventually would have become painful. Fusing the joint creates a potential for added vascularity, but this was not the primary reason for immediate fusion. (*E*), The postoperative AP view shows a 6.5-mm compression screw and a Kirschner wire in the body of the talus and the hindfoot in neutral alignment. (*F*), An AP view taken six weeks postoperatively reveals early signs of osteoporosis in the talus, consistent with the partial vascularity found in the talar body. (*G*), A lateral view x-ray film of a Hawkins type III talus fracture shows fracture healing and fairly uniform disuse osteoporosis in the body fragment and in the head and neck fragment. Disuse osteoporosis indicates that vascularity is probably restored in both fragments. This case dramatically demonstrates the value of keeping the deltoid ligament attached to the talus, because in this instance it was the only remaining source of blood to the body of the talus.

the screws have been placed. This wire should remain in place for approximately four weeks and then be removed so that motion may be initiated. However, if direct observation reveals that the articular surfaces of the subtalar joint are severely damaged, a primary arthrodesis may be carried out using screw fixation.

Some avascular necrosis is to be expected in very displaced talar neck fractures, but the vascular loss is rarely complete. If part of the deltoid ligament and its branch of the posterior tibial artery remain attached to the medial body of the talus, and the blood supply is not interrupted, the medial vascularity may gradually spread and maintain normal anatomy of the talus even after partial weight bearing is begun.

Subchondral bone begins to show evidence of vascularity at approximately six weeks following injury. At that time, roentgenograms of the talus should be examined for Hawkins' sign, i.e., evidence of disuse osteoporosis. Osteolysis is an excellent indication of revascularization and confirms that more weight bearing may be initiated. Osteolysis may appear only in the medial half of the body of the talus, but even this is an optimistic sign. Union of a talus fracture is usually demonstrated approximately eight weeks postoperatively, and the patient may proceed to full weight bearing at that time.

If Hawkins' sign is not evident eight weeks after ORIF but the patient is not experiencing any painful symptoms, my experience has been that no amount of discouragement will keep the patient from gradually increasing weight bearing. Fortunately, good function is usually restored despite partial collapse or minor arthrosis.

FRACTURES OF THE BODY OF THE TALUS

The lateral and medial approaches described previously may not adequately expose fractures in the midbody or in the posterior body, and other approaches should be used to avoid dissecting or jeopardizing the blood supply at the fracture site. A fracture in the midbody is visualized best through a medial transmalleolar approach. A posterolateral approach, either vertical or transverse, is a better choice for a posterior body fracture. A vertical incision that begins just lateral to the heel cord and continues behind the sural nerve provides very good visualization of the posterior body after the posterior fat is removed. Screws inserted from here may be directed anterior and slightly medial, following the normal anatomy of the head and neck of the talus (Fig. 53–5).

In a high-energy type III or IV fracture, in which the body is extruded posteromedially, a long vertical posteromedial incision provides the best access. As mentioned earlier, the deltoid ligament's attachment to the medial body must not be severed in order to preserve blood supply.

The size of the fracture fragments and the density of the bone determine the diameter of the screws to be inserted and the size of the holes to be drilled. Large fragments require 6.5-mm screws to compress and immobilize the fracture and a Kirschner wire to prevent rotation. Small fragments are adequately secured with 3.5-mm screws inserted through 3.5-mm gliding holes in the proximal fragment and 2.5-mm thread holes in the anterior talus. Dense bone may require 4.5-mm cortical screws to maintain reduction after a 4.5-mm gliding hole and a 3.2-mm or a 3.5-mm thread hole are

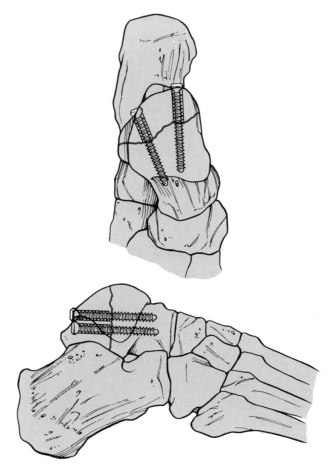

Figure 53–5.

A fracture near the midbody of the talus is fixed with two 3.5-mm cortical screws inserted from behind. This area may be approached either through a vertical lateral incision near the heel cord or through a vertical medial incision behind the neurovascular bundle. The first screw is placed under direct vision through the main incision, and the second screw may be placed either through the same incision or through a lateral stab wound.

drilled. As explained previously, the screws are allowed to self-tap.

FRACTURES OF THE HEAD OF THE TALUS

Fractures of the head of the talus are less common but may occur with axial load or high-energy injuries such as motor vehicle accidents. When these fractures occur, they are usually part of other, more complex injuries in which the talus is partially dislocated or subluxated. Capsular and ligamentous injuries frequently occur with subluxation or dislocation and are often present in fractures of the talar head.

The approach to treating fractures and dislocations in the head of the talus is similar to that for other talar fractures. Large fracture fragments are secured to the head of the talus with 3.5-mm cortical or Herbert screws perpendicular to the fracture line, and the screws are countersunk into the cartilage. Fragments that are too small to replace and hold securely may be excised. By themselves, fractures in the head of the talus do not threaten vascularity in the body, although dislocations associated with fracture may present this risk. A dislocation is treated by pinning the talonavicular joint in its anatomic position with a thick, axial Kirschner wire and suturing the capsule in place to ensure stability. A fracture or dislocation of the talar head usually heals in five or six weeks in a partial or full weight-bearing cast.

OSTEOCHONDRAL FRACTURES

Small osteochondral fractures of the talus are not always seen on standard roentgenograms and may be missed on examination, as their symptoms may mimic those of a sprain syndrome. However, the presence of fracture fragments should be suspected in all third-degree ankle sprains and in all partial or complete subtalar fracture dislocations. The diagnosis of osteochondral fragments may be confirmed by Brodèn's views on roentgenograms and careful palpation of the ankle during a clinical examination. If left untreated, even small undisplaced fragments may result in secondary subtalar arthritis that may eventually require a subtalar fusion. Scintigraphy and magnetic resonance imaging (MRI) have recently been shown to be very helpful in making difficult diagnoses.[1]

Small osteochondral fractures of 5 mm in diameter or less may occur on the medial or lateral dome or around the head. These fragments are usually composed primarily of cartilage and should be removed using either an open technique or arthroscopy, and the subchondral bone should be drilled. Larger fractures, which may include a significant portion of the talonavicular joint, should be anatomically repositioned and secured with 2.7-mm or 3.5-mm cortical or Herbert screws as soon as possible after injury, and the screws should be countersunk under the articular surface.

Osteochondral fractures on the undersurface of the talus are more difficult to diagnose and treat in an acute situation. Arthroscopy is not possible in this area, and fragments here usually lead to late arthrosis in the subtalar joint, which eventually requires a subtalar arthrodesis.

FRACTURES OF THE LATERAL PROCESS

The lateral process or "shoulder" of the talus forms the posterior wall of the sinus tarsi and the anterolateral corner of the posterior facet of the talus. Osteochondral fractures of the lateral process result from axial load injuries with dorsiflexion and eversion and are larger than most osteochondral fractures. Although these fractures usually can be seen on plain films, a computed tomographic (CT) scan may be warranted in this kind of injury to detect an undisplaced body fracture. When osteochondral fractures are large and not comminuted, they should be anatomically fixed and compressed with one or two small screws. Smaller or comminuted fragments should be excised, especially when an undisplaced body fracture is present.

POSTOPERATIVE CARE AND REHABILITATION

Postoperatively, talus fractures are treated in the same manner as other major injuries in the foot. The foot is either wrapped in a bulky compression dressing or placed in a cast for two to three days and is elevated slightly while the patient is confined to complete bed rest.

The patient should actively wiggle the toes and begin isometric exercises in the ankle and other foot muscles very soon to stimulate circulation and to control swelling. After three days, a walking cast is applied and weight-of-leg weight bearing is allowed if the fixation can tolerate the weight. The foot must be elevated frequently for two and one-half to three weeks postoperatively, at which time the original cast and the sutures are removed and a well-molded cast is applied. Weight-of-leg weight bearing and active motion of the toes should be continued until healing, which may be expected at approximately eight weeks postoperatively.

Early motion is extremely important for a satisfactory result, and a bivalve cast or a commercially made removable walker, which may be removed to gently exercise the ankle and the subtalar joints two or three times a day, are preferable to casting. However, a bivalve cast may be used on a patient who will reliably follow the exercise regimen and replace the cast afterward. At night, the cast must be firmly applied in a neutral position to prevent the foot from drifting into talipes equinus during sleep.

Roentgenograms of all fractures that are susceptible to avascular necrosis should be taken six weeks postoperatively to look for Hawkins' sign. Disuse osteoporosis that is associated with retained vascularity is sometimes found only in the medial half of the body of the talus. When this condition occurs, the patient should continue partial weight bearing until obvious signs of either healing and increased vascularity or slight collapse occur.

Some surgeons rely on a patellar tendon–bearing brace to guarantee protected weight bearing, but a brace is not always a reliable solution, as patient compliance is difficult to ensure and adequate orthotic services are not always available. Keeping a patient on crutch-protected weight bearing for a sufficient period of time is also difficult. My experience has been that unless partial weight bearing produces significant discomfort, the patient usually ceases to cooperate with partial weight bearing instructions after approximately three months and proceeds to normal weight bearing. If this is the case, I prescribe a bivalve right-angled cast at night for at least three months so that an equinus contracture does not develop.

Vigorous active subtalar exercises should be initiated as soon as the cast is removed. Active but nonresisted eversion and inversion exercises are best at first, followed by eversion and inversion exercises using rubber tubing for resistance. By looping a length of rubber tubing over the toes of both feet, one foot can work against the other in eversion. By wrapping the loop of tubing around a solid object such as a table leg, the foot may be inverted against resistance. The return of normal motion in the foot is very gradual and may take up to a year.

Our experience, confirmed by Szyszkowitz et al.[35] and others,[9] has been that total avascular necrosis is unusual if very early reduction and compression-fixation are followed by an active but low-impact postoperative course. Although patient compliance with a long and uncomfortable rehabilitation period is difficult to ensure, enough vascularity usually remains in the body fragments to heal the fracture even when a patient does not strictly adhere to weight-bearing restrictions. Anatomic reduction, secure fixation, and early motion produce excellent results in most talus fractures and allow us to anticipate near-normal function after the fracture has healed.

Fractures of the Os Calcis

Os calcis fractures are common among foot injuries. They can produce serious functional disabilities.

ETIOLOGY

An os calcis fracture is frequently caused by a work-related injury and can result in chronic disability that is debilitating to the patient and very costly to society. This fracture is usually sustained by a sudden, high-velocity impact to the heel. A motor vehicle accident is the most common cause of injury, but fracture may also occur when landing from a fall of six feet or more or standing on a floor that explodes from below. An os calcis fracture may be extraarticular or intraarticular, but the articular surface of the subtalar joint is involved

approximately 75% of the time. Os calcis fractures frequently occur bilaterally and occasionally occur together with other axial compression fractures, such as vertebral fractures.

FRACTURE PATTERNS

Palmer,[24] and later McReynolds[21] and Burdeaux,[5] described the common patterns of os calcis fractures before modern imaging techniques were available. Currently, advanced technology using CT scans reveals fracture patterns very clearly and has verified the fracture patterns described earlier. More recently, Carr et al. have published an excellent study that identifies primary fracture patterns in the os calcis in three-dimensional imaging.[8]

Several distinctive component injuries characterize an os calcis fracture. A triangular-shaped sustentacular fragment, which varies in size and comminution, usually remains in place medially. The anterior portion of the posterior facet may be impacted much farther into the body than the posterior portion. As a result, the posterior facet may appear to be rotated 30° to 60° plantarward and hinged at its posterior extent. A long posterior extension of the posterior body may be fractured and rotated upward, producing a tongue fracture. The lateral wall of the body may burst and be displaced laterally under the fibula and the peroneal tendons. This makes the heel appear wider than normal. The force of a vertical fracture occurring lateral to the sustentaculum may cause the body of the os calcis to be angled in a varus direction or to be displaced laterally. In this latter case, the laterally displaced heel appears to have a valgus deformity.

The distortion caused by an os calcis fracture is not always limited to the subtalar joint. Sagittal fractures, for example, may originate in the subtalar joint and continue anteriorly into the calcaneocuboid joint. If left unreduced, an os calcis fracture may heal in a very incongruous manner and create major deformities in the subtalar joint and in the foot in general. The heel and the arch may be flattened, the talus may be dorsiflexed in the ankle mortise, and the body of the heel may be tilted in a varus direction and displaced laterally.

Minimally displaced nonarticular os calcis fractures of any size may be treated nonoperatively. As in other foot fractures, large displaced fragments should be repaired, but small fragments may be excised. Small nonarticular fractures usually occur as posterosuperior beak fractures. They do not involve the Achilles tendon and may be excised. Operative reduction may be indicated in larger nonarticular fractures in which the Achilles tendon is involved.

The symptoms of an anterior beak fracture of the calcaneus, which involves the calcaneocuboid joint, are often identical to those of a chronic ankle sprain. Therefore, such a fracture must be suspected when a patient complains of continuing pain in the region of the calcaneocuboid or the sinus tarsi.

Closed Reduction

Closed reduction usually does not restore normal anatomy and may leave a patient with serious functional disabilities. Most os calcis fractures that are treated nonoperatively heal after 12 to 18 months with a tolerable level of residual pain, but because subtalar motion is either decreased or absent, the patient rarely returns to a normal level of activity and retains a permanent limp. Painless joint motion in the hindfoot cannot be restored without anatomically reducing the subtalar and calcaneocuboid joints. Some related injuries, such as soft tissue damage to the heel pad, may not be treatable and may create disability regardless of whether joint motion is restored.

A final note of caution concerns treatment of the posterior heel in elderly patients, in whom there is a high incidence of complication with wound healing. Treating both displaced and undisplaced fractures in a plantarflexed cast without surgery is advisable in these patients. Even though the fracture might heal in a slightly displaced position, the patient is not exposed to risk from surgery and usually is satisfied with the resulting level of function.

Open Reduction and Internal Fixation

Until fairly recently, ORIF was not a routinely successful procedure. The technique was associated with infection and wound breakdown and was thought to be dangerous. In recent years, several trauma centers have established clinical protocols for using ORIF in os calcis fractures and have reported far better results with this technique than with nonoperative treatment.[3,4,19,28,34,40] The amount of function that can be anticipated after ORIF is directly related to how accurately the talocalcaneal joint is restored, to what degree the normal height, width, and alignment of the heel are reestablished, and to how close to normal the midfoot and the forefoot are aligned.

Several technologic advances explain why ORIF is currently more successful than in previous years. Better operative equipment and imaging techniques, particularly computed tomography, allow fracture patterns to be evaluated more accurately and anatomic reduction to be planned efficiently, and new techniques handle damaged soft tissues without inflicting more harm.

After increasingly successful results with ORIF, musculoskeletal traumatologists now suggest that associated infections were the result not of the open technique itself but of the lack of skill in handling injured tissues.

Incisions

Open reduction is increasingly accepted as the best treatment for intraarticular os calcis fractures, but no general agreement exists as to the best surgical approach to use. Various incisions are advocated by prominent surgeons: Palmer,[24] Letournel,[18] and Bèzes et al.[4] endorse open reduction from the lateral approach; McReynolds[21] and Burdeaux[5] favor the medial approach; Romash[28] and Zwipp et al.[40] recommend a primary approach from a medial position, moving to the lateral side as needed; Ross and Sowerby[29] and Sclamberg and Davenport[32] prefer a sinus tarsi approach from a lateral position and add a medial approach when needed; Harding and Waddell[14] use a very small but more posterior lateral approach. Regazzoni[26] and Benirschke[3] have independently developed an L-shaped lateral incision through which the entire fracture may be visualized and anatomic reduction may be performed. This incision was described earlier by Gould,[13] who attributed it to Seligson. All these authors advocate minimal but stable internal fixation and have reported good results and a low incidence of complications.

Although good arguments may be presented for stabilization from the medial side, where there is a major weight-bearing medial wall and where fracture patterns are usually simple, I believe the soft tissue approach from this side is more difficult and may threaten the medial neurovascular structures. I prefer to use the lateral approach, because it is safer for the soft tissues and provides better visualization of the large, depressed posterior facet fragments. Another advantage of this approach is that it can be extended anteriorly to reduce fractures that extend into the calcaneocuboid joint.

Hardware

The choices of hardware for internal fixation of the os calcis are just as varied as the choices of incisions. Plates supporting the lateral wall must have a low profile so that they do not protrude from the area, and they must be narrow so that they allow the greatest possible contact between the injured bone, the adjacent soft tissues, and the blood supply.

Some surgeons prefer to use a long H plate or a 3.5-mm reconstruction plate. Both Benirschke[3] and Regazzoni[26] use screw fixation and reconstruction plates from the lateral side. Bèzes et al.[4] have developed a technique with flattened one-third tubular plates, either using them alone or crossing them and forming a Y configuration to stabilize the fracture. A Y plate is especially useful in a tongue fracture or in a comminuted fracture of the posterior body, because it may be angled backward and upward while the posterior screws are angled downward into the body of the heel. The screw in the middle section of the plate is aimed straight across into the sustentacular fragment, and the anterior screw is directed at an angle going upward into the anterior body behind the calcaneocuboid joint. A thinner, more malleable reconstruction plate is needed to stabilize the lateral side of the os calcis. A Y plate of this design would be ideal when the fracture in the posterior body of the heel is comminuted.

Operative Management

The primary goal of open reduction of the os calcis is to restore the anatomic surfaces of the joints, most often the posterior facet and occasionally the os calcis portion of the calcaneocuboid, under direct vision.

In our institution, we use the approach advocated by Regazzoni[26] and Benirschke[3] to expose the fracture (Fig. 53–6). At first impression, this incision appears to harm the damaged soft tissues, but in fact it has proved to be very safe when the soft tissues are handled gently. The incision is composed of two limbs meeting at a right angle. The first is vertical and is carried downward, just anterior and parallel to the heel cord, where it forms a juncture with the horizontal limb just above the sole skin near the lower body of the os calcis. The horizontal limb extends from posteroinferior to the calcaneocuboid joint. Both incisions are carried straight down to bone and deep tissue, leaving the subcutaneous fat, the fascia, the sural nerve, the peroneal tendons, and the lateral ligaments intact in the soft tissues as the entire flap is elevated subperiostially. The flap must be lifted gently with skin hooks until the lateral wall of the os calcis and the subtalar joint are exposed. The incision may be extended to visualize the entire upper body of the heel. If the calcaneocuboid joint must be visualized, the peroneal tendons may be separated from the flap anteriorly and pulled toward the plantar surface for better visualization.

When the posterior body is distracted downward, the medial portion of the posterior facet and the sustentaculum of the talus may be visualized, and joint fragments in the posterior facet may be replaced. A Kirschner wire and either one or two 3.5-mm screws are inserted under the posterior facet and extended straight across into the medial side of the posterior facet and the sustentacular fragment. The Kirschner wire provides provisional fixation that holds the joint in place while the screws align the joints anatomically. The medial wall is reduced indirectly by placing a trans-

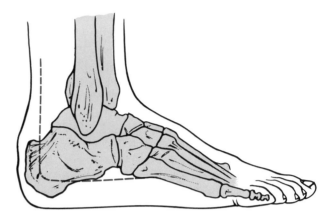

Figure 53–6.

The extensile lateral incision advocated by both Regazzoni and Benirschke is carried straight through the soft tissues, deep into the subperiosteal layer. The incision may be extended anteriorly to the calcaneocuboid joint and then posteriorly superior to the top of the os calcis. The flap containing the sural nerve and the peroneal tendons is lifted up intact. This incision is safe and allows complete reconstruction under direct vision when the flap is elevated correctly.

verse Kirschner wire or a Schanz screw in the heel, pulling it downward, and rotating the heel out of varus alignment while translating it medially if necessary (Fig. 53–7).

After the articular surface of the posterior facet is anatomically reconstructed, the body of the heel and the calcaneocuboid joint may be inspected, anatomically positioned, and fixed. Reduction of the medial wall should be confirmed on postoperative roentgenograms, and the entire flap is then carefully laid back in place and sutured with Allgöwer-Donati sutures. A small suction drain may be placed under the flap for two or three days postoperatively (Fig. 53–8).

Bone Grafting

Some surgeons favor grafting the defect that results from reducing an os calcis fracture, and others think bone grafting is unnecessary. Once the lateral wall is narrowed and returned to its anatomic position, os calcis fractures frequently heal well without grafting. However, because the posterior facet occasionally settles without a graft, we graft the defect if taking the graft does not threaten the patient with morbidity. Most young patients heal with very little defect once the fracture fragments are replaced, and for these patients, grafting may not be necessary. In older patients, whose healing potential is less certain, a tricortical block of bone may be fitted under the elevated posterior facet to fill in the defect with cancellous bone and to provide structural support.

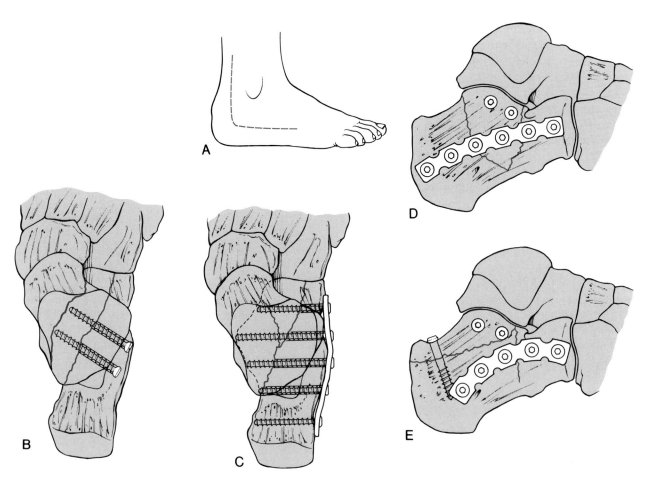

Figure 53–7.

Various methods of applying orthopedic hardware through an extensile lateral approach to an os calcis fracture are illustrated in a composite drawing. Screws or Kirschner wires were placed from just under the articular surface of the posterior facet into the medial triangular (sustentaculum) fragment in all examples. A tongue fracture must be stabilized posteriorly and superiorly to inferiorly. The lateral wall may require a variety of neutralization devices to ensure that the os calcis will maintain its length and that the lateral wall will be held securely in place, narrowing the os calcis. Indirect reduction of the sustentacular fragment on the medial side is maintained by screws that extend through the plane and across the fragment's inferior portion.

Timing

Whereas the amount of function that may be expected after ORIF is directly related to the accuracy of reduction, the accuracy of reduction is directly related to the timing of the operation. Reduction is easiest and soft tissue complications are rare when surgery is done within 6 to 12 hours of injury, before major swelling develops. However, when surgery is not possible immediately after injury, it should be postponed for approximately four to seven days if swelling becomes well established. During this interval, the foot is elevated, ice and compression dressings are applied, and the patient is encouraged to move the toes and forefoot to decrease the swelling.

Surgery must be postponed further if fracture blisters develop. Primary reduction is still possible after a delay of three or four weeks but becomes progressively more difficult. By this time, the wiser course of action may be to allow the fracture to consolidate for 3 to 12 months and to reconstruct the os calcis later with an osteotomy and a subtalar joint fusion.[7]

COMPARTMENT SYNDROME

Approximately 2% to 5% of severe os calcis fractures develop compartment syndrome from significant hemorrhaging in the sole of the foot. Although potentially dangerous, a compartment syndrome is easily recognized and may be decompressed by running a longitudinal incision along the body of the abductor hallucis muscle and bluntly opening the tissue in the sole of the foot (Fig. 53–9).

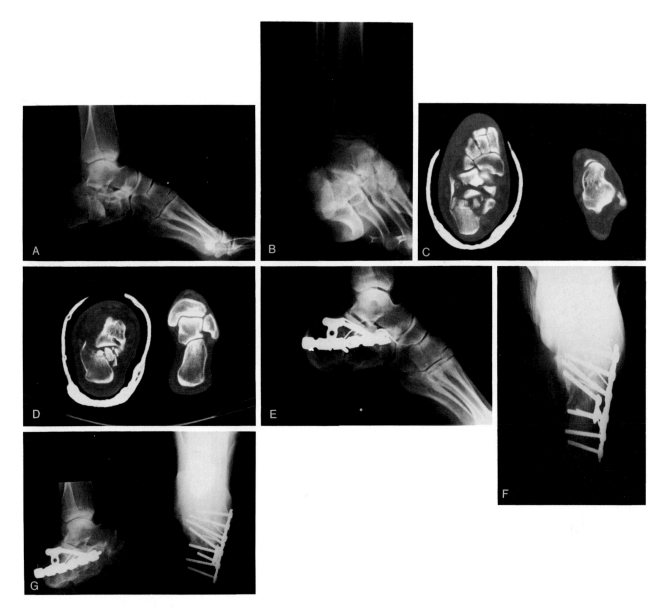

Figure 53–8.

(*A*), A lateral view on x-ray film of a comminuted os calcis fracture shows a significant depression in the lateral posterior facet and secondary fracture lines in the sagittal and transverse planes. (*B*), Distortion in the subtalar joint is seen in a Brodèn's view. (*C*), A computed tomographic (CT) scan taken in a transverse plane reveals comminution in the midbody and shortening along the long axis of the os calcis. (*D*), A CT scan taken in the frontal plane shows the lateral translation of the os calcis and comminution in the posterior facet.

(*E*), Postoperatively, the anatomically restored joint surface is seen on roentgenogram. The joint surface was restored with Kirschner wires and screws that support the articular surface. A small H plate was added under the reconstruction plate to provide better mechanical support of the posterolateral os calcis. Length was restored and maintained by the long reconstruction plate. (*F*), An axial view x-ray film of the os calcis shows the heel, which has been realigned and narrowed. The entire exposure was done through an extensile lateral approach, and the overall position is excellent, even though small fragments on the nonexposed medial side were not reduced. (*G*), A roentgenogram taken four months postoperation shows solid union. Some articular cartilage space has been lost, but the overall structural anatomy of the hindfoot has been maintained. Clinically, the patient experienced a 50% loss in motion but had little or no discomfort, and the foot had a normal appearance.

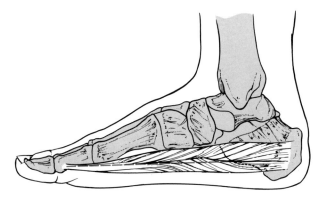

Figure 53–9.

A compartment syndrome secondary to an os calcis fracture may be released by a simple medial incision made over the abductor hallucis. Usually caused by hemorrhage into the muscles in the sole of the foot, a compartment syndrome may be diagnosed initially by symptoms of intense swelling and significant pain and, in later stages, by numbness in the toes. The diagnosis may be confirmed by measuring the compartment pressure. A long incision is made over the abductor hallucis muscle and the sole of the foot is opened with a long blunt curved clamp. This incision relieves pressure and pain by allowing hemorrhage to evacuate. Delayed primary closure may be done at four or five days.

POSTOPERATIVE CARE AND REHABILITATION

Postoperatively, a soft compression dressing is applied under a short-leg cast or splint. The patient is confined to complete bed rest with the leg elevated for two to three days and is instructed to do active and isometric exercises of the toes. Once out of bed, the patient may bear very limited weight on crutches while the foot is immobilized in a short-leg cast. The sutures are removed and a very close-fitting short-leg cast is applied two to three weeks postoperatively. At that time the patient is allowed to go to weight-of-leg weight bearing for another three weeks and to gradually increase weight bearing until eight weeks postoperatively, when the second cast is removed. After the cast is removed, vigorous subtalar exercises are begun, and partial weight bearing on crutches is continued for two or three more weeks. Full weight bearing may be initiated approximately three months postoperatively.

Alternatively, the patient may be treated without a cast. In this case the patient is non–weight bearing, on crutches, and wears elastic hose. Exercises for inversion, eversion, and dorsiflexion must be performed daily and a 90° splint must be worn at night. Weight bearing is begun after approximately 12 weeks, provided that evidence of union is seen on roentgenograms.

Tarsal Navicular, or Scaphoid, Fractures

ANATOMY

The tarsal navicular, or scaphoid, is the keystone of the medial arch of the foot. A thick, ovoid, saucer-shaped bone, it articulates with the very important talonavicular joint on its posterior or proximal concave surface. Distally, it articulates with the first, second, and third cuneiforms in three separate facets, all of which are relatively immobile. In some instances, a small lateral facet may articulate with the cuboid.

The only muscle that attaches into the tarsal navicular is a variable portion of the posterior tibial tendon (called the "anterior component" by Sarrafian), which inserts into the inferomedial tuberosity.[31] The strong inferior calcaneonavicular ligament originates on the os calcis and attaches to the inferior surface of the navicular. Just medial to this attachment is the superomedial calcaneonavicular ligament, which also connects the calcaneus and the navicular. These ligaments, together with the posterior surface of the navicular and the anterior facet of the os calcis, form the acetabulum pedis for the head of the talus.

Restoring the anatomic integrity of this complex joint is essential for maintaining normal gait mechanics after an injury. The talonavicular articulation is the key joint that allows pronation, which cushions heel strike, and supination, which strengthens push-off. It works in concert with the subtalar (talocalcaneal) and calcaneocuboid joints and is crucial for inversion and eversion of the hindfoot as the foot adapts to sloped surfaces.

ETIOLOGY

The tarsal navicular is prone to three main types of fractures: stress fractures, which commonly occur in running or jumping athletes; acute fractures, which result from high-energy injuries (usually motor vehicle accidents); and avulsion fractures, which may be part of a major fracture complex or may occur as isolated injuries.

STRESS FRACTURES

Stress fractures of the tarsal navicular often occur in running or jumping athletes who increase the intensity of their training too rapidly. The etiology of stress fractures in the navicular is unclear, although several theories have been proposed. Stress fractures may occur with more frequency in patients who have a cavus foot deformity or in those who have abnormal motion and stresses on a fibrous or osseous calcaneal navicular coalition, conditions that restrict normal motion in the navicular. Several factors seem to aggravate stress fractures, but how these conditions relate to the causes of stress fractures is not certain.

Diagnosis

A stress fracture almost always occurs in the sagittal plane in the midthird of the bone and generally starts on the dorsal surface. The presenting symptom is usually pain in the dorsomedial and medial mid-arch, and the stress fracture is often misdiagnosed as anterior tibial tendinitis. An accurate early diagnosis is expedited by being suspicious of the origin of the pain and by localizing it clinically or with scintigraphy. Plain x-ray films may not reveal a fracture in the early stages, and if scintigraphy and clinical examination suggest that a stress fracture might exist, a CT scan may be indicated. A CT scan will reveal whether the fracture is partial or complete.

Secondary changes such as cystic degeneration, partial avascular necrosis (especially in the lateral fragment), sclerosis in the margins of the fracture, and secondary arthritis in the talonavicular joint commonly occur in chronic, complete, or separated fractures. Clearly, a stress fracture of the navicular can end an athlete's career if it is not diagnosed and treated early.

Nonoperative Management

Torg et al. studied these injuries and noted that in the very early stages, when injury is pending or is still incomplete, they may be successfully treated in a short-leg cast with non–weight bearing for a period of four to six weeks, followed by gradual resumption of activity over the next six weeks.[36] This treatment regimen differs from the traditional method of treating incomplete stress fractures in the lower extremity, which simply calls for training to be discontinued for a period of time and then to be resumed gradually. If an early diagnosis of an incomplete stress fracture is missed and the tarsal navicular goes on to become a complete or displaced fracture, surgical treatment is advised.

Operative Management

Meticulous operative technique is required to reduce a navicular stress fracture absolutely anatomically and to restore the very important motion in the talonavicular joint. Dissection must be kept to a minimum to preserve the blood supply going to the navicular and to prevent avascular necrosis.

The superior end of the fracture is exposed through a dorsomedial incision, and a short talonavicular capsulotomy is performed to visualize the joint surface on the posterior side. A stab incision is made over the upper tuberosity, and a small linear incision is made just over the lateral navicular. After the fracture site is debrided with a very small curette, the medial and lateral sides of the bone are gripped with large, pointed (Weber) forceps that are inserted through the small incisions, and the fracture is compressed together with force applied perpendicular to the fracture line.

Once the fracture site is anatomically aligned and reduced, several small holes are drilled across the fracture site from a lateral to a medial direction, especially if the fracture edges are sclerotic. Following this, two 3.5-mm cortical screws are placed in compression perpendicular to the fracture using image intensifier guidance (Fig. 53–10). The screws are placed from the

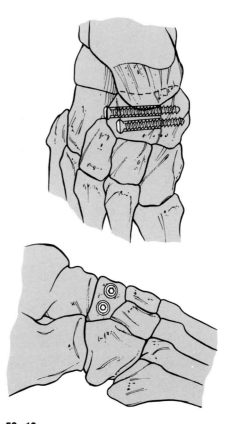

Figure 53–10.

In this navicular stress fracture, a fracture line is seen in the sagittal plane in the midportion of the navicular bone. The ideal placement of screws for this type of fracture is lateral to medial. A 3.5-mm gliding hole is drilled into the lateral fragment and a 2.5-mm thread-gripping hole is drilled into the medial fragment.

small lateral incision over the lateral fragment through holes drilled with a 3.5-mm drill and are continued into the medial fragment through 2.5-mm drill holes. The screws self-tap in this dense, cancellous bone. In large bones, a 4.5-mm screw may be used as one of the two screws, and in this case, the near fragment is drilled with a 4.5-mm drill, whereas the far fragment is drilled with a 3.2-mm drill.

Postoperative Care and Rehabilitation

A short-leg cast is applied postoperatively, and the patient is confined to bed rest with the foot elevated for two days. Once out of bed, the patient is limited to weight-of-leg weight bearing for approximately six weeks. The cast is then removed, but protected weight bearing is continued for an additional four weeks. Vigorous range-of-motion exercises should be done for supination and pronation during this time. After bony union is confirmed by roentgenograms, a more strenuous walking training program may be initiated, gradually progressing to a running training program.

If the stress fracture was originally caused or aggravated by a fibrous coalition or by an abnormality that may have precipitated the stress fracture, that abnormality should be addressed and treated appropriately.

If diagnosis of a tarsal navicular stress fracture is missed and significant posttraumatic arthritis develops, some form of fusion may be indicated. A tricortical block of iliac bone may be inserted into the injured joint to appropriately align and lengthen the medial column. Stiffness in the hindfoot and lack of normal pronation, supination, eversion, and inversion, which result from fusion, are permanently disabling.

ACUTE DISPLACED INTRAARTICULAR FRACTURES

Little has been published about traumatic tarsal navicular fractures, because isolated fractures are relatively rare. Most reports include very few cases or just one case report.

Classification

Sangeorzan et al. reported on 21 displaced intraarticular fractures of the tarsal navicular, reviewed the existing literature, devised a classification according to the type and direction of displacement, and related this classification to treatment.[30] They classified displaced tarsal navicular fractures into three types of injuries.

A type 1 navicular fracture is caused by a centrally directed axial force along the foot. The fracture line is located in the transverse plane and separates the dorsal and plantar sections of the navicular, but it is not significantly comminuted.

A type 2 fracture is the most commonly seen tarsal navicular fracture and results from axial compression with a dorsomedial force on the forefoot. The resulting fracture line runs from dorsolateral to plantar-medial. The talonavicular joint is often subluxated or dislocated, and the larger, relatively intact, dorsomedial navicular fragment is dorsomedially displaced.

A type 3 fracture is caused by an axial and laterally directed force. The naviculocuneiform joint is disrupted, and the navicular is compressed centrally or laterally. The fracture is usually comminuted and disrupted. Associated fractures may exist in the cuboid, anterior calcaneus, or calcaneocuboid joint.

Displaced intraarticular fractures of the navicular should be treated with anatomic and stable internal fixation in the same manner as for all other displaced intraarticular fractures. Open reduction is recommended for displaced fractures, because it allows anatomic reduction of the joint surface without posing a significant risk to the blood supply. The navicular is unique among bones with large areas of articular surface, however, in that its proximal or posterior articular surface is located in a joint where maintaining mobility is critical. The joint facets on its distal or anterior surfaces are much less important to restore, because these joints have little mobility and may be transfixed or eventually fused with little residual disability.

Surgical Technique

Type 1 fractures are the most easily treated and heal with the best prognosis. An anteromedial incision is made between the anterior and the posterior tibial tendons, and a small capsulotomy is performed in the talonavicular joint to visualize the fracture and the talonavicular articular surfaces. Note that navicular fractures may easily be reduced indirectly by placing a small external fixator or a distractor between the talus or medial malleolus and the base of the proximal metatarsal.

After the fracture is exposed, it may be reduced with longitudinal traction and large, sharp-pointed reduction forceps that grip the major fragments perpendicular to the fracture line through two stab incisions. Two compression screws are inserted through dorsal stab incisions to hold the fracture tightly compressed. Adequate fixation may be achieved with 4.0-mm cancellous screws, but 3.5-mm cortical screws are a better choice in this situation. The larger root diameter of the 3.5-mm screws is stronger and minimizes the chances of screw breakage. The dorsal and plantar fragments of displaced intraarticular navicular fractures are usually not very comminuted and are sufficiently intact to hold screws securely. Extending a screw from the tarsal navicular to the distal cuneiforms is usually not necessary.

A type 2 fracture presents a more difficult problem, because the lateral plantar fragment is often comminuted and the dorsomedial fragment is dislocated at the talonavicular joint. The dorsomedial fragment may have to be reduced with screws aimed obliquely into the second or third cuneiform (Fig. 53–11). This procedure is effective and is well tolerated, but it requires the talonavicular joint to be fixed separately in its reduced position with smooth Kirschner wires.

The same type of problem that is described in type 2 tarsal navicular fractures also applies to type 3 fractures: the central or the plantar lateral fragment is usually comminuted and cannot be held securely with screws. Again, the solution is to fix the large medial or dorsomedial fragment in its anatomic position by anchoring the screw in the cuneiforms. This fixation reduces both the navicular fracture and the naviculocuneiform joint disruption. Any injury that extends into the calcaneocuboid joint should be fixed separately in anatomic position with small screws or a Kirschner wire.

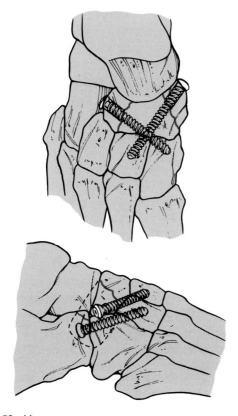

Figure 53–11.

Screws placed in a comminuted navicular fracture utilize the very dense bone in the subchondral area and the cuneiforms to fix the fragmented navicular. The goal of the reduction is to restore the anatomic articular surface of the talonavicular joint.

Postoperative Care and Rehabilitation

Postoperatively, the patient is confined to bed rest with the foot elevated for two days, and the foot is immobilized in a short-leg cast for seven to ten weeks. The amount of weight bearing that is allowed depends on the strength of fixation. Limited weight bearing may be tolerated in type 1 fractures, and the patient may gradually proceed to full weight bearing by week six or seven of an eight-week period in a cast. For a type 2 or a type 3 fracture, in which the joint is disrupted and the comminuted fragment is fixed with minimal fixation, only touch-down weight bearing is allowed for seven to eight weeks. Kirschner wires that were placed through the joints may be removed at that time, and range-of-motion exercises may be initiated while the patient continues only partial weight bearing until 10 to 12 weeks postoperatively. Weight bearing is gradually increased when roentgenograms show evidence of union.

Partial avascular necrosis, late partial collapse of the bone, or narrowing of the joint cartilage are not unusual in type 2 and type 3 navicular fractures, even after optimal treatment (Fig. 53–12). In displaced fractures, such as stress fractures, these complications may become severe enough to require later bone block fusion or even a triple arthrodesis.

A syndrome of late progressive hindfoot varus deformity is occasionally seen after collapse of the lateral navicular, and if this is the case, a talonavicular fusion or a triple arthrodesis is indicated. The sequelae of hindfoot varus deformity and the subsequent breakdown of shoes sometimes become a more significant problem than the original posttraumatic arthritis. The goal of a talonavicular fusion or a triple arthrodesis is not only to fuse the involved joints but also to correct the varus deformity by re-creating the talocalcaneal angle prior to fusion.

AVULSION FRACTURES

Avulsion fractures of the navicular are caused by excessive flexion or eversion in the midfoot. A dorsal flake of bone may be avulsed by the capsule when the foot is hyperdorsiflexed, or the inferomedial tuberosity may be avulsed by the posterior tibial tendon in a hypereversion injury. Small nonarticular fracture fragments of the dorsal lip or the medial tubercle may be excised. If the fragment is large, the capsule or the posterior tibial tendon may be reattached with a compression screw (Fig. 53–13).

Accessory Navicular Injury

Kidner suggested that injury to an accessory navicular, a nonunited ossification in the plantar medial tuberos-

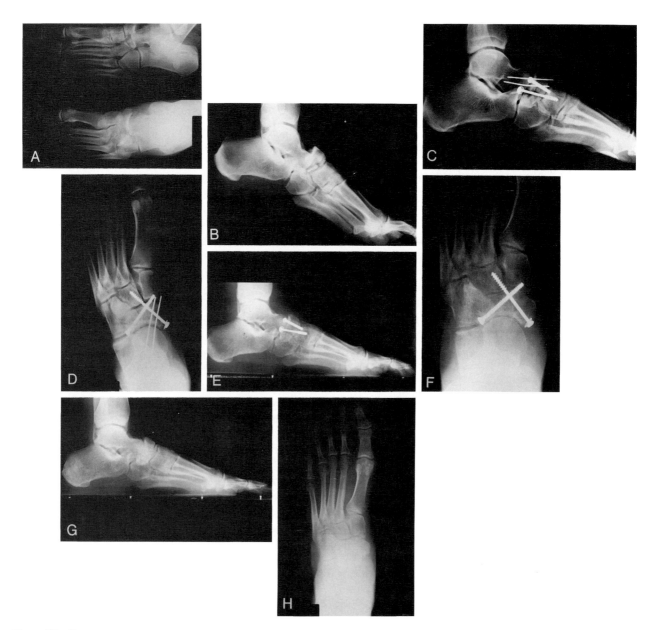

Figure 53–12.

AP and oblique (*A*) and lateral (*B*) roentgenograms show the dislocated talonavicular joint of a 24-year-old man who was injured when he fell from a roof. The patient experienced immediate pain, dorsomedial swelling, and deformity in his left foot. The dislocated talonavicular joint reveals a large intact dorsomedial fragment riding over the head of the talus and a comminuted inferolateral fragment from a crushing type-II injury.

Postoperative lateral (*C*) and AP (*D*) views of the fracture after open reduction, internal fixation show the large dorsomedial fragment held in position by screws attached to the distal tarsal row. Note that the large medial tubercle fragment is fixed by a screw that extends into the second cuneiform. The second screw, placed from a lateral stab wound, crosses the comminuted lateral fragment and enters the intact medial portion after crossing the first naviculocuneiform joint. Two Kirschner wires placed across the talonavicular joint hold the reduction intact while the capsular attachments heal. A congruent joint seen on the AP view at the end of the procedure indicates that the talonavicular joint was successfully restored.

Lateral (*E*) and AP (*F*) view x-ray films taken approximately 10 weeks postoperation show a well-healed fracture. The Kirschner wires were removed six weeks postoperation. The patient was out of cast approximately 8 to 10 weeks postoperation and was actively moving the joint with minimal weight bearing. Although the talonavicular joint space is within normal bounds, the navicular is slightly subluxated dorsally on the head of the talus.

One year postoperation the lateral (*G*) and AP (*H*) views reveal narrowing of the talonavicular joint and slight collapse, both of which are probably the result of avascular necrosis in the middle and inferior portions of the body. Approximately 80% of normal motion has returned, and the patient has good function for everyday activities, although athletic activity produces discomfort. In spite of a good initial result, the patient may need a talonavicular fusion in the future for complications caused by the avascular necrosis.

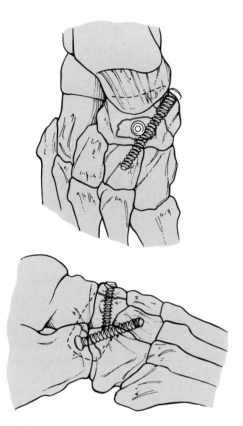

Figure 53–13.

The methods of placing screws in a dorsal avulsion fracture and a tuberosity avulsion fracture are illustrated. In the latter example, the screw is placed across the navicular and into a cuneiform bone for resistance. A small plastic washer can be used on the screw to secure the posterior tibial tendon.

ity where the anterior component of the posterior tibial tendon normally attaches, may be associated with a weak arch or flatfoot.[17a] In some instances, nearly the entire posterior tibial tendon is attached to this tubercle, and if it is excised, the foot collapses in a manner similar to the ruptured posterior tibial tendon syndrome.

If the accessory navicular is symptomatic after an injury, I recommend performing an augmented Kidner procedure. In this procedure, the accessory bone and any other excessive plantar medial tuberosity is excised, and the posterior tibial tendon is reattached to the navicular. The flexor digitorum communis is transected at the master knot of Henry and is reinserted through a drill hole in the plantar surface of the first cuneiform. An augmented Kidner procedure restores normal posterior tibial tendon dynamics to the arch without producing noticeable weakness in the plantar flexion of the toes.

Postoperative rehabilitation of avulsion fractures is similar to that for acute fractures.

Tarsometatarsal (Lisfranc's), Tarsal, and Intertarsal Fracture-Dislocations

ETIOLOGY

The five tarsometatarsal joints of the foot are very stable and immobile and are injured only by high-energy forces. Isolated injuries are often sports related and may occur, for example, when a runner stumbles into a hole or when a football player falls on the heel of another player's dorsiflexed foot. Traumatic injuries in the tarsometatarsal joints, which are usually part of a larger complex of injuries, may be caused by high-energy motor vehicle or industrial accidents. These traumatic injuries are usually open fractures and are occasionally further complicated by degloving.

CLASSIFICATION OF INJURY

Several systems for classifying tarsometatarsal fractures have been proposed, but none of the existing classifications are particularly helpful for determining treatment. The Quenu and Kuss system, for example, describes several commonly occurring combinations of injuries, but it neither classifies the injuries according to severity nor indicates optimal treatment or prognosis.[25]

A useful classification for tarsometatarsal injuries is difficult to create because of the many possible fracture combinations. The amount of displacement in a tarsometatarsal disruption may vary from a very subtle pure dislocation, which is often difficult to diagnose, to a severe displacement, which may involve fractures in the bases of the metatarsals, the cuneiforms, or the distal metatarsals. An injury to the tarsometatarsal joint may also involve a fracture or dislocation of the tarsal cuneiform bones and the cuboid.

DIAGNOSIS

Most tarsometatarsal fractures are clearly seen on standard anteroposterior (AP) and lateral roentgenograms. When no fracture is seen, a tarsometatarsal fracture should still be suspected if the base of the second metatarsal reveals a small fracture on an AP view or if the second or third metatarsals exhibit dorsal displacement on the lateral view, even if the amount of displacement is minimal. When only slight displacement is seen on roentgenograms but tenderness or swelling is present on clinical examination, diagnosis should be pursued with a stress roentgenogram view. The manipulation necessary to take a stress view can be quite painful, but pain itself is indicative of fracture or sprain. A stress roentgenogram should be done under a regional (ankle block) or a general anesthetic, the same as for an ankle sprain. The forefoot should be held in abduction with pressure for an AP view and in plantar flexion against a neutral hind- and midfoot for the lateral view. Operative treatment should be considered if the tarsometatarsal joint is displaced by 2 mm or more.

TREATMENT

Historically, the treatment of tarsometatarsal fractures has progressed from closed reductions treated with casting or percutaneous Kirschner wire fixation to open reductions fixed with either smooth or threaded Kirschner wires and screw fixation. No general consensus exists about optimal treatment, but most recent evidence demonstrates that a good final result is directly related to how accurately the reduction is accomplished and how well the reduction is maintained throughout healing.[2,24] For this reason, we recommend treating all tarsometatarsal fractures and dislocations with ORIF.

Some surgeons have expressed concern over the possibility of complications when ORIF is performed in closed tarsometatarsal fractures and dislocations. They argue that screw fixation stiffens the joints and that the risks of doing additional surgery to remove the screws three or four months after the initial surgery far outweigh any advantages ORIF may offer. In my opinion, the disadvantages of closed reduction are considerably more significant than the supposed complications from ORIF. Many patients treated with closed reductions suffer from postdislocation deformities, marked disability from secondary arthritis, and shoe-fitting problems when the original reduction was not accurate or when reduction was lost during rehabilitation. Conversely, when normal anatomy is restored, normal function for routine activities and even function required for demanding sports activities usually returns.

Stiffness from screw fixation is not a major concern in tarsometatarsal joints because they normally have very little motion; even arthrosis seen on roentgenograms does not correlate with functional disability or discomfort in the tarsometatarsal joints. We recommend that at least the medial two or three joints of all tarsometatarsal (Lisfranc's) joint dislocations or fracture-dislocations be secured with screws, while the fourth and especially the fifth metatarsals may be fixed with Kirschner wires. Surgery to remove the screws three months after the initial operation constitutes an expense, but the risks related to this procedure are very minor, and the disability time from surgery for screw removal is short.

Less disagreement exists over doing stable anatomic fixation in open or markedly displaced fractures. The advantages of ORIF in these fractures are clear: ORIF protects soft tissues, helps with general healing, and controls pain.

Timing

Timing of the operation for tarsometatarsal joints is of major importance in an open injury or in one in which the soft tissues are severely damaged. In these situations, treatment is recommended within the first 4 to 6 hours after injury, when reduction is easiest to accomplish. A dislocation in the foot may easily damage the arterial and venous circulation, and reestablishing good circulation early in this dependent limb is a critical factor in promoting soft tissue and bony healing.

The dorsalis pedis is frequently disrupted in tarsometatarsal injuries, but breakdown of this arterial flow alone is not a significant problem, as this artery is only one of many branches of the anterior and posterior tibial arterial system. However, a severe vascular injury, which may occur when the distal bony and soft tissue structures are crushed, may destroy all sources of blood to the tarsometatarsal region, and unless blood flow can be restored, an amputation may be required at the midfoot level.

OPERATIVE MANAGEMENT

The surgical approach for an isolated tarsometatarsal fracture-dislocation is carried out through two longitudinal incisions, one in the first/second metatarsal interspace and the other in the third/fourth interspace. The incisions should be approximately 4 to 6 cm long and, as in all foot approaches, should go straight down to the bone, undermining the tendons and neurovascular structures as little as possible (Fig. 53–14).

Beginning with the first and second joints, all the metatarsal joints should be explored before any fixation devices are applied. On direct observation, the capsules of the first and second metatarsal joints are often more damaged than expected, and an oblique fracture may be found at the base of the second metatarsal, where the ligamentous attachments are very firm. The first and second tarsometatarsal joints are relocated to their anatomic positions during the exploration through the first incision but are not yet fixed.

Next, the third and fourth tarsometatarsal joints are examined and relocated through the second incision. Any soft tissues or fragments of bone or cartilage that prevent anatomic relocation but are not large enough to be repaired are removed. After the third and fourth tarsometatarsals are explored and realigned, attention

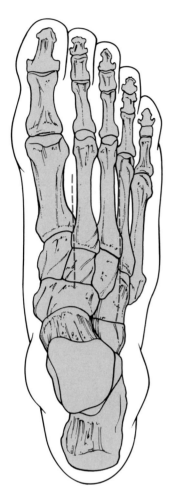

Figure 53–14.

Two dorsal incisions are usually needed to completely stabilize a tarsometatarsal (TMT) fracture-dislocation, and the parallel incisions shown here are safe. The incisions are carried straight down to bone and do not undermine or separate the skin or the subcutaneous tissues from the fascia.

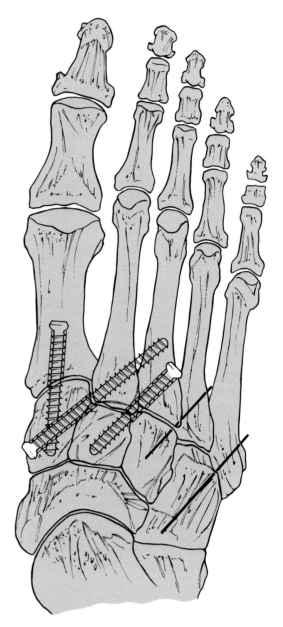

Figure 53–15.

Screw placement for the treatment of acute TMT fracture-dislocations, delayed treatment of acute fractures, and realignment and fusion of old TMT fracture-dislocations are illustrated. One screw is placed from the base of the first metatarsal into the first cuneiform through a notch in the dorsum of the metatarsal. The most important screw is placed from the proximal medial first cuneiform into the bases of the second and third metatarsals. It is angled from a gliding hole in the cuneiform directly into the proximal medial corner of the base of the second metatarsal, which has been predrilled with a 2.5-mm drill. This screw provides extremely firm fixation by compressing the base of the second metatarsal into the notch between the first and second cuneiforms as it is tightened.

Another screw can be placed at the same angle from the dorsolateral surface of the third metatarsal into the second cuneiform through the more lateral dorsal incision. It will also push the bases of the second and third metatarsals snugly into their corrected positions. Either Kirschner wires or screws may be used in the fourth and fifth metatarsals, but they must be angled from lateral to medial and must be directed slightly upward to avoid missing the more shallow cuneiforms on the plantar side.

is turned to reducing and applying fixation to the first and second. The base of the second tarsometatarsal may be reduced first if it is intact.

The key to successful internal fixation in a tarsometatarsal joint is correct placement of the screws. Small holes are drilled into the metatarsal bases and cuneiforms to allow sharp-pointed forceps to grip and reduce them accurately. The base of the second metatarsal may thus be pulled very snugly into its anatomic position against the lateral first cuneiform and the distal second cuneiform. To fix the second tarsometatarsal joint, a screw may be inserted percutaneously from the medial side of the first cuneiform and directed obliquely through a gliding hole into the base of the second metatarsal (Fig. 53–15). This screw enters the base of the second metatarsal at the proximal medial corner and angles across into the lateral cortex at approximately 45°. A longer screw may be extended through the base of the third metatarsal for even more stable fixation. This technique is extremely useful in late reductions and in Charcot (neuropathic) tarsometatarsal joint dislocations.

After the second tarsometatarsal joint is reduced, the first may be fixed. The size of the screw to be used for the first tarsometatarsal depends on the size of the bone; a 4.5-mm cortical screw should be used in large bones, and a 3.5-mm cortical screw should be used in smaller patients. The gliding holes for these two screw sizes are 4.5-mm and 3.5-mm, respectively. A small notch is made in the dorsal cortex of the first metatarsal 1.5 to 2 cm distal to the joint (Fig. 53–16). This notch serves two purposes: to prevent the screw head from hitting the inclined surface of the metatarsal and breaking out through the dorsal cortex of the proximal portion and to provide an indentation in which to countersink the head of the screw. A gliding hole, aimed at the middle of the joint, is drilled through the upper half of the notch (not through the base of the notch) to a level in the joint that is parallel to the sole of the foot. The thread hole is extended into the first cuneiform with smaller 3.2-mm or 2.5-mm drills. After gliding and tap holes are appropriately drilled through the upper portion of the notch, a screw is inserted and allowed to self-tap in the relatively dense cancellous

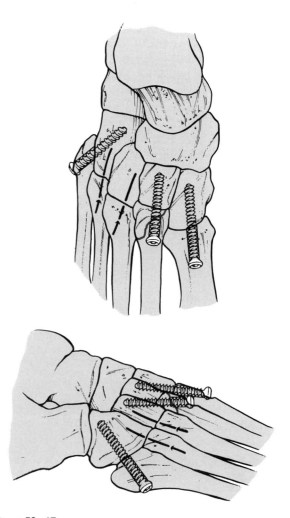

Figure 53–17.

The following alternative techniques are also used to reduce acute TMT fracture-dislocations. The first and second metatarsals are fixed with screws that are placed through notches in the dorsum of the metatarsals and that extend into their respective cuneiforms; the third and fourth metatarsals are fixed with Kirschner wires inserted from dorsolateral to medial into the third and fourth cuneiforms and the cuboid; the fifth metatarsal is fixed with a screw that is inserted upward from its base and angled medially.

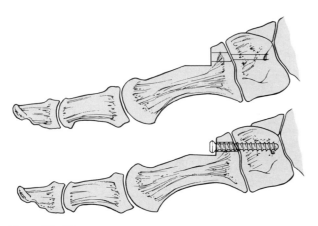

Figure 53–16.

The techniques of notching and drilling the proximal metatarsal and the cuneiform bones are seen in an enlarged view. A notch made in the base of a metatarsal must be at least 1 cm away from the joint. A hole is drilled across the base of the metatarsal to the joint with a 3.5-mm drill and is continued into the cuneiform with a 2.5-mm drill. The hole is drilled not at the bottom of the notch but rather up from the base of the notch. The screw may then be inserted without its head hitting the metatarsal shaft and angulating to split the dorsum of the base of the metatarsal. The screw head is simultaneously countersunk so that it will not protrude from underneath the skin.

bone. The screw must be applied without force so that it does not crush the joint cartilage.

If the naviculocuneiform joint is unstable or subluxated, a longer threaded hole and screw may be necessary to carry the fixation proximally into the navicular to permit stabilization of both joints. The naviculocuneiform joint, like the tarsometatarsal joint, normally has little motion, and placing a screw across this joint for 12 to 16 weeks does not compromise function.

Screws or threaded Kirschner wires may then be placed across the third and fourth tarsometatarsal joints under direct vision (Fig. 53–17). The angle of entry is different from that used in the first and second tarsometatarsals, because the transverse arch slopes downward laterally in the third and fourth tarsometatarsal joints. Fixation is easier to apply from a lateral and slightly dorsal position, and the screw is angled in a medial direction through the base of the metatarsal into the tarsus. The bones of the lateral tarsus are more shallow than the first cuneiform, and this approach prevents missing the tarsus on the plantar side.

Although I prefer to use a screw to secure the third tarsometatarsal joint, a Kirschner wire is not only an acceptable alternative for fixation in the fourth tarsometatarsal but is also a good choice in the fifth. The fifth tarsometatarsal joint is usually fixed percutaneously unless it must be opened for anatomic reduction. If it is opened, the screw or Kirschner wire must enter from a lateral direction and angle slightly upward into the medial cuboid and tarsus.

Any dislocations that are found between the other tarsal bones should be fixed either with additional screws or with longer screws in the metatarsal bases so that they cross the affected areas of both joints.

Metatarsal fractures at any level should be fixed either by intramedullary Kirschner wires or small plates. In the larger first and second metatarsals and in comminuted fractures, 2.7-mm or 3.5-mm plates are the best choice of fixation. Distal metatarsal fractures, which often occur with tarsometatarsal fracture-dislocations, must also be fixed anatomically (see metatarsal fracture section).

CUBOID AND CUNEIFORM FRACTURES AND DISLOCATIONS

Injuries in the midfoot tarsal bones may occur in combination with fractures in the hindfoot or the metatarsals. For example, a tarsometatarsal fracture may be associated with separation of the first and second cuneiforms, or a compression-fracture in the cuboid may occur with a laterally displaced tarsometatarsal fracture, a subtalar fracture-dislocation, a type III navicular fracture, or a Chopart dislocation. Roentgenograms of any major injury in the midfoot should be closely inspected for these injuries, but midfoot tarsal fractures may be apparent only on CT scans, which should be taken to diagnose occult or complex fractures of the foot.

Lateral dislocations of the forefoot are reduced by placing a small distractor laterally from the os calcis to the base of the fifth metatarsal. In addition to reducing the fracture, the distractor also helps to dislodge impacted fractures in the cuboid region and to regain length and normal alignment. Regaining length in a compressed cuboid is essential to reestablishing normal

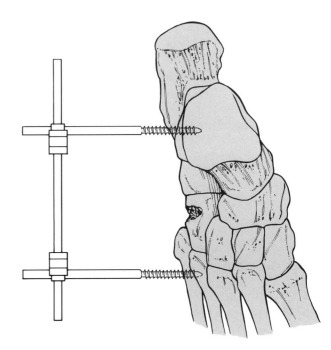

Figure 53–18.

A small external fixator is applied laterally to open and regain length in a compressed cuboid fracture. Depending on the nature of the fracture, this device may be left in place for three or four weeks while a small screw secures a bone graft in place. An external fixator also may be used as an indirect reduction device to realign the fragments.

alignment of the foot and preserving the arch (Fig. 53–18).

Bone grafting may be required to fill gaps in a tarsal bone that was compressed by fracture and later reexpanded. Screws placed between cuneiforms to maintain position cause little or no symptomatic arthrosis later, as the cuneiforms normally have very little motion.

POSTOPERATIVE CARE AND REHABILITATION

Postoperatively, a right-angled splint or a padded cast is applied to the foot if further swelling is anticipated. A soft compression dressing and a posterior plaster slab may be used, but I prefer to apply a regular padded short-leg cast with a minimal amount of plaster. When the cast is dry, a 1.0-cm strip is removed from the anterior section of the cast on the dorsum of the foot and expanded slightly over the instep. This strip reduces constriction and allows the underlying soft dressing to be cut open to examine the wound.

The patient is confined to bed rest with the leg slightly elevated for two full days. After two days, the cast is overwrapped lightly, and the patient is instructed to bear limited weight (15 or 20 pounds or weight-of-leg weight bearing) on crutches, supporting most of the weight on the hindfoot. The cast is changed and the sutures are removed between two and three weeks postoperatively, and a very well-molded short-leg walking cast is applied. The amount of weight bearing is gradually increased, and more weight is transferred to the anterior part of the foot over the next eight to ten weeks. A pure tarsometatarsal dislocation must remain in a cast for at least ten weeks. Fractures of the metatarsal bases unite more quickly, and the cast for these fractures may be removed approximately eight weeks postoperatively.

After the cast is removed, any Kirschner wires are removed and the patient returns to partial weight bearing on crutches while wearing elastic hose. Nonresistive range-of-motion exercises are begun in the ankle and the foot at this time. Full weight bearing may be initiated two weeks after the final cast is removed, and the screws are removed shortly thereafter to avoid breakage secondary to joint motion. Two weeks after the screws are removed, resistive exercises are begun to strengthen the ankle and subtalar joint, and the patient is allowed to gradually return to more demanding activities.

Metatarsal Fractures

Metatarsal fractures are common injuries, but the disability they can produce is often underrated, especially in high-performance athletes in whom a fifth metatarsal stress fracture may ruin performance. The five metatarsals all function differently from one another and must be treated differently in order to expect a good prognosis. Fractures of the first metatarsal, the middle three metatarsals, and the fifth metatarsal will be considered in separate sections so that the differences in treatment may be discussed adequately.

Skin Grafts

Crushing injuries or degloving of the overlying skin require special coverage techniques. When degloving occurs, the procedure originally described by Ziv et al. for applying skin grafts to the dorsum of the foot is appropriate.[38] This technique entails tacking the avulsed skin into position and removing thin split-thickness grafts from the areas of questionable viability. Viability of the avulsed skin is demonstrated by bleeding. If the graft donor site bleeds, it may be left in place; if a portion does not bleed, it must be removed and replaced by the split-thickness skin graft harvested from the questionable area.

When a free graft is needed, the temporoparietal fascia free-flap technique described by Sherman is recommended.[33] This flap is very vascular and may be covered with a simple split-thickness skin graft after it is applied. The greatest advantage of applying this graft to the foot is that it heals with a normal contour, allowing the foot to fit into a shoe without difficulty.

FIRST METATARSAL

Anatomy

The first metatarsal is unique in several ways. It is considerably wider in diameter but shorter in length than the lesser metatarsals. It may also be slightly more mobile than the lesser metatarsals, because the ligamentous supports attaching into its base are less extensive.

Two powerful extrinsic muscles that attach into the first metatarsal influence its position as well as that of the entire forefoot. The first is the anterior tibial tendon, which attaches to a tubercle on the anteromedial base of the first metatarsal and is responsible for elevating the first metatarsal and supinating the forefoot. The second is the peroneus longus, which attaches to a tubercle on the proximal lateral base of the first metatarsal. The peroneus longus plantarflexes the first metatarsal and pronates the forefoot.

The first metatarsal bears approximately one third of the body's weight through the forefoot on two subjacent sesamoid bones. The sesamoids are secured under the head of the first metatarsal by the medial and lateral flexor brevis muscles, which originate in the ligaments and tendon sheaths under the cuneiforms. Two heads of the adductor hallucis muscle attach into the lateral or fibular sesamoid laterally, and the abductor hallucis inserts part of its attachment into the medial or tibial sesamoid medially. More important, the sesamoids are tethered to the deep transverse intermetatarsal ligament, and their relationship to the lesser metatarsals is fixed.

Injuries to the first metatarsal are usually open or comminuted fractures that are sustained by directly applied force. If the first metatarsal head is displaced in any direction, the major weight-bearing complex of the anterior portion of the foot is significantly disturbed, and forefoot function is impaired.

Musculoskeletal trauma protocols call for anatomic fixation of all open fractures and of all fractures that threaten joint function either directly or indirectly. Displaced fractures of the first metatarsal are included in this category and have the best prognosis when they are anatomically reduced with plate and screw fixation.

The goal of ORIF for a first metatarsal fracture is to maintain normal distribution of weight under the rest of the metatarsal heads. In ideal circumstances, the body's total weight is equally distributed over six contact points: the two sesamoids and the remaining four metatarsal heads. However, individual proportions may vary from this generalization, and the second and third metatarsals often bear more weight than the fourth and the fifth.

Operative Management

The anatomy of the first metatarsal limits the types of fixation that are suitable for a fracture in this area. The diaphysis of a first metatarsal is small in relation to the long bones, and its thin overlying tissues require a low-profile device. Therefore a one-third tubular plate with four or five holes and 3.5-mm cortical screws is the best choice of fixation (Fig. 53–19).

The position of the plate on a metatarsal is determined by the kind of injury that has been sustained and by the type of incision that will inflict the least possible additional harm. Placing a plate on the tension side of a metatarsal bone is not always feasible.

Postoperatively, casting and early active and passive motion of the metatarsophalangeal (MTP) joint are indicated. Applying a cast helps to control dependent edema and the position of the ankle. Distally, the dorsal trim line of the cast must not limit MTP dorsiflexion.

SECOND, THIRD, AND FOURTH METATARSALS

Etiology

A traumatic fracture in the middle metatarsal is usually sustained by direct application of force to the foot. The resulting fracture is usually slightly comminuted, transverse, and may be open. Indirect force, such as twisting, may also fracture a middle metatarsal and generally produces a spiral fracture. Because a fracture in a middle metatarsal is usually not very displaced and generally heals well, the complications that may result are often underestimated. Problems occur only months later, when metatarsalgia or intractable plantar keratoses may develop in the metatarsal heads that are still bearing weight; these can occur from just 2 to 4 mm of elevation or shortening of the injured metatarsal.

Operative Management

For a metatarsal fracture to heal with a good prognosis, anatomic reduction must be achieved, and the length, rotation, and declination of the metatarsal must be maintained throughout healing. Casting usually maintains reduction effectively in closed, undisplaced, or

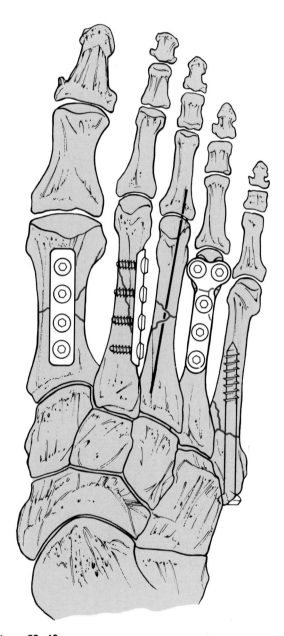

Figure 53–19.

Various fixation devices for metatarsal fractures are illustrated. A one-third tubular plate, placed either straight dorsally or slightly dorsomedially is suitable for a displaced fracture of the first metatarsal. A quarter-tubular plate may be used in fracture fixation or osteotomy fixation on a significantly displaced second metatarsal. It can be placed straight dorsally or dorsolaterally, as depicted here. Kirschner wires are ideal for middle shaft fractures of the lesser metatarsals. A quarter-tubular T plate and 2.7-mm screws can be used to fix an extremely distal neck fracture in a lesser metatarsal. A straight quarter-tubular plate with four holes is often used to fix osteotomies. A malleolar screw, seen here in the fifth metatarsal, can be used for a typical Jones fracture, for a delayed union, or for acute fixation in a high-performance athlete.

minimally displaced lesser metatarsal fractures. Intramedullary Kirschner wire fixation is frequently used in open fractures and, when done precisely, produces good results. When used in open or displaced fractures in a middle metatarsal, a Kirschner wire is inserted into the medullary canal of the distal segment, run through the metatarsal head and the base of the phalanx, and passed out through the plantar skin at the base of the toe. It is drilled back into the proximal fragment when the fracture is reduced (Fig. 53–20).

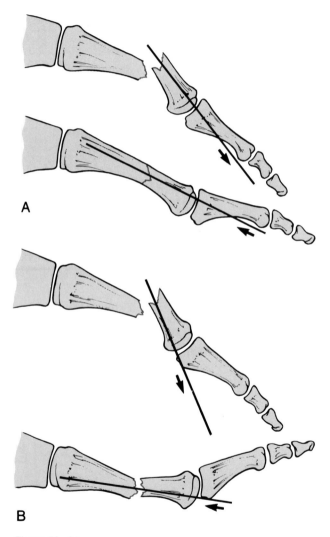

Figure 53–20.

(A), A Kirschner wire reduces a metatarsal fracture. Note that the metatarsal head is not elevated. (B), The Kirschner wire elevates the distal metatarsal head when it is drilled back into the proximal fragment. This situation commonly occurs when the surgeon tries to miss the phalanx in the metatarsophalangeal (MTP) joint and inadvertently angles out too far to the plantar side in the distal fragment. Fixation in this position causes a malunion that will result in metatarsalgia and a transfer lesion under the adjacent metatarsals.

Some problems are inherent in this technique. If the Kirschner wire is angled too far plantar in the distal fragment, it may overreduce and elevate the head of the metatarsal when it is drilled retrograde into the proximal fragment. Excessive angling and overreduction may be avoided by running the Kirschner wire distally just within and parallel to the dorsal cortex, through the MTP joint, and out the plantar surface of the proximal phalanx. To assure that the fixed position of the metatarsal head is not elevated or depressed in relation to the other metatarsal heads, the forefoot must be palpated carefully at the end of the operation.

Stress Fractures

A very important consideration in treating a stress fracture is knowing the cause of the injury. If the second metatarsal sustains a significant stress fracture, a short or hypermobile first metatarsal must be ruled out as the cause of the injury. Conversely, a metatarsal that bears an excessive amount of weight, possibly because it is overlong, also may cause a stress fracture, and it should be shortened slightly at the time internal fixation is applied.

If a stress fracture is undisplaced, restricted activity in a molded cast or in an orthosis is advised. If a stress fracture is complete or displaced, it should be treated with anatomic reduction and internal fixation, as for any acute fracture. A stress fracture may heal more slowly than an acute fracture, but only anatomic reconstruction will ensure normal distribution of weight in the forefoot. Intramedullary callus should be removed, and the bone should be grafted to encourage early union.

FIFTH METATARSAL FRACTURES

Etiology

The most common fracture of the fifth metatarsal is an avulsion fracture of the proximal apophysis. Until recently, it was believed that this type of injury was caused when the fifth metatarsal was avulsed by the peroneus brevis. Richli and Rosenthal[27] examined the mechanism of this injury and suggested that the avulsion is caused instead by the lateral plantar aponeurosis. The cause of injury is usually an acute inversion, often in plantar flexion, and is the same mechanism that causes an anterior talofibular ligament injury or a sprain or avulsion fracture of the anterior tubercle in the os calcis. The proposed mechanism explains why fifth metatarsal fractures are seldom displaced. When diagnosing an inversion injury, the lateral foot and ankle should be palpated to help determine whether to take an x-ray film of the foot or the ankle and whether to search for an avulsion fracture or an occult fracture on the anterior beak of the os calcis.

Avulsion Fractures

An avulsed fifth metatarsal fracture is usually treated without surgery with a walking cast or with strapping and a walking boot if it is displaced less than 2 mm. Internal fixation with a small tension band or a lag screw should be considered only if the fracture is significantly displaced. Occasionally, a very proximal transverse fracture involves the cuboid/fifth metatarsal joint, and in this case, internal fixation is indicated if the fifth metatarsal fracture is displaced more than 2 mm (Fig. 53–2C).

Jones Fracture

A fracture in the proximal shaft near the metaphyseal junction of the fifth metatarsal is called a Jones fracture. Unfortunately, many fractures in the proximal fifth metatarsal are sometimes grouped under the term "Jones fracture." Dameron,[10] and later, Kavanaugh et al.[17] and Torg,[37] pointed out that injuries in the proximal shaft of the fifth metatarsal can be significantly different. Treatment of a fracture in this area varies according to whether the fracture is caused by an acute traumatic injury or is a stress fracture. Related to the origin of injury is the time at which the fracture is seen (i.e., acutely or delayed) and whether it is a nonunion. With so many variables, calling all these fractures by one name can cause confusion. The term "Jones fracture" will probably persist, but a better description should be added when an individual case is discussed. For example, the description of the fracture should include information about whether it is an acute traumatic fracture, an undisplaced stress fracture, or a chronic nonunion of the metaphyseal-diaphyseal junction.

Operative Management

An acute traumatic injury of the fifth metatarsal's proximal metaphysis is usually not caused by the same type of inversion force that produces an avulsion at the base of the fifth metatarsal. An acute fracture is the result of an upward force or a direct blow on the planted fifth metatarsal. A stress fracture in an athlete, on the other hand, may result from a mild biomechanical abnormality such as genu varum or a varus heel and, if this is the original cause of the stress fracture, the abnormality should be treated as well as the fracture itself.

Nonoperative management of stress fractures requires a long period of inactivity and rehabilitation, and a surgical approach may be warranted in patients who must remain active, especially high-performance athletes. Torg et al. pointed out that if sclerosis or intramedullary callus develops in stress fractures, the potential for healing without surgery is significantly reduced.[36] They recommend a surgical approach that reestablishes the medullary canal of a delayed union or a nonunion by drilling or burring the bone and inserting an inlay graft. Kavanaugh et al.[17] and DeLee et al.[12] recommend intramedullary screw fixation for a fracture with sclerosis or a history of stress fracture or for one that has a poor prognosis because of delayed union or nonunion (Fig. 53–19).

We recommend short-leg casting for acute, traumatic fifth metatarsal fractures. Non–weight bearing is advised for approximately six weeks, followed by gradually increased weight bearing for two weeks. Union occurs in most cases treated with this regimen.

In a high-performance athlete or for a chronic fracture, we suggest doing very careful intramedullary screw fixation and adding a *strain-relieving bone graft* on the dorsomedial surface of the bone. A 4.5-mm malleolar screw is used in an average-size patient, but in a very large athlete, a 6.5-mm screw may be necessary. Placing the screw requires precision and image intensifier guidance to ensure that the screw is of the appropriate size and that it is placed directly down the canal from the tip of the base of the fifth metatarsal (Fig. 53–19).

The technique for a strain-relieving bone graft is to drill a short dorsomedial segment of hard cortical bone on both sides of the fracture line with a small, spherical, 5- to 8-mm bur and filling the gap with cancellous bone taken from the os calcis or from the base of the fifth metatarsal.

Postoperatively, the foot is immobilized in a short-leg cast, and protected weight bearing is prescribed for six weeks. Following this, a walking cast is applied for two to four weeks, after which the patient may gradually return to normal function.

Acute Fractures in the Diaphysis of the Fifth Metatarsal

Traumatic fractures are common in the diaphysis or the distal portion of the fifth metatarsal and may be treated in the same manner as that used for other lesser metatarsal fractures. They require internal fixation only if they are significantly displaced, as the fifth metatarsal is quite flexible and is not as crucial to weight bearing as the medial lesser metatarsals or the first metatarsal. Most distal fifth metatarsal fractures that are not markedly displaced are treated in a walking cast and tend to heal successfully without later complications. Some are simply treated in a stiff-soled boot, and in areas of the country where rigid-soled hiking boots are commonly worn, this treatment may be adequate.

Fractures and Dislocations in the MTP Joints, Phalanges, and Sesamoids

Normal gait and a comfortable forefoot are largely attributable to mobility of the MTP joints. Mobility may be sacrificed in the tarsometatarsal joints or in the interphalangeal (IP) joints without losing function, but every effort should be made to salvage motion in the MTP joints. The first MTP joint should be fused only under extraordinary circumstances as a salvage procedure, and the lesser MTP joints should never be fused.

FIRST METATARSOPHALANGEAL JOINT

Anatomy

The first MTP joint differs from the lesser MTP joints in several ways. It is larger than the others, and several strong muscles (the abductor hallucis, the extensor brevis, the adductor hallucis, and the two flexor brevis tendons) attach into the base of its proximal phalanx. The abductor and medial short flexor attach medially into the MTP joint, and the adductor and lateral short flexor attach laterally, often as conjoined tendons.

Management of Injuries

One of the several types of fractures that occur in this area is an avulsion fracture. The force of a traumatic injury may avulse the lateral conjoined tendon along with a large section of the lateral base of the proximal phalanx. The resultant fracture may be displaced by several millimeters and should be opened and fixed with a lag screw or a tension band device (Fig. 53–21). If left unreduced, the muscle imbalance will allow the great toe to drift into a varus position.

Osteochondral fractures may also occur from traumatic injuries. If the osteochondral fragments are small, they should be excised; if the fracture fragments are large enough to be reduced, they should be fixed anatomically. Although Kirschner wires are sometimes used to stabilize large osteochondral fractures, small compression screws or double-threaded Herbert screws are preferred when attempting to restore an anatomic joint surface.

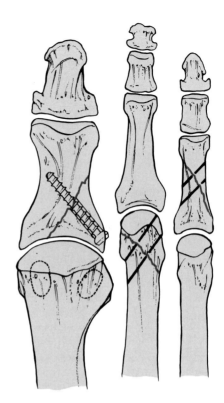

Figure 53–21.

Fixation techniques for MTP and proximal phalangeal fractures are shown. Screws are usually used to fix fractures in the proximal phalanx of the great toe and in the first metatarsal head, but Kirschner wires may be more appropriate in the smaller heads of the lesser metatarsals. Phalangeal fractures need not always be fixed, but if they tend to angulate or if they are open fractures, Kirschner wire fixation similar to that used in the hand may be helpful. Note that this screw is placed from the lateral side but that the lateral base of the first proximal phalanx is usually more plantar-lateral than depicted here. In that case, the screw would be placed through a gliding hole in the dorsomedial surface of the proximal phalanx and angled perpendicular to the fracture line, compressing the plantar lateral fragment in its anatomic position.

Fractures may occur in the base of the proximal phalanx or in the head of the first metatarsal, and all acute displaced fractures and dislocations should be reduced as soon after injury as possible.

Some dorsal dislocations cannot be reduced using a closed technique, because the head of the first metatarsal "buttonholes" through the sesamoid–short flexor mechanism. When an open reduction of the first MTP joint is necessary, the approach is made through a dorsal incision and is combined with a short linear incision through the intersesamoid transverse ligament to allow visualization and reduction. After open reduction, the foot and the great toe are casted in a neutral position for two to three weeks, and following this, the joint is gradually rehabilitated.

Compression injuries, sprains, and hyperextension injuries (turf toe) may all potentially occur in the first MTP joint. Cartilage injuries are very common in this area and may lead to hallux limitus and eventually to hallux rigidus, or a so-called "dorsal bunion." Operative treatment of hallux rigidus usually consists of cheilectomy and careful remobilization of the sesamoid complex. Nonoperative treatment consists of immobilization of the foot in a stiff, rocker-sole shoe.

LESSER METATARSOPHALANGEAL JOINTS

Anatomy

Anatomically, the lesser MTP joints are very similar. Each has simple collateral ligaments, a volar plate mechanism, and intrinsic tendons that attach to the dorsal hood. The long flexors attach to the bases of the distal phalanges, the short flexors attach to the middle phalanges, and the long extensors attach extensively along the dorsal hoods and dorsally into the distal phalanges. The plantar fat pads of the MTP joints are properly positioned under the metatarsal heads when the proximal phalanges are in a neutral or a slightly flexed position in relation to the metatarsal heads.

The actions of the intrinsic and extrinsic flexor tendons complement each other during normal gait. Gait mechanics require the toes to passively dorsiflex about 30° to 40° as the foot continues past heel-off and rolls forward. The toes may require between 60° and 90° of passive dorsiflexion for kneeling or squatting. When they function normally, the intrinsic and extrinsic flexor tendons flex the toes, elevate the metatarsal heads slightly, and assume weight from the MTP joints during stance and early push-off.

Management of Injuries

A dislocation, a sprain, or a fracture in a lesser MTP joint must be treated in a manner that maximizes motion in the joint after healing. Early reduction of a dislocation usually may be done with a closed technique, but reduction may not be possible if the metatarsal head "buttonholes" through the plantar plate mechanism. In this situation, a straight dorsal incision may be needed over the base of the phalanx and the metatarsal head to divide the mechanism in line with the metatarsal before it can be relocated under the metatarsal head.

Because the MTP joint does not bear weight through its articulating surface, anatomic reduction and early passive and active motion during rehabilitation restore adequate motion for most activities. Small Kirschner wires and screws are used in metatarsal head fractures to achieve the best possible anatomic reduction (Fig. 53–21).

Motion in the MTP joint is initiated two to three days postoperatively, beginning with gentle passive dorsiflexion with the foot in a neutral splint. Active motion and more vigorous passive motion are started after three to four weeks, when signs of early bony healing are evident.

FIRST PHALANGEAL AND INTERPHALANGEAL JOINT FRACTURES

The first toe proximal phalanx and the first interphalangeal (IP) joint will be discussed separately, as they are anatomically different from the lesser toe phalanges.

First Proximal Phalanx

Diaphyseal fractures in the first proximal phalanx are treated more aggressively than are fractures in the lesser toes. Because the short flexor complex is stronger than the short extensor complex, it can cause plantar angulation in an unstable proximal phalanx fracture, which later may result in keratosis formation and shoe pressure problems. For these reasons, unstable fractures in the proximal phalanx should be treated with anatomic reduction and Kirschner wire or lag screw fixation rather than with simple splinting.

First Interphalangeal Joint

It is not necessary to fix fractures in the first IP joint with open reduction and perfect anatomy. This joint does not require a range of motion greater than 20° for normal function, and an ankylosed first IP joint produces little disability in most situations. Motion in the IP joint should be salvaged only if the MTP joint is so severely injured that it is ankylosed or will require later fusion. Under these circumstances, mobility in the IP joint will compensate somewhat for stiffness in the MTP joint.

LESSER PHALANGEAL AND INTERPHALANGEAL JOINT FRACTURES

Motion in the proximal IP joints and the distal IP joints is not essential for normal toe function, a fact that is evidenced by the frequent use of IP joint fusions to treat claw toes.

Diaphyseal fractures of the proximal and middle phalanges are usually closed injuries and are generally treated with a closed technique (i.e., simple splinting or "buddy taping"). A piece of gauze or lamb's wool is placed between the injured toe and the adjacent toe, and the two are lightly taped together. The tape must not be applied with excessive pressure during the first two or three days postinjury, when swelling is likely to be significant. Fractures that extend into the IP joints are usually splinted together with the shaft fractures in a straight position. They are not operated on unless they are markedly displaced or open.

If a lesser toe cannot be aligned anatomically by closed means, it may require open reduction and Kirschner wire fixation. Much of the stiffness that results from fusing the IP joints can be prevented by fixing the major fracture fragments early with Kirschner wires. A relatively serious complication of allowing the toes to heal in an angulated position is that a lateral prominence may rub against an adjacent toe and form an interdigital corn, which in turn may become macerated. In addition to being painful, a macerated corn can easily become infected and may require later surgery to eradicate the infection and eliminate any deformity.

DISTAL PHALANX AND NAIL BED INJURIES

Etiology

Injuries to the distal tuft and the nail bed are fairly common. In the fingers, they are caused by a blow (as from a hammer) or from trapping the fingers in a door. In the toes, these injuries are often caused by dropping a heavy object on the foot or by catching the toes under a power mower. The latter injury may not be limited to the nail bed and may produce a much more severe injury that involves the entire forefoot.

Nail bed problems frequently occur in long-distance runners. Runners may completely dislodge their toenails by subjecting them to repeated trauma when running downhill in loose shoes.

Management of Injuries

The simplest nail bed injury results only in a subungual hematoma. The hematoma may be very painful and tender at first and may result in loss of part of the nail bed, but completely normal recovery is usually expected. As in the fingers, a hematoma in a toe may be drained after the area is prepped in a sterile manner, and the blood may be evacuated by boring a round hole through the nail into the middle of the hematoma with a heated paper clip or a small bur. The area should be kept clean and sterile to prevent infection in the nail bed and the distal tuft.

Crushing Injuries

Crushing injuries sustained from high-energy trauma may damage the nail bed and the nail matrix more severely and, like all crush injuries, must be treated with meticulous care. A disrupted nail bed or matrix must be carefully cleansed and debrided, even if the injury appears to be merely a laceration, and the nail bed must be very carefully reapproximated with an absorbable suture if normal nail growth is to be expected.[39] The nail tuft area must be protected against possible hematoma by wrapping the foot in a bulky, soft compression dressing and elevating it for two or three days postinjury. Subsequent protection is provided by a bunion shoe, with the end protruding beyond the toes, or by a cast with an extended toe plate.

In contrast to the fingers, severe proximal injuries to the nail matrix in the toes may result in significantly disordered nail growth, which may require complete excision or a matricectomy.

SESAMOID INJURIES

Anatomy

The sesamoids are a very important component of the two-headed short flexor mechanism in the great toe and serve a function similar to that of the patella in the quadriceps mechanism in the knee. They protect the underside of the metatarsal heads and the MTP joints from the pressure of weight bearing and provide leverage to the short flexors as they pull on the proximal phalanx.

The sesamoids are approximately 7 to 10 mm long and are slightly oblong shaped. Their dorsal surfaces articulate with the underside of the first metatarsal head. A midline crista on the undersurface of the head divides the medial and lateral articular surfaces and keeps the sesamoids in position under the head. A strong intersesamoid ligament connects the two sesamoids and extends into the deep transverse intermetatarsal ligament. The extensions of the medial and lateral short flexors become conjoined tendons with the abductor and adductor muscles and attach to the inferior medial and lateral bases of the first proximal phalanx.

Etiology

Injury to a first MTP sesamoid is rare, but may be quite painful and disabling. Dancers who wear light or thin-soled shoes are most susceptible to this injury, which may occur when they land on a hard surface with the toes dorsiflexed. Both dancers and runners are susceptible to traumatic stress fracture in the sesamoids as a result of subjecting the sesamoid bone to repeated impact and tension.

Sesamoiditis

The syndrome of pain, tenderness, inflammation, and possible cartilage injury in the metatarsal head–sesamoid articulation is called sesamoiditis. Sesamoiditis is similar to chondromalacia in the patellofemoral joint, which in turn is very similar to traumatic chondritis or chondrosis and arthrosis. This condition may be aggravated by improper tracking of the sesamoids under the metatarsal head or by progressive metatarsus varus, either with or without the presence of an atavistic tarsometatarsal joint. A plantarflexed metatarsal or an overactive long peroneal tendon may overload the sesamoids and may produce pain that is similar to that of sesamoiditis. These problems must be recognized and treated.

Sesamoid Fracture

A sesamoid fracture not only causes discomfort, but it can also significantly disrupt half of the flexor mechanism/conjoined tendon by allowing the great toe to drift or angulate to the opposite side. For example, if the medial sesamoid–short flexor complex is disrupted, the great toe will drift laterally into a hallux valgus position. The crista that normally separates the medial and lateral articular surfaces on the anterior metatarsal head is worn away as the medial sesamoid moves under it and as the head shifts medially. Sesamoiditis often progresses to complete dislocation of the fibular or lateral sesamoid and to a painful condition in which only the tibial sesamoid lies under the metatarsal head.

Management

Traditionally, acute sesamoid fractures or suspected stress fractures of the sesamoid have been treated conservatively by placing soft padding under the arch and the first metatarsal head and by strapping the MTP joint in a neutral or slightly flexed position. The foot was kept in a cast or a bunion shoe for four to eight weeks. This nonoperative treatment should be attempted in acute cases. If casting does not lead to healing (and it often does not), and if pain persists, a sesamoidectomy should be performed.

Sesamoidectomy

Sesamoidectomy is an extremely delicate procedure in which the broken bone must be shelled out while the tendon is left intact. Once the bone is enucleated, the tendon is repaired or imbricated, and the wound is closed. The toe is splinted in a protected position for four to six weeks before rehabilitation with dorsiflexion exercises and full weight bearing is begun. Night splinting may be continued for several months to protect the great toe from potentially drifting out of position. Depending on individual anatomy, this operation is sometimes not feasible.

Unfortunately, a sesamoidectomy does not restore painless, normal function. Every attempt should be made to save the sesamoids, as very serious problems are associated with removing them. Excision of the lateral sesamoid causes medial drift and a cock-up deformity called hallux varus, a well-known complication of the McBride bunionectomy, in which the lateral sesamoid is excised.

Even if the injured flexor mechanism remains intact and continues to function after a sesamoidectomy, the remaining sesamoid may become painful from the extra weight it must support, and a transfer lesion may result. Occasionally the second sesamoid must also be removed but before this procedure is carried out, the surgeon must be absolutely sure that neither a plantarflexed first metatarsal nor a hyperactive or over-strong peroneal tendon is causing the excessive load on the sesamoids and the first metatarsal head.

Bone Grafting

Grafting sesamoid fractures that resist healing is a new approach that may result in a higher rate of union than does splinting alone. To perform a graft, a small bur hole is drilled into the center of the fracture site, and the hole is filled with cancellous bone. Postoperatively, the great toe and the short flexor mechanism are splinted in a neutral position (the same as would be done for routine nonoperative treatment). This procedure is a variation of a strain-relieving bone graft and appears to produce excellent results.

REFERENCES

1. Anderson, I.F.; Crichton, K.J.; Grattan-Smith, T.; et al. Osteochondral fractures of the dome of the talus. J Bone Joint Surg 71A:1143, 1989.
2. Arntz, C.T.; Veith, R.G.; Hansen, S.T. Fractures and fracture-dislocations of the tarsometatarsal joint. J Bone Joint Surg 70A:173, 1988.
3. Benirschke, S.K. Results of operative treatment of os calcis fractures. Paper presented at AAOS, New Orleans, Feb 8–12, 1990.
4. Bezes, H.; Massart, P.; Fourquet, J.P. Die Osteosynthese der Calcaneus-impressionsfraktur. Unfallheilkunde 87:363, 1984.
5. Burdeaux, B.D. Reduction of calcaneal fractures by the McReynolds medial approach technique and its experimental basis. Clin Orthop 177:87, 1983.
6. Canale, S.T.; Kelly, F.B. Fractures of the neck of the talus: Long-term evaluation of seventy-one cases. J Bone Joint Surg 60A:143, 1978.
7. Carr, J.B.; Hansen, S.T.; Benirschke, S.K. Subtalar distraction bone block fusion for late complications of os calcis fractures. Foot Ankle 9:81, 1988.

8. Carr, J.B.; Hansen, S.T.; Benirschke, S.K. Surgical treatment of foot and ankle trauma: Use of indirect reduction techniques. Foot Ankle 9:176, 1989.

9. Comfort, T.H.; Behrens, F.; Garthe, D.W.; et al. Long-term results of displaced talar neck fractures. Clin Orthop 199:81, 1985.

10. Dameron, T.B. Fractures and anatomical variations of the proximal portion of the fifth metatarsal. J Bone Joint Surg 57A:788, 1975.

11. DeLee, J. Fractures of the calcaneus. In: Mann, R.A., ed. Surgery of the Foot. St. Louis, C.V. Mosby, 1986, pp 592–808.

12. DeLee, J.C.; Evans, J.P.; Julian, J. Stress fractures of the fifth metatarsal. Am J Sports Med 5:349, 1983.

13. Gould, N. Lateral approach to the os calcis. Foot Ankle 4:218, 1984.

14. Harding, D.; Waddell, J.P. Open reduction in depressed fractures of the os calcis. Clin Orthop 199:124, 1985.

15. Hawkins, L.G. Fractures of the neck of the talus. J Bone Joint Surg 52A:991, 1970.

16. Inman, V.T.; Ralston, H.J.; Todd, F. Human Walking. Baltimore, Williams and Wilkins, 1981.

17. Kavanaugh, J.H.; Brower, T.D.; Mann, R.V. The Jones fracture revisited. J Bone Joint Surg 60A:776, 1978.

17a. Kidner, F.C. The prehallux (accessory scaphoid) in its relation to flatfoot. J Bone Joint Surg 11A:831, 1929.

18. Letournel, E. Open reduction and internal fixation of calcaneus fractures. In Spiegel, P.G., ed. Techniques in Orthopaedics— Topics in Orthopaedic Trauma. Baltimore, University Park Press, 1984, p. 173.

19. Leung, K.S.; Chan, W.S.; Shen, W.Y.; et al. Operative treatment of intraarticular fractures of the os calcis—the role of rigid internal fixation and primary bone grafting: Preliminary result. J Orthop Trauma 3:232, 1989.

20. Mann, R.A. Surgery of the Foot, Ed. 5. St. Louis, C.V. Mosby, 1986, pp 1–30.

21. McReynolds, I.S. Fractures of the os calcis involving the subastragalar joint: Treatment by open reduction and internal fixation with staples using a medial approach. J Bone Joint Surg 58A:733, 1976.

22. Müller, M.E.; Allgöwer, M.; Schneider, R.; et al. Manual of Internal Fixation, Ed. 2. Berlin, Springer-Verlag, 1979.

23. Myerson, M.A.; Fisher, R.T.; Burgess, A.B.; et al. Fracture-dislocations of the tarsometatarsal joints: End results correlated with pathology and treatment. Foot Ankle 6:225, 1986.

24. Palmer, I. The mechanism and treatment of fractures of the calcaneus. J Bone Joint Surg 30A:2, 1948.

25. Quenu, E.; Kuss, G. Etude sur les luxations du metatarse. Rev Chir 39:1, 1909.

26. Regazzoni, P. Technik der stabilen osteosynthese bei calcaneusfrakturen. Hefte Unfallheilkd 200:432, 1988.

27. Richli, W.R.; Rosenthal, D.I. Avulsion fracture of the fifth metatarsal: Experimental study of pathomechanics. Am J Radiol 143:889, 1984.

28. Romash, M.M. Calcaneal fractures: Three-dimensional treatment. Foot Ankle 8:180, 1988.

29. Ross, S.D.K.; Sowerby, M.R.R.. The operative treatment of fractures of the os calcis. Clin Orthop 199:132, 1985.

30. Sangeorzan, B.J.; Benirschke, S.K.; Mosca, V.; et al. Displaced intra-articular fractures of the tarsal navicular. J Bone Joint Surg 71A:1504, 1989.

31. Sarrafian, S.K. Anatomy of the Foot and Ankle. Philadelphia, J.B. Lippincott, 1983.

32. Sclamberg, E.L.; Davenport, K. Operative treatment of displaced intra-articular fracture of the calcaneus. J Trauma 28:510, 1988.

33. Sherman, R.; Wellisz, T.; Wiss, D.; et al. Coverage of type III open ankle and foot fractures with the temporoparietal fascial free flap. Presented at the Orthopaedic Trauma Association Meeting, Philadelphia, Oct 18–21, 1989.

34. Stephenson, J.R. Treatment of displaced intra-articular fractures of the calcaneus using medial and lateral approaches, internal fixation, and early motion. J Bone Joint Surg 69A:115–130, 1987.

35. Szyszkowitz, R.; Reschauer, R.; Seggl, W. Eighty-five talus fractures treated by ORIF. Clin Orthop 199:97, 1985.

36. Torg, J.S.; Pavlov, H.; Coolly, L.H.; et al. Stress fractures of the tarsal navicular. J Bone Joint Surg 64A:700, 1982.

37. Torg, J.S. Fractures of the base of the fifth metatarsal distal to the tuberosity. A review. Contemp Orthop 19:497, 1988.

38. Ziv, I.; Zeligowski, A.; Mosheiff, R.; et al. Split-thickness skin excision in severe open fractures. J Bone Joint Surg 70B:23, 1988.

39. Zook, E.G. Treatment of nail bed injuries. Surg Rounds Orthop 3:20, Dec. 1989.

40. Zwipp, H.; Tscherne, H.; Wülker, N. Osteosynthese dislozierter intraartikulärer calcaneusfrakturen. Unfallchirurg 91:507, 1988.

READING LIST

Arntz, C.; Hansen, S.T. Dislocations and fracture-dislocations of the tarsometatarsal joints. Orthop Clin North Am 18:105, 1987.

Carr, J.B.; Hansen, S.T.; Benirschke, S.K. Surgical treatment of foot and ankle trauma: Use of indirect reduction techniques. Foot Ankle 9:176, 1989.

Enna, C.D. The denervated great toe. A review of anatomy and functions as they relate to the deformity. Orthop Rev 6:29, 1977.

Grob, D.; Simpson, L.A.; Weber, B.G.; et al. Operative treatment of displaced talus fractures. Clin Orthop 199:88–96, 1985.

Hansen, S.T.; Clark, W. Tendon transfer to augment the weakened tibialis posterior mechanism. J Am Podiatr Med Assoc 78:399, 1988.

Heckman, J.D.; MacLean, M.R. Fractures of the lateral process of the talus. Clin Orthop 199:108, 1985.

Hulkko, A.; Orava, S.; Pellinen, P.; et al. Stress fractures of the sesamoid bones of the first metatarsophalangeal joint in athletes. Arch Orthop Trauma Surg 104:113, 1985.

Jones, R. Fracture of the base of the fifth metatarsal bone by indirect violence. Ann Surg 35:697, 1902.

Lowrie, I.G.; Finlay, D.B.; Brenkel, I.J.; et al. Computerized tomographic assessment of the subtalar joint in calcaneal fractures. J Bone Joint Surg 70B:247, 1988.

Markowitz, H.D.; Chase, M.; Whitelaw, G.P. Isolated injury of the second tarsometatarsal joint. Clin Orthop 248:210, 1988.

Mayo, K.A. Fractures of the talus: Principles of management and techniques of treatment. Tech Orthop 2:42, 1987.

Munro, T.G. Fractures of the base of the fifth metatarsal. J Can Assoc Radiol 40:260, 1989.

Pavlov, H. Radiology for the orthopaedic surgeon. Contemp Orthop 13:41, 1986.

Pennal, G.F. Fractures of the talus. Clin Orthop 30:53, 1963.

Pennal, G.F.; Yadav, M.P. Operative treatment of comminuted fractures of the os calcis. Orthop Clin North Am 4:197, 1973.

Peterson, L.; Goldie, I.; Irstam, L. Fracture of the neck of the talus: A clinical study. Acta Orthop Scand 48:696, 1977.

Peterson, L.; Goldie, I.F.; Lindell, D. The arterial supply of the talus. Acta Orthop Scand 46:1026, 1975.

Ross, S.D.K. The operative treatment of complex os calcis fractures. Tech Orthop 2:55, 1987.

Sanders, R. Talonavicular Joint Subluxation Presenting with Hindfoot Varus. American Orthopaedic Assoc., Colorado Springs, June 12–15, 1990. Submitted to J Bone Joint Surg.

Sangeorzan, B.J.; Hansen, S.T. Early and late post-traumatic foot reconstruction. Clin Orthop 243:86, 1989.

Tile, M. Fractures of the talus. In: Schatzker, J.; Tile, M., eds. The Rationale of Operative Fracture Care. Berlin, Springer-Verlag, 1987, p. 407.

Wilson, P.D. Fractures and dislocations of the tarsal bone. South Med J 26:833, 1933.

Wiss, D.A.; Kull, D.M.; Perry, J. Lisfranc fracture-dislocations of the foot: A clinical kinesiological study. J Orthop Trauma 1:267, 1988.

Index

Note: Page numbers in *italics* refer to illustrations; page numbers followed by (t) refer to tables.

C

D

F

Healing *(Continued)*
   granulation phase of, *81–84,* 81–85, 330
   inflammatory phase of, 79–81
   repair of specialized tissues in, 87–91, *87–92*
   scar formation in, 85, *85, 86*
   of tendinous injury, 88–89
   of tibial fracture, 1839, 1841, *1842, 1843*
      callus formation in, 1775, *1775*
   of wound. See *Healing, of soft tissue injury.*
   by secondary intention, 330
Heart disease, risk of pulmonary embolism with, 447
Heavy work, 572
Helmet-wearing injured patient, examination of, 593
Hematogenous osteomyelitis, 457
Hematoma, epidural, spinal surgery and, 658, 661
   fracture and, 456
   paraspinous, midthoracic vertebral fractures and, *606*
   postoperative formation of, 456
      in patient treated for spinal injury, 658, 661
   infection associated with. See *Infection, fracture surgery and.*
   subungual, 1003
Hemiarthroplasty, for femoral head fracture, 1382, *1382*
   for femoral neck fracture, 1412–1428, *1419–1427*
      problems with, 1400, 1400(t), 1434–1435
      vs. internal fixation treatment, 1399–1401
   for intertrochanteric fracture, 1461, 1473–1474, *1474,* 1477
Hemorrhage. See also *Arterial injury* and *Vascular injury.*
   pelvic fracture and, 866–867, 893
   shock due to, 135, 137
Henry approach, to decompression of compartment syndrome of forearm, *298, 299*
   to radius, 1098, 1099, 1099(t), 1100, *1100*
Heparin, in prophylaxis against deep venous thrombosis, 450
Hepatic function, effect of gut bacteria and toxins on, *454*
   effect of Kupffer cell activation on, *455*
Herbert screw fixation, for proximal humeral fracture, 1256, *1256*
   for radial head fracture, 1130, *1131*
   for scaphoid fracture, *1031,* 1031–1032, *1032, 1052*
   for transscaphoid perilunate dislocation, *1052,* 1052–1053
Herniation, of intervertebral disc(s), and spinal cord compression, 791, *792*
   in lumbar spine, 790–791, 793
   in thoracic spine, 790–791, *792,* 793
   in Scheuermann's disease, 791
Heterotopic bone induction, 47
Heterotopic ossification, femoral head fracture and, 1371
   indomethacin for, 921, 1364, 1380
   proximal humeral fracture and, 1283
   surgery and, 921–922, 1364, 1383, 1632
High-angle fixation, for intertrochanteric hip fracture, 1458
High-energy injuries, 312–313
High extension transcolumn fracture, of distal humerus, 1168, *1169*
High flexion transcolumn fracture, of distal humerus, 1168, *1169*
High single-column fracture, of distal humerus, *1151,* 1152

High T pattern bicolumn fracture, of distal humerus, 1154, 1158–1159, *1159*
High transcolumn fracture, of distal humerus, 1168, *1169*
Hill-Sachs fracture, of proximal humerus, 1218, *1223,* 1266
   reverse, 1218, 1266–1267
Hip, anatomy of, 1329–1333, *1330–1333, 1486–1488*
   anterior dislocation of, 1340–1341, *1342,* 1342(t), *1343*
   anterior surgical approach to, 1352–1353, *1379–1380, 1417*
   anterolateral surgical approach to, 1353, *1354,* 1356, *1405*
   anteversion of, 1331–1332, 1334, 1334(t), 1443–1444
   capsule of, 1331
   direct lateral surgical approach to, 1353, *1355,* 1356, 1415, *1418*
   dislocation of, 1329–1364
      Allis technique of reduction of, *1348,* 1348–1349
      anterior, 1340–1341, *1342,* 1342(t), *1343*
      anteversion of hip in, 1331–1332, 1334, 1334(t)
      arthritis following, 1335, 1360–1361, *1361,* 1371, 1384
      avascular necrosis of femoral head following, 1336, *1336,* 1360, 1371, 1384
      causes of, 1329, 1333
      classification of, 1337–1341, *1338–1342,* 1340(t), 1342(t), 1371–1372
      closed reduction of, 1347–1349, *1348, 1349,* 1378
         management following, 1349–1356
      complications of, 1360–1363
      computed tomographic assessment of, 1344–1345, *1345, 1346,* 1351
      consequences of, 1335–1336
      diagnosis of, 1341–1347
         delayed, 1362–1363
      foot injuries associated with, 1337
      fracture associated with, acetabular, 1357, 1358, 1361, 1362(t)
         femoral, 1337
         femoral head, 1334, *1335,* 1339, *1339,* 1359, *1359,* 1362(t), 1370. See also *Femur, head of, fracture of.*
         femoral neck, 1335, 1358
      gravity technique of reduction of, 1349, *1349*
      iliofemoral ligament tethering in, 1356, *1357*
      imaging studies of, 1343–1347, 1374
      in polytrauma patient, 1347, 1377
      initial management of, 1347–1349
      injuries associated with, 1336–1337, 1363, 1383–1384
      knee injuries associated with, 1337
      management of, 1347–1359
         delayed, 1362–1363
         initial, 1347–1349
         postreduction, 1349–1356
         surgical, 1351–1359
            complications of, 1363–1364
      mechanisms of injury in, 1329, 1333–1335
      motor vehicle accidents and, 1329, 1333–1334, *1334*
      MRI following reduction of, 1351
      nerve injuries associated with, 1337, 1363, 1383–1384
      open reduction of, 1378–1379
      pathology of, 1329–1337

Hip *(Continued)*
   patient history in, 1341
   peroneal nerve injury associated with, 1337
   physical findings in, 1341–1343, 1372, 1374
   posterior, 1340, 1340(t), *1341, 1343*
   postreduction management of, 1349–1356
   radiographic assessment of, 1343–1344, *1344,* 1350, *1350*
   recurrent, 1361–1362
   reduction of, closed, 1347–1349, *1348, 1349*
      management following, 1349–1356
      open, 1378–1379
   results of, 1359–1360, 1360(t), 1362(t)
   sciatic nerve injury associated with, 1337, 1363, 1383–1384
   Stimson gravity technique of reduction of, 1349, *1349*
   surgery for, 1351–1359
      complications of, 1363–1364
   traction for, 1350–1351, 1356
   type I, 1356
   type II, 1356–1358
   type III, 1358
   type IV, 1358–1359
   type V, 1359
fracture of, 1369–1436. See also *Femur, head of, fracture of* and *Femur, neck of, fracture of.*
   deep venous thrombosis following, 1478
   falling and, 103, *103,* 1446
   in elderly patient, 1443, *1444*
   intertrochanteric, 1443–1479. See also *Intertrochanteric hip fracture.*
      femoral shaft fracture and, 1564, 1569, *1569, 1570*
      gunshot wound and, 386–387, *388,* 389
      pathologic, 411, 416, 1455
   intracapsular, 1369–1436. See also *Femur, head of, fracture of* and *Femur, neck of, fracture of.*
   mortality rate associated with, 1475–1476
   nonunion of, *531*
   osteoporosis and, 432, 433, 1387
   pathologic, 411, 416, 1455
   pressure sores associated with, 1479
   pulmonary embolism following, 1478
   risk factors for, 102–104
   stable, 1457, 1463
   unstable, 1458–1459, 1463
function of, and intertrochanteric fracture, 1454, 1477(t)
   scales for rating, 1430(t), 1475, 1517, *1518*
gunshot wound of, 394, *394–395*
Hardinge approach to, *1418*
heterotopic ossification of, following femoral head fracture, 1371
   following surgery for femoral head fracture, 1383
   surgery for hip dislocation and, 1364
instability of, following treatment of femoral head fracture, 1383
intertrochanteric fracture of, 1443–1479. See also *Intertrochanteric hip fracture.*
   femoral shaft fracture and, 1564, 1569, *1569, 1570*
   gunshot wound and, 386–387, *388,* 389
   pathologic, 411, 416, 1455
intracapsular fracture of, 1369–1436. See also *Femur, head of, fracture of* and *Femur, neck of, fracture of.*
Kocher-Gibson approach to, *1416*
Kocher-Langenbeck approach to, 904, *905,* 906, 1351, *1352–1353*

U